The Breast Cancer EPIDEMIC

AF327898

About the Author

Dwight Thomas, Ph.D.,

is an experienced medical writer who specializes in translating bewildering terminology into plain English for intelligent laypersons. An objective commentator, he has neither financial nor personal reasons to promote any particular preventive, diagnostic, or therapeutic strategies. Rather he is concerned to identify the limitations of the currently available interventions as well as their merits.

Dr. Thomas attended Emory University in Atlanta, where he studied biology, the history of science, and English and American literature. During the Vietnam War he served in the United States Army, being stationed overseas in West Germany. Subsequently he pursued graduate studies at the University of Pennsylvania in Philadelphia. He has long been following new developments in breast cancer medicine. In 1990 he participated in the influential Consensus Development Conference hosted by the National Institutes of Health in Bethesda, Maryland, which endorsed lumpectomy as the preferred surgical therapy for early-stage breast cancer. In 1994 he became a charter member of the Information Associates Program of the National Cancer Institute.

Dr. Thomas has been the subject of biographical sketches in *Who's Who in America* and *Contemporary Authors*, and of a feature article in the *Wall Street Journal* of November 21, 2005.

The Breast Cancer Epidemic

The
Breast Cancer Epidemic

Dwight Thomas, Ph.D.

MONTEREY SQUARE PRESS

SAVANNAH, GEORGIA USA

Copyright © 2006 by Dwight Thomas

First Edition

All rights reserved. With the exception of brief quotations for inclusion in reviews or scholarly articles, no portion of this book may be reproduced in any fashion without written permission from the publisher:

MONTEREY SQUARE PRESS
P. O. BOX 366
SAVANNAH, GEORGIA 31402

Library of Congress Control Number: 2006921631

ISBN   0-9743892-1-8

An Important Disclaimer

This book deals with diverse neoplasms which may arise in the mammary gland. It is published as a work of responsible journalism. While it necessarily deals with diagnosis and treatment, it is not intended as a guide to self-diagnosis or as an individualized prescription for any particular prophylactic or therapeutic intervention. No guarantee can be given that this book is free from error, nor any liability accepted for errors which have been inadvertently introduced into the text.

TABLE OF CONTENTS
The Breast Cancer Epidemic

INTRODUCTION   1

1. Cancer: The Last Epidemic   7

2. Inside a Cell's Nucleus   32

3. Looking for Oncogenes   42

4. The Human Breast:
Anatomy, Hormones, Carcinogens   55

5. Epidemiology:
Identifying the Risk Factors
for Breast Cancer   79

6. Estrogen Replacement Therapy   119

7. "The Pill": Hormonal Contraception   140

8. A Lump in the Breast   152

9. The Office Visit:
Palpation, Ultrasound,
Needle Aspiration   173

10. Diagnostic Mammography   180

11. Biopsy Becomes a Friend   200

12. Pathology Report:
Understanding the Varieties
of Breast Cancer   214

13. Dealing with a Cancer Diagnosis   246

TABLE OF CONTENTS
The Breast Cancer Epidemic

14. Staging:
The Evolving Art of Prognosis — 256

15. Breast Cancer Surgery:
From Antiquity to the NSABP — 288

16. Making a Decision:
Lumpectomy or Mastectomy? — 315

17. Undergoing Surgery
and Recovering from It — 323

18. Breast Reconstruction — 342

19. Radiation Therapy
after Lumpectomy — 363

20. The Threat of Recurrence — 378

21. Alternative Medicine:
Vitamins, Diet, and
Positive Thinking — 394

22. Hormonal Therapy:
The Triumph of Tamoxifen — 412

23. Breast Cancer Chemotherapy — 448

24. Undergoing Chemotherapy — 472

25. High-Dose Therapy
and the Taxoid Drugs — 488

TABLE OF CONTENTS
The Breast Cancer Epidemic

26. Stage Four:
The Management of
Metastatic Disease — 515

27. The Emerging Immunotherapies — 556

28. Screening Mammography — 588

29. Breast Self-Examination — 615

PATIENT RESOURCES — 619

NOTES — 624

INDEX — 681

LIST OF ILLUSTRATIONS
The Breast Cancer Epidemic

{1} Germ Cells, A Somatic Cell — 13

{2} A Normal Breast Duct — 20

{3} Hyperplasia in a Breast Duct — 21

{4} Ductal Carcinoma *in situ* — 23

{5} Infiltrating Ductal Carcinoma — 25

{6} Looking for Tumor Dissemination: The Role of Sentinel Node Sampling — 27

{7} Chromosomes Visible during Mitosis — 34

{8} The Mammary Gland — 57

{9} Lymphatic Drainage of the Breast — 61

{10} Alveoli in a Lobule — 70

{11} The Breast Quadrants — 155

{12} The "Mobility Criterion" for the Evaluation of Breast Masses — 157

{13} A Typical Cyst — 160

{14} Duct Ectasia — 163

{15} Skin Dimpling — 168

LIST OF ILLUSTRATIONS
The Breast Cancer Epidemic

{16} Benign Mammographic Appearance 185

{17} Malignant Mammographic
        Appearance 187

{18} Clustered Calcifications 191

{19} Branching Calcifications 193

{20} Ductography 197

{21} Handheld Core Needle 207

{22} "Cribriform"
        Ductal Carcinoma *in situ* 236

{23} "Micropapillary"
        Ductal Carcinoma *in situ* 237

{24} "Solid" Ductal Carcinoma *in situ* 239

{25} "Comedo" Ductal Carcinoma *in situ* 241

{26} Lobular Carcinoma *in situ* 244

{27} The Three Levels of Axillary Nodes 328

{28} Elliptical Mastectomy Incision 335

{29} A Tangential Field for
        Breast Irradiation 367

{30} A Mature Dendritic Cell 577

The Breast Cancer Epidemic

INTRODUCTION

Who would want to read a book about breast cancer? Obviously, *nobody!* It's not a pleasant subject, and no one would pursue it as a hobby. Notwithstanding these facts, every year millions of Americans find themselves forced **to get interested** in this topic; they will in one way or another be drawn into the complex and often bewildering world of breast cancer medicine. To begin with, there are those 200,000-plus women—as well as a thousand or so very surprised men—who must listen to a solemn-faced physician ominously pronouncing a diagnosis of "breast cancer" in their particular case. Numerically speaking, that's just the tip of the iceberg. If we are to properly count the number of our fellow citizens involved with this subject, we must certainly count those tens of millions of asymptomatic women who faithfully troop to the radiologist's office for the ritual of annual mammograms. Then there are all those millions of women (no one knows how many) who must rush off to their personal physicians because they have noticed a breast symptom which awakens fears of cancer. Most men are at very low risk for malignant transformation in the breast, but they can hardly be said to be "uninvolved" when their wives or mothers, their sisters or daughters, must struggle with this diagnosis. If you do not have breast cancer, the odds are quite good that someone near and dear to you is—or shortly will be—a patient. But even if you are not involved on a personal level, you are being financially penalized if you must pay for health insurance or if you pay taxes to the federal government

or to any local or state government. Either directly or indirectly we must all foot higher bills because medical science has failed to discover an easy solution to this problem.

Simply as intelligent adults and as responsible citizens, we should welcome any opportunity to learn about beast cancer, with a view to reducing those tremendous costs exacted by the actual disease or by the fear of it. These costs are much higher than they should be, whether measured in terms of dollars and cents, or of needless worries and anxieties, or of imprecise diagnoses and less than optimal therapies. If more American laypersons could comprehend the basic issues of breast cancer medicine, perhaps the aforementioned costs might come down a little. Unfortunately, in our society it has never been easy for laypersons to obtain sophisticated information on this subject. Back in the 1950s and 1960s, American newspapers and magazines shied away from discussing human malignancy generally and from breast cancer in particular. There terrible matters were to be left to professional physicians; they were not often mentioned in sources of information to which laypersons had ready access. If we must assign a date for the dissolution of this conspiracy of silence, then surely it would be the fall of 1974. In September and October—within a period of three weeks—both Betty Ford and Happy Rockefeller underwent radical mastectomies for the treatment of breast cancer. The television and newspaper coverage given these operations hitherto considered "of a private nature" was extraordinary but not at all surprising, because these women were the wives respectively of President Gerald Ford and Vice-President Nelson Rockefeller. Our Presidential families, the nation's most public, have been singled out by breast malignancies. In October 1987 Nancy Reagan underwent a mastectomy for early-stage breast cancer; in January 1994 Virginia Kelley, mother of Bill Clinton, died from metastatic (disseminated) disease. The publicity accorded these "First Family" patients raised our awareness of breast cancer, but more importantly it removed the veil of hushed embarrassment which earlier generations of Americans had drawn around the entire subject. The social stigma attached to the diagnosis faded away, and prominent patients from other walks of life shared their personal experiences with the public. In July 1992 the rock singer Olivia Newton-John, who had played a frisky teenager in the hit movie "Grease," announced that she had undergone a mastectomy and was receiving chemotherapy. Her courageous disclosure reminded us that a significant minority of breast cancer patients are people who would otherwise seem much too young and energetic to be ill.

The era in which breast cancer was a tabooed topic for the mass media has long since been superseded by an era in which it is a staple commodity. Our newspapers, magazines, and TV newscasts are positively overflowing with little stories and reports about this subject. Unfortunately, today's intense media coverage tends to be fragmentary and superficial; with regard to helping laypersons understand basic issues, it is not much better than yesterday's embarrassed silence. Little snippets of data are constantly being presented out of context and without meaningful editorial comment. The daily newspapers are not blameless, but television is the worst offender. Those thirty-second reports on the nightly TV news are typically read by highly articulate and very photogenic announcers who know no more about cancer research than anybody else. And the reports usually manage to convey an erroneous impression. Unwary viewers might conclude that broccoli has been proven to prevent breast cancer, or that a therapeutic revolution is imminent because some researcher cured an induced tumor in an immunodeficient mouse. The newspapers and newscasts are by their nature consigned to present brief excerpts and fleeting images. For in-depth coverage we remain largely dependant on bound volumes. Are there no books specifically written to convey sophisticated medical information to literate laypersons? Ah, there's the rub! The standard textbooks on breast cancer are unsuitable, either with regard to their length or their price or their readability. These volumes can run a thousand pages or more in length, and they cost anywhere from $100 to $300. The separate chapters are written by groups of specialists who are exclusively addressing their fellow specialists, with no thought whatsoever of translating technical terms into plain English. Now there have been many books about breast cancer aimed at a popular audience; but most of them seem to have been composed in a personal vein, with titles like ***Why Me?*** or ***First, You Cry***. These books often do a splendid job of recording individual experiences, which may perhaps move the reader to tears, or to become angry with the insensitive physicians therein depicted; but they do not convey balanced information about diagnosis and treatment. Men with prostate cancer are sometimes urged to "male bonding" with other sufferers, but this hardly compares to the constant showers of sisterly sentiments which fall upon breast cancer patients. Quite a few books on breast cancer intended for laypersons carry gender much too far, by seeming to reduce diverse biological phenomena brought about by complex genetic mutations to the simplistic matter of sexual discrimination.

Let me be perfectly frank. As an author I have no truck with tears or anger, with male bonding or feminist solidarity. These emotional postures are an entirely comprehensible response to a cancer diagnosis, but they do not help us to understand that diagnosis or to select an appropriate treatment. In fact, they pose a barrier to understanding, and I cannot be concerned with them. I am interested in two things—*what scientists know and what physicians do*. And my book may be viewed as a short history of recent trends in biomedical research and in medical practice. It is written in the spirit of awestruck admiration and of amused skepticism. Admiration is in order, because the story deals with impressive advances in knowledge and technology. But skepticism is also indicated. If this history teaches us anything, it is that our understanding of disease mechanisms can often be wrongheaded, that our diagnostic assays can often be inconclusive or misleading, and that the treatments given patients may often be determined by outdated traditions or by local customs, by the self-interest of practitioners or by economic considerations of one kind or another.

History does repeat itself; but in breast cancer medicine, ignorance is not always bliss. This is one area in which naive patients have historically been exposed to great harm, and there is no reason to suspect that this circumstance will necessarily be altered in the future. It is more important than ever that patients be knowledgeable, because now they are expected to confer with various specialists about the available treatment options. Yet the misconceptions that breast cancer patients and their family members bring to a consultation can amount to monumental ignorance and make any meaningful dialog with a physician exceedingly problematic. I would like to take a moment to destroy the greatest and most dangerous of these misconceptions—*namely,* the belief that there is a single disease called *breast cancer*. Oh no! There is no such disease! The subject we are concerned with can be properly described only in the plural. It is **BREAST CANCERS**. Many decades ago pathologists using light microscopes divided malignant breast tumors into two or three dozen distinct subtypes; they recognized that there were considerable differences in behavior and growth rates between these subtypes. Nowadays we still classify breast malignancies by their characteristic features as seen under a light microscope, but we are more concerned with the invisible genetic mutations which have occurred in the nuclei of cancer cells. There are dozens of genes implicated in mammary carcinogenesis, and they can mutate in many different ways. The upshot is that instead of recognizing a mere two or three dozen tumor species, we now find ourselves confronted by **a thousand and one diseases**. The particular "mix" of aberrant genes in each individual tumor represents its **genetic profile** and will dictate its future behavior, which could be essentially benign, chronically progressive, or rapidly metastatic. This tremendous genetic and behavioral diversity explains why breast malignancies constitute such a fertile field for errors in diagnosis and treatment. That convenient singular term *breast cancer* has been indiscriminately applied to cellular proliferations which do not need treatment (e.g., lobular carcinoma *in situ*), to small noninvasive cancers whose malignant potential cannot be accurately predicted, and to invasive tumors whose malignancy is certain but which can nonetheless be cured by adequate local therapy (i.e., surgical excision with or without irradiation). Other invasive tumors will demonstrate the ability to spread throughout the body, and sooner or later they will tend to produce complications which result in death. These metastasizing tumors constitute an ever-shrinking minority of the breast cancer cases currently being diagnosed.

Fortunate is the patient whose highly knowledgeable and very kind physician will take the time to explain what **"breast cancer"** really means in her particular case. Fortunate is the patient who is not <u>over</u>-treated or <u>under</u>-treated, whose therapy may be said to correspond to her actual condition. Were these fortunate circumstances always to prevail, there would be little need for a book like *The Breast Cancer Epidemic*. As things stand, however, I believe that a concise textbook written especially for intelligent laypersons should fulfill a great need. Back in the 1980s the National Cancer Institute published a modest paperback volume entitled *The Breast Cancer Digest*. This book aimed to provide reliable information on diagnosis and treatment to the general public, and it was buttressed with citations of seminal articles published in leading medical journals. My intent and my methodology in *The Breast Cancer Epidemic* are much the same, but my scope is considerably broader.

It has become a formidable task simply to list all those learned professionals, both pure scientists and practicing physicians, who are engaged in the pursuit of additional knowledge about breast malignancies or of improved therapies for them. Your crying babies may be handed over to pediatricians, and your aching feet presented to podiatrists, but who's taking care of the mammary neoplasms? Just about everybody, it would seem. There are the **epidemiologists** trying to identify the risk factors which predispose to disease development, and the **geneticists and molecular biologists** looking at the DNA mutations which put cells on the road to malignancy. And then there are the **immunologists and pharmacologists** designing new drugs and biological response modifiers, and verifying the ways in which these agents act upon cancer cells and upon the human body generally. Any family physician, any gynecologist, or any internist might be asked

to evaluate a breast lump or other clinical symptom noticed by a patient. But these days the real work of diagnosis and treatment is left to more highly focused specialists—the **diagnostic radiologist** (mammographer), the **pathologist**, the **cancer surgeon**, the **reconstructive surgeon** (plastic surgeon), the **radiotherapist** (radiation oncologist), and the **medical oncologist**. The number of professionals who might be called upon to provide supportive services to breast cancer patients is not negligible—**nurses and social workers, psychologists and political activists, hospice caregivers**.

As a mere author I cannot be expected to be an expert in all of these scientific disciplines and therapeutic vocations. Frankly, I would not claim to have more than a nodding acquaintance with any of them, yet they all deserve inclusion in a breast cancer book aspiring to completeness. I have tried to compile and edit wisely, so as to depict the valuable role played by each of the aforementioned disciplines and professions. I believe that the information in this book is reliable; but because it is intended for intellectually curious laypersons rather than for highly trained professionals, it is necessarily condensed and simplified. Readers desiring more detailed information or an evaluation of their individual status are referred to the experts. Insofar as the leading American scientists and physicians involved with breast malignancies have expressed themselves in print, they are likely to be named, cited, and quoted in this book. I do not wander too far afield from what the experts are saying; in fact, my principal goal has been to present these expert opinions verbatim or nearly so, supplying only that minimal editorial apparatus needed to make them intelligible to a wider audience.

In 1988, when I first began to study breast cancer medicine, I foolishly dreamed of writing a little book which would cover all the pertinent topics and which would be totally up-to-date. The intervening years have taught me that any inclusive book on this subject cannot be brief, and that by the time it is finished, it will be more of a retrospective chronicle than a news bulletin. Absolute "up-to-date-ness" is no longer possible in books about cancer, and perhaps not so necessary. A reader with a firm grasp of the fundamentals can obtain instantaneous updates by calling one of the toll-free numbers hosted by the National Cancer Institute, by the American Cancer Society, or by various support groups. The Internet has become an unparalleled source of up-to-date information. The NCI and ACS websites are trustworthy, as are those hosted by the National Library of Medicine, by the large cancer hospitals, and by many universities. Continuing education may be recommended to any patient who wishes to avoid the ravages both of uncontrolled disease and of ill-considered treatments. In breast cancer medicine it has never been clear whether the sum total of suffering is increased more by pathological complications or by inappropriate interventions. As an unbiased writer with no financial interest in any therapeutic strategy, I will counsel awareness and caution. Trust in God—learn as much as you can—*and get a second opinion!* If the fundamental knowledge presented in ***The Breast Cancer Epidemic*** can assist some readers in locating, consulting, and understanding other sources of information, I will have accomplished my mission as an author.

Dwight Thomas, Ph.D.
American Medical Writers Association

ACKNOWLEDGMENTS
And a Note on the Text

This book is based on multitudinous published documents. From my point of view, anyone who publishes something worthwhile about breast cancer has created a valuable historical document which can be precisely cited and which really ought to be quoted. I have thus become indebted to hundreds and hundreds of authors, far too many to name individually at the front of an overlong book. These cherished collaborators—physicians, patients, and scientists—are acknowledged in my text and in my notes. Here I have only space to acknowledge four indispensable serials whose pages I have been quarrying for over a decade and which figure largely in my documentation: the *New England Journal of Medicine*, the *Journal of the National Cancer Institute*, *JAMA* (the *Journal of the American Medical Association*), and the *Journal of Clinical Oncology*.

I must apologize to many fine authors for minor editorial liberties I have taken in the interest of brevity or of readability. I have consistently shortened long rosters of contributing authors to *et al* (Latin for "and others"). And very often I have condensed the longish titles of journal articles to briefer "running titles," which would convey a sense of content without testing the lay reader's patience. Normally I am horrified by the prospect of making surreptitious alterations to quoted material, but I must confess that I have occasionally made enhancements in spelling and punctuation to achieve maximum clarity. Any layperson who wants to read a book about breast cancer medicine probably has enough to contend with, and I did not wish to make matters worse by producing a text saturated with brackets and ellipses.

D. T.

Chapter One

Cancer: The Last Epidemic

Cancer. The word sends shivers of fear down our spines. It gives us precisely the same sensation we would have if we were to hear—while swimming far out in the ocean—an excited cry from some distant beach consisting of the single word *SHARK!!* Cardiovascular disease, with its "heart attacks" and strokes, is easily the foremost cause of mortality in contemporary America; but cancer alone evokes the sort of terror which our grandparents and great-grandparents felt when confronted with recurrent epidemics of cholera, yellow fever, typhoid, and polio. Of course, our anxieties about cancer are tempered with the hope—yea, even with *the expectation*— that "a cure" will be found. The newspapers and TV newscasts are always reporting the most promising research; surely progress is being made, yet the death rates for many types of cancer seem to remain fairly constant, revealing little change from one decade to the next.

Our fears are overwrought, if not exactly unwarranted. Our therapeutic optimism is probably premature, but certainly understandable. In the past century and a half, medical science has achieved results unprecedented in any previous era of history; its accomplishments dwarf those of most other fields of human endeavor. Let's use life expectancy to prove this point. In 1900 a newborn American could expect a life span of about 47 years. By the 1980s life expectancy at birth was up to 75 years or more. Within the timeframe of two or three generations, American longevity had been *increased by over one-third*. If we look only at the female sex, the actuarial statistics are even more impressive. In 1900 baby girls had a typical life expectancy of 48 years; in 1984 the figure stood at 78 years—a round gain of thirty years.[1]

Where are the dread diseases of yesteryear? Gone to the history books, mainly. In 1900 the two leading causes of death were tuberculosis and pneumonia, which often killed vigorous young people. Today neither disease poses a major threat in American society, except to the elderly and other persons with weakened immune systems. Who could have envisioned, a century ago, that American physicians could pass their entire professional careers without ever seeing a case of diphtheria—or hearing a child with whooping cough—or watching a young woman die during childbirth? A century ago surgery of any kind, even simple appendectomy, was a dangerous undertaking. Today surgery is so safe that we submit to general anesthesia and the scalpel solely for the sake of appearance—to tuck in protruding tummies or to smooth out facial wrinkles. Open-heart operations are now routine, and even such wonders as heart-lung transplants are no longer deemed newsworthy.

Surgery is not, however, the principal reason why so many of us are living so much longer. The reason is that we have achieved a significant understanding of **infectious diseases** and that we can therefore control them, either by preventing them in the first place or by curing them when they occur. We've already mentioned a few infectious diseases; we could in fact make a thick catalog of potentially deadly afflictions which don't bother us as they once did. Those ancient scourges of leprosy and bubonic plague still exist, but only in remote areas of the Third World. Smallpox, an eighteenth-century terror, has been totally eradicated. Today not many Americans are likely to die from rabies or tetanus—from syphilis or gonorrhea—from scarlet fever, strep throat, rheumatic fever, or meningitis—from dysentery, malaria, measles, or typhus.

How many millenniums did it take the human race to understand the nature of infectious diseases? Only in the last half of the nineteenth century, with the work of European scientists like Louis Pasteur and Robert Koch, did the shades of darkness start to fall from our eyes. To simplify matters, we can say that each of these diseases can be traced to—and is caused by—a single infectious agent, either a bacterium or a virus. **Bacteria** are one-cell organisms capable of independent existence; they can often be seen under a conventional light microscope, and they can often be cultured (grown) in a Petri dish or test tube. **Viruses** are little bits of genetic material, much too small to be seen under a light microscope. Unlike bacteria, viruses are obligate parasites. They have no energy-generating metabolisms, and consequently they must enter the cells of a host animal and usurp the cells' genetic machinery to accomplish reproduction. Once we understood how bacteria and viruses caused their mischief, we could take steps to combat them. Diseases caused by waterborne bacteria—dysentery,

typhoid, cholera—soon yielded to water purification systems and better sewage disposal. Pasteurization of milk stopped the transmission of tuberculosis bacilli from cattle to humans. In the 1920s diphtheria was vanquished by mass vaccination. In the 1930s and 1940s the discovery of the sulfonamides and subsequently of such improved antibiotics as penicillin and streptomycin heralded the *Age of the Wonder Drugs*—and an era of unparalleled trust in the knowledge and powers of physicians. Suddenly our doctors could not merely diagnose bacterial illnesses; they could *cure* them, painlessly, quickly, and inexpensively. Pneumonia, syphilis, and tuberculosis ceased to be mortal terrors; and young mothers no longer died after childbirth from puerperal fevers, those raging infections which result when streptococci or other bacteria are introduced into an open, raw uterus.

Viral diseases failed to respond to the new antibiotics, but some of them could be prevented by vaccines. As early as 1796 the English physician Edward Jenner had stumbled across a crude but effective immunization for smallpox. In the 1880s Louis Pasteur developed laboratory techniques for attenuating (weakening) the virulence of bacteria and viruses; he thus created safe strains of these microorganisms which, when injected into animals or humans, would induce immunity without causing disease. In 1886 Pasteur used an attenuated vaccine to save the life of a boy who had been bitten by a rabid dog. American scientists in the late 1890s paid particular attention to yellow fever, an epidemic viral disease which had periodically ravaged cities on the eastern seaboard, and which was then hampering work on the Panama Canal. The discovery that the disease was spread by mosquitoes led to a means of control—infected persons were isolated in buildings with window screens so that the insects could not bite them and thus acquire the virus for further transmission. Yellow fever had vanished from the American scene long before the preparation of an effective vaccine in 1941. The most famous antiviral vaccines were those named after Jonas Salk and Albert B. Sabin. Introduced in 1954 (Salk) and 1961 (Sabin), these two vaccines put a stop to paralytic polio, which had crippled President Franklin Delano Roosevelt as well as large numbers of American children and teenagers. Other viral diseases now preventable by vaccination include chicken-pox, measles, mumps, rubella (German measles), and hepatitis B.

If our war against infectious diseases has been largely *won*, it is not—and probably will never be—*over*. Bacteria, through genetic mutation or other means, tend to become resistant to our antibiotics, continually forcing us to invent new drugs. And some viral infections have yet to be prevented by vaccination. The most prevalent of these are those upper respiratory infections which we usually lump together as "the common cold." In this case, so many different viruses are involved that a single vaccine has yet to be feasible. Vaccines have been only partially successful in curbing influenza epidemics: the causative viruses frequently undergo minor structural alterations, so that last year's vaccine may not protect against this year's flu. In the 1970s and 1980s American society experienced a large increase in **sexually transmitted diseases** (STDs) caused by viruses. Neither genital herpes nor *condylomata acuminata* (genital warts) was quite as fearful as the old bacterial STDs (syphilis and gonorrhea), but both these viral infections could be unsightly and recurrent. No cures or vaccines were at hand. In late 1980 a far more serious STD made its appearance among male homosexuals and intravenous drug users: **AIDS**, or the "Acquired Immune Deficiency Syndrome," caused by **HIV**, the "Human Immunodeficiency Virus." According to one hypothesis, HIV originally infected certain monkeys in

Africa, presumably undergoing a nasty mutation or two before making its way into human populations. Whatever its origin, HIV proved to be one of the most lethal infectious agents in history. It was all the more troublesome because it had a long incubation period, during which asymptomatic victims could continue to infect others. Future generations may look on the AIDS epidemic as merely a short episode in the annals of medicine. At least it should remind us that miracle drugs and vaccines are not produced overnight, and that biomedical technology cannot substitute for public education and private restraint.

HEY! WHAT ABOUT CANCER?

Some readers may be puzzled to find a book about cancer beginning with a capsule history of the conquest of infectious diseases. In self-defense, the author will suggest that a little bit of historical awareness is necessary to put the cancer epidemic and our attitudes toward it in a proper perspective. Today the only Americans likely to die from infections are either very elderly or extremely reckless. Cancer has become a major threat because it predominately afflicts people who are over the age of 50, and most of us can expect to live two, three, or even four decades beyond the half-century mark. An American born in 1900 had a life expectancy of about 47—and consequently little risk of developing cancer. A newborn in 1985 could typically anticipate 75 or more additional years, and—horrors!—a whopping 35% chance of eventually developing cancer.[2] Our tremendous victory over the infectious diseases of childhood and youth has left us to confront a bewildering array of geriatric malignancies. That victory has also conditioned us to expect pharmacological miracles—some sort of penicillin which would painlessly cure cancer, or a Salk vaccine to prevent it. So far the untold millions spent on cancer research have not led to such facile solutions.

BUT WHAT IS CANCER?

Cancer is very different from the aforementioned infectious diseases, each of which represents a well-defined malady caused by an identifiable microorganism. The **etiology** (cause) of malignancies tends to be much more complex. Cancer is not a single disease in the sense that syphilis and tuberculosis are single diseases, whatever their myriad manifestations may be. Most writers on this topic will refer loosely to "a hundred types of human cancer," but we could easily offer much higher estimates. A textbook on breast cancer, the most prevalent malignancy among women, informs us that there are "about thirty different types of breast cancers, based on pathologic criteria."[3] Thus the term *breast cancer* by itself does not define a single disease with a predictable course; it principally serves to name an anatomical location where many dissimilar diseases can arise. Other broad designations in human cancer—e.g., brain, lung, or skin—are similarly descriptive in an anatomical sense: they require additional nomenclature before they begin to identify the diverse pathological conditions that may be involved.

Cancer is not limited to *Homo sapiens*. All mammals, from tiny shrews to giant whales, are subject to cancer. So are birds, fish, insects, and plants—in fact, just about every living organism on earth. Traces of cancer have been discovered in ancient Egyptian mummies and in dinosaur bones. Cancer is a universal biological enigma. We are hard pressed for a good definition of it; the medical dictionaries offer feeble attempts which seem to revolve around the word *malignant*. What do they mean by "malignant"? Before we can understand that term, we must consider the thing which becomes malignant—which manifests cancer and which serves (so to speak) as the agent of disease. Let us begin with the primal entity of life—**the cell**.

Omnipotential Zygote

The human body is much more complicated than anything that men can construct or, indeed, even dream of constructing. In the United States we take pride in our feats of engineering and technology, in our space shuttles and towering skyscrapers. A brief reflection on the body should remind us that such inventions are only crude imitations of natural physiology. Compared to the central nervous system, the electrical wiring in a space shuttle is but a tinkertoy that any child could piece together. The plumbing systems in all the skyscrapers of Manhattan can hardly be compared, in terms of design complexity, to the intricate system of blood vessels—arteries, arterioles, capillaries, veins—found in the body. To build things we make use of metals and plastics. To construct a human body, nature relies on a variety of living cells. All that we are as physical beings consists either of cells or of substances secreted by cells. There are several hundred types of specialized cells in the body. The number will not surprise us if we reflect on the body's varied characteristics—the **hardness** of our tooth enamel (a cellular secretion), or the **strength** of our bones (a matrix of cells and their secretions), or the **flexibility** of our muscles, or the exquisite **sensitivity** of those cellular gatherings which give us our senses of sight, hearing, smell, taste, and touch. Some biologists have speculated that the human body contains a total of *one hundred trillion cells*, though no one has taken the time to count them all. The closest approach to any precise enumeration of our cells is represented by the **Complete Blood Count**, or

CBC, a routine laboratory procedure which records the number of white cells (thousands) and red cells (millions) in a tiny drop of blood.

Human cells are far too small to be seen with the naked eye. Hippocrates, the Greek father of medicine, knew nothing of them. The body's cellular construction did not become evident to medical researchers until the 1830s, following the invention of improved microscopes with compound lenses. It was not widely appreciated by physicians before the 1870s and 1880s, when the development of chemical staining techniques provided a way to highlight the individual cells in messy tissue specimens. To convey some idea of the complexity of our cells, we can profitably begin with their female progenitor—the **ovum** (Latin for "egg"). About once a month, in women of childbearing age, a swelling follicle on the surface of an ovary bursts open to release a gigantic ovum, which is almost as large as the period at the end of this sentence. Like those chicken eggs we're all familiar with, the human ovum consists mainly of nutrients, or yolk. The genetic material it contains is very small, occupying less than a hundredth part of the cell's volume. That material is incomplete, being **haploid**—i.e., with only half of the necessary instructions for the creation of human life. By itself the ovum cannot grow or reproduce; unless it is fertilized, it soon shrinks and shrivels, passing away unnoticed during menstruation.

The male germ cell, or sperm, is minuscule compared to its female counterpart. Unlike the ovum, it carries no nutrients or other excess baggage; it's just a spear-like piece of genetic material propelled by a wildly thrashing tail. This cell is also haploid; it cannot grow or reproduce, and typically dies shortly after leaving the male body. However, if a sperm should chance to encounter and penetrate an ovum, the haploid bits of genetic material carried by each are quickly merged. At that moment ovum and sperm cease to exist; they are replaced by a new cell called **the zygote**, from the Greek word for "paired" or "yoked." Unlike the germ cells from which it arose, the zygote is **diploid**—it possesses a full complement of genetic material, and it's capable of the most marvelous reproduction and growth. As the zygote drifts down a fallopian tube, it undergoes several elementary self-reproductions, yielding in each instance another copy of itself. If by some accident this growing sphere of zygotic cells were now to split in two, the end result would be identical twins: two human beings who are genetically uniform and physically duplicates of each other. Such twinning is relatively rare; usually the ball of cells arrives intact in the uterus, where it implants in the receptive uterine lining and obtains the blood supply necessary for oxygen and nutrients.

As we've noted, the zygote's earliest growth pattern resembles that of a primordial bacterium: one cell, then two, four, eight, sixteen. Within a week after conception, the pattern of simple duplication is replaced by one of **differentiation**. We can discuss the process of differentiation—to some extent, even observe it happening when an embryo is formed—but we do not understand it. None of the machines we make is capable of self-duplication, much less differentiation. By way of defining this term, let's consider the astonishing fate of the zygotic cells; suddenly they've vanished—or at least undergone an incredible number of metamorphoses. A month-old embryo displays no recognizable human features, but reveals the most intense cellular activity. Cells of all types seem to be rushing about, trying to find their proper place in the emerging drama of creation—positioning themselves to become blood, bone, brain, ears, eyes, heart, kidneys, liver, lungs! By the end of the third month of pregnancy, all organ systems are in place, albeit undeveloped. The embryo has become **a fetus**—clearly a human being, although in extreme miniature.

How can one zygote give rise to such multitudinous complexity in only ninety days? How do the daughter cells (the zygotic offspring) know to transform themselves into brain cells or kidney cells or lung cells, and how do these cells in turn know to unite themselves into separate organs, and how do all the diverse cells and organs work together in such perfect harmony that they ultimately create a life form capable of rational thought, passionate love, and spiritual ecstasy? If we could understand the zygote and its power of differentiation, we could certainly understand and cure cancer. But there is no parallel to the zygote even in our wondrous computer technology. The invisible genetic matter in a zygotic cell contains the complete instructions ("programming") for a unique human life. These specifications dictate the color of eyes and hair, the shape of ears and nose, even the minute tracing of loops and whirls to be shown on each fingerprint. The zygote's genetic material is smaller than any speck of dust you might see floating in a sunbeam, yet in it the Lord God (or Mother Nature) has packaged more information than could be stored in the largest computer owned by the Internal Revenue Service.

Somatic Cells

The end products of the differentiation occurring during embryogenesis are **somatic cells**. The term comes from the Greek word *soma*, meaning "body"; and it refers to those differentiated cells which comprise the body's organs and tissues, and which perform highly specialized functions. The zygote, in contrast, was undifferentiated and unspecialized but fully potential; its function was simply to evolve into—more correctly, *to differentiate into*—any and all succeeding somatic cells. These resulting cells have surrendered the zygote's youthful potential for evolution and movement. They are instead the productive adults in the complex cellular society of the body—very good and sound citizens if much less exciting, being tied (as it were) to particular locales and repetitious jobs.

Somatic cells vary greatly in shape, size, and overall appearance; but they tend to follow a basic structural arrangement. Typically, each cell reveals a distinct **nucleus** bounded by a thin membrane. The nucleus is surrounded by the **cytoplasm**, which is in turn bounded by the thicker and somewhat porous **plasma membrane**, this being the cell's outer boundary and serving to separate it from other cells as well as from bodily fluids. The nucleus contains the cell's genetic material and functions, so to speak, as its operations center or command post. The cytoplasm is best described as a workshop or factory; it contains numerous small structures called **organelles** which turn out proteins and accomplish other essential tasks. The number and type of organelles vary according to the particular somatic cell's function. The cells lining the stomach and secreting gastric juices have a different set of organelles from those found in the eye's retinal cells, whose role is to process visual images from the outside world.

Nuclei tend to be more uniform in appearance and chemical composition than cytoplasms; in fact, the genetic material carried in any somatic cell is identical to that in all other somatic cells. The original "blueprint" created at zygogenesis (conception) is preserved in the nucleus of every cell in the body.[4] However, the cells in different organs and tissues do not follow the same sections of this general blueprint. It is as though the bone cells were doing their construction work using the specifications found in one part, while the nerve cells were following the directions

Germ Cells

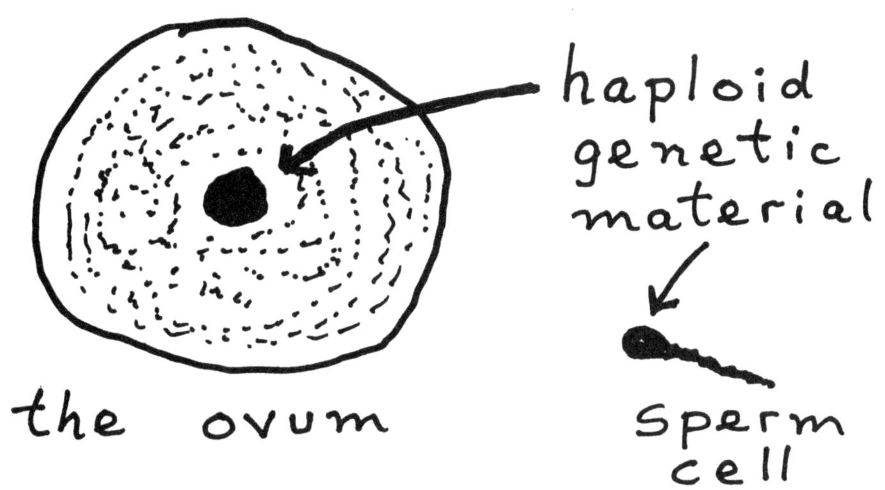

A Somatic Cell

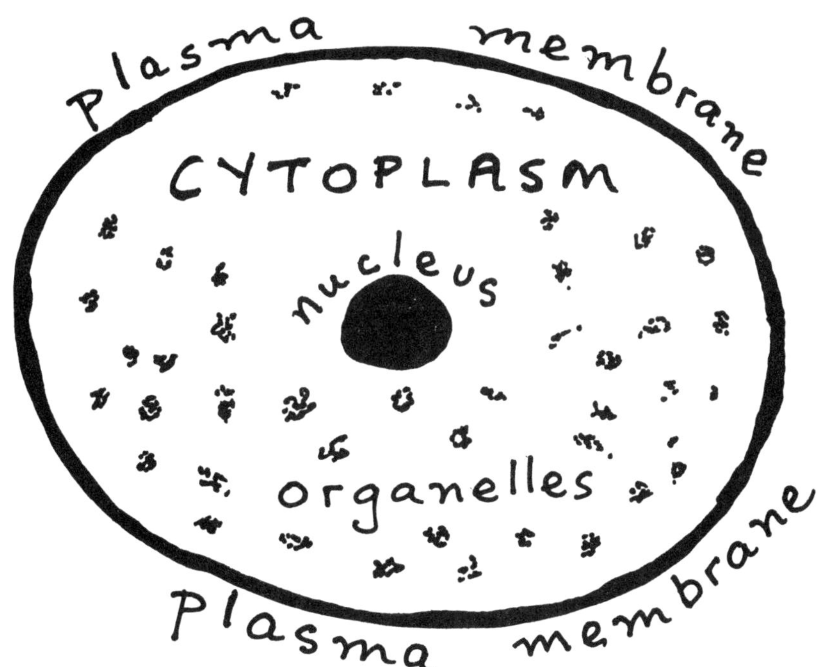

found in another. This state of affairs is not difficult to understand. When our architects and engineers design a skyscraper or other large building, they will prepare a comprehensive set of specifications , which is made available to all the construction workers involved. While the various carpenters, electricians, plumbers, masons, painters, welders, et al are thus using the very same text, they need comply only with those portions of it which pertain to their particular trades.

Our genetic blueprint should not be too extensively compared to those drawn up by architects, because it contains fantastic provisions calling not only for spontaneous growth and development, but also for perennial self-maintenance and self-repair. By and large the body takes care of itself in ways we hardly comprehend and rarely notice. The trillions of cells live in total harmony, each in its proper place and working solely for the good of the whole. Lung cells do not invade the liver; pancreatic cells do not spread into the gallbladder; the genitals never migrate to the brain. Somatic cells multiply only when there is reason to do so. For example, if you should cut or scratch your finger, the cells surrounding the wound will immediately begin rapid multiplication as your body undertakes a small self-repair. Within a few days the cut will have vanished, cellular division ceased, and the skin surface returned to normal—all this without any conscious effort on your part! If you live at sea level in San Francisco and then move to mile-high Denver, your blood will soon contain a larger number of oxygen-carrying red cells. Within hours your body will have automatically adjusted itself to the thinner atmosphere at Denver's higher altitude. When you become ill because of invading bacteria or viruses, a sample of your blood will reveal increased numbers of infection-fighting white cells: they have hurriedly multiplied in response to the foreign micro-organisms. As soon as the invaders are subdued, your immune system will automatically "switch-off," and your white-cell counts return to normal.

We could cite many more examples of the body's inscrutable mechanisms of regulation and regeneration, but they would not be especially pertinent. Such abilities characterize the body in health; and this book deals with disease, with those cases when the body proves unable to defend, regulate, or repair itself. We've already touched on infectious diseases; our physicians can usually fix us up, or at least identify the cause of the trouble. We now need to consider an entirely different category of human disease, and one which medical scientists have just recently begun to understand. For most of the resulting illnesses, we have no cures, and sometimes not even treatments which can effectively control symptoms and prolong longevity. The many varieties of human cancer fall under our next topic heading, as do to some extent such widespread afflictions as Alzheimer's disease, cardiovascular disease, diabetes, and osteoporosis.

Genetic Diseases

Errors in the zygotic blueprint created at conception are much more common than most of us realize. A serious error does not usually result in childbirth, but in spontaneous abortion (miscarriage), often so soon after conception that a woman never knows that she has been temporarily pregnant. Nature allows only the very smallest mistakes to be perpetuated, but some of them will sooner or later result in devastating illnesses. These **genetic diseases** are caused by misprints or malfunctions in the genetic material carried in the nucleus—by (as it were) "monkey wrenches" thrown into the cell's delicate operational machinery. A century ago medicine hardly recognized the existence of these diseases; today we can name thousands, both commonplace and rare, and the list is growing. Most diseases are now believed to have a genetic component—even infectious ones, because an individual's ability to resist particular bacteria or viruses tends to be genetically determined.

Genetic diseases can be subdivided into two broad categories: firstly, those resulting from errors which are present at the instant of conception, and secondly, those resulting from mutations which occur much later in previously normal somatic cells. The conceptional errors are often called **germline**. They can arise either by **inheritance of a defect** (one being passed on to an embryo from the father or from the mother or from both), or by **a totally new mutation occurring during zygogenesis**. A germline error would be repeated in every cell in the body, but it would adversely affect only those cells which must try to do their work following that flawed portion of the genetic blueprint. By way of illustration, we can cite three diseases which have been frequently discussed in our mass media. Cystic fibrosis, a hereditary disease found among Americans of European descent, results from a small error which affects the cells lining the lungs. As a consequence, the lungs fill with a thick, sticky mucus: this makes breathing difficult and leads to chronic bacterial infections. Another hereditary disorder, muscular dystrophy, results from a germline mutation which severely limits the production of an essential protein (dystrophin) by muscle cells. Without this protein muscles throughout the body gradually weaken and cease to function; the disease victims, almost all young boys, are soon confined to wheelchairs and usually die before age thirty. Sickle-cell anemia is prevalent among Americans of African descent; in this case the genetic misprint causes the red blood cells to produce an abnormal hemoglobin. As a result these cells can't transport

sufficient oxygen; and they assume a contorted "sickle shape," making it difficult for them to travel through tiny capillaries.

The preceding three examples can be described as **single-gene, early-onset diseases**. In each case, if the small error is present in the zygote, the disease will inevitably appear, and at an early age. Genetic illnesses of this type are quite different from those which typically afflict adults—e.g., cancer, heart disease, diabetes, and so forth. These adult diseases can be described as **late-onset** and **multifactorial**. They arise from a number of minor genetic imperfections, whose eventual expression as serious illness is often considerably influenced by personal lifestyles (e.g., factors like stress, obesity, or poor nutrition), by environmental agents (e.g., cancer-inducing chemicals), and by the inevitable effects of aging. By the 1990s our scientists had identified—and had come to understand—the genetic mistakes behind cystic fibrosis, muscular dystrophy, and sickle-cell anemia. There has yet to be a comparable understanding of those adult diseases which involve multiple genetic errors and various contributing factors.

CANCER:
A Genetic Disease of Somatic Cells

Cancer is the best example of our second category of genetic diseases—that is, those arising from new mutations in fully differentiated cells. While one or more germline errors may predispose an individual to this or that type of cancer, full-fledged disease will occur only after additional errors have thoroughly disrupted the normal functions of the somatic cell population involved. Such mutations typically creep in when our cells are duplicating their genetic material prior to dividing in two. As a rule of thumb, we can say that the more cells divide, the more likely they are to give rise to cancer. Some cells in the adult body no longer divide, and for all practical purposes they never become malignant. Who ever heard of "cancer of the nerves" or "cancer of the heart"? The cells in question have largely lost the ability to reproduce themselves—a fact which explains why damage to the heart muscle or the spinal cord tends to be irreversible. The cells of the adult liver divide only rarely; but if the organ is damaged, they can resume active reproduction to repair it. Still other groups of cells remain in a constant state of division and reproduction. Our blood cells, both red and white, are always reproducing themselves because they are short-lived. Billions die and disintegrate every day; and if the body is to stay healthy, billions of replacements must be born. However, blood cells are not the cellular species responsible for most adult cancers; that dubious distinction belongs to **epithelial cells**. Briefly defined, epithelial cells are those which cover the surface of the body, which line its internal cavities, and which form the productive portions of secretory glands like the adrenals, breasts, ovaries, pancreas, prostate, and testicles. Epithelial cells also wear out and die; therefore they too exhibit frequent reproduction. A general explanation for their tendency toward malignancy lies in the fact that they are often directly exposed to **carcinogens**—external substances which can produce mutations in genetic material.

Let's consider a few obvious examples. The skin represents the most accessible epithelium; since it's constantly being rubbed or worn away, the underlying cells are always dividing, and during that intricate process, exposing their genetic machinery to carcinogens. In this case the principal mutagenic agent is solar radiation, as demonstrated by the geographic distribution of skin cancers. The incidence is significantly higher in our Sunbelt cities (e.g., Dallas, Texas) than in those farther north (e.g., Detroit, Michigan). While skin cancers occur much more frequently than any other kind, they usually can be arrested by simple excision, and with the exception of melanomas, rarely become life-threatening.

In contrast, the epithelial cells lining our internal body cavities give rise to cancers which are potentially lethal. The best chance for survival rests on early detection and prompt treatment; but timely intervention often proves difficult, because most of these cavities are hidden from sight. They include the oral and nasal cavities, trachea (windpipe), esophagus, lungs, stomach, small intestine, colon, rectum, bladder, uterus, and vagina. We might be stretching the definition of "cavity" if we were to cite the tiny ducts of the milk-producing mammary glands; but the cells lining breast ducts display the relevant characteristics of other epithelial cells, namely frequent replication and susceptibility to mutation. Of course, the body cavities associated with the respiratory system and the gastrointestinal tract are those most likely to come in direct contact with carcinogens. Whatever we eat, drink, or breathe in, if it contains a mutagenic agent, can do damage. Since our cells possess considerable powers of self-repair, a prolonged exposure to the agent is usually necessary before cancer develops. A twenty-year habit of cigarette smoking—that is, of constantly inhaling the carcinogenic byproducts of burning tobacco—has often sufficed for malignant transformation in the larynx or lungs. The likelihood of colon and rectal cancers is probably increased by diets which are high in animal fat and low in vegetable fiber. The fat seems to be converted into a mild carcinogen during the digestive process, while the lack of fiber promotes constipation, ensuring that any mutagens in the stool are kept in prolonged contact with the colorectal epithelium.

Stomach cancer has been a major killer in Japan and some other countries, but the incidence in the United States has been steadily declining since the 1930s. The carcinogens behind the high Japanese rate of stomach cancer have been found in a traditional diet emphasizing smoked fish, pickled vegetables, and other salted or cured foods. The nitrates used to preserve these staples are converted into mutagenic nitrosamines during digestion. In less affluent nations, poor sanitary conditions and a lack of refrigeration often lead to infection with the intestinal bacterium *Helicobacter pylori*, which not only can produce chronic stomach inflammation, but may also predispose that organ to malignancy. Several viruses have been identified as *de facto* carcinogens. The hepatitis B virus has long been known to be associated with elevated rates of liver cancer, and three varieties of sexually-transmitted papillomavirus are now strongly linked to cervical cancer. This is not to imply that any kind of cancer is an infectious disease, but simply to acknowledge that some viral infections can destabilize our cells' genetic machinery and thus facilitate the development of tumors.

Variations in Susceptibility

Perhaps we have inched a little closer to a basic understanding of malignant transformation. The many forms of human cancer follow a common pattern. This or that group of somatic cells begins to multiply without reason and without restraint—and otherwise behave abnormally—because of multiple mutations which have accumulated in their nuclear genetic material. The chances of obtaining sufficient mutations are dependent on the aging process generally, as well as on the frequency with which the cells involved divide and with which they are exposed to carcinogens. While this scenario is as true as

any which could be penned in a sentence or two, it leaves a great deal unsaid and unexplained. We have identified the culprit carcinogens for some cancers (e.g., tobacco smoke for lung cancer), but for other tumors we can't point to any particular carcinogens which would adequately explain the incidence of disease. Cancers of the bladder, brain, breast, kidney, ovary, pancreas, and prostate may be said to lack a well-defined etiology, in that only occasionally do we have plausible "causes" for individual cases of disease.

We also have yet to understand the wide variations in genetic susceptibility to carcinogens. Why do most sunbathers remain free of melanoma? And why do many smokers fail to develop lung cancer or some other malignancy affecting the respiratory passages? Our methods of predicting an individual's risk for cancer generally, or for any one type of cancer, remain less than optimal. We do know that certain tumors seem to run in certain families. And we are working to catalogue those hereditary genetic defects which, when passed on from parent to child, virtually guarantee the subsequent development of a particular malignancy. The family of former President Jimmy Carter has provided an especially poignant illustration of a **familial cancer syndrome**. Carter's father, his two sisters, and his brother all died prematurely from pancreatic cancer. Some cases of breast cancer are hereditary; in Chapter Three we'll consider the recent findings in this area. But next we need to learn the working vocabulary of cancer-oriented physicians and researchers.

Basic Definitions in Oncology

The field of medicine devoted to cancer is called **oncology**, from the Greek word (*onkos*) for a mass or tumor. The term **oncologist** refers to a physician who treats many types of cancer using a variety of drugs. These days radiotherapists (who principally deal with cancer patients) sometimes appropriate the designation and identify themselves as **radiation oncologists**. The many types of human cancer are divided into three main groups, which correspond to the particular tissues where malignancies can originate. Cancers arising from epithelial cells are called **carcinomas**; they are by far the most numerous. **Sarcomas** originate in connective tissues, such as muscle or bone; they are relatively rare, but they sometimes occur in adolescents who are experiencing rapid growth of muscles and bones. The **leukemias and lymphomas** constitute an important third group; they typically arise from the hematopoietic ("blood-producing") tissues found in the bone marrow. These malignancies involve the overproduction of immature or otherwise dysfunctional white cells, which may be present throughout the circulatory system (as in the leukemias) or be initially confined to the lymph nodes (as in the lymphomas).

Not all abnormal growths are malignant. The vast majority are benign, as amply illustrated by the moles or warts which we all have somewhere on the skin, by the most common tumors of the breast (fibroadenomas) and of the uterus (fibroids), and in case of the white blood cells, by infectious mononucleosis. Benign tumors normally stop growing or regress after they reach a certain size; their constituent cells never invade the surrounding tissues. At worst these tumors may cause trouble through the mechanical processes of expansion and compression; they are not likely to be life-threatening unless they happen to develop within the confines of the skull, where they would dangerously compress the brain.

Malignant tumors, in contrast, have many ways of doing damage. They have three characteristics which set them apart from benign cellular proliferations and which provide as good a definition of the word **malignancy** as we will ever have. The first characteristic is **unrestrained growth**; they do not stop growing or regress. The second characteristic is **invasion**; their constituent cells will sooner or later infiltrate into the surrounding tissues. The third and most striking characteristic is **metastasis**. The word comes from the Greek, meaning a change (*meta*) in standing or position (*stasis*). However, the best English word for the relevant process is simply **colonization**. During metastasis, a tumor's malignant cells enter the nearby lymphatic or blood vessels, and are thus carried to other parts of the body. When these cells come to rest in distant tissues or organs, they take root and start to multiply, creating secondary tumors (metastases) which tend to be more aggressive and proliferative than the original (primary) tumor. For some malignancies, metastasis alone imparts a lethal potential. Breast tumors which remain confined to the breast may become extremely disfiguring, but they will never become life-threatening. A breast tumor whose cells metastasize to essential organs like the lungs, the liver, the brain, or the skeleton will soon start to interfere with functions essential for life; and eventually it will prove fatal.

BREAST CARCINOMAS:
Steps in Malignant Transformation

Writers on cancer often hypothesize that tumors begin with just a single cell which turns malignant. Whether this is true or not, we can safely say that as the zygote demonstrates the creative power of a single cell, the individual cancer cell could provide an equally impressive demonstration of destructive power. Unlike zygotes, however, cancer cells are not created overnight; their development in solid tumors involves an extended multistep process. For some malignancies, notably those of the breast, colon, lung, and prostate, the transformation would often seem to require twenty years or more. Let's consider the most obvious steps in this transition of normal epithelial cells to frankly cancerous cells, as these steps might be identified by a skilled pathologist using a light microscope. While our hypothetical tissue specimen is based on a milk duct in the breast, our discussion of general concepts is applicable to other epithelial tissues which can become malignant.

(1) normal breast epithelium

The cells which line breast ducts are, like other epithelial cells, arranged neatly in thin layers, only several cells deep. These cells rest on a **basement membrane**, which separates them from the surrounding supporting tissues known as **the stroma** (from the Greek word for "bed"). The stroma reveals numerous capillaries, which supply blood to the ductal cells above the basement membrane. It also contains lymphatic drainage vessels, and it's crisscrossed with fibers made from the protein **collagen** (an extracellular secretion). Under a microscope, normal epithelium appears as a model of order and uniformity. The individual cells resemble each other in size and appearance, with only a very occasional cell undergoing **mitosis** (the process of division). Their nuclei are quite regular, and small in comparison with the surrounding cytoplasms.

(2) hyperplasia

This Latinate word signifies an excessive (*hyper*) development or formation (*plasia*). In pathology, it refers to an increase in the number of cells, which remain as yet reasonably normal in appearance and function. David L. Page and Jean F. Simpson, pathologists at Vanderbilt University, define

this term as it pertains to the breast ducts: "Hyperplasia may be considered to represent an increased number of cells above the basement membrane, and because this number is normally two, then three or more cells above the basement membrane constitutes hyperplasia."[5] Hyperplasia is not cancer, but simply a benign overgrowth which may sometimes indicate an increased risk of subsequent malignant transformation. There are degrees of hyperplasia, the most suspicious being designated ***highly atypical*** and being characterized by numerous excess cells of different sizes and with irregular nuclei. In one study, women diagnosed with atypical hyperplasia who had as well a family history of breast cancer were found to have eleven times the usual risk of developing invasive carcinoma.[6] Most women who receive a diagnosis of hyperplasia after biopsy have a considerably lower risk; usually the only course of action recommended is observation—e.g., follow-up examinations by the physician and regular mammograms.

(3) ductal carcinoma *in situ*

The Latin term *in situ* means "in place." Pathologists use it to refer to cells which seem to have undergone malignant transformation, but have not yet begun to invade the surrounding tissues. As applied to the breast, a diagnosis of ductal carcinoma *in situ* (DCIS) means that the milk ducts examined are largely or totally filled up with apparently malignant cells, but that the basement membranes are intact and continue to separate these cells from the surrounding stroma. The cells themselves are no longer organized in neat layers, but jumbled together and crowding each other. However, it is their nuclei which give the clearest evidence of transformation. The nuclei are typically ***pleomorphic*** (revealing diverse shapes) and ***hyperchromatic*** (staining brightly with the applied

A Normal Breast Duct

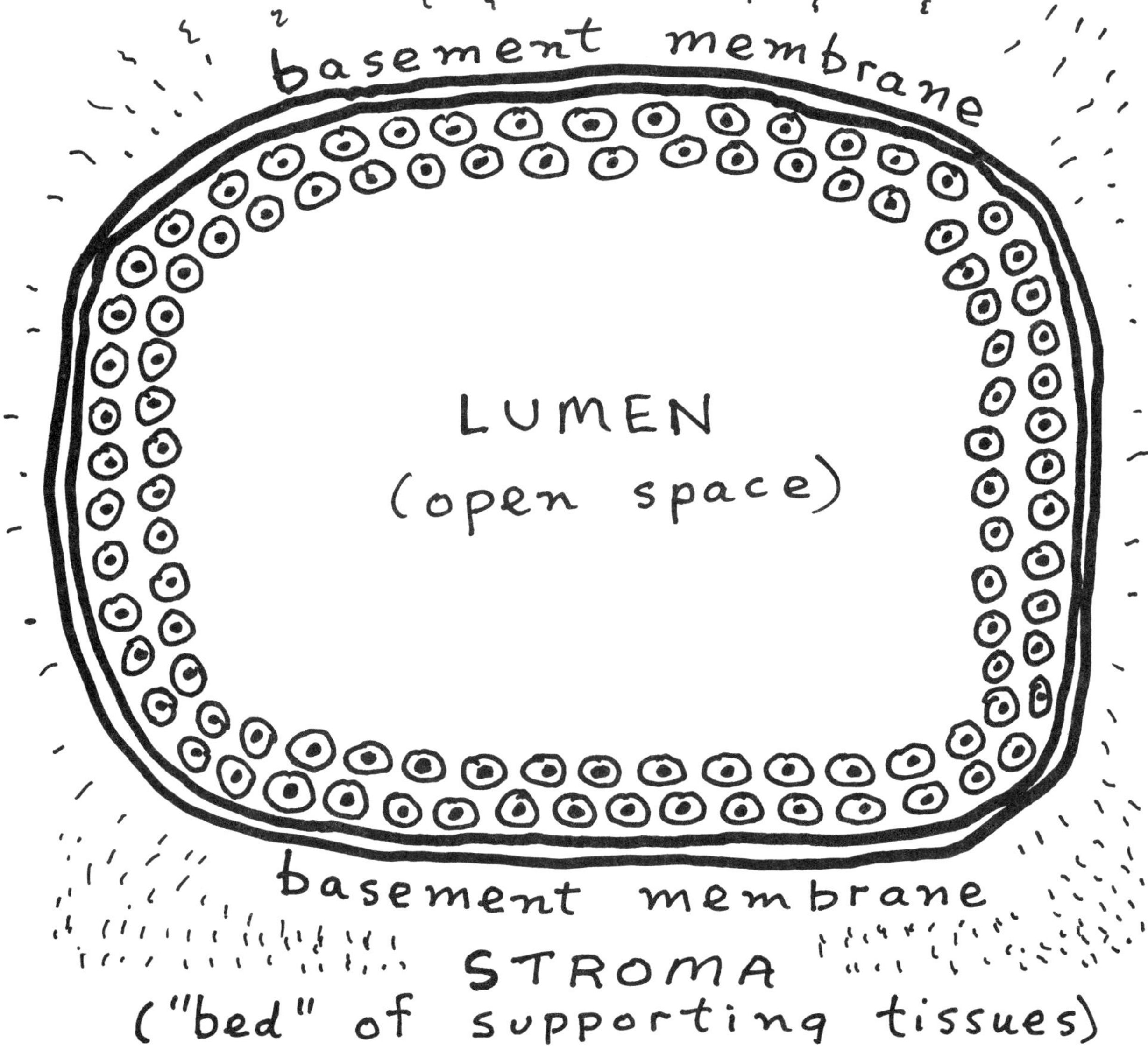

The normal duct is characterized by a well-defined **basement membrane** on all sides and by a **thin layer of small regular cells** above that membrane. The largely fibrous **stroma** ("bed") surrounds and supports the duct, which has a distinct **lumen** (central open passageway).

Hyperplasia in a Breast Duct

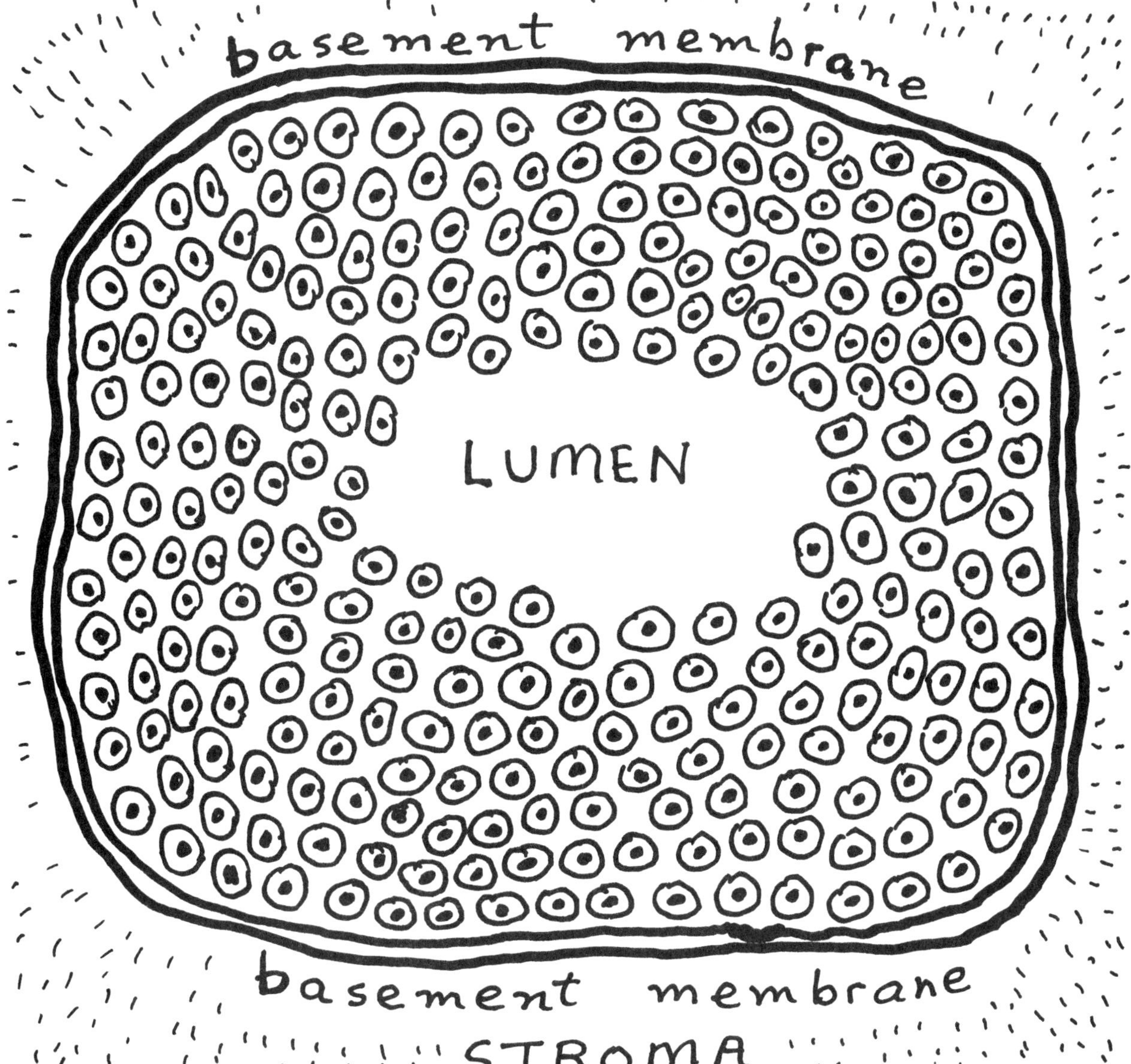

Hyperplasia is a pathological term used to denote a benign proliferation of the epithelial cells lining a breast duct. But if these cells reveal variations in the size and shape of their nuclei, the risk of malignant transformation must be assumed to be elevated, and the term **"atypical hyperplasia"** would be used.

chemical stains). They have also grown considerably larger—the cytoplasms often seem to have shrunken so much that they resemble thin rims or "halos" around these transformed nuclei.

Ductal carcinoma *in situ* is also referred to as **intraductal carcinoma**. By either designation DCIS is still not the feared disease we think of as "cancer." Yes, the genetic machinery of DCIS cells has gone haywire, as indicated by their enlarged, pleomorphic nuclei; but the principal characteristic of malignancy—invasion of other tissues—is not present. When does DCIS progress to an invasive carcinoma? And what particular alterations in cellular function lead to this progression? At the moment we do not have really useful answers to these prognostic queries. Even the diagnosis of DCIS often leaves something to chance and to subjective interpretation. On the one hand, pathologists can't always be sure of the fine distinction between highly atypical hyperplasia and true DCIS. On the other, when they agree on the diagnosis of DCIS, they cannot always rule out the possibility of occult invasion of a basement membrane—and such subtle unnoticed infiltration could be the key event which marks the beginning of a potentially deadly tumor. While atypical hyperplasia is only an indicator of increased risk, DCIS must be presumed to be the forerunner of invasive disease, and physicians will always recommend that it be treated. Yet because the patient is in no immediate danger either of local invasion or of metastasis, the treatment will probably be limited to the removal (surgical excision) of the involved duct or ducts, which could be accomplished either by a simple mastectomy or by a breast-preserving lumpectomy. There would be no need for systemic chemotherapy. If a patient with extensive DCIS opts for breast preservation, whole-breast irradiation may be advisable to control any cancer cells which have escaped

the surgeon's scalpel.

(4) <u>infiltrating</u> <u>ductal</u> <u>carcinoma</u>

This is frank malignancy; no conscientious pathologist will err in the diagnosis. The basement membrane has vanished, and the transformed ductal cells are present in the stroma. These cells will henceforth secrete lytic enzymes called **proteases**, which not only accomplish the disintegration of basement membranes, but also dissolve the collagenous bonds holding the stromal elements together. With these barriers removed, the growing mass of malignant cells is free to expand in all directions; but its growth will be limited to a millimeter or two unless it can obtain an additional blood supply. Unfortunately, an expanding malignant tumor—like a growing embryo in the uterus—possesses the power of **angiogenesis**; it can stimulate the creation of those new blood vessels which are needed to nourish rapid growth.

Hyperplasia and DCIS, the first two steps toward breast malignancy, usually do not produce any **clinical symptoms** (outward signs) that a woman or her physician could detect during a routine physical examination. In contrast, the more an invasive tumor progresses, the more likely it is to produce noticeable symptoms. The tumor becomes a focus of metabolic activity, with tissue dissolution, ongoing angiogenesis, and frequent mitoses. The involved area consequently tends to be slightly warmer than the adjacent normal tissues; the temperature difference can sometimes be recorded by a test called **thermography**. However, what typically brings a growing breast carcinoma to medical attention is the formation of a hard lump, which is usually (but not always) painless. The lump does not consist of cancer cells; instead it represents a **stromal reaction**, which occurs as the connective cells in the stroma (fibroblasts) churn out large quantities of collagen

Ductal Carcinoma *in situ*

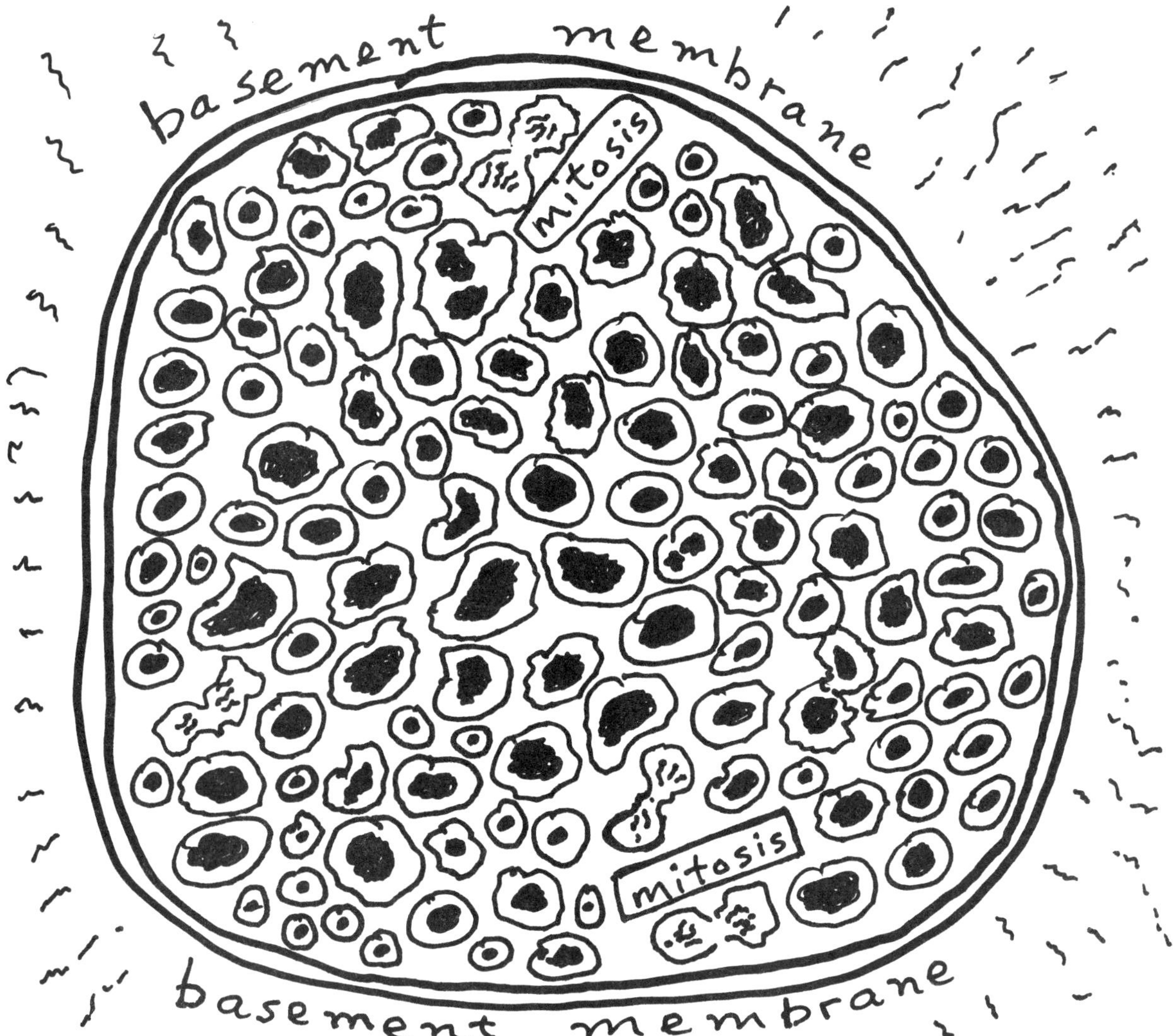

In **ductal carcinoma *in situ*** (DCIS) the orderly arrangement of epithelial cells into thin layers has vanished. To a greater or lesser degree, the individual ductal cells will reveal enlarged and irregularly shaped nuclei, visible **mitoses** (cells in the act of division), and other changes characteristic of malignancy. But as long as the basement membrane remains intact, these cells cannot spread outside of the involved duct.

fibers in response to the infiltrating malignant cells. This reaction can be viewed as a defensive mechanism: the body is trying to encapsulate (seal off) the tumor in the same way that it often encapsulates foreign objects (e.g., silicone breast implants) or bacteria (e.g., the tubercles of tuberculosis). In the case of breast carcinoma, such fibrous encapsulation does not work very well. The proteases secreted by the cancer cells dissolve portions of the newly erected collagen barrier, permitting the tumor to send out "tendrils" in different directions.

(5) <u>metastasis</u>

The invasion of the basement membrane and the subsequent dissolution of the underlying matrix are ominous events, not so much because they allow local expansion of a tumor, but because they give its malignant cells ready access to the capillaries and lymphatic vessels in the stroma. Once these cells enter the bloodstream or lymph fluid, they will be carried to other parts of the body, where they may—or may not—give rise to metastases. Solid tumors vary widely in their ability to metastasize. Some, including small-cell lung cancer and testicular cancer, do so regularly and rapidly. Other malignancies, including those of the prostate and thyroid, tend to remain localized to the organ of origin for an extended period, and then to metastasize slowly. We cannot generalize about breast cancers. Some mammary tumors can grow to grotesque sizes and still never acquire the ability to metastasize; others seem to metastasize as soon as they cross the basement membrane, long before their presence can be consistently detected either by physical exam or by mammography. Since the majority of breast cancer patients die of causes unrelated to cancer, we may safely conclude that even those tumors which metastasize do not always behave aggressively. But a few

breast cancers, most notably those designated "inflammatory," behave with considerable aggressiveness and sometimes will prove fatal within a year or two after diagnosis.

The possibility of metastasis needs to be taken into account in all cases of invasive carcinoma. While breast cancers do spread through the bloodstream, an initial dissemination through the lymphatic system is more obvious—and more easily verifiable. Most of the lymphatic vessels draining the breast pass through a battery of filtering lymph nodes located in the **axilla** (Latin for "armpit"). When a primary tumor in the breast reveals evidence of local invasion, the axillary nodes need to be biopsied (surgically sampled) and examined by a pathologist. If one or more of these nodes should contain cancer cells, we will have strong circumstantial evidence—*but not proof*—that other malignant cells are circulating throughout the body. The more **positive nodes** found in the axilla, the greater the likelihood of distant metastases. But involved axillary nodes are only a plausible indicator of a tumor's metastatic potential. The fact of metastasis can never be established before the symptoms of malignant colonization are documented in some distant organ or tissue.

The Biology of Metastatic Cells

A main goal of cancer research is to understand the mechanisms of metastasis, so that someday we may devise a drug to prevent or to arrest this process. The characteristics of cancer cells have been intensively studied *in vitro*: these Latin words, literally meaning "in glass," refer to laboratory experiments carried out on living cells cultivated in a test tube or (more commonly) in a flat Petri dish. Normal human cells are difficult to keep alive *in vitro*; they will reproduce only a limited number of

Infiltrating Ductal Carcinoma

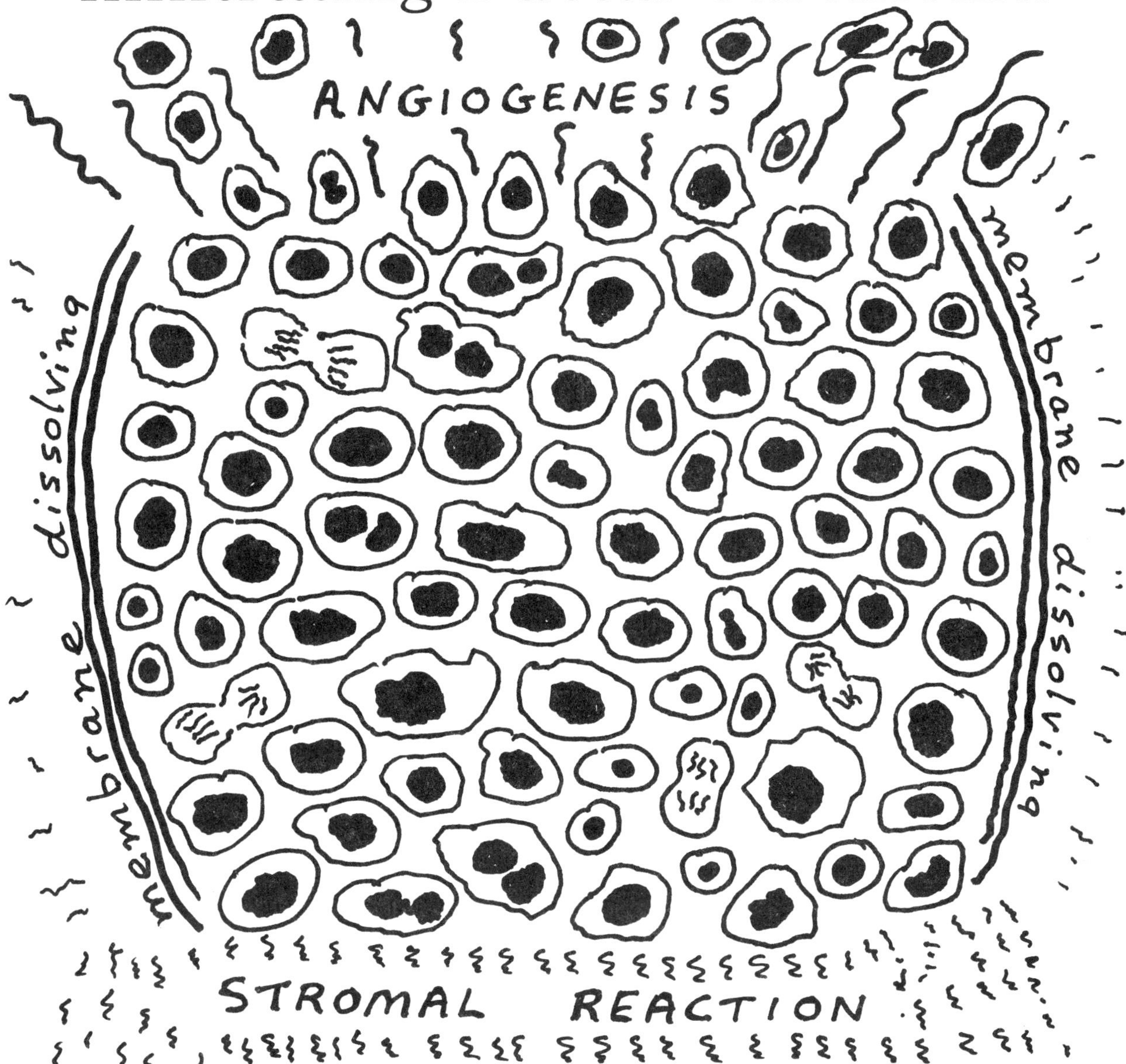

The complete or partial absence of the duct's basement membrane is the hallmark of invasive cancer. Obviously "transformed" cells with highly irregular nuclei typically indicate an aggressive malignancy which will stimulate **angiogenesis** (the growth of new blood vessels) and provoke a **stromal reaction** (fibrous thickening) in the adjacent tissues.

times and then die. Cancer cells are different: they have become immortal. Properly cared for, they will multiply endlessly in Petri dishes. Because of this **immortalization**, we can conduct inexpensive experiments on numerous **cell lines**—that is, on living cancer cells taken from a wide range of tumors and made available to qualified researchers. From such experiments we have learned that cancer cells usually divide about as rapidly as do the normal cells in the organs or tissues from which the respective malignancies arose. For example, leukemic blood cells multiply rapidly, as do normal blood cells. Malignant liver or pancreatic cells reproduce slowly, as do the normal cells in these organs. An acute leukemia, untreated, could overwhelm the body and produce death in a few weeks; but while cancers of the liver and pancreas also tend to be deadly, they require years of growth before they become life-threatening. Newly diagnosed cancer patients often worry that their malignant cells are proliferating explosively; this is not often the case. While cancer cells reproduce without the customary restraints, the frequency of their reproduction can vary greatly; consequently, the prognosis in disseminated disease can vary greatly. There is tremendous variation in the reproductive rates seen in breast carcinomas. Fortunately, we now have tests which can estimate a breast tumor's rate of cellular proliferation. As explained in Chapter Thirteen, physicians should consider this rate before making treatment recommendations involving chemotherapy.

Besides immortalization, two other characteristics distinguishing malignant cells from normal ones can be clearly demonstrated in laboratory experiments—**anchorage independence** and **loss of contact inhibition**. These two attributes are also prerequisites for tumor growth and metastasis. Normal epithelial cells are anchorage dependent—to live and reproduce, they must be "anchored" to a basement membrane or to other cells. *In vitro*, they will grow only in thin layers one-cell deep, the bottom of a Petri dish serving as a substitute for the basement membrane. Malignant epithelial cells no longer require anchorage; they can live and multiply while suspended in a liquid gel medium. If they did not have this characteristic, they could hardly survive extended transport floating in the bloodstream or in lymph fluid. Normal epithelial cells also exhibit contact inhibition: that is, they tend not to reproduce if their outer membranes are touching each other. But malignant cells have no scruples about crowding their neighbors and multiply even when hemmed in. A colony of these cells growing in a Petri dish soon starts to resemble a tumor in the body; it becomes a jumbled mass of cells heaped haphazardly on top of each other.

Metastatic Progression

While malignant cells possess reproductive advantages over normal ones, many factors may limit their ability to multiply and metastasize. Even in those tumors which give rise to metastases, it is probable that only a few cells are capable of establishing distant colonies. Mark E. Sobel, a pathologist at the National Cancer Institute, calls our attention to this heterogeneity: "Metastatic propensity is distinctly separate from tumorigenicity alone. Metastatic potential varies among particular cells of a tumor."[7] Unfortunately, those cells which metastasize seem to be the most aggressive and rugged. They are of necessity hardy colonists—as well as biological outlaws, pirates, and squatters. Cut loose from all anchorage and void of restraint, they penetrate into lymphatic and blood vessels, evade challenge by the white cells guarding these passageways, and manage to survive a long, mechanically stressful journey in fluids

Looking for Tumor Dissemination: The Role of Sentinel Node Sampling

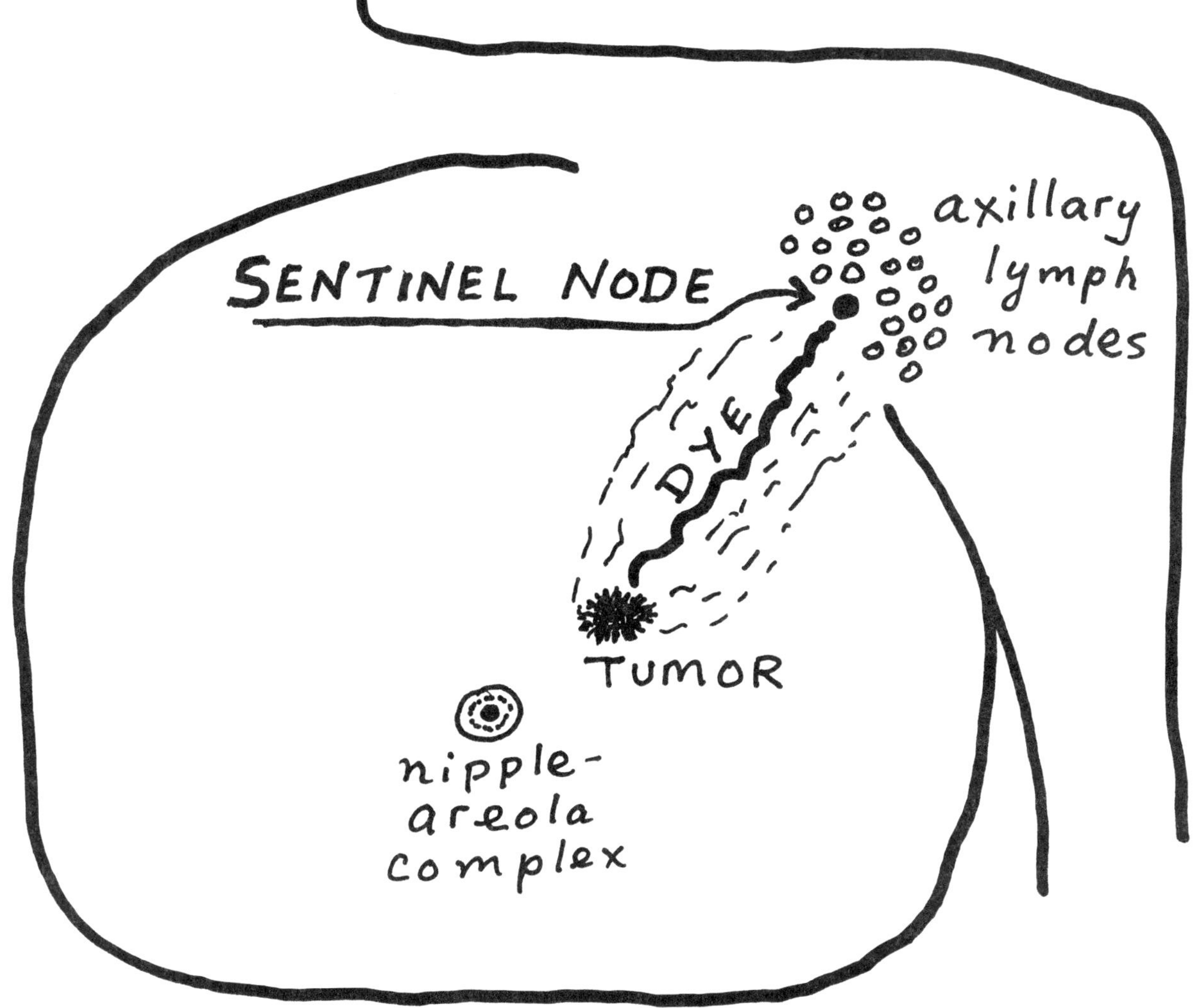

Breast cancer cells spread first through the nearby lymphatic vessels to the nodes in the axilla, later entering the bloodstream and being carried to the bone marrow and other organs. Colored dye injected in the tumor area highlights the draining lymphatic vessels and usually permits the identification of a **single sentinel node**, which would normally contain cancer cells if tumor dissemination has taken place.

that are to them strange and hostile. When these metastatic cells finally lodge in distant parts of the body, they must adapt to—and learn to flourish in—foreign environments quite unlike their original locales. Unfortunately, the metastatic colonies they create will be dedicated to exploitation. The processes of invasion and angiogenesis are continually repeated, ensuring malignant growth while destroying normal tissues.

Metastatic cells can spread to virtually any site in the body, but the different varieties of human cancer tend to follow fairly predictable patterns of metastasis to certain locations. For example, colorectal carcinomas will spread first to regional lymph nodes, and then secondly to the liver. Breast cancers, like those of the prostate, reveal a strong tendency to metastasize through the bloodstream to the bone marrow. Here the metastatic colonies supplant the normal marrow and thus reduce the production of blood cells. More ominously, they interfere with the work of neighboring osteoblasts (bone-forming cells) and slowly dissolve the bone matrix, sometimes causing pathologic quantities of calcium and other minerals to be released into the blood. An early symptom is increasing bone pain, which often serves as a harbinger of impending fractures, typically of such weight-bearing structures as the hip or femur (thighbone). The lungs may also be involved with metastatic breast cancer. Sometimes their mucosal linings will be studded with small nodules of tumor. Malignant breast cells often implant on the pleura, a lubricated membrane separating the lungs from the surrounding rib cage. In either case, the eventual result is a loss of respiratory function. When a breast tumor spreads to the liver, the probable consequences include pain, jaundice, and digestive disorders. Metastases to the brain, spinal cord, or cerebrospinal fluid may be temporarily managed with chemotherapy or irradiation; but they are likely to prove fatal, regardless of whether they emanate from a breast tumor or from some other malignancy.

End-stage metastatic cancer bears a perverse resemblance to embryogenesis; it is a second childhood of sorts. Malignant cells seem to be moving about freely, establishing colonies at will throughout the abdominal and chest cavities. As we recall, a zygote's cellular offspring demonstrate a comparable freedom of movement in early pregnancy. But the evolution of zygotian cells is toward a productive differentiation, resulting in creation and stability. Malignant cells evolve from an initial differentiation to a total lack of differentiation, producing physiological chaos. First they abandon their roles as mature somatic cells; finally they have—like garden weeds or insect pests—no function except that of self-serving multiplication. And the more malignant cells divide, the more the genetic machinery in their nuclei will run amuck. These cells can become so misshapen—*so undifferentiated*—that a pathologist examining them under a microscope could not positively identify the source of the primary tumor. He or she could not say offhand whether the cells originated from the breast or the bladder, from the lungs or the liver.

When metastatic cells are present in sufficient numbers, they will begin to derange the body's metabolism, leading to **anorexia** (loss of appetite) and **cachexia** (wasting away). These two conditions are easily recognizable by those of us who have lost a family member or friend to terminal cancer. Eventually the body is so weakened that the immune system ceases to function, leaving a patient vulnerable to pathogenic microorganisms. In many cases of advanced metastatic disease, the precipitating cause of death will be an infection like bacterial pneumonia rather than cancer *per se*.

CURABLE CANCERS
Why We Still Need Research

At present there are no painless and totally efficient "miracle drugs" for breast cancers—or for any other human malignancies. Yet our hopes for therapeutic breakthroughs are high, because our knowledge of the genetic malfunctions leading to malignancy has been expanding by leaps and bounds. All manner of **designer drugs** which would selectively target and in effect nullify these mutations are under development. Some of these drugs have already reached the market, most notably **Gleevec**, which produces seemingly miraculous remissions in chronic myelogenous leukemia, and **Herceptin**, which occasionally achieves a stunning response in breast cancers whose growth is prompted by the HER-2/*neu* oncogene. These successes should not blind us to the fact that there are still no designer drugs for most types of cancer. Moreover, it is probably unreasonable to expect that a single pharmaceutical will ever cure a broad spectrum of malignancies in the same way that penicillin once cured a broad spectrum of infectious diseases. For the time being, cancer patients and their physicians must continue to rely upon three imprecise therapies which treat the aberrant nuclei of malignant cells by simply attempting wholesale destruction, inevitably damaging normal tissues in the process. These therapies are **surgery**, which came of age in the early decades of the last century, and **radiotherapy** and **chemotherapy**, both of which matured considerably in the 1970s and have since undergone additional refinements. Proponents of unconventional treatments often refer sarcastically to these mainline therapies as "Cut, Burn, and Poison." Admittedly, these modalities involve a degree of mutilation or toxicity, but either singly or in combination they can consistently cure some cancers. The "cures" produced by unorthodox methods

(wacky diets, coffee enemas, positive thinking) are anecdotal; they are not reproducible under controlled conditions. Let's confine our discussion to the verifiable cures.

Surgery can always cure a tumor which remains localized to a nonvital organ. Early-stage cancers of the breast, colon, and prostate are usually curable by careful surgical excision, as is the occasional lung cancer which has not spread beyond a single lobe. The most dramatic reductions ever seen in cancer mortality rates have been brought about by timely surgery for two gynecological malignancies, those of the endometrium (uterine lining) and the cervix. Endometrial cancers typically afflict postmenopausal women, and they "present" (as the doctors say) with unexplained vaginal bleeding. This early symptom leads to early diagnosis, which is usually made before the tumor penetrates through the muscular uterine wall. Hysterectomy is always curative for localized endometrial cancers. While cervical cancers do not produce early symptoms, widespread screening with the famous **Pap smear** has led to their timely discovery in most cases. A simple surgical procedure can always cure localized disease.

Radiotherapy is often used in conjunction with surgery. Sometimes irradiation serves to shrink an overly large tumor to operable size; at other times it's used postoperatively, to destroy any cancer cells which may have been left behind when the surgeon removed the primary tumor. Both pre- and postoperative applications are playing an increasing role in the initial treatment of breast cancers. Occasionally, radiotherapy will be used by itself as the sole modality, either to cure an especially radiosensitive cancer or to control a tumor whose location makes resection (surgical excision) impractical. Early-stage Hodgkin's disease (a form of lymphoma) is an example of a potentially lethal malignancy which can be cured by radiation alone. Radiotherapy finds its most varied applications in the management of advanced cancers. It's used to alleviate the pain and slow the progression of bone metastases—to shrink metastatic tumors which may be obstructing the bowel, or blocking airways (bronchial tubes) in the lungs, or pressing against the spinal cord—and to reduce the edema and excessive intracranial pressure which result from brain metastases.

Both surgery and radiotherapy are local treatments: they are used to destroy cancer cells which are causing a problem at a specific site. **Chemotherapy**, in contrast, is a systemic treatment: it's aimed at cancer cells which have spread—or are presumed to have spread—throughout the body. Surgery for cancer dates back to antiquity; radiotherapy was first attempted around 1900. Chemotherapy with cytotoxic ("cell-killing") drugs is much more recent. The first attempt to treat a human malignancy with chemo did not occur until 1942; in the 1960s this modality was available only at the larger American medical centers, and it was used almost exclusively for the treatment of leukemias and lymphomas. The 1970s and 1980s brought revolutionary changes. Complex multidrug regimens were developed for commonplace solid tumors—notably, for malignancies of the breast and lung—and chemo became readily available at community hospitals and in oncologists' offices. By the 1990s **adjuvant chemotherapy** was standard for most cancer patients with positive lymph nodes or other indications of possible metastatic progression. That puzzling term "adjuvant" is more precisely used if expanded to **surgical adjuvant**. It simply means that the drugs are given after—and as an aid to—surgery (the initial therapy). The curative potential of adjuvant chemotherapy remains the subject of much debate and controversy, especially in the case of breast carcinomas. Oncologists will argue that even those breast cancer patients who will eventually develop metastatic disease

stand to benefit from a judicious regimen. The drugs usually delay the appearance of metastases, and for some patients they can significantly extend life expectancy. But the proper test for a systemic modality would be its ability to cure established systemic disease. Judged by this rigorous criterion, the existing chemo regimens can be said to cure only a few malignancies, most notably the acute leukemias afflicting children and teenagers which had hitherto been universally fatal. Chemotherapy cannot cure metastatic disease arising from the solid tumors which typically afflict older adults. Indeed, of all the solid tumors, cytotoxic drugs can unequivocally cure only three—testicular cancer, the very rare choriocarcinoma (which arises from the placenta during pregnancy), and germ-cell ovarian carcinoma (which needs to be distinguished from the more prevalent epithelial ovarian tumors). These three cures are real but terrible; they involve repeated cycles of intravenous drug administration, with all the side effects we've learned to associate with chemo (nausea, vomiting, hair loss, reduced libido and fertility). Why does chemo work with these particular tumors, even in the presence of distant metastases? The answer lies in the uniform aggressiveness of the three cancers. Their cells divide with a rapidity approaching that of the childhood leukemias; consequently they are vulnerable to our cytotoxic drugs, which act most efficiently on rapidly dividing cells. The other solid tumors grow more slowly, and they are not nearly so chemosensitive. Attempts at curing them have been stymied by the main deficiency of cytotoxic chemotherapy—that is, the drugs lack sufficient specificity for malignant cells; they will kill normal cells as well as the cancerous ones. Thus for the vast majority of solid tumors, the dose required to eradicate established metastases would also suffice to kill the patient.

Fortunately, most breast cancer patients

are not candidates for intensive chemotherapy, either because their tumors are **node-negative** (i.e., presumably localized to the breast) or because they are **hormonally responsive**. Generally speaking, hormonal manipulations play only a minor role in cancer medicine, but there are three important exceptions. These involve malignancies of the prostate and endometrium, as well as selected breast cancers. The normal cells of these organs are extremely responsive to the steroid sex hormones, with testosterone (an androgen) acting upon the prostate, and estrogen and progesterone stimulating the uterine lining and the mammary gland. When a malignant tumor arises from one of these tissues, its transformed cells frequently retain their hormonal responsiveness; and their ability to multiply can often be hindered for many years through hormonal manipulations. Not long ago, the initial manipulation was likely to be surgical ablation—removal of the testicles to end the supply of testosterone fueling the growth of metastatic prostate cancers, or removal of the ovaries to reduce estrogenic stimulation of metastatic breast tumors. In the 1980s ablative surgery yielded ground to several drugs which effectively block the action of sex hormones on cancer cells. Foremost among these antagonist agents is **tamoxifen**, a powerful antiestrogen. As explained in Chapter Twenty-two, the systemic agent used most often in breast cancer treatment has been tamoxifen, not chemo. It's given both as an adjuvant (to prevent or delay the appearance of metastatic disease) and in the management of recurrent disease. While tamoxifen probably does not eradicate many cases of breast cancer, it has few side effects; and it demonstrably delays the progression of well-differentiated, slow-growing, hormonally responsive tumors. Such tumors are common among postmenopausal women, who constitute a majority (75% or more) of breast cancer patients.

Chapter Two

Inside a Cell's Nucleus

Oddly enough, the first step toward an understanding of the nuclear genetic material was taken not with a microscope, but with a gardener's trowel. In the year 1856 Gregor Mendel, a Catholic priest living in a monastery in Moravia (later Czechoslovakia), began to conduct a series of experiments which would do much to reveal how this genetic material dictates the physical characteristics of living organisms. Mendel had no cell lines or laboratory animals; he used garden peas, painstakingly crossbreeding different strains of peas, and meticulously recording the attributes of the resulting hybrids. Any college textbook on genetics will give you the details of Mendel's experiments—for example, how he crossed round-seed pea plants with those yielding wrinkled seeds, or green-pod plants with yellow-pod plants. We need be concerned only with the revolutionary conclusions Mendel reached. In a paper published in 1866, he postulated that the characteristics of peas—and by implication, of other living things—are determined by discrete hereditary factors, and that these factors are transmitted intact from one generation to the next, in a mathematically predictable fashion. Mendel did not use the word **genes** to describe these units of heredity; that term became current only after 1900. What his work on peas demonstrated so clearly was, however, the fundamental distinction between **dominant and recessive genes**.

Let's briefly consider how Mendelian principles might apply to human inheritance, by imagining a single gene which would control eye color. But if your mother had brown eyes and your father had blue, and your own eyes are brown, does that mean you received your mother's eye-color gene but not your father's? Hardly. You would have received two copies of the eye-color gene, one from your mother and one from your father. Such paired copies of a gene coding for a single characteristic are called **alleles**. You have brown eyes because the eye-color allele (gene) you received from your mother is dominant, and it is therefore "expressed" (as the geneticists say) in your **phenotype** (physical make-up). The blue-eye allele you received from your father is recessive; and while it is not expressed, you are a carrier for it. Recessive alleles normally remain unexpressed, except when two carriers of the same recessive allele have children together. In this case, there is a 25% chance that any given offspring will receive two copies of the recessive allele, which would then be fully expressed. The result is not always a matter of pretty blue eyes; many hereditary diseases are transmitted recessively, among them cystic fibrosis and sickle-cell anemia. The parents of afflicted children are healthy carriers, being **heterozygous**—that is, each has a dominant normal allele which suppresses the recessive disease-producing allele. Any children with disease are **homozygous**—that is, they have inherited two copies of the defective allele.

Most people carry a number of quiescent but potentially troublesome recessive alleles. When close relatives marry and have children, the risk of homozygosity and subsequent disease is significantly increased. From time immemorial, human societies have tried to discourage such unions, not from any knowledge of genetics, but simply from observing the mental and physical deficiencies which often result from inbreeding. Mendel's experiments gave us the first clues to genetic transmission; but however suitable Mendelian principles may be to garden peas, they do not explain all the vagaries of human inheritance. Our genetic inheritance is far more complex than that of the pea; most of our characteristics and traits are determined not by single genes, but by subtle interactions among large numbers of genes.

CHROMOSOMES
The Carriers of Genes

The next advance in understanding our genetic material was accomplished by German **cytologists** (i.e., scientists investigating the structures and functions of cells). Normally no structures can be seen in a cell's nucleus, even with a powerful microscope. However, in the late 1870s Walther Flemming observed that when a cell begins to duplicate itself, certain threadlike structures gradually become visible in its nucleus. These "threads" grow denser; and then they appear to engage in a choreographed dance of sorts, each pairing off with another. Finally, as the original cell prepares to divide in two, the threads separate into two equal groups, which are pulled in opposite directions by invisible fibers. Each

of the two daughter cells will receive the same number of threads for its nucleus. Once the act of duplication has been completed, the threads grow thinner and again vanish from sight.

The early cytologists who witnessed these events under their microscopes coined two words which we need to add to our permanent vocabulary. **Mitosis**, meaning the division of one cell into two, refers to those threadlike nuclear structures, drawing upon the Greek words for "thread" (*mitos*) and "a condition" (*osis*). Since these structures stained so deeply with colored dyes, Wilhelm Waldeyer proposed in 1888 that they be called **chromosomes**, from the Greek words for "color" (*chroma*) and "body" (*soma*). The term was promptly adopted, while the function and chemical composition of these "colored bodies" remained unknown.

Mammalian cells, especially human ones, are difficult to study; in the early twentieth century, American researchers looked closely at the chromosomes in cells from lower organisms. Beginning in 1910 Thomas Hunt Morgan, a zoology professor at Columbia University, confirmed and elaborated Mendelian principles by experiments with the fruit fly *Drosophila*. Morgan and his co-workers not only demonstrated that the chromosomes of *Drosophila* carried its genetic information, but they were able to map particular genes to individual chromosomes. More significantly, they revealed the role of the sex chromosomes in determining gender. For *Drosophila* as for *Homo sapiens*, two "X" chromosomes characterize the female of the species; and one "X" and one "Y" identify the male. The new knowledge led to the first assignment of human genes to an individual chromosome; from patterns of disease occurrence in related families, geneticists could infer that the mutant alleles causing color blindness, hemophilia, and muscular dystrophy were located on the X chromosome. In

Chromosomes Visible during Mitosis

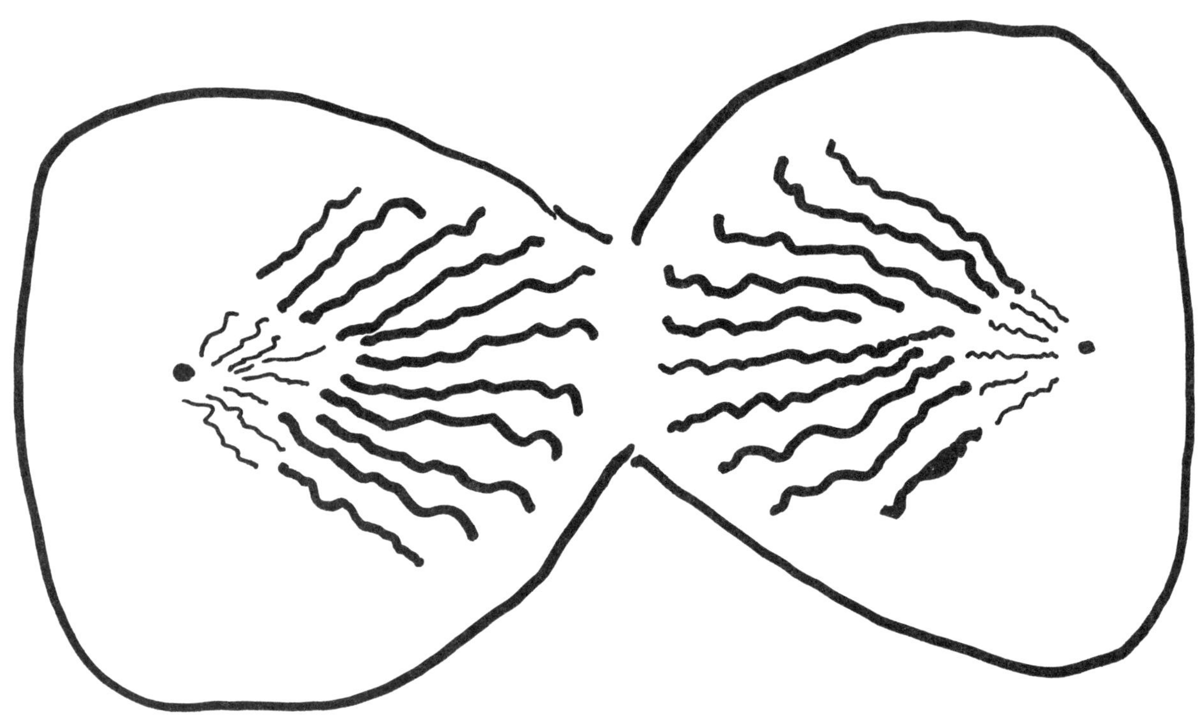

The chromosomes in a cell's nucleus are not normally visible under a microscope. But during **mitosis** (the formal division of a cell into two identical daughter cells), these highly condensed structures become the most prominent cellular feature. The illustration above depicts a **mitotic figure**, that characteristic event in which two sets of chromosomes are drawn apart into two newly-forming daughter cells.

such X-linked recessive disorders, the healthy carrier is always a female; there is a 50% chance that any given son will be afflicted, and that any given daughter will be a carrier.

Morgan and other early proponents of Mendelian genetics envisioned genes and chromosomes as relatively stable elements. In the late 1920s and early 1930s Barbara McClintock, a botanist at Cornell University, conducted experiments with corn which emphasized the mutability of genetic material. The chromosomes of corn proved to be subject to frequent breakage, whereby a piece of one chromosome would be transferred to another, and vice versa. These translocations, clearly visible under the microscope, caused changes in the phenotype of the mature plant. For example, a new chromosomal arrangement might result in a different number of kernels, or in kernels of a different color. McClintock thus provided additional evidence that an organism's chromosomes carried its genes; more importantly, she established that changes in the chromosomal location of genes were common and that they could dramatically alter the way in which genes were expressed.[1] As we shall see, chromosomal translocations have been implicated in the development of some cancers.

DNA

Such Stuff as Genes Are Made Of

While the role of chromosomes had been clarified by 1940, the biochemical composition of genetic material remained a mystery. What were genes made of, and how exactly did they transmit hereditary information and so determine the phenotypes of living things? In 1869 a Swiss chemist named Friedrich Miescher had isolated a new chemical substance from the nuclei of white blood cells; he called it "nuclein." This substance was later identified as a nucleic acid. By the 1920s it had a formal name—**deoxyribonucleic acid**, abbreviated simply as **DNA**. Chromosomes were now known to be composed of DNA and associated proteins; but most researchers believed that the proteins carried the genetic information, DNA being seen as a type of glue which held all the genes together. Chemically speaking, DNA was a simple substance, consisting of four bases (cytosine, thymine, adenine, guanine) attached to a sugar-phosphate chain. Proteins seemed far more plausible as the transmitter of genetic instructions; these complex and varied molecules provided the body's building materials as well as the enzymes needed for its chemical reactions. In 1944, however, an experiment performed at the Rockefeller Institute in New York overturned the prevalent theory of chromosomal substances. Oswald Avery and his co-workers transformed a harmless strain of pneumococci into an extremely virulent one, merely by exposing the inoffensive bacteria to purified DNA taken from a lethal variety of pneumococci. DNA alone, therefore, carried the genetic instructions which dictated an organism's appearance and behavior. Genes were made of DNA—those chromosomal proteins were just the glue!

In the late 1940s and early 1950s, scientists hastened to investigate the chemical and physical properties of DNA. The most important discovery occurred in 1953, when the American James Watson and the Englishman Francis Crick announced the molecular structure of DNA in the weekly journal *Nature*. As they explained in the May 30 issue, that structure was a **double helix**. It consisted of "two chains," both of which were "coiled around a common fibre axis" and held together "by hydrogen bonds between the bases." Lest nonspecialist readers should miss the point, Watson and Crick spelled out the significance of this double-helix arrangement: it revealed how DNA "might carry out the essential operation required of a genetic material, that of exact self-duplication." When DNA duplicates itself, "the hydrogen bonds are broken, and the two chains unwind and separate. Each chain then acts as a template for the formation on to itself of a new companion chain." Watson and Crick's discovery marked the beginning of modern molecular biology.[2]

By the early 1960s the genetic code of DNA, used by all living things on earth, had been completely deciphered. The four bases of DNA could be joined in 64 different combinations, more than enough to code for the 20 amino acids which go to make up a seemingly infinite variety of proteins. DNA was a template which could not only reproduce itself in a cell's nucleus, but which could send instructions (messenger RNA) for the creation of proteins to the appropriate workshops (ribosomes) in the cytoplasm. We now had a biochemical definition of the word **gene**—viz., a discrete sequence of DNA molecules which directs the manufacture of a particular protein. Within the next two decades we were to learn how to synthesize DNA and how to manipulate genes.[3]

KARYOTYPING
Human Chromosomes Revisited

In the early 1950s cytologists still knew far more about *Drosophila* chromosomes than human ones. The precise number of our chromosomes had not been established, though the erroneous figure of 48 was widely accepted. Researchers had no reliable way of isolating and studying the individual chromosome, much less of investigating any genes which it might carry. Human chromosomes were so tiny and so intertwined, and only visible during cellular duplication. How could mitosis be stopped at midpoint, and the

jumbled mass of chromosomes be untangled and then extracted from the cell? Two innovations in laboratory techniques achieved this feat. First it was noticed that the chemical treatment of cells with colchicine (an alkaloid) can stop cellular division in metaphase. At this stage of the mitotic process, the chromosomes are highly condensed and neatly aligned on the cell's "mitotic spindle"—that is, aligned on the submicroscopic fibers which will soon pull them apart into two equal groups. In the early 1950s T. C. Hsu of Houston's M. D. Anderson Cancer Center discovered that adding a hypotonic salt solution to metaphase-arrested cells has the effect of dissolving their mitotic spindles, swelling their cytoplasms with fluid, and allowing the condensed chromosomes to float free.[4]   By 1956 other cytologists had used Hsu's technique to determine the total number of human chromosomes—*46!* More precisely, we have **23 paired chromosomes**, each of us receiving at conception 23 maternal chromosomes and 23 paternal chromosomes. We all receive one X chromosome from our mothers; whether we develop as male or female depends on whether we receive an X or a Y from our fathers.

Detailed images of human chromosomes finally became available in the late 1950s, by virtue of **karyotyping**. In this technique, a photograph is taken of a cell's metaphase chromosomes after they've been separated by treatment with colchicine and hypotonic solution. Then the individual chromosomes are clipped out of the photograph and arranged according to their size and structural similarities, thereby creating a visual composite of all 23 pairs. Each chromosome is naturally divided into a long arm and a short arm by its centromere, a constricted region where the thin fibers of the mitotic spindle had been attached. The centromere is located at different positions on different chromosomes, a circumstance which greatly aided the early attempts to identify individual chromosomes. However, because human chromosomes often resemble each other outwardly, their definitive identifications came only with the development of **banding techniques** in the late 1960s. The separate chromosomes stain with highly distinctive patterns of light and dark bands, probably because some segments have more active genes than others. By the early 1970s the properties of the two standard stains (Giemsa and quinacrine mustard) had been adequately studied, and the catalogue of our chromosomes was complete. Each chromosome had been assigned a definite number and subdivided into large regions and smaller bands.[5]

Medical journals now began to publish frequent karyotypes, with little arrows pointing to chromosomal abnormalities in this-or-that region and band of the long or short arm of this-or-that chromosome. No doubt many physicians were as mystified as their patients; but even the earliest karyotypes had proven their worth, by revealing the true nature of some enigmatic disorders. In 1959 cytologists announced the cause of **Down's syndrome**, which had been inappropriately called "Mongolism." An infant born with Down's is destined to lifelong mental retardation, but not (as previously suspected) because of vices or degradation on the parents' part. Down's results from **trisomy 21**—that is, an affected infant will have received three copies of chromosome 21 at conception. Normally an extra chromosome means fetal death and spontaneous abortion, but trisomies with certain smaller chromosomes (13, 18, 21) can result in the live births of severely handicapped children. Nature is considerably more forgiving of conceptional accidents involving the sex chromosomes. The earliest karyotypes also explained **Klinefelter's syndrome** (a male receives two X chromosomes at conception as well as the necessary Y) and **Turner's syndrome** (a female receives only one X chromosome at conception instead of the necessary two). Both these syndromes occur with some frequency; persons affected tend to be sterile, but may have normal intelligence.

Trisomies and other chromosomal accidents occurring at conception can now be detected prenatally. The amniotic fluid surrounding a fetus contains a number of its cells, which can easily be sampled by needle aspiration (amniocentesis). A karyotype of a single cell will tell us whether the fetus has Down's syndrome. Unfortunately, it's not so easy to understand and diagnose the myriad chromosomal abnormalities which characterize human cancers.

The Karyotypes of Cancer

Before 1960 the cancer cell was viewed as a black box; no one had any clues to its inner workings. We finally glimpsed inside that box in 1960, when Peter C. Nowell of the University of Pennsylvania and his graduate student David A. Hungerford karyotyped the white cells taken from seven patients with **chronic myelogenous leukemia**, a fairly common adult malignancy. The finished karyotypes held a surprise! All the patients had the same chromosomal abnormality—a segment from the long arm of chromosome 22 had been relocated to the long arm of chromosome 9. The shortened chromosome (number 22) soon became known as **the Philadelphia chromosome**, because of the location of Professor Nowell's institution. It became famous because—for the first time—someone had looked inside a cancer cell's nucleus and identified a malfunction which had led to malignancy.[6] In the 1970s and 1980s, after the refinement of the Giemsa and quinacrine staining techniques, chromosomal abnormalities were identified in other hematopoietic malignancies. Perhaps the best known examples have been the translocations in Burkitt's lymphoma (a segment lost on chromosome 8 is gained on 14) and in follicular lymphoma (segments are exchanged between chromosomes 14 and 18). With the leukemias and lymphomas, characteristic chromosomal abnormalities visible on karyotypes often prove helpful in making the proper diagnosis and in selecting the best treatment. For example, the Philadelphia chromosome usually points toward chronic myelogenous leukemia—but not *acute* myelogenous leukemia, which tends to reveal a loss on chromosome 7 and a gain on chromosome 8. In chronic B-cell leukemia, a loss on chromosome 13 has been associated with an improved prognosis, while a gain on 14 generally spells for shortened survival.[7]

Chromosomal analysis has been less useful in diagnosing and treating the solid tumors. With the leukemias it's easy to obtain malignant cells (a drop of blood from a finger prick will suffice) and to culture them for karyotyping. With the solid tumors, sampling and culturing are much more difficult. But the greatest obstacle to meaningful karyotyping lies in the appalling number of chromosomal aberrations. A leukemia or lymphoma will typically have a single prominent abnormality, which is found in all the malignant cells and which remains reasonably constant throughout the course of disease. In a solid tumor, the chromosomal defects in one malignant cell might be entirely different from those in another; and the sum total of aberrations seems to rise exponentially as the disease progresses. The nuclei of metastatic tumor cells may exhibit such gross errors as **monosomies** (one chromosome where there should be two), **trisomies** (three instead of two), and **aneuploidies** (two or more times the normal complement of chromosomes, owing to a cell's duplication of genetic material without a subsequent division into two

daughter cells). Errors like these are of a different order of magnitude from the modest deletions and translocations which we find in the leukemias and lymphomas. Solid tumors are not usually karyotyped in clinical practice. As Emil J. Freireich and Noreen A. Lemak of the M. D. Anderson Cancer Center explain, "the cytologic pictures are so complex as almost to defy analysis."[8] There are a few exceptions. Researchers at New York's Memorial Sloan-Kettering Cancer Center have reported that the duplication of the short arm of chromosome 12 indicates a poor prognosis in testicular cancer, with resistance to chemotherapy which would otherwise be curative.[9] Melanoma patients with structural abnormalities on chromosomes 7 and 11 do not survive as long as patients without these defects.[10]

While karyotypes of breast and ovarian cancers have documented many chromosomal aberrations, they have failed to demonstrate those recurrent patterns which physicians might use in making treatment decisions. An early study of breast cancers indicated that the long arm of chromosome 1 often revealed a loss, but that the missing segment went to different chromosomes in different patients. These inconsistent rearrangements of chromosome 1 have also been reported in over 80% of epithelial ovarian tumors.[11] Both breast and ovarian cancers frequently have deleted segments on chromosomes 6 and 11. In ovarian malignancy, the short arm of chromosome 19 may gain genetic material; in breast cancers, deletions and other rearrangements also occur on chromosomes 3, 7, 13, 16, and 17. Researchers at the National Cancer Institute found that breast tumors which had lost DNA segments from the short arm of chromosome 11 were more likely to metastasize.[12]

Any genetic abnormality visible on a karyotype is a very large mistake. However, the varied chromosomal anomalies found in cancer cells—all those deletions, translocations, inversions, and duplications—are not *per se* the cause of disease. They are better understood simply as the outward signs of malignancy—that is, as the very smallest signs which we can actually see and photograph. Chromosomes serve as the carriers of multitudinous genes, which we cannot see or photograph. Like other genetic diseases, cancer is ultimately a matter of genes—of genes which are missing—or defective—or active when they should be quiet—or inactive when they should be functioning. And the significance of chromosomal rearrangements lies in their effect on genes. Typically, the fracture of one or more chromosomes during cell division has somehow resulted in the improper activation or inactivation of one or more genes. To illustrate this point, let's return briefly to the Philadelphia chromosome, which has been intensively studied since its discovery in 1960. The malignancy involved—chronic myelogenous leukemia— begins in the bone marrow with a single blood cell which accidentally exchanges DNA segments between chromosomes 9 and 22. By the late 1980s researchers had learned that this particular accident transfers a gene called *abl* from chromosome 9 to 22, where it is improperly joined to another gene called *bcr*. The two genes then produce an abnormal hybrid protein, which fuels the proliferation of these defective granulocytes (white cells). The protein (the gene product) actually causes this leukemia, not the chromosomal translocation. A few patients will not display the Philadelphia chromosome on their karyotypes; with our current tools for molecular analysis, we can demonstrate that such cases have either a submicroscopic transfer of the *abl* gene or a substantial mutation in the *bcr* gene.[13]

Molecular Analysis of Genes

The deciphering of the DNA genetic code in the early 1960s, in itself a remarkable feat, was a prelude to even more wondrous achievements. The evolving technology for the analysis and manipulation of genes is too complex to be discussed at length in this book, but we do need to be aware of a few seminal innovations and of their impact on the practice of medicine. By 1968 Nobel Prize laureate Arthur Kornberg and his associates had produced "a completely synthetic DNA, made with natural DNA as a template," which had "the full biological activity of the native material."[14] In the mid-1970s methods for sequencing DNA—that is, of determining the precise order of chemical bases in genes— were developed independently by Frederick Sanger of Cambridge University and by Walter Gilbert at Harvard. Learning how to sequence and synthesize DNA was like learning how to read and write, the "language" being that of the universal genetic material, with genes serving (so to speak) as individual words, and linked base-pairs appearing as the letters in a chemical alphabet.

These basic skills were soon to find medical applications. Unwieldy strands of DNA extracted from cells could be sliced (or "scissored") into smaller, more manageable fragments through the addition of restriction enzymes (endonucleases). In 1975 the English biologist E. M. Southern developed the technique of gel electrophoresis, popularly known as the **Southern blot**, to separate masses of enzyme-digested DNA. In this laboratory procedure, DNA fragments are placed atop a viscous gel, which is then subjected to a low electric current. The pieces of DNA migrate in response to the current, conveniently arranging themselves according to size, with the smaller fragments moving to the bottom of the gel, and the larger ones remaining at the top. Later the gel can be blotted onto a nylon filter, thereby creating a permanent record of an individual's DNA.[15]

In the late 1970s the use of gene probes began to revolutionize the diagnosis of genetic diseases. Once we had isolated a gene and deciphered its chemical message, we could prepare a synthetic copy of it. This "gene probe" would hybridize (bind tightly) to the natural gene hidden away among multitudinous spirals of DNA. A probe could be "labeled with"—i.e., attached to—radioactive or fluorescent material; and—*presto!*—a Southern blot or a single chromosome would *light up*, revealing the presence of the gene in question. Depending on how the probe and the laboratory test were designed, they could detect a normal gene or a disease-causing gene or the absence of a gene. In the 1980s carrier identification and prenatal diagnosis through DNA testing became more or less routine for some X-linked and recessive single-gene disorders, including sickle-cell anemia, hemophilia, muscular dystrophy, and cystic fibrosis.[16] Diagnosis was easy if a gene probe existed; an adequate number of cells could be obtained by sampling either the peripheral blood of children and adults, or the amniotic fluid surrounding fetuses.

The growing power of DNA analysis to predict future disease raised a variety of troublesome questions, not the least of which being whether affected fetuses would be aborted, and whether employers and insurance companies would discriminate against persons known to be susceptible to hereditary illnesses. Huntington's disease poignantly illustrated the dilemmas of medical prophecy: this devastating neurological disorder develops late in life, in previously healthy middle-aged persons who have inherited a single dominant gene (disease-causing allele) from one of their parents. As no cure or effective treatment is available, a positive result on a gene probe looms like a death sentence. Some individuals at risk—among them Arlo Guthrie, son of the Depression-era folk singer Woody Guthrie—have declined to be tested for the Huntington's disease allele. Others have welcomed the test, asking to be relieved from the anxiety of not knowing their fate.

Drugs from Recombinant DNA

The greatest benefits which we might anticipate from our new biotechnologies will not be diagnostic, but therapeutic. DNA is common to all living things—this fact has enabled us to produce some much-needed drugs. During the 1980s scientists became increasingly adept at isolating and cloning human genes which carried the instructions for essential proteins. These DNA segments were native to *Homo sapiens*; but if they could be transferred to the cells of other organisms, the encoded proteins would be produced by these cells. In **recombinant DNA technology**, a chromosome of a lowly bacterium like *Escherichia coli* (a harmless resident of mammalian intestines) is sliced open by restriction enzymes. A cloned human gene is then added to the test tube. Assuming a successful transfer, the bacterial chromosome will mend itself while incorporating the human gene into its DNA. The bacterium then multiplies—and multiplies—and multiplies, all the while reproducing the human gene and turning out vast quantities of a hitherto unobtainable human protein.

Recombinant DNA has been a boon for patients as well as a bonanza for pharmaceutical companies. Suddenly, beginning in the mid-1980s, diabetics had an inexhaustible supply of recombinant human insulin, whereas formerly they had been dependent on extracts for animal pancreases. And hemophiliacs had recombinant blood-clotting factors, reducing their dependence on donated blood which might be contaminated with the viruses causing hepatitis B or AIDS. And unusually short children had a chance to be taller, thanks to recombinant growth hormone. Of course, these new "natural" products were not exempt from drug abuse. Recombinant erythropoietin, which stimulates the bone marrow to produce more red blood cells, was intended as a remedy for severe anemia. But some athletes took it just to improve their performance in endurance sports, without considering the potentially lethal side effects like heart attacks or strokes which might result from the blood's increased viscosity.

In the 1990s our mass media paid the most attention to **recombinant cytokines**. These elusive proteins stimulate the immune cells to fight off bacterial and viral infections. But the various **interferons** and **interleukins** were also supposed to have wondrous properties as cancer drugs. Eventually they did find therapeutic applications in a few malignancies, but they were not consistently beneficial, and they could not predictably cure any type of cancer. In this instance, performance lagged far behind the newspaper and TV publicity. There were no major indications for the interferons and interleukins in the treatment of the most common solid tumors, those of the breast, colon, lung, and prostate.

Polymerase Chain Reaction

The significance of gene probes, gene transfers, and recombinant DNA cannot as yet be said to lie in miracle cures. These innovations are better understood as signposts indicating a fundamental change in the direction of modern medicine. *In the 1980s medicine went molecular!* Henceforth our research on cancer and other genetic diseases would attempt to understand—and ultimately learn to counteract—the minuscule errors distorting the messages carried by the patients' DNA. In 1985 Kary Mullis, a biochemist employed by the Cetus Corporation, invented a laboratory procedure called the **polymerase chain reaction** (PCR), which has greatly simplified DNA research. In essence, PCR allows the rapid amplification of DNA fragments which have been placed in a test tube with a polymerase (an enzyme promoting molecular replication) and then subjected to variations in temperature. One formidable barrier to the analysis of individual genes had been the difficulty in obtaining adequate quantities of the relevant DNA segments. Cloning these segments in bacteria can require several weeks; PCR does the same task in a few hours. Moreover, PCR works fine on long-dormant DNA, which has been preserved between a pathologist's glass slides, or even buried during the last Ice Age. A single cell could theoretically provide an unending supply of DNA segments.[17]

The implications of PCR for cancer diagnosis are profound. The DNA in a few malignant cells, aspirated from a tumor by hypodermic needle, can now be tested to reveal which genes have gone haywire and are fueling the abnormal growth. But PCR makes the most headlines for its uses in forensic pathology. A drop of blood or semen left at a crime scene can provide conclusive evidence of guilt. The criminal's DNA, amplified by PCR, will yield a distinctive pattern of bands on a Southern blot; that pattern constitutes a "DNA fingerprint," which is now accepted as evidence in courts of law.

Chapter Three

Looking for Oncogenes

ancer is God's gift to molecular biologists who are writing applications for funding grants. Our research aimed at discovering the mutated genes which cause cancer has been intensive, prolonged, and—*unfinished!* The first important clue came from the observation that certain retroviruses can rapidly induce tumors in some lower species—mice, rats, chickens, cats, monkeys. The famous Rous sarcoma virus, which produces sarcomas in chickens, was isolated in 1911 by Peyton Rous of New York's Rockefeller Institute. In the next six decades, dozens of other animal-tumor viruses were identified, provoking curiosity among researchers. What devastating genes did these tiny viruses carry? Robert A. Weinberg of the Massachusetts Institute of Technology (MIT) has marveled at the minute quantities of aberrant DNA which can ignite a malignancy: "An infecting tumor virus brings into an animal cell only a very small amount of DNA, perhaps a millionth of that which is present in the cell's own chromosomes."[1]

By the late 1970s most of these retroviral oncogenes had been isolated, analyzed, and named. Geoffrey M. Cooper of the Harvard Medical School reminds us that the three-letter names given these genes "usually refer either to the type of neoplasm [cancer] induced by the virus, to the species of animal the virus infects, or to the scientist who first

isolated the virus."[2] Thus, *src* designates the oncogene carried by the Rous sarcoma virus to chickens, and *abl* recalls Herbert Abelson's discovery of a mouse leukemia virus. The oncogene extracted from a simian (monkey) sarcoma virus was dubbed *sis*. Those called *erb* and *myc* were originally isolated from viruses afflicting chickens with erythroblastosis ("leukemia" of red blood cells) and myelocytomatosis (myelocytic leukemia). But the most widely studied viral oncogene was ***ras***—several variations of this gene were isolated from rat sarcomas.

The power of malignant transformation possessed by these oncogenes was convincingly demonstrated through the technique of **transfection**, developed by Dutch researchers in the mid-1970s. In laboratory experiments, viral DNA segments were coated with calcium phosphate, which allowed them to penetrate normal cells being cultured in Petri dishes. The "transfected" cells soon displayed the standard test-tube indications of malignancy: loss of contact inhibition, anchorage independence, and immortality. A solitary oncogene, just a tad of unadulterated DNA, could induce cancer all by itself—at least under highly controlled conditions and in certain lines of mouse cells.

The next logical step would be to isolate cancer-causing genes from human tumors. In 1981 researchers from three American labs were engaged in a race to extract and clone the relevant oncogene from cell lines cultured from human bladder carcinomas. Michael Wigler's lab at Cold Spring Harbor on Long Island found the gene a few days ahead of its competitors. When this first human oncogene was sequenced in early 1982, it yielded a surprise no one expected. It proved to be "homologous" (essentially identical) with the *ras* gene extracted from rat sarcomas.[3] How could this be? What, exactly, were these oncogenes?

To begin with, such cancer-inducing genes, whether found in retroviruses afflicting rats or in human tumor cells, do not represent direct attempts by Mother Nature to create pathological agents. Oncogenes actually derive from life-giving genes which play crucial roles in regulating cell growth, differentiation, and reproduction. So important are these genes that they are broadly conserved— and pretty much identical—across many dissimilar species, from yeast to chickens, from mice to men.[4] They become agents of carcinogenesis only when they malfunction, but they malfunction in various ways. In the case of retroviral infections afflicting lower animals, these crucial genes have somehow become incorporated in viral DNA, where they don't belong and where they are consequently improperly activated. After an affected retrovirus enters an animal cell, it will insert its oncogene into the cell's DNA. The transferred gene will henceforth turn out proteins which stimulate cellular proliferation. In the case of the *ras* gene discovered in human bladder cancers, the defect leading to malignancy proved to be a single point mutation. Of the 6,600 base-pairs of DNA in this lengthy gene, only one had been incorrectly transcribed, causing the amino acid valine to be substituted for glycine. That tiny error resulted in the production of an abnormal, inflexible protein, which permanently kept the cells in a reproductive mode.[5] As previously

mentioned, any kind of chromosomal disruption may cause genes to malfunction. In the well-known translocation seen in Burkitt's lymphoma, a normally quiescent *myc* gene is moved from its usual position on chromosome 8 to chromosome 14, where it is placed among very active immunoglobin genes and consequently begins to be rapidly expressed like its new neighbors.

Proto-Oncogenes

The discovery of the true nature of oncogenes prompted a revision in terminology. The genes from which oncogenes derive came to be called, somewhat infelicitously, **proto-oncogenes**, as though these DNA segments had no other purpose except to wait for an opportunity to promote cancer. It would be more appropriate (if rather wordy) to call them **growth genes prone to mutations which can lead to malignancy**. In any event, molecular biologists doing cancer research were elated by the breakthroughs of the early 1980s, which decisively shifted their field from chicken and rat sarcomas to the more relevant human carcinomas. Robert A. Weinberg of MIT reflected this buoyancy in a 1983 essay: "From the perspective of a molecular biologist, cancer is no longer more than a hundred diseases, each of them characterized by a different tumor type. Instead it begins to look as if there are only a small number of molecular mechanisms, which are common to all tumor types. The molecular mechanisms underlying cancer should be well defined by the end of this decade."[6]

Weinberg's timetable was optimistic. By the early 1990s we had identified many of the genes which are improperly activated in human cancers, but we knew relatively little about how the resulting gene products functioned in malignant cells. Were these proteins growth factors? Or were they receptors for growth factors? Did they concentrate in a cell's nucleus, or were they active on its outer plasma membrane? Did they perhaps reside in the cytoplasm and transmit proliferative signals from the outer membrane to the genes in the nucleus? Our new tools for DNA analysis could not readily unravel the Gordian knots which are protein structures, or map the intricate pathways that proteins followed in cells, or define the numerous biochemical reactions induced by proteins. Some molecular biologists cautioned that the transfection of oncogenes into cultured cells, while informative in certain respects, bore little resemblance to the development of tumors in the human body. Colon cancer was often cited by way of illustration. The progression from a benign colonic adenoma to an invasive malignancy had been well studied; it typically required "at least eight mutational events."[7] A single gene, or even two or three, cannot be held responsible. Various and sundry genes must malfunction to achieve the end effect we know as colon cancer.

Stratagems to Tame *ras*

Our efforts to develop antidotes to oncogenes and their protein products have progressed slowly. An early target was *ras*, which had been implicated in a wide variety of human cancers, including some 50% of colorectal tumors and about 90% of pancreatic tumors. Significantly, the function of the *ras* proteins had also been deciphered. They migrate to the inner surface of a cell's outer membrane, where they serve to relay external growth signals to the nucleus. The cancer-causing versions of *ras* proteins are almost normal, usually revealing the effects of only a point mutation or two in the coding DNA. But these mutant proteins will send proliferative signals to the nucleus *even when no growth factors are present*. Any affected cell would thus enter upon a relentless cycle of pathological reproduction.

Knowledge of the *ras* pathway lets pharmacologists design novel compounds which might prevent these proliferative signals from reaching the nucleus. Researchers from the firms Genentech and Merck reported that they had used designer drugs to reverse malignant growth patterns in several cell lines transformed by *ras*.[8] A team at the National Cancer Institute experimented with a different strategy—vaccination. Laboratory mice were injected with a purified solution of mutant *ras* proteins; subsequently they received implants of malignant cells taken from human tumors, some of which were known to express the *ras* oncogene. Those mice challenged with *ras*-positive tumors did not develop cancer, but those challenged with other tumors soon died of the disease. Larry A. Feig, a biochemist at Tufts University, explains this intriguing result: "To the nonimmunologist, it seems quite perplexing how cytotoxic T cells can detect mutated *ras* protein inside tumorigenic cells. Apparently, intracellular proteins are processed to short peptides and presented on the cell surface. These findings suggest that tumor cells containing oncogenic *ras* could be targeted directly by the immune system by virtue of the altered structure of mutant *ras* proteins."[9]

While the preliminary experiments with *ras*-specific agents have been encouraging, the road from a successful laboratory demonstration involving cell lines or mice to a practical therapy for human patients tends to be long—very long indeed. In cancer medicine it is not often traversed. We need to remember that *ras* is but one oncogene of many, and moreover, that oncogenes are not the only genes which have been implicated in human cancer.

TUMOR SUPPRESSOR GENES

The Case of Retinoblastoma

Oncogenes act to accelerate cell growth. Through point mutations, gene relocations, or other errors, they have begun to instruct the cellular workshops in the cytoplasm either to manufacture abnormal proteins, or to produce excessive quantities of normal ones. Under either circumstance, cells will be stimulated into improper reproduction. To use an obvious automotive analogy, we might say that "the accelerator" has somehow been "pressed to the floor—and gotten stuck there!" But there are other genes which act as *brakes* to unnecessary cellular proliferation. And the development of most solid tumors involves not only the activation of oncogenes, but also the loss or inactivation of cellular braking devices. These anti-proliferation genes were originally called "anti-oncogenes"; they are now known as **tumor suppressor genes**.

The first clue to the existence of these genetic brakes came from cell fusion experiments carried out in the late 1960s and early 1970s. When malignant cells were made to combine with normal ones *in vitro*, the resulting hybrids did not display the full attributes of malignancy. Cancer cells, for example, will induce tumors when they are injected into "nude" (immunodeficient) mice. The hybrids produced by the fusion of malignant and normal cells were unable to induce tumors in mice. This observation seemed to indicate that the normal cells carried one or more genes which acted to restrain malignant growth.[10] However, we did not learn much about suppressor genes before the 1980s, a decade in which researchers devoted considerable time and effort to a rare juvenile cancer called **retinoblastoma**.

Unlike the solid tumors which afflict adults, retinoblastoma is a single-gene, early-onset disease. It develops from the retina in the back of the eyeball; and it almost always begins before the age of three, by which time the retinal cells have matured and ceased to divide. Retinoblastoma is hardly typical of human malignancy; but it has been instructive as to the nature and function of tumor suppressor genes, and as to the way in which inherited defects in these genes can lead to familial cancer syndromes. Roughly 40% of all retinoblastoma cases are hereditary, arising from a germline mutation present at conception. These cases tend to appear very early, sometimes even before birth, and they typically involve multiple tumors in both eyes. Sporadic (nonhereditary) cases occur a little bit later, and they usually involve only a single tumor in one eye.

What happens in retinoblastoma? First of all, something is lost. Karyotypes made from the tumor cells of retinoblastoma patients often revealed a deletion involving a locus (band q14) on the long arm of chromosome 13. We now know that this locus carries the *Rb* (retinoblastoma) tumor suppressor gene. In 1971, before the era of DNA manipulations, the medical geneticist Alfred G. Knudson, Jr., formulated a **two-hit theory** which aptly explained the differences between hereditary and sporadic retinoblastoma.[11] If we assume that this cancer arises from the absence of a protein encoded by a single gene, and if we recall that we receive two copies (alleles) of each gene from our parents, we will readily comprehend Knudson's proposition. Before a tumor can develop, both copies of the *Rb* gene must somehow be lost or inactivated or malfunctioning. In hereditary retinoblastoma, the affected infants begin life with one functional *Rb* allele and one defective or missing *Rb* allele. This germline mutation could be either inherited from a parent or newly created by an accident during conception; it would be present in all somatic cells. Only one additional mutation would therefore be required to produce a retinal cell without any functional *Rb* allele—that is, to produce a cell which will proliferate into a tumor. During fetal development and early infancy, when the retinal cells are rapidly dividing, mutations can easily occur; and in hereditary retinoblastoma, they tend to result in multiple eye tumors. The sporadic version of this malignancy presents with a solitary eye tumor, because these patients begin life with two normal *Rb* alleles. That both gene copies in any given retinal cell would be deleted, or "hit," is an unlikely event. Fortunately, just one child in 20,000 develops retinoblastoma; it's a potentially lethal disease which until recently had to be treated by enucleation—the surgical removal of the affected eye or eyes.

Familial Cancer Syndromes

N. R. Dennis, an English geneticist, has succinctly explained a mechanism by which defective alleles of tumor suppressor genes can give rise to familial cancer syndromes. He observes that although such alleles would be "transmitted dominantly," they probably would "act recessively." That is, they could spur a cell toward malignancy only when "their paired normal allele is removed."[12] In contrast, defective alleles of proto-oncogenes may well act dominantly—one bad allele turning out a mutant protein might suffice to transform a cell.

Tumor suppressor genes would seem to play a larger role in hereditary cancers than oncogenes. To inherit a defective suppressor allele could be like inheriting a time bomb: just a single mutation to the normal allele might end a cell's supply of growth-restraining protein, and (as it were) light a fuse which eventually would lead to an explosion of malignant growth. But persons with this unfortunate genetic legacy do not always develop tumors at a young age. Retinoblastoma occurs unusually early because of the intense early activity of retinal cells, and because only one gene has to be disabled. Most cancers arising from defective suppressor genes occur much later, and they probably require synergetic mutations in oncogenes. Surprisingly, the *Rb* gene has also proven to be an instructive model for these more typical malignancies. While the gene's protein plays a crucial role in modulating retinal differentiation, it is needed as well by cells in other tissues. Survivors of hereditary retinoblastoma—that is, persons with a defective *Rb* allele in all their cells—are at an extremely high risk of subsequently developing other tumors. One study of these survivors found that, compared to the general population, they had thirty times the risk of dying from cancer.[13] Teenage survivors are especially prone to osteosarcoma (bone cancer), because the protein issued by the *Rb* gene helps to direct bone growth. Other malignancies which occur at elevated rates in hereditary retinoblastoma survivors include melanomas, soft-tissue sarcomas, and brain tumors. The chromosomal locus of the *Rb* gene is sometimes deleted in advanced breast cancers. Researchers have found that both *Rb* alleles are defective or missing in some 20% to 25% of the cell lines cultured from mammary carcinomas.[14] This gene probably doesn't play a pivotal role in starting breast cancers, but the absence of its protein may be associated with increased tumor aggressiveness.

Retinoblastoma, while not a major cause of cancer mortality, taught us much about the molecular mechanisms behind carcinogenesis. Moreover, it was the first solid tumor we were able to fully understand. We now understand retinoblastoma in the same way that we understand such single-gene diseases as cystic fibrosis and sickle-cell anemia. In 1986 the *Rb* gene was cloned by Robert A. Weinberg's lab at MIT; two years later researchers at Wen-Hwa Lee's lab at the University of California in San Diego were able to reverse the malignant behavior of retinoblastoma cells by giving them copies of the cloned gene.[15] David Abramson, a cancer specialist at New York Hospital, believes that this terrible juvenile malignancy might be controlled by a drug which would serve as "an analogue of the natural protein missing in retinoblastoma cells."[16]

A Gene in the Limelight: *p53*

During the 1990s tumor suppressor genes moved to the center stage of cancer research, occupying that limelight which had formerly shone on oncogenes like *ras* and *myc*. Some of these suppressor genes seemed to play limited roles in human cancer; they were principally implicated in just one or two tumor types. Among these bit players we might list obscure suppressor genes like **NF1** (implicated in neurofibrosarcoma) and **WT1** (disabled in Wilms' tumor, a juvenile kidney cancer), as well as such decidedly acronymic DNA segments as **DDC** (Deleted in Colon Cancer) and **MCC** (Mutated in Colon Cancer). However, one tumor suppressor gene was found to be missing or nonfunctional in an amazingly broad spectrum of human malignancies, including the leukemias and lymphomas, and solid tumors of the bladder, bone, brain, breast, cervix, colon, esophagus, liver, lung, prostate, stomach, and skin. This gene, located on the short arm of chromosome 17, came to be called *p53* because it encodes a **protein** with a molecular weight of **53 kilodaltons**. It is not the long-sought-after "cause" of human cancer, but it is the most frequently involved gene, playing a leading or supporting role in perhaps 50% of all cases. Writing in *Science*, Robert A. Weinberg pondered this versatility: "Why is *p53* such a popular actor? To begin, it may be a centrally important growth regulator in many cell types. But its genetic and biochemical traits are important as well. Point mutations create carcinogenic *p53*, and such simple genetic changes occur readily."[17] Indeed, Mother Nature should have labeled this gene *EXTREMELY* *FRAGILE*   *Handle with Care!* It is terribly prone to mutate. The several varieties of *ras* are typically subject to only two or three point mutations which can lead to cancer. In contrast, no fewer than 280 point mutations of *p53* have been identified in specimens of human tumors, and these were found to be distributed over 90 codons.[18] A codon is, of course, a set of three consecutive bases which codes for an amino acid; the *p53* gene contains 393 codons. The mutations most likely to occur in *p53* are called **missense**: in these cases the substitution of a single base causes the wrong amino acid to be incorporated in the finished protein. Some of these changes appear to be innocuous; others result in a mutant protein which no longer works or which works in the wrong way. The effect can vary not only according to the particular mutation, but also according to the type of cell in which it occurs.

Unfortunately, the *p53* gene does not necessarily need to lose both alleles before it begins to make trouble. Mutant *p53* proteins have a much longer half-life than the normal ("wild-type") protein, and they therefore tend to accumulate in the cell. Sometimes the abnormal protein encoded by a single mutated allele can negate the effects of any normal protein present in the cell, thus permitting improper reproduction to occur. Neither the functions of the wild-type protein nor the ways in which mutant versions of it impede these functions have been as clearly understood as we would like. We do know that normal *p53* protein remains in the nucleus; apparently it binds to certain segments of DNA containing growth genes, preventing their active expression.

Like the *Rb* gene, *p53* has been implicated in familial cancer syndromes. The rare

Li-Fraumeni syndrome is the best-known example: affected family members have almost a 50% risk of developing an invasive cancer by age 30. By age 70 over 90% of the family members who carry the defective *p53* allele will have developed cancer. While the Li-Fraumeni syndrome can involve a wide variety of malignancies, its hallmark is the occurrence of relatively uncommon sarcomas (bone and soft-tissue) at an early age. But the tumor which occurs most frequently in Li-Fraumeni families is a commonplace one—carcinoma of the breast. A survey of 43 families affected by this syndrome turned up 60 cases of breast cancer, and an astonishing 82% of these cases were diagnosed before age 45. The havoc wrought in Li-Fraumeni families is usually caused by a single germline mutation in a single *p53* allele. One family revealed the same mutation at codon 248 throughout three generations: the base cytosine had been replaced by thymine, causing the amino acid tryptophan to be substituted for arginine.[19]

Some mutations in *p53* are more "penetrant"—i.e., likely to cause cancer—than others. Arnold J. Levine, a molecular biologist at Princeton, observes: "An inherited *p53* mutation is not a sure predictor of the occurrence of cancer at a young age, since some family members with these mutations are free from cancer well into their 50s."[20] We might add that the vast majority of *p53* mutations found in tumor specimens are not inherited, but have occurred in somatic cells, and that of themselves, they are insufficient to cause cancer. The *p53* gene is not a solitary culprit like the *Rb* gene of childhood retinoblastoma; it's usually implicated with a few oncogenes and possibly another suppressor or two. The most thoroughly studied example of this carcinogenetic collaboration has been colorectal cancer. In the first stage of tumor development, the oncogene *ras* is activated while the suppressor gene *MCC* is lost,

leading to the formation of a benign adenoma. Subsequently the suppressor *DCC* is also lost. Finally, when *p53* ceases to function, an invasive cancer of the colon or rectum will result.[21] The inactivation of *p53* cannot be said to cause colorectal cancer; it is better described as a crucial turning point—or a "point-of-no-return"—on the long road to malignancy. Thanks to the efforts of Bert Vogelstein at Johns Hopkins and many other scientists, we have a good idea of the sequential genetic mutations which ineluctably lead to colon cancer; and at least in the laboratory, we can reverse the chain of events. When the normal *p53* gene is transfected into colorectal tumor cells being cultivated *in vitro*, these cells cease to divide; and they lose their ability to form malignant colonies.[22] Experiments like these demonstrate the importance of the wild-type *p53* protein in controlling cellular reproduction and, needless to say, raise our hopes that someday we'll find a practical way to supply malignant cells with that protein.

nm23
An Anti-Metastasis Gene

Another tumor suppressor gene on chromosome 17 may also be involved in a variety of human cancers. Patricia S. Steeg and her colleagues at the National Cancer Institute discovered a "novel gene" while experimenting with melanoma cell lines. Melanoma cells expressing this gene were able to produce local tumors in mice, but not metastases. Cells which failed to express the gene not only induced local tumors, but metastasized freely. When the cloned gene was transfected into these metastatic melanoma cells, they lost their ability to produce metastases.[23]

This gene came to be called *nm23* ("nm" standing for "nonmetastatic"). Cancer researchers were curious to learn whether it really prevented malignant cells from metastasizing. Studies in breast malignancies gave intriguing results. Steeg and her NCI team analyzed *nm23* expression in specimens of invasive ductal carcinomas taken from both node-positive and node-negative patients. Of course, the presence of cancer cells in the axillary (underarm) lymph nodes remains the most plausible indicator we have of a breast tumor's ability to metastasize. The NCI team discovered that *nm23* expression was uniformly lower in node-positive breast tumors. And among the node-negative tumors, there was less *nm23* protein in those tumors which were poorly differentiated and hormonally unresponsive.[24] A group of English surgeons and pathologists looked at *nm23* expression in the breast tumors of 71 patients: a high level of gene activity, shown by messenger RNA, was strongly correlated with the absence of lymph node involvement and longer survival.[25] Another English study measured the levels of *nm23* protein in ductal carcinoma *in situ* (DCIS) as well as invasive breast tumors. The authors reported that "*nm23* negativity was significantly associated with worsening invasive ductal carcinoma grade and advancing lymph node stage." DCIS specimens of the unpropitious *comedo* variety were uniformly *nm23* negative, while other types of DCIS were uniformly positive—"a finding consistent with the fact that *comedo* histology is known to have a higher likelihood of becoming invasive."[26]

Perhaps measurements of *nm23* activity will eventually provide us with a tool to determine which cases of DCIS are going to become invasive breast tumors. At the moment the functions of this protein are poorly understood. Patricia S. Steeg suspects that *nm23* is "modulating signal transduction" (i.e., controlling the signals sent from the cell's outer membrane to its nucleus); but she adds, "I don't know how."[27]

HER-2/*neu*

The Breast Cancer Oncogene

The development of breast cancers, like that of colorectal tumors, presumably involves the sequential malfunction of several genes, both oncogenes and tumor suppressors. Yet for breast malignancies we cannot presently outline a plausible sequence of molecular events in the same way that we can for colorectal tumors. Perhaps the only thing we can bet on is that any gene even remotely implicated in breast malignancies will be intensely studied by molecular biologists. Breast cancer represents the Great Sphinx of differential diagnosis in oncology; physicians have long been driven to distraction in their attempts to predict the future course of newly discovered tumors. On the one hand, there are those small breast tumors, ostensibly node-negative, which defy conventional prognostic wisdom by quickly metastasizing. On the other, large tumors with numerous positive nodes do not always produce evident metastases or otherwise appear to shorten the customary life expectancy. Hence any gene whose activation or inactivation consistently promotes breast cancer aggressiveness would have immediate relevance for the practice of medicine: it would give physicians a marker to distinguish between the truly dangerous and the relatively benign. The gene most frequently mentioned as such a prognostic marker has been **HER-2/*neu***, also known as ***erb*B-2**. Both the gene and its two names require a bit of explanation.

The oncogene ***neu*** was isolated in 1980 from chemically-induced rat neuroblastomas by a researcher in Robert A. Weinberg's lab. The name *neu* alludes to these infrequent tumors originating in immature cells (neuroblasts) of the nervous system; however, this oncogene began to attract attention only when its role in breast cancers became apparent. It is a powerful agent of mammary transformation. In one experiment the *neu* oncogene was inserted into fertilized mice ova (zygotic cells). All of the new-born mice which expressed the transplanted gene eventually developed breast cancers—and the resulting malignancies completely replaced the animals' mammary tissues.[28] When molecular biologists analyzed the DNA of *neu*, they found that it was homologous (almost identical in its sequence of chemical bases) to *erb*, a previously discovered oncogene which induces erythroblastosis (red-cell "leukemia") in chickens. At first *neu* and *erb* looked like different versions of the same thing. The latter oncogene derives from a proto-oncogene named *erb*B, whose protein product serves as a receptor for the **epidermal growth factor** (EGF). Cancer researchers had long been curious about possible links between the EGF, its receptors, and malignant transformation. EGF, a small molecule found in the blood, stimulates the proliferation of many kinds of cells, including those of the skin and breast. Normally it acts by binding to EGF receptors present on a cell's outer membrane; this union brings about a biochemical chain reaction, sending a signal to divide through a cell's cytoplasm to its nucleus. In the case of the *erb* oncogene, a mutated gene in the nucleus results in truncated EGF receptors on the cell's outer membrane; these shortened receptors will send proliferative signals to the nucleus even in the absence of EGF—and thus prompt malignant transformation. The *neu* oncogene was so similar to *erb* that cancer researchers concluded that the normal version of *neu* must also encode a growth factor receptor.[29]

Was the *neu* proto-oncogene just a variant allele of *erb*B, or was it a gene proper? By 1985 we had the answer: the *neu* proto-oncogene was a different gene from *erb*B, and it encoded a protein of a different molecular weight from the EGF receptor.

Moreover, these two genes—that is, the normal human counterparts of the rat *neu* proto-oncogene and the chicken *erb* proto-oncogene—resided on different chromosomes. The human *neu* gene was mapped to the long arm of chromosome 17; the human *erb*B gene encoding the EGF receptor lay on the short arm of chromosome 7. Notwithstanding these disparities, the two names chosen for the human *neu* gene reflected a strong belief that it was similar in function, as in DNA sequence, to *erb*B. Many cancer researchers refer to it as **HER-2** (indicating that it is <u>H</u>omologous to <u>E</u>GF <u>R</u>eceptor), while others prefer ***erb*B-2**. With either name the "2" simply serves to remind us that the gene in question, like *erb*B, encodes a growth factor receptor for the cell's outer membrane.[30]

Some Assays for HER-2/*neu*

As we've observed with the oncogene *ras* and the suppressor gene *p53*, point mutations in DNA are a frequent cause of genetic malfunctions leading to malignancy. With both *ras* and *p53*, such minuscule errors in the DNA sequence can result in an **abnormal protein product**; and it is an abnormal protein which typically causes the uncontrolled cellular proliferation. HER-2/*neu* illustrates a different mechanism of tumorigenesis. In this case both the gene and its protein product are usually normal; there are no structural alterations either in the DNA or in the protein's amino acids. What is abnormal is simply an **excessive quantity of the protein**. In the 1980s researchers at the National Cancer Institute demonstrated that high levels of normal HER-2 protein were all that was needed to induce malignancies in cultivated mouse cells.[31] Such a surfeit of a gene product is referred to as **overexpression**; it is most often caused by **gene amplification**—that is, by having too many copies of the gene. We're not always sure how or why gene amplification occurs, but the condition sometimes shows up on karyotypes which reveal chromosomes with **homogeneously staining regions**. The fact that these chromosomal regions stain with a peculiarly uniform intensity suggests that the same sequence of DNA is being repeated over and over again.[32]

Our standard assay for gene amplification remains that workhorse of DNA analysis, the **Southern blot**. In this procedure DNA isolated from a pathology specimen is first fragmented with restriction enzymes. Then the fragments are placed in a gel and separated by electrophoresis. The gel is subsequently blotted onto a nylon filter. A radioactive probe for the gene under investigation would hybridize (bind tightly) to the corresponding DNA sequence on the filter. When the filter is placed against a photographic plate, an **autoradiograph** will be created. A single copy of the gene would produce a thin dark line or a small smudge (i.e., a slight photographic exposure) on an autoradiograph; multiple copies would leave a much thicker line. The more copies of the gene present, the greater the amount of radioactive probe that binds to the DNA sequence, and consequently the larger and darker the line or smudge on the photographic plate.

A Southern blot can tell us if a gene is amplified and give us a rough idea (not an exact count) of the number of extra copies. In the case of HER-2/*neu*, amplification generally correlates quite well with overexpression. The more gene copies, the more protein likely to be present in the cell—and the more likely that the cell will be stimulated to divide. But it is not always sufficient just to test for gene amplification, because protein overexpression can occur in the absence of amplification. One mechanism which can cause this phenomenon is a mutation in a DNA promoter sequence (or "control switch") adjoining the

gene in question. A single copy of that gene could be (as it were) permanently switched on, constantly issuing instructions for the manufacture of more protein. In this instance the amount of HER-2 protein present in a cancer cell would be a far more plausible indicator of tumor aggressiveness than gene amplification.

Three laboratory tests are commonly used to screen for protein overexpression. The first two rely (like the Southern blot) on gel electrophoresis and probe hybridization. The **Northern blot** assays the other nucleic acid, **ribonucleic acid** or **RNA**. Of course, messenger RNA carries a gene's instructions for building a protein from the cell's nucleus to the relevant cytoplasmic workshops. Thus the quantity of HER-2/*neu* messenger RNA recorded on a Northern blot would be a good (albeit indirect) measure of cellular protein levels. The **Western blot** measures that protein directly. In this case electrophoresis is used to separate proteins of different molecular weights; a radiolabeled antibody would then bind to the protein of interest, producing that telltale exposure on an autoradiograph. For many applications the Western blot is now being replaced by a simpler and faster technique, **immunohistochemistry**. This third test utilizes traditional pathology procedures as well as the more recent innovation of monoclonal antibodies. We can profitably shorten the name to **immunostaining**. In essence, antibodies reacting to the protein under investigation are blended with a staining agent. When applied to a cross section of tissue containing the protein, these antibodies will leave a stain visible under a microscope. The more protein present in a cell, the heavier the stain. In the case of the HER-2 protein, any immunostaining would tend to be concentrated on the cell's outer membrane—the usual location of growth factor receptors.

HER-2/*neu* in Prognosis

The increasing acceptance of HER-2/*neu* as a prognostic indicator for breast malignancies owes much to the work of Dennis J. Slamon and his colleagues at the University of California at Los Angeles. By the mid-1980s the gene was known to be amplified in several cell lines derived from human mammary carcinomas. Slamon's team at the UCLA School of Medicine tried to find out whether this amplification had any effect on survival rates; they used Southern blotting to screen tissue samples from 189 breast tumors. On January 9, 1987, *Science* published the results of their study with much fanfare. Slamon et al had found evidence of amplification in approximately 30% of the specimens; the degree varied from an estimated two gene copies to more than twenty. Looking at the case histories of the patients assayed, Slamon et al concluded that HER-2/*neu* "was a significant predictor of both overall survival and time to relapse in breast cancer." The more the gene was amplified, the worse the prognosis; patients with five or more copies fared especially poorly. The correlation with outcome was most pronounced in node-positive patients; for this subgroup, Slamon et al asserted, "amplification of HER-2/*neu* has greater prognostic value than most currently used prognostic factors."[33]

Talking about breast cancer before an audience of scientists and physicians is usually tantamount to igniting a controversy. HER-2/*neu* was no exception to this rule. The debate on the gene began in earnest when other groups of researchers failed to duplicate the results of Slamon et al. Foremost among the skeptics were Iqbal Unnisa Ali and his coworkers at the National Cancer Institute: they analyzed 122 breast tumors, detected HER-2 amplification in 12, but found no evidence that the extra copies of this gene were associated with increased tumor aggressiveness or poorer patient outcome.[34] Slamon et al were undaunted. They attributed the contradictory results obtained by other laboratories to flaws in technique, pointing out that improper handling of tumor specimens can cause DNA deterioration and thus invalidate any oncogene assay by Southern blotting. This test will also be compromised if the specimen analyzed contains too many nonmalignant cells—for example, too many lymphocytes (white blood cells) which have infiltrated the tumor, or too many fibroblasts (connective cells) from the stromal tissues surrounding the breast ducts.[35]

In 1989 Dr. Slamon and his colleagues published a more detailed study of HER-2/*neu* amplification and overexpression, which helped to remove doubts. They had tested 345 breast tumors from node-positive patients, as well as 181 tumors from node-negative patients. To demonstrate the reproducibility of their findings, they subjected the tumor specimens to four different assays: Southern blotting for gene amplification, Northern blotting for messenger RNA, Western blotting and immunostaining for elevated protein levels. There was a high degree of correlation between the tests; and as in the 1987 study, HER-2 amplification pointed toward a poorer prognosis for node-positive patients. Both the **disease-free survival** or **DFS** (i.e., the period after the original surgery before any disease recurrence is detected), and the **overall survival** or **OS** (i.e., the total time surviving after the original surgery), were noticeably shorter in node-positive patients with multiple copies of the gene. Follow-up of the node-negative breast patients still did not reveal any association between HER-2 amplification and outcome. However, Slamon et al found a striking association between increased amplification and decreased survival when they analyzed 87 cases of ovarian cancer. Long-term follow-up of these ovarian patients revealed "median survivals of 1879, 959, and 243 days for patients having one copy, two to five copies, and more than five copies of the gene, respectively."[36] If it was not clear exactly what role HER-2/*neu* played in cells, it seemed entirely probable that the gene somehow became amplified in about 25% of breast and ovarian cancers, increasing the likelihood of rapid metastatic dissemination and early mortality.

The effect of HER-2 overexpression on breast tumors was now investigated by the influential **National Surgical Adjuvant Breast and Bowel Project** (NSABP). The NSABP researchers preferred immunostaining to Western blotting; they did not attempt to quantify protein levels, but simply judged specimens positive or negative depending on whether the individual tumor cells revealed "distinct membrane staining" on microscopic examination. Specimens from 292 invasive breast cancers were tested, and 62 judged positive for excessive HER-2 protein. Overall survival in both node-negative and node-positive patients was found to be noticeably shortened by overexpression. The assay's prognostic power proved greatest for those tumors whose constituent cells had **good nuclear grade**—that is, well-defined, nearly normal nuclei. This is a favorable prognostic finding; but in the NSABP study, node-negative patients whose tumor cells were of good nuclear grade yet overexpressed HER-2/*neu* experienced five times the mortality rate of comparable patients without protein overexpression.[37]

IMMUNOSTAINING
Molecular Analysis Enters the Clinic

HER-2/*neu* does not begin to represent the whole story of genetic malfunctions in breast malignancies. It has merited detailed discussion in this book because it was the first **genetic tumor marker** to prove unquestionably useful. A flurry of studies on *p53* suggest that this gene is also likely to become a valuable prognostic marker, especially for node-negative patients.[38] If the pathology work-ups of breast tumors routinely take into account the status of HER-2/*neu*, *p53*, *nm23*, and other pertinent genes, it will probably be due largely to the ease and simplicity afforded by immunohistochemistry. As previously stated, this assay relies on monoclonal antibodies which bind to the protein products of genes. When tumor cross sections are stained with appropriate reagents, the antibody-protein complexes become visible under the microscope, showing us things about individual cells which we were never able to see before. Mutant, nonfunctional *p53* protein tends to accumulate in the nuclei of cells; and if present, it will produce nuclear staining of varying intensity. An excess of HER-2 protein results in strong membrane staining, while low levels of *nm23* protein would be indicated by weak cytoplasmic staining.[39]

Immunostaining offers several practical advantages. First of all, it requires only the smallest sliver of specimen tissue: this is important in an era when newly discovered breast tumors tend to be quite small (as a result of early diagnosis), and numerous assays are expected to be performed on them. Secondly, unlike the Southern blot and related tests based on electrophoresis, immunostaining isn't subject to false readings caused by the presence of nonmalignant cells in the specimen. A pathologist can *see* the malignant cells and the way in which the staining affects them. Thirdly, immunostaining is relatively inexpensive and uncomplicated; it requires no elaborate apparatus.

A major drawback to immunostaining is that it is not precisely quantitative. Estimates of the degree of staining may vary from pathologist to pathologist. While this technique works on archival tumor specimens embedded in paraffin, it is considerably more reliable on freshly frozen specimens. Dennis J. Slamon and his colleagues caution that almost all proteins suffer some loss of "antigenic immunoreactivity" during chemical fixation and paraffin embedding: "This phenomenon is particularly significant in tumors expressing moderate levels of the gene product. Data generated from archival material should be interpreted with this caveat in mind, since it could significantly reduce both the incidence and intensity of immunostaining."[40]

Chapter Four

THE HUMAN BREAST
Anatomy, Hormones, Carcinogens

Why is the breast so prone to malignancy?

To begin to answer that question, we need to forget everything that Hollywood has ever tried to teach us about "breasts" in all those fluffy films with the chesty leading ladies—Mae West, Marilyn Monroe, and Jayne Mansfield! First of all, we might reflect that other species have the same problem. Why are cats and mice so prone to breast cancers?

The human breast is not simply an ornament of sexual attraction, or some kind of peacock-like appendage designed to excite men who—(their number is legion)—remain perpetual sophomores. Amorous advertisement is at best a secondary and incidental function of the breast. Its principal role is to serve as **a protective carrier for the mammary gland**. That gland is sometimes referred to as a "sexual organ, but it would be much more logical to use the term **reproductive organ**. In *Homo sapiens* as in all mammals, the mammary gland provides milk for the newborn of the species. Since these newborn are not mature enough to tolerate any other form of nourishment, the gland and its milk are essential to the reproduction of—

indeed, to the very survival and continuance of—the species. Lactation (the secretion of milk) and breast-feeding have always been necessary and commonplace aspects of human life, at least until the development and marketing of infant formula products in the twentieth century.

Breast-feeding is still the best method of infant nourishment. The milk is ready to serve day or night, and constantly at the right temperature; it contains the exact nutrients an infant needs, as well as maternal antibodies which protect against infections. In Third World countries, many nursing mothers cannot afford to buy infant formula, nor do they have ready access to the refrigerators and uncontaminated tap water required for its preparation and preservation. Under these circumstances breast-feeding remains what it has been since time immemorial—a life-and-death matter for newborn humans. In the United States we tend to lose sight of this elemental function of the breast, bombarded as we are by the aforementioned frivolous images that Hollywood continues to give us, and by even sillier insinuations churned out by the advertising agencies of Madison Avenue.

The mammary gland is, so to speak, the "active ingredient" of the breast; and it's also the part of the breast—*the only part!*—which is likely to undergo malignant transformation and give rise to a cancerous tumor. Accordingly, we need to consider its form and function in some detail. We have been speaking of this gland in the singular, and shall continue to do so; but for the record, there are two—one in each breast. The gland is **a paired organ**.

Before puberty the human breast is inchoate, with no appreciable difference between boys and girls. Puberty brings a torrent of growth hormones to both sexes. In the female, rising levels of estrogen in the blood stimulate breast development, resulting first in enlarging nipples, and then (after several years) in the rounded contours of adulthood. The breast may thus be said to be the last anatomical feature which appears on the human body. The mammary gland is even more tardy, being nonexistent before puberty, and remaining immature until after pregnancy and childbirth. The gland has something of a will-of-the-wisp character—"now you see it, now you don't." Its subtle structures are not normally visible to the naked eye, nor can they be demonstrated by the anatomical dissections carried out in medical schools. However, if we were to conduct a microscopic examination of the mammary gland in a nursing mother, we would see that its milk production is concentrated in some 15 to 20 **lobes**, irregularly spaced throughout the breast. Each lobe is in turn subdivided into numerous **lobules**. The epithelial cells secreting most of the milk are those found lining tiny indentations or crevices in the lobules, which are called **alveoli** (Latin for "small hollows").

These secretory elements (alveoli, lobules, lobes) are connected with the nipple by a system of progressively larger **ducts**. The minuscule ducts leaving the individual lobules join together to form a single larger duct, which carries all the milk produced in a lobe to the nipple. Thus **the nipple** serves as the collection point and outlet for some 15 to 20 of these larger ducts, each of which drains one lobe. Of course, we can call these ducts "large" only in comparison to the intralobular ducts. They're really quite small. Unless they become dilated (greatly expanded) due to infection, obstruction, or malignancy, they cannot be palpated (felt by an examiner's hand). The nipple and the surrounding heavily-pigmented **areola** are the only features related to the mammary gland which we can readily see and feel. In males, the nipple remains undeveloped, relatively insensitive, and totally functionless. But the female nipple is marvelously sensitive, being rich in nerve endings; it's most important function is that of a dinner bell. An infant suckling at the nipple sets off a series of complex signals, both nervous and hormonal, which tell the mammary gland—"Make more milk and send it quick!"

No Two Breasts Are Alike

Even the most casual observer could not fail to notice that there are enormous variations in the size and shape of human breasts. Mother Nature obviously did not set a norm for breasts, yet many young women are distressed when their own breasts don't measure up to some imaginary or idealized standard. On the one hand, women may feel less feminine because their breasts seem "too small." On the other, such vague feelings of inadequacy can hardly be compared to the real pains, both physical and psychological, endured by women with very large and very heavy breasts. The added weight on the chest predisposes to nagging aches in the neck and upper spine. A brassiere begins to resemble an instrument of medieval torture when its shoulder straps bite too deeply into the wearer's flesh. An excessive endowment

The Mammary Gland

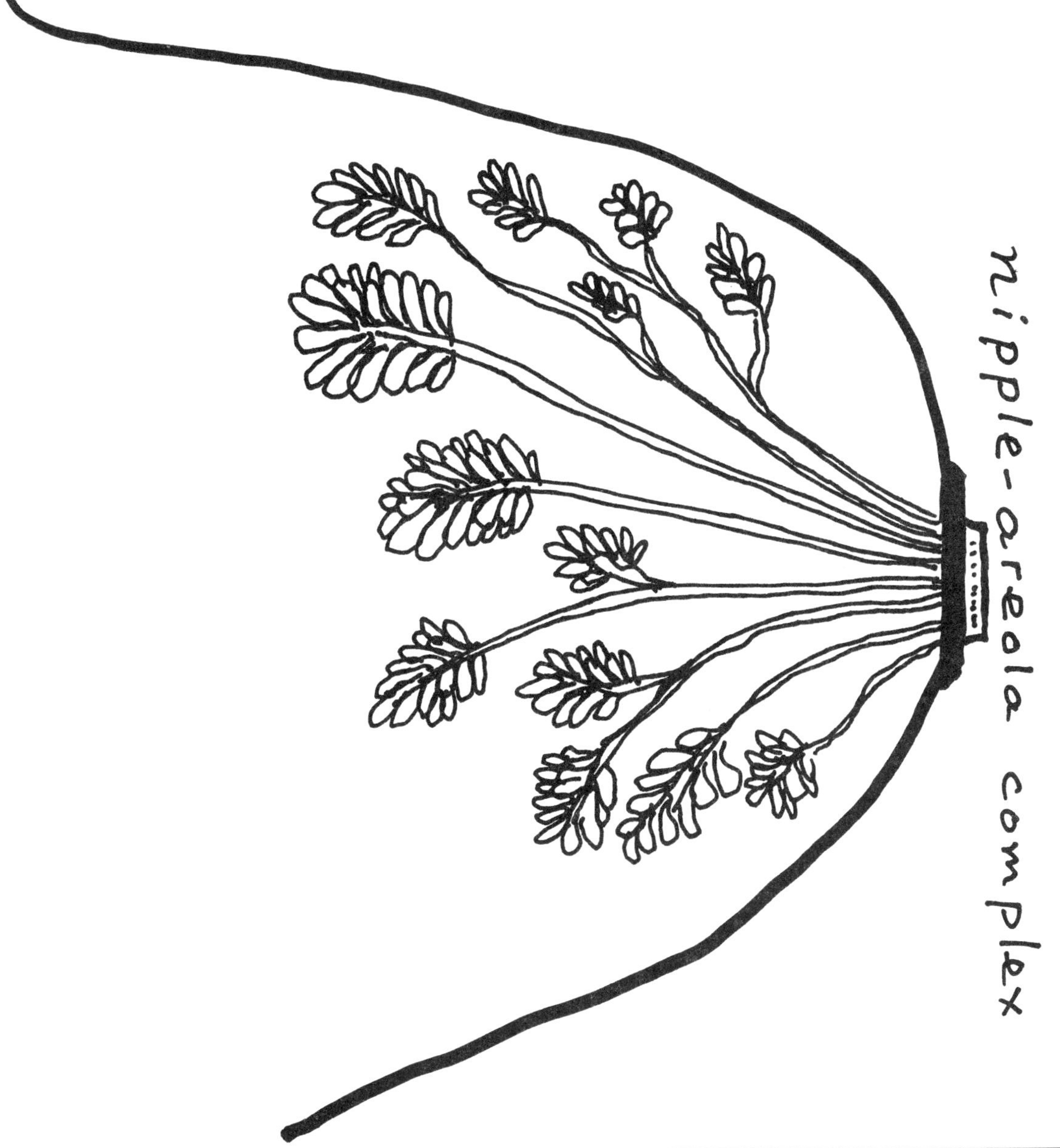

The mammary gland contains some **15 to 20 lobes**. Each of these lobes consists of a cluster of **milk-producing lobules**. Those small **terminal ducts** draining the individual lobules connect with larger milk ducts, which then exit the gland at the nipple.

of breasts—too much of a good thing—makes participation in active sports (tennis, jogging, horseback riding) next to impossible, and turns a shopping trip for well-fitting clothes into the proverbial Grail quest.

The variations in size, as in shape, have little to do with the mammary gland. Women with small breasts or asymmetrical ones nurse infants quite as well as the women who pose for *Playboy* centerfolds. Breast size and shape are largely determined by a woman's genetic inheritance; the genes transmitted by her father may be every bit as important as those she received from her mother. Size in particular is related not to the mammary gland, but to—dare we say it?—the total volume of **subcutaneous fat**. Indeed, this relatively inert fatty tissue, which lies just beneath the skin and serves as padding for the gland, constitutes the largest component of the breast. The gland itself occupies considerably less space. One recent estimate suggests that the epithelial (glandular) cells typically take up "less than 15% of the volume of the breast" in premenopausal women, and that "this decreases to less than 5% by age 60 years."[1] During pregnancy the mammary gland undergoes rapid, florid growth; during lactation it achieves its maximum volume, being filled with milk. With the advent of menopause it atrophies: the lobules wither and shrink, leaving behind the system of ducts as the most prominent relics of a defunct biological factory.[2]

The Supporting Structures

The breast does not contain any muscles to speak of; but it rests upon, and is intimately connected with, two chest muscles which play important roles in moving the arm and shoulder. These muscles are the **pectoralis major**, which extends from the sternum (breastbone) to the humerus (the arm bone between the shoulder and the elbow), and the **pectoralis minor**, which lies beneath the pectoralis major and which extends from the sternum to the scapula (shoulder blade). These pectoral (chest) muscles are covered with a sheet of durable fibrous tissue called the **fascia** (Latin for "a band" or "a sash"). The breast is firmly anchored to the pectoral fascia by a large number of thin fibrous strands known as **Cooper's ligaments**. These connective fibers start in the superficial layers of the dermis (skin), and travel down through the breast, weaving around the ducts and lobes of the mammary gland. Cooper's ligaments suffice to hold the breast erect and keep it from sliding downward; at the same time they are flexible enough to allow freedom of movement.

All elements of the mammary gland (ducts, lobes, lobules) are surrounded by the **stroma**, dense supportive tissue which is richly supplied with blood and lymph vessels, with nerves, and with collagen fibers. Stromal tissue separates the different lobes from each other, and even provides thin partitions between the numerous lobules in each lobe. As we've previously noted, most malignancies of the mammary gland begin in the milk ducts, usually in the **small terminal ducts** which drain the lobules.[3] But other breast cancers (a minority) begin in the lobules proper. In either case, when malignant cells move from a duct or lobule into the stroma, an invasive (infiltrating) tumor will have begun. After this event there are two ways in which the cancerous cells can spread to distant regions of the body—either through the lymphatic vessels or through the bloodstream. The second mode of transport should be fairly obvious; the first requires some explanation for those readers who have never studied medicine.

A Word about Lymphatics

The visible fluid in the body is blood. Prehistoric peoples recognized the existence of blood vessels, although the true nature of the circulatory system was not demonstrated until 1628, with the experiments of the English physician William Harvey. That the human body has a second pervasive fluid and a second circulatory system of sorts escaped the observation of the ancients; even today most laypersons are unaware of the fact. The existence of lymph and of lymphatic vessels was discovered in the seventeenth century, by early anatomists using crude microscopes.

The differences between blood and lymph are profound. Blood serves to carry nutrients and oxygen to individual cells in all parts of the body; it also removes carbon dioxide and other byproducts resulting from cellular metabolism. Blood moves through the body with considerable force and speed, being massively pumped by that most tireless of muscles, the heart. Our blood vessels—arteries, arterioles, capillaries—are the broad rivers, rustling streams, and bubbling springs which carry absolutely essential commerce. If the bloodstream should be impeded or stopped, even for a few minutes, the body will die. The lymphatic system is also essential; without it the body would perish in a few days—but its innumerable tiny vessels do not lend themselves to poetic descriptions. Our lymph vessels, if we should not think of them as sewers, may be appropriately likened to drainage ditches. The lymphatic system has to do with drainage, waste disposal, and detoxification.

The word **lymph** comes from the Latin *lympha*, meaning "clear water"; it refers to the colorless fluid extract of blood which escapes from the smallest capillaries and accumulates in tissues throughout the body. Lymph bathes the individual cells and picks up any solid debris in their vicinity; it then gathers in tiny channels which run alongside the blood vessels. Lymph moves sluggishly, being propelled by the occasional contraction of nearby muscles. Like blood veins, the smallest lymphatics flow into larger ones, which join up with still larger ducts. Unlike blood, however, lymph flows only in a single direction—from the extremities (arms, legs, head) to two central ducts located just behind the right and left collarbones. At these junctures (one on each side of the body), lymph reenters the bloodstream; the large lymphatic ducts merge seamlessly with the subclavian blood veins. By virtue of the lymphatic system, any fluid which may have seeped from the bloodstream is effectively drained from the tissues and returned to the circulation; but first that fluid must undergo filtration and purification in one or more lymph nodes.

The Lymph Nodes

If we can compare lymphatic vessels to drainage ditches, surely we may be pardoned for referring to the nodes as **sewage treatment plants**. Once again our analogy is unpoetic, but quite apt. While the structure of lymph nodes is complex, their function is easy enough to understand. Every lymphatic vessel passes through at least one node before it empties into a main duct merging with the bloodstream. The nodes, little bits of soft sponge-like tissue, serve as filters which remove debris and bacteria from lymph. They also function as the watch posts and front-line fortresses of the body's immune system. Each node carries a varied contingent of white cells to defend against possible invaders. Those large omnivorous cells called **macrophages** literally devour bacteria and pieces of particulate matter. **Lymphocytes**, smaller cells taking their name from lymph, likewise abound in the nodes.

Classified either as **B cells** (which produce antibodies) or as **T cells** (which can kill other cells), lymphocytes stand ready to fight elusive or disguised aliens like viruses or virus-infected cells, which might not alert the less discriminating macrophages.

Most of the time we are blissfully oblivious of our busy lymph nodes; we can't feel them unless we've got a problem. For example, a boil or other bacterial infection on the scalp or face is likely to result in a few palpable nodes, perhaps around the ear or under the jaw. Usually the enlarging nodes will be felt as small tender masses, slightly painful to the touch; they appear suddenly but fade away after a day or two, as the body's white cells quickly rout the offending bacteria. The symptoms are more insidious, and the outcome much more problematic, when lymph nodes become involved with malignancy. Almost all solid tumors spread to some degree though the lymphatic system. Typically, cancer cells arriving in a lymph node will cause a slowly enlarging mass, painless to the touch, which continues to grow until it becomes a hard rubbery lump. This process may take a few months or many years; but once enlarged and palpable, an involved node does not subside. The nodal white cells have obviously failed to recognize the intruding cancer cells as foreign, and the node itself has probably become a seedbed of malignant dissemination.

The Breast's Drainage System

The breast is well supplied with small blood vessels, and the very active mammary gland accumulates excess fluid both in itself and in its surrounding tissues. As we might expect, the breast contains multitudinous lymphatic vessels. These vessels flow toward various regional lymph nodes, which are almost never of concern to women in good health, but whose importance to women diagnosed with breast cancer can hardly be overstated. Any recommendation regarding chemotherapy is likely to be based on the status of the regional lymph nodes; it is prudent to know something about them. In their weighty textbook William L. Donegan and John S. Spratt remind us that "lymph nodes tend to cluster in fatty tissue near the bifurcation of great veins."[4] The exact number of nodes clustered in the fatty tissue of the axilla (armpit) varies from person to person. The estimates found in textbooks also vary; most authors give a ballpark figure of 25 to 30, while some go as high as 40. What is certain is that the overwhelming majority of lymphatic vessels draining the breast pass through the axillary nodes. An experiment done in the 1950s traced the movement of a radioactive isotope injected into breasts; about 97% to 99% of the measurable radioactivity was subsequently detected in the axilla, demonstrating the predominance of this pathway.[5] The axillary nodes are doubly important because they also filter all lymph draining from the arm.

The breast has several secondary pathways which we need to be aware of. The **internal mammary nodes** are clustered in two separate chains, one on each side of the sternum (breastbone), usually about an inch or so from mid-sternum, and perhaps three-quarters of an inch beneath the skin. On the average, each chain contains about seven or eight nodes; these are located in the "intercostal spaces"—i.e., between the ribs. While the aforementioned experiment with a radioactive tracer suggested that less than 10% of the lymph draining from the breast passed through the internal mammary nodes, another study found that perhaps 20% of the lymph flowed through these nodes.[6] Their role is clearly secondary to that of the axillary nodes; but they do help to drain the breast, especially its "inner quadrants"—that is, the

Lymphatic Drainage of the Breast

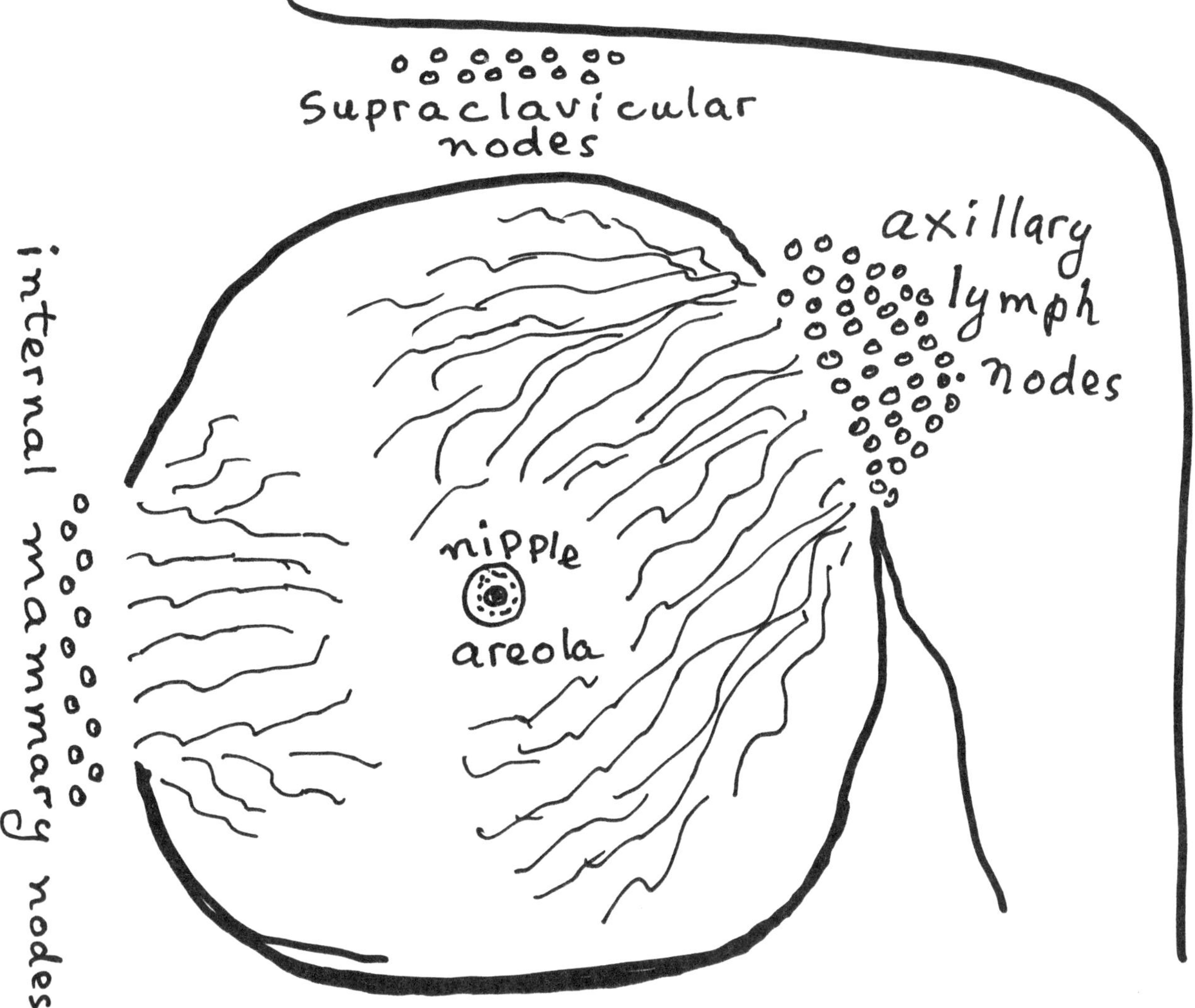

Most lymphatic fluid draining from the mammary gland is filtered through the **axillary nodes**. But a little fluid coming from the breast's inner quadrants is filtered through the **internal mammary nodes** located under the ribs, near the sternum (breastbone). The **supraclavicular nodes** above the collarbone are not directly involved with the breast's lymphatic drainage, and consequently they are unlikely to harbor malignant cells in early-stage breast cancer.

inner half bordering the sternum.

The chest muscles underneath the breast have their own lymphatic vessels and nodes. Lying between the pectoralis major and minor muscles are a number of very tiny nodes called **Rotter's nodes**, after a German surgeon who described them in 1899. These interpectoral nodes would seem to filter lymph coming from the chest muscles rather than from the mammary gland; but in cases of advanced breast cancer, they are sometimes found to harbor malignant cells, a fact which implies at least a possible connection between the pectoral lymphatic vessels and those draining the gland.[7]

The **supraclavicular nodes** above the collarbone can become as large as golf balls in advanced malignancies, including those of the breast. In the 1890s pioneering surgeons like William Steward Halsted often pondered the role of these nodes in breast cancer. Today we know that lymph from the mammary gland never flows directly to the supraclavicular nodes, and that their involvement during breast malignancy indicates a tumor of long duration and extensive regional spread, one which has very probably metastasized.

Most breast cancers currently diagnosed in the United States are detected early; and consequently when our physicians talk about "the nodes," they mean the axillary nodes. The other nodal groups (internal mammary, interpectoral, supraclavicular) are not usually involved in early-stage disease; they are almost never found to be positive when the axilla is negative. Today's surgeons and radiotherapists do not often see a need to dissect or irradiate these other nodal groups, but this has not always been true. Controversies regarding the proper treatment of the regional lymph nodes have been raging for over a century, with diverse schools of thought ranging from *"Leave 'em alone"* to *"Get 'em all out!"* The side effects brought about by the latter philosophy were always substantial and irreversible. A full axillary dissection will invariably hinder the lymphatic drainage of the arm, causing it to swell up with fluid. To be certain of removing Rotter's nodes, both pectoral muscles have to be stripped from the chest. The internal mammary nodes can't be removed without resecting the sternum (cutting open the breastbone), a risky operation for all but the most experienced surgeons. Such drastic interventions, appropriate for the few, were once indiscriminately applied to several generations of breast cancer patients.

HORMONES!
a short answer to a tough question

Our review of basic anatomy is finished; we can now consider that intriguing question posed in this chapter's opening sentence. Why is the breast—more accurately, *the mammary gland*—so prone to malignancy? Strangely enough, this is one of the very few questions in breast cancer which admits of an emphatic single-word answer—*hormones!* The mammary gland contains some of the most hormonally responsive tissues in the human body. From puberty until menopause it remains in a state of constant activity. Its ductal and lobular cells are forever reproducing themselves—dividing in two, dying off, and then dividing again—in response to the surging or receding waves of hormones (estrogen and progesterone) produced by the ovaries. Thus stimulated, these epithelial cells amply fulfill the first prerequisite for malignant transformation—**frequent cellular division**. The more cells divide, the more likely they are to undergo mutations leading to cancer. Of course, the sex hormones acting on the mammary gland are not *per se* mutagenic; they are not carcinogens which by their very nature tend to damage DNA and disrupt the genetic code. But these hormones are *highly mitogenic*—they cause responsive cells to undergo mitosis (division), creating that condition of genetic flux in which mutations can occur.

Our bodies are the end products of millions of years of evolution, of trial-and-error biological experimentation. Unfortunately, our reproductive systems, being geared up for maximum fertility, are much better suited for the Stone Age than for modern industrialized society. In those dark prehistoric days, the average life expectancy probably did not approach 30 years, and infant mortality was horrendous. The human species needed constant reproduction just to maintain existing populations. These days our fecundity has proven to be both a nuisance and a danger. In a book about cancer there should be no more than parenthetical references to the social havoc caused by unplanned teenage pregnancies in urban America, or to the exploding population growth in less developed nations, or to the rapid depletion of the earth's natural resources by an excessively prolific *Homo sapiens*. But we can certainly reflect on the ways in which our ingrained reproductive traits predispose us to malignancy. In any given year the cancer statistics for the United States will begin with two tumors of the reproductive organs—breast cancer in women, prostate cancer in men. Among serious malignancies, these two are the clear front runners in the number of cases (incidence), though not in mortality. Both originate from exocrine glands which produce fluids essential for human reproduction— milk in the case of the mammary gland, seminal fluid in that of the prostate. The glands themselves are notable as target organs for the hormones secreted by the gonads (ovaries and testicles). And they are always active in fertile humans. The mammary gland is always getting ready for lactation, even if pregnancy and childbirth do not transpire. The prostate is always making seminal fluid, unless prevented by accident, disease, or extreme old age.

If perhaps some readers have found that one-word explanation for the breast's susceptibility to cancer too simplistic, the author can assure them that not only is "hormones" an acceptable answer, but it is a profound one which could be experimentally verified. Women who undergo early menopause, either naturally or through oophorectomy (surgical removal of the ovaries), have a substantially reduced risk of postmenopausal breast cancer. Stop the flow of ovarian hormones which stimulate the mammary gland, and you'll lower the odds of getting breast cancer! Of course, *all* risk could be eliminated by removing or irradiating the ovaries before puberty. In this case the breast and its enclosed gland would simply not develop. Similarly, men who undergo castration as children fail to develop such secondary sexual characteristics as beards (facial hair), deepening voices, and gradually encroaching baldness. Men deprived so early of the testicular hormone testosterone have no risk of developing prostate cancer or that benign enlargement of this gland which causes difficulty in urination. While marvelously effective, timely castration is not a remedy that many people would choose to prevent malignancies of the breast and prostate.

The remainder of this chapter will deal largely with the effects of estrogen and progesterone on the mammary gland, and with the ways in which these effects vary according to the different phases of a woman's reproductive life (menstrual cycle, pregnancy, lactation, menopause). This overview of breast endocrinology is a necessary prelude to Chapter Five, on the risk factors for mammary cancer, and to Chapters Six and

Seven, on the controversies surrounding estrogen replacement therapy and birth control pills. As we shall see, hormonal stimulation explains a great deal about the risks, which will generally be found to increase when the levels of estrogen and progesterone in the blood increase, and to decrease when these levels fall.

Cellular Hormone Receptors

The human body reveals systems of interlocking and interactive communications far surpassing the most futuristic products of our telephone companies. The nervous system handles those split-second reactions between brain and muscles—for example, when you inadvertently place your hand on a hot stove and have only two seconds to remove it before a burn occurs. Hormones also represent a system of communications, although the messages sent travel much slower and are far more subtle than those electrical impulses relayed by the nerves. It is this endocrine system which enables reproduction and which (so to speak) keeps the ovaries, uterus, and breast in constant communication from ovulation through pregnancy and childbirth to lactation.

At this juncture we might offer a brief definition of a hormone—"a biochemically active molecule which is secreted into the blood by an endocrine gland and which produces effects on target organs and tissues elsewhere in the body." Some hormones act on—and are needed by—virtually all bodily tissues. Insulin secreted by the pancreas and growth hormone from the pituitary have such broad effects. The action of the sex hormones is considerably more focused, though not limited to the reproductive organs. While the female hormone estrogen acts most noticeably on the uterus, vagina, and breasts, it's also necessary for the bones and skin.

How do the individual cells in the target organs and tissues manage to recognize and react to hormones? Typically, the outer plasma membranes of the affected cells are studded with **receptors**, little bits of protein which unite with (bind to) the appropriate hormone molecules in the blood and, by so doing, initiate a biochemical chain of events called **signal transduction**. The end result is mitosis (cell division) or some other important cellular activity. Different types of cells display different types of receptors, depending on the hormones they need for their respective jobs. Receptors for sex hormones like estrogen and progesterone are located in the cytoplasms of cells, rather than on the outer membranes. Unlike other hormones, the sex hormones are not proteins but **steroids**, lipid-soluble molecules derived from cholesterol. These smaller molecules easily diffuse through plasma membranes; they then bind to and activate the receptors in the cellular cytoplasms. D. J. Weatherall of Oxford University has concisely described the next event: "In the bound configuration, receptor proteins acquire an affinity for DNA that leads to their accumulation in the nucleus. Here the complex binds to chromatin and regulates the transcription of a number of different genes."[8]

The nature of estrogen receptors and their crucial role in the cells of the mammary gland did not become evident until the late 1960s and early 1970s, following the seminal experiments of Elwood V. Jensen and his co-workers at the University of Chicago. The new knowledge soon found applications in breast cancer medicine. In the late 1970s and early 1980s, William L. McGuire, Marc E. Lippman, and other researchers demonstrated that the quantity of estrogen receptor protein present in the cytoplasms of breast cancer cells could be used to predict tumor aggressiveness and the likely response to systemic therapy. Generally speaking, higher levels of estrogen receptor protein are associated with reduced tumor aggressiveness and a favorable response to hormonal manipulations. Lower levels usually point toward a more aggressive tumor which probably won't respond to hormonal therapy, but which should react to cytotoxic chemotherapy.[9] By the mid-1980s it was clear that the measurement of progesterone receptors was also valuable in breast cancer prognosis.[10] The old division of patients into node-negative and node-positive groupings now began to be supplemented with a secondary division into groups that were hormone receptor-positive (prognosticly good) or hormone receptor-negative (prognosticly bad). Controversies persisted as to whether estrogen or progesterone receptors constituted the better indicator of prognosis, and as to the most accurate assays for measuring them; but the fundamental importance of hormone receptors was conceded by physicians and scientists alike.

The Menstrual Cycle

The reproductive urge in male mammals tends to be constant; with females it is generally periodic. For lower mammalian species we use the term **estrus** to describe the time just after a female animal has released one or more ova (eggs) into the uterus, and is therefore fertile and receptive to mating. When the first ovarian hormone was isolated in 1923, the name selected for it (estrogen) pointedly alluded to these episodes of sexual frenzy in the barnyard. Females of the most intelligent order of mammals, the primates, do not exhibit estrus; but they do reveal a unique monthly pattern of fertility known as **the menstrual cycle**. The most noticeable sign of this cycle is the **menses** (Latin for "months") or **menstruation**—that is, the shedding of the dense cellular lining from a uterus which has failed to receive a fertilized

ovum. This phenomenon, marked by loss of blood, is observed only in *Homo sapiens*, the great apes, and Old World monkeys. Ovulation occurs rather predictably at midpoint in a menstrual cycle of 28 days, typically 14 days after the last menses and 14 days away from the next.[11] We need to look more closely at the menstrual cycle, paying special attention to the changes taking place in the uterus and the breast.

By convention, the first day of menstruation is referred to as "day one" of the menstrual cycle. Menstruation usually lasts three to five days, during which time the estrogen and progesterone circulating in the blood fall to their lowest levels. The depressed levels of these ovarian hormones trigger a new cycle of ovulation and endometrial replenishment, involving a complex interaction among several endocrine glands. The initial response comes from the **hypothalamus**, located at the base of the brain; it responds to the hormonal ebbtide by secreting **gonadotropin-releasing hormone**, or **GnRH**. This hormone acts on the neighboring **pituitary**, once known as the body's "master gland" because it plays a central role in many endocrine processes. The first gonadotropin ("gonad nutrient") secreted by the pituitary is called **follicle-stimulating hormone**, or **FSH**. As its name implies, it stimulates the development of egg-bearing follicles on the surface of the ovaries. In some lesser mammals (rabbits, pigs, cats, dogs), many follicles mature in response to FSH, producing and then releasing the multiple ova which result in the birth of large litters. In *Homo sapiens*, usually only one follicle on one ovary matures during each monthly cycle. The cells inside that swelling follicle, spurred on by FSH, begin to secrete estrogen into the blood. This hormone acts most noticeably on the endometrium (lining of the uterus), which has been reduced to a thin layer of epithelial and stromal cells, just a millimeter or two thick, by the preceding menstruation. Under the influence of estrogen, these cells multiply rapidly. During this time—roughly from day four or five to day 14 of the menstrual cycle—the endometrium is said to be in its "proliferative phase": it doubles in thickness. Estrogen also has proliferative effects on the vagina and the fallopian tubes, preparing these structures for their respective roles in the transport of sperm to the ovum, and of the fertilized ovum to the uterus.

In marked contrast to the uterus, the breast remains relatively quiescent during the first half of the menstrual cycle, which we call the **follicular phase**. The rising levels of estrogen associated with a developing follicle do not spur the mammary gland into the furious mitotic activity that is seen in the endometrium. Some cellular division occurs in the milk ducts, but the lobules are hardly affected.[12] The estrogen surge does not, however, escape the notice of the hypothalamus. Around day 12 of the cycle, that sensitive monitor issues a second releasing hormone, directing the pituitary to produce **luteinizing hormone**, or **LH**. This gonadotropin acts on the ovarian follicle, which has by now swollen to a diameter of some 25 millimeters (almost an inch). Within 28 to 36 hours after LH levels peak in the blood, the follicle will rupture, setting the ovum free.[13]

Ovulation marks the beginning of the second half of the menstrual cycle, known as the **luteal phase**. The ruptured follicle is now referred to as the **corpus luteum**—Latin for "yellow body"—because the cells lining this open cavity assume a yellowish color, owing to their high lipid (fat) content. These cells have plenty of work to do: under the continuing stimulus of LH, they produce increasing quantities of **progesterone**. This second ovarian hormone has a more specialized function than estrogen. As its name

suggests, it is peculiarly a pregnancy hormone, being "pro-gestation"; and it exerts the most striking effects both on the uterus and on the breast.[14] Rising levels of progesterone serve initially as an endocrine alarm bell, warning that a pregnancy is—or could be—in progress, and that ovulation and conception must be temporarily avoided. When this hormone is elevated, the hypothalamus will not issue GnRH, and the pituitary will not issue FSH and LH. Hence ovulation does not occur. Progesterone also causes the mucus filling the cervical opening (the narrow passage into the uterus) to become thick and sticky, effectively barring sperm from entering. Needless to say, these two hormonally-mediated effects (prevention of ovulation and exclusion of sperm) explain why a progestin (a synthetic version of the hormone) is the active ingredient in birth control pills.

But progesterone's role in averting additional conceptions is secondary to its function in sustaining the pregnancy which, in the natural scheme of things, would have typically begun shortly after ovulation. Progesterone is to the endometrium what fertilizer is to unturned, dry soil in which a seed must be planted. The endometrial cells have already repopulated themselves during the follicular phase, and progesterone does not spur further cellular proliferation. Its task is rather to promote cultivation. Under its influence the cytoplasms of these cells fill with fats, proteins, sugars, and minerals. And tiny blood vessels appear among the cells, linking them together. In short, progesterone turns the endometrial lining into a dense, soft, well-vascularized "bed," which has been specially prepared to allow the ovum's implantation and to provide nutrients for the developing embryo. During this time of high progesterone levels—roughly days 15 through 28 of the menstrual cycle—the endometrium is said to be in its "secretory phase."

The breast, which remains relatively dormant during the first half of the menstrual cycle, will awaken in the second. Estrogen, the predominant hormone of the follicular phase, is not particularly efficient in stimulating cellular division in the mammary gland. Yet the combination of estrogen with another hormone can be highly mitogenic, as demonstrated by the rapid development of the adolescent breast in response to estrogen and growth hormone. The luteal phase of the menstrual cycle is characterized by rising levels of both estrogen and progesterone, which peak at around day 21—that is, at the beginning of the fourth week. The cells of the mammary gland, especially those in the lobules, respond with mitotic activity. More cellular divisions occur in the lobules during the fourth week of the cycle than in the first three weeks combined.[15] This fact does much to explain why the cycle's last week has long been associated with those symptoms of hormonal surfeit and glandular instability which physicians and patients lump together under the heading **PMS** (premenstrual syndrome). In the breast the lobular activity of the late luteal phase often results in the accumulation of fluid and consequent swelling, in tenderness, and in generalized lumpiness. The breast may increase in size during the last half of the cycle, sometimes by as much as 20%.

Conception, if it is to occur, does so most advantageously early in the luteal phase, within a day of ovulation. Once an ovum leaves its follicle, it ages rapidly; the older it is, the less likely that conception will lead to a successful pregnancy. The regression of the corpus luteum is nature's way of preventing tardy fertilization. If a fertilized ovum has not implanted in the endometrial lining within a week or ten days after ovulation, the corpus luteum will sense the situation and begin to shut down. The level of progesterone in the blood will then fall precipitously; and as it does, the small blood vessels in the endometrial lining will constrict, depriving the newly built-up tissues of oxygen and nutrients. Within a day or two, the outer layer of the endometrium will die and slough away, passing through the cervical opening as menstrual discharge.[16]

The breast's response to the end of the menstrual cycle is less apparent than that of the uterus, but it is nonetheless significant. Mitotic activity slows down, and any swelling or tenderness subsides. Unnoticed, large numbers of cells in the lobules and in the small terminal ducts will have undergone **apoptosis** (programmed cell death). The sum total of breast cells being born and dying off during each cycle has never been calculated, but the figure probably runs into the billions. John S. Meyer, a pathologist at Washington University in Saint Louis, has estimated that in a 20-year-old woman the epithelial cells lining the lobules and the terminal ducts have a turnover time of about 22 days. In teenagers and women in their early twenties, these cells would thus replace themselves once a month—that is, *with every menstrual cycle*.[17] This tremendous rate of cellular division does much to explain why the breasts of very young women are so terribly sensitive to carcinogens (e.g., ionizing radiation). Fortunately, the mitotic rate drops sharply with increasing age. At age 30, the typical turnover time is 70 days; at age 40, it's 147 days. Dr. Meyer points out that "the rate of cell renewal decreases toward the menopause and is markedly diminished after the menopause. This helps explain the well-known atrophy of the lobules that occurs at this time."[18]

Pregnancy and Childbirth

Parity is a Latinate term—(from *parere*, to bear or bring forth)—that physicians use to describe the state of having carried a pregnancy to term. A woman who has experienced a full-term pregnancy is said to be **parous**, regardless of whether the infant was born alive or not. The first childbirth may sometimes be a profound spiritual event; it is always a profound physiological one, bringing permanent changes to both the uterus and the breast.

Pregnancy requires that the menstrual cycle be suspended for the nine-month duration of gestation and for at least a few weeks afterward. Even as implantation is taking place, a fertilized ovum will begin to secrete **human chorionic gonadotropin**, or **hCG**. This powerful chemical messenger is very similar to luteinizing hormone (LH); its principal function is to rescue the corpus luteum. Instead of shutting down and atrophying, the corpus luteum will now turn out increasing quantities of estrogen and progesterone. Menstruation does not occur, and the lush endometrial tissues not only allow the fertilized ovum's implantation, but secrete additional nutrients to support its rapid growth into an embryo. By the beginning of the second trimester, the level of hCG in the maternal blood has fallen considerably; but the corpus luteum is no longer needed to sustain the pregnancy. Its functions have been taken over by a much more powerful endocrine organ, the **placenta** (Latin for "a flat cake"). Attached to the uterine wall, the placenta is a curious hybrid structure which develops partly from maternal endometrial cells and partly from the outer layer (trophoblastic cells) of the fertilized ovum. This organ serves the fetus as a nutrient warehouse, holding and distributing proteins, fats, sugars, minerals, and electrolytes. But its most crucial role is as a blood exchange. In the placenta the mother's circulatory system comes into intimate contact with that of the fetus. Although blood itself does not pass between mother and fetus, the oxygen carried by the maternal blood easily diffuses across the thin membranes into the fetal circulation. Carbon dioxide, urea, and other waste products from the fetal blood diffuse into the mother's circulation, eventually to be exhaled by her lungs or excreted in her urine. These two placental functions—nutrient storage and circulatory exchange—have little or no impact on the mammary gland; it is as an endocrine organ that the placenta transforms the breast. In the second and third trimesters of pregnancy, the placenta pours massive, unprecedented quantities of estrogen and progesterone into the maternal blood. The skyrocketing levels of these hormones dwarf those present during the menstrual cycle. Advanced pregnancy may reveal a hundred times the normal level of estrogen and ten times the normal level of progesterone.

In many women the breasts actually double in size during pregnancy. The first trimester brings **cellular proliferation** to the mammary gland, not unlike that which occurs during the menstrual cycle, but understandably much greater. In the second and third trimesters, the tremendous waves of placental hormones propel the glandular epithelium beyond mere proliferation into **final differentiation**. By the time of childbirth, the mammary gland will have assumed its mature form as an endocrine organ which can, given the proper stimuli, manufacture and release appreciable amounts of milk. The process of differentiation during pregnancy may be observed in the small terminal ducts, which spread out in all directions like tree branches in early spring, reaching deep into the lobules. An even more dramatic blossoming occurs in the lobules themselves, which open up like flowers in the summer sunshine. The **alveoli**—the individual secretory units in the lobules—become more numerous and more pronounced. The cytoplasms of the alveolar cells fill with droplets of lipids and other raw materials needed for the production of milk. When the alveoli are thus primed for secretion, they are sometimes referred to as **acini** (the Latin word for "grapes").

The pathologist Irma H. Russo and her co-workers at the Michigan Cancer Foundation in Detroit have documented the extent of the lobular expansion brought about by pregnancy. When they examined mammary tissue specimens obtained from breast reduction surgery or from autopsies, Russo et al discovered that a lobule in a nulliparous woman (one who has never had a full-term pregnancy) typically contains no more than five or six alveoli, but that a lobule in a parous woman contains on the average 81 alveoli.[19] The expansion of the mammary gland is substantial and reasonably permanent, but it's not the most intriguing alteration brought about by the first full-term pregnancy. The glandular cells have not merely multiplied themselves; they are intrinsically different. Through mechanisms which we do not fully understand, the mammary epithelium has become far more stable and much less sensitive to carcinogens. Naturally these cells will still respond to estrogen and progesterone, but they will not do so as dramatically as before. In subsequent menstrual cycles and in any future pregnancies, they will exhibit lower mitotic rates.

As we shall see in Chapter Five, the differentiation of the mammary gland occasioned by parity tends to significantly reduce the risk of postmenopausal breast cancer. While estrogen and progesterone play the foremost roles in achieving this differentiation, they are not the only hormones which come into play. The process is probably

initiated by human chorionic gonadotropin in the earliest days of pregnancy. When sufficient doses of hCG are administered to virgin rats, the mammary glands of these lab animals undergo growth and differentiation comparable to that achieved by pregnancy; and they become resistant to carcinogens which normally induce breast tumors in this rodent species.[20] Another essential stimulus to breast differentiation is almost certainly **prolactin**, the "pro-lactation" hormone which stimulates milk production. Issued by the pituitary in late pregnancy, prolactin brings about internal changes in the lobular cells, preparing them for subsequent milk secretion. No milk is actually released during pregnancy itself, because prolactin's activity is being offset by the high levels of estrogen and progesterone.

Parturition (childbirth) signals the mammary gland to release the pent-up milk stored in the alveolar cells. The complex phenomenon of birthing is governed by both mechanical and hormonal factors. By the ninth month of pregnancy, the uterus has swollen to many times its usual size, affecting virtually every organ in the maternal body. The mother's stomach, intestines, diaphragm, and bladder all suffer from compression, while her abdominal muscles are stretched taut. Also a muscle, the uterus has been stretched to its limit, and it now begins to rebound. The first sign of the impending contractions is typically the repositioning of the fetal head (the largest body part) in the lowest portion of the uterus, directly above the cervical opening into the vagina. This maneuver establishes **the basic stretch-and-contraction relationship of childbirth**. On the one hand, the cervix is to be stretched open—or dilated—by the fetal head; on the other, the upper portion of the uterus will naturally contract in response to the cervical

Alveoli in a Lobule

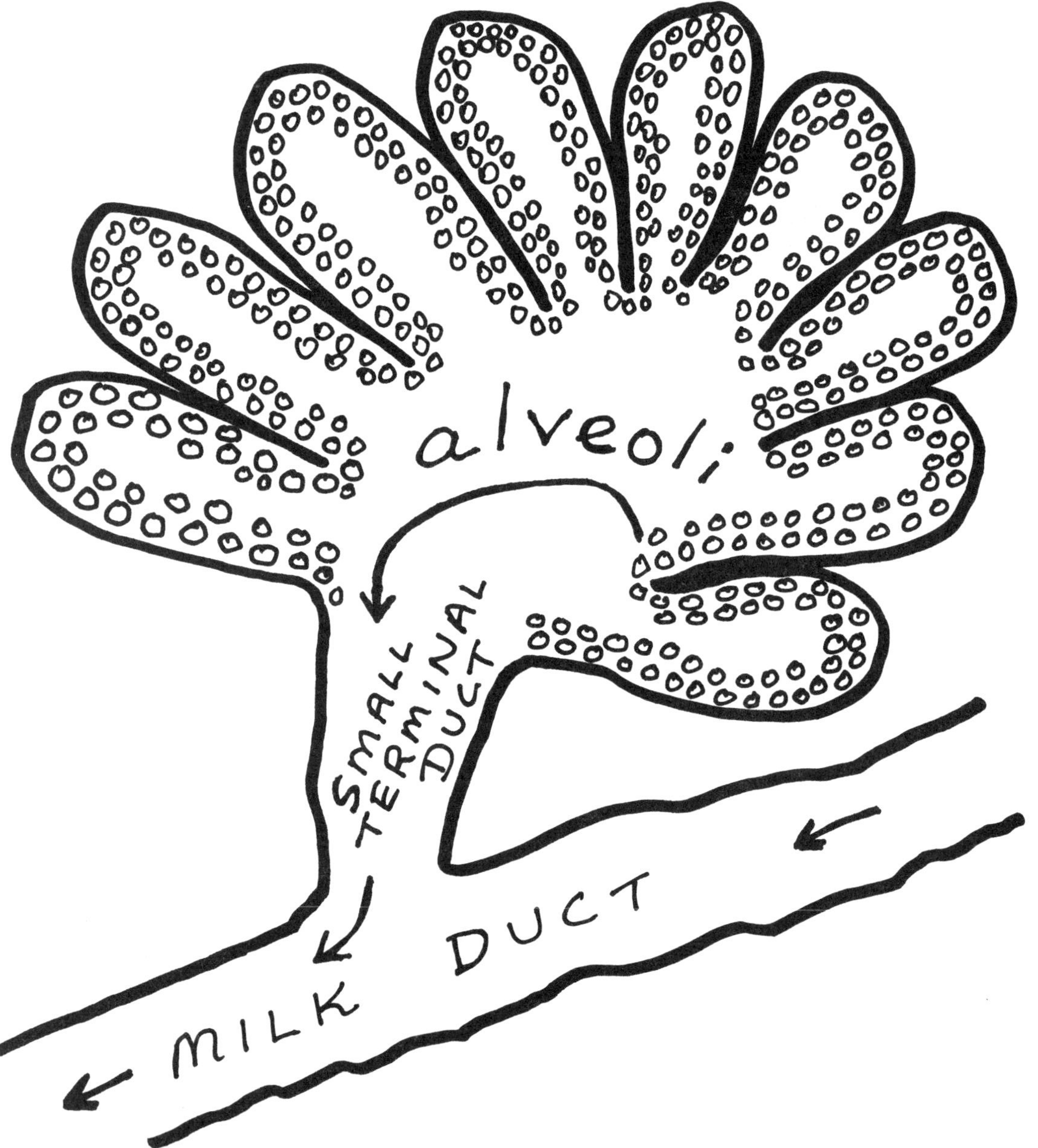

Alveoli are indentations or pockets in the lobules lined with milk-producing cells. Full-term pregnancy vastly increases the number of alveoli. Each lobule is drained by **a small terminal duct**, which in turn merges with a larger milk duct leading to the nipple.

stretching. Together these mechanical pulls and pushes work to propel the baby into the light of day; they are aided by a hormonal environment which has been recently altered. While progesterone acts to prevent uterine movements, the placental production of this hormone levels off a few weeks before term. **Oxytocin** now comes into play. This pituitary hormone specifically promotes uterine contractions; it appears in the blood shortly before labor begins. To each contraction during labor, the pituitary will respond by secreting still more oxytocin, which cannot fail to stimulate still another contraction. The series of contractions thus becomes stronger and faster, each one more powerful than the last, and occurring more quickly than before. Eventually these parturient forces become irresistible; childbirth happens whether the mother is ready or not, in the safety of a hospital room or on the back seat of a taxi.

Within a few minutes after delivery, the placenta will be expelled from the uterus, which has now begun to rebound toward its original position. The expulsion of the placenta precipitates an enormous change in the mother's hormonal environment. The levels of estrogen and progesterone quickly plummet, leaving prolactin and oxytocin to act unopposed on the mammary gland. Milk secretion will be established in a day or two, but the quantity produced and delivered depends largely upon the degree of physical stimulation given the nipples. Each time an infant suckles at a nipple, the nerves relay signals to the pituitary, commanding that gland to release more prolactin and oxytocin. During lactation the latter hormone brings about contractions of the myoepithelial cells surrounding the alveoli, causing milk to be expressed into the terminal ducts. Sometimes physical stimulation of the nipples is not necessary to send the appropriate neuro-hormonal messages to the pituitary—milk

secretion can occur when the mother just hears her baby crying.

Childbirth typically delays a young woman's return to regular ovulation for no more than several months. But breast-feeding, if performed constantly and on demand, can often postpone the resumption of the menstrual cycle for well over a year. This lactational suppression of fertility is nature's way of preventing a second baby from intruding too soon on a mother preoccupied with nursing a prior infant. As we'll discover in Chapter Five, there is considerable evidence that diligent breast-feeding could also reduce the risk of breast cancer. The menstrual cycle entails the proliferation and apoptosis of mammary cells, with ever increasing opportunities for genetic mutation. From the standpoint of breast cancer prevention, any decrease in the number of monthly cycles tends to be protective.

The Menopausal Changes

Menopause, the cessation of the menses, marks the end of a woman's reproductive years; it also brings irreversible changes to her hormonal environment. The cause of the menopause is commonly cited as "ovarian failure": this term refers to the gradual depletion of undeveloped oocytes (egg cells) which can be hormonally stimulated to mature into ova capable of being fertilized. For most American women the menopause will occur somewhere between the ages of 45 and 55. It is preceded by a variable time— perhaps a year, perhaps several—of inconsistent and unpredictable ovarian function which physicians call the **perimenopause** (the Greek prefix *peri* means "about" or "near"). In the perimenopause the estrogen-producing follicles are slow to develop. The hypothalamus, sensing the low estrogen levels, now produces large quantities of gonadotropin-releasing hormone (GnRH) to stimulate the pituitary. That gland in turn secretes large quantities of follicle-stimulating hormone (FSH) and luteinizing hormone (LH) in an attempt to prod the ovaries into action. Usually the growth of follicles and ensuing ovulations will take place during the perimenopause, but only at irregular intervals. The aging ovaries can no longer maintain the 28-day menstrual cycle established in youth. The cycles become longer and occasionally anovulatory (without ovulation). Besides irregular menstruation, another common indication of the approaching menopause is provided by those vasomotor symptoms popularly known as "hot flashes." The sudden feelings of intense heat on the face or neck last only a minute or two, being followed by profuse perspiration. These annoying episodes are related to the combined effects of estrogen deprivation and the extraordinarily high levels of FSH and LH. The body's internal thermostats for regulating skin temperatures have been disordered, and they must now be reset in accord with the new hormonal environment. The menopause itself brings relief from the menstrual cycle, from hot flashes, from worries about pregnancy, and from various other problems related to the ovarian hormones (e.g., breast tenderness and swelling, uterine fibroids, endometriosis). Currently physicians regard a woman as postmenopausal when she has gone twelve consecutive months without menstruating. The chances of any future ovulation and pregnancy are now extremely remote.

During a woman's reproductive years the circulating sex hormones derive almost entirely from the cyclical maturation of egg-bearing follicles. With the menopause this source of hormones vanishes. The ovaries become much smaller and can no longer be palpated (felt) during a pelvic examination.

Their production of estrogen and progesterone is negligible, although they do turn out small quantities of androgens. The two adrenal glands, located on top of the kidneys, produce larger quantities of androgens. We traditionally associate these hormones with the male of the species; but in postmenopausal women the androgens secreted by the ovaries and adrenals are eventually converted into estrogen by a biochemical process known as aromatization, which takes place in fatty tissues throughout the body. Generally speaking, the more adipose (fat) tissue a postmenopausal woman has, the more circulating estrogens she is likely to have. Her estrogen levels would nonetheless be low compared to those of a premenopausal woman.

Since the 1950s American women have had the option of taking hormone replacement therapy to offset some of the negative effects caused by the menopause. Short-term estrogen supplementation can be good medicine for hot flashes, vaginal dryness, and feelings of fatigue and depression. A much more controversial issue has been whether long-term estrogen therapy can help prevent osteoporosis and cardiovascular disease without overly increasing the risk of breast cancer (the evidence is reviewed in Chapter Six). As yet, no one has proposed a hormonal regimen to combat those changes which occur in the menopausal breast. The loss of ovarian hormones affects not only the epithelium of the mammary gland, but also the adjacent supporting structures. The breast's connective tissues undergo degenerative changes, with a marked decrease in the number of stromal cells and collagen fibers. As a result the ligaments responsible for the breast's mobility and elasticity (Cooper's ligaments) become thinner and weaker; and the breast may tend to **ptosis** (the Greek word for "dropping" or "drooping"). Quite a few body parts sag with advancing age; the breast is no exception. Many women are distressed because their breasts become smaller after the menopause. This is largely due to the loss of subcutaneous fat, a side effect of estrogen deprivation. On the other hand, breasts can sometimes grow larger if they receive additional fat deposits, as may happen during postmenopausal weight gain.

The atrophy of the mammary gland is an important but unseen phenomenon of the menopause. Deprived of progesterone, the lobes and lobules start to shrink, and the milk-secreting alveoli wither and disappear. But the estrogen-responsive ducts are considerably more resilient. The ductal system was the first glandular element to develop at puberty, and it passes through the menopause with minimal alterations. Indeed, the cells lining the larger ducts continue to reproduce long after the menopause. This fact does much to explain why so many ductal carcinomas arise in postmenopausal breasts. As the pathologists John S. Meyer and Robert E. Conner observe, "carcinogens that act preferentially on proliferative cellular populations will generate new carcinomas in the ducts of postmenopausal women, even at advanced ages."[21] Fortunately, tumors which originate in postmenopausal ducts can usually be detected early by regular mammography. The premenopausal breast with its dense glandular tissues often looks like a tangled thicket of impenetrable vegetation on a mammogram. In contrast, the postmenopausal breast tends to be radiographically lucid, because most of the lobular tissues have been replaced by fat. The ducts—and any abnormal changes in them—can be seen clearly.

Can We Learn from Men?

Some of our best clues to the hormonal etiology of female breast cancer come from our studies of *male* breast tissue and *male* breast cancer. This will not astonish us if we reflect on the fact that human gender is not an absolute, but mostly a proper mix of hormones. Daniel D. Federman of the Harvard Medical School reminds us that both sexes need the very same hormones, and that "the ovary and testis both make the same androgens and estrogens." Dr. Federman points out that androgens are "obligatory intermediates in the biosynthesis of estrogen. Thus, the hormonal difference between males and females is quantitative, not qualitative: the male makes a lot more testosterone and converts a minute fraction to estradiol; the female makes much less testosterone but converts a much larger fraction to estrogen."[22]

Sexual differentiation is determined *in utero* by the mix of hormones in the fetal body. Gender will develop as female, save for a few genes on the short arm of a Y chromosome. Abnormalities caused by small genetic defects have helped us to understand the biological processes behind normal sexual development. One instructive aberration is called **testicular feminization**—or **androgen insensitivity**. Afflicted individuals are genetic males; they have XY sex chromosomes, but owing to a tiny mutation their cells lack functional androgen receptors and therefore cannot respond to this hormone. As a consequence their fetal development will follow the female pattern; and the testicles created by the XY chromosomes will remain undescended, hidden in the pelvic cavity like ovaries. While conceived as boys, babies with this rare syndrome will be born as girls, with female external genitalia; and they will be raised as girls. Indeed, they *are* girls, both physically and psychologically. But as teenagers they will fail to menstruate, because they lack ovaries, fallopian tubes, and uteri. The gynecological investigation occasioned by the amenorrhea (absence of menses) will quickly unmask the cruel jest resulting from an ineffectual ingredient in the hormonal recipe for maleness.

An even rarer syndrome in the male is **estrogen insensitivity**. The *New England Journal of Medicine* once published a case history of a virile 28-year-old man who was over six and a half feet tall, weighed 280 pounds, and wore a full beard. Unfortunately, he had a disease which we normally associate with elderly women—*severe osteoporosis*. DNA analysis revealed a disruptive mutation in both alleles of the gene which encodes for estrogen receptor protein. None of the cells in this young man's body could respond to estrogen. The investigators who described this case in the *Journal* concluded that "estrogen is important for bone maturation and mineralization in men as well as in women."[23]

If men need a little estrogen to stay healthy, they certainly don't want a lot. Among other problems, excessive estrogen will cause them to develop breasts, a condition that (in men) is called **gynecomastia**. In affected men as in normal women, the hormone acts most notably in promoting nipple enlargement, the deposition of subcutaneous fat, and the growth of the ductal system. Yet in large quantities estrogen can stimulate the male breast to develop lobules and alveoli— and these milk-producing structures are microscopically indistinguishable from those in the mature female breast. Does that mean that men could develop full-fledged mammary glands and eventually start secreting milk? Well, yes, they could—but as with women, other hormones besides estrogen would be needed, notably progesterone and prolactin. Moreover, according to the famed medical physiologist Arthur C. Guyton, these hormones would have to be administered during "the first two decades of life."[24]

Male Breast Cancer

Male lactation, while theoretically inducible by the proper mix of hormones, has no practical significance. But male breast cancer is a real problem; it's not exactly commonplace, but then neither is it all that rare. The rudimentary glandular tissues in the male breast can and do give rise to potentially deadly malignancies. In the United States less than one percent of reported breast cancer cases involve men; yet that small percentage means that about one thousand American men will be diagnosed each year. Almost all these tumors are invasive (infiltrating) ductal carcinomas. By in large, men do not get lobular carcinomas (they do not normally have lobules), nor do they undergo the periodic mammography which turns up so many cases of ductal carcinoma *in situ*. Male breast cancer patients tend to be slightly older than female patients—they are typically well into middle age or elderly.[25] For men as for women, a family history of the disease (genetic inheritance) can sometimes play the most striking role in etiology. A large survey found that American men whose mothers or sisters were breast cancer patients ran risks of 2.33 times normal (mothers affected) or 2.23 times normal (sisters affected). The more relatives affected and the closer the relation, the higher the risk. With a history of breast cancer among *male* relatives, a man's risk of eventually incurring this diagnosis was four times that seen in the general male population.[26]

But most male patients—like most female patients—have no obvious family history; and etiological studies have usually sought to link male breast cancer with hormonal imbalances, specifically with excessive estrogen. There have been scattered reports of cases among men who were given estrogen to combat prostate cancer, and of cases among male transsexuals who were given estrogen after surgical operations to change their gender. We have more convincing data for Klinefelter's syndrome, in which afflicted males have an XXY chromosomal constitution. That extra X chromosome leads to high estrogen-to-androgen ratios in the blood. With more estrogen than they need, Klinefelter's sufferers exhibit twenty times the normal risk for male breast cancer.[27] Another sizable group of men with elevated levels of estrogen has historically been found in Egypt, where **schistosomiasis** (infection with flukes of the genus *Schistosoma*) was once extremely prevalent. These parasites damage the liver, the organ which removes excess estrogen from the blood. Infected men will tend toward estrogenemia as the hormone gradually accumulates in their bodies. At one time about 6% of Egyptian breast cancer cases occurred in men, a rate much higher than found in other countries.[28] In the United States men with impaired liver function—for example, those with chronic liver disease or alcoholic cirrhosis—have noticeably higher rates of breast cancer than the general male population, presumably because of their inability to metabolize estrogen. Any casual observer will notice that obese men often display gynecomastia; they also have a slightly increased risk of male breast cancer, presumably owing to their higher estrogen levels. In men as in women, androgens are readily converted to estrogen by the body's fatty tissues.

Estradiol, Estrone, Estriol

The research on possible hormonal imbalances in female breast cancer has naturally been more extensive than that done on male disease. While scientists have sometimes considered the possible contribution of prolactin, progesterone, and other hormones, most research on female breast cancer has

been similarly focused on apparent irregularities of estrogen metabolism. The human body manufactures three distinct types of estrogen. **Estradiol**, produced by the ovaries, has by far the greatest biological activity; it is the predominant estrogen in premenopausal women. Most of the estrogen in postmenopausal women is **estrone**, synthesized from adrenal and ovarian androgens in lipid-rich cells containing the enzyme aromatase. The liver converts both estradiol and estrone into a third estrogen, **estriol**, which has little biological activity and a short half-life. The potent estradiol as well as the somewhat weaker estrone are mitogenic—that is, they goad cells containing estrogen receptor protein to divide—and hence they are the estrogen varieties principally suspected in the etiology of breast cancer. Accurate measurements of estrogen levels in blood or urine present numerous methodological problems, not the least of which being that the hormone levels of premenopausal women vary widely from day to day. Nonetheless, most studies indicate that breast cancer patients and groups of women known to be at higher risk for the disease tend to have elevated estrogen levels. An early finding was that women with breast cancer excrete more estradiol and estrone in their urine than they do estriol; they would thus seem to have an imbalance favoring the mitogenic estrogens. Another well-designed study compared postmenopausal breast cancer patients in Los Angeles to a control group without cancer. The patients had almost 15% more estradiol in their blood than the controls, and 10% more estrone. The total estrogen content of the patients' urine was 37% higher than the controls. Leslie Bernstein and Ronald K. Ross of the University of Southern California, the principal researchers in this study, offer a judicious appraisal of current knowledge: "Although there is general agreement that estrogens are involved in the etiology of breast cancer, there is no general consensus as to the precise estrogen environment that defines risk. The association between postmenopausal obesity and breast cancer risk appears to be mediated by the effect of obesity on estrogen profiles."[30]

Where Are the Carcinogens?

By now attentive readers of this chapter should be thoroughly aware of the underlying reason for the breast's proclivity toward cancer, both in humans and in lesser mammalian species. As we have seen, the mammary gland contains hormonally sensitive cells which constantly reproduce themselves, beginning several years before puberty and—at least in the case of the ductal cells—continuing long after the menopause. This prolonged mitotic activity vastly increases the chances that genetic errors (mutations) will appear spontaneously in cellular nuclei, and betters the odds that any exposure to carcinogens will efficiently induce such errors. Carcinogens do the most damage when cells are synthesizing new DNA just prior to mitosis; the uncoiled chromosomes are vulnerable targets.

It is nonetheless easier to prove that the mammary gland is susceptible to carcinogens than to demonstrate exactly what those carcinogens might be. The latter issue has prompted hundreds of scientific studies. Even seemingly implausible carcinogens have been extensively investigated. For example, laboratory tests indicated that the **chemicals in hair dye** can damage DNA, yet massive surveys of tens of thousands of women who dye their hair failed to establish an association with breast cancer. Perhaps some survey participants didn't tell the whole truth about this matter! Are **electromagnetic fields** an unseen culprit? One study found

that women who were employed as "telephone installers, repairers, and line workers" had "approximately twice the number of breast cancer deaths expected."[31] These results, if confirmed by subsequent studies, may conceivably deter some of the many young women aspiring to become telephone linemen. **Electric blankets?** It may be too soon to pull the plug on these appliances. A study done in New York state found only a "slightly elevated" risk of breast cancer, even among women who used electric blankets "continuously throughout the night."[32]

Pesticide residues in agricultural products represent a more likely agent of carcinogenesis in breast cancer and other human malignancies; but it hasn't been possible to assess how much damage they have actually done or not done. We do know that virtually everyone in our society has been exposed to at least trace amounts of pesticides, and that these chemicals can linger in the human body and in the environment for many decades. The best-known example of such lingering toxicity has been provided by **DDT**. Introduced in the 1940s and touted as a cure-all for pests and vermin, this powerful chemical was extensively used in American agriculture during the 1950s and 1960s. Only gradually did the problems associated with DDT come to light. First of all, there was drug resistance, as certain crop-destroying insects became immune to the pesticide and then could multiply without restraint, creating a farmer's nightmare. But a more threatening problem was the way in which DDT spread throughout the natural environment and the food chain. The birds which fed on DDT-exposed insects absorbed quantities of the chemical, and soon began to have reproductive difficulties. Either their young failed to hatch, owing to abnormally thin eggshells; or the hatchlings emerged deformed. DDT seemed to get into everything—fruits, vegetables, cow's milk, meat, ground water. In 1972 the federal government banned its use in the United States.

In the early 1990s, two decades later, researchers began to look closely for a relationship between breast cancer and previous exposure to **organochlorines**, a class of fat-soluble compounds which includes DDT as well as PCBs (the polychlorinated biphenyls used for electric insulation and other industrial applications). The human body cannot metabolize organochlorines completely, with the result that byproducts of these pollutants are stored indefinitely in fatty tissues. Traces of them can be detected a lifetime later in the subcutaneous fat of the breast, in close proximity to the mammary epithelium. One study done at New York University found that women with elevated DDT residues in their blood had "a fourfold increase in relative risk of breast cancer." Mary S. Wolff and her co-workers on this study observed that "diminishing rates of breast cancer in Israel have paralleled a precipitous decline in environmental contamination with DDT." They suspect that American women who were exposed to DDT from foodstuffs between 1945 and 1972 could constitute a population group at especially high risk.[33] A more reassuring conclusion was reached by Nancy Krieger and allied researchers, who studied 150 breast cancer patients and 150 matched control subjects drawn from the Kaiser Permanente Medical Care Program in the San Francisco area. No significant differences were found between patients and controls in serum (blood) levels of DDT and PCB residues.[34]

Our scientific juries have yet to return unanimous verdicts against pesticide residues, electromagnetic fields, and other potential carcinogens that are virtually unavoidable in our industrialized society. We may suspect that these agents lie behind the increased incidence of certain cancers, but we are hard pressed to demonstrate any cause-and-effect relationships. In the case of breast cancer, perhaps the main thing we should remember is that the mammary gland does get exposed to carcinogens or their metabolites. It is not so directly exposed as the respiratory system (lungs) or the gastrointestinal tract (stomach, colon); but anything consumed or inhaled—alcohol, nicotine, traces of pesticides—could possibly have an effect.

Radiation as a Carcinogen

A century ago scientists did not realize that exposure to radiation could induce cancer. That fact became apparent only after large numbers of radiologists and other workers dealing with radioactive materials began to sicken and die from all kinds of malignancies. The effects of high-dose radiation on the mammary gland and the consequent elevation in breast cancer risk have been thoroughly documented; but the most famous large-scale experiments involving humans cannot be said to have been either controlled or precise, since they were designed principally as acts of war. The atomic bombs dropped on Hiroshima and Nagasaki in August, 1945, provided a gruesome opportunity to record the ways in which excessive radiation can affect the body. As a group the bomb survivors suffered sharply increased rates of various cancers, especially the leukemias, for years afterward. Some of the Japanese girls and women who survived were prone to develop breast cancer—*but not all.* Women who were mature adults at the time of the bombings, particularly those aged 40 or older, were not affected; they had the same incidence rate for breast cancer as their contemporaries who were not exposed to atomic radiation. On the other hand, survivors who were in their teens and twenties in 1945, especially those right around puberty, eventually experienced an incidence rate significantly higher than that of their unexposed contemporaries. Yet these younger survivors still did not start to develop breast malignancies before middle age, typically some twenty or thirty years later.[35]

What can we conclude from the tragic case of the atomic bomb survivors? It is reasonable to generalize that the developing mammary glands of preteens and teenagers are exceptionally vulnerable to radiation (and presumably to other carcinogens), that this sensitivity diminishes with age, and that several decades are likely to elapse between any exposure to carcinogens and the appearance of breast cancer. In the case of radiation, a strong dose-and-effect relationship exists: the higher the dose, the more mutations and the greater the risk of breast cancer. We can demonstrate this relationship by analyzing the medical histories of women who have received substantial radiation for the diagnosis or treatment of other conditions. For example, girls with scoliosis (severe curvature of the spine) typically undergo numerous diagnostic X-rays during childhood and adolescence; as adults they reveal "a nearly twofold increased risk" of breast cancer.[36] Far greater elevations of risk can result from the massive doses of therapeutic radiation historically used to arrest Hodgkin's disease. This malignant lymphoma usually begins in a few lymph nodes located in the thoracic (chest) cavity. As previously noted, the early stages of Hodgkin's disease can be arrested by irradiating the affected nodes in the chest, but this therapy is not without risk. A large study done at Stanford University found that girls who were under age 15 when irradiated for early-stage Hodgkin's later revealed a breast cancer incidence rate 136 times higher than that seen in the general population. But female Hodgkin's patients who were over age 30 when irradiated had no increased risk for breast malignancies.[37] These findings do much to explain why the same medical authorities can caution against mammograms or unnecessary chest X-rays for younger women, yet have no qualms when recommending that older women have regular mammograms or possibly consider radiotherapy as a breast-preserving treatment for mammary carcinoma.

Radiation is the breast carcinogen we understand best. Yet only a very small percentage of the human population is likely to be exposed to large doses of manmade radiation. Most of the radiation we're constantly receiving comes from natural sources, originating as cosmic rays from outer space or coming from radioactive elements (like radon) in the earth itself. We can only make general estimates as to how much natural radiation any given individual will receive over the course of a lifetime. How many cancer cases, particularly those involving the breast, are induced by this largely unavoidable radiation? We might speculate that it plays a considerable role in mammary carcinogenesis, but then we have never devised a means of testing this hypothesis.

Chapter Five

EPIDEMIOLOGY
Identifying the Risk Factors for Breast Cancer

The branch of science which attempts to identify the risk factors for disease is called **epidemiology**. This term has the same derivation from the Greek as "epidemic"; but while it literally refers to the study of epidemics, it has come to have broader connotations. When the human species is troubled by a disease whose cause is unknown and whose cure remains undiscovered, **epidemiologists** (the practitioners of this discipline) are sure to find steady employment. In this instance, the best we can hope for is that epidemiologists will identify behavioral patterns associated with the malady's development. Thus, by avoiding the implicated behaviors, we would stand a chance of lowering disease incidence.

Epidemiologists are playing an ever-growing role in shaping public health policies in the United States. In certain areas they have served us extremely well. Thanks to epidemiological research, we all know—or *should* know—that cigarette smoking vastly increases the likelihood of lung cancer and emphysema, and that a diet rich in saturated fats and cholesterol can predispose some individuals to cardiovascular disease, and that obesity and physical inactivity are strongly associated with adult-onset diabetes. Hurried epidemiological studies performed in the early 1980s provided the initial clues that the mysterious immune deficiency which had suddenly afflicted male homosexuals, heroin addicts, and hemophiliacs was caused by a virus present in bodily fluids (blood and semen), and transmitted through intimate sexual contact or transfusions. It should be emphasized that if we seriously followed the advice epidemiologists have given us, we could end the epidemics of lung cancer and AIDS, and greatly reduce the incidence of cardiovascular disease and diabetes. That tremendous American mortality from heart attacks and strokes has already begun to decline, as more and more of us are learning to avoid the modifiable risk factors (e.g., high blood pressure, obesity, smoking, high-fat diet, stressful sedentary lifestyle).

Epidemiologists have also devoted much time and effort to breast cancer, but this field cannot be counted as one of their triumphs. At present we can't say that we know of any behavioral modifications—simple, down-to-earth, feasible changes in lifestyle—which would sharply lower the incidence of breast malignancies. Epidemiological studies have given us lots of hints about etiology, but so far most of the behavioral modifications proposed tend to be unproven or impractical. While we are waiting on a coherent and efficacious preventive strategy, we should be grateful to our epidemiologists for identifying certain subgroups of women who are at increased risk and who may wish to be especially vigilant.

John Snow's Demonstration

Like geneticists and molecular biologists, epidemiologists are scientists rather than physicians. They wear no white coats, carry no stethoscopes, write no prescriptions. They do not see or counsel patients, yet their published research will often determine the advice that physicians offer to patients in the confidentiality of examining rooms. Epidemiologists have little to do with genes and DNA; they are much more concerned with statistics. The principal tools of today's epidemiological trade are those lengthy questionnaires filled out by thousands of patients and healthy controls, and those large computers which electronically record and analyze these masses of data, eventually yielding a relative risk for each behavioral factor. In a typical epidemiological study, that risk would be neatly expressed in a numerical figure with two digits behind the decimal point. All this sounds so precise and scientific, just like pure truth falling straight out of the computer—but things are rarely that simple.

Fortunately, when their data or their methods or their conclusions come under attack, epidemiologists have a patron saint to whom they can pray: **John Snow** (1813-1858). This English physician can hardly be compared to innovators of the stature of Gregor Mendel (the geneticist's patron) or of Watson and Crick (heroes of molecular biology); but he demonstrated the importance of asking questions of persons afflicted with disease and of looking for telltale similarities or patterns in their answers. In 1854 a cholera epidemic was raging in the slums of London; more than 500 people had died within a few days. Dr. John Snow took it upon himself to question the cholera victims and their families; he quickly found the telltale pattern he was looking for. All the victims had obtained their drinking water from the public pump on Broad Street. Even those victims who lived in distant parts of the city shared this risk factor, either by visiting the Broad Street area and using its water supply, or (in a few cases) by sending jugs to that pump because they preferred the water's taste. In September 1854 Dr. Snow advised the London municipal authorities: "Remove the handle from the Broad Street pump!" That handle was removed, and the epidemic ceased. An effective strategy for managing cholera epidemics had been discovered, but no one knew why it worked. This happened 29 years before Robert Koch proved that cholera was caused by the waterborne bacterium *Vibrio cholerae*.

Bias upon Bias
And Confounded Too?

These days the published results of major epidemiological studies command banner headlines in our newspapers, conveying the impression of issues resolved. Most laypersons are blissfully unaware of the heated controversies which generally erupt in the professional journals following such "definitive" publications. Few epidemiological findings are as clear and authoritative as John Snow's prototypical demonstration. In retrospect, we can see that Snow had an easy task, because he just had to identify a single overwhelming risk factor. Today's epidemiologists, particularly those investigating cancer, must contend with numerous factors—diet, exercise, genetics, hormones, microbes, and cosmic radiation, you name it! Apart from the inherent difficulty of assessing and quantifying intertwined and almost inseparable risks, epidemiological studies are often critiqued for methodological shortcomings. Studies involving a small number of subjects are said to "lack statistical power": while the findings may be suggestive, they do not permit a conclusion to be drawn because they could have resulted from chance alone. Virtually no study is immune from the suspicion of **bias**. We're not talking about that conscious bias of dishonest researchers who design studies rigged to support their hypothesis rather than to test it. Culpable fraud is rare; but subtle, unintentional bias seems inescapable. Questionnaires may be worded so as to preferentially solicit this or that reply from study participants. Then there is **selection bias**. Did the researchers conducting a study recruit an excessive proportion of subjects at high risk for the disease? Or did persons volunteer for the study because they believed themselves to be at high risk? In either case we would have a selection bias which would probably lead to inflated, exaggerated findings. **Surveillance bias** can also distort epidemiological results. Were more cases of breast cancer detected because the study participants were kept under surveillance and given free mammograms? **Recall bias** presents an intrinsic problem in studies of a retrospective nature—as, for example, when middle-aged breast cancer patients are asked to recall the varied diet they consumed as teenagers, or perhaps an intermittent use of oral contraceptives during their college years.

Bias is a Hydra-headed beast, displaying one or more horrid physiognomies in every study; but it's not the most dreaded monster lurking in the epidemiological labyrinth. **Confounding factors** are worse. To illustrate what is meant by "a confounding factor," we might imagine a hypothetical study designed to test whether the synthetic hormones in oral contraceptives (OCs) increase the risk of cervical cancer. By asking cervical cancer patients to recall their use of OCs in previous decades, we might discover a strong association between cervical cancer and "The Pill." *So it's the hormones, right?* Hardly. Nobody thinks that OC hormones play a causative role in the etiology of cervical cancer, but we do know that infection with certain strains of human papillomavirus (HPV) is a prelude to this malignancy. And the probable reason for our positive results would be a change in sexual behavior raising the odds of HPV exposure. Some young women taking the Pill, freed from worries about pregnancy, may have experimented with multiple sexual partners while simultaneously abandoning the use of those barrier contraceptives (condoms, diaphragms) which offer protection against sexually transmitted diseases like HPV. In our hypothetical study, sexual behavior predisposing to viral infection would therefore be our hidden **confounding factor**.[1] And epidemiologists designing this study today would make the necessary allowances for—"control for," as they say—the possibility of altered sexual behavior, because they would know about HPV's role in cervical cancer. The problem with confounding factors is that usually they are not recognized, at least not at the time of the study. Do Japanese women have much lower rates of breast cancer than Americans or Europeans because they consume a low-fat diet (as has been frequently asserted), or are there one or more confounding factors we don't know about? Perhaps the water supply in the Japanese islands contains an elusive mineral which retards mammary carcinogenesis. Perhaps Japanese women are at lower risk because they're genetically programmed for lower estrogen levels (this is one hypothesis), or because they eat fairly large quantities of tofu or other soy products which have antiestrogenic properties (this is a recent theory).

All those revelations about diet and breast cancer constantly blazoned in the supermarket tabloids—e.g., *BROCCOLI CUTS BREAST CANCER RISK IN HALF*—are peculiarly vulnerable to accusations of bias and confounding. Is it the low-fat diet which seems to reduce the risk, or maybe the fact that the dieters greatly upped their intake of vitamin-rich fruits and vegetables when they abandoned their steaks and milkshakes? If there's a protective component in diet, we're hard pressed to sort it out, especially when the results of one epidemiological study are contradicted by the next one that comes along.

Teeny-Weeny Risk Factors

The central problem of breast cancer epidemiology is not that the risk factors are so large, but that they are so small. Unless a woman has received substantial irradiation to the chest as a child or teenager, or comes from a family troubled by hereditary breast cancer, she cannot be said to have any large risk factor on the order of the Broad Street pump for the London cholera victims or of tobacco smoke for lung cancer patients. For breast cancer we can identify numerous small risks which, if taken together, begin to add up to a larger likelihood—but because these risks are small, we cannot with confidence express them as exact percentages, or say that any particular factor or combination of factors typically precedes the development of disease. Samuel Shapiro, an epidemiologist at Boston University, frankly acknowledges the limitations of his science: "Epidemiological methods can only yield valid documentation of large relative risks. Relative risks of low magnitude (say, less than 2) are virtually beyond the resolving power of the epidemiologic microscope. We can seldom demonstrably eliminate all sources of bias, and we can never exclude the possibility of unidentified and uncontrolled confounding."[2] Assuming that the general population has a baseline risk of 1.0 for breast cancer, most of the factors known to increase that baseline seem to hover between 1.5 (a 50% increase) and 3.0 (a 200% increase). For illustration, we might consider postmenopausal obesity, the risk factor which could be most easily modified. In one analysis, obese postmenopausal women were found to have a relative risk of 1.6 compared to leaner postmenopausal women, a 60% increase.[3] Now 60% may sound like a large jump upwards in risk; but epidemiologically speaking, it's just a small step, as we'll realize if we momentarily recur to the **Great American Carcinogen**. Compared to nonsmokers, American men who smoke cigarettes have a relative risk of 22.36 of dying from lung cancer, and 27.48 of dying from oral cancer. These handy statistics from the American Cancer Society also inform us that women smokers have relative risks of 11.94 for lung cancer mortality and 5.59 for oral cancer mortality.[4] Risks of this magnitude—say, a 500% or a 2,000% increase—are almost certain to be detected in any epidemiological study, regardless of how poorly designed it may be. For the smaller risk factors linked to breast cancer, the way a study is designed may well determine whether it detects a positive association or no association or a negative association. Even when repeated epidemiological studies consistently yield positive associations for a particular risk factor, the numerical estimate of risk may vary considerably from study to study. Statistics and percentages are glibly quoted in all areas of breast cancer research and therapeutics; but much depends upon whose study and whose calculations you'd like to cite.

A Clue from the Convent

The oldest epidemiological observation about breast cancer is still the most intriguing. In the year 1700, a century and a half before John Snow demonstrated that such observations could lead to disease prevention, the Italian writer Bernardino Ramazzini pointed out that nuns were especially prone to breast cancer: "You seldom find a convent that does not harbor this accursed pest, cancer, within its walls."[5] No doubt Ramazzini's findings were confounded by clerical longevity. In an era when so many women either perished during childbirth, or died prematurely due to the hardships of constant childbearing and childrearing, a higher percentage of celibate nuns would have lived to those ripe old ages when breast cancer claims most of its victims. By the mid-twentieth century modern medicine had greatly diminished that longevity gap between nuns and other women; yet in 1969, when Joseph F. Fraumeni and his co-workers at the National Cancer Institute compared 31,658 American nuns with an equal number of controls from the general population, they reached the same conclusion that Ramazzini had in 1700. Beginning as early as age 39, American nuns revealed a noticeably higher risk of dying from breast cancer. That risk increased dramatically in the oldest age brackets. Nuns aged 60 through 69 had a risk 50% higher than the general population; for those aged 70 through 79, the mortality risk was 110% higher, and 180% higher for those over age 80. Some characteristic of convent life is therefore a fairly strong risk factor for postmenopausal breast cancer. Ramazzini waggishly attributed the increased incidence of disease to the nuns' celibacy; today we recognize its cause as **nulliparity**, the absence of full-term pregnancies.[6]

Parity is one of the few breast cancer associations that all epidemiologists agree upon. In general, we may say that giving birth at a young age (teens or early twenties) is protective, while never having a baby or having one at a late age (30 or older) will increase the likelihood of postmenopausal breast cancer. The numerical expression of this risk factor has varied; more recent studies tend to show weaker associations. The most frequently cited estimates seem to be those given by the Harvard epidemiologist Brian MacMahon and his international collaborators, which are worth repeating here. MacMahon's group postulated a breast cancer risk of 0.5 for women who have a first child before age 20, and a 1.4 risk for women who do so after age 35. The oldest first-time mothers would thus have roughly three times the risk of the youngest; their risk is probably even higher than that of women who remain nulliparous. At approximately age 28 the protective effect of full-term pregnancy vanishes, becoming a positive risk factor within a year or two.[7]

Throughout most of human history, pregnancy and motherhood soon after puberty represented the natural order of things. Today protection from breast cancer may look like the solitary good thing to derive from teenage maternity, which often creates problems in our complex society. We should stress that only early parity is protective, and that it protects against late-onset disease. In 1994 two large epidemiological studies revealed that not only does childbirth fail to protect against early-onset breast cancer, it actually increases the odds. The influential **Nurses' Health Study**, conducted by Walter C. Willett and other epidemiologists at the Harvard School of Public Health, analyzed the reproductive histories of 91,523 female nurses, "who were followed for fourteen years (1,212,855 person-years and 2,341 incident breast cancers)." The mountains of data yielded a surprising result. For some twenty to thirty years after experiencing their first childbirth, the parous nurses actually had a higher incidence of disease (more cases of breast cancer) than their nulliparous colleagues. Yet when these statistics were carried forth into the postmenopausal years, early parity's protective effect became apparent. The cumulative incidence up to age 70 was "about 20% lower, 10% lower, or 5% higher" for the parous nurses, depending upon whether the first birth occurred "at age 20, 25, or 35 years, respectively." The Nurses' Health team concluded: "Pregnancy is associated with a transient increased risk of breast cancer . . . followed by a lifetime reduction in risk."[8]

These findings were corroborated by a Swedish study of parity published in the *New England Journal of Medicine*. The Swedish epidemiologists compared 12,666 patients with breast cancer with 62,121 age-matched control subjects, hoping to achieve "a data set large enough to generate high statistical power." A first full-term pregnancy had essentially the same effect on this nationwide cohort in Sweden as on the American nurses. The parous women "were at higher risk of breast cancer than nulliparous women for up to fifteen years after childbirth and at lower risk thereafter." Both the risks and the protective effects were modest. For illustration we might cite the Swedish estimates for two age-matched women—one being nulliparous and the other having a first child at age 25. At age 30 the risk of breast cancer for the nulliparous woman could be expressed as 1.0 while the parous woman's risk would be 1.18 (i.e., 18% higher). At age 40 the risk for both women would be 1.0—identical. Of course, relatively few cases of breast cancer occur in women aged 30 or 40; the Swedish estimates for age 59, a time of high disease incidence, indicate why early parity must be classified as a definite protective factor. At age 59, while the nulliparous woman's risk would still be expressed as 1.0, that of the

parous woman would have dropped to 0.71—that is, 29% lower.[9] We can't predict exactly how parity will affect any individual woman's chances of developing breast cancer; but whenever we compare large numbers of parous and nulliparous subjects, the parous group never fails to have a lower lifetime incidence.

Parity's Protective Mechanism

As stated in Chapter Four, the first full-term pregnancy brings about the differentiation, or maturity, of the mammary gland. The cells of the breast epithelium subsequently divide at a slower rate and display a greater resistance to carcinogens. Before protective differentiation occurs, however, these cells must undergo the tremendous mitotic activity characteristic of advancing pregnancy. It is this unprecedented cellular multiplication which offers the best explanation of our epidemiological findings about parity. If a few of the mammary cells already harbor deleterious mutations at the time pregnancy begins, or if an incipient malignancy is already present, these months of constant hormonally-stimulated mitosis can only serve as an efficient tumor promoter. So in the years immediately following childbirth, more cases of breast cancer naturally turn up among parous women than nulliparous women. Pregnancy starts to become a risk factor after age 28, because the older the mammary cells are, the greater the chances that they will harbor pre-existing mutations or incipient tumors. Hence the higher rate of breast cancer seen in women who become first-time mothers in their thirties or forties.

While the preceding account of parity's biological mechanisms gives us a convenient and plausible concept to retain in memory, it doesn't explain all the changes wrought by childbirth. For one thing, there would seem to be significant differences in hormone levels between parous and nulliparous women. Leslie Bernstein and other epidemiologists at the University of Southern California have measured the estrogen concentrations in the blood and urine of premenopausal women, contrasting the parous with the nulliparous. A group of nuns served as the nulliparous subjects; their biological sisters who had given birth were chosen as the parous counterparts, thus minimizing any confounding due to innate genetic differences between different families or races. Bernstein et al found that the parous women had shorter menstrual cycles than the nuns, as well as lower estrogen levels in both blood and urine. Most notably, the serum (blood) estradiol of the parous subjects was 22% lower than that of the nuns on the eleventh day of the menstrual cycle, a time of peaking estrogen levels just prior to ovulation.[10] The USC researchers suggested that a reduction in "estrogen bioavailability" could be an important mechanism for parity's protective effect, but estrogen is not the only hormone affected. An Emory University study appearing in the *New England Journal of Medicine* concluded that "a first pregnancy leads to a long-term decrease in serum prolactin secretion, lasting at least twelve to thirteen years."[11] The breast ducts of premenopausal women normally secrete small amounts of hormone-rich fluid at all times, even in the absence of pregnancy or lactation. For several years after any pregnancy, this ductal fluid reveals lower concentrations not only of estradiol and estrone, but also of cholesterol.[12]

As previously mentioned, microscopic examinations can show us how full-term pregnancy changes the fine structures of the mammary gland, producing a flowering of the lobules and a vast multiplication of alveoli. Yet we don't know how or why parity alters the ovarian secretion of estrogens or reduces the cholesterol levels in breast ductal fluid, or causes the pituitary to issue less prolactin once lactation is finished. Suffice it to say that the metabolic and physiologic aftereffects of childbirth are profound—and not adequately understood. Our lack of knowledge has thwarted any meaningful attempts to exploit parity's mechanisms for disease prevention. Theoretically, it should be possible to prevent most breast cancers by giving pubertal girls a nine-month hormonal regimen which would produce the mammary differentiation associated with full-term pregnancy. Hormonal pseudo-pregnancies have been shown to accomplish breast differentiation and to deter malignancy in laboratory experiments done with mice and rats. The idea of a pseudo-pregnancy prophylaxis for *Homo sapiens* has often been pondered, yet the road to any practical intervention is likely to be very long indeed. We have no hormonal regimens known to be both safe and effective for this purpose. And testing the pseudo-pregnancy hypothesis in humans would require thousands of adolescent girls (trial subjects too young to give informed consent), as well as a follow-up period of forty or fifty years. This strategy works fine in rodents; the ethical, legal, and organizational problems facing any human trial of it currently seem insurmountable.

Abortion and Other Variations

Epidemiological curiosity also extends to the variations on parity. If having one baby is protective, will having a dozen be much more so? Does giving birth to twins or triplets raise—or lower—the risk of breast cancer? And then there is the question of pregnancies terminated before term, either spontaneously through miscarriage or through induced abortion. What does that do to the risk of subsequent breast malignancies?

The effects of **multiparity** (several full-term pregnancies) have not been investigated as thoroughly as those of **uniparity** (one completed pregnancy). Yet most studies indicate that additional pregnancies further reduce the risk of postmenopausal breast cancer, although the degree of reduction is not as great as that accomplished by the first completed pregnancy. The data released by the **Cancer and Steroid Hormone Study** (CASH), a large project conducted by the Centers for Disease Control and other government agencies, show a graduated risk reduction for additional births. According to CASH, if American women with one prior childbirth are assumed to have a lifetime risk of 1.0, then women with three childbirths would have a risk of 0.9—that is, an additional 10% reduction from the uniparous level. Having five full-term pregnancies drops the breast cancer risk to 0.7—30% lower than the uniparous women—and having seven or more gets the risk down to 0.6, a full 40% reduction.[13] The biological mechanism bringing about this added protection probably involves the suppression of ovulation and the menstrual cycle.

A few epidemiological studies have tried to evaluate the potential effect of a multiple birth—that is, having twins or triplets—but so far the results don't permit firm conclusions to be drawn. A woman having twins, especially dizygotic (nonidentical) twins, tends to have higher estrogen levels during pregnancy; conceivably, this might lead to a slightly elevated risk of breast cancer. But Herbert I. Jacobson and his colleagues at the Albany Medical College (New York state) have reached the opposite conclusion. They point out that twin pregnancies also produce higher levels of alpha-fetoprotein, which is secreted into maternal blood from the livers of developing fetuses.

According to Jacobson et al, this fetal protein may well be mediating protection against mammary carcinogenesis.[14]

The unresolved issue of multiple births is unlikely to excite anyone who is not a professional epidemiologist or the mother of twins. But when epidemiologists attempt to establish whether abortion increases the risk of breast cancer, they are venturing upon a topic which excites many people in American society. Before proceeding with any discussion of abortion, perhaps we should make a sharp distinction between scientific investigations and religious beliefs. Given a sufficient number of well-designed epidemiological studies, the relationship of induced abortion to breast cancer risk will eventually be clarified. The political controversy which pits a developing embryo's "right to life" against a woman's "freedom of choice" cannot be resolved by science. It is true that the 1973 Supreme Court decision which legalized abortion, and the ensuing increase in documented pregnancy terminations, have made epidemiological investigations of this topic both feasible and urgent.

Experiments with laboratory rats did much to teach us how pregnancy accomplishes the differentiation of the mammary gland; they also revealed that when pregnancy is interrupted, this protective differentiation does not take place. Pregnant rats given hysterectomies before term are as susceptible to carcinogen-induced breast cancers as virgin rats.[15] Malcolm C. Pike and his colleagues at the University of Southern California conducted a preliminary epidemiological study which found that women who had an abortion before age 33 were 2.4 times more likely to develop premenopausal breast cancer. The USC team reasoned that since the early months of human pregnancy involve a tremendous multiplication of mammary cells, and since protective differentiation of these cells does not occur until the final months, an abortion in the first or second trimester could accomplish only a risky stimulation of the gland. It would amount to proliferation without the ensuing differentiation. Any existing genetic mutations would probably be enhanced, and new ones might be created. The risk of breast cancer ought to go up.[16]

While this hypothesis sounds plausible enough, not all studies have supported it. Researchers in Sweden, a country which permitted abortion long before the United States, were curious to see whether the growing frequency of this procedure had somehow contributed to a national "increase in the incidence of breast cancer of about 40% in women aged 20 to 44." The Swedish epidemiologists examined the medical records of 49,000 women who had undergone a first-trimester abortion before age 30; by and large, they found no increased risk of breast cancer. But like other studies, this analysis had its limitations. One of them was its short follow-up, as only 10% of the women were followed for more than eleven years after their abortions.[17]

In November 1994 the question of abortion's effect on breast cancer incidence suddenly became a popular topic on the TV talk shows, after Janet R. Daling and other epidemiologists at Seattle's Fred Hutchinson Cancer Research Center published a case-control study bubbling over with positive associations. Daling and her colleagues compared 845 women in Washington state with early-onset breast cancer (diagnosis before age 45) with 961 age-matched controls. The overall results revealed a 50% elevation in breast cancer risk for women who had ever had an induced abortion. Now a 50% increase isn't much to shout about at epidemiological conferences, but some subgroups of patients had noticeably higher risks for early-onset breast cancer. Women undergoing abortions before age 18 had a 2.5-fold

increase in risk, and those doing so after age 30 had a 2.1-fold increase. The most stunning elevation in risk was observed in women under age 18 who terminated a pregnancy that had lasted more than eight weeks: their risk was eight-fold higher than the comparable controls.[18]

Notwithstanding the considerable publicity given the study by Daling et al, it was hardly definitive, either with regard to the statistical assessment of abortion risks or to any explanation of the biological mechanisms creating these risks. At the moment the only broad conclusions we can draw are that the induced termination of pregnancy is a serious matter and should not be used as a routine means of birth control. Nobody knows if a history of induced abortions could have an effect on the more typical cases of breast cancer, which present in women over age 50. While Dr. Daling and her co-workers did not address this question, they did consider the possible relationship between spontaneous abortion (miscarriage) and the risk of breast cancer. Their finding was reassuring: a history of miscarriages did not increase the risk, even seemed to lessen it a tad (down 10%). Daling et al reasoned that most embryos destined to abort will die or stop growing early in pregnancy. "Either way," Dr. Daling told a reporter from *Time*, "breast-cell development doesn't really have a chance to get going, as it would in a healthy pregnancy."[19]

Breast-Feeding Controversies

You might suspect that breast-feeding would be as uncontroversial as Motherhood and Apple Pie—ah, but please remember that almost everything about breast cancer is controversial! In the case of breast-feeding, there has been a large discrepancy between epidemiological studies conducted in China and Japan, which seem to reveal the practice as marvelously protective, and comparable studies conducted in the United States and other Western nations, which have usually reported that it has little or no effect on breast cancer incidence. Let's consider the Nurses' Health Study as representative of American epidemiological findings. In July 1990 the Harvard researchers published their analysis of the questionnaires submitted by "a cohort of 89,413 parous registered nurses," providing information on "total duration of lactation" between 1976 and 1986. What were the results from the Study's whopping "785,958 person-years of follow-up"? A complete blank! The Harvard team found "no independent association between lactation and the risk of breast cancer." Most of the nurses (63%) had lactated, 35% "for up to 7 months" and 6% "for 24 months or more"; but regardless of how long they breast-fed, they accrued no protective benefits, either against premenopausal disease or postmenopausal.[20]

The Nurses' Health findings stand in sharp contrast to those from a case-control study of Chinese women in Shanghai, which was conducted by officials of the Shanghai Cancer Institute in collaboration with three epidemiologists from the University of Southern California (Mimi C. Yu, Ronald K. Ross, Brian E. Henderson). Since virtually all Chinese women breast-feed, the Sino-American team looked mainly at the duration of lactation. And the results? "Increasing duration of nursing," the team reported, "was significantly associated with decreasing risk of breast cancer." Women who had breast-fed for more than nine years revealed a 63% lower risk than those whose lifetime nursing totaled less than three years. And breast-feeding appeared to be protective against both premenopausal and postmenopausal disease.[21] Similar findings emerged from a case-control study conducted in Japan.

Comparing parous women who had breast-fed with mothers who had never done so, the Japanese researchers found that overall the breast-feeding subjects had a 38% lower risk of breast cancer. The risk did not seem to be greatly affected by the number of children breast-fed, but it decreased markedly with increasing duration of nursing. Women who had never nursed were assigned a risk of 1.0. The risk for women who had nursed from four to six months proved to be 0.75 (a 25% reduction), and this dropped to 0.53 (a 47% reduction) for women whose lifetime breast-feeding totaled thirteen months or more.[22]

In 1993 and 1994 epidemiological studies from England, Canada, and the United States finally began to corroborate the results from Asia, at least in respect to lactation's protection against premenopausal disease. The United Kingdom National Case-Control Study focused on young women diagnosed with breast cancer before age 36. Comparing 595 parous patients with 616 matched controls, the English researchers found that breast-feeding for as little as one to three months lowered the risk for early-onset breast cancer by 17%.[23] A study done in British Columbia, Canada, compared 1,018 patients with 1,025 controls selected from the provincial voters list. No association with lactation was detected in postmenopausal women; but a protective effect was seen among the premenopausal subjects, which became stronger as the total lifetime duration of nursing increased. Premenopausal women who had nursed for two or three months were assigned a breast cancer risk of 1.0. Those who had nursed from four to six months were found to have a risk of 0.7—a 30% reduction apparently achieved by a slight increase in duration. The Canadian team acknowledged that their results were "plausibly within the bounds of chance."[24] A multicenter American study published in the *New England Journal of*

Medicine had considerably more statistical power, contrasting 5,878 parous breast cancer patients with 8,216 parous controls. Polly A. Newcomb of the University of Wisconsin and her numerous collaborators found no association between lactation and postmenopausal breast cancer, but they detected "a slight reduction" in the risk for premenopausal disease. Overall, young women with any history of lactation had a relative risk of 0.78 for early-onset breast cancer (a 22% reduction) when compared to parous women who had never breast-fed. This protective effect became noticeably stronger if the breast-feeding had commenced at a young age and continued for at least half a year. Newcomb et al discovered that "the relative risk among women who first lactated at less than 20 years of age and breast-fed their infants for a total of six months was 0.54"—that is, 46% below that of comparable controls who had never breast-fed.[25]

American Lactational Vagaries

Thanks to the work of Dr. Newcomb and her colleagues, we may reasonably surmise that early lactation could add an independent protective benefit against premenopausal breast cancer to the substantial protection which early maternity offers against post-menopausal disease. And since breast-feeding naturally goes hand-in-hand with motherhood, the combination of these two factors at a young age might confer a lifetime of protection for many women. Unfortunately, we can't evaluate the full prophylactic potential of lactation, because women in the United States and other industrialized countries tend to be casual and inconsistent breast-feeders. To lower the subsequent risk of mammary carcinogenesis, breast-feeding has to be done in a constant and prolonged fashion. The reason for this will become clear when we consider the biological mechanisms which might conceivably confer the desired protection.

Some epidemiologists have speculated that milk secretion could protect the mammary gland simply by "flushing out" any accumulation of carcinogenetic substances. This theory is not implausible; but of the current explanations, the only one which has been proven involves a well-documented phenomenon—**lactational suppression of ovulation**. As stated in Chapter Four, the menstrual cycle with its surging levels of estrogen and progesterone leads the mammary cells through repeated bouts of mitotic activity; any respite from the monthly routine therefore diminishes the opportunities for genetic mutation. Breast-feeding stops ovulation by virtue of its endocrine demands on the pituitary gland. Presumably the pituitary gets so busy manufacturing the milk hormone prolactin that it neglects to issue the gonadotropic hormones which bring about the menstrual cycle.

Breast-feeding is not the most reliable contraceptive because it must be done round-the-clock to achieve and maintain ovulatory suppression. Once lactation ceases or becomes infrequent, the menstrual cycle quickly re-establishes itself. In Western societies where young mothers typically alternate between breast-feeding and infant formula, lactation has little or no contraceptive value. In some African countries where the vast majority of mothers rely exclusively on breast-feeding, lactation is reasonably effective. One study of African women found that only 5% of those who breast-fed became pregnant within nine months after childbirth, whereas 75% of those who did not became pregnant again. But even in undeveloped African nations there are lactational vagaries. Another study found that urban women in Rwanda became pregnant after childbirth some twelve to sixteen months earlier than women living in rural areas. Evidently the rural mothers in this central African country nursed their infants more faithfully than the city dwellers. Breast-feeding cannot indefinitely postpone the resumption of ovulation, but its effects are clear. Without lactation, ovulation will quickly resume, often as early as one or two months after delivery. But with constant lactation it may be delayed for as long as two years. In the absence of the menstrual cycle, the body's estrogen levels are low; rigorous breast-feeders may even experience meno-pausal symptoms like hot flashes and vaginal dryness. Needless to say, mitotic activity in the mammary gland is greatly reduced owing to the diminished supply of estrogen and progesterone.[26]

If we assume that the protection that breast-feeding confers against subsequent malignancy is mediated largely through ovulatory suppression, we can readily ex-plain the differences between American epidemiological findings and those coming out of Asia. First of all, American profes-sional women—for example, the registered nurses monitored by the Nurses' Health Study—might be the worst cohort in the world to demonstrate lactation's protective benefits. The mothers in Africa who sup-pressed ovulation for a year or more typically nursed their infants *every hour* during the day, and at periodic intervals during the night. How could American nurses adhere to such a schedule? We're talking about women who work shifts of eight or ten hours at the hospital, then must rush to the bank or supermarket, and at night really need their sleep. Most of the African mothers nursed their infants for two or three years, but only 6% of the subjects in the Nurses' Health Study breast-fed for two years. Stephanie J. London, an epidemiologist who worked on this study, suggests that the nurses were

influenced by "the ideal of five feedings per day" held out by pediatric guru Benjamin Spock in his popular manual *Baby and Child Care*.[27] Unfortunately, Dr. Spock's pro-nouncements are not the only barrier to the kind of prolonged, on-demand breast-feeding which might help reduce the rising incidence of mammary carcinoma. Our stressful American culture is singularly inhospitable to lactation. Young mothers who work outside the home cannot take their infants to their places of employment, much less breast-feed them there. In many cultures public breast-feeding is regarded as a natural occurrence. In the United States any open display of breasts goes against ingrained attitudes which combine prudery with las-civiousness. Woe to the young mother who decides to nurse her baby on a public bench at a shopping mall or department store! If this action does not result in a citation for indecent exposure, it's sure to provoke aston-ished stares from passers-by and a quick admonition from a store manager—"You can't do *that* here!"

Menstrual History

A girl's first menstrual period is called her **menarche**. That word comes from the Greek and literally means the beginning of the menses (*men* for "month" and *arche* for "beginning"). Menarche stands in contrast to menopause, the end of the menses. Between these two events lie a variable number of menstrual cycles and ovulations. Our epi-demiologists have made great strides in determining how a woman's total number of ovulations affects her risk of developing breast cancer. There is universal agreement about the general trend associated with men-strual history. Early menarche and late menopause indicate increased risk; late menarche and early menopause are highly protective. While the attempted quantifications of these risk factors vary from study to study, we can give a ballpark estimate which shouldn't be too far off base. Girls who experience menarche at age 12 or younger have approximately a 50% higher risk of subsequent breast cancer than girls whose menarche occurs at age 14 or 15. Women who experience menopause in their early forties probably have a 50% lower risk than women who do so in their early fifties. Menstrual history is hardly an overwhelming risk factor; nonetheless, as a group, women in the high-risk pattern (early menarche and late menopause) have about the twice the odds of developing breast cancer as women in the low-risk pattern. Pubertal years, when the adolescent mammary gland is most active and most sensitive, count much more heavily than perimenopausal years. According to recent estimates, the risk of adult breast cancer is reduced as much as 15% "for each year that menarche is delayed."[28]

Unfortunately, the average age of menarche has been steadily falling in the United States and other industrialized countries. In the nineteenth century menarche typically occurred around age 15. In the 1990s the average American girl reached that milestone at 12.8 years.[29] Human biology has not been altered in the past hundred years, but the circumstances of our daily lives have changed drastically. Alterations in diet are the main culprit behind the declining age of menarche. A century ago Americans consumed a diet relatively low in fats and animal proteins, and relatively rich in complex carbohydrates, especially in cereal products which did not require refrigeration for preservation. Over the decades those bowls of porridge and bags of oats gave way to iceboxes groaning with high-fat, high-calorie items—whole milk, butter, cheese, bacon, eggs, ice cream. On such nutritious fare teenagers tended to grow taller and

heavier; they also achieved sexual maturity much sooner, thanks to the dietary fat which their bodies so readily converted into the steroid sex hormones. International epidemiological surveys have discovered strong associations between a country's per capita fat consumption and the national age at menarche—as the former increases, the latter declines.[30] But diet is not the only determinant of pubertal timing. Rigorous physical activity can delay menarche; young girls who are very active in ballet or gymnastics may arrive at this turning point a year or two later than their more sedentary classmates.[31] From the standpoint of breast cancer prevention, those radiant high school girls of the 1950s and 1960s were doing all the wrong things when they spent their afternoons chatting away at the soda fountains, while munching on cheeseburgers and sipping milkshakes. Their leaner and plainer grandmothers, deprived of these caloric excesses as adolescents and kept busy with household chores, had better odds of escaping this disease.

Perils of Regular Ovulation

Women who experience early menarche tend to have higher estrogen levels in their blood and urine throughout their teens and twenties.[32] In the 1980s some researchers tried to explain the elevated risk associated with early menarche and late menopause by postulating an **"estrogen window" hypothesis**. In this scenario, stimulation of the mammary gland by estrogen without progesterone was seen as especially risky. This condition occurs just before and after menarche, when regular ovulatory cycles have not yet been established, and again during the perimenopause, when the cycles become irregular and often anovulatory (without ovulation). Of course, progesterone is not present until after ovulation, as it is the ruptured ovarian follicle (corpus luteum) which principally secretes this hormone. Yet the ingenious "estrogen window" hypothesis, like most ideas in medical history, proved to be mistaken; it rested upon the false assumption that progesterone would stall mitotic activity in the mammary gland as it does among the cells of the endometrium (uterine lining).[33] The opposite is true. In the breast progesterone acts synergistically on cells previously primed by estrogen; by far the greatest proliferation of mammary cells occurs in the luteal phase of the menstrual cycle, when both hormones are present in abundance.

In 1985 Brian E. Henderson and his colleagues at the University of Southern California formulated a more straightforward explanation of menstrual risks, focusing simply on the total number of ovulations and on the synergetic effects produced by progesterone after each ovulation. They observed that girls with early menarche established regular menstrual cycles in less time and more predictably than girls with later menarche, and that these cycles were more likely to be ovulatory and of short duration. Then the USC team released a statistical bombshell from their recent investigations: "A woman with early menarche (age 12 or younger) and rapid establishment of regular cycles has an almost four-fold increased risk of breast cancer when compared with a woman with late menarche (age 13 or older) and long duration of irregular cycles." The plausibility of this finding should be apparent to readers of this book. The more cells divide, the greater the risk of mutation—and in young fertile women the mammary epithelium typically reproduces itself with each menstrual cycle. Hence, the sooner the cycles begin and the more regular they are, the more cellular division and the greater the risk! The USC epidemiologists offered an additional reason why shorter cycles would be associated with higher risks: "The major part of the variation in cycle length is in the length of the follicular phase. Women with shorter cycles will therefore have more of their menstrual life in the luteal phase."[34] Thus a woman with regular 28-day cycles would spend approximately 182 days per year in the highly mitogenic luteal phase—a woman with regular 33-day cycles, only about 154 days. Other epidemiological studies have corroborated the USC hypothesis. Whatever their age at menarche, breast cancer patients are more likely than controls to have established a regular menstrual pattern early and to have maintained it throughout their reproductive life.[35]

Prevention Remains Academic

The USC epidemiologist Malcolm C. Pike has neatly tied together several strands of pertinent epidemiological knowledge. He contrasts the reproductive and menstrual histories of an average eighteenth-century woman with those of her modern counterpart. According to Dr. Pike, a woman two or three centuries ago usually experienced menarche around age 17, had her first pregnancy not long thereafter, and gave birth to as many as eight children, which she faithfully breast-fed. During her entire reproductive life she may have ovulated 150 times. In contrast, the typical modern woman has a longer but much less prolific reproductive life. She begins menstruating around age 12 or 13, then delays pregnancy for a decade or two, and finally has one or two children, which may (or may not) be rather haphazardly breast-fed. Consequently, she may ovulate 450 times during some forty years of fertility.[36]

We now know that this modern reproductive pattern is intrinsically associated with a much higher risk of breast cancer than the traditional pattern, which was presumably as prevalent in ancient Babylon or the Roman Empire as in colonial America. What can we do about all those ovulations? Some epidemiologists have pondered the advisability of delaying menarche. Brian E. Henderson stresses that regular ovulation and short menstrual cycles most effectively elevate the lifetime breast cancer risk early in a woman's reproductive life: "During your adolescent years, if you miss half your cycles, you'll reduce your risk by 50%. That's when the most risk accrues—before your first pregnancy or age 25."[37] These days we do have pharmaceutical agents capable of delaying menarche—notably, **synthetic agonists of the gonadotropin-releasing hormone**—but the wisdom of using them for this purpose is questionable. GnRH agonists can completely shut down the ovarian production of estrogen and progesterone, and the long-term effects of giving them to pubertal girls, especially on bone formation, are entirely unknown. But the biggest obstacle to any pharmaceutical postponement of menarche could well be patient resistance. American girls aged 11 or 12 want desperately to be grown-up women with rounded breasts and curvy silhouettes. Any drug regimen designed for the express purpose of delaying sexual adulthood, in the hope of preventing a disease which may (or may not) transpire forty or fifty years later, would be a bitter pill for preteens to swallow, and about as popular as a cancellation of the senior prom.

The induction of early menopause is not likely to be any more palatable than the postponement of puberty. Still it would unquestionably reduce the risk of postmenopausal breast cancer. One cohort study found that bilateral oophorectomy (the surgical removal of both ovaries) before age 40 reduced the risk of breast cancer by 75% for both nulliparous and parous women.[38] The physiological changes brought about by the menopause are not welcomed by all women; but the main difficulty with induced menopause as a preventive strategy is that while it would lower the risk of mammary carcinoma, it would considerably raise the risk of osteoporosis and cardiovascular disease. And regardless of how much fear that breast cancer engenders, the two latter diseases represent greater health hazards. Far more American women die from heart attacks, from strokes, or from the complications of hip fractures than they do from breast malignancies.

* * *

Possibly the preceding commentary has left a few readers with the impression that a pattern of timely menarche, short regular cycles, and late menopause is somehow unhealthy. To the contrary! This pattern is actually the healthiest one, conducive to physical and mental well-being as well as longevity. The pattern would not entail a noticeably increased risk of mammary carcinogenesis if women adhered to the natural reproductive mode which can be seen even today among primitive tribes living in remote jungles and rain forests. Unfortunately, that natural mode—early motherhood, lots of subsequent pregnancies, prolonged lactation—no longer seems either desirable or practical. Men and women alike, we lead lives dictated by economic exigencies and societal imperatives rather than by the rhythms of nature. And all too often we pay a stiff price for our deviation by developing late-onset chronic diseases.

CLUES FROM ABROAD
Some International Variations

Many cancers could be prevented. The incidence rates for the different malignancies are not constant. Enormous variations occur from country to country, and among separate groups of people living in the same country. These variations demonstrate that some humans are doing things which strongly protect against certain malignancies, while others have adopted lifestyles which tend to promote these same malignancies. Prostate cancer provides a striking example of variation by race and nationality. The incidence rate among American men of African descent, the world's highest, is roughly thirty times as great as that among Chinese and Japanese men.[39] Several decades ago Denis Burkitt, the famed English surgeon whose career was spent in Africa, observed that colon cancer was virtually nonexistent among African tribes like the Bantu. These tribal peoples consumed a high-fiber diet, mainly fresh vegetables and cereal grains; and they were never troubled by constipation, having several bowel movements each day. Stomach cancer has long plagued the Japanese, mainly because of their excessive use of nitrates for food preservation. Even today their incidence and mortality rates for this malignancy are roughly seven times those of Americans.[40]

Breast cancer also reveals substantial variations from nation to nation. For decades women in China and Japan had an incidence rate only one-fourth or one-fifth as great as that of women in the United States and western Europe. But the breast cancer rates within the United States and the European Community are hardly uniform. Women living in East Midlands, England, revealed a yearly mortality rate of 29.0 per 100,000 population; women living in southern Italy's Basilicata, a rate of only 9.6—a threefold reduction.[41] Denmark and Holland, two high-risk nations, have recorded breast cancer mortality rates of 28.3 and 26.8 per 100,000 population, respectively—these figures are almost twice the 15.4 rate seen in Greece, a low-risk nation.[42] The incidence and mortality rates for breast cancer also vary noticeably within the United States. Geographically speaking, urban areas are riskier than rural locations. Melting-pot California has given epidemiologists a splendid opportunity to study the variations among different ethnic groups. In the late 1980s white women living in California had an annual incidence rate of 110.6 per 100,000 population; black women, 96.3; Hispanic women, 59.2; and women of other races (mostly Asian descent), only 52.8—less than half the elevated Caucasian rate.[43]

Epidemiologists are understandably excited by these variations between nations, regions, and cultural or racial groups. Yet it is relatively easy to count the cases of a disease—identifying the behavioral patterns lurking behind high incidence rates usually proves more difficult. Nonetheless, few epidemiologists would doubt that dietary patterns are implicated in the etiology of colorectal cancers. The generous per capita incomes of Americans and Europeans allow culinary excesses far beyond the means of the simpler Bantu. Vegetable fiber and cereal roughage get replaced by red meat, dairy products, refined flour, highly processed foods (canned or frozen), and all manner of delicacies laced with sugar, salt, fatty oils, and artificial preservatives. In short, a recipe for constipation with potentially mutagenic fecal matter! Insofar as a dietary pattern tends to raise the levels of steroid sex hormones, it's sure to be a main suspect in cancers of the breast, endometrium, and prostate. Consumption of dietary fat, especially that originating in red meat, has been rather consistently linked with elevated testosterone levels in the male and with a consequently increased risk of prostate cancer. Epidemiologists usually attempt to explain international variations in the incidence of breast malignancies by pointing out differences in diet, again looking closely at the consumption of fat and protein derived from animal sources. Nobody thinks that diet is the complete answer to the riddle; as we've seen, differences in reproductive, lactational, and menstrual histories do much to explain the variations in breast cancer rates. Yet if we add "diet" to the aforementioned "histories," we will have largely covered the known risk factors, save for the unavoidable one of genetic inheritance (which lies behind familial breast cancer).

Learning from the Japanese

International comparisons won't be meaningful if they are based on inaccurate data. The low incidence rates for breast malignancies announced by many nations could simply be artifacts of fragmentary and haphazard reporting. Third World countries do not have the pervasive distribution of hospitals and physicians that Americans enjoy; and organizations which collect data on malignancies seem irrelevant in societies still plagued by infectious diseases, malnutrition, and infant mortality. For a number of reasons, American epidemiologists looking at international variations in cancer incidence have focused on Japan. This Asian nation is one of the world's most sophisticated and technologically advanced societies, with a disciplined, literate, and largely homogeneous population. The Japanese keep adequate medical records; and they have extremely low rates of breast, prostate, and colon cancers. Since the Second World War the economic ties between the United States and Japan have been

constantly expanding. But long before the war Japan was exporting "raw material" for future epidemiological studies: a goodly number of its citizens emigrated to Hawaii and California. In the United States these immigrants and their children retained a distinct cultural identity; what they did not retain were the low cancer rates characteristic of the Japanese islands. Adult immigrants weren't significantly affected; but their children tended to reveal incidence rates halfway up to the American level, and their grandchildren exhibited pretty much the same rates as the general American population. As the immigrants and their descendants gradually adopted the American lifestyle, they were presumably abandoning those habits and practices which served to protect their relatives in Japan proper.[44]

Epidemiologists naturally suspected that differences in American and Japanese dietary patterns were responsible for the tremendous variations in cancer rates between the two nations. In the 1950s and 1960s the typical Japanese diet was low in calories and quite unlike the customary American fare. It was characterized by the virtual absence of red meat and by only very limited quantities of dairy products, but it featured copious portions of rice, fish, vegetables, and vegetable products like tofu. These dietary peculiarities are readily explained by reference to Japan's geography and history. With around a hundred million people occupying a land area smaller than California, this island nation had no space for cattle ranches and little room for dairy farms. Beefsteak, necessarily imported, cost the proverbial king's ransom; not many Japanese could afford it at a time when the country was recovering from the social upheavals wrought by the Second World War. Even chicken and pork were expensive. Fish, so abundant in the surrounding seas, therefore supplied most of the protein consumed by the Japanese.

Those dietary statistics generated in the 1950s are truly eye-opening. Somewhere between 40% and 50% of the calories in the American diet then came from fat, derived mostly from animal sources. Only about 10% of the calories in the Japanese diet came from fat, derived mostly from vegetable sources. Ernst L. Wynder of the American Health Foundation and his colleagues in Japan have given us pertinent comparisons for the years 1955 through 1959. During this period the average American consumed 254 grams of red meat per day; the average Japanese, 14 grams. The American ate or drank 532 grams of milk products daily; the Japanese, only 25 grams. In the cereals category, however, the average Japanese proved a much better consumer, eating 422 grams daily (mostly rice), compared to the American's 186 grams. Fish consumption was no contest: the Japanese ate 124 grams daily, versus the American's meager 17 grams.[45]

Dietary fat emerged as the chief carcinogenetic suspect highlighted by these investigations, the typical American diet of the 1950s being notoriously high-fat, and the typical Japanese diet being astonishingly low-fat. In the 1960s Americans consumed a little less fat, and the Japanese consumed a little bit more, but a wide gap remained between the cuisines in these two industrialized nations. Americans now got 39% of their calories from fat, the Japanese only 11%—not quite a fourfold variation. Yet if the analysis is confined to **saturated fat** (the kind considered most suspicious in cancer epidemiology), a sixfold variation becomes apparent. Americans in the 1960s got 18% of their calories from saturated fat; only 3% of Japanese calories came from this source. By and large, the Japanese continued to avoid premature deaths from coronary heart disease and breast cancer. In the 1960s American men died before age 65 from

heart attacks at an annual rate of 189 per 100,000 population, while Japanese men had a rate of 34. American women died before age 65 from breast cancer at an annual rate of 22 per 100,000 population, while Japanese women had a rate of 4—less than one-fifth the American mortality.[46]

In the 1970s prosperity descended on the Japanese islands. The consumption of dietary fat increased; and the incidence rates of breast, prostate, and colon cancers began to inch upwards, while remaining well below American and European levels. In 1964, for example, Japan's rate of breast cancer mortality stood at 3.8 per 100,000 population; by 1978 the per capita fat intake had doubled, and that mortality rate had risen to 5.2—a 37% increase.[47] Was dietary fat the sole factor behind this increase? One epidemiological study from the late 1970s pointed an accusatory finger at meat, a staple that more and more Japanese could now afford. Wealthy Japanese women who ate meat daily were found to have a breast cancer risk 8.5 times greater than that of poorer women who never ate meat.[48] Findings like these must surely try the souls of cattle ranchers and meat packers! By the 1980s these businessmen were actively displaying their succulent products in Japanese supermarkets, and the unique dietary patterns which had attracted epidemiologists to this nation were rapidly becoming a thing of the past. By the early 1990s dietary fat accounted for some 25% of the Japanese caloric intake; and the mortality rate for breast cancer stood at 6.0 per 100,000 population—noticeably higher than in previous decades, but still far below the relatively stable rate of 22 per 100,000 population being reported by the United States.[49]

Possible Confounding Factors

Cancers of the breast, like those of the colon and prostate, often seem to be diseases of financial affluence and nutritional excess. Internationally, the incidence of these tumors correlates rather well with a country's per capita income and caloric intake. But not all the explanations offered for the low rates of breast cancer among Japanese and other Asian women have been dietary. Genetics has been mentioned as a possible confounding factor. Nicholas L. Petrakis, an epidemiologist at the University of California in San Francisco, pointed out that the vast majority of Asian women have dry-type cerumen (earwax), while most Caucasian women in western Europe and the United States have wet-type cerumen. Does the genetic variant which dictates a wet, sticky consistency for earwax somehow predispose women to breast cancer? Dr. Petrakis argued that it might, correlating national mortality rates for breast cancer with national frequencies of the "wet earwax gene." For example, 85% of American whites and 100% of American blacks were presumed to carry a dominant wet-type gene, but only 9% of the Japanese were apparent carriers. A relationship between earwax and the mammary gland was plausible, Petrakis explained, "since the ceruminous, mammary, and certain axillary sweat glands are histologically of the apocrine type, and their secretions are biochemically similar."[50] To save readers a trip to a medical library, we should note that the cells of **apocrine glands** secrete particulate granular matter as well as fluids. While not confirmed in breast cancer etiology, the earwax hypothesis does suggest that genetic factors could be subtly interacting with reproductive and dietary patterns to increase or reduce those national incidence rates.

Besides drier earwax, Asian women tend to have lower estrogen levels in their blood and urine than American women, whether of European or African descent. Sometimes the differences are substantial. One study pitted Caucasian women living in Boston against recent Asian immigrants (Vietnamese, Japanese, Koreans) living in Hawaii. The premenopausal Caucasians had "30% to 75% higher plasma estrone and estradiol levels" than their age-matched Asian compeers in Hawaii; the postmenopausal Caucasians had "threefold higher plasma levels of estradiol" than their Asian compeers. In this study as in others, it was difficult to separate any genetic contribution from the effects of nutrition, because the Caucasian women in Boston consumed more dietary fat, especially the saturated variety so readily converted into the steroid sex hormones.[51]

The smaller statue and lower weight of Asian women have also been cited as likely confounding factors. Larger body size and greater weight are consistently associated with higher rates of postmenopausal breast cancer. Three European nations—England, Denmark, Holland—have long had the world's highest rates of breast cancer, and possibly the world's tallest and heaviest women; but how could anyone sort out the relative contributions of genetics and nutrition? For centuries these countries have been famed as lands of beefeaters and beer drinkers, of dairy farms and copious cheeses. The three national cuisines are slanted toward saturated fats and animal proteins. Moreover, we might postulate that the larger body size of some European women not only involves longer legs and arms, but a greater length of intestines, possibly allowing more nutrients to be absorbed and turned into sex hormones. There may well be an element of truth in this intestinal hypothesis, but clearly the quantity and the quality of nutrients entering the oral cavity are of paramount importance. During the Second World War the citizens of England, Denmark, and Holland were forced to adopt low-calorie, low-fat diets. Beefsteak, butter, and cheese got temporarily replaced by garden vegetables and whole-wheat bread; and for some years afterward the cancer rates in these nations actually declined. In England food rationing during the war "correlated with a reduction in breast cancer mortality two decades later."[52]

THE "DIETARY FAT" BATTLE
Consensus Becomes Controversy

By the early 1980s the hypothesis that the frequent consumption of dietary fat increases breast cancer risk appeared to be one of the few self-evident, universally accepted truths in a field otherwise fraught with controversy. Who could dispute this theory? To begin with, animal experiments from the 1940s onward had yielded a consistent result—female mice and rats given high-fat diets develop lots of breast cancers, while comparable rodents put on fat-restricted diets stay free of these tumors. Firm conclusions about human malignancies cannot be drawn from animal models, but the striking statistics coming from international epidemiological studies looked like powerful corroborative evidence. A comparison of 39 countries found that breast cancer mortality was five to ten times higher in nations where the per capita fat intake was 140 to 150 grams per day, than in those where fat intake was only 50 grams or less per day.[53] Several studies of dietary interventions involving human subjects also produced supportive data. A group of postmenopausal American women experienced a 17% reduction in blood estradiol levels when their daily fat intake was reduced from an average of 68.5 grams to 29.5 grams. The researchers conducting this small trial hypothesized that "a fourfold to fivefold reduction in breast cancer risk eventually may result from the effects of fat reduction on plasma estradiol."[54] Jacques Brisson and his co-workers at Quebec's Laval University reported that the effects of saturated fat consumption could actually be seen on mammograms. Women whose diets were high in saturated fat revealed dense glandular patterns on radiographs of their breasts. Presumably, these "parenchymal densities" indicated increased mitotic activity in the mammary gland—and therefore an increased risk of subsequent carcinogenesis.[55]

The growing epidemiological and experimental evidence implicating dietary fat in breast cancer etiology did not escape the notice of our health care strategists. In 1982 the National Research Council, composed of distinguished scientists, recommended that Americans reduce the percentage of fat-derived calories in their diet from the prevalent 40% to 30%. Conceding that evidence existed "to justify an even greater reduction," the Council members explained that the one-quarter reduction was proposed because "it is a moderate and practical target, and likely to be beneficial."[56] In 1986 the National Cancer Institute (NCI) published a widely circulated monograph entitled *Cancer Control Objectives for the Nation*, which boldly ventured to estimate the mammary benefits to be gained from this moderate alteration: "A reduction of dietary fat from 40% to 30% of calories could reduce the death rate from breast cancer by 25% in ten years."[57] Since 1983 the NCI had in fact been making plans for a large clinical trial which would demonstrate the effectiveness of restricting fat consumption in breast cancer prevention. The study in question, dubbed the **Women's Health Trial**, was just getting under way in the mid-1980s—32,000 subjects were to be followed for "an average of eight years," long enough to demonstrate the anticipated benefits.[58]

Unfortunately, the shimmering bubble of consensus burst on January 1, 1987, suddenly making dietary fat as controversial as almost everything else pertaining to breast cancer. The *New England Journal of Medicine* for this date published an impressive analysis prepared by Walter C. Willett and his Harvard University colleagues, who had examined the relationship between dietary fat consumption and breast cancer risk in a cohort of 89,538 registered nurses. These new results from the **Nurses' Health Study** shook epidemiologists' preconceptions about the role of dietary fat as thoroughly as Galileo's telescope had once shaken the medieval belief in planet earth as the immobile center of the universe. Willett et al had divided the nurses responding to a food questionnaire into five subgroups, or quintiles, depending upon the percentage of daily caloric intake derived from fat. The highest quintile got approximately 45% of their calories from fat. The lowest quintile, drawing only 30% or so of their calories from fat, pretty much fulfilled the aforementioned guidelines promoted by the National Research Council and the National Cancer Institute. After a four-year follow-up, the highest quintile of nurses proved to have a breast cancer risk which was—*SURPRISE!*—0.82 relative to the nurses in the lowest quintile. Risk-wise, the high-fat eaters were 18% *lower* than the low-fat eaters! Even when Dr. Willett and his colleagues based their calculations solely upon the consumption of that devilish saturated fat, the results were much the same. The highest quintile had a relative risk of 0.84 compared to the lowest.[59]

The Harvard epidemiologists acknowledged that their analysis could not answer two crucial questions. Does a high-fat diet adversely affect the developing mammary glands of preteens, teenagers, and young women in their twenties? Would reducing fat intake to levels well below 30% of the total calories have an impact on breast cancer incidence? The first question could not be addressed because the nurses studied ranged in age from 34 to 59; the second, because very few people in the American population have a fat intake below that 30% marker. What Willett et al did conclude from their analysis would have been unsettling enough to the health strategists—*viz.*, a modest 25% reduction in fat consumption by adult women isn't likely to decrease the incidence of breast cancer.

Just as the NCI'S long-awaited Women's Health Trial was finally gaining momentum, it seemed to stall, and then—*it stopped!* In January 1988 officials at the National Cancer Institute announced that they had decided "to discontinue full-scale implementation of the trial," citing concerns about a lack of statistical power and the problem of verifying "long-term compliance to a diet radically different from the norm in this country."[60] Privately, the NCI powers-that-be must have had reservations about spending millions of taxpayer dollars on a prevention demonstration which might not work at all. In the meantime, those epidemiologists who had devoted so much time and effort to elaborating the dietary fat hypothesis were busy looking for shortcomings in the Nurses' Health Study. One correspondent to the *New England Journal of Medicine* wondered if those adult nurses consuming a low-fat diet (the bottom quintile) were doing so because they had previously been overweight as teenagers. If this should be the case, and if fat consumption does the most damage during adolescence, the findings by Willett et al might be seriously confounded and quite misleading. Other correspondents to the *Journal* questioned whether the dietary fat hypothesis could be properly tested in any cross section of the American population.

Virtually everybody in the United States would be classified as a high-fat eater if judged by worldwide standards. James R. Hebert and Ernst L. Wynder of the American Health Foundation pointed out that increasing the dietary lipids fed to laboratory animals results in cancer promotion "up to a threshold in the range of 20 to 30 percent of calories as fat." If a similar threshold exists in humans, we might look in vain for any protective effects from a dietary intervention which did not restrict fat consumption to 20% or less of the total caloric intake.[61]

In 1989 Arthur Schatzkin and three other NCI epidemiologists threw down a gauntlet in the *Journal of the American Medical Association*. Schatzkin et al argued that few, if any, inferences should be drawn from the Nurses' Health Study. While international comparisons have revealed more than fivefold variation in fat consumption and breast cancer incidence, countries where dietary fat comprises about 45% of the average caloric intake—that is, in the highest quintile of the Nurses' Health Study—have only a 1.5 relative risk of breast cancer mortality when compared to countries where dietary fat comprises about 30% of the caloric intake (as in the Nurses' lowest quintile). The risk differential between these two levels of fat consumption is small—just 50%—and only a very large and well-designed epidemiological study could detect it. Schatzkin et al doubted that the food frequency questionnaires used by the Harvard team were sophisticated enough to measure nuances in fat consumption: "It is difficult to reconstruct precisely how often particular foods were eaten over an extended period." Dr. Schatzkin and his colleagues endorsed the dietary fat hypothesis because it explained a vast body of epidemiological evidence and offered women a feasible way of reducing their breast cancer risk.[62]

Fiber's No Good Either?

Dr. Willett and his Harvard team were in no way deterred by the slings, arrows, and arguments coming from epidemiologists wedded to the dietary fat hypothesis. In 1992 Willett et al published updated results from the Nurses' Health Study, now based on an eight-year follow-up and "an expanded, 121-item semiquantitative food frequency questionnaire."[63] Once again, analysis of the nurses' responses yielded no evidence of a positive association between fat consumption and the incidence of breast cancer, either for premenopausal or postmenopausal women, and regardless of whether the fat was saturated, polyunsaturated, or monounsaturated. Higher fat intake actually tended to have "weak inverse associations" with risk. This remained true even when Willett et al compared the tiny subgroups at the furthermost ends of the dietary spectrum. Those nurses getting over 49% of their calories from fat had 0.86 the relative risk (14% lower) of those nurses who received less than 29% of their calories from fat. Could fat possibly be good for you? The data indicated only that fat consumption by middle-aged women did not significantly increase their risk of subsequent breast cancer. Dr. Willett and his colleagues cautioned that "the positive association between intake of animal fat and risk of colon cancer provides ample reason to limit this source of energy." What about all those international comparisons linking fat consumption to breast cancer? Willett et al were not impressed: they observed that while American fat intake has "steadily decreased since the early 1950s," the reported incidence of breast cancer has "increased by about 40%."

The updating of the Nurses' Health Study also cast a stone at another sacred cow—**dietary fiber**. Fat and fiber usually get scrambled together in the epidemiological literature on diet and cancer. When dieters reduce fat consumption by cutting back on meat and dairy products, they almost inevitably increase their fiber consumption by eating more fruits, vegetables, and cereals. There has been much research attempting to identify specific compounds in fruits and vegetables which might prevent DNA damage and thus retard malignant transformation. But some studies have suggested that fiber pure and simple could be protective against breast and prostate cancers. Barry R. Goldin of Boston's New England Medical Center and allied researchers compared the blood estrogen levels in omnivorous premenopausal women with those in premenopausal women who were strict vegetarians. Goldin et al offered a simple explanation for the 19% lower levels found in the latter group: "Vegetarian women have an increased fecal output, which leads to increased fecal excretion of estrogen and a decreased plasma concentration of estrogen."[64] Presumably the same vegetable fiber which softens stools, makes them larger, and speeds them through the intestines may also act to remove excess hormones which might otherwise be reabsorbed into the bloodstream. Cereal fiber would seem to confer comparable protection. David P. Rose and his colleagues at the American Health Foundation looked at the cancer rates and per capita food consumption in 39 countries, finding that mortality from malignancies of the breast, colon, ovary, and prostate was inversely associated with cereal intake.[65] Researchers at this foundation based in Valhalla, New York, later conducted an animal experiment to see whether cereal fiber could counteract the tumor-inducing effects of a high-fat diet. Sure enough, the female rats given wheat bran along with a high-fat menu developed 24% fewer breast tumors than control rats given just the fatty fare.[66]

The middle-aging nurses followed so closely by Dr. Willett and his colleagues seemed blissfully unaware of the aforementioned evidence. Regardless of how much dietary fiber they consumed, their incidence of breast cancer remained constant. Willett et al concluded: "Our data suggest that a protective effect of total dietary or crude fiber intake in humans, if any, is not likely to be large. However, because dietary fiber encompasses a heterogeneous group of substances, we cannot exclude the possibility that some specific fraction may be related to risk of breast cancer."[67]

Dr. Willett Not a Nihilist

The controversy over the value of a low-fat, high-fiber diet in breast cancer prevention will probably continue. What the Nurses' Health Study has demonstrated is simply that we don't know nearly as much about fat and fiber as we thought we did, and that ballyhooed proposals to slash cancer rates with dietary interventions may represent leaps of faith by prestigious health organizations or excesses of enthusiasm by nutrition-oriented researchers. We would be doing a disservice to leave the impression that Walter C. Willett and his Harvard co-workers are nutritional nihilists. On the contrary! Dr. Willett in particular has been a very active interventionist. He is simply concerned—as we all should be—that there be scientifically reproducible evidence to support the proposed dietary interventions. Willett's thoughts are worth noting. He argues that both animal and human studies of fat intake have been confounded by energy intake—i.e., by total caloric consumption—"because fat is the most energy-dense macronutrient."[68] To explain the low rates of breast cancer in Japan and other Asian countries, he replaces the fat-intake hypothesis with one of "energy restriction," especially if it occurs early enough in life "to limit adult stature."[69] While plausible, this theory seems unlikely to lead to practical preventive measures. How many preteen girls want to limit their height? On the topic of red meat and its high saturated fat content, Willett is as much a scourge of the cattle barons as other epidemiologists, only he focuses on the plausible associations with colon cancer and cardiovascular disease rather than on the more speculative links to breast and prostate cancers.[70] After all, the same Nurses' Health Study which failed to implicate dietary fat in breast cancer found that women "who ate beef, pork, or lamb as a main dish every day" had 2.49 times the risk of colon cancer as "those reporting consumption less than once a month."[71]

Dr. Willett believes that the emphasis on total fat intake, typical of epidemiological studies in the 1970s and 1980s, is wrongheaded. Some varieties of fat might be bad for you, others possibly helpful. Willett argues that we need to look more closely at the fatty acid composition of individual foods; he points out that the questionnaires hitherto used by epidemiologists have not been detailed enough to elicit worthwhile data on the intake of specific fats.

Generally speaking, we can divide fats into three main categories. **Saturated fats** in the American diet come principally from meat and whole-milk dairy products like butter and cheese; these foods derived from land-dwelling mammals also provide **cholesterol**, a lipid which is never present in vegetable products. The human body can manufacture its own saturated fats and cholesterol, and really doesn't need much more. Plausible evidence linking excessive consumption of these nutrients to cardiovascular disease has been provided by the Framingham Study, that famous epidemiological project begun in 1948 to chronicle the heart attacks and strokes suffered by the citizens of a small Massachusetts city.[72] **Polyunsaturated fats**, derived from vegetables and fish, are sometimes called "essential," because they provide fatty acids that the human body can't make on its own. **Monounsaturated fats**, liberally supplied by nuts and some vegetable oils (notably olive oil), have recently begun to look like friends; their consumption seems to reduce cholesterol levels and may possibly retard some cancers.

Lessons from the Greeks

By the mid-1990s Greece had replaced Japan as the most revered national model in our literature on diet and cancer. This Mediterranean country featured traditional dietary patterns which not only looked healthy, but which might prove more palatable to Americans than the rice-and-fish staples of Japan. Our interest in the so-called "Mediterranean diet" stems from the **Seven Countries Study** begun in the 1960s, which discovered that citizens of the Greek islands Crete and Corfu were remarkably free from cancer and cardiovascular disease, and outlived even the Japanese. Ancel Keys, the epidemiologist who headed this study, recalls that the Greek islanders devoured vast quantities of olive oil and whole-grain bread, "these two alone accounting for 50 to over 60 percent of their total calories." Fresh fruits and vegetables were constants in their cuisine, but eggs and dairy products were consumed in moderation, and red meat infrequently.[73] Perhaps the most striking element of this diet was its fat content. The total fat intake approached the American level, but very little of it consisted of saturated fat. The Greeks got most of their lipids from olive oil, which is rich in monounsaturated fat.

Dr. Willett reminds us that the consumption of monounsaturated fat appears to have a beneficial effect on cholesterol profiles, reducing the "low-density lipoprotein" (LDL) which is associated with cardiovascular risk, without greatly affecting the "high-density lipoprotein" (HDL) which seems protective.[74] But factors other than monounsaturated fat almost certainly played important roles in the Greek islanders' liberation from heart disease. The islanders stayed physically active from dawn to dusk, being employed as shepherds, farmers, or fishermen; and they lived in an environment free from the stresses of traffic jams, telephones, air pollution, and urban crime. They drank a glass or two of wine each day, and by and large they did not smoke.

Does consumption of monounsaturated fat somehow contribute to the low breast cancer rates seen in Greece? And if so, through what mechanism? A team of Greek and American epidemiologists published a case-control study of breast cancer risk in Greece, making olive oil sound like the next best thing to ambrosia. Greek women consuming olive oil "more than once a day" had a 25% lower risk of breast cancer than those who reported consumption just once a day. As these researchers pointed out, the monounsaturated fat in olive oil doesn't promote mammary tumors in laboratory rats with the same efficiency as saturated fat. In some animal experiments it has even seemed to protect against breast carcinogenesis.[75] Olive oil is consumed daily by many people in Greece, Spain, and southern Italy; no doubt Americans would be well advised to use it for culinary applications where they have previously relied on butter (high in saturated fat). But like butter, olive oil is marvelously fattening. Unless you burn up calories like those shepherds roaming up and down the Greek hillsides, you'd be wise to use it sparingly.

Epidemiologists, cancer specialists, and cardiologists all agree that Americans would be less likely to develop chronic diseases if they were leaner and more active, if they consumed red meat and high-fat dairy products only in moderation, and if they followed diets emphasizing a variety of fruits, vegetables, and whole-grain cereals. But there is no consensus on more specific dietary strategies; no one has discovered a magic foodstuff sure to ward off atherosclerosis and malignancy. Epidemiological studies lauding the protective qualities of broccoli, olive oil, or tofu ought not to be dismissed out of hand; but they may be taken *cum grano salis* ("with a grain of salt") owing to the large number of possible confounding factors. The best lesson we can learn from Greece is summarized by a pithy inscription placed on the ancient temple at Delphi—*"Nothing in excess."*

The Women's Health *Initiative*

The cancellation of the abortive Women's Health Trial in 1988 did not stop the officials at the National Cancer Institute from dreaming of a splendid experiment—that is, *a clinical trial*—which would clarify the role of diet in breast cancer etiology. But after the negative findings from the Nurse's Health Study, the NCI powers-that-be were leery of concentrating exclusively on dietary fat and breast cancer. Plans were soon afloat for a trial testing the hypothesis that dietary fat restriction can reduce the incidence of both breast *and* colon cancers, but doubts about the project's cost and methodology were hard to extinguish. The trial seemed to get started one month, then put on hold the next. All this hesitation ended in 1991, when Bernadine Healy became the first woman ever to serve as director of the National Institutes of Health (NIH). By training a cardiologist, Dr. Healy was appalled that research on coronary heart disease had been largely restricted to men; and she felt the absurdity of trying to find a dietary prophylaxis simply for breast cancer, when in fact far more women die from the aftereffects of coronary occlusions and osteoporotic bone fractures. Why not design a really big trial which would simultaneously resolve a wide range of important questions in women's health? Under Dr. Healy's promptings, the dietary intervention experiment which the NCI people had been mulling around for a decade got bigger—*much, much bigger*—and finally began in 1993 with a slightly modified name: **The Women's Health Initiative**. Touted as the largest clinical trial ever organized in the United States, this monumental project under NIH auspices offered mind-boggling numbers: a $600 million price tag, a projected enrollment of 160,000 subjects aged 50 to 79,and a fifteen-year follow-up.[76] The long-proposed restriction of dietary fat remained a central component in the Women's Health Initiative, but any ensuing benefits were to be assessed for cardiovascular disease as well as for breast and colorectal cancers. Another arm of the trial aimed to resolve the simmering debate about hormone replacement therapy. Do the reputed benefits of supplemental estrogen for the postmenopausal heart and bones outweigh its apparent dangers to the breast and uterus? The Initiative was also to test a frequently advocated prophylactic measure for osteoporosis. Do calcium supplements and extra vitamin D really do any good?

The NIH imprimatur has not protected the Initiative from brickbats. Epidemiologists interested in breast cancer, including Brian E. Henderson and Walter C. Willett, were quick to point out that this trial did not address the most plausible tenet of the dietary fat hypothesis—namely, that high intake of saturated fat by preteens and adolescents establishes a lifetime elevated risk of breast cancer, by inducing early menarche and possibly by causing other deleterious effects on the developing mammary gland. Critics have complained that any reduction in disease risk which may be found in the trial's low-fat intervention group will be hard to interpret, because these women were rigorously counseled to eat more fruits, vegetables, and grain products. Thus the effects of fat restriction *per se* might be confused with those due to increased consumption of these other foodstuffs. If there's a benefit, how can we be sure what caused it?

* * *

Diet is the very devil to figure out! Perhaps we'll have verifiable answers in a decade or two. At the moment let's put these controversies behind us, and move on to four topics for which we can reach reasonably definite conclusions—obesity, exercise, smoking, and alcoholic beverages.

Obesity—The Modifiable Risk

Most Americans are overweight, being a few pounds above those ideal weights for sex, age, and height proposed by the actuaries and insurance companies. It's hard to say when mere overweight-ness stops and obesity begins, but physicians usually employ the latter term for individuals whose body weights are 25% or more above the actuarial guidelines.

Obesity is an undisputed risk factor for postmenopausal breast cancer. A survey of 400,000 women made by the American Cancer Society found that obese postmenopausal women had a 50% greater chance of dying from breast cancer than their thinner contemporaries.[77] Some epidemiologists give higher estimates of the risk level. Basil A. Stoll of London cautions that an obese postmenopausal woman "carries twice the risk of breast cancer compared to a similar-age woman of normal weight."[78] Needless to say, there are *degrees* of obesity and of risk elevation. The heavier a person becomes, the greater the risk—the trend is clearly linear and upward, although its precise quantification may be difficult.

We have a good understanding of the mechanisms through which obesity alters breast cancer risk. As previously mentioned, the predominant estrogen in postmenopausal women is estrone, synthesized principally from adrenal androgens in adipose (fatty) tissues. Obese postmenopausal women not only have larger amounts of estrone in their blood, but they also have more estradiol, the most mitogenic estrogen. All this estrogen tends to be biologically active, because obese women have lower concentrations of **sex hormone-binding globulin** (SHBG) in their blood. The hormonal surfeit sharply elevates the risk of endometrial cancer in postmenopausal women, because the cells lining the uterus are very responsive to estrogen. It modestly elevates the risk of breast cancer, because the cells lining the mammary gland's ductal system are moderately responsive to estrogen.[79]

Obesity influences cancer risk through its effects on hormone production and hormone bioavailability. We are still learning how this risk may vary in different subgroups of women. Researchers associated with the American Health Foundation reported that heavy women who were "lean at age 18" and later gained enough weight to be "in the upper tertile [top third] of body mass" had a breast cancer risk of 2.6 (i.e., a 160% increase) compared to women who stayed lean throughout their lives.[80] The dangers of a thin-to-fat transition have not been so widely publicized as those associated with abdominal fat deposition. Some epidemiologists believe that the overall quantity of adipose flesh doesn't matter quite as much as the

location where that excess baggage is carried. According to this hypothesis, heavy women with a pear-shaped silhouette (adiposity around the hips) are less likely to develop breast cancer and cardiovascular disease than heavy women with an apple-shaped figure (abdominal adiposity). A survey of 41,837 postmenopausal women in Iowa found that heavier women with a high waist-to-hip ratio had "greater than a twofold excess relative risk" of breast cancer.[81] David V. Schapira and his colleagues at the University of South Florida have produced case-control studies linking that apple shape to elevated rates of both breast and endometrial cancers.[82] Not all studies have implicated abdominal obesity in cancer etiologies, but this hypothesis seems plausible enough. Women naturally tend to fat deposition around the hips; there is nothing natural about the masculine beer-belly pattern, which derives from excessive consumption of high-calorie foods and inadequate exercise. Such abdominal girth in postmenopausal women has been consistently associated with higher levels of adrenal androgens and lower levels of SHBG. The former imbalance leads to an increased production of estrogen, and the latter means that the hormone circulates in a non-protein-bound form and is readily bioavailable.

Obesity is <u>not</u> a risk factor for premenopausal breast cancer. It is somewhat protective against early-onset disease. The best statistics we have for premenopausal obese women may well be those from the Nurses' Health Study, which reported that "the risk of breast cancer decreased significantly with increasing relative weight." In other words, the fatter young women are, the less likely they are to develop breast cancer in their thirties and forties. Yet the risk reduction is modest: the heaviest of the 115,534 nurses surveyed had 0.6 the risk (a 40% reduction) of their thinner colleagues.[83]

How does obesity manage to reduce the premenopausal risk of breast cancer when it so surely raises the postmenopausal risk? To explain this apparent paradox, we will need to recall our previous discussions of the menstrual cycle and of regular ovulation as a risk factor. Obese women, young and old alike, have considerable non-ovarian production of estrone and estradiol. In premenopausal women that extra estrogen acts like hit-or-miss hormonal contraception—a kind of "on-again, off-again" birth control pill. Presumably the hypothalamus and the pituitary get confused by the constantly elevated estrogen levels. In any event, during many menstrual cycles the mid-cycle surge of luteinizing hormone (LH) does not occur, and consequently ovulation does not take place. Without ovulation there is no ruptured follicle (*corpus luteum*) to produce progesterone. As we've seen, mitotic activity in the premenopausal mammary gland peaks during the last half of the cycle—in the luteal phase which commences with ovulation and which is characterized by an abundance of both estrogen and progesterone. Those anovulatory cycles to which young obese women are prone are characterized by the absence of progesterone and by reduced mitotic activity in the mammary gland. This situation understandably reduces the chances of mutations in the mammary cells and lowers the risk of breast cancer in the immediately ensuing years.

Young women with an unfortunate genetic condition known as the **polycystic ovary syndrome** are also prone to anovulatory menstrual cycles. Like premenopausal obesity, this syndrome is associated with abnormal hormonal profiles—elevated estrogens and androgens, irregular secretion of pituitary gonadotropins (FSH and LH), deficient progesterone—and with a reduced risk of early-onset breast cancer. One study found that women with polycystic ovaries have a 48% lower risk for premenopausal breast cancer.[84] But neither obesity nor polycystic ovaries can be recommended as a preventive measure. These morbid conditions are ultimately associated with higher rates of postmenopausal breast cancer. Yet cancer would seem to be the least of an obese person's worries. In men and women alike, prolonged obesity strongly predisposes to an array of serious health problems—diabetes, hypertension, heart disease, arthritis, gallstones, and renal (kidney) failure.

The Benefits of Exercise

Moderate exercise on a regular basis, daily or at least every other day, is a mighty weapon against creeping obesity. Physical activity is inversely associated with the incidence and severity of cardiovascular disease and other late-onset maladies where adopted lifestyle and genetic inheritance surreptitiously conspire to hasten mortality. It is quite probable that a lifetime pattern of physical activity would also reduce the incidence of breast cancer, though the scientific demonstrations of this theory are as yet scanty, and the optimal regimens entirely speculative.

We do know that preteen girls who train rigorously for ballet or gymnastics often experience delayed menarche, and that young women who participate in strenuous college sports often experience irregular menstrual cycles.[85] Both these exercise-induced phenomena are inversely associated with breast cancer risk, but are they otherwise healthy? Physical exercise sufficient to delay or disrupt the menstrual cycle for years on end may interfere with bone maturation in adolescent girls, and it can cause a loss of bone mass in young adult women. The rail-thin gymnast who spends her days on the parallel bars is not a practical model for our public health programs. Still, there is something to be said for exercise in breast cancer prevention. Rose E. Frisch, emeritus professor at the Harvard School of Public Health, has long been a leading advocate of this strategy. In the 1980s Frisch and her colleagues surveyed large numbers of college alumnae, finding that those who had been athletes during their school years had a much lower incidence of breast cancer.[86] Leslie Bernstein and other epidemiologists at the University of Southern California did a case-control study focusing on women aged 40 and younger. Bernstein et al discovered that the women who spent "3.8 or more hours per week" doing physical exercise had a breast cancer risk of 0.42 (a 58% reduction) relative to the inactive women in the study.[87]

Hormonal modulation is the most obvious mechanism by which physical activity could reduce breast cancer risk. Whether a woman is premenopausal or postmenopausal, regular exercise would tend to work against an estrogen surfeit by reducing the body's adipose tissue. Possibly physical activity has other subtle effects which may slow or prevent malignant transformation in the breast and elsewhere—but we really don't know what these effects could be, any more than we know the amount and type of dietary fat which we should optimally consume. We do know that the **avoidance of obesity** and **regular exercise** constitute reasonable preventive strategies, which can be enthusiastically recommended.

Smoking *Prevents* Cancer?

For several decades cigarette smoking has been **Public Health Enemy Number One**, damned and double-damned by the American Cancer Society, the American Heart Association, and the Surgeon General. Cigarette addicts may be comforted to learn that smoking is not an appreciable risk factor for breast cancer. There would actually seem to be inverse associations between heavy smoking and malignancies of the breast and endometrium. A case-control study published in the *New England Journal of Medicine* found that postmenopausal women who smoked 25 or more cigarettes per day had half the risk of developing endometrial cancer as comparable nonsmokers.[88] John Laszlo of the American Cancer Society has succinctly explained the biological basis of this protective effect: "Cigarette smoking changes normal metabolism of estrogen. Smokers experience menopause at an earlier age."[89] By lowering estrogen levels in the blood, smoking offers a definite degree of protection against endometrial cancer—and possibly a little bit of protection against breast cancer. But this "protection" is not worth having. We must stress that those malignancies induced by smoking, notably lung and esophageal cancers, are extremely lethal, with relatively few long-term survivors. In contrast, the malignancies inversely associated with smoking (breast and endometrial) can usually be cured outright or at least effectively managed.

Smoking remains a bad bet for women of any age, but perhaps especially for very young ones. Some epidemiologists have wondered whether the carcinogens in cigarette smoke could adversely affect the developing mammary glands of adolescent girls. A joint American and Canadian study found that women smokers who adopted the habit before age 16 had an elevated risk of breast cancer, approximately 70% to 80% above that of nonsmokers.[90] If smoking affords any protection against breast malignancies, the benefits would seem to be confined to older women. The Nurses' Health Study, focusing mainly on premenopausal women, reported that smoking did not influence the incidence of breast cancer either one way or the other.[91] This same study bubbled over with positive associations linking smoking with coronary artery disease and cerebrovascular incidents. Compared to nonsmokers, those nurses who smoked 25 or more cigarettes daily had five-and-a-half times the risk of a fatal heart attack, and better than three-and-a-half times the risk of a premature stroke.[92] Cancer is not the only reason for "kicking the habit."

Alcohol Consumption

Alcohol is by far the most prevalent drug on the planet. In one form or another, whether as wine, beer, or potent spirits, it has been publicly consumed in human societies from early recorded history down to the computer age. Given the tremendous popularity of alcoholic beverages and their daily consumption by the majority of adults, it is surprising that only in the 1980s did epidemiological studies finally begin to demonstrate how alcohol affects the risk of developing certain cancers and cardiovascular disease. Within a few years we also had some good clues to the biological mechanisms through which this drug may act to increase or decrease the probability of these diseases.

Alcohol consumption represents **a risk factor for breast cancer**, although not a very great one. Epidemiological investigations of this topic gained momentum after the appearance in 1982 of a sizable case-control study by Lynn Rosenberg of Boston University and numerous collaborators. Rosenberg et al reported that "women who drank alcoholic beverages experienced a rate of breast cancer about one-and-a-half to two times that of women who never drank. Each type of alcoholic beverage was associated with breast cancer."[93] For several years informed opinion wavered, with some subsequent studies finding a positive association while others did not. On May 7, 1987, the publication of two cohort studies in the *New England Journal of Medicine* tipped the balance in favor of a positive association. The Nurses' Health Study offered a four-year follow-up on 89,538 American women. The risk of breast cancer appeared to escalate with increasing consumption. Compared to nondrinkers, those nurses who drank from five to fourteen grams of alcohol daily— "about three to nine drinks per week"—had a relative risk of 1.3 (a 30% increase). And those who drank fifteen or more grams daily had a relative risk of 1.6 (a jump of 60% over the teetotalers).[94] In the *Journal*'s second cohort study, Arthur Schatzkin and his co-workers at the National Institutes of Health analyzed a ten-year follow-up of 7,188 women ranging in age from 25 to 74 years: "The results suggest that moderate alcohol consumption is associated with an elevation in the risk of breast cancer of 50 to 100 percent."[95] Both these studies indicated that drinking seemed to be riskier for younger women than for older ones. Another major study published in 1987 specifically highlighted the dangers of youthful indulgence. Using data from a national case-control project, epidemiologists at the National Cancer Institute confirmed that the consumption of "one or more alcoholic beverages per day" was associated with a slightly elevated risk of breast cancer (about 50% above that of nondrinkers). The NCI team emphasized that "the adverse effects appeared related to drinking practices prior to 30 years of age."[96]

Controversy came swiftly. Randall E. Harris and Ernst L. Wynder of the American Health Foundation cast a skeptical eye on the new risk factor in the *Journal of the American Medical Association*, their objections appearing under the irreverent heading **"Breast Cancer and Alcohol Consumption: A Study in Weak Associations."** Harris and Wynder worried about confounding factors. Did the frequent social drinkers come from the upper economic brackets, and were they consequently more likely to postpone that first full-term pregnancy until their late twenties or early thirties? Were the nondrinkers more health conscious, and thus more likely to watch their weight and exercise regularly? No one knew how alcohol might adversely impact the mammary gland. "Human studies and animal models," Harris and Wynder observed, "have failed to reveal a mechanism by which moderate alcohol intake might either induce or promote the disease."[97]

The Cardiovascular Benefits

Before we consider potential mechanisms through which alcohol might elevate breast cancer risk, we can profitably review this drug's well-documented effects on the incidence of cardiovascular disease. Autopsies performed on alcoholics sometimes produce an astonishing finding: while the liver shows irreparable cirrhotic damage, the coronary arteries nourishing the heart muscle may be virtually free from atherosclerotic plaque, that awful sludge of solidified cholesterol and calcium which slowly narrows blood vessels and eventually closes them altogether.[98] Arteriosclerosis, popularly known as "hardening of the arteries," remains the leading cause of mortality in America. It kills by gradually or suddenly disrupting the flow of blood to the heart (as in angina and coronary occlusions) or to the brain (as in senile dementia and strokes). Taking a cue from the autopsied alcoholics, epidemiologists sought answers. Did the drug alcohol delay or lessen that atherosclerotic clogging of the coronary arteries? If so, since excessive alcohol consumption is extremely dangerous, at what dose level may the cardiovascular benefits be obtained and the risks avoided? Most studies have focused on male subjects, since men die from heart disease

at a much faster rate than women. For ten years the Health Professionals' Follow-Up Study kept track of 51,529 men employed principally as dentists and veterinarians. The published results strongly supported "the hypothesis that the inverse relation between alcohol consumption and risk of coronary disease is causal." Men whose alcohol consumption averaged 30.2 grams per day (about two good drinks) had 0.55 the relative risk (a 45% reduction) of those men who totally abstained from alcohol. The Harvard epidemiologists who conducted this study emphasized alcohol's effect on high-density lipoprotein (HDL), the "good cholesterol," as the most plausible explanation for the significant benefit detected: "When given in experimental studies, even reasonable amounts of alcohol, such as 39 grams per day for six weeks, increased HDL by 17%. A change in HDL of this magnitude could account for a reduction in risk of perhaps 40%, which is similar to our findings."[99] Writing in the *New England Journal of Medicine*, Walter C. Willett and his colleague Frank M. Sacks confidently asserted that alcohol is "the only dietary factor consistently associated with the risk of coronary heart disease" and that it has a "powerful protective effect."[100] In 1994 a team of Harvard researchers headed by the cardiologist Paul M. Ridker announced a second biological mechanism by which alcohol might reduce the risk of coronary heart disease. Moderate alcohol consumption tends to raise blood levels of **tissue-type plasminogen activator** (t-PA). This enzyme has considerable fibrinolytic activity—in other words, it acts to dissolve those tiny blood clots which might otherwise begin to clog up arteries and veins.[101]

Does moderate alcohol consumption by women produce the same cardiovascular benefits seen in men? Nobody seems to to have designed a clinical trial just to answer this question. Fortunately, the questionnaires sent out by the Nurses' Health Study have inquired about the consumption of alcoholic beverages; and an analysis of the nurses' responses yielded even stronger evidence for alcohol's protective effects than the data generated by the all-male Health Professionals' Follow-Up Study. Compared to their nondrinking colleagues, those nurses whose alcohol consumption averaged 25 or more grams per day (about two drinks) had a relative risk for coronary disease of 0.4 (a 60% reduction). The protection appeared to be dose-related: those nurses consuming five to fourteen grams of alcohol per day achieved only a 40% reduction from the abstainers' risk level. The Nurses' Health data for cerebrovascular incidents probably reflects the fibrinolytic activity associated with t-PA. The drinking nurses experienced fewer ischemic strokes (i.e., those caused by narrowing of the brain's blood vessels or by clots forming in these vessels), but they experienced more hemorrhagic strokes (i.e., those caused by bleeding from ruptured blood vessels).[102]

Should women worried about breast cancer refrain from drinking? The answer has to be left to the individual. From the available evidence, we may plausibly conclude that for most people moderate drinking will slightly raise the risk of breast cancer and slightly lower the risk of coronary heart disease and ischemic strokes. More women die from cardiovascular events than from breast malignancies; this probably holds true even for women previously diagnosed with *in situ* and small node-negative tumors. On the other hand, excessive drinking always wreaks havoc on the body and on human relationships. The dose level at which the risks start to outweigh any possible benefits will no doubt vary from individual to

individual. The massive cohort studies performed by the Harvard epidemiologists suggest that most people could safely consume 25 to 30 grams of alcohol (about two drinks) per day. In 1995 an updated analysis from the Nurses' Health Study looked at the relationship between alcohol consumption and overall mortality. Nurses who engaged in "light-to-moderate drinking" had a death rate from all causes ranging from 12% to 17% lower than their nondrinking colleagues. But this reduction in mortality was largely confined to "women with risk factors for coronary heart disease and those 50 years of age or older." Moreover, the benefit vanished altogether in that subgroup of nurses whose alcohol consumption averaged more than 30 grams a day. Their death rate proved to be 19% higher than that of the abstaining nurses.[103]

What's the biological mechanism causing the risk elevation? Alcohol consumption very probably alters breast cancer risk by raising estrogen levels. Marsha E. Reichman and other government researchers conducted a little experiment which does much to explain the finding that drinking is more risky for younger women than for older ones. They measured the hormone levels in the blood and urine of premenopausal women who alternately practiced total abstinence or drank exactly 30 grams of alcohol per day. The women's estrogen levels were found to vary considerably, depending on whether they were consuming alcohol. When drinking, the trial subjects revealed higher plasma levels of estrogen—estrone up 21.2%, estradiol up 27.5%--in the middle of the menstrual cycle, right around the time of ovulation.[104] Presumably the additional mid-cycle estrogen would tend to increase mitotic activity in the luteal phase.

Alcohol's effect on plasma estrogen levels would seem to be less pronounced in postmenopausal women. In the cohort of 41,837 postmenopausal women followed by the Iowa Women's Health Study, drinking was associated with an increased risk of breast cancer only among those subjects who consumed alcohol while taking estrogen replacement therapy. The excess risk ranged from a 13% elevation for women on hormone replacement who consumed less than five grams of alcohol daily, to an 83% elevation for women on hormone replacement who consumed more than fifteen grams of alcohol daily.[105] A case-control study done in New York state found that alcohol consumption was associated with an increased incidence of breast cancers, but only for tumors judged estrogen receptor-positive. The elevation in risk was modest—up 35% for women drinking fifteen or more grams of alcohol per day.[106]

Hereditary Breast Cancer
Steps Forward in Understanding

Heredity is now recognized as the most dangerous risk factor for breast cancer. With some familial cancer syndromes, the probability that a given individual will eventually develop a mammary carcinoma can approach one hundred percent. With other syndromes that probability may be considerably lower. Cancer researchers continue to try to define these syndromes, to discover the genetic mutations which cause them, and to devise screening tests which will distinguish between family members at high risk and those who did not inherit the causative mutation and whose risk is no greater than that of the general population. Our growing awareness and knowledge of familial cancer syndromes owes much to the prolonged efforts of **Henry T. Lynch** of the Creighton University School of Medicine in Omaha, Nebraska. Dr. Lynch

remembers that when he first began to investigate hereditary cancers in the 1960s, human malignancies were regarded almost entirely as environmental diseases caused by exposure to carcinogens. Heredity was not seen as an important factor. Older, established physicians pooh-poohed the idea, as Lynch recalls: "They put their hand on my shoulder and said, 'You are young—this isn't going to pan out. Very few cancers have a hereditary etiology.'"[107] Today, of course, we recognize over 200 familial cancer syndromes, involving all sorts of tumors. And the Hereditary Cancer Institute at Creighton University has become an internationally known center for genetic research and the counseling of persons from afflicted families.[108]

Notwithstanding our new understanding of hereditary factors, the vast majority of breast cancers must still be classified as "sporadic" (nonhereditary). The standard textbooks usually say that perhaps five to ten percent of all cases are hereditary; yet for this topic as for most others, much depends upon whose statistics you would like to cite. The Nurses' Health Study has downplayed the role of inheritance, reporting that no more than six percent of the breast cancer cases recorded in the cohort of 117,988 nurses were "attributable to a positive family history."[109] However, researchers relying on the Utah Population Database estimated that "approximately 17% to 19% of breast cancer could be attributed to family history," with an increased risk of disease "even if the nearest relative with breast cancer is a third-degree relative."[110] The Utah statistics, being generated by genealogy-conscious Mormons, would seem to slightly overstate the effect of genetic inheritance. Perhaps the Nurses' Health analysis slightly undervalues it.

What techniques do physicians use to identify familial cancer syndromes? The traditional, time-honored method has relied on information provided by family members; this is then used to construct a **pedigree** (family tree), which would illustrate how malignant tumors have cropped up over several generations. When geneticists look at the pedigrees of breast cancer families, they usually detect a pattern consistent with **autosomal dominant transmission**. "Autosomal" means that the genetic defect presumed to cause disease is not located on a sex chromosome and that hereditary transmission is consequently not in the X-linked pattern which disproportionately affects males. "Dominant" means that if the defect is inherited from either parent, it has the potential to cause disease. With autosomal dominant transmission, children typically have a 50% chance of inheriting the genetic defect. Pedigree analysis usually cannot tell us for a fact that a troublesome mutation has been inherited, and it is even less able to predict if and when an inherited defect will cause the associated disease. But these days **DNA analysis** can often address these troubling questions with considerable accuracy.

What are the distinguishing characteristics of hereditary breast cancer? The fact that several family members have developed breast tumors does not necessarily mean that a family suffers from hereditary breast cancer. Multiple cases in a single family can result purely from chance, or because family members share common risk factors (e.g., diet, obesity, nulliparity). Ideally, we'd make the diagnosis of hereditary disease by demonstrating the particular genetic defect which lies behind the elevated disease incidence in a particular family; but often neither the identification of the defect nor a screening assay for its presence can be easily accomplished. Physicians interested in hereditary breast cancer have therefore learned to look for **three characteristics** which tend to point toward a familial cancer

syndrome. They are:

(1) Two or more first-degree relatives (mothers, daughters, sisters) have been diagnosed with breast cancer.

(2) The disease developed at an early age, typically in the patients' thirties or forties.

(3) The disease was bilateral—it eventually affected both breasts. Bilaterality is the most telling characteristic, because it suggests that all the cells in the mammary epithelium are carrying a defect predisposing them to malignant transformation. This does not mean that the bilateral tumors must appear simultaneously; the second breast might not be affected until years after the initial diagnosis.

Does heredity ever play a role in postmenopausal breast cancer? Physicians naturally suspect a hereditary etiology in early-onset bilateral disease. Heredity almost certainly contributes to the more typical cases diagnosed in postmenopausal women, but its effects are more subtle, and its role largely undefined. To date, neither epidemiologists nor molecular biologists have any firm answers to give a woman whose mother and aunt developed breast cancer in their sixties and who wants to know whether her own risk may be elevated. A study of 9,000 Chicago women found that a family history of breast cancer was associated with increased risk, but only in women under age 60.[111] In other words, if there's a genetic defect being transmitted from one generation to the next, it would tend to cause early-onset disease. Family members who are free from disease at age 60 probably did not receive it. But the Nurses' Health Study, with considerable statistical power, indicated that even women in their sixties and seventies might be at some risk from inheritance. All the nurses whose mothers had developed breast cancer proved themselves to be at higher risk for the disease, but the degree of risk varied significantly according to the age at which the parent was diagnosed. Those nurses whose mothers developed breast cancer before age 40 had approximately double the risk—a 100% increase—compared to nurses whose mothers never had breast cancer. Those nurses whose mothers developed breast cancer after age 70 still displayed an elevated lifetime risk, but it was only about 50% greater than that seen in nurses whose mothers stayed cancer-free.[112]

What can we conclude from epidemiological studies? The diagnosis of breast cancer in a family member, even a mother or sister, is not in itself sufficient to warrant a dire prognostication for other family members. But the diagnosis in any relative, even a distant one, may well be associated with increased risk. We may safely conclude that the closer the relative and the younger the age at diagnosis, the greater this risk is likely to be—but unfortunately we can't conclude much more. Big epidemiological projects like the Nurses' Health Study can give us broad clues but not specific directions. We must look to molecular biology for assistance in understanding the genetic mutations behind hereditary breast cancer and in assessing the particular level of risk which this or that family member may actually face.

The Hereditary Gene: *BRCA1*

In the 1970s **Mary-Claire King**, a geneticist at the University of California at Berkeley, began to search for a gene whose malfunctions might play a pivotal role in mammary tumorigenesis. She collected DNA specimens (blood samples) from patients thought to have hereditary breast cancer, because she believed that any involved gene or genes would be easier to track down in hereditary

cases than in sporadic ones. For years the DNA specimens remained in cold storage; in the late 1980s the development of the polymerase chain reaction (PCR) enabled King, the biochemist Jeff M. Hall, and other Berkeley researchers to scan these samples for genetic defects. Using a technique called **linkage analysis**, they discovered that almost half of these hereditary cases shared an abnormal marker on the long arm of chromosome 17. The linkage to this chromosomal locus was especially strong in early-onset tumors occurring before age 45. Dr. King and her colleagues published their findings in *Science* in December 1990. The announcement of "a gene for inherited susceptibility to breast cancer," neatly traced to a single area of one chromosome, set off an international race to isolate *BRCA1*, as it came to be called (in allusion to "<u>BR</u>east <u>CA</u>ncer").[113]

Mark H. Skolnick's team, drawing on scientific talent at the University of Utah and the pharmaceutical company Myriad Genetics, crossed the finish line before anybody else. In October 1994 they published the pertinent DNA sequence in *Science*, along with a brief explanation: "Like many other genes involved in familial cancer, *BRCA1* appears to encode a tumor suppressor, a protein that acts as a negative regulator of tumor growth."[114] As mentioned in Chapter Three, mutant alleles of such suppressor genes are typically transmitted dominantly but act recessively. An affected cell in a person who has inherited a normal ("wild-type") allele from one parent and a mutant allele from the other might be compared to an airplane flying with a single engine when there should be two. If the cell should somehow lose the good allele (this could happen during mitosis), a nose dive toward malignancy may ensue. The remaining defective copy of the gene cannot produce the protein which restrains cellular proliferation.

Mary-Claire King and many other

researchers had hoped that *BRCA1* would shed light upon genetic mutations in sporadic breast cancer, which is far more common than hereditary disease. But the attempts to identify *BRCA1* mutations in late-onset, nonhereditary tumors came up empty-handed.[115] Andrew Futreal, a molecular biologist at the National Institute of Environmental Health Sciences, believes that germline mutations in *BRCA1* are probably most dangerous in the adolescent mammary gland: "The lack of mutations in sporadic cancers is telling us that it's really bad to have a mutant copy of the gene sometime during growth and development."[116] Writing in the *New England Journal of Medicine*, Barbara L. Weber of the University of Pennsylvania estimated that no more than one American in every 200 or 400 carries an inherited *BRCA1* mutation, but that affected women "have an astonishing 85 percent lifetime risk of breast cancer," with most tumors developing "before the age of 50 years."[117]

Nobody is finished with *BRCA1*. The gene is gigantic, covering approximately 100,000 base-pairs of DNA and encoding a protein consisting of 1,863 amino acids. A hasty survey of *BRCA1*-positive tumors turned up 38 different mutations; presumably some are more dangerous than others. We know that most of those which cause trouble result in the production of a truncated, nonfunctional protein.[118] A few researchers have suggested that a screening assay for truncated *BRCA1* protein could be developed as a test for hereditary breast cancer, but at present we know relatively little about this protein's role in various types of cells. Moreover, *BRCA1* is not the only gene implicated in hereditary breast cancer. As we've seen, p53 mutations lie behind the Li-Fraumeni syndrome with its frequent mammary tumors. In 1994 a team of international researchers used linkage analysis to track another susceptibility gene

to a locus on the long arm of chromosome 13. *BRCA2*, as this second gene was hastily named, is responsible for some hereditary breast cancers which reveal no trace of a *BRCA1* mutation. Unlike *BRCA1*, this second gene has often been implicated in familial cancer syndromes which involve *male* breast cancers as well as the usual female cases.[119] Mary-Claire King and her colleagues actually studied one family in which the men afflicted with hereditary breast cancer outnumbered the women by a four-to-three ratio. But while the women in the family developed the disease in their thirties, the men were not diagnosed until their sixties.[120]

Multiple Cancer Syndromes
The Ovarian-Prostate Connections

Thanks to the pedigree studies of Henry T. Lynch and others, we know that familial breast cancer may sometimes be accompanied by a clustering of other, nonmammary tumors. The best known example is the **breast-ovarian syndrome**. Breast cancer patients reveal about twice the incidence of ovarian cancer seen in the general population; conversely, ovarian cancer patients reveal about three times the expected incidence of breast cancer.[121] Many of these cases might be attributed to common risk factors—the incidence rates of both breast and ovarian tumors are elevated by nulliparity and by frequent ovulation. In some families, however, pedigree analysis points to the breast-ovarian syndrome, in which an inherited genetic defect is presumed to cause the distinctive clustering of these two malignancies. Before *BRCA1* was tracked to its chromosomal locus, we had no clue to the mutations which gave rise to this syndrome. In the 1990s, however, Douglas F. Easton and other English researchers applied the technique of linkage analysis to DNA samples taken from 153 families affected by hereditary breast cancer and from 57 families affected by the breast-ovarian syndrome. The results were eye-opening! Only 45% of the families suffering from breast tumors alone revealed linkage to the *BRCA1* locus on chromosome 17, but virtually all the families suffering from both breast and ovarian tumors did so.[122] The *BRCA1* gene would thus seem to be responsible for much familial clustering of breast and ovarian cancers. Fortunately, it is also clear that not all mutations in this gene lead to the breast-ovarian syndrome. Some researchers feel the region of the gene where the mutation occurs is the determining factor. According to this hypothesis, mutations in one region might spell trouble for both breast and ovarian cells, while those in another would affect only the mammary gland.[123]

Do men with *BRCA1* mutations get off scot-free? Needless to say, half the carriers of deleterious *BRCA1* alleles are male—women can inherit that terrible predisposition to breast and ovarian cancers from their fathers equally as well as from their mothers. And while not so endangered as female carriers, affected men do face an elevated risk of several tumors. Epidemiological studies have suggested the existence of a **breast-prostate syndrome** in some cancer-prone families. A large cohort study done in Iceland found that male relatives of breast cancer patients ran a 50% greater risk of prostate cancer than that seen in men who had no affected female relatives.[124] The Iowa Women's Health Study collected data from 30,883 women aged 55 to 69 to assess the risk factors for postmenopausal breast cancer. Those subjects with a family history of breast cancer revealed a 45% elevated risk compared to those subjects without a family

history. But subjects with a family history of *both breast and prostate cancers* were found to have a risk for postmenopausal breast cancer 110% greater than subjects without a family history of either malignancy.[125] Such population studies imply that breast and prostate tumors can arise from the same genetic defects, without telling us what genes might be involved. But DNA linkage analysis of seven Icelandic families affected by hereditary breast cancer would seem to implicate the *BRCA1* locus in prostatic as well as in breast malignancies. Of sixteen men identified as the paternal carriers of a deleterious *BRCA1* allele, seven (44%) developed prostate cancer; and these tumors behaved in an uncharacteristically aggressive fashion, "all metastasizing."[126] The penetration of *BRCA1* mutations in prostatic malignancies appears to be significant, though not nearly so great as in breast cancer. An epidemiological study of 33 families thought to harbor *BRCA1* defects found that the male family members had a relative risk of 3.33 for prostate cancer—that is, 233% greater than men in the general population. Surprisingly, these families also revealed an elevated risk of colon cancer—311% greater than the general population.[127] The functions of *BRCA1* in the prostate gland and colonic mucosa need further clarification. We do know that mutations in this gene can sometimes affect other organs besides the mammary gland and the ovaries.

To Test or Not to Test?

Women at high risk for early-onset, hereditary breast cancer constitute a small minority, probably less than one percent of all women. Their tragic plight, not their numbers, claims our attention. All too often a woman in this tiny subgroup has been forced to watch a mother or a sister die prematurely from metastatic breast cancer, which destroyed a family's sense of well-being as surely as it ravaged the patient's body. Readers who wish to experience the human impact of familial breast cancer are referred to the touching memoirs by Nancy Brinker (*The Race Is Run*) and by Gayle Feldman (*You Don't Have to be Your Mother*). These books can be highly recommended, though with the caveat that the breast cancer cases depicted tend to follow an aggressive pattern quite unlike most late-onset cases of disease.

Today our understanding of hereditary breast cancer is advancing by leaps and bounds. Once we have identified the causative mutation in a particular family, we can soon predict any family member's risk level with reasonable accuracy. The dilemma posed by DNA assays for hereditary breast cancer, as for other inheritable diseases, grows out of the fact that our ability to predict future disease currently exceeds any abilities we might have either to prevent it before it develops or to cure it after it develops. True, a mutation detected in the *BRCA1* susceptibility gene is not so much a death warrant as the diagnosis of impending Huntington's disease; it nonetheless presents a woman with some hard choices. One strategy after a positive test result would emphasize **intensive surveillance**, with a view to discovering any breast tumors before they have a chance to metastasize. The problem here is that our early detection methods for breast cancer, as for other malignancies, are not nearly as sensitive or as accurate as we would like. Screening mammography, while greatly improved in recent decades, cannot detect malignant changes in the individual cells; and its proven ability to detect small tumors is often hampered by the glandular densities characteristic of premenopausal breasts. Manual breast exams, whether performed by physicians or by the women themselves, are considerably less sensitive

than mammography. With these current methods, even the most rigorous surveillance cannot guarantee that family members at risk will not develop disseminated breast cancer.

A second strategy offers a much better assurance that mammary tumors will not develop, though at a psychological price that many women find awfully steep. This solution is simple and permanent: **prophylactic mastectomy of both breasts.** Having first-hand experience of disease and death, young women from high-risk families often request this option—and cancer surgeons, after they have reviewed the relevant family histories, generally comply with the request. The problem here is that if we assume autosomal transmission of the causative allelic defects, 50% of these mastectomies have hitherto been performed needlessly. Half the young women did not inherit the predisposing defects, and thus were not at increased risk. Sophisticated DNA analysis stands to eliminate this type of Russian roulette, where women and their medical advisors are torn between fear of deadly disease and apprehension of unnecessary mutation, and have not the slightest clue to the proper decision. For many family members, a negative test result will remove the specter which has overshadowed their lives. For others, a positive result will at least ensure that unpleasant strategies like constant surveillance or preventive mastectomies are adopted only to counter a real threat.

GROWING OLDER
The <u>Unavoidable</u> <u>Risk</u> <u>Factor</u>

Some silly things are said about breast cancer. Probably the silliest is the oft repeated observation that "most patients have no known risk factors." This trite remark would seem to betray a blissful ignorance of a vast body of epidemiological investigation which has conclusively demonstrated a goodly number of risk factors. As we've seen, these risks are relatively small; but when added together, they begin to represent significantly increased odds of tumor development. Women in the United States and other industrialized countries have largely abandoned those traditional patterns of child-bearing and lactation which serve to protect the mammary gland. At the same time many of them have been consuming high-calorie fatty foods, getting too little exercise, and drifting toward obesity. Our chapter on risk factors is already overlong, yet it presents no more than a cursory survey of epidemiological findings. And we are just now arriving at the most important risk factor of all—the sole danger shared by almost all patients. That inevitable risk is simply **aging, the natural process of growing older**.

The average age at diagnosis for American breast cancer patients hovers somewhere in the early sixties.[128] But you'd never suspect this fact from glancing at the articles about breast cancer in newspapers and popular magazines, whose full-color illustrations typically depict lithesome, semi-nude models in their late twenties or early thirties undergoing mammography or practicing breast self-examination. Of course, relatively few women in this age bracket will receive the diagnosis. Let's briefly refer to some incidence statistics released by the National Cancer Institute. According to this NCI data, only 2.4% of breast cancer cases occur in women under age 35. The incidence rate starts to climb in the next two decades of life, women aged 35 to 44 accounting for 11.4% of diagnosed cases, and those aged 45 to 54 for 16.8%. But altogether only 13.8% of breast cancer cases can be firmly classified as "early-onset"—that is, occurring in women under age 45. And postmenopausal women probably account for about 75% of

disease incidence. The NCI reports that 69.3% of cases are diagnosed in women aged 55 or older. The most dangerous years fall between the ages of 65 and 74; approximately one quarter of all cases—25.4%—occur in this decade.[129]

It is not surprising that growing older is the predominant risk factor for breast cancer, as it is for most malignancies. The effects of aging are clear enough. Our individual cells lose their marvelous powers of self-repair and flawless duplication. We might speculate that both aging and cancer occur largely because our cells can no longer repair errors in their DNA. Mutations would thus gradually accumulate in an aging population of susceptible somatic cells, becoming ingrained parts of the genetic repertoire. Eventually the cells' nuclear machinery would spin out of control; and the affected cellular population would enter that second childhood we call cancer, a "senile dementia" characterized by needless reproduction and disorderly new growth.

The above scenario is applicable to all late-onset malignancies. But there are two ways in which breast cancers tend to differ from other adult tumors. First of all, regardless of whether the patients are young or old, mammary tumors display wide discrepancies in clinical behavior. Two tissue specimens examined under a pathologist's microscope may look identical; but the deformed cells from one tumor will behave in an almost benign fashion, with limited invasion and no metastasis, while the similar-looking cells from the other tumor will prove devastatingly metastatic. Secondly, unlike malignancies of the colon and prostate, breast cancers claim a substantial number of younger patients. Given the high prevalence of these tumors, that small government statistic for early-onset cases (13.8%) means that upwards of 30,000 American women under age 45 are currently being diagnosed *each year*. The disease strikes a few women in their twenties, and as we've seen, the incidence rate rises steadily in women over age 35.

Valid generalizations about breast cancer are hard to come by; but we may tentatively state that early-onset cases usually follow a more aggressive pattern than those which present later. This rule admits of endless individual exceptions. Patients in their thirties may have curable node-negative tumors, while those in their seventies may have metastatic disease as an initial presentation. As a group, however, patients aged 35 and younger have the lowest five-year survival of any age bracket. The percentage surviving five years after diagnosis (70.3%) is quite high compared to patients with some other serious malignancies—(if only the five-year statistics for brain, lung, and pancreatic cancers were half as good!)—but this percentage is *low* for breast malignancies.[130] The increased aggressiveness of early-onset tumors may be partially due to the fact that mammary cells, like other cells, duplicate more rapidly in younger bodies, and that this greater mitotic activity stands to be sustained after any malignant transformation. But early-onset tumors often reveal adverse genetic alterations, notably those inherited mutations in *p53* and *BRCA1*, which are seen less frequently in late-onset cases. Younger patients are also more likely to have tumors which are hormone receptor-negative. The nature of the mutations which deprive mammary cells of their receptor proteins for estrogen and progesterone is not fully understood; we do know that receptor-negative tumors will grow even in the absence of these hormones and that they tend to behave more aggressively than receptor-positive tumors.[131]

Breast cancer in younger women is tragic. In various ways the disease exacts disproportionate tolls among this patient minority. More potential years of life stand to be lost, and that loss stands to be felt more deeply by family, friends, and society.

Chapter Six

Estrogen Replacement Therapy

When speaking of hormones, physicians and researchers frequently use the modifiers **endogenous** and **exogenous**. The former term indicates that the hormones in question are generated by the human body itself (from the Greek *endon*, "within"); the latter, that the hormones or hormone-like substances are not made by the body, but are being consumed as drugs or foodstuffs (from the Greek *exo*, "without"). A century ago medical science knew very little about hormones; adrenalin, the first to be characterized, was not isolated until 1901. The discovery of hormones and of ways to produce them ranks as one of the greatest pharmaceutical success stories, rivaling the development of antibiotics. Initially we learned how to extract natural hormones from the organs, blood, or urine of lesser mammals, and then how to synthesize the chemical equivalents of various hormones in the laboratory. More recently, recombinant DNA technology has enabled us to insert the genes encoding for human hormones into colonies of receptive bacteria, which will evermore secrete the requisite molecules.

No one would quibble about some prescriptions for exogenous hormones. Insulin, available from animal sources (pig pancreases) since 1922, has saved the lives of millions of diabetics. Recombinant growth hormone, available since the late 1980s, has helped thousands of abnormally short children to grow taller. Of course, relatively few people in the general population are destined to be insulin-dependent diabetics or dwarfs. The market for exogenous hormones was to expand exponentially when it came to include hormonal therapy to relieve those menopausal symptoms caused by estrogen deficiency, and hormonal contraception to prevent unwanted pregnancies. Pharmaceutical companies, sensing profits, have long concentrated their promotional efforts on these two interventions. Almost all women could be potential customers, from puberty onward. But estrogen replacement therapy and birth control pills were sure to be more controversial than insulin injections, because neither pregnancy nor the menopause is a disease of any kind, certainly not a lethal one. Epidemiologists have understandably worried about carcinogenesis, because cancers of the female reproductive system—those of the breast, ovaries, and endometrium—are clearly related to hormonal stimulation. When exogenous estrogens are given to laboratory mice, mammary tumors are the usual result, and not just in females. Male mice given estrogens also develop breast cancers.

DES Ought to be "A Caution"

Estrogen and progesterone were not isolated and studied until the 1920s. In the 1930s estrogen extracts taken from animal ovaries were already being used to combat menopausal symptoms, but not widely. These natural estrogens had severe limitations— they were expensive to obtain, and since they could not survive a passage through the acidic stomach, they had to be injected. In 1938 a nonsteroidal chemical compound with pronounced estrogenic activity was synthesized in England. This new drug **diethylstilbestrol**, popularly known as **DES**, looked like a major breakthrough. It was cheap to manufacture and considerably more potent than the natural estrogens, and it could be taken by mouth, in convenient tablets.[1] DES was soon used to treat hot flashes and other menopausal symptoms; unfortunately, it became famous for another application, which proved to be particularly ill-conceived.

In the early 1940s researchers speculated that estrogen supplementation might be helpful in human pregnancy, preventing spontaneous abortions and premature labor. They had observed that pregnancies which end in miscarriage are typically characterized by low estrogen levels, rashly concluding that hormonal deficiencies were the probable cause of gestational failure. Today we know that the low estrogen levels are simply a symptom of distressed pregnancies; they do not cause the difficulties. But this mistaken hypothesis gained much currency in the 1940s; and it led some researchers, notably George and Olive Smith, a prominent husband-and-wife team at the Harvard University Medical School, to give DES to pregnant women. The Smiths quickly published several studies which seemed to indicate that DES prevented miscarriages. Today we would charitably characterize these studies as biased, confounded, and devoid of statistical

power; at the time they looked like scientifically sound experiments demonstrating the benefits of yet another wonder drug. In 1947 the Food and Drug Administration approved the use of DES to prevent the "accidents of pregnancy." Aggressive marketing ensued, as various pharmaceutical companies offered the drug under competing brand names. The postwar Baby Boom was already underway, and DES meant easy profits.

By the early 1950s better designed studies than the ones the Smiths had conducted began to provide evidence that DES therapy had no value in preventing miscarriages. The pharmaceutical companies naturally preferred to believe the earlier research. DES marketing continued unabated, sometimes including totally unsubstantiated claims. In 1957 an advertisement in a leading gynecological journal urged DES as "routine prophylaxis in ALL pregnancies," the sure-fire way to "bigger and stronger babies."[2] Busy obstetricians, when they found time to read the medical literature, weren't sure which studies to believe. The drug companies not only kept the doctors' mailboxes filled with brochures touting DES, but they sent out teams of glib salesmen who relentlessly pitched this product to the unsuspecting practitioners. In the 1950s and 1960s DES was liberally prescribed for millions of pregnant American women; no one knows exactly how many.

The drug's hidden dangers did not come to light until 1970 and 1971, when alert physicians in Boston and New York noticed a highly unusual clustering of clear-cell adenocarcinoma of the vagina. All these new cases had occurred in young women in their teens and twenties. Hitherto this extremely rare cancer had almost exclusively afflicted postmenopausal women. Epidemiologists rushed to the hospitals reporting this strange epidemic; and within a few days they had— like John Snow—found the solution to the puzzle. The mothers of the unfortunate young women had taken DES during pregnancy; at least in these cases, the drug had adversely affected the developing genital organs of female embryos. Suddenly the former wonder drug began to look like a dangerous carcinogen—did the children exposed to DES *in utero* carry silent time bombs ticking away toward malignancy?

Cancer researchers and public health officials now questioned the wisdom of other DES applications. For over two decades, cattle ranchers and poultry producers had been feeding the inexpensive estrogenic compound to their livestock, finding that it made for juicier beef and plumper, tenderer chickens. No one really knew how much DES remained in the processed meat, or whether these residues would in any way affect consumers. On college campuses DES tablets had gained popularity as a "morning-after" contraceptive, a postcoital medication which could sufficiently disrupt the endometrial surface so as to prevent implantation by a fertilized ovum. No one really knew how effective DES was for this purpose, or whether it would have unanticipated side effects which might not appear until years later.

By 1980 DES had been banned, both in human pregnancies and in animal husbandry. The drug remained in use principally as a second-line hormonal therapy for metastatic prostate cancer. It is doubtful that a single pregnancy was helped by DES; the tally of persons harmed by its indiscriminate administration may never be complete. In the mid-1980s DES daughters—(i.e., young women who had been exposed to the drug *in utero*)—were estimated to have one chance in a thousand of developing vaginal carcinoma by age 35. These women also had a much higher incidence of reproductive tract abnormalities, including strange "T-shaped" uteri and misshapen fallopian tubes. As a

group they were more likely to have difficulties becoming pregnant and in carrying their babies to term.[3] DES mothers (those who took the drug during pregnancy) have a slightly elevated risk of breast cancer, about 40% or 50% higher than other women, which does not become apparent "until at least twenty years after exposure."[4] In 1995 a survey of DES sons born at the Chicago Lying-in Hospital in 1951 and 1952 found that they were as fertile as other men, but were three times more likely to have genital malformations.[5] At present we do not know whether DES daughters and sons will eventually reveal elevated rates of late-onset breast and prostate tumors.

THE FOUNTAIN OF YOUTH?
Premarin® and Dr. Wilson's Book

DES has given us a cautionary example of a hormonal intervention which was officially approved by regulatory agencies and aggressively marketcd before we had any knowledge of the drug's long-term effects. Unlike DES, estrogen replacement therapy and oral contraceptives involve hormonal medications which actually work for the indicated applications. They do what they're supposed to do—that is, relieve menopausal symptoms and prevent unwanted pregnancies—and they do it quite effectively. But like DES these products were governmentally sanctioned, widely advertised, and liberally prescribed for many years before scientists had acquired sufficient knowledge of their long-term effects, especially those pertaining to the induction of malignancies. Fortunately, with these products we seem to have been lucky, perhaps more lucky than we should have expected. Let's begin by reviewing the history of estrogen replacement therapy.

In the 1950s American medicine cabinets bulged with a plethora of estrogenic products—pills, nasal sprays, nostrums, facial creams. Nobody worried much about dosage or side effects. Estrogen was supposed to be good for middle-aging women—get it where you could and stay young! Considering this jumbled grab bag of remedies, we can perhaps appreciate the single product which began to dominate the American market in the 1960s. **Premarin**, a trademark of Ayerst Laboratories (later Wyeth-Ayerst), offered **conjugated equine estrogens** in convenient pills. For our purposes it's enough to say that "conjugated" means that the estrogens have been processed so that they could be taken by mouth and still retain some biological activity after the harsh gastrointestinal passage. "Equine" refers to the source of these estrogens; they were extracted from the urine of pregnant mares, an undeniably natural if not exactly aesthetic origin. In 1995, as Wyeth-Ayerst's patent for its popular product expired, the company tried to fend off cheaper generic versions by advertisements reminding physicians that there was nothing like Premarin: "A complex blend of estrogens . . . unique manufacturing process . . . costs the patient only about 36 cents a day." Estrogen replacement therapy could hardly be simpler; one of the familiar maroon-colored pills in the 0.625 milligram dosage, taken daily, sufficed for most patients' complaints. But Wyeth-Ayerst also produced Premarin pills in four other dose levels (0.3, 0.9, 1.25, and 2.5 mg), as well as a Premarin vaginal cream "in a nonliquefying base." By 1995 the company could boast that over thirty billion pills had been manufactured "without a single recall."[6]

The growing popularity of estrogen replacement therapy in the 1960s owed much to the new ease of administration and a standardized product, as exemplified by Premarin; but a Brooklyn gynecologist named

Robert A. Wilson also had a lot to do with it.[7] Dr. Wilson emerged as America's leading propagandist for estrogen replacement. For him, the menopause was a deficiency disease caused by a shortage of this hormone. Not only could it be alleviated by exogenous estrogen, it could be in effect *cured*. Wilson advocated hormone therapy beginning as early as age 30; by age 40 almost every woman should be medicated. In a stream of articles churned out for *Look*, *Vogue*, and other popular magazines, Wilson reported that supplemental estrogen made for mental alertness and emotional equilibrium, that it banished acne and the blues, that it kept the skin lovely and the hair radiant, and put the torso in good form. The highpoint of his crusade came in 1966 with the publication of *Feminine Forever*. In this bestselling book Wilson depicted the menopause as "the death of femininity." Postmenopausal women seemed to be shuffling along, gray, tired, and unobservant. But once they took estrogen, they were "restored" and strode boldly into the future.

Wilson's writings reeked of the pitchman's hyperbole, oversimplifying the aging process and overstating the benefits of estrogen replacement; but they persuaded many women. Other women, then as now, were skeptical of self-confident male physicians who urged estrogen on their female patients, but who would never dream of taking hormones themselves. This suspicion of paternalistic complacency is not altogether warranted. Aging men lose testicular function and testosterone production gradually, over a period of several decades. Aging women lose ovarian function and the associated hormones fairly rapidly, within several years. When men are suddenly deprived of their sex hormones through accident, castration, or drug therapy, they also experience vasomotor symptoms (hot flashes).

Estrogen replacement therapy cannot

serve as a fountain of youth. Claims by Dr. Wilson and others that it could keep the skin and hair radiantly youthful were excessive, as was the idea that it could prevent depression and the loss of intellectual acumen. It can control hot flashes, and it does prevent the rapid atrophy of the female genital tract. Deprived of estrogen, the cellular lining of the vagina quickly becomes thin, inelastic, and fragile. Nature really did not intend that postmenopausal women would engage in reproduction, and for them the reproductive act (sexual intercourse) becomes increasingly difficult. Estrogen therapy helps to relieve the ensuing vaginal dryness and itching, and to maintain an adequate degree of lubrication and elasticity. The cells of the adjacent urinary tract are also negatively affected by estrogen deprivation. Those postmenopausal women who have low estrogen levels are more prone to urethral and kidney infections, as well as to loss of bladder control. Supplemental estrogen helps to prevent these problems.

Endometrial Cancer:
The Most Likely Carcinogenesis

Dollar sales of estrogens increased fourfold between 1962 and 1973, principally owing to a growing use of Premarin. At the time no one had any firm evidence that conjugated estrogens could promote human malignancies. Today it seems incredible that scientists and physicians could have overlooked the obvious danger that estrogen therapy poses to the endometrium, the lining of the uterus. As we've seen in Chapter Four, estrogen spurs endometrial cells into mitotic activity. In premenopausal women the endometrium doubles in thickness during the estrogenic follicular phase (first half) of the menstrual cycle. Such a proliferation of normal cells is

called **hyperplasia**: this condition often predisposes to subsequent malignant transformation. But endometrial cancers do not usually occur in premenopausal women, because rising progesterone levels during the luteal phase (second half) of the menstrual cycle slow down the mitotic activity and stabilize the endometrium. Then at the end of the cycle, as the levels of both estrogen and progesterone fall sharply, the thickened cellular lining degenerates and sloughs away as menstrual discharge. Menstruation thus removes the endometrial hyperplasia on a monthly basis, preventing any progression of these cells toward malignancy. Postmenopausal women no longer have this protective mechanism; and for them estrogen, whether endogenous or exogenous, tends to promote unrelieved hyperplasia.

By the early 1970s American tumor registries had begun to report a mysterious increase in the number of endometrial cancers. Suspecting the recent boom in estrogen replacement therapy, epidemiologists quickly went to work. Two case-control studies published in the *New England Journal of Medicine* on December 4, 1975, alerted physicians—and greatly alarmed estrogen users. A study done at the University of Washington found that postmenopausal women who took estrogen had a risk of endometrial cancer four-and-a-half times greater than that of age-matched nonusers. The second study, coming from the Kaiser Permanente Medical Center in Los Angeles, pointed out that the risk rose considerably with longer durations of therapy. Compared to nonusers, postmenopausal women who took conjugated estrogens from one to 4.9 years had a relative risk of 5.6 for endometrial cancer. Women who took estrogens for seven years or more had a risk almost fourteen times greater than comparable nonusers.[8] In 1976 the Food and Drug Administration issued a warning citing the danger of endometrial cancer when estrogen is given to postmenopausal women with intact uteri. Additional epidemiological investigations simply confirmed the salient finding—viz., estrogen therapy constitutes a large risk factor for endometrial cancer, of a magnitude comparable to the risk that cigarette smoking poses for lung cancer. In 1995 a "meta-analysis" of prior studies reported a relative risk of 9.5 after ten years or more of unopposed estrogen supplementation.[9]

Estrogen-Progestin Combos

In the late 1970s hormone replacement therapy was at an impasse. Estrogen could be given safely only to those postmenopausal women who had undergone hysterectomies and thus could not develop endometrial cancer. What could physicians do for other postmenopausal women? The answer seemed clear—add a progestin (a synthetic version of progesterone) to the exogenous estrogen, and thereby create a regimen which would mimic menstruation and efficiently remove endometrial hyperplasia. By the early 1980s such combo therapy became commonplace, the progestin element often being supplied by 10 milligram tablets of **Provera**, Upjohn's brand name for medroxyprogesterone acetate. As in the natural menstrual cycle, the estrogen (usually Premarin) came first, then the progestin, and then several days without hormones to induce withdrawal bleeding (endometrial shedding). But there was no standard regimen, nor any general agreement as to how often the "menstruation" needed to be induced. Was it sufficient to give a progestin every three months, or did you have to do it monthly? A British study published in the *New England Journal of Medicine* in 1986 recommended twelve or thirteen days of progestin administration every month as "the optimal duration

to protect against endometrial abnormalities"; the authors cautioned that "a dose of progestin that is adequate for one person may be insufficient for another."[10] Brian W. Walsh and Isaac Schiff of the Harvard Medical School remind us that the most common American regimen consisted of conjugated equine estrogens, "0.625 mg given daily," and medroxyprogesterone acetate, "10 mg given for the first 13 calendar days of each month." Most women taking this regimen experienced withdrawal bleeding by the twentieth calendar day.[11]

Not everybody was thrilled by the new therapy. The progestin addition often produced the same unpleasant effects that natural progesterone causes in many premenopausal women. Older patients on a combo regimen might complain of breast swelling and tenderness, abdominal bloating, headaches, and generalized malaise. Quite a few patients with intact uteri were appalled that hormone replacement therapy now began to look like "menstruation forever" rather than the promised "femininity forever." However tactfully physicians might convey the necessary information—("You will continue to cycle")—many women in their fifties and sixties did not relish the prospect of shopping for tampons. But the estrogen-progestin regimens worked; they greatly reduced the danger from endometrial cancer. In the 1980s the incidence of this malignancy fell sharply as physicians became more cautious about hormone replacement, shying away from the higher dosages of estrogen or prescribing a progestin combination. Evidence of the combo's effectiveness came from a cohort study done in Sweden which had kept track of 23,244 postmenopausal women receiving hormone replacement. Those who took a progestin along with the estrogen did not reveal an elevated risk of endometrial cancer. For those who took estrogen alone, the risk jumped "twofold to threefold after three or more years of use."[12]

Estrogen and Breast Cancer:
Pinning Down a Small Risk

The cancer risk which estrogen replacement therapy poses to the mammary gland is not nearly as great as that which it poses to the endometrium. We know this for a fact. But when the pharmaceutical companies and gynecologists began to promote supplemental estrogen in the 1960s, no one had any plausible data on the question of mammary carcinogenesis. The first study laying claim to even modest statistical power did not appear until 1976. Robert Hoover of the National Cancer Institute headed a team of researchers who followed 1,891 Kentucky women "given conjugated estrogens for the menopause." Compared to the general population, this cohort proved to have an overall risk of 1.3 for breast cancer, a modest 30% elevation. But Hoover et al observed that the risk rose progressively with longer durations of therapy: after fifteen years it stood at 2.0, a 100% increase.[13] In 1980 Ronald K. Ross and other epidemiologists at the University of Southern California looked at the breast cancer incidence among postmenopausal women living in two retirement communities near Los Angeles. Women with intact ovaries whose lifetime consumption of conjugated estrogens totaled more than 1,500 milligrams—(that is, slightly over six-and-a-half years of the daily 0.625 mg pills)—had a relative risk of 2.5, up 150% compared to nonusers. A considerably higher risk was detected among longtime estrogen users who not only had intact ovaries but also had "a history of surgically confirmed benign breast disease." In this subgroup "the risk ratio rose to 5.7 relative to nonusers with normal breasts."[14] These findings indicate that

exogenous estrogen can amplify the effects of hormones produced by the body's endocrine glands, and that it may be more risky to breasts prone to abnormal proliferative growths.

In 1981 Louise A. Brinton and other epidemiologists at the National Cancer Institute published a noteworthy case-control study of postmenopausal estrogen use and breast cancer risk. The study population of 881 diagnosed cases and 863 controls was drawn from the 280,000 women enrolled in the nationwide Breast Cancer Detection Demonstration Project. The overall risk among ever-users of estrogen proved to be quite small—1.24, up only 24% compared to nonusers—but it rose among women who had consumed larger doses for extended periods. The risk associated with the 2.5 mg Premarin pills seemed to be about twice as great as that associated with the 0.625 mg dosage. Like Ross et al, Brinton and her co-workers detected increased risk among estrogen users who had undergone prior breast biopsies, but their most striking finding pertained to bilateral oophorectomy. The surgical removal of both ovaries had long been recognized as protective, reducing breast cancer risk by perhaps 50% to 100%. However, the oophorectomized women in this study who took estrogen had an overall relative risk of 1.54, a 54% elevation. Their risk climbed sharply with increasing durations of therapy, reaching elevations of 100% to 200% after ten years or more.[15]

In the late 1980s the most compelling evidence that exogenous hormones can directly affect the mammary gland came not from epidemiologists, but from radiologists. Paul C. Stomper led a team of these physicians who followed fifty postmenopausal women recruited at Boston's famed Brigham and Women's Hospital. High-resolution mammograms were taken of the patients' breasts just before they began hormonal replacement therapy, and then "at approximately one-year intervals thereafter." For twelve of these patients (24%), the hormones produced decided changes which were visible on successive mammograms. The translucent breasts characteristically seen on postmenopausal mammograms soon began to resemble the dense glandular breasts of premenopausal women. Cysts formed in the breasts of three subjects—"a premenopausal phenomenon." Noticeably increased density of the mammary epithelium developed in several women given estrogen alone, but the combination of estrogen and a progestin proved more effective in bringing about the glandular flowering. One 69-year-old woman whose before-treatment mammograms were translucent showed progressive increases in density on mammograms taken at 13 and at 27 months after starting estrogen-progestin therapy.[16] The radiological experiment conducted by Stomper et al demonstrates that low-dose exogenous hormones can induce mitotic activity in the postmenopausal mammary gland, even in women nearing age 70.

How Risky Is that Combo?

Epidemiological studies trying to determine the impact of estrogen-progestin regimens on breast cancer risk lagged a good decade behind those focusing solely on estrogen replacement. In the 1980s many researchers continued to speak casually of progestins "opposing" the effects of estrogen. The implication of opposition was altogether misleading. We now know that while progesterone counteracts estrogen's mitotic stimuli in the premenopausal endometrium, it strongly reinforces them in the premenopausal breast. But at the time the effect of conjugated estrogens on the postmenopausal mammary gland had not been adequately

assessed, and even less was known about what progestins might do.

The first sizable study to consider the estrogen and progestin combination held nothing but good news. R. Don Gambrell, Jr., and his co-workers looked at the breast cancer incidence among 5,563 postmenopausal women seen at the hospital of Lackland Air Force Base, Texas, between 1975 and 1981. In 1983 Gambrell et al enthusiastically reported that the use of conjugated estrogens did not increase the risk of breast cancer in this cohort, and that estrogen-progestin therapy reduced that risk by 70%! These researchers recommended that a progestin be routinely included in estrogen replacement regimens, even in those prescribed for "patients who have had a hysterectomy."[17] Naysayers quickly detected all manner of epidemiological sins in the Gambrell study, alleging that it failed to control for confounding factors and that it was subject to selection bias. Moreover, argued the critics, the estrogen-progestin arm lacked sufficient size to generate statistical power, and the follow-up was much too short.[18] Obviously, no conclusions about the hormone combo's relation to breast cancer risk should have been based on the flawed study by Gambrell et al, but for the rest of the decade it remained a source of information frequently cited in textbooks and medical journals. By 1990 the proportion of American women on hormone replacement whose regimens included a progestin had risen to 30%; the combo was becoming popular.[19]

A major study disputing the conclusions reached by Gambrell et al did not appear until six years later. In 1989 the *New England Journal of Medicine* published a cohort study of 23,244 women living in or near Uppsala, Sweden, who had been receiving hormone replacement therapy. The breast cancer risk detected for estrogen users proved to be very similar to that reported by several American studies. It started out small—1.1 for ever-users, up only 10%—and it grew with increasing duration of treatment. After nine years it stood at 1.7, elevated 70% above the nonuser baseline. But the Swedish study detected a much larger risk among women who had used estrogen and a progestin in combination. After six years or more these women had a relative risk of 4.4, up 340% above the baseline. The authors concluded that the breast cancer risk associated with estrogen therapy "is not prevented and may even be increased by the addition of progestins."[20]

In 1995 the venerable Nurses' Health Study reported weighty data which tended to corroborate the Swedish findings. Graham A. Colditz and his Harvard colleagues could claim an impressive follow-up on postmenopausal nurses receiving hormone replacement therapy—89,427 person-years on those taking only conjugated estrogens, and 28,946 person-years on those taking estrogens plus a progestin. The relative risk of breast cancer among current hormone users was modestly elevated—1.32 (up 32%) for those taking estrogen alone, and 1.41 (up 41%) for those taking the combination. As in other studies, the risk increased with long-term use. Women aged 55 to 59 who had taken hormone replacement therapy for five years or more revealed a relative risk of 1.54 (up 54%). For women aged 60 to 64 with five or more years of therapy, that risk was 1.71 (up 71%). While adding a progestin to the estrogen did not reduce the breast cancer risk, neither did the addition appear to triple that risk as the Swedish study had implied. Colditz et al cautiously observed that their findings "do not support the use of progestin by women who have undergone hysterectomy."[21]

Any Benefits for the Heart?

The therapeutic benefits of supplemental estrogen for hot flashes and vaginal dryness become rapidly apparent; but since no one dies of menopausal symptoms, this application cannot be said to extend life expectancy. Estrogen replacement therapy would have greater utility if it helped to prevent cardiovascular disease, the principal killer of postmenopausal women. In 1991 Elizabeth Barrett-Connor and Trudy L. Bush reviewed the growing body of epidemiological literature in the *Journal of the American Medical Association*, concluding that "most, but not all, studies show around a 50% reduction in risk of a coronary event in women using unopposed oral estrogen." Barrett-Connor and Bush judiciously recommended that, "until better data are available," the prescription of estrogen solely as cardiovascular prophylaxis might be reserved for "women at high risk—particularly women who have high LDL cholesterol or low HDL cholesterol."[22]

The idea that estrogen could prevent cardiovascular disease grew out of the elementary observation that before the menopause women are only about one-fifth as likely to suffer heart attacks as age-matched men, while after the menopause they quickly catch up, so that the incidence rate for both sexes becomes similar. In animal experiments done in the 1950s, chickens fed high-cholesterol diets did not develop clogged, atherosclerotic coronary arteries if they were also given estrogen. However, a human trial conducted in the late 1960s spectacularly failed to support the hypothesis. Men who had suffered previous heart attacks were given high-dose conjugated estrogens (2.5 mg per day) in the hope of preventing recurrences. But not only did these men fail to achieve a reduction in the number of coronary events, but they experienced a greatly increased number of thromboembolic events (blood clots), especially in the lungs. Estrogen was no vascular Drano. Brian W. Walsh and Isaac Schiff of the Harvard Medical School remind us that estrogens taken orally, whether natural or synthetic, have noticeable effects on hepatic (liver) metabolism. The beneficial actions include "increasing HDL production and increasing LDL catabolism." One negative effect is the increased production of blood coagulation factors.[23] High-dose estrogen can promote pathological coagulation in susceptible persons, as amply illustrated by the excess pulmonary (lung) embolisms and occlusive strokes recorded back in the 1960s by the male coronary patients and by young women taking the early hormone-rich oral contraceptives. Thus any liver disorder which might hamper that organ from metabolizing estrogen, or any history of abnormal blood clotting, are definite counterindications to estrogen replacement therapy.

There has never been a big clinical trial which demonstrated that exogenous estrogen reduces the incidence of cardiovascular disease in postmenopausal women. In the 1990s we were still drawing tentative conclusions based on epidemiological studies which counted the heart attacks and other vascular events among different groups of estrogen users and nonusers. Whatever their methodologies, these studies had pronounced limitations. They were dependent on recall data, provided after the fact by the subjects themselves. The estrogen users were not randomly assigned to therapy, but self-selected or encouraged by their physicians. The type of estrogen used, the dose, and the duration of treatment varied widely. Verification of details was difficult, but the main problem with these epidemiological comparisons lay with suspected confounding factors. Aren't estrogen users less prone to cardiovascular

disease for reasons unrelated to hormone replacement therapy? To begin with, the users are more likely than nonusers to be lean and under a physician's regular care (obesity and the lack of medical care being powerfully associated with elevated disease incidence). It has also been suggested that estrogen users are better educated, more affluent, and more health conscious—that they exercise more—and that they are less likely to have diabetes. Any one of these factors, or any combination of them, could account for the protective effect supposedly generated by estrogen pills—and only an epidemiological Solomon could design a study which would adequately control for all of them.

On October 24, 1985, the *New England Journal of Medicine* published reports from two major epidemiological enterprises, whose contradictory findings demonstrated the numerous pitfalls inherent in this science. The famous Nurses' Health Study reported that postmenopausal women currently taking estrogen had a relative risk of 0.3 for coronary disease, 70% lower than nonusers.[24] The equally famous Framingham Heart Study reported that postmenopausal women who had previously taken estrogen revealed "over a 50 percent elevated risk of cardiovascular morbidity and more than a twofold risk for cerebrovascular disease."[25] *Talk about controversy!* In the next decade, however, subsequent studies of various kinds tipped the balance of medical opinion in favor of estrogen supplementation. Researchers at the University of Pittsburgh kept track of "541 healthy, initially premenopausal women 42 to 50 years of age," seeking to determine how the menopausal transition affected their risk factors for cardiovascular disease. Blood tests on women who had recently experienced a natural menopause revealed declining levels of high-density lipoprotein cholesterol (the HDL thought to be protective) and rising levels of low-density lipoprotein cholesterol (the LDL thought to predispose to disease). In newly menopausal women who took estrogen, the levels of HDL and LDL did not change; they remained similar to those found in age-matched premenopausal controls.[26] Estrogen therapy thus appeared to forestall the unfavorable effects that menopause has on lipid metabolism.

Some researchers felt that estrogen exerted a protective effect by acting directly on the endothelial cells which line the blood vessels. Jay M. Sullivan and other cardiologists at the University of Tennessee tried to determine how estrogen use might affect the risk of **stenosis**, the gradual closing of blood vessels (from the Greek word *stenos*, meaning "narrow"). Sullivan et al kept track of 2,188 postmenopausal women who had undergone diagnostic angiography at a Memphis hospital. Angiograms are X-rays of the coronary arteries made after an injection of an opaque contrast agent—they reveal the location of any stenosis or blockage. In this group the women who had been taking estrogen proved 56% less likely to have coronary artery stenosis than comparable nonusers.[27] Among the women diagnosed with coronary stenosis, those who took estrogen had significantly longer survival than comparable nonusers.[28]

The Harvard epidemiologists conducting the Nurses' Health Study stayed busy, continually re-analyzing their growing mountains of data. In 1987 they issued a revised report stating that estrogen replacement therapy did not significantly alter the cardiovascular risk level of those nurses who had experienced a natural menopause, but that it was protective for those who had undergone bilateral oophorectomy (removal of both ovaries and hence immediate menopause).[29] A ten-year follow-up on the study was published in 1991. This time the Harvard team concluded that estrogen replacement therapy did indeed reduce cardiovascular risk factors,

both for "women with either natural or surgical menopause," though the anticipated benefit proved to be smaller than that which was originally proposed in 1985. Compared to nonusers, postmenopausal women currently taking the hormone had a relative risk of 0.56 for coronary disease, a 44% reduction.[30] In an editorial accompanying the Nurses' Health analysis, Lee Goldman and Anna N. A. Tosteson of the Brigham and Women's Hospital commented: "It is disappointing that we in medicine collectively have not made more progress toward resolving the clinical conundrum of postmenopausal estrogen replacement." Goldman and Tosteson emphasized that a definitive solution could save lives, citing current mortality estimates to make their point. American women between the ages 50 and 94 had approximately a 31% chance of dying from heart disease, but only a 2.8% chance of dying from breast cancer and a 0.7% chance of dying from endometrial cancer. Thus if estrogen replacement therapy really reduced cardiovascular mortality by 50%, it would still be a potent lifesaver for postmenopausal women even if it doubled the odds for fatal breast cancer and caused a fivefold increase in mortality from endometrial cancer.[31]

Subsequent analyses of data from the Framingham Heart Study also tended to support a role for estrogen in coronary disease prevention. In 1992 William Castelli, the study's director, told a reporter from *Time* magazine that he now regarded the evidence favoring estrogen supplementation as "overwhelming."[32] But no one knew what the best regimen might be, and some scientists were beginning to worry that adding a progestin to estrogen therapy might counteract the beneficial effects on lipid profiles. Unlike estrogen, progestins tend to lower the beneficial HDL cholesterol. Since the combined hormonal regimens did not become popular until the 1980s, the first studies attempting to define their effects on lipid profiles were not published until the following decade. In 1993 a survey of American women taking hormone replacement found that the estrogen-progestin combination "appears to be associated with a better profile than the use of estrogen alone."[33] And a Swedish study focusing on hormone users in the Uppsala area reported that added progestins did not seem to reduce the benefits associated with estrogen alone.[34] These epidemiological surveys lacked the mantle of scientific authority which can invest a well-designed clinical trial. Fortunately, the first results from the **Postmenopausal Estrogen/Progestin Interventions Trial** became available in 1995. The PEPI trial was randomized, double-blinded, and placebo-controlled. Neither the trial investigators nor the carefully screened participants knew who was taking what regimen, as all the pills looked alike. The objective of the PEPI trial was to document the effects of selected hormonal interventions on cardiovascular risk factors—HDL and LDL cholesterol, blood pressure, insulin levels, and fibrinogen (a blood protein which promotes clotting). PEPI tested a placebo (no hormonal intervention) against daily conjugated estrogens (Premarin in the 0.625 mg dose) and against three different estrogen-progestin combinations. The first of these combinations was the prevalent cyclic therapy—daily Premarin plus 10 mg medroxyprogesterone (MPA), supplied by Upjohn's brand Provera, for twelve calendar days each month. The second combination consisted of daily Premarin plus 2.5 mg of MPA daily, a regimen whose constant low-dose progestin minimizes withdrawal bleeding, breast tenderness, and other menstrual symptoms. The third combination consisted of a new cyclic therapy—daily Premarin as usual, but instead of the synthetic MPA, **micronized progesterone** (capsules supplied by Schering Plough) was

was taken on twelve calendar days.

The PEPI results, published after three years of follow-up, established that hormonal replacement therapy has beneficial effects on several standard indicators used to assess the risk of cardiovascular disease. The subjects' blood pressure and insulin levels were not affected by treatment assignment, whether to placebo or to one of the four hormonal regiments. But while the levels of the unfavorable markers LDL cholesterol and fibrinogen tended to rise in the placebo arm of the trial, they fell noticeably on all of the hormonal regimens. The PEPI investigators paid especial attention to HDL cholesterol, which they regarded as "the best predictor of coronary disease risk in women." HDL levels fell in women assigned to the placebo arm—an indication of increasing risk. But while these levels rose in all women receiving hormonal replacement, the degree of elevation varied among the four regimens. HDL levels rose the highest in women receiving estrogen alone; they did not rise nearly so high in women receiving the progestin MPA along with the estrogen. However, women receiving micronized progesterone (MP) with their estrogen fared almost as well as the women receiving estrogen alone—the difference in HDL levels between these two regimens was small. The PEPI investigators concluded that there are "significant losses with regard to HDL cholesterol when MPA is added to estrogen therapy." For postmenopausal women with intact uteri, "estrogen plus MP appears to spare the endometrium and to preserve the bulk of estrogen's favorable effects."[35]

Bernadine Healy, former director of the National Institutes of Health, hailed the report from the PEPI trial as "a wonderful beginning." At last there was solid evidence that "estrogen reduces key cardiovascular risk factors in women at a time when they become especially vulnerable to heart disease, namely, after fifty years of age."[36] It remained to be seen whether the favorable short-term improvement in lipid profiles would eventually be translated into a long-term reduction in mortality.

Estrogen Fights Osteoporosis

In the 1990s researchers were beginning to investigate whether exogenous estrogen could reduce the incidence of Alzheimer's disease and colon cancer. But there was only one disease for which estrogen replacement therapy had won general acceptance as a preventive measure—**osteoporosis**. What happens at a cellular level in this complex pathological disorder is not fully understood. However, the epidemiological signposts pointing toward osteoporosis are easy to read: familial (genetic) tendency, loss of the sex hormones at menopause, and aging, as well as such modifiable factors as faulty diet and inadequate exercise. The disease is also easy to diagnose—"porous bones" (just as the Latinate name clearly states), bones which have become thin, weak, and brittle. On X-rays osteoporotic bones seem abnormally translucent, owing to a loss of mineral content. But no one need be a radiologist or skilled clinician to recognize the symptoms of this disease in elderly people. Loss of height and a distorted spinal curvature result as the weakened osteoporotic vertebrae in the backbone yield to gravity's compressive forces or to a series of small asymptomatic fractures. Elderly women with osteoporosis are prone to **kyphosis** (Greek for "humpback"), that convex protuberance of the thoracic (upper) spine known in English as "the dowager's hump." Men also suffer from osteoporosis, but not as often, because they usually begin with larger and denser bones, and because they experience no abrupt curtailment of the sex hormones in midlife.

Most laypersons visualize bones as dry, dead, and inert, a misconception no doubt fueled by Halloween skeletons or by dusty fossils seen in museums. Bone is in fact moist, living tissue, built by and around several varieties of indwelling specialized cells called **osteocytes**. Like other connective tissues, bone is crisscrossed with collagen fibers, which endow it with tensile strength and resilience. Its hardness is due to its mineral deposits, principally of calcium and phosphate. There are two major categories of bone. **Cortical bone** is dense and compact; it provides the hard, smooth outer shell which we can feel beneath the skin. **Trabecular bone**, softer, fills the interior ; it is not solid, but resembles a kind of latticework or piece of Swiss cheese. Bony spicules known as **trabeculae** (Latin for "little beams") create a tiny labyrinth with innumerable vacant spaces. These spaces are soon filled with **bone marrow**, the stuff which continually manufactures the body's red and white cells.

Bones constitute the body's self-renewing framework or scaffolding; they also serve as its mineral reservoir, a savings bank in which deposits and withdrawals are constantly being made. In youth we all have favorable bank statements: the formation of new bone exceeds the resorption of the old, and mineralization (deposits) far surpasses demineralization (withdrawals). Peak bone mass is obtained around age thirty; thereafter we begin to run a deficit, losing perhaps half a percent of accumulated mass each year Trabecular bone is particularly affected; in adults about 25% is resorbed and replaced each year, as compared to a 3% turnover for cortical bone.[37] Numerous hormones come into play during bone formation and remodeling; estrogen has an indispensable role for both sexes. Women are adversely affected when the ovarian production of estrogen ceases. Immediately after the menopause, they may lose bone mass at a rate of 2% or 3% annually. The rate of loss varies from individual to individual, but the disintegrative process is inescapable.

What we know about the complications of osteoporosis was ably summarized by a Consensus Development Conference sponsored by the National Institutes of Health in 1984. That conference opened with a sobering statistic. Of those Americans who live to be ninety years old, 32% of the women and 17% of the men will suffer hip fractures, "most caused by osteoporosis." Only a few persons with osteoporotic hip fractures will recover normal mobility, and "mortality within one year approaches 20%."[38] Another common event is Colles' fracture—a transverse break in the radius (the smaller of the forearm bones), which typically occurs when an elderly person attempts to brake a fall with outstretched hands. Osteoporotic bones, once broken, do not heal well. These fractures lead to prolonged immobilization, which in turn promotes an additional loss of bone mass and a greatly increased likelihood of future fractures. In time, with repeated fractures and immobilizations, other vital bodily systems (heart, lungs, kidneys, immune response) will malfunction and hasten the patient's death. Osteoporosis is thus inevitably—although indirectly—lethal.

The Consensus Development Conference emphasized two probable causes of osteoporosis: "deficiency of estrogen and deficiency of calcium." The conference panelists displayed a remarkable unanimity regarding prophylaxis: "Estrogen replacement therapy is highly effective for preventing osteoporosis in women. Estrogen reduces bone resorption and retards or halts postmenopausal bone loss." The panel recommended that estrogen be given to women "whose ovaries are removed before age 50," and considered as an option for women who experience a natural menopause. Even low

doses, "such as 0.625 mg of conjugated equine estrogen," were deemed to provide significant protection: "The duration of estrogen therapy need not be limited." The conference panelists sang a comparable paean to calcium. Premenopausal women and postmenopausal women taking estrogen appeared to have "a daily requirement of about 1,000 mg of calcium," but postmenopausal women not taking estrogen were thought to need "about 1,500 mg daily." Recommendations for modest weight-bearing exercise to stimulate bone formation, and for vitamin D to facilitate intestinal absorption of calcium, rounded out the preventive strategies endorsed by this important conference.[39]

The 1984 consensus statement on osteoporosis was based on numerous epidemiological studies, but of course, there had been no clinical trials which conclusively demonstrated that estrogen therapy and calcium supplements really stave off the disease. Writing in the *New England Journal of Medicine* in 1993, Robert P. Heaney of Creighton University counted 43 studies of calcium intake and osteoporosis. Of these studies, 26 reported that added dietary calcium helped to preserve bone mass, but 16 failed to find an association. "In a Presidential election," Dr. Heaney observed, "such a majority would be considered a landslide; but for scientists, the 16 negative studies leave a nagging doubt. No one questions that if those 43 studies had involved the use of estrogen in postmenopausal women, all 43 would have been positive."[40] Estrogen is no wonder drug which mandates the formation of new bone, but at least it acts directly on the osteocytes which must do this work. Calcium is only a building material (one of several) used in bone construction. If the osteocytes aren't stimulated to the task, then all the added calcium will not accomplish much, except to increase the risk of painful *calculi* (kidney stones) lodging in the urinary tract.

Some plausible data on estrogen's protective effects came out of the long-running Framingham Heart Study, which recruited a cohort of 2,873 women between 1948 and 1951. By the mid-1980s a sizable portion of the Framingham cohort had reached those advanced ages when osteoporotic fractures begin to occur. The Framingham investigators now attempted to relate the incidence of hip fractures in this cohort to estrogen use. The mean age for a first hip fracture proved to be 75. Compared to nonusers, women in the cohort who had ever taken estrogen had a relative risk of 0.65 for hip fracture, a 35% reduction. But women who reported estrogen use "within the previous two years" had a risk of only 0.34, down 66% from the nonuser baseline. The Framingham team concluded that estrogen use appeared to protect against hip fractures, regardless of the type of menopause (natural or surgical). "Our findings also suggest that administering estrogens to older women, at least up to the age of 74, may be protective."[41]

In 1993 the Framingham investigators issued a report describing how past estrogen use had affected bone mineral density in 670 women from the cohort, whose ages ranged from 68 to 96 (mean age, 76). Only those women who had taken estrogen for seven years or more had noticeably increased bone density compared to nonusers. Long-term users under age 75 had on the average 11.2% greater bone mass, as measured in the spine, femur, and radius. But even seven years of previous therapy did not offer much protection to users over age 75: their bone density was "only 3.2% higher than in women who had never taken estrogens."[42] These findings seemed to indicate that the postmenopausal loss of bone mass quickly resumes once

estrogen is discontinued, and that short-term therapy to relieve menopausal symptoms will not affect the eventual probability of developing osteoporosis. In 1995 a report from the Osteoporotic Fractures Research Group, based on a survey of 9,704 American women aged 65 or older, implied that estrogen therapy cannot restore bone mineral density which has already been lost. In this cohort the protection against fractures was largely restricted to "current users who initiated estrogen replacement therapy early in menopause." Compared to nonusers, current users who began early achieved a 71% reduction in the risk of wrist fractures; but current users who began "more than five years after menopause" recorded only a 23% reduction. The study's authors recommended that estrogen replacement therapy be initiated early in the menopause and continued indefinitely.[43]

High-water Mark for Estrogen

The mid-1990s represented a high-water mark for exogenous estrogen in the United States, a time when the benefits of postmenopausal hormonal replacement seemed very great and the risks very small. American epidemiologists did not doubt that estrogen therapy tended to increase the risk of late-onset breast cancer, but there was no consensus as to the degree of risk elevation. The estimates given varied from study to study, with some reporting higher risks than others, or finding the risk elevation to be mainly confined to this or that subgroup. With a view to resolving these divergent assessments, Karen K. Steinberg and her colleagues at Atlanta's Centers for Disease Control performed a "meta-analysis," pooling the data from sixteen case-control studies of estrogen use and breast cancer. Their results can only be described as *reassuring*— there was no detectable increase in breast cancer risk until "after at least five years of estrogen use," and only a 30% increase after fifteen years of use.[44] Epidemiologists naturally wonder whether the consolidation of data from different studies, with contrasting methodologies and diverse groups of subjects, actually generates higher statistical power or really overcomes the ubiquitous specters of bias and confounding. But at least such pooling of data gives us a better grasp on the salient fact which has emerged from several decades of investigation—viz., postmenopausal estrogen therapy represents a risk factor for breast cancer, but it's not like pouring gasoline on a fire. The 1995 update from the Nurses' Health Study also yielded modest assessments of the risk involved, ranging from 32% to 71%. Elevations of this magnitude are similar to those associated with obesity and with alcohol consumption.[45] Since all three factors would seem to be principally mediated by estrogenic stimulation of the mammary gland, the long-term estrogen user who is considerably overweight and frequently consumes alcohol is no doubt compounding her small risks for breast cancer, piling one on top of another. But by themselves those low-dose pills of conjugated estrogens do not constitute a major risk factor, because they provide only a small fraction of the hormonal stimulus naturally provided by the ovaries of premenopausal women. Moreover, the epithelial cells in the postmenopausal breast do not respond to hormonal stimulation as vigorously as those in the premenopausal breast—mitotic rates diminish with age. Even the accumulated dosage of decades of estrogen therapy would appear to add only a small increment to the lifetime risk of breast cancer. As we've seen in Chapter Five, that risk is determined largely by the number of ovulatory cycles during adolescence and early adulthood.

In the mid-1990s health professionals began to speak about estrogen replacement with unprecedented assurance. The statisticians designing the **Women's Health Initiative** estimated that the thousands of trial participants assigned to its estrogen treatment arm would experience "annual increases of 2.1 deaths from breast cancer and 1.2 deaths from endometrial cancer" as well as "annual decreases of 25.6 deaths from heart disease and 14.7 cases of hip fracture."[46] The odds of mortality, *as calculated before the trial began*, were most heavily weighted in favor of hormone replacement! There had never been a stronger counterindication to estrogen therapy than a previous diagnosis of breast cancer. Every textbook and every Premarin flier cautioned against prescribing the hormone in cases of "known or suspected mammary carcinoma." Did not everybody know that estrogen would spur the malignant cells to divide, and possibly even to metastasize? But in the 1990s some cancer specialists began to argue that this prohibition was excessive. One reason for the turnabout in opinion lay in the growing numbers of young patients—women in their thirties and forties—being given adjuvant chemotherapy. Most chemo regimens induced ovarian failure, sending these patients into the menopause a decade ahead of schedule. Did the treatment better the odds of surviving breast cancer, only to increase overall mortality by placing patients at the highest risk for premature heart attacks and hip fractures? In 1992 oncologists at Houston's M. D. Anderson Cancer Center initiated a clinical trial in which previously diagnosed breast cancer patients were randomly assigned to daily estrogen (Premarin pills in the 0.625 mg dosage) or to no intervention (control group). Admission to this trial was restricted to subjects with estrogen receptor-negative tumors and "no evidence of disease for at least two years."[47] In 1994 physicians affiliated with the Eastern Cooperative Oncology

Group leaped on the barricades in the *Journal of the American Medical Association*, calling for a large clinical trial ("thousands of women") to resolve this issue.[48] Intelligent decision making was, as usual in breast cancer therapeutics, caught in a bind between the time-honored taboo and enthusiastic revisionism. Physicians in private practice were still reluctant to prescribe estrogen for breast cancer patients: if fears about hormone-fueled metastatic disease had diminished somewhat, worries about malpractice litigation remained quite strong.

New Pharmaceutical Wrinkles

The wave of optimism in the early 1990s brought with it several products which promised to make hormone replacement therapy more convenient and more effective. The CIBA Pharmaceutical Company pioneered an estrogen patch which adhered to the skin and delivered a steady dose of hormone for days at a time. Touted as an "estradiol transdermal system," **Estraderm®** was promoted with slick advertisements depicting elegantly dressed older women who radiated youthful desirability. The ideal held out by Robert A. Wilson's *Feminine Forever* seemed to have been realized! "Now the change of life doesn't have to change yours," proclaimed one Estraderm advertisement in 1990. "Throughout the menopausal years you can, and should, expect to be as vital, healthy and attractive as ever."[49] The new estradiol patches were more expensive than the familiar Premarin pills; but since the absorbed hormone went directly into the bloodstream, they possibly affected hepatic (liver) metabolism less than conjugated estrogens taken by mouth. Estraderm might thus have been a better choice for those postmenopausal women with less than optimal liver function or with a tendency toward blood clotting.

Wyeth-Ayerst, the maker of market-leading Premarin, did not rest on past laurels. In the spring of 1995 this firm began to promote its new product **Prempro®** as hormone replacement therapy for postmenopausal women with intact uteri. The brand was distinguished for its convenience rather than for pharmaceutical innovation. Prempro offered a continuous estrogen-progestin regimen. The daily Premarin pills (0.625 mg) were packaged together with daily low-dose tablets of medroxyprogesterone (MPA, 2.5 mg). The pills came in little "blister packs" marked with the days of the week, so that it was easy to remember to take them. And the regimen was noticeably safer for the uterus. Wyeth-Ayerst emphasized that with Prempro the incidence of endometrial hyperplasia—this would predispose to malignant transformation—was less than 1%, compared to the 20% incidence observed when Premarin is given to postmenopausal women who retain their uteri. While Prempro did not increase the beneficial HDL cholesterol as much as Premarin, Wyeth-Ayerst believed strongly in the regimen's long-term benefits for both the heart and the skeleton. At the time this product seemed to represent state-of-the-art therapy, and it was chosen as one of the hormonal replacement regimens to be tested in the Women's Health Initiative. If that mammoth clinical trial had in fact documented significant cardiovascular benefits brought about by Prempro, the product's sales might have soared beyond all expectations. But this was not to be.

The Great Debunking!!

Anyone who follows developments in contemporary medicine will soon be struck with the rapidity with which cherished articles of faith can sometimes be overturned. In 1995 everyone "knew" that estrogen replacement therapy could reduce the incidence of cardio-vascular disease in postmenopausal women, but within five or six years that belief began to look like an outdated folly. What happened? To be brief, we can say that the results from several clinical trials actually testing this hypothesis were finally tallied, and that they tended to topple a tower of data generated by earlier case-control and cohort studies. The **Heart and Estrogen/progestin Replacement Study** (HERS) randomly assigned 2,763 postmenopausal women with intact uteri and diagnosed coronary artery disease to receive daily Prempro (estrogen plus a low-dose progestin) or a placebo. Deborah Grady, who worked on the HERS trial, recalls that the epidemiologists conducting it had difficulty in believing the results: "We actually went out and had the pills tested to make sure we hadn't mixed them up."[51] The coronary patients assigned to Prempro did indeed have improved lipid profiles—11% less LDL cholesterol and 10% more HDL cholesterol—but this did not translate into improved outcomes. Not only did these subjects have more coronary events than those taking the placebo, but they also suffered from increased rates of deep-vein thrombosis (blood clots) and gallbladder disease.[52]

Prempro did not fare much better in the **Women's Health Initiative**, that much larger trial which sought to define the effects of hormone replacement therapy on healthy postmenopausal women. The Initiative had randomized 16,608 subjects with intact uteri to receive either daily Prempro or a look-alike placebo; neither the trial participants nor their physicians knew who was actually receiving the hormones. But the effects of therapy soon became apparent. On May 31, 2002, the safety board monitoring this trial announced that it was being terminated ahead of schedule, after an average follow-up of only 5.2 years, because the regimen tested

was causing more harm than good. There had been 166 cases of invasive breast cancer in the Prempro group, but only 124 in the placebo group (a 26% elevation linked to the intervention). The Prempro group suffered 164 events due to coronary artery disease, the placebo group only 122 (a 29% elevation linked to the intervention). Other vascular parameters were similarly unfavorable: 41% more strokes in the Prempro group, and 113% more pulmonary embolisms (blood clots lodging in the lungs). On the positive side, treatment with Prempro did indeed help to preserve bone strength. While there had been 44 hip fractures recorded for those women taking the hormonal regimen, 62 occurred in women taking the placebo (a 34% reduction favoring the drug). Prempro did not elevate the risk of endometrial cancer (22 cases recorded compared to 25 cases detected in the placebo group). And for reasons no one fully understood, the estrogen-progestin regimen seemed protective against colorectal cancer: the incidence was down 37% in the Prempro group (45 cases recorded compared to 67 cases in the placebo group). Notwithstanding these benefits, the researchers conducting the Women's Health Initiative chose to emphasize the risks when they announced the trial's results in the *Journal of the American Medical Association* on July 17, 2002. The regimen tested, they counseled, "should not be initiated or continued for the primary prevention of coronary heart disease." And the regimen's demonstrated reduction in the risk of fractures should be weighed against "the substantial risks for cardiovascular disease and breast cancer." The Initiative researchers observed that their findings "do not necessarily apply to lower dosages of these drugs, to other formulations of oral estrogens and progestins, or to estrogens and progestins administered through the transdermal route. It remains possible that transdermal estradiol with progesterone, which more closely mimics the normal physiology and metabolism of endogenous sex hormones, may provide a different risk-benefit profile."[53]

Reconciling the Contradictions

Following the disclosure of the results from the Women's Health Initiative, not a few epidemiologists who had endorsed estrogen replacement therapy wondered how their data on cardiovascular disease could have been so mistaken. After all, dozens of prior case-control and cohort studies had consistently pointed to protective benefits conferred by postmenopausal estrogen use. The best explanation anyone had was that previous observational or survey-type studies did not adequately "control for" (as the epidemiologists say) a major confounding factor—viz., **the phenomenon of the healthy user**. In the United States the woman who took conjugated estrogen pills for years on end tended to be healthier and wealthier than most of her contemporaries. Presumably, she was more likely to watch her weight, to exercise, to refrain from smoking, and to see a doctor regularly. These habits, not exogenous estrogen use *per se*, probably accounted for that reduced risk of coronary artery disease and strokes detected in the observational studies.

Of course, not all the estrogen proponents adopted an apologetic posture, humbly seeking to explain their errors. Some of them went on the offensive, looking for flawed methodology in the Women's Health Initiative. In spite of its imprimatur from the National Institutes of Health, this trial drew its share of brickbats. A common objection was that its participants, with a mean age of 63 at enrollment, were too old to properly benefit from hormone replacement therapy. If the therapy is to prevent cardiovascular disease, the estrogen proponents argued, it should be begun as soon as menopausal symptoms appear. For most American women, that would be in the early fifties. Commencing it a decade later with women in their early sixties might actually be dangerous, because some of these subjects would have already developed atherosclerotic narrowing of the arteries. Frank E. Speizer of the Harvard Medical School worried that "women with increased susceptibility to the prothrombotic effects of estrogen may have acute coronary events in the first few years of therapy." In monkeys, Dr. Speizer observed, "estrogen reduces atherosclerosis when started at oophorectomy" (removal of the ovaries), "but not when started later." Other skeptics complained that assigning all treated subjects to the same estrogen-progestin regimen, regardless of their age or weight or symptoms, was overly simplistic and hardly represented optimal therapy. Beverley E. Pearson Murphy, a Montreal physician, argued that the hormonal dosages used in the trial were too high: "Surely it is not surprising that there should be an increase in the incidence of strokes and cardiac events caused by giving two drugs that are both known to increase the incidence of thrombo-embolism at high doses."[54]

The researchers running the Women's Health Initiative paid no heed to the fault-finders. Instead they published a steady stream of reports which portrayed hormone replacement therapy in an unfavorable light. In the 1990s an increasing number of epidemiological surveys had hinted that estrogen use might convey some protection against Alzheimer's disease, memory loss, and other forms of age-related intellectual decline. But when the Initiative researchers analyzed the neurological outcomes among 4,532 trial participants older than age 65, they found the opposite to be true. Of those 61 participants later diagnosed with "probable dementia,"

66% had been taking the estrogen-progestin regimen while only 34% had been assigned to the placebo. There was also no evidence that the regimen offered any protection against the milder forms of cognitive impairment, such as memory loss.[55] The newspapers and TV newscasts naturally sensationalized the Initiative's findings, conveying the impression of a causal relationship between hormonal replacement therapy and intellectual decline. "Hormones Linked to Dementia," said the headlines and the talk-show hosts. In vain did the Initiative's critics argue that the progestin in the tested regimen might have nullified any protective effects from the estrogen; the damage had been done.

The Food and Drug Administration, always sensitive to changes in the prevailing climate of opinion, quickly moved to require stronger warning labels on Prempro. Henceforth a black-bordered message accompanying each package would state that the regimen should not be used to prevent cardiovascular disease, and that it had been linked to "increased risks of myocardial infarction, stroke, invasive breast cancer, pulmonary emboli, and deep vein thrombosis." Physicians were cautioned to "prescribe estrogens and progestins at the lowest effective dose and for the shortest duration."[56] Women who had been taking hormone replacement therapy, or who were considering doing so, could not fail to be affected by the sudden flood tide of negative publicity. A report in the *Journal of the American Medical Association* pointed out that while "hormone therapy prescriptions increased from 58 million in 1995 to 90 million in 1999," there was a precipitous decline between the first six months of 2002 and the first six months of 2003: "prescriptions declined by 66% for Prempro and 33% for Premarin." Vaginal creams were the only estrogen-containing products which experienced a significantly increased demand: the number of prescriptions rose from 2.8 million in 2001 to 3.3 million in 2003.[57]

The Premarin-Only Results

The Women's Health Initiative will not have the last word on hormone replacement strategies. This trial simply tested the effects of the two most widely used pharmaceuticals—Prempro and Premarin—on the risks of developing certain chronic diseases. As we've seen, the results published in 2002 indicated that Prempro's estrogen-progestin formula slightly increases the risk of coronary artery disease, venous thrombosis, and breast cancer. For comparable data on the effects of conjugated estrogens alone, we had to wait until the National Institutes of Health ended the Premarin arm of the Initiative in February 2004, after an average follow-up of 6.8 years. This trial arm had randomized 10,739 healthy postmenopausal women who had undergone prior hysterectomies to take either the familiar Premarin pill (0.625 mg daily) or a look-alike placebo. The results appeared in the *Journal of the American Medical Association* on April 14, 2004. Unlike Prempro, Premarin did not elevate the incidence of coronary artery disease. In fact, the subjects taking the daily estrogen pills recorded 9% fewer coronary events than those taking the placebos, but this risk reduction did not achieve statistical significance. The incidence rates for strokes and for pulmonary embolisms were elevated in the Premarin group by 39% and 34% respectively, demonstrating that the regimen has the potential to induce excess thrombotic (clotting) events in susceptible individuals. Its favorable impact on bone strength was equally clear: the Premarin group suffered 39% fewer hip fractures than the placebo group. These findings are entirely in line with our expectations and our long-term experience, which assure us that low-dose conjugated estrogens definitely help to preserve postmenopausal bone mass while slightly increasing the risk of blood clots. But one finding from the Initiative's estrogen-only arm was totally unexpected. The women taking daily Premarin experienced 23% fewer cases of invasive breast cancer than the women taking the placebos. The Initiative researchers observed that "this comparison narrowly missed statistical significance."[58] No one has identified a mechanism by which conjugated estrogens might *reduce* the risk of postmenopausal breast cancer; and as the Initiative researchers commented, this trial result "requires further investigation." Yet the novel finding ought to be counted as one more piece of evidence that low-dose estrogen replacement does not greatly increase the incidence of—or the mortality from—postmenopausal breast cancer, and that our fears on this point have been overwrought.

Waiting on a Better Solution

Unfortunately, the development of pharmaceuticals in the United States is more likely to be determined by economic considerations than by pure science or humanitarian concerns. Like other manufacturers, the drug companies must look for products which can be attractively packaged and then marketed at a profit. This business is not without its potential for abuse, especially when the estimates of a drug's therapeutic value are based on biased epidemiological studies or on poorly designed clinical trials, and when

the drug's long-term side effects are largely unknown. The marketing of the synthetic estrogen DES as a pregnancy adjuvant gave us a notorious example of abuse. The conjugated estrogens in Wyeth-Ayerst's Premarin derived exclusively from a natural source, the urine of pregnant mares. When first introduced, this product represented a decided advance in the management of menopausal symptoms. Over the decades, however, Premarin began to illustrate a lamentable but understandable trait in our profit-driven pharmaceutical industry. The drug was so successful and profitable that it removed any incentive for research on more sophisticated estrogenic pharmaceuticals.

Premarin has shown us that even a crude estrogen replacement can favorably affect the lives of postmenopausal women, alleviating hot flashes and vaginal dryness, slowing urogenital atrophy, and preserving bone mass. But the results from the Women's Health Initiative clearly indicate that conjugated estrogens in convenient pill-form are not going to be a broad-spectrum prophylaxis for cardiovascular disease and neurological deficits. Conceivably, pharmaceuticals which acted more like the body's own estrogen might well help to stave off atherosclerotic clogging of the arteries and Alzheimer's disease. No current drugs have been proven effective for these purposes. And the era in which many people facilely assumed that equine estrogens would be helpful had definitely drawn to a close by early 2004, when newspapers throughout the United States reported that the herds of horses used in Premarin manufacture were being auctioned off due to reduced product demand.

Chapter Seven

"The Pill": Hormonal Contraception

To many young women of childbearing age, the oral contraceptive (OC), popularly known as "The Pill," is the best thing that happened since the invention of the wheel. This hormonal product works splendidly. The Pill stops ovulation, and therefore removes any chance of pregnancy, by virtue of gonadotropin suppression. The mechanism involved will be easy enough to understand if we refer to the outline of the menstrual cycle given in Chapter Four. The cycle is initiated anew each month by the hypothalamus (a well-defined region in the brain), which senses the low hormone levels during menstruation and responds by producing gonadotropin-releasing hormone. GnRH acts on the pituitary gland, which responds by secreting follicle-stimulating hormone (FSH) and luteinizing hormone (LH) into the bloodstream. As we've seen, both these gonadotropins powerfully stimulate the ovaries. FSH brings about follicle development and increasing estrogen production in the first half of the menstrual cycle (follicular phase), while LH ensures ovulation at mid-cycle and then spurs progesterone production in the second half (luteal phase).

Hormonal contraception significantly alters the menstrual cycle. Today's OC regimens consist of 21 tablets, each of which contains a fixed dosage of synthetic hormones with biological activity approximating that of natural estrogen and progesterone. Typically, a young woman going on The Pill will take her first tablet on the first day of menstruation, or within several days thereafter; she then takes one tablet daily until all 21 are consumed. The first few tablets serve to elevate the levels of estrogen and progesterone in the bloodstream; as a result, the hypothalamus does not sense any hormonal depletion and does not produce GnRH. Without GnRH, the pituitary issues no FSH and no LH; and the ovaries remain quiet, in a state of suspended animation. Follicle development and subsequent ovulation do not occur. The ovaries also aren't turning out the hormones associated with these reproductive events; but as the daily OC tablets are supplying the estrogen and progesterone exogenously, a young woman on The Pill will not experience symptoms of hormone deficiency (e.g., hot flashes). Hormonal contraception creates a kind of reversible menopause: the ovaries are shut down, and their hormones artificially supplied. What's missing in an OC cycle is, of course, the endocrinal cascade (GnRH, FSH, LH) which leads to ovulation. Endometrial shedding, popularly known as "a period," is provided for. After consuming 21 daily tablets, the OC user will have seven days in which she takes no pills—and therefore no hormones—thus mimicking the precipitous drop in estrogen and progesterone which occurs in a natural cycle right before menstruation. Pharmaceutical companies also offer OCs in 28-day regimens; but here the last seven pills in the package are always dummies—placebos with inert ingredients intended only as reminders to help the OC user stay on schedule. With either a 21-day or a 28-day regimen, withdrawal bleeding (the menstruation effect) occurs at the same time, during the week after the hormones are discontinued. The OC user would then begin a new cycle—that is, a new package of pills!

Women taking hormonal contraception are supposed to have the impression that their bodies are functioning pretty much as before, but this is hardly the case. That apparent "menstrual cycle" has been created by the regulated administration of synthetic hormones. Medical science, by learning how to fool the hypothalamus and the pituitary, has given women a convenient and reliable method of avoiding unwanted pregnancies. Should pregnancy be desired, an OC user just needs to discontinue the daily tablets. Within a month or two the menstrual cycle and ovulation will resume as before. But control of reproductive function is not the only benefit of OCs. The monthly periods tend to be shorter and more predictable; they can even be postponed during weekends or vacations, by the simple expedient of taking a few extra pills. Blood loss is usually much less; premenstrual symptoms (breast tenderness, abdominal cramps) are less frequent or less severe. OC users do not experience **mittelschmerz** (pain at ovulation), and they are less likely to develop benign breast disorders ("fibrocystic disease"). The synthetic progestin in The Pill makes the cervical mucus thicker and less permeable; for this reason OC users have a lower incidence of pelvic inflammatory disease, that dire infection which results when gonococci or other bacteria swim up through the uterus and begin to

breed in the fallopian tubes.

Different Recipes for The Pill

Today's OC is the product of many decades of research and experimentation. The details of the menstrual cycle were not deciphered, nor ovarian hormones isolated, until the 1920s. In the 1930s ovulation in rabbits was successfully prevented by injections of natural progesterone. In the 1950s researchers learned that synthetic progestins, given orally, could prevent ovulation in humans; but the preliminary clinical trials with progestin OCs revealed significant problems. The use of progestins as single contraceptive agents often led to menstrual abnormalities, including **spotting** (a slight loss of blood between periods) and **breakthrough bleeding** (menstrual flow at the wrong time). When OCs were first marketed in the early 1960s, they therefore contained two hormones, estrogen and progestin, in order to mimic the natural menstrual cycle more faithfully and to ensure punctual withdrawal bleeding. Two synthetic estrogens have been used in American OCs, ethinyl estradiol and the somewhat weaker mestranol. Both these compounds are much more potent than the conjugated estrogens given in postmenopausal hormone replacement. Because of their considerable effects on hepatic (liver) metabolism, their prescription is largely limited to healthy premenopausal women. Dosage has been traditionally expressed in micrograms (mcg) rather than in milligrams (mg). The first OCs were highly estrogenic, containing as much as 100 mcg of ethinyl estradiol or 150 mcg of mestranol. All this estrogen was not prudent. Since the high-dose estrogen increased the liver's production of coagulation factors, a few susceptible women taking the early OCs developed blood clots in the lungs (embolisms), brain, or coronary arteries. Law suits followed on the heels of the inevitable fatalities. The dangers associated with the estrogen component were intensified by the **sequential OCs** put on the market in the mid-1960s. Touted as "more natural," sequential regimens featured fourteen days of high-dose estrogen (in simulation of the follicular phase), followed by seven days of estrogen and progestin (as in the luteal phase). These pills worked better in theory than in practice; they were soon withdrawn. In the 1970s epidemiological studies began to link OC use with a higher incidence of premature strokes and heart attacks; a warning about blood clots now accompanied every package. And physicians were beginning to recognize the kind of OC user who might be at significant risk for vascular complications: a woman over age 35 who smoked cigarettes, or one with a personal or family history of early-onset diabetes, hypertension, or circulatory disorders.[1]

The pharmaceutical companies soon responded to the documented side effects by slashing the amount of ethinyl estradiol in their OCs. After 1974 no American OC was introduced which contained more than 50 mcg per tablet; prescriptions for first-time users typically called for pills providing 30 or 35 mcg daily, roughly one-third the dosage given in the 1960s. By 1987 only 3% of the OCs consumed in the United States held more than 50 mcg. The risk of thrombosis was greatly reduced; most physicians felt that the lower-dose OCs could be taken safely by women in their forties, so long as they did not smoke or have other risk factors for cardiovascular disease.[2]

In the 1990s over thirty different brands of The Pill were available in the United States. This product variability had more to do with the progestin component than with estrogen dose levels. Six types of progestin were being used, including the prevalent norethindrone and the very potent levonorgestrel. No two compounds had exactly the same effects, a fact which let the prescribing physician tinker with different formulations until a suitable OC for a particular patient was discovered. If a patient developed acne while taking one OC, it was probably time to substitute another OC with a different progestin whose androgenic side effects might be less pronounced.

Triphasic OCs, introduced in the mid-1980s, offered even more flexibility. In triphasic regimens all the 21 tablets still combined estrogen with a progestin, but the hormonal dose varied according to the day of the cycle. Sometimes the estrogen content was slightly raised or lowered; but most of these new OCs emphasized a three-step increase in the progestin component, thus paralleling the gradual rise of progesterone during the natural menstrual cycle. Ortho Pharmaceuticals brand **Ortho-Novum 7-7-7** exemplified this approach: all the pills had 35 mcg of ethinyl estradiol, but the first seven had 0.5 mg of norethindrone, the second seven 0.75 mg, and the last seven 1.0 mg. Those side effects principally associated with progestins, such as breast tenderness and swelling, tended to be minimized on triphasic regimens, because the accumulative monthly dosage of these agents was lower than with conventional OC formulations. Manufacturers hinted that their triphasic OCs also reduced spotting and breakthrough bleeding. But consumers needed a keen memory and an eye for colors to adhere to the 21-day schedule, as a triphasic package typically featured pills in three different colors. The 28-day regimens with their seven placebos began to look like floral bouquets—the pills came in four colors!

The Pill and Cancer

We quickly learned about the thrombotic dangers related to the estrogen component of OCs, because the induced blood clots did not take long to develop; they could appear after only a few days on The Pill. Any assessment of the risk of induced malignancies was bound to take a lot more time—cancers usually don't appear until several decades after exposure to the implicated carcinogens. As The Pill was not widely used before the mid-1960s, epidemiological studies conducted before the mid-1980s could hardly claim to have considered the possible effects of long-term exposure. Moreover, The Pill itself was not a constant, and women tended to use it in an irregular fashion. Different OCs contained different compounds in different doses; the formulations shifted radically over the years. The low-dose OCs introduced in the mid-1970s could not be expected to have the same effect on cancer risks as the estrogen-rich OCs of the 1960s. Cigarette smokers and beer drinkers often exhibited remarkable loyalty to this or that brand-name product, but a woman who stayed on the same OC for years and years was an exception. A more representative pattern seemed to be a year on The Pill, then a year off, then back on again, with several switches between OC brands and formulations. How could epidemiologists conclude anything from such inconstant data? By and large, they have relied on case-control methodology, pitting cancer patients against healthy controls, and asking both groups for information on their past use of OCs. The possibility of recall bias can never be entirely eliminated from studies of this type. Would not the cancer patients probe their memories more deeply than the controls, and might not the studies consequently produce misleading findings?

One of the first case-control studies of breast cancer risk got underway in the San Francisco area in 1970, not long after OCs began to be widely used. The results, published in 1975, indicated an elevated risk only among women who had taken OCs for "not less than two nor more than four years." The study's authors speculated that OCs might "accelerate the growth rate of pre-existing subclinical malignant lesions, with these lesions reaching the level of clinical recognition only after two years of drug usage and all being diagnosed within two additional years."[3] Subsequent investigations have not confirmed this hypothesis, but one finding from the early San Francisco study did make its way into the textbooks as gospel truth. OC usage proved to be associated with a lower incidence of benign mammary lesions—cysts, fibroadenomas, and intraductal papillomas. After eight years or more on The Pill, users in the San Francisco study had only one-fifth the incidence of benign lesions that was detected in the nonusers.

For two other gynecological cancers, the earliest case-control studies yielded remarkably accurate results about the effects of OC usage. In 1979 researchers at the University of Southern California reported that OC use, like pregnancy and other factors which suppress ovulation, confers significant protection against ovarian cancer. The USC team observed that "the ovarian surface epithelium incurs minor trauma each time an ovum is released," and that it is moreover "exposed to estrogen-rich follicular fluid."[4] After ovulation the cells near the ruptured follicle must proliferate rapidly to repair the damage. This mitotic activity inherently raises the risk of DNA mutations—and of subsequent malignant transformation. It does not occur in women taking The Pill, a fact which sufficiently explains the well-documented protective effect against ovarian tumors. In 1980 two case-control studies published in the *New England Journal of Medicine* reported that combined OCs—i.e., those providing daily doses of both estrogen and a progestin—offered substantial protection against endometrial cancer. A study done in Washington state found that OC users "had only 50 percent of the incidence of endometrial cancer of nonusers."[5] Several months later epidemiologists affiliated with Boston University, Harvard, and other eastern institutions reached the same conclusion. Women who had used combined OCs for one year or more had "about half the risk of endometrial cancer experienced by other women." The risk declined further with increasing duration of use, and the protective effect "appeared to persist for at least five years after use had stopped."[6]

The biological mechanisms through which combined OCs work to prevent endometrial malignancies are obvious. As we've seen, endometrial proliferation occurs mainly in the follicular phase, in response to rising levels of unopposed estrogen. That proliferation is muted with combined OCs, because the daily tablets provide a synthetic version of progesterone along with the estrogen. Not only is mitotic activity reduced, but the prompt shedding of hyperplastic endometrium is encouraged by the total cessation of both hormones on day 22. Sequential OCs, which were removed from the market in 1976, offered no protection against endometrial cancer; in fact, by providing fourteen days of unopposed high-dose estrogen, they promoted more endometrial proliferation than would occur in a natural menstrual cycle. The Washington State study found that some sequential OC users had a risk of endometrial cancer almost six-and-a-half times greater than that of women who never used any OCs.

By the early 1980s, two decades after The Pill was introduced, we were beginning to have solid evidence that certain OC regimens could serve as valuable preventive measures against two serious malignancies. Epithelial ovarian tumors, while not nearly so common as those of the breast, often prove fatal; they usually have spread throughout the abdominal cavity before they are discovered. Endometrial cancers pose a risk of mortality among poorly educated patients who ignore the early symptoms (e.g., unexplained vaginal bleeding). In these two instances, both our pharmacologists and our epidemiologists served us well. Unfortunately, for the most important gynecological malignancy, we knew virtually nothing about how OCs might affect disease incidence. Knowledge about breast cancer does not come easy.

The CASH Findings
Too Good to be True?

In the mid-1980s one study of The Pill and cancer possessed a unique aura of statistical power and governmental imprimatur. The findings from the **Cancer and Steroid Hormone Study**, principally conducted by the Centers for Disease Control, looked authoritative, maybe even definitive. This major case-control study, abbreviated as **CASH**, recruited patients and controls from population centers throughout the United States. Trained interviewers visited the thousands of participants in their homes, recording the answers to detailed questionnaires. On March 25, 1983, the *Journal of the American Medical Association* published a three-part report from CASH examining the relationships between OC use and cancers of the breast, ovary, and endometrium. The CASH researchers found no association between The Pill and breast cancer—women who had taken OCs at one time or another actually had a 10% lower risk than nonusers.

For both ovarian and endometrial malignancies, CASH reported substantial reductions in risk: ovarian incidence down 40% in OC users, endometrial down 50%. An editorial accompanying the report observed that "the *Journal*'s readership should be reassured."[7] Not everybody was. For one thing, CASH's initial analysis of breast cancer risk was based upon only a small percentage of the women eventually recruited by the study— just a mere 689 cases and 1,077 controls.

Rose Kushner, the writer and activist, fueled public skepticism with the 1984 edition of her book on breast cancer, which contained a chapter entitled "The Problem of The Pill." Kushner faulted physicians and pharmaceutical companies alike for failing to inform patients about possible risks: "I could not find a single scientist involved in breast cancer research who believes OCs are safe."[8] Malcolm C. Pike and his fellow epidemiologists at the University of Southern California sought to translate such vague suspicions into believable data. Pike et al looked at certain subgroups of OC users who might be especially sensitive to exogenous hormones. In 1981 they published a case-control study of 163 breast cancer patients diagnosed before age 33. Long-term use of OCs seemed to be a major risk factor for early-onset disease in young nulliparous women. Eight or more years on The Pill before that first full-term pregnancy elevated the risk 252% above the nonuser baseline.[9] By 1983 Pike et al had expanded their study to include 314 breast cancer patients diagnosed before age 37, but this time their report focused on the possible effects of different OC formulations rather than on nulliparity. OCs with a high progestin content seemed especially risky: five years of use before age 25 increased the odds of early-onset breast cancer fourfold. Pike et al suggested that other case-control studies absolving The Pill of blame probably relied too heavily on patients who "were much older than our patients and, hence, were unlikely to have used combination-type OCs for a long enough time at young ages."[10]

The USC reports of 1981 and 1983 possessed a certain element of biological plausibility. The breast epithelium of young women, especially nulliparous ones, reveals higher mitotic rates and a greater sensitivity to carcinogens. Progesterone acts synergistically with estrogen on mammary cells. Conceivably, the same OCs which protected the endometrium by providing the two hormones simultaneously could have the opposite effect on the breast—and the more potent the progestin component, the more the risk could be elevated. But the CASH researchers paid little heed to these hypotheses. In 1986 they published an expanded analysis in the *New England Journal of Medicine*, now based on 4,711 breast cancer patients between the ages of 20 and 54, and 4,676 matched controls. Once again The Pill seemed blameless—CASH found no elevated risk of breast cancer, regardless of the user's age bracket or the duration of OC use, and "regardless of the progestin content." In an accompanying editorial, Samuel Shapiro of Boston University commented that the benefits of OCs outweighed the risks: "the vast majority of users will experience only the benefits."[11] In 1987 CASH released updated analyses of The Pill's effect on endometrial and ovarian cancers. Compared to nonusers, women who had taken OCs for just one year experienced a 40% reduction in the incidence of both malignancies. And the protective effect persisted for at least fifteen years after OC use was discontinued.[12] In the 1990s ongoing analyses of the massive CASH database indicated that OCs might serve as a prophylactic for women at high risk for hereditary ovarian cancer. Ten years of OC use by women with a positive family history appeared to reduce their risk level below that of nonusers with no family history.[13]

Are Young OC Users at Risk?

The worries about long-term OC use by young women and the possible induction of early-onset breast cancers, argued so persuasively by the USC epidemiologists, did not fade away. In early 1989 these concerns flared into a controversy which, being widely reported by the newspapers and on TV, alarmed OC users quite a bit.[14] Donald R. Miller of Boston University and his colleagues released the results from a case-control study of The Pill and breast cancer before age 45. Any OC use, even less than three months, seemed associated with an elevated risk (up 100%) for early-onset disease; and ten years or more on The Pill raised the risk 310% above the nonuser baseline. The study by Miller et al was small (407 patients, 424 controls), and the authors acknowledged that either selection bias or recall bias could have influenced their findings.[15] But subsequent studies done in England and Sweden appeared to corroborate Miller et al. The United Kingdom Case-Control Study had interviewed 755 breast cancer patients diagnosed before age 36, and it reported "a highly significant trend in risk with total duration of OC use." After eight years or more the risk rose to 74% above the nonuser baseline.[16] The Swedish researchers focused on a slightly older group of premenopausal patients, some of whom had begun to use OCs back in the 1960s. The risk of breast cancer was elevated principally among users who began at an early age—five years on The Pill before age 25 upped it 430% above that of nonusers.[17]

Nobody wanted to give too much weight to the Swedish study because of its small size (174 cases) and retrospective nature (old high-dose OCs from the 1960s). The results from the Nurses' Health Study provided much more statistical power, but the Harvard researchers sidestepped the troublesome issues of OC use in the teenage years or before a first pregnancy. They explained that in their cohort "the number of women who used OCs for a long duration in early reproductive life was too small to permit firm conclusions." Yet the follow-up of 118,273 nurses from 1976 to 1986, with 1,799 cases of breast cancer confirmed in the interval, tended to acquit The Pill of any major role in mammary carcinogenesis. Past users of OCs did not have a significantly increased risk—it was up only 6% above the nonuser level. Current users revealed a slightly increased risk, 53% above the nonuser baseline. The Harvard team tentatively concluded that "oral contraceptives could act as a late-stage promoting agent of susceptible precancerous lesions."[18] In other words, OCs probably don't cause cellular damage, but they might accelerate the growth of pre-existing abnormalities. The San Francisco researchers had said much the same thing back in 1975.

The Food and Drug Administration, worried by the flurry of risk-finding studies, debated whether a stiffer warning about breast cancer should be required in OC packages, but eventually refrained from making changes. The FDA advisory committee explained: "The studies are conflicting and inconsistent, so it is difficult to draw a conclusion."[19] Three prominent epidemiologists at Harvard—Isabelle Romieu, Jesse A. Berlin, and Graham Colditz—attempted to impose a semblance of order on the medley of divergent methodologies and results. They performed a "meta-analysis," pooling and analyzing the data from 27 case-control studies of OC use and breast cancer incidence. Their analysis was generally reassuring: "Overall there is no increase in the risk of breast cancer for women who ever used oral contraceptives, even after a long duration of use." However, when Romieu et al looked specifically for a relationship between OCs and premenopausal breast cancer, they found slightly elevated risks with longer durations of use. On the average, ten years on The Pill upped the risk for early-onset disease by 46%: "This risk was predominantly among women who used OCs before their first full-term pregnancy." Indeed, just four years of OC use by nulliparous women increased their risk by 72% above the nonuser baseline.[20]

CASH Finally Finds a Risk

Like the FDA, the Centers for Disease Control (CDC) had been bothered by the new studies reporting an association between OCs and early-onset breast cancer. The CDC responded to the controversy by re-examining the old CASH data which had been used to give The Pill such a clean bill of health in 1986. This time the CASH investigators sought to identify possible "age-specific differences" in risk. They divided the study's 4,711 breast cancer patients and 4,676 controls into three groups based on "age at diagnosis or interview." The revised CASH analysis, published in 1991, held a surprise or two. For the women aged 45 to 54, a history of OC use proved to be associated with a 10% reduction in risk. For those women aged 35 to 44, past OC use led neither to a risk elevation nor to a reduction. And for those women aged 20 to 34, the risk for past OC users was 40% above that of nonusers. After a decade of defending The Pill against all comers, CASH had to admit that, *yes*, OC use seemed to involve a slightly increased risk of breast cancer before age 35. But the CASH investigators cautioned against "over-interpretation" of their findings, seeing "no reasons for changes in prescribing practices."[21] In 1993 CASH published a second re-examination of its data, focusing on women who began using OCs

before age 25. For those women reporting first OC use as teenagers, the risk of early-onset breast cancer was up 40% above the nonuser baseline. For those women first taking The Pill between the ages of 20 and 24, the CASH investigators detected a 50% elevation in risk. After age 25 the timing of first use hardly seemed to influence disease incidence.[22]

Several groups of epidemiologists hastened to conduct case-control studies specifically designed to detect any breast cancer risks that long-term OC use might pose to young women. Emily White and her co-workers at Seattle's Fred Hutchinson Cancer Research Center compared 747 breast cancer patients diagnosed between the ages of 21 and 45 with 961 age-matched controls. Long-term OC use proved to be associated with "a small increased risk of breast cancer." After ten years or more on The Pill, the overall risk of premenopausal breast cancer went up 30% above the nonuser baseline. But for those users aged 35 or younger, the risk went up 70%. White et al also found risk elevations among OC users who began "within five years of menarche" (up 30%) or who had taken pills containing a potent progestin (up 50%).[23] Louise A. Brinton of the National Cancer Institute and ten other epidemiologists examined the effects of OC use in 1,648 breast cancer patients diagnosed before age 45 and in 1,505 age-matched control subjects. Overall, the risk of breast cancer before age 35 was elevated for OC users, "the relative risk rising to 2.2 for users of ten or more years." However, for users who began before age 18 and then continued for ten years or more, the relative risk of breast cancer before age 35 was 3.1, up 210% above the nonuser baseline. Brinton et al concluded that the association between OC use and early-onset disease "appears to have a biologic basis rather than to be an artifact."[24]

The Progestin-Only Pills

Either estrogen or progesterone, if administered in sufficient quantities, can inhibit ovulation. Pharmaceutical companies have not rushed to produce single-hormone contraceptives, because their side effects tend to be greater than those produced by combined OCs. Nonetheless several types of progestin-only contraceptives have long been available in the United States. While they account for only a small fraction of the market, they need to be discussed here, in the interest of completeness and because they have received considerable publicity. OCs containing just a low-dose progestin were introduced in 1973; they immediately gained the nickname **Mini-Pills** (the tablets are very small), but never acquired popularity.   They are prescribed principally for women who have severe reactions (e.g., nausea or headaches) to the estrogen component of combined OCs, or for women who are breast-feeding (combined OCs reduce milk production and expose infants to two exogenous hormones). Mini-Pills do not reliably inhibit ovulation; they are effective contraception because the daily progestin keeps the cervical mucus thick and impenetrable, preventing sperm from reaching the uterus and fallopian tubes. The main drawback with Mini-Pills, as with other progestin-only contraceptives, is an erratic menstrual cycle with a higher incidence of spotting and breakthrough bleeding. American women have been quick to discontinue Mini-Pills, and consequently epidemiological data on them has been limited.   Several previous studies found no association between their use and the risk of breast cancer.[25]

Progestin-only contraceptives can be remarkably long-acting. **Norplant**, the implant system introduced by Wyeth-Ayerst in 1991, featured six permeable capsules containing levonorgestrel. These capsules resembled little matchsticks; they were inserted under the skin of a patient's upper arm, where they slowly released small but constant doses of the potent progestin into the bloodstream. As one implantation provided reliable contraception for five years, Wyeth-Ayerst promoted Norplant as "an excellent option for women desiring a long-term method," readily reversible but with "effectiveness comparable to tubal ligation."[26] The implants worked regardless of the user's intelligence or motivation; hence they were urged as a birth control method for substance abusers, teenagers, and other fertile but feckless women. Most Norplant users seem to have been satisfied with this product. Those users who were not increasingly sought assistance from attorneys. By the mid-1990s a tidal wave of litigation threatened to end the distribution of Norplant. The law suits typically alleged that patients were not informed of possible side effects, including irregular or prolonged menstrual bleeding, headaches, and weight gain, and that the implants were difficult to remove.

Depo-Provera, Upjohn's brand of depot medroxyprogesterone acetate, has been studied more extensively than Norplant, but still remains controversial. This injectable contraceptive was finally approved for American distribution in 1992, after years of debate centering around its possible effects on mammary carcinogenesis (breast tumor induction reported in beagles), on bone mineralization (a loss reported in some users), and on those rare pregnancies which may occasionally occur in women taking this drug.[27] But Depo-Provera has been around for decades; it's been widely prescribed in many countries, with a good safety record. A single injection every three months is all that is required; the system is quick, reliable, and inexpensive.

Epidemiological studies of Depo-Provera's effect on breast cancer risk are not numerous. An important case-control study came from New Zealand, where this contraceptive was introduced in 1969 and subsequently "used more extensively than in any other developed country." The results have a familiar ring about them, being similar to the findings from studies of combined OCs. The New Zealand epidemiologists reported "no overall association" between Depo-Provera use and breast cancer incidence—but, *yes*, they found that young women who used this hormonal contraceptive for long periods before age 25 were indeed at increased risk of disease before age 35. For use after age 25, there was no risk detected; but two to five years use before age 25 elevated the risk for early-onset disease 360% above the nonuser baseline.[28] The World Health Organization (WHO) subsequently released results from a larger study done in Kenya, Mexico, and Thailand, comparing 869 breast cancer patients with 11,890 age-matched controls. Like the New Zealanders, the WHO epidemiologists detected an association between early Depo-Provera use and breast cancer before age 35; but the risk elevation was modest—up only 21% among the youthful users.[29]

In 1995 the New Zealand and WHO teams collaborated on "a pooled analysis" of their two studies, attempting to iron out inconsistencies and to generate statistical power. The new review of data from 1,768 breast cancer patients and 13,905 controls pointed to current or recent Depo-Provera use as "the key factor." With any use beginning "within the previous five years," breast cancer risk was elevated 100% above the nonuser baseline. After five years had elapsed since first use, the elevated risk faded away. The two teams of epidemiologists agreed that Depo-Provera does not induce breast tumors in humans; they speculated that in susceptible women it may "accelerate the growth of pre-existing tumors."[30]

Our scientific juries remain out on progestin-only contraceptives. These products probably will not reduce the risk of ovarian cancer as effectively as combined OCs, because they do not always suppress follicle development and ovulation. Their impact on the incidence of endometrial cancers remains to be defined. Their effect on breast cancer incidence would seem to be very small.

Combined OCs:
Weighing the Risks and Benefits

No pharmaceutical product is completely safe. But the combined oral contraceptive supplying low-dose estrogen with a trace of progestin, the prevalent variety of The Pill in American society, has an extremely good safety record. For most women taking OCs, side effects will not be a problem, and the benefits can be said to outweigh the risks. Not only do combined OCs prevent unwanted pregnancies, but they significantly reduce the incidence of ovarian and endometrial cancers. Several decades of diligent epidemiological investigation have generally given The Pill a clean bill of health in regard to mammary carcinogenesis. In 2002 Polly A. Marchbanks of the Centers for Disease Control and other American epidemiologists published a big case-control study in the *New England Journal of Medicine*, reporting that "current or former use of OCs did not significantly increase the risk of breast cancer." This finding held true even "with longer periods of use or with higher doses of estrogen."[31] Such an unalloyed paean to The Pill had not been heard since the old CASH reports of the 1980s. But a few epidemiologists continued to worry that OCs could be a risk factor for young women whose mammary glands had not yet undergone the protective differentiation achieved by a full-term pregnancy. A portion of the literature had long since put warning signs before the very young and the nulliparous; as we've seen, the venerable CASH study eventually said as much.[32]

Why should the same hormonal regimens which protect against ovarian and endometrial cancers tend to promote early-onset breast tumors? Thomas J. Anderson of the University of Edinburgh and other pathologists did a ground-breaking study which suggests an answer to this query. With a view to defining the effects of OC regimens on "breast epithelial proliferation," Anderson et al measured the mitotic rates in the excised glandular tissues of 347 women ranging in age from 14 to 48 who had undergone biopsy for benign breast lesions. They discovered that these rates were consistently higher in OC users than in nonusers. And different formulations had different effects: OCs with 50 mcg of ethinyl estradiol elevated the mitotic rates far more than those with 35 mcg or less. In contrast to a prevalent hypothesis, Dr. Anderson and his colleagues found that the quantity of progestin in the OCs, whether low or high, did not greatly affect breast mitotic rates. They reasoned that "estrogen facilitates progestin action by increasing progesterone receptor levels," and that with sufficient estrogenic stimulation, even low doses of progestin could have "maximal effect." Two findings by Anderson et al are marvelously apropos to those repeated epidemiological findings indicating an increased risk for nulliparous women under age 25. The breast mitotic rates in OC users under age 20 were much higher than in older users; only after age 25 did these rates start to decline. Parity emerged as an even more important determinant of proliferation: "The nulliparous breast was very responsive to OC use, whereas the parous breast was almost unaffected."[33]

The study by Anderson et al would seem to indicate that combined OCs, by supplying estrogen and a progestin together, can induce more mitotic activity in the immature mammary gland than would occur during a natural menstrual cycle. The Pill might also elevate the risk of breast cancer in younger women simply by creating an artificial cyclic regularity. As we've seen in Chapter Five, long, irregular cycles tend to reduce the risk. These cycles are common in teenagers, who would naturally lose this protective effect by going on The Pill at such a young age. Combined OCs ensure short, regular cycles; and for the immature mammary gland at least, they probably create a kind of "extended luteal phase" with both hormones present and stimulating breast cells.

The increased risk of early-onset breast cancer reported for very young and nulliparous OC users does not appear to be an artifact, but an understandable and verifiable response to certain regimens of exogenous hormones. Because the incidence of breast malignancies remains extremely low in women under age 35, that risk elevation cannot be said to represent a grave threat. Nonetheless, any nulliparous woman under age 25 who has a family history of early-onset breast cancer might be wise to consider some other means of birth control, because at the moment we cannot predict how the existing regimens for hormonal contraception would affect her individual risk of developing premenopausal disease. On the other hand, any young woman with a family history of epithelial ovarian cancer might be well advised to use combined OCs throughout her entire reproductive life, because we know for a fact that this method of birth control can substantially reduce her risk of a potentially lethal malignancy which does not lend itself to early detection.

Insofar the risk of breast cancer is concerned, our epidemiologists have been pretty much unanimous in declaring combined OCs to be safe for women who are parous or over age 25. The main health risk posed by OCs continues to be venous thrombosis—that is, a tendency toward the formation of blood clots in the slower moving venous circulation, which might eventually travel to the lungs or brain. This risk exists because in susceptible individuals the estrogen component of combined OCs tends to stimulate the liver's production of coagulation factors. Naturally the risk associated with the newer low-dose OCs is not nearly as great as that associated with the high-dose OCs of the 1960s, and it principally applies to individuals with a demonstrated susceptibility to thrombotic events. Writing in the *New England Journal of Medicine* in 2003, Diana B. Petitti observed that the risks of OCs outweigh the benefits for women with a history of strokes, occlusive heart disease, or thromboembolism. "Oral contraceptive use," advised Dr. Petitti, "should be discouraged among women older than 35 years of age who smoke, because they clearly have an increased risk of arterial vascular disease."[34]

Chapter Eight

A Lump in the Breast

Just a little knowledge can be a dangerous thing. In the case of breast cancer, a modicum of knowledge offered gratis by the American Cancer Society (ACS) has occasioned needless concern in untold numbers of women. Many decades ago the Society embarked on a most extensive campaign to educate the public about **"Cancer's Seven Danger Signals"**—one of which was identified as **"A Lump or Thickening in the Breast."**[1] This particular danger signal has been mentioned so often that it's ingrained in everybody's consciousness. How many American women, feeling a breast lump or thinking that they felt one, have rushed off to their doctors' offices in stark terror? Nine times out of ten, this kind of anxiety proves to be completely unwarranted. That catch-all term *lump* is so vague and imprecise that it cannot be said to depict any pathological condition, much less serve as an alarm bell for cancer. If the ACS will persist in talking about breast lumps, its public service messages should at least include a qualifying sentence along these lines: "Any persistent mass must be evaluated by a qualified physician, but please remember that the overwhelming majority of breast lumps *are not malignant and do not evolve into cancer*."

As we've seen in Chapter Four, the human mammary gland is a complex and dynamic organ, constantly active throughout a woman's reproductive years. Therefore it is not surprising that all sorts of disorders and malfunctions can and do occur in the breast, from puberty onward. Mammary carcinoma is a relatively rare event, which tends to happen late in life. Notwithstanding the ACS fervor for early detection, there is no danger signal or warning sign which specifically indicates the presence of malignancy. All those scary symptoms, even hard lumps and bloody nipple discharges, can also be produced by benign, easily treatable conditions. More often than not, these symptoms *are* the result of benign processes. Physicians recognize this fact, which sometimes leads them to complacently dismiss growing malignancies as "nothing to worry about." Usually there is nothing; but cancer must always be ruled out because the breast offers a broad field for biological mimicry. Benign conditions may mimic cancer, and vice versa. The eminent clinician William L. Donegan cautions that "physicians must appreciate that any sign of disease in the breast is potentially attributable to cancer until proved otherwise."[2] Breast specialists like Dr. Donegan can often arrive at the correct diagnosis with a touch of the hand or a quick glance. But often the symptoms are equivocal, and the diagnosis can only be established by putting a sample of the questionable tissues under a microscope.

This chapter focuses largely on benign conditions which commonly affect the breast, while succeeding chapters explore the techniques physicians use to distinguish them from malignancies. Chapter Nine deals with the exams readily conducted in a doctor's office—Chapter Ten deals with diagnostic mammography, and Chapter Eleven with methods of biopsy.

Where Do the Cancers Arise?

Having emphasized that most breast lumps are not malignant, we need to concede that most breast cancers have historically presented as lumps or—as the doctors would say—**dominant masses**. There is no typical presentation for breast tumors, but a certain scenario of discovery repeats itself so often that we may declare it commonplace. In this scenario a woman a few years past the menopause discovers a hard painless lump in her breast while taking a bath or shower. Before the advent of screening mammography, perhaps 80% or 90% of all breast cancers were detected in just this fashion—viz., lumps (masses) being found by the women themselves. Of course, a lump is not always present; and if one is present, it is not necessarily hard and painless. In a minority of cases, breast cancers may be associated with noticeable pain at the tumor site.

Malignancies can develop anywhere in the breast, but they most frequently appear in the **upper outer quadrant**. For convenience physicians customarily speak of the breast as if it were divided into four portions—or quadrants—with the nipple being the point where the vertical and horizontal dividing lines meet. A few textbooks assert that 50% of breast cancers develop in the quadrant nearest the axilla (armpit), but this figure is a trifle inflated. Dr. Donegan gives us a more precise estimate, stating that 37% of tumors develop in that upper outer quadrant, and 15% around or behind the nipple. The other quadrants have a much lower incidence: 12% in the upper inner, 8% in the lower outer, and 5% in the lower inner. Dr. Donegan adds that approximately 23% of tumors appear in two or more quadrants, or on the midlines between quadrants.[3] The reason why more than half of all breast malignancies develop either in the upper outer quadrant or in the nipple area is simply that the glandular tissue tends to be concentrated in these locations. The mammary gland typically stretches from the nipple towards the axilla—comparatively little milk-producing epithelium is found in the lower quadrants. In most women the left breast tends to be a tad larger than the right one, and to contain slightly more glandular tissue. The cancer statistics reflect this disproportion, tumors being 5% to 10% more likely to occur in the left breast than in the right. This left-breast predominance transcends gender: one study of *male* breast cancer found that tumors developed 7% more often on the left side than on the right.[4]

Any reader of this book who might feel a lump in the upper outer quadrant of the left breast should not yield to sensations of panic. The locations where breast cancers arise most frequently are the very same locations where all those benign problems arise—cysts, fibroadenomas, infections, dilated milk ducts. The potential trouble spots simply follow the spatial expansion of the mammary gland; but whatever the symptom may be and wherever it may occur, the odds generally favor a benign etiology over a malignant one. L. E. Hughes and his colleagues in the breast clinic at the University Hospital of Wales, Cardiff, assure us that benign conditions "account for 90% of clinical presentations related to the breast."[5]

Tumors as Hard as Stone

The phenomenal hardness of some breast carcinomas is proverbial. Why do tumors arising in the mammary gland occasionally achieve the consistency of rocks, while soft-tissue tumors elsewhere in the body do not? In Chapter One we observed that invasive breast cancers typically provoke a strong reaction in the surrounding stroma, with excessive production of collagen fibers by the stromal connective cells (fibroblasts). The malignant epithelial cells are not hard, but the induced mesh of collagen tends to become increasingly mineralized and inflexible. Pathologists literally have to saw or file their way through some breast tumor specimens, which can feel as gritty as coarse stones. The particular designation applied to these cases, **scirrhous ductal carcinomas**, denotes their unusual solidity (from the Greek *skirrhos*, meaning "hard").

Harold F. Dvorak, a pathologist at Boston's Beth Israel Hospital, has likened the stromal fibrosis seen in breast carcinomas to "wound healing gone awry."[6] The biological processes which ensue when the body heals an injury are not unlike those which occur when malignant epithelial cells invade the neighboring stroma. And both events—injury as well as carcinoma—can result in a hard lump. Trauma (a vigorous blow or whack) to an area of soft tissue such as the breast, buttocks, or thigh, will cause the tiny blood vessels to rupture or leak. The body reacts immediately to stop internal bleeding. Within minutes a temporary closure of these leaking vessels will be accomplished by a solidifying mixture of platelets and the protein fibrin. A few days later the wound area, originally tender, will appear as a hard lump—the body has (as it were) built a sturdy collagen scaffolding to immobilize the area and thus facilitate the extensive repairs needed on the injured vessels and tissues.

This fibrous mass which arises in response to leaking blood vessels is called a **hematoma** (Greek for "blood tumor"). Usually it is quite firm, has an irregular outline, and appears to be attached to the surrounding tissues. Hematomas in the breast can mimic—and be clinically indistinguishable from—those indurate masses caused by infiltrating ductal carcinomas. This is not surprising because both types of dominant mass begin with an "injury" (whether caused by impact or by malignant infiltration), and because both owe their hardness, irregular outline, and lack of mobility to a copious production of the same material (collagen). The important difference between hematomas and scirrhous carcinomas is resolution. Within a week or two any breast mass resulting from trauma should begin to fade away, growing smaller and smaller, and then vanishing altogether. The body's repair job having been completed, the collagen scaffolding is quickly dissolved and reabsorbed.

A woman with a hard breast lump which "just popped up" needs to search her memory for possible trauma. Was there a collision with a door last week, or a half-forgotten bruise from a fall? No diagnostic procedures are indicated when a hematoma resolves of its own accord. On the other hand, a persistent mass often necessitates a diagnostic biopsy, even if there is a history of trauma to the area. Blows to the breast do not induce malignancies, but sometimes they can serve to conceal them by providing a false explanation for a mass which would otherwise be deemed suspicious. The lumps caused by trauma are almost always of short duration. When one seems to persist for many months, a biopsy may sometimes reveal a benign condition called **fat necrosis**. Monica Morrow, a surgeon at the University of Chicago, points out that fat necrosis often presents as "a painless mass in the breast that is firm, ill-defined, and poorly mobile," and

The Breast Quadrants

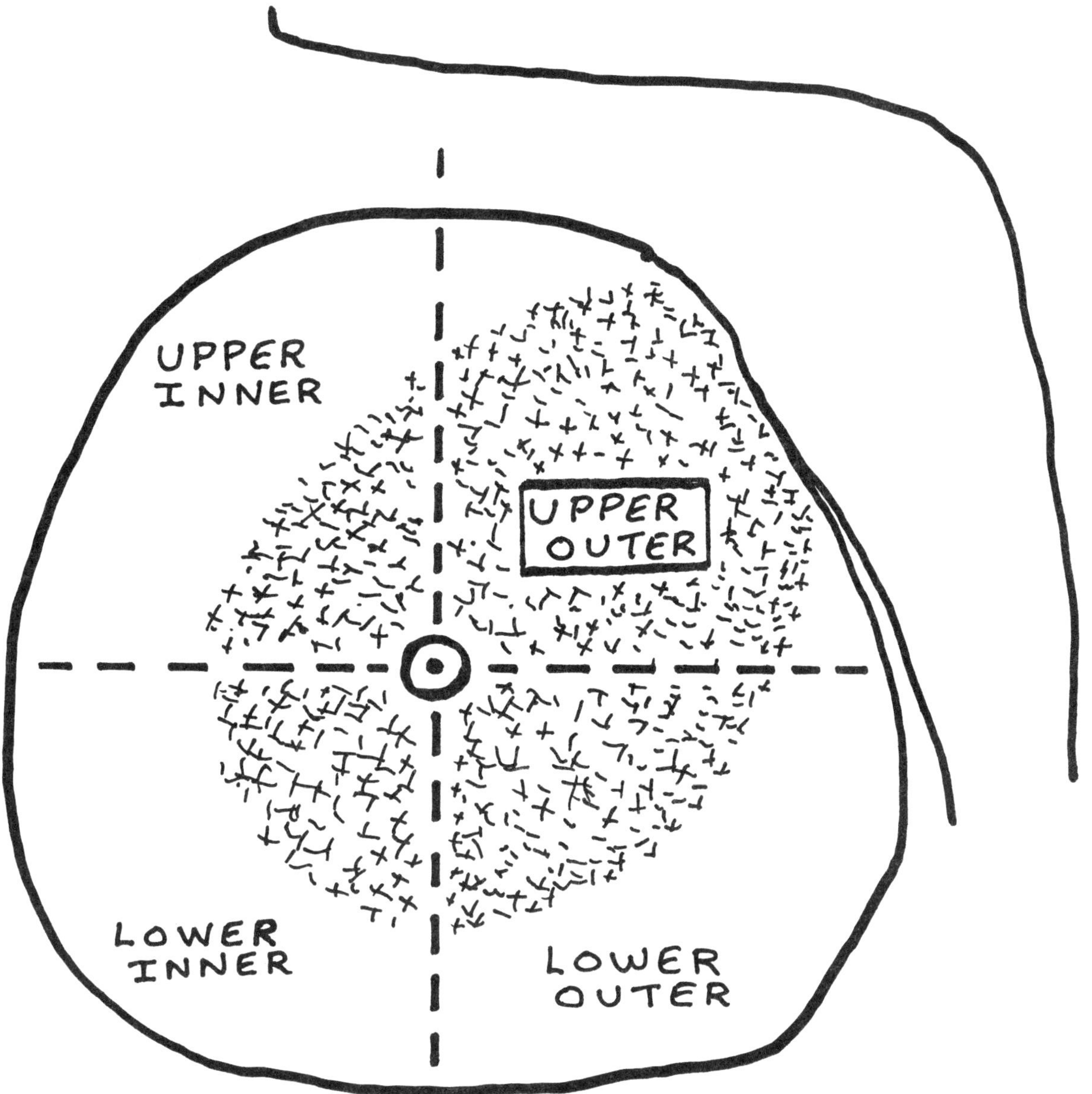

For convenience, breast specialists will speak of the breast as if it were divided into **four quadrants**, with the nipple at the center. The concentration of glandular tissue, represented here by the hatched areas, is most pronounced in the upper outer quadrant and around the nipple.

that "it is difficult to distinguish from carcinoma on both physical examination and mammography."[7] While not a frequent finding, fat necrosis can occur when the flow of blood to the fatty tissues cushioning the mammary gland has been interrupted for an extended period of time. Usually the resulting mass is located superficially, right below the surface of the skin; and it may produce thickening or retraction of the overlying skin, symptoms which understandably raise a suspicion of malignancy.

FIBROADENOMAS
Mobile, Regular, and Benign

The two characteristics which most strongly suggest a benign etiology for breast masses are **mobility** and **regularity of outline**. Cancers typically infiltrate into the surrounding tissues. The outlines of the resulting tumors are indistinct and difficult to determine, and the masses lack mobility—they don't roll about freely when palpated by an examiner's hand. There are exceptions to these rules; as we've seen, the benign lumps resulting from hematomas or fat necrosis generally follow the carcinoma pattern, with indistinct margins and deficient mobility. But **fibroadenomas**, the most prevalent benign tumors, would seem to have been designed just to embody the rules; they have exceptionally regular outlines and a remarkable degree of mobility. According to L. E. Hughes and his colleagues at the University Hospital of Wales, a fibroadenoma is nothing more than a "gross hypertrophy" of one or more lobules in the developing breast. These tumors primarily afflict teenage girls and women in their twenties; after age 35 they occur less frequently. Microscopic examination of fibroadenomas will usually reveal abnormal proliferation of both epithelial and stromal cells. Dr. Hughes and his colleagues emphasize that "the fibrous stromal element is the key to classification and behavior."[8] The epithelial cells are encapsulated by a fibrous shell which rolls around like a loose marble or pea, and which feels like hard rubber.

Fibroadenomas are typically self-limiting. They will grow to a certain size, commonly from one to three centimeters (maybe an inch or so), and then either stop growing or slowly regress. Occasionally one will continue growing until it occupies a large portion of the breast; such a "giant fibroadenoma" is a rare phenomenon of the teenage years. Fibroadenomas do not occur after the menopause. When they are discovered in postmenopausal breasts, they will usually be found to contain considerable calcification, suggesting that they are mineralized relics which actually developed much earlier.

In young women fibroadenomas are wondrously easy to diagnose—the tumors are so distinctive, and the chances of cancer are so remote. In older women mammography generally reveals a well-defined mass surrounded by a halo of compressed fat, a finding which bespeaks a benign and noninvasive entity. Surgical excision is curative, but there is no consensus regarding which fibroadenomas need to be excised. Hughes et al believe that typical fibroadenomas "can safely be left untreated" in women under age 25. For older women they recommend biopsy to rule out the possibility of occult cancer. If a young woman decides to leave a fibroadenoma untreated, she should remember its approximate location in the breast: this might prevent unnecessary diagnostic procedures in later years, should the very same tumor be rediscovered on some future mammogram or physical examination.

The "Mobility Criterion" for the Evaluation of Breast Masses

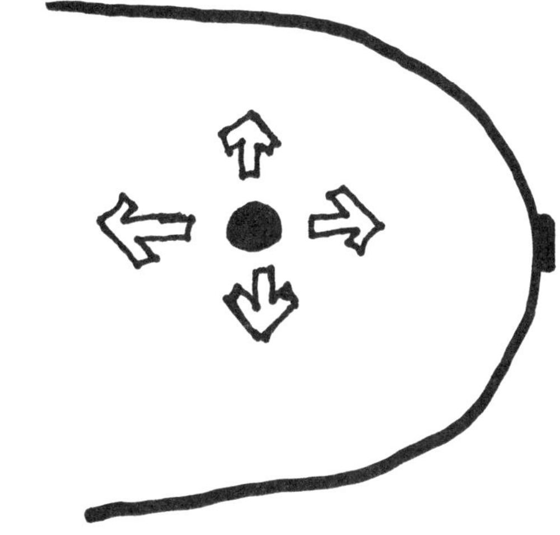

**freely mobile
in all directions
&
regular outline
(usually benign)**

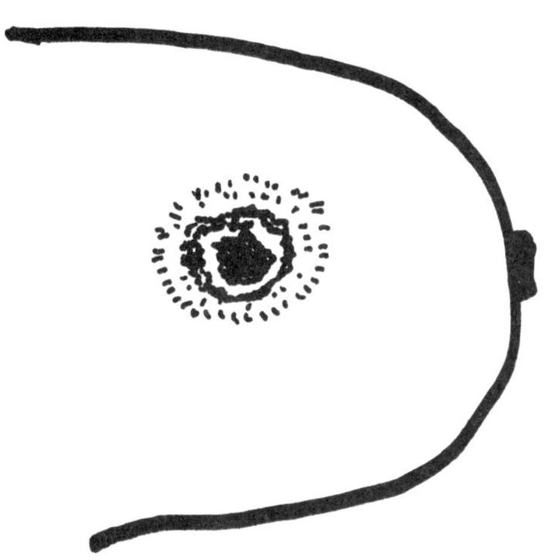

**seemingly attached
to surrounding tissues
&
indistinct outline
(usually suspicious)**

The **palpation of breast masses** can often provide clues to their nature. Masses which have well-defined outlines and which roll about freely under the examiner's hand are **usually benign**. Masses which have indistinct outlines and which seem attached to the surrounding tissues normally raise **suspicions of malignancy**, unless a history of recent trauma suggests a diagnosis of hematoma or fat necrosis.

Those Exuberant Lobules

Two other benign conditions of the breast also involve excessive development of the milk-producing lobules, and like fibroadenomas, display abnormal proliferation of the surrounding stromal cells as well as the glandular epithelial cells. Unlike fibroadenomas, these two lesions often mimic malignancy and are the very devil to diagnose. Fortunately, they are relatively rare.

Phyllodes tumors are closely related to fibroadenomas, so much so that pathologists have long been battering their brains trying to agree on criteria demarcating the two species. The term **phyllodes** denotes a leaf-like appearance (from the Greek word for leaf, *phyllon*). The French pathologist Monique Trojani observes that the fibroblasts (connective cells) and the collagen they secrete will assume "an arrangement like the veins of a leaf."[9] Phyllodes tumors are usually larger than fibroadenomas, grow faster, lack the distinctive fibrous capsule, and afflict an older patient population (Dr. Trojani cites a mean age of 45 at diagnosis). The stromal component provides the main identifying feature of a phyllodes tumor; it tends to hypercellularity, with an abundance of cells which may display irregularly shaped nuclei and increased mitotic activity. The stroma would seem to be well on the road to malignancy; but only occasionally will a phyllodes tumor evolve into a metastatic cancer, which would then be called a sarcoma in recognition of its origin from connective tissues. Surgical excision is not always curative. Because these tumors lack the isolating fibrous shells characteristic of fibroadenomas, it's easy to leave abnormal cells behind in the breast. Local recurrence at the tumor site is common, but most patients are spared extensive regional spread.[10]

Sclerosing adenosis has gained notoriety as the benign condition which most perfectly mimics an infiltrating carcinoma. The name may sound forbidding to laypersons; but **adenosis** simply refers to a glandular enlargement (from the Greek *aden*, "gland," and *osis*, "condition"), and **sclerosing** simply indicates an excessive growth of fibrous tissue (from the Greek *skleros*, "hard"). The glands involved—the tiny lobules—not only reveal hyperplasia but assume all manner of strange shapes because they are being compressed by proliferating connective cells in the surrounding stroma. Sclerosing adenosis can have a wide range of presentations. David L. Page and Jean F. Simpson, pathologists at Vanderbilt University, observe that it usually occurs as "a microscopic lesion," which is nonpalpable and asymptomatic.[11] Unfortunately, when detected on a mammogram, this condition may appear as an ill-defined area of abnormal density, which is liberally sprinkled with small calcifications.[12] In short, it's the very thing to set off all the alarm bells in your radiologist's office! Sclerosing adenosis can also present as an irregularly shaped mass (lump) which will seem affixed to adjacent tissues and which may even be painful. According to Page and Simpson, "a palpable mass may be created by aggregations of microscopic foci."[13] Biopsy does not always remove the suspicion of cancer. If the tissue specimen has been frozen or if it is too small, sclerosing adenosis may be extremely difficult to distinguish from malignancy. This condition may afflict women of any age from the teens through the postmenopausal years, though the vast majority of patients are in their thirties and forties.[14]

Cysts—A Common Problem

Cysts are the breast masses most frequently diagnosed in older premenopausal women; they usually afflict women over age 35 but under age 50. Cyst formation is rare in teenagers and women in their twenties, and does not occur after the menopause except in women taking hormone replacement therapy. Cysts are nothing more than lobules which have been expanded by entrapped breast fluid. There is considerable size variation: most cysts are too small to be felt, but some may grow to two or more inches in diameter.

The tremendous incidence of cysts in the 35-to-50 age bracket suggests that they are created by the combined effects of hormonal stimulation and aging. With each menstrual cycle, fluid is produced and retained in the mammary gland, especially during the late luteal phase. Postmenopausal women taking estrogen, especially in combination with a progestin, may also experience fluid retention. Normally this breast edema resolves when the hormonal stimulation is removed, either at menstruation or by discontinuance of the progestin. The smallest ducts—also known as **ductules**—drain the accumulated fluid from the lobules; it is then returned to general circulation by the surrounding lymphatic vessels. Cysts occur when the involutional changes associated with aging obstruct the ductules draining the lobules, or otherwise impair the body's ability to reabsorb breast fluid. We may speculate that the ductules may become clogged with cellular debris, or that with aging they lose their flexibility and resilience, becoming more prone to kinking which could result in an obstruction. The increased fibrosis seen in the aging breast almost certainly plays a large role in cyst formation. The proliferating stroma tends to impinge on the ductules, narrowing them or shutting them altogether. The dense collagen in the stroma also makes it difficult for breast fluid to diffuse through the thin walls of the lobules, further impeding lymphatic drainage. The term **fibrocystic disease**, long used as an omnibus diagnosis for breast problems,

correctly implies an association between fibrosis and cyst formation, while wrongly conveying the impression that these processes somehow constitute a pathological condition (a "disease"). Most women would seem to develop at least microscopic, nonpalpable cysts. But in other women the fluid retention will continue until one day a distended lobule suddenly becomes a palpable mass.

Cysts are usually easy to diagnose. The breast surgeon Susan Love observes how a touch of the examiner's hand may suffice to identify a cyst which is superficially located: "It's smooth on the outside and 'ballottable'—squishy—on the inside, so that if you push on it, you can feel that it's got fluid inside."[15] Of course, palpation will not be very revealing when a cyst is taut with fluid and buried deep in a large breast; the examiner may feel a remote mass, but can't tell whether it has a regular outline or whether it's solid or fluid-filled. In this instance, diagnostic mammography would typically reveal the well-defined margins associated with cysts and other benign lesions; and ultrasound would typically tell us whether the buried mass was solid or fluid-filled. Mammography and ultrasound are less accurate when applied to the engorged breasts of women who have been breast-feeding. Fortunately, the **galactoceles** (milk cysts) which may develop after a period of lactation usually appear close to the nipple, where they can be readily palpated. In these cases the entrapped fluid happens to be milk.[16]

Treating a cyst is possibly the most gratifying thing that breast specialists may be called upon to do. The remedy is so simple, swift, and painless—and the patient's relief and gratitude are so apparent. Most cysts will vanish when they are aspirated with a hypodermic needle. Typically the physician will immobilize the cyst with the left hand while inserting a needle into it with the right.

A Typical Cyst

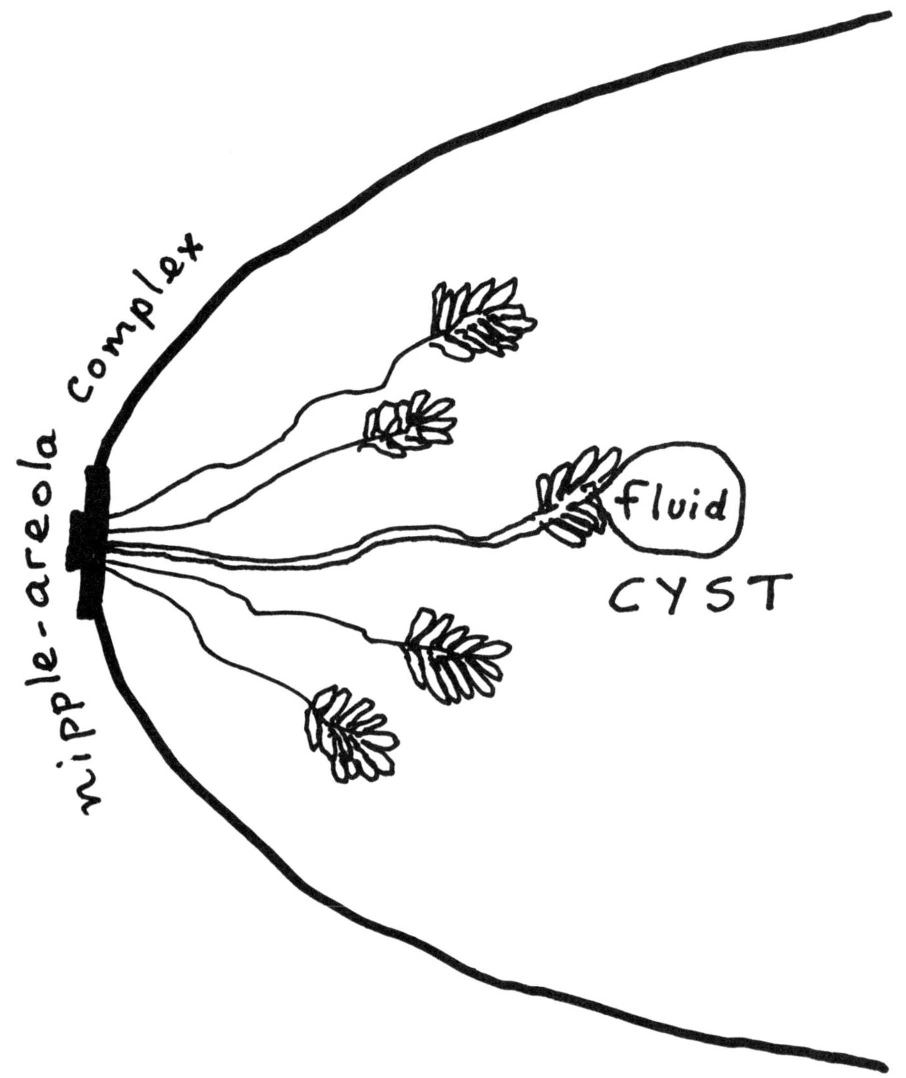

Cysts are the most frequent breast complaint reported by older premenopausal women. Fluid accumulates in the lobules during the menstrual cycle, but then fails to drain out because age-related fibrosis in the surrounding tissues has obstructed the small terminal ducts. Eventually a fluid-swollen lobule will present as a palpable mass.

The process takes only a minute or two. The withdrawn fluid, ranging from a few drops to several ounces, never resembles mountain spring water. Textbooks employ a spectrum of unappetizing hues in describing cystic breast fluid—dirty brown, toad green, sickly yellow—but these sordid colors indicate staleness, not malignancy. Cysts do not require additional diagnostic procedures, unless the aspirated fluid proves to be tinged with blood, or the underlying mass remains palpable after its fluid has been withdrawn. In these cases, any bloody aspirate would need to be sent to the pathology lab and checked for the presence of malignant cells—and the area of any residual mass would need to be attentively radiographed, preferably with focused **magnification mammography**. Cysts would not seem to increase breast cancer risk, but this is not to say that they would not occasionally be found in proximity to an occult tumor.[17]

Some women are never troubled by cysts—some may experience only a single cyst—and others will be downright plagued. Both breasts can be affected, as cysts spring up one after another over a period of years. This constant affliction should be viewed as a nuisance like acne, athlete's foot, or dandruff. **Recurrence**—that is, the refilling of a cyst previously aspirated—is emotionally distressing, but not a threat to health. L. E. Hughes and his colleagues in Wales assure us that cyst recurrence is not related to cancer: "We have seen no carcinoma associated solely with refilling of a cyst without blood-stained fluid. We treat a recurrent cyst by repeated aspiration, and are not particularly concerned at the number of aspirations required."[18] Fortunately, multiple recurrences of the same cyst are relatively uncommon. According to William L. Donegan, "less than 20 percent of simple cysts will refill, and less than 9 percent will refill after two or three aspirations."[19]

Postmenopausal Duct Ectasia

Consciously or unconsciously, physicians bring certain preconceptions to the evaluation of breast masses. If the patient with a lump is in her teens or twenties, they'll initially suspect a fibroadenoma, by far the most likely cause in that age bracket. If the patient is in her thirties or forties, they'll think about a cyst, the prevalent diagnosis in those two decades. When a woman aged 50 and older presents with a dominant mass in the breast, physicians understandably suspect carcinoma and will take pains to rule out—or confirm—this possibility. But even with postmenopausal women, suspicious lumps often prove to have a benign etiology. **Duct ectasia**, one syndrome which can produce a hard mass mimicking carcinoma, is rarely seen before age 40 and principally diagnosed after age 50. The venerable breast specialist C. D. Haagensen pronounced duct ectasia "a lesion of the inactive and aging breast."[20] The term **ectasia**, from the Greek, simply means "dilation"; the ducts dilated to abnormal widths may be found anywhere in the breast, but are most frequently encountered right below the nipple. Autopsy studies have revealed some degree of duct ectasia in almost half those women over age 60—but most cases are not severe enough to produce symptoms.[21]

The origins of duct ectasia are open to question. The subareolar ducts may dilate to five millimeters or more, several times their normal width of about half a millimeter, and become palpable. Upon microscopic examination these expanded ducts will prove to be clogged with a sticky mixture of dead cells, cellular debris, and fatty secretions. But dilated clogged ducts are only part of the problem; the other factor is **periductal mastitis**, a persistent inflammation in the stroma around the affected ducts. Numerous white cells are sometimes detected in the periductal area, suggesting that the mastitis (breast inflammation) could result from a bacterial infection. Alternately, it might represent a response to irritant substances leaking from the clogged ducts. Pathologists continue to debate whether ductal dilation leads to periductal mastitis (this is the traditional view), or whether stromal inflammation comes first and produces duct ectasia as a late effect. We do need to remember that both duct ectasia and periductal mastitis are accompanied by stromal fibrosis, often resulting in a hard lump with irregular outlines. This growing fibrotic mass can shorten the subareolar ducts and pull on the subcutaneous ligaments, causing a suspicious retraction of the nipple or changing the contour of the skin. Symptoms like these always set off the alarm bells for breast cancer! In advanced duct ectasia, a nipple discharge may develop which is so copious as to be socially embarrassing. The discharge can range from an off-color fluid which oozes out at the nipple, to a gummy white substance resembling toothpaste which literally has to be squeezed out of the affected duct. A duct which has become ulcerated may yield a bloody discharge.[22]

Duct ectasia can imitate breast carcinoma with considerable verisimilitude, but usually it's not difficult to arrive at the correct diagnosis. In many cases involving nipple retraction, the thickened duct or ducts can be palpated beneath the areola. A specimen taken from any nipple discharge will often reveal the presence of bacteria, but no malignant cells will be detected.[23] Diagnostic mammography can provide significant clues, showing smoothly dilated ducts filled with pulpy material as well as the surrounding calcification and fibrosis.[24] Biopsy is necessary to confirm the diagnosis of ductal ectasia, which is sometimes reported in men as well as in women. Of course, men are not subject to lobular disorders like cysts or fibroadenomas, because lobules do not develop in the male breast. But the rudimentary ductal system would seem to be prone to duct ectasia—one study found 30 ectatic ducts among a hundred men examined at autopsy—yet the vast majority of male cases will remain asymptomatic. The cancer-mimicking symptoms are similar in both sexes (subareolar mass, nipple retraction, nipple discharge), and the treatment is the same. Mild cases of duct ectasia sometimes resolve spontaneously, but persistent ones require excision of the offending duct or ducts. Barbara L. Smith, an instructor in surgery at the Harvard Medical School, recommends that broad-spectrum antibiotics be given prior to any operation to lessen the possibility of abscess formation.[25]

FOCUS ON THE NIPPLES
Unilaterality as a Warning Sign

The simplest guideline we can use in distinguishing benign presentations in the breast from those which might be malignant is **unilaterality**. There is no reason why cancer could not appear simultaneously in both breasts, but such a bilateral presentation would be an extremely rare event. For all practical purposes, therefore, **bilateral means benign**. Symptoms which are equally affecting both breasts almost certainly do not have a malignant etiology—this rule will prove true at least 99% of the time. In contrast, persistent unilateral symptoms (those affecting only one breast) always need to be investigated with a view to ruling out cancer. Most unilateral symptoms will also prove to be caused by nonmalignant conditions, but not all.

The principle of unilaterality is especially applicable to the nipples. A lingering problem affecting one nipple but not the other demands the definitive diagnosis which

Duct Ectasia

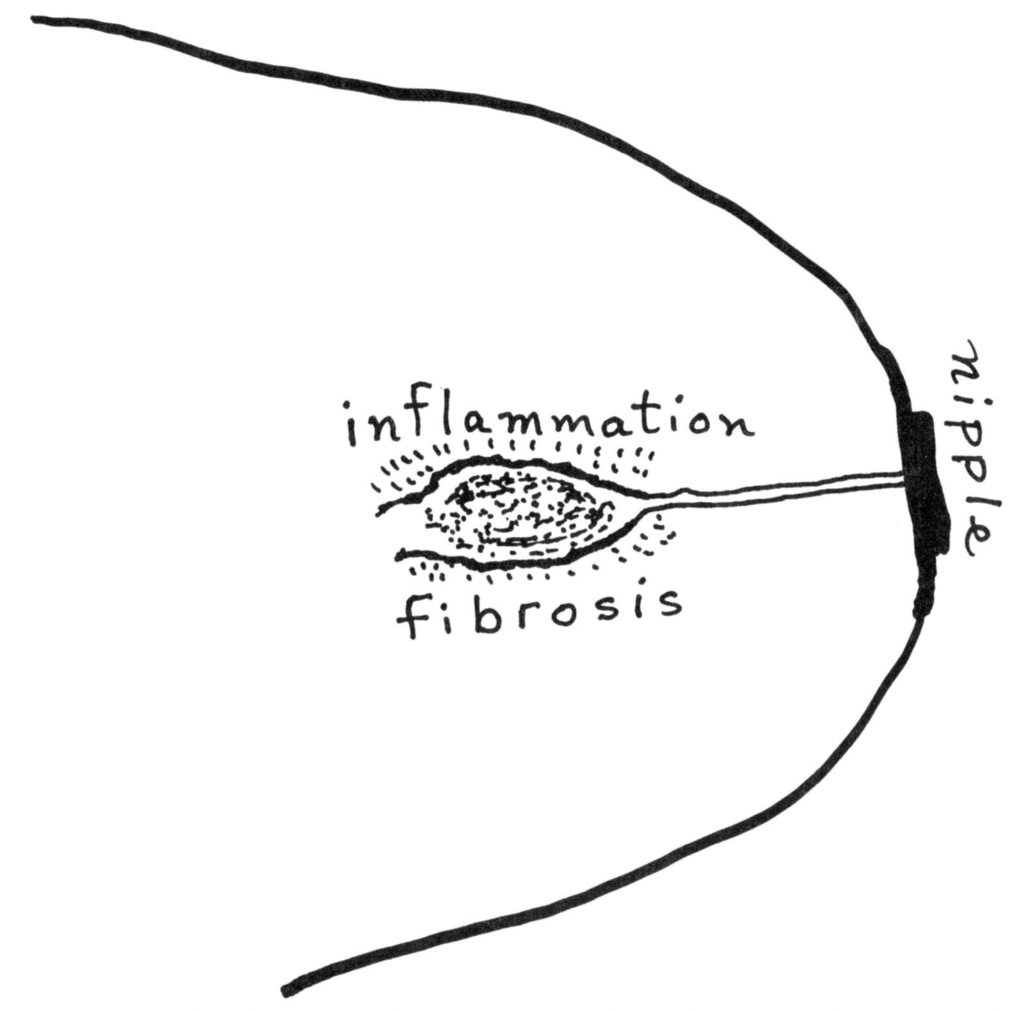

Duct ectasia is a benign postmenopausal disorder which can mimic an infiltrating ductal carcinoma. One of the large ducts beneath the nipple typically becomes dilated (expanded), with inflammation and fibrosis in the surrounding stroma. The clinical presentation consists of a hard immobile mass, which may be accompanied by retraction of the nipple and of the adjacent breast contour.

can only be had by putting a tissue specimen under the pathologist's microscope. The symptoms commonly seen in the nipple and its surrounding areola are nonspecific. On the basis of clinical observation, we cannot be sure whether the problem results from eczema, from infection, from an irritation caused by tight clothing, or from malignancy in the underlying breast. Tissue sampling is therefore indicated for any symptom which does not promptly respond to treatment.

The **nipple-areola complex** should be viewed as a part of the mammary gland—that is, as the gland's external terminus. L. E. Hughes and his colleagues in Wales remind us that "the nipple has an extensive network of smooth muscle whose fibers are mainly arranged in circular fashion." The heavily pigmented areola "contains the glands of Montgomery which provide a protective lubrication during lactation."[26] The tiny muscles hold the nipple erect during sexual arousal; they also facilitate the flow of milk during breast-feeding. Normally a nipple will begin to protrude from the areola at puberty. A nipple which fails to protrude during adolescence is said to be **inverted**; this condition may sometimes impair a woman's ability to breast-feed, but it has no relation to cancer. **Retraction** is another matter. Physicians use this term when a previously everted nipple (one that has normally protruded) recedes back into the areola. Retraction suggests a pathological process in the subareolar breast, possibly cancer; but as we've just seen, duct ectasia can produce the same effect. In the premenopausal breast, fibroadenomas or cysts which displace the large milk ducts can sometimes cause retraction. In the postmenopausal breast, nipple regression can be brought about by a generalized involutional fibrosis which tends to shorten the milk ducts and pull on ligaments. Like all other breast symptoms, retraction is not *per se* a sign of malignancy; but any unilateral change in nipple position, either a withdrawal back into the breast or a protrusion outwards, should be brought to a physician's attention. We need to know what caused that repositioning.

A breast cancer which first appears on the nipple-areola complex will be called **Paget's disease**, after the English physician James Paget who described the characteristic symptoms in 1874. Paget's disease typically begins with slight sensations of itching or burning in the nipple-areola complex, which later becomes red and irritated. Other changes gradually ensue. The nipple may flatten out or seem to wither away. The areola seems to expand, encroaching on the surrounding skin; the affected area can be either extremely dry or unusually moist and sticky. The scenario of Paget's disease varies from case to case, but the point of origin is constant. Paget's originates as a carcinoma (typically occult) in the large milk ducts beneath the nipple; the malignant cells then migrate upward and outward. William L. Donegan observes that "the spread of Paget's disease is centrifugal from ductal orifices on the nipple."[27] In some cases a physical examination or a mammogram will reveal a mass right below the nipple, suggesting that the malignant cells came from an infiltrating ductal carcinoma. When no mass is detected, we may suspect that the disease originated more subtly, perhaps from a small focus of ductal carcinoma *in situ*.

Because the early stages of Paget's resemble a benign eczema, the disease is often initially misdiagnosed as "dermatitis," and the patient given a dose of reassurance and a mild ointment for topical (local) application. Francis E. Rosato and R. S. Boova, surgeons at Philadelphia's Jefferson Medical College, lament that "frequently the delay in diagnosis exceeds one year due to continued treatment for eczema." The distinctions between these two conditions need to be emphasized. Eczema is likely to be bilateral, while Paget's would be unilateral. Minor skin irritations usually clear up after a few days; Paget's will not respond to topical lotions or ointments. Rosato and Boova recommend "a two-week trial with keratolytic or steroid creams," to be promptly followed by biopsy "if complete cure does not ensue."[28]

Nipple Discharges

An unwanted discharge from one or both nipples is a common breast symptom. Bilateral discharges (those coming from both nipples) fall under the aforementioned principle of unilaterality, and cancer may be ruled out almost automatically. A bilateral discharge could be caused by an endocrine abnormality, by drug consumption, or as Dr. Donegan points out, by "diffuse fibrocystic changes" in both breasts.[29] Some unilateral discharges are entirely harmless. A milky discharge encountered in a parous woman who has recently been breast-feeding should not raise suspicions of any kind. It is not uncommon for a premenopausal woman to secrete a few drops of breast fluid, especially if a nipple is massaged or otherwise stimulated. The expressed fluid could come in various pastel colors (clear, amber, pale yellow), but no investigations are needed— this is a normal phenomenon.[30] A few secretions from the nipple suggest pathological conditions other than cancer. Prolonged milky discharges unrelated to recent lactation point toward an excessive production of prolactin, possibly owing to a pituitary tumor. Thick, sticky discharges approaching the consistency of toothpaste suggest duct ectasia rather than malignancy.

Cancer enters into the differential diagnosis only with nipple discharges which are unilateral and spontaneous. Textbooks on breast cancer usually describe the suspect secretions as **serous** (like serum) or **sanguineous** (containing blood). The former adjective allows a wide range of colors— clear, brownish, greenish, yellowish, opalescent. The latter term is straightforward enough—indeed, when a hidden breast cancer presents with a nipple discharge, that discharge is more likely to be bloody or bloodstained than serous. Bloody discharges thus demand rigorous investigations to rule out (or confirm) cancer, but the absence of blood is no guarantee of benign etiology. An analysis of nineteen breast cancers presenting with nipple discharges yielded the following breakdown: six bloody discharges and seven "serosanguineous" (bloodstained), while four were deemed "serous" and two "watery."[31]

Bloody or blood-tinged discharges are frightening; in most cases, however, the underlying condition will be found to be benign, usually either a ductal papilloma or an ulceration resulting from duct ectasia. **Ductal papillomas** are probably the most frequent cause of unexplained bleeding from the nipple. Papillomas, whether in the breast or elsewhere in the body, are small fingerlike projections of hyperplastic epithelial cells. In the breast, papillomas typically begin as little protuberances on the sides of the larger milk ducts. They gradually develop into thin elongated growths of a centimeter or more in length, but only two or three millimeters in diameter. Often a mature papilloma will completely fill the lumen (passageway) of a duct. Bleeding from the nipple is not uncommon since the point at which the papilloma is attached to the duct wall can become ulcerated. While papillomas can occur at any age, they seem most prevalent in women between the ages of 40 and 50.

There is no evidence that papillomas routinely progress toward malignant transformation, yet pathologists need to exercise caution in distinguishing them from their more dangerous cousins, the **papillary carcinomas.** Paul Peter Rosen of New York's Memorial Sloan-Kettering Cancer Center has defined these latter lesions as "a variant of intraductal carcinoma" exhibiting a "frond-forming or papillary growth pattern."[32] Both papillomas and papillary carcinomas begin as tiny fingerlike growths from the duct walls; but while the former remain confined to the ducts, the latter will progress to stromal invasion and possibly to eventual metastasis.[33] Papillary carcinomas are relatively rare and mainly afflict women over the age of 60.

Physicians begin their investigation of all nipple discharges with a manual examination. Can a firm mass, a cyst, or an abscess be palpated beneath or around the areola? Even if no mass is detected, a physician can sometimes locate the diseased duct or ducts by gently applying pressure to the breast in a circular fashion. The problem may be presumed to originate at the spot where point pressure seems to produce or increase nipple secretions. A sample of the discharge might be placed on a glass slide and sent to the pathology lab for **cytology**. That is, the pathologist would study any individual cells which have been shed into the sample. The presence of malignant cells would indicate cancer, while inflammatory (white) cells would suggest an ongoing infection.[34] Mammography usually proves helpful both in locating the abnormality and in diagnosing it. A mammogram might reveal a nonpalpable mass beneath the areola, or an occult cyst draining into the ductal system, or a distended duct filled with the minute calcifications characteristic of ductal carcinoma *in situ*. If one of the larger ductal orifices on the nipple is actively discharging fluid, radiologists can perform a mammographic procedure called **ductography** or **galactography**. The ductal orifice involved is gently

cannulated—expanded with a thin tube (a cannula)—and then a nontoxic contrast medium is injected into the duct. A subsequent mammogram would clearly reveal any obstruction caused by a papilloma, by a papillary carcinoma, by duct ectasia, or by any other pathology. Of course, it would not necessarily distinguish the type of lesion responsible.

Treatment of a persistent nipple discharge usually requires surgical excision of the diseased areas of the affected duct or ducts. Excision may be needed not only to stop the discharge but to rule out cancer, which is detected less often than you might think. One survey of 270 patients undergoing surgery for nipple discharges found that papillomas were the most frequent problem, followed by duct ectasia (second most frequent), fibrocystic disease (third), and cancer (fourth).[35] We should caution that in three subgroups a nipple discharge is much more likely to be associated with breast cancer, mandating a precise pathological diagnosis in all cases. These subgroups are (1) postmenopausal women who have a serous or sanguineous discharge, (2) women of any age who have a discharge accompanied by an unidentified breast mass, and (3) men who have any nipple discharge whatsoever. Some writers assert that "spontaneous bleeding" from the male nipple is "almost invariably due to carcinoma"; but as men are also subject to ectasias and papillomas, perhaps a few cases of sanguineous discharge in the male are due to these benign conditions. The bilateral bleeding from female nipples which may occur during pregnancy results from the rapid expansion of the mammary gland; it requires no treatment and normally resolves soon after childbirth.[36]

SCARY SKIN SYMPTOMS
Infection or Inflammatory Cancer?

By and large, the surface of the breast is not a sensitive indicator of changes taking place in the mammary gland. Nonetheless the skin should be regularly inspected, because occasionally it will give the initial clinical (outward) symptom of a growing breast cancer. While the principle of unilaterality also applies to the skin, the fact that one breast differs slightly from the other is no cause for alarm. No two breasts are exactly alike. Diagnostic investigations are indicated only when one breast appears *newly different* from the other. A recent change visible on the outer surface of one breast, but not the other, always merits our attention. A woman who practices monthly breast self-examination will have a great advantage in this matter, since she will have learned how her breasts normally look and thus can detect unilateral changes in a timely fashion. The necessary visual inspection requires no more than average attention to detail and average eyesight, whether performed by a physician or by a layperson looking in a mirror.

Has one breast recently grown larger or smaller than the other? Malignancy can alter breast size in either direction. Some carcinomas, notably those classified as mucinous and medullary, can cause the entire breast to swell up; on the other hand, tumors with abundant fibrosis often cause a breast to become smaller and firmer.[37] Has the contour of one breast recently changed, bulging out here or there? As previously mentioned, red eczematous patches on the nipple-areola complex might be a sign of Paget's disease. Changes in skin coloration or texture anywhere on the breast should be regarded seriously, though eczema is a far more likely diagnosis than cancer. Superficial veins which become unusually visible at this or that spot on the breast suggest underlying

pathology, possibly a developing tumor which draws an increased blood supply. An equally suspicious symptom is an area revealing what the textbooks call "dimpling" or "retraction." In this instance the breast's contour is pulled inward, typically because a hidden mass is pulling on or otherwise dislocating Cooper's ligaments beneath the skin. Infiltrating carcinomas often produce such ligamental retraction; but since fibroadenomas, cysts, and duct ectasias can also cause this symptom, it is not a specific indicator of malignancy.

Inflammatory symptoms visible on the breast's surface are often due to bacterial infection. Early signs may include erythema (redness), painful tenderness, swelling, and skin thickening. Untreated, a bacterial infection will often cause considerable tissue destruction and progress to become an ugly abscess filled with purulent fluid and pus. Breast infections are commonly referred to under the cover-all term **mastitis** (literally "breast inflammation," from the Greek word for breast, *mastos*). Infections can occur at any time; but they are far more common during or shortly after periods of lactation, and most likely to afflict new mothers who lack experience in breast-feeding and fail to keep the nipple-areola complex clean and dry. Infant suckling can produce small cracks or fissures in the nipple, providing bacteria with entry to the ductal system. Dr. Hughes and his Welsh colleagues remind us that the invading bacteria, most frequently *Staphylococcus aureus*, would find "an ideal culture medium" in breast milk.[38] Staphylococci and other bacterial species also can gain access to the breast through skin abrasions or by transport through the bloodstream. Antibiotic therapy alone may cure an uncomplicated mastitis; but once an abscess has formed, surgical debridement and postoperative drainage are usually needed for resolution.

Skin Dimpling

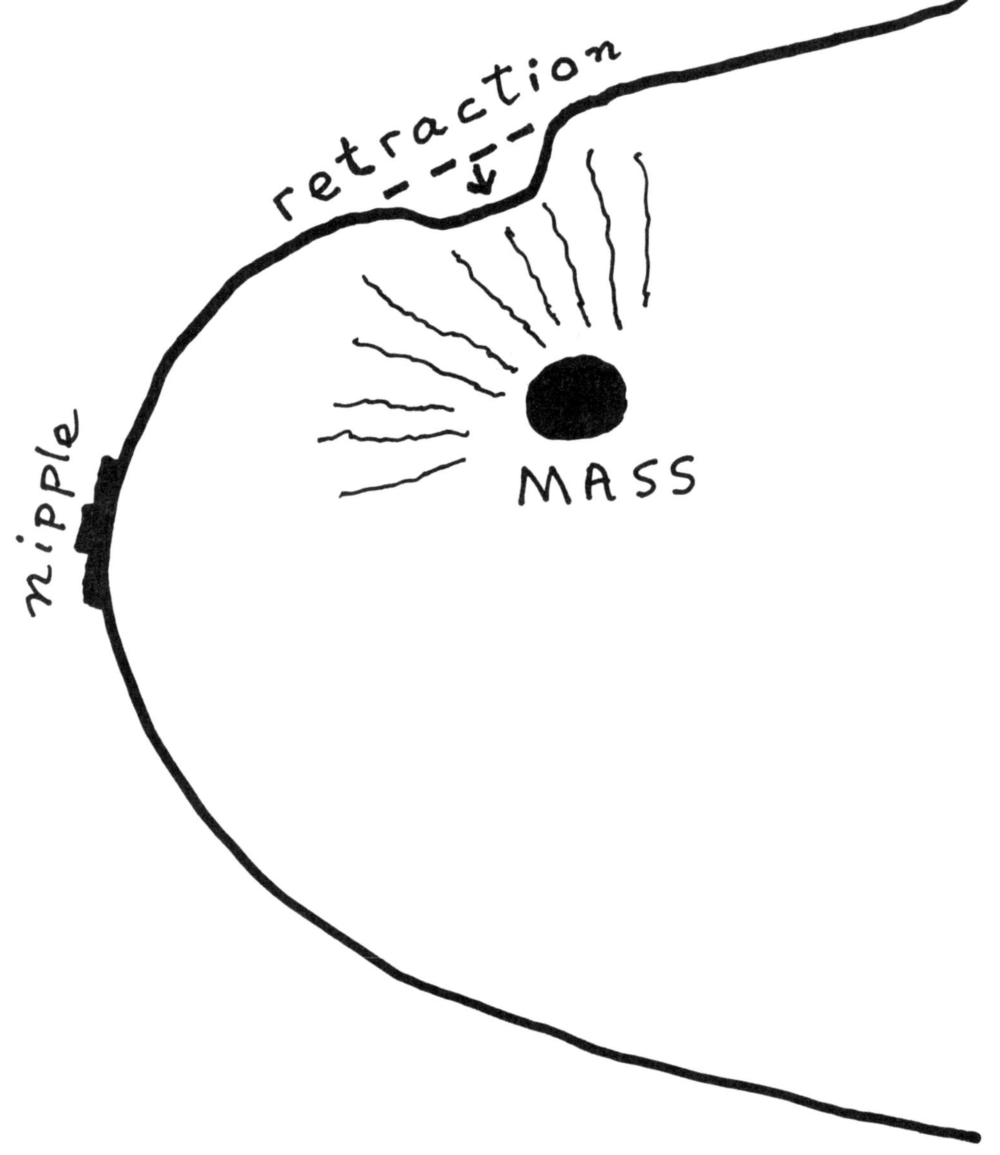

"Skin dimpling" refers to an inward retraction of the breast's contour; it suggests the presence of an underlying mass pulling on the breast's ligaments. This symptom is not specific for malignancy, since benign masses like cysts or fibroadenomas can also produce it.

One time in a thousand, those inflammatory symptoms characteristic of bacterial infection will be a harbinger of a far more serious condition—**inflammatory carcinoma of the breast**. This is breast cancer at its worst. Edward J. Wilkinson and his colleagues in the pathology department at the University of Florida remind us that inflammatory breast cancer "is not a specific tumor type, but rather a distinctive clinical presentation."[39] Most cases would be classified simply as infiltrating ductal carcinomas—that is, as the prevalent variety of breast malignancy. They are distinguished by a presentation and a clinical course which is so aggressive that it mimics acute mastitis, with the rapid onset of redness, swelling, and painful tenderness. An underlying mass may or may not be present; the affected breast usually grows larger. The defining feature of inflammatory breast cancer can be seen only by a pathologist—the tiny lymphatic vessels draining the dermis (skin) are filled with malignant cells. Since these lymphatics are clogged up and nonfunctional, the temperature of the skin will rise, producing sensations of heat; and fluid will accumulate under the skin, leading to localized **edema** (swelling). The involved breast may reveal a side effect of subcutaneous fluid retention known as *peau d'orange* (French for "orange skin"): the pores become highly visible, and the skin develops a pitted surface like an orange.

Inflammatory breast cancer is always locally advanced at presentation, with a high probability of subclinical distant metastases. Surgery hardly slows this disease; by itself mastectomy leads to a distressing result known as carcinoma *en cuirasse*, whereby new malignant lesions crop up along the operative scar and mock the surgeon's skillful handiwork. Traditionally, a measure of local control could be obtained by irradiating the affected breast prior to surgery, but few patients lived more than a year or two after

diagnosis. In recent years, however, potent chemotherapy has enabled some patients to enjoy disease-free remissions. Early diagnosis and prompt referral to an up-to-date oncology center are essential if a patient is to have a chance of long-term survival. Unfortunately, the diagnosis is often delayed for months on end, while unwary practitioners regard the condition simply as a recalcitrant infection. An initial error in diagnosis is understandable, as inflammatory breast cancer looks just like a commonplace mastitis. But any breast "infection" which does not respond to antibiotic therapy is suspect and demands a diagnostic procedure. A needle aspiration done in the doctor's office can sometimes provide an identification of the pathology involved, either by extracting the pus indicative of an abscess, or by yielding the malignant cells indicative of cancer. William L. Donegan cautions that a "full-thickness ellipse" (punch biopsy) taken from the edematous skin is necessary to demonstrate malignant invasion of the dermal lymphatics.

Painful Lumpy Breasts

Most visits to breast clinics by premenopausal women are prompted by vague "lumpiness" rather than by definite "lumps" (dominant masses). Experienced physicians can almost recite the relevant complaints before the patients reveal them. One textbook on breast diseases has summed up the clinical picture in this fashion: "Symptoms are monotonously similar, consisting of pain, nodularity, and tenderness. Both breasts are usually involved and the symptoms are either sporadic (usually premenstrual) or continuous."[41] Attentive readers of this chapter will recognize that symptoms which are bilateral and intermittent are not caused by cancer. This kind of generalized breast discomfort is due to repeated hormonal stimulation of the lobules—the lumpiness and painful tenderness are most pronounced in the late luteal phase of the menstrual cycle, and subside with the menses. Some women are more troubled than others; but even when severe this syndrome does not arise from any pathological condition and should be referred to as **cyclical nodularity** rather than as "fibrocystic disease." Diagnostic uncertainties arise because after twenty or more years of monthly menstrual cycles the breast tends to develop areas of persistent nodularity which can mimic dominant masses. The gradually increasing lumpiness is caused by progressive fibrosis in the stroma surrounding the lobules; this is a natural phenomenon of the aging breast, most often affecting women in their thirties and forties.

Areas of nodularity which wax and wane with the menstrual cycle are harmless. The most frequent challenge faced by physicians is to distinguish such nodularities from the dominant masses which require biopsy. A reasonable initial strategy is to examine or re-examine the suspicious area early in the menstrual cycle (follicular phase), when the hormones acting on the mammary gland are at ebb tide. Is the lump which seemed so apparent a few days before menstruation still palpable a few days afterward? Palpation of both breasts simultaneously often reveals that the area of suspicious lumpiness in one breast is mirrored by a comparably lumpy area at the same spot on the opposite breast. Such bilateral symmetry suggests widespread nodularity rather than a unilateral mass. If doubts persist after the physical examination, a mammogram focusing on the suspicious area may help to resolve them. We should caution that mammography will occasionally fail to detect a dominant mass, even an obviously palpable one, in a densely glandular premenopausal breast. Nonetheless, if neither palpation nor mammography indicates the presence of a mass, we have no target for a surgical biopsy or a needle-aspiration procedure; and the patient should be spared the anxiety and expense which tissue-sampling always entails.

A patient who questions the diagnosis of cyclical nodularity and continues to feel a breast lump would be wise to request a re-examination by her physician—or to seek a second opinion from another physician. The dividing line between pronounced nodularity and dominant mass is not always clear; sometimes an informed patient can be a better judge than her physician. John S. Spratt and other leading specialists recommend monthly breast self-examination for its educational value, so that "a woman with lumpy breasts" will "become familiar with the palpatory consistency of her own breast tissue," and therefore learn to "concentrate not on the lumpiness but on *changes* in consistency or appearance."[42]

The management of painful lumpy breasts relies largely on the alleviation of anxiety and a hoped-for placebo effect. Home remedies abound, but scientific proof of their effectiveness is lacking. Avoidance of foods and beverages containing caffeine (coffee, tea, colas, chocolate) would seem to be the most prevalent recommendation. Salt, nicotine, and emotional stress are sometimes cited as possible aggravating factors, while vitamin E is lauded as a preventive agent.[43] The use of a softer, more supportive bra is a commonsense remedy that certainly won't do any harm. Both the lumpiness and any associated pain typically disappear after the menopause.

Where's the Cancer Risk?

While it's quite clear that most lumps and other clinical presentations in the breast will prove to have a benign etiology, it's much less certain which benign conditions might produce an elevated risk of subsequent breast cancer. Inquiries from patients about the degree of risk often meet with evasive or indefinite answers. Prior to the 1980s no one had been counting the vast number of cysts and fibroadenomas, much less systematically following the discharged patients for twenty or thirty years to assess their risk for breast malignancies. Recent research indicates that the degree of risk has less to do with the particular diagnosis than with the hard-to-assess degree of abnormality of the constituent epithelial cells. In 1985 the biostatistician William D. Dupont and the pathologist David L. Page of Vanderbilt University published a seminal study in the *New England Journal of Medicine*, reporting a seventeen-year follow-up on 3,303 women biopsied for various benign conditions in three hospitals in Nashville, Tennessee. The risk of subsequent breast cancer was noticeably elevated in those patients whose biopsies revealed **atypical hyperplasia** (also called **atypia**) of the cells lining the ducts and lobules.[44] Simple hyperplasia of these cellular populations resulted only in a modest risk elevation, up 50% compared to women whose biopsies revealed nonproliferative lesions.[45] Dupont and Page defined atypical hyperplasia as a cellular proliferation "meeting some but not all the criteria for a diagnosis of carcinoma *in situ*"; in their study it resulted in 330% risk elevation. Women with both atypia and a family history of breast cancer proved to have eleven times the risk of women with no epithelial proliferation and no family history.[46]

In 1988 Christine L. Carter and her coworkers at the National Cancer Institute surveyed 16,692 women "with biopsy-diagnosed benign breast disease." Atypical hyperplasia again emerged as the principal indicator of breast cancer risk in benign conditions. Compared to normal subjects,

women with atypia had three times the risk. Youth compounded the danger—women diagnosed with atypia before age 46 were found to have 5.7 times the risk.[47] The Nurses' Health Study has released neatly corroborative findings, based on its poll of 121,700 registered nurses. Overall, those nurses with atypical hyperplasia had 3.7 times the breast cancer risk of "women with no proliferative disease." But youthfulness again upped the odds a bit more, those nurses diagnosed with atypia while premenopausal having 5.9 times the risk.[48]

We may reasonably conclude that atypical hyperplasia detected in connection with any benign condition indicates a significantly increased risk of subsequent breast cancer, especially in premenopausal patients or in patients with any family history of this disease. While atypical hyperplasia is thus an established risk factor, its diagnosis requires an attentive microscopic examination of the tissue specimen. Everybody agrees that abnormal epithelial proliferation spells increased risk.[49] But benign conditions without this proliferation are much less risky. **Fibroadenomas** illustrate this point. Results from both the National Cancer Institute survey of benign disorders (1988) and the Cancer and Steroid Hormone Study (1992) indicated that a history of one or more fibroadenomas involved a 70% elevation in risk.[50] In 1994, however, a Vanderbilt University team headed by William D. Dupont looked more closely at fibroadenomas, studying the case histories of 1,835 patients diagnosed with these tumors between 1950 and 1968. Dupont et al found that two-thirds of the fibroadenomas did not involve an elevated risk of subsequent breast cancer . Only those fibroadenomas exhibiting hyperplastic epithelial changes were associated with increased risk. Dupont et al emphasize that fibroadenomas do not represent a precisely uniform entity, but "exhibit a wide range of cytologic and histologic patterns; the epithelial component can vary from an absence of hyperplastic activity to carcinoma *in situ*."[51] Needless to say, the risk of subsequent breast cancer could be expected to vary between fibroadenomas, depending on the degree of proliferation in that epithelial component. Most of these lesions do not pose a threat.

We would expect **sclerosing adenosis** to entail a higher risk of subsequent breast cancer, since this benign condition is characterized by proliferation of both epithelial and connective cells. Some plausible data came out of the Nashville study done by Dupont and Page. Of the 3,303 women followed in the study, 349 had sclerosing adenosis. The Vanderbilt team found that patients with this diagnosis had an overall risk of 2.1 for invasive breast cancer, but that this estimate needed to be adjusted upwards or downwards in the individual cases, depending on the degree of epithelial hyperplasia. For those few patients with atypical hyperplasia, the relative risk rose to 6.7; it decreased to 1.7 when the analysis was limited to patients without atypia.[52]

Ductal papillomas also involve a proliferation of epithelial cells, this time in the ducts rather than in the lobules. But a solitary papilloma would seem to foreshadow no more than a modest elevation in breast cancer risk. Dupont and Page cite "an approximate twofold increase in risk."[53] This estimate has been corroborated by Carol A. Bodian of the Mount Sinai Medical Center and other researchers in New York City, who found ductal papillomas to be associated "with approximately a 2.5-fold excess risk, as compared with population incidence rates."[54] **Papillomatosis**, the widespread occurrence of multiple papillomas in both breasts, probably entails a higher risk. Fortunately, this condition is rare.

Cysts occasion much anxiety and multitudinous visits to doctors' offices; but since their formation depends more on stromal fibrosis than on epithelial proliferation, any risk of subsequent breast cancer would seem to be quite small, even for patients plagued by recurrent cysts. The Vanderbilt pathologists David L. Page and Jean F. Simpson state flatly that "there is no proven linkage of cysts alone to breast cancer risk. Cysts are more common in high-risk geographical groups, but are not determinants of cancer risk within geographical groups."[55] We are constrained to point out that the Nashville study by Dupont and Page, as updated in the 1990s, did find a slight elevation in risk (up 50%) for women diagnosed with cysts. This became a substantial risk elevation (up 200%) for those women who had both cysts and a family history of breast cancer.[56] Carol A. Bodian of Mount Sinai argues that cysts, while nonproliferative lesions, "are usually accompanied by other epithelial changes," and that "gross cystic disease" with the formation of multiple cysts may be a sign of epithelial instability and an increased risk for breast cancer. The study she headed linked cysts to an 80% elevation in risk, although this finding was only "of borderline statistical significance."[57] The literature on cysts and breast cancer is inconsistent; we may speculate that the elevated risk reported by some studies may be partially due to surveillance bias. Women troubled by cysts probably see physicians and have mammograms more often than other women; being so closely observed, they would naturally stand to have more malignancies detected. Cysts are no cause for alarm, and nothing would be gained by worrying about them.

Chapter Nine

THE OFFICE VISIT
Palpation, Ultrasound, Needle Aspiration

Lest any readers of Chapter Eight be tempted to perform self-diagnosis, the author has to say—*Don't do it!* You really ought to visit a doctor instead: there is no substitute for that clinical wisdom which comes from being constantly involved with patients and their symptoms over a period of many years. Unfortunately, finding an experienced breast clinician is not always easy. Back in the 1980s the writer and activist Rose Kushner lamented that "most general practitioners do not know enough about breast cancer to do a proper examination." She found that even gynecologists lacked sufficient training, reporting that young OB/GYNs had to memorize just "two paragraphs about examining breasts" before becoming board-certified.[1] Things have been getting better; but we must keep in mind that doctors are only human—and as subject to errors caused by deficient knowledge, by fatigue, or by haste as everybody else. Physicians usually score high in the knowledge department, but are more likely than other professionals to be troubled by fatigue or forced to work hastily. Errors made by physicians sometimes have grave consequences, which may serve to bring about prolonged litigation. In the face of these unpleasant realities, the patient's duty is quite simple: **TRUST YOUR DOCTOR—** *but not too much!* If the breast symptom which prompted your visit to the doctor's office persists, you should insist on further diagnostic procedures—or see another physician and get a second opinion. All those "failure-to-diagnose" lawsuits are not commenced by informed patients who know something about breast cancer and recognize the limits of our medical technologies. These suits are invariably commenced by naive patients who have placed complete trust in a single physician and permitted themselves to be reassured even as their symptoms worsened. Under these circumstances the eventual cancer diagnosis seems less like a misfortune than a betrayal of trust; and the patient's disillusionment quickly turns into anger, directed against the physician who had so confidently assumed the posture of superior knowledge.

The Doctor's Breast Exam

An initial breast examination performed by a physician, whatever his or her specialization might be, will consist of three distinct parts. The first is **oral**, and largely the responsibility of the patient, who must fully recount the history of the presenting symptom or symptoms. When did the problem begin? Where is the lump (mass) located? Is it painful? Ideally the patient will have anticipated the questions and prepared her responses beforehand, facilitating this interview. If she has a family history of breast cancer or a personal history of benign breast problems, she should provide her physician with the pertinent details.

The **visual examination** typically begins with the patient sitting or standing upright in a well-lighted room, as the physician looks for possible irregularities of color or texture on the skin or on the nipple-areola complex, and for possible inconsistencies of contour or size between the two breasts. The patient is then asked to raise both arms overhead—this movement would accentuate any changes in contour in the lower quadrants of the breast, and reveal any skin alterations along the inframammary fold (the line in the skin where the lower breast meets the chest wall). The patient is next requested to place her hands on her hips, akimbo-fashion, and to press down forcefully. This action flexes the pectoralis major muscle (the big chest muscle) and would accentuate any area of skin dimpling (contour retraction) caused by an underlying mass.

While the ensuing **palpatory examination** is essential, physicians have slightly different methods of accomplishing it. The surgeon David W. Kinne and the radiologist Daniel B. Kopans suggest that "palpation of the breast with the patient still sitting upright may allow detection of subtle lesions that would be more difficult to palpate if she were supine."[2] But most physicians seem to have preferred the supine position, often placing a pad or pillow beneath the patient's back so as to elevate the breast being examined. William L. Donegan finds that palpation in the upright position is "least informative," since the breast may be "pendulous and folded on itself." In the supine position he adds, "the breast is flattened and thinned on the chest wall," making it easier to detect small masses or densities.[3] Palpatory sensitivity is also enhanced if the examiner's fingertips are slightly lubricated with a thin film of oil or lotion—Kinne and Kopans recommend talc for this purpose.

If the patient is aware of a dominant mass or an area of increased density, she should point to it. Otherwise, the physician's palpation would usually proceed in overlapping concentric circles, either beginning on the periphery and working toward the nipple, or vice versa. The axilla (armpit) and the clavicular regions (above and beneath the collarbone) should be carefully examined for enlarged lymph nodes—palpation of these areas is best accomplished with the patient sitting or standing upright. Some authorities recommend that the examiner gently manipulate and compress the nipple, to see if any discharge can be expressed. Since we discussed the evaluation of nipple discharges in the last chapter, we need not enter on this topic here. However, we should again stress that with premenopausal women the palpatory examination is likely to be most informative if performed about a week after the onset of menstruation, when breast engorgement is minimal. Premenopausal women may wish to take this fact into account when scheduling a doctor's appointment, especially if the symptom to be investigated is a small, barely palpable mass.

Ultrasound and Other Tools

Sometimes a patient and her physician will not agree about the presence of a dominant mass. For one reason or another the examiner may not feel the lump—or there will be doubt as to whether a palpated mass is cystic (filled with fluid) or solid. Our medical technologies can resolve uncertainties of this kind. Of course, the most important tool remains X-ray mammography; but since this procedure involves specialized equipment and requires a radiologist to interpret the exposed film, it is not routinely done in the offices of gynecologists and internists. We'll discuss diagnostic mammography in the next chapter; at the moment we need to consider several tools for the visualization of breast masses which could be used in almost any doctor's office.

Transillumination, the simplest procedure, is also referred to as "light scanning" and "diaphanography." It's been around since the 1920s. In the old days the physician would first turn off the lights in the examining room and pull down the window shade. A flashlight would then be applied to the breast; in the near-total darkness its rays might effectively illuminate a suspect mass or other abnormality. Flashlights have been superseded by powerful halogen lights on the ends of curved fiber-optic rods, and the resulting images can now be recorded on infrared film. Even with these enhancements, rays of light have a limited ability to penetrate tissues. Transillumination is useful only in examining lesions near the surface of the breast. Cysts appear translucent, while solid masses are revealed as areas of markedly decreased luminosity. While sometimes helpful in identifying cysts, the technique cannot tell us which solid masses might be malignant.

Thermography is an office procedure which was formerly touted for the early detection of breast cancers. It is based on the perfectly correct idea that growing malignant tumors tend to be "hot spots" of metabolic activity, with angiogenesis and frequent cellular mitoses, and that as these areas would be slightly warmer than the surrounding tissues, they could be detected by measuring subtle variations in the breast's surface temperature. Easier said than done! But back in the 1970s, when many women were unduly concerned about radiation exposure from X-ray mammography, thermography machines had a great vogue. OB/GYNs rushed to buy them, hoping to acquire new capabilities in breast cancer screening. Thermography represented a safe noninvasive procedure which did not require special credentials on the operator's part. The exam itself was simple. Stripped to the waist, the patient sat motionless in a cool room, while the machine's sensors recorded the heat emitted from her breasts and displayed the temperature patterns as visible images on a TV screen of sorts. In the 1980s thermography fell into disrepute, as it became evident that the machines caused more problems than they solved. There were too many false positives, with suspicious readings for healthy breasts, and too many false negatives, whereby small malignancies went unnoticed. By and large this technique is inferior to mammography, but we must concede that conscientious thermography can indeed detect metabolically active cancers. In 1974 a thermographic exam indicated the invasive tumor in Rose Kushner's breast which had been missed on a previous mammogram.[4]

Ultrasound has become one of the most widely used technologies in American medicine. It has revolutionized obstetrics by providing a means of seeing the developing fetus without incurring exposure to X-rays. Almost everyone is familiar with the typical ultrasound exam in prenatal care, whereby a hand-held scanner is pressed against a pregnant abdomen while images of the fetus flicker across a viewing screen. This superb imaging tool grew out of the technical know-how acquired from **sonar**, developed to locate enemy submarines during the Second World War. Like sonar, ultrasound relies on sound waves bouncing off an object and then returning to a receiver. In this case the high-frequency waves are transmitted into the human body and reflected from the interfaces between different organs and tissues; the "echoes" are immediately processed by a computer, which converts them into recognizable images. Ultrasound works best on hollow and relatively quiescent organs like the uterus or the bladder; it is less effective on the breast, which is full of vibrations from the beating heart and the bellowing lungs. Ultrasound has never proven useful as a screening tool to detect early breast cancers; it cannot reliably image masses smaller than one centimeter, and it cannot depict minute clusters of telltale calcifications. In one important application, however, ultrasound is superior to mammography—it is virtually 100% effective in distinguishing fluid-filled cysts from solid masses. Occasionally this ability will save a patient from an unnecessary biopsy when a suspicious lump deep in the breast turns out to be a harmless cyst. Sometimes ultrasound can serve as a complement to mammography in examining premenopausal women with dense glandular breasts, which are poorly imaged on mammograms. It also helps to identify fibroadenomas in teenage girls, whose breasts should not be casually exposed to radiation. Ultrasound is usually very good in identifying abscesses (because of their cystic character), and it can often distinguish hematomas from ill-defined masses which might be malignant.[5]

Back in the 1960s ultrasonography of the breast was a complicated affair. The patient had to lie motionless upon a table, while suspending her breasts into a tank of water beneath. These days an exam can be performed in a few minutes. The breast is coated with a thin film of lubricating jelly, and then a hand-held "transducer" (scanner) is moved over the area of interest, producing an instantaneous image.[6]

Fine-Needle Aspiration

Neither mammography nor ultrasound nor any other imaging modality can actually diagnose breast cancer—or establish that a solid mass of indeterminate nature is not malignant. Cancer is a disease of individual cells, and in all cases diagnostic certainty can only be obtained by submitting a sample of cells for the pathologist's microscope. And there is only one routine office procedure which can be said to provide such a sample: **fine-needle aspiration**.

The sticking of hypodermic needles into breast masses has long been common practice. No one would quibble about it when cysts are involved, because inserting a needle and withdrawing the fluid is exactly the remedy that's needed. Unfortunately, American physicians have been in the habit of rather casually sticking needles into lumps *whose nature is unknown*. The explanation traditionally offered is that needle insertion offers the easiest and fastest way to determine whether a mass is solid or cystic. But in these days when both mammography and ultrasound are readily available, it would seem prudent to request an imaging examination before resorting to an invasive procedure, even one so modest as a probing needle. A patient is always relieved when a cyst is deflated; but she will experience a different emotion when a needle is inserted into a breast mass and no fluid comes out, especially if her doctor has not taken the time to explain the procedure beforehand.

In the 1980s fine-needle aspiration began to play a much larger role in the identification of breast cancers and many other types of tumor. The needle was no longer merely an instrument for deflating cysts or determining a tumor's solidity. Thanks to our pathologists' growing knowledge of cytology, it became the most convenient diagnostic tool in cancer medicine, likely to be employed anywhere in the body where a suspicious mass or lymph node could be found. We should explain that an ordinary "fine" (thin) hypodermic needle to which gentle suction has been applied by a syringe will not only withdraw fluid, but also a number of loose cells. The pathologist Edward J. Wilkinson and the surgeon Kirby I. Bland estimate "that the lumen of a single needle can retain as many as 100,000 cells."[7] Our attempts to obtain cellular specimens by fine-needle aspiration are generally successful, especially in the case of malignant tumors because here the customary adhesiveness between individual cells has been greatly diminished. If cancer is present, needle aspiration will generally tell us so. Any diagnosis of malignancy would be made largely on cytological features—that is, on morphological abnormalities of the aspirated cells such as enlarged and hyperchromatic nuclei, or irregular spacing between nuclei in cell clusters. Aspirates from malignant tumors tend to be hypercellular (lots of cells), with conspicuous variations in cellular size and arrangement. Aspirates from benign lesions tend to be hypocellular (only a few cells); but today's pathologists can often identify the type of benign lesion (e.g., fat necrosis or fibroadenoma) just by studying those few cells. Cytology is still not as informative or as accurate as the traditional histological examination. Even such dedicated cytologists as Edmund S. Cibas of the Harvard Medical School and his colleague Barbara S. Ducatman are quick to admit this technique's limitations. They point out that the cytological analysis of breast aspirates is "generally quite sensitive in detecting ductal carcinomas," but that "it cannot distinguish between an infiltrating ductal carcinoma and a ductal carcinoma *in situ*. It cannot identify the presence of lymphatic or vascular invasion." The dividing lines between malignancy and some benign conditions aren't

always apparent. Cibas and Ducatman observe that cytological examinations of aspirated cells may fail to distinguish benign papillomas from papillary carcinomas, and that they cannot be used to evaluate phyllodes tumors.[8]

The main advantage of fine-needle aspiration is that it can often give us a reasonably definitive diagnosis before any surgical biopsy or excision, and that in many cases it may eliminate the need for a surgical intervention. This procedure can be performed in the doctor's office without anesthesia or even sedation; it is fast and relatively inexpensive. Its biggest drawback is that it is heavily dependent on physician expertise. Needless to say, the pathologist who looks at the aspirate must be a skilled cytologist who's familiar with all the benign and malignant disorders of the breast and with the ways in which isolated cells and the accompanying cellular debris can yield diagnostic clues. But deficiencies in the pathology lab are not the only pitfall. Aspiration cytology assumes that we have an adequate sampling of cells from the suspect lesion, and getting such a sample depends on the skills of the examining physician. If the needle point is moved a millimeter or two beyond the lesion being probed, the resulting aspirate may well consist of the wrong type of cells. Either mammography or ultrasound could provide directional guidance, helping to center the needle point in the lesion; but then the necessary imaging equipment and skilled technicians to operate it are not universally available. With a view to ensuring adequate cellular sampling, most textbooks have emphasized a scattergun method—that is, the needle point would be moved through a lesion at several different angles while multiple aspirations are made. George W. Mitchell, Jr., a professor of gynecology at the University of Texas in San Antonio, gives representative instructions for sampling a solid breast mass: "By a tangential approach, the needle is passed to and fro eight to ten times through the tumor in various planes while constant suction is maintained. The material thus aspirated is squirted on at least six separate slides, fixed, and sent immediately to the laboratory."[9] Taking aspirates from different areas of a breast mass betters the odds that the pathologist will be able to render a conclusive diagnosis.

In recent years American physicians have become so convinced of cytology's utility that many are ready to perform needle aspirations even when a subsequent surgical biopsy is anticipated. Writing in the *New England Journal of Medicine*, William L. Donegan pronounced fine-needle aspiration "a routine part of evaluating a palpable breast mass"—and recommended that it be performed as the first step in this process, before mammograms are taken.[10] While we have the highest regard for Dr. Donegan, we must emphasize that insofar as mammograms are expected to provide information of diagnostic import, they should *precede* any attempt at needle aspiration. The radiologists Karen K. Lindfors and Lydia P. Howell observe that needle aspiration may tend to distort the contour of a breast mass and thus may "sacrifice the diagnostic accuracy" of any ensuing mammography: "Hematomas or edema created by fine-needle aspiration can appear as masses with ill-defined margins, which are suggestive of cancer." Lindfors and Howell point out that mammograms taken within a week after fine-needle aspiration are 36% more likely to yield false-positive results, setting off alarm bells for spurious "malignant findings."[11]

A Warning for Young Women
Reassurance Is Not Diagnosis

The movies and television have given us pervasive dramatizations of physicians as godlike figures who are constantly making life-and-death decisions. The reality is often very different. Most Americans today are essentially healthy; and perhaps the principal activity of our physicians is neither diagnosis nor treatment, but simply **reassurance**. In many cases all we need is to be told that our symptoms are not serious—not the forebodings of grave disease—and that they will resolve of their own accord. Some medical specialties lean more toward the reassurance business than others, but we may be sure that the most active traffickers in this commodity are those doctors who must listen to the breast symptoms described by young women in their thirties or early forties. There are oodles of complaints, and at least 90% of them are due to harmless and largely untreatable conditions—creeping fibrotic lumpiness, premenstrual edema, cyclical nodularity. In this instance the problem is that physicians become so accustomed to providing younger women with reassurance about breast symptoms that they do it automatically, almost as a kind of knee-jerk reaction from overworked professionals who have heard too many sound-alike stories. And what happens to those few young women who actually have breast cancer? All too often the conclusive diagnostic investigations which would be ordered immediately for the 50-year-old woman with a breast symptom are overlooked in the case of a 35-year-old. Mammograms are not taken, fine-needle aspirations not performed, and any legitimate worries about breast cancer are rather casually dismissed as pointless anxiety.

One 37-year-old breast cancer patient described rather typical experiences in a letter to advice columnist Abigail van Buren: "I went to my OB/GYN doctor. She felt the lump and said, 'Don't worry. It's nothing.' I trusted her judgment and ignored the lump for eight months, until I started to feel a dull pain in that area." This patient then saw another physician, who wisely ordered the mammograms which "showed a definite growth."[12] An eight-month delay seems short compared to some of the postponements which have been recorded for premenopausal patients. A physician who has already diagnosed "nothing" could have an entirely understandable tendency to defend that original judgment, and may simply repeat it if the patient returns on subsequent visits with the same complaint.

Diane Craig Chechik, a young breast cancer patient from Madison, Wisconsin, wrote a book about experiences which should serve as a cautionary tale for physicians and patients alike.[13] One day in March 1982 Ms. Chechik consulted her personal physician of seventeen years standing, a trusted friend, about a lump in her right breast. Her doctor promptly resorted to the needle, attempting to aspirate the mass. When no fluid came out, he did nothing except write "mammary hyperplasia" (an unverified diagnosis) in her file. Of course, this doctor's action violated the cardinal rule of fine-needle aspiration. If no fluid is withdrawn, or if the fluid is bloody or blood-stained, or if a residual mass remains after aspiration, you've got to take steps to positively diagnose that mass or suspicious area. Minimally, if no fluid comes out, the physician should attempt to aspirate loose cells for cytological analysis.[14]

Ms. Chechik revisited her doctor several times during the next year and a half, always with the same lump. He gave her kindly reassurances ("You don't have cancer") and downplayed the growing indications for biopsy ("I would not cut into your beautiful breasts"). By December 1983,

some 21 months after her initial consultation, Ms. Chechik not only had a large firm lump in her breast, but also a palpable axillary lymph node (a likely indication of malignant dissemination). At this time her cancer was finally diagnosed—not by her physician in Madison, but by a breast specialist in New York City. It was now too late to think about breast preservation. Diane Craig Chechik had to endure a mastectomy and several courses of toxic chemotherapy, and finally thirty radiation treatments after her cancer recurred along the surgical scar. Disillusioned, she sued her longtime physician for malpractice. In 1985 a Patient Compensation Panel in Wisconsin handed down a decision displaying the wisdom of Solomon. Needless to say, Ms. Chechik's physician was found to have been negligent in providing medical services; but she was also found to have been negligent in that she waited too long before seeking a second opinion. The panel assessed the blame in this unconscionable failure-to-diagnose case as follows: physician 80% negligent, patient 20% negligent.

Health care cannot be entrusted solely to the doctors, any more than we can leave matters of justice solely to the lawyers or religious observance solely to the clergy. This is not to say that credentialed professionals, be they doctors of medicine, law, or divinity, aren't entitled to the proper degree of respect; but we must resist that tendency to regard them as infallible founts of wisdom. Whatever their age, women with breast symptoms should recognize that there is an enormous difference between diagnosis and reassurance—and they should know when they are being served with the latter commodity instead of the former.

Chapter Ten

Diagnostic Mammography

A mammogram is an X-ray of the breast. Today mammography represents the single most important modality in breast imaging. While far from perfect, it is indispensable. The diagnosis and treatment of breast disorders without frequent recourse to this tool would seem inconceivable. Mammographic investigations should be divided into two distinct categories, which have to do with the reasons for which the X-rays are taken. The first category is **diagnostic mammography**—that is to say, mammograms are taken to help in locating and diagnosing the cause of a patient's symptoms. Strictly speaking, we cannot call mammography "diagnostic," because the final verdict on a breast disorder can be made only by the pathologist who examines a tissue specimen under a microscope. Yet mammography can often tell us whether or not a needle aspiration or a surgical biopsy has to be performed. The numerous benign and malignant disorders of the breast tend to have characteristic appearances on mammograms, so much so that sometimes we can be reasonably certain of their identity without tissue sampling. The radiographic image, considered together with the patient's age and with the findings from a physical examination, may lead us to conclude that the lump (breast mass) is a cyst, a fibroadenoma, or a lipoma (harmless fatty tumor) rather than an infiltrating ductal carcinoma. Occasionally a mammogram may indicate the proper diagnosis with a probable accuracy rate of 99% or better; but even in these cases, the radiologist's report would shy away from emphatic terminology, prefacing the diagnostic verdict with an expression like "consistent with" or "compatible with" (a cyst, a fibroadenoma, a carcinoma, and so forth). Usually diagnostic mammograms are suggestive rather than indicative. Under certain circumstances they may be uninformative or misleading.

The second category of radiological investigation is **screening mammography**—that is to say, apparently healthy women with no breast complaints are mammogramed periodically in the hope that these regular exams will detect any early cancers before they have a chance to metastasize. Screening mammography has been much more controversial than diagnostic mammography. Everybody agrees that mammograms can help in the evaluation of symptoms, but the utility and cost-effectiveness of examining asymptomatic individuals are constantly being debated. The evidence for (and against) screening mammography will be considered in a later chapter. For the present we need to review the scientific principles upon which mammography is based—and to assess its inherent strengths and weaknesses.

How Mammography Works

Medical X-rays, whether of the breast or of other bodily structures, depend upon differences in the density of the tissues being imaged. Softer tissues allow X-rays to pass through, while denser tissues impede their passage. When an exposed X-ray film is developed, the denser structures will appear as white areas while the softer tissues will be dark, thus producing a recognizable image of the body's internal parts. X-rays work best on bones, which are heavily mineralized and much denser than the surrounding soft tissues, and on foreign objects like bullets or needles, which are also radiologically opaque. Wilhelm Roentgen produced the first X-ray in 1895, imaging the bones in his wife's hand; within several years the emergent technology was widely employed to diagnose fractures and to locate embedded bullets. In the 1930s and 1940s X-rays proved useful in the detection of pulmonary tuberculosis: once expanded with a good breath of air, the lungs are much less radio-opaque than other chest structures and can be visualized on film. Chest X-rays remain a standard imaging exam, invariably required before any surgical operation involving total anesthesia.

At first the human breast looked like an improbable object for X-ray examinations. This body part had neither bones nor inflatable air sacks—all its structures consisted of pliable tissues, seemingly without significant variations in density. How could we produce that contrast so necessary for photographic images? Fortunately, the breast contains one element which is just a trifle less dense than its other tissues—and that element is **fat**. Carl J. Vyborny and Robert A. Schmidt, radiologists affiliated with the University of Chicago Hospitals, explain how the adipose tissue interspersed throughout the breast enables the production of mammographic images: "The fibrous, glandular, and ductal elements attenuate X-rays as soft tissue and cannot be differentiated by their radio-opacities. On the other hand, the presence of fat in most breasts allows the soft tissue elements to be seen in relief, providing the representation of breast anatomy." The breasts of premenopausal women often appear as a tangle of fibrous and glandular tissues, sometimes without enough interspersed fat to provide the necessary contrast. Vyborny and Schmidt remind us that a mammogram of a youthful breast largely devoid of adipose tissue would be "a monotonous gray, conveying essentially no information."[1] Mammography works much better on postmenopausal breasts, in which the residual glandular elements are set off—highlighted as it were—by a gradually increasing fat content.

Technological advances in breast imaging came but slowly. As early as 1913 a surgeon in Berlin, Albert Salomon, published a report describing the X-rays he had taken of numerous mastectomy specimens (breasts amputated because of malignant tumors). Salomon found that the resulting films often allowed him to distinguish between highly invasive cancers and those circumscribed tumors which the surgery might have cured. In 1930 Stafford L. Warren, a radiologist at the Rochester Memorial Hospital in upstate New York, described the preoperative breast X-rays taken of 119 symptomatic women who were about to undergo surgical biopsies. These films, Dr. Warren reported, could usually distinguish between cancers and benign conditions. In 111 of the 119 cases, the radiological interpretations made before surgery were confirmed by the pathological examinations made afterwards.[2] These initial reports outlining mammography's potential went unheeded. The first book about breast imaging did not appear until 1953, and the scientific foundations of mammographic cancer detection were laid only in the 1960s.

Robert L. Egan, long a faculty member at the Emory University School of Medicine, has a strong claim to being America's first professional mammographer. Egan devoted himself to breast imaging from 1956 onward; in the 1960s he began to catalogue the mammographic appearances of benign and malignant lesions, doing much to establish the reproducibility of these observational criteria. Egan and other researchers also demonstrated how the calcifications which show up so clearly on breast films often point to a diagnosis. The 1970s were noted for massive clinical trials which reported that regular mammographic screening could reduce breast cancer mortality in postmenopausal women by about one-third. The enthusiasm for mammography was briefly dampened, in the mid-1970s, by widely publicized reports about radiation carcinogenesis; these fears soon proved to be unwarranted. Mammography truly came of age in the 1980s. Manufacturers were now producing "dedicated" machines—that is, X-ray equipment specifically designed to image the breast. Equally important to mammographic accuracy was the growing number of highly trained specialists, which included the technicians who operated the machines as well as the radiologist physicians who interpreted the developed films. The radiation scares of the previous decade led to the introduction of improved photographic films, which not only gave clearer images but required much lower levels of X-ray exposure. A typical mammogram in the 1960s required a dosage of eight rads; by the 1980s the necessary dose had been reduced fortyfold, usually being no more than one-fifth rad. Philip Strax, a leading proponent of mammography screening, observed that any radiation hazard from this small exposure, even if repeated at frequent intervals, was "probably not measurable."[3]

Getting a Good Mammogram

Diagnostic mammograms are absolutely indicated before any surgical biopsy; and as emphasized in the last chapter, they may be advantageously taken before an attempt at fine-needle aspiration. There are several important reasons why both breasts should be attentively mammogramed whenever a patient has a clinical symptom, be it a lump, nipple discharge, or asymmetrical density. The first reason is, of course, that the mammograms stand to tell us something about the abnormality causing the symptom. The second reason is that the mammograms may reveal unsuspected subclinical abnormalities, either in the same breast with the presenting symptom or in the opposite breast. Is there another smaller mass, or perhaps another suspicious density? Mammograms usually provide worthwhile information about the size, shape, and location of breast masses and other lesions; but this information does not necessarily correlate with that gained from visual inspection and palpation. A malignant tumor is apt to appear larger on physical examination, because the physician's hand would respond to any edema or fibrotic reaction surrounding the central mass. In this instance the mammograms would give us a better idea of the tumor's actual size.

Most breast imaging centers continue to rely on **film-screen mammography**. The breast image is captured on film, which is developed and then placed over a light source (illuminated box) to be viewed. In 1972 the Xerox Corporation introduced an alternative technology called **xeromammography**, which captured the breast image on a specially-treated sheet of paper. This system worked much like the familiar Xerox copying machines, and it was quite the vogue in the late 1970s. Xeromammography proponents praised its ability to image the entire breast with one exposure and its sensitivity in depicting the tiniest calcifications.[4] Other radiologists argued for film-screen mammography, which required a lower dose of radiation and which could better portray subtle variations in tissue density. The film-screen technology eventually won out. In 1989 the Xerox Corporation announced its decision to stop manufacturing the xeromammography machines.[5]

Radiologists conduct ongoing debates over the optimal number of mammographic exposures and the proper positioning of the breast when these exposures are made. In the United States there is a broad consensus that at least two exposures from different angles should be made of each breast. Frequently a tumor or other lesion which is obscured by fibrous or glandular tissues on one exposure will be better visualized on another. There are three standard positions in American mammography. The first is called **craniocaudal**, or top-to-bottom (from the Latin *cranium*, skull, and *cauda*, tail). Here the patient sits or stands upright, while the radiation source is placed over the breast and the film beneath it. The **mediolateral** position offers a side view of the breast—Robert L. Egan suggests that the best results may be obtained when "the patient lies comfortably on her side." Large numbers of radiologists swear by a third position, the **mediolateral oblique**. Here the radiation source is placed in front of the shoulder to allow better imaging of the "axillary tail," that part of the mammary gland stretching toward the axilla, which is often poorly visualized in the first two positions. Dr. Egan observes that good mediolateral oblique exposures can be taken with the patient standing, sitting, or lying down, "with as many variations as there are mammographers."[6]

Positioning is always open to modification, to suit the individual patient's body configuration. But the need for rigorous

breast compression is common to all angles and positions—it cannot be compromised in any way. Without compression there is no mammography. The breast must be firmly compressed so as to remain motionless, lest the mammographic image be blurred by the constant heaving of the lungs and rib cage. The uneven contours of the breast pose a considerable obstacle to X-ray imaging. But adequate compression smoothes out all those hills and valleys; and it ensures a uniform exposure of the breast, avoiding a situation where some imaged areas would be either overexposed or underexposed. When the breast's tissues are flattened and spread out, X-rays have a shorter distance to travel through them—therefore we can use a lower radiation dose and reduce the exposure time. Compression is the thing patients like least about mammography; if not exactly painful, it necessarily involves momentary discomfort. Unfortunately, the woman who experiences no discomfort probably isn't getting a good mammogram.

Like other diagnostic procedures, mammography is somewhat dependent on patient compliance. A woman undergoing mammography needs to recognize the possibility of **radiological artifacts**. Moles or scars on the skin can sometimes look like breast masses on a mammogram. A previous biopsy or a penetrating trauma can leave scar tissue in the breast itself, which may mimic malignancy on a mammogram. Therefore if a patient has any superficial moles or scars, any patches of irregular skin, or a history of breast biopsy or trauma, she should mention the fact beforehand to the person taking the mammogram. Most radiologists advise against the use of underarm deodorants or talcum powders on the day mammograms are to be taken. The fine mineral particles in these products can create distracting artifacts, showing up on mammographic films as vague densities or as ill-defined shadows.

At the radiologist's office a patient needs to display patience and stoicism. Since human bodies do not come in standard sizes, each breast must be individually positioned. This may require more time in some cases than in others. Stoicism (the stiff upper lip) is always in order as the breast is sandwiched between this or that compression device, which is slowly tightened like a medieval vise. Premenopausal women will experience less discomfort if the mammograms are taken during the week after menstruation, when breast engorgement is minimal.

Interpretation of Mammograms

The analysis of the breast images captured on mammograms is not a precise science, but the basic guidelines which enable radiologists to distinguish between obviously benign "lumps" and presumably malignant ones are easy to understand. Robert L. Egan sums up the radiological characteristics of benign masses in a single sentence: "The homogeneous, smooth-bordered, rounded lesion with a radiolucent rim pushing the normal breast tissue aside fulfills the criteria for a benign lesion."[7] Sometimes a benign mass in the breast may be oval or slightly lobulated, rather than truly round; it would usually be homogeneous (uniform) in its consistency and density. However, the most important feature used in diagnosing a benign mass is neither shape nor consistency, but the status of the border or edge. In this instance the margins are well-defined and visible in their entirety. The thin "halo" which encircles benign masses is likewise characteristic. Often it is produced by a rim of compressed fat being shoved outward by the benign mass; it may also result from an optical effect created by the sharp transition from one tissue type to another. In all cases, well-defined margins and an encircling halo are indicative of a rigorous demarcation. The mass is set apart from the surrounding tissues; there is no evidence of infiltration.

Only occasionally will a breast mass with the preceding characteristics, even if large, prove to be malignant. Myron Moskowitz of the University of Cincinnati and other radiologists analyzed the data from a sizable series of mammographic examinations. Smoothly contoured round masses over one centimeter in diameter, "with margins visible in their entirety," were found to contain cancer cells about 2% of the time. Dr. Moskowitz pointed out that these breast tumors tended to be minimal, "either small cancers intimately attached to or within fibroadenomas, or intracystic papillary carcinomas."[8] Of course, most fibroadenomas and cysts do not harbor foci of malignant cells; the ability of mammography to identify these commonplace benign lesions may vary from case to case, but it is generally very high. Fibroadenomas in the postmenopausal breast often contain clumps of coarse calcifications, which show up as white flags indicating a lack of aggressiveness.[9] Cysts can usually be identified by mammography, though in a few cases either fine-needle aspiration or ultrasound would be required to confirm the diagnosis. Lipomas represent another type of benign lesion which is easily recognizable on mammography. They are little bits of fatty tissue which get entangled in the breast's ligaments and after a while start to feel like dominant masses. But mammograms reveal lipomas as radiolucent masses with distinct borders, clearly indicating their self-contained nature and homogeneous fat content.

The radiological hallmarks of malignant tumors are the opposite of those associated with benign entities. Breast cancers are typically neither rounded nor homogeneous; they are seen on mammograms as irregularly shaped masses of uneven density, which are

Benign Mammographic Appearance

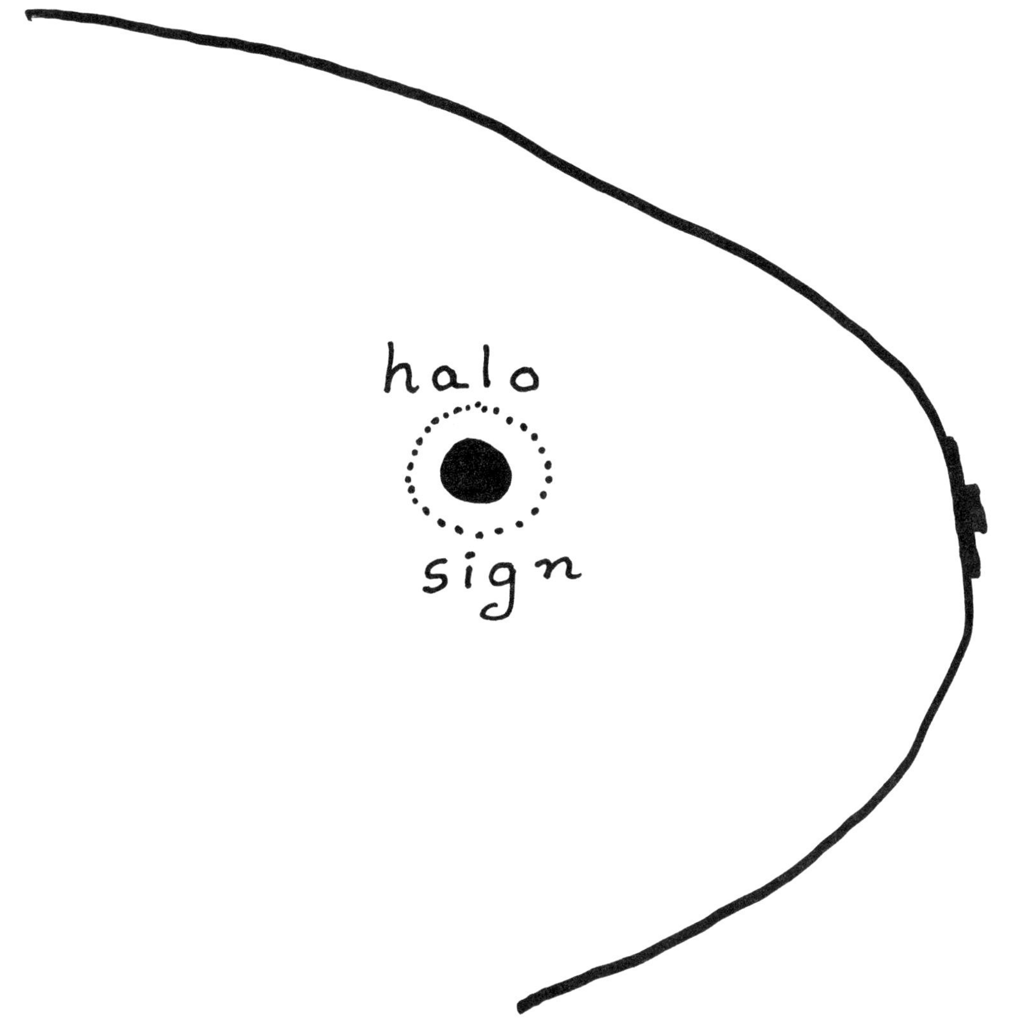

When viewed on mammograms, benign masses like cysts, fibroadenomas, and lipomas will tend to appear homogeneous in texture and to reveal distinct borders on all sides. The radiological **"halo sign"** is characteristic—it results from the abrupt transition from one type of tissue to another, and it assures us that no malignant infiltration has taken place.

often sprinkled lightly with clusters of tiny calcifications. As with benign tumors, the border or edge provides the most important clue. The margins of malignant tumors have often been described as "stellate" (shaped like a star) or "radiating," but the term currently preferred is **"spiculated."** The tumor outline is not smoothly contoured, but consists of numerous small projections (spicules) suggestive of encroachment or invasion. This mammographic appearance reflects what is actually happening in the breast—tendrils of malignant cells are migrating outward from the tumor center, provoking discernible fibrotic activity in the surrounding stroma. Invasive breast cancers do not often merit the adjectives "circumscribed" or "well-defined"; usually it's hard to tell where the tumor might stop and where normal tissue might begin. That thin halo or radiolucent rim characteristic of benign lesions is not seen. Instead the mammogram may reveal a largish area of encircling tissue disturbance, which could be either edematous (marked by fluid accumulation) or fibrotic (commonly seen with scirrhous carcinomas).

The likelihood that any spiculated mass will prove malignant is substantial. With a palpable spiculated mass—one that would be detected on physical examination—that likelihood would probably be 90% or better. Even with nonpalpable lesions the odds strongly favor malignancy. In the mammographic series analyzed by Dr. Moskowitz and his colleagues, 74% of the nonpalpable spiculated lesions proved to be malignant when biopsied. And those spiculated masses which produced any clinical sign typical of breast cancer, such as fixation to the overlying skin, had essentially a 100% likelihood of proving malignant.[10] Spiculation at the margins is as close as Mother Nature gets to running up a red flag which says "breast cancer." Lesions bearing this mammographic clue must always be biopsied, but

at least a few of them will be due to benign conditions. As mentioned in Chapter Eight, sclerosing adenosis often assumes a spiculated appearance on mammograms—and so does a slightly less notorious mime known as **radial scar**. This latter term is applied to little areas of fibrosis which sometimes develop at the bifurcations of the smaller milk ducts; they may show up as stellate images on breast films, but have nothing to do with cancer.[11] A previous biopsy or other breast surgery can leave internal scarring in the proper sense, which may resemble a spiculated mass on mammographic films. Jacquelyn P. Hogge of Georgetown University and other radiologists remind us that fat necrosis produced by breast trauma can wear many mammographic disguises, possibly appearing as "a spiculated area of increased opacity" whose minute calcifications are "indistinguishable from those of malignancy."[12] Under certain circumstances fat necrosis can mimic an infiltrating breast carcinoma with great verisimilitude; even Dr. Egan concedes that mammography is "rarely of reliable help" in diagnosing these cases.[13]

Differential Diagnosis

So far the mammographic presentations we've discussed have been offered largely as illustrations of certain general principles. In reality, however, breast lesions as seen on mammograms do not always fall into neat groupings of the benign (rounded, homogeneous, circumscribed, haloed) and the presumably malignant (irregular and spiculated). Sometimes those telltale margins seem generally well-defined, but are not visible in their entirety. Does this partial loss of margination identify a focus of malignant infiltration, or is it merely an artifact? The lesion's outline could be simply obscured by surrounding tissues, especially in a dense

Malignant Mammographic Appearance

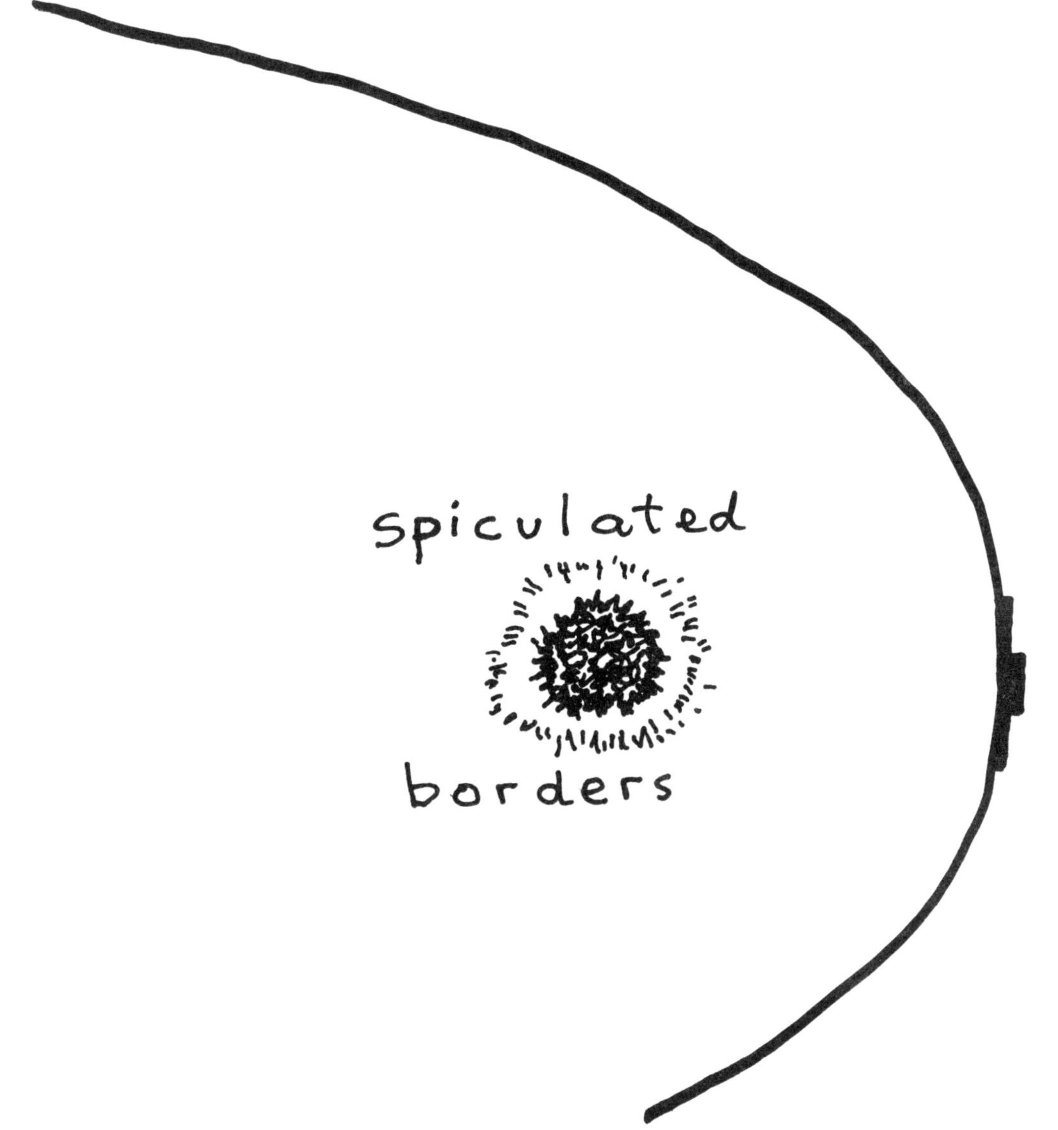

The characteristic radiological presentation of an infiltrating (invasive) ductal carcinoma consists of **an irregularly shaped mass with spiculated ("ragged") borders**. As the tumor grows larger, an edematous or fibrotic reaction in the surrounding tissues can usually be observed.

premenopausal breast. Sometimes a benign mass will not be uniform and nodular, but uneven and lobulated. Eva Rubin, a radiologist with the University of Alabama at Birmingham, estimates that breast masses with mixed characteristics, "such as partial loss of margination and prominent lobulation," have an intermediate likelihood (20% to 40%) of being malignant.[14] The mammographic series followed by Moskowitz and his colleagues gave slightly better odds—relatively circumscribed masses "with partial loss of border" proved to be malignant about 5% of the time if they were nonpalpable, and about 11% of the time if palpable.[15]

The evaluation of mammograms is further complicated by the fact that several of the rarer subtypes of breast cancer can begin as benign-looking masses, seemingly circumscribed and marginated. Those tumors designated **medullary** or **mucinous** are slow-growing cancers which may mimic cysts or fibroadenomas. The medullary subspecies typically presents as a rounded mass; the margins can appear intact, though a closer inspection may reveal a vague lack of definition or a minuscule spiculation. Mucinous breast cancers, also known as "colloid" cancers, secrete large quantities of mucin, so much so that the malignant cells appear to be floating in this jelly-like solution. Mucin-secreting tumors tend to be softer and much less dense than other infiltrating carcinomas; they can be mistaken for cysts both on physical examination and on mammography.[16]

In their earliest stages breast malignancies do not produce masses that we can detect in any way, either by palpation or by mammography. The development of a mass is a late event in the natural history of breast cancer, one that often occurs after malignant cells have spread to other parts of the body. Good radiologists are therefore continually looking for the subtler signs of cellular transformation, which might reveal tumors before they have a chance to progress. Unfortunately, if palpable masses and other clinically apparent symptoms sometimes pose difficulties in evaluation, the more subtle radiological signs always do so. They constitute a gray area where suspicious findings have a relatively low yield in terms of the malignancies actually detected. The most important of these lesser clues are the tiny calcifications which stand out like white dots on mammographic films—we'll discuss them at length in succeeding paragraphs. The other signs involve distortions in breast architecture. Asymmetry between the two breasts is suggestive, but biopsies done for this reason alone usually reveal a benign process rather than cancer. Dr. Moskowitz points out that "asymmetric areas of fibrosis occur frequently in the general population."[17] Isolated increases in breast density are also more often the result of harmless fibrosis rather than malignancy, but many radiologists might advise biopsy in these cases to be on the safe side. Neovascularity (the formation of new blood vessels) is an ominous sign, since it suggests increased cellular activity in the area. Dr. Egan points out that an unexplained expansion in the caliber (width) of existing blood vessels can be as suspicious as the formation of new ones.[18]

With subtle findings like asymmetries, calcifications, or slight increases in density, it's often helpful to compare past and present mammograms before venturing upon a tentative diagnosis. Are these radiological signs really indications of pathologic change, becoming more pronounced on each successive mammogram, or are they merely idiopathic—just peculiar to the individual? If the findings remain unchanged on sequential mammograms taken over a period of several years, they may reasonably be presumed to be benign, perhaps warranting continued observation but not a rush to biopsy. Subtle mammographic abnormalities, even when suspicious enough to demand biopsy, are more likely to have benign etiologies than malignant ones. A University of Virginia study of 1,464 breast biopsies performed for "nonpalpable abnormalities" found that only 18% proved to be malignant; and the majority of the cancers thus detected, 67%, were *in situ* lesions which could be easily cured.[19]

Explaining the Results

You might think that the radiologist's role in diagnostic mammography would be simply to evaluate the films of this or that breast problem which has come to medical attention. But evaluation is only half of the mammographer's task—the other half, just as important, is **COMMUNICATION**. Concise information and recommendations must flow from the radiologist's office to the referring physician and ultimately to the patient. Good communication about mammograms, like their judicious interpretation, is not always easy. Many radiologists rely on written reports, often to the chagrin of the referring physicians who must read them. William H. Hindle, a gynecologist at the University of Southern California, has commented on a deplorable state of affairs: "Why do mammographers dictate long, confusing reports? It's because of the fear of missing breast cancer. And the physician doesn't understand the mammography reports and doesn't know what to do when he gets them."[20] Detailed written reports have been flourishing of late as a kind of legal defense mechanism. In these days when pathology labs are monumentally sued for having misread Pap smears, who knows what mountains of malpractice litigation might fall upon a dull-eyed mammographer? A written report is thus valuable as a permanent record of the radiologist's work in examining and interpreting breast films, forever retrievable by physicians, patients, and—in the worst scenario—by lawyers! The problem is that in an effort to be comprehensive and technically correct, breast radiologists tend to compose long-winded documents which are pure gobbledygook to anyone except other breast radiologists. The essential recommendations may sometimes get lost in a welter of extraneous details.

Patients should be encouraged to question their mammographers directly and with some persistence. After all, it is the patients who must foot the bill and whose very lives could be at stake. A word or two of *real* information given informally can often get to the crux of the matter. Ideally, any discussions between radiologist and patient would take place before a lighted viewing box, with both looking at the same breast films while any apparent abnormalities are pointed out. With just a little coaching, an intelligent layperson can understand the imaged abnormality and weigh the odds that it may (or may not) represent malignant transformation. And with just a little understanding, she might be more likely to comply with the radiologist's recommendation, be it for a timely biopsy or simply for follow-up mammograms to verify a lesion's benign nature.

CALCIFICATIONS
The Tiniest Clues

The accumulation of calcium deposits in tissues throughout the body is a natural consequence of aging. The breast is especially prone to minute calcium depositions which are prominently visible on mammograms Most of them are harmless byproducts of the aging process or are associated with benign lesions like cysts or fibroadenomas. But a few of them are produced by newly developing carcinomas. Because the calcifications caused by malignancies tend to appear in certain characteristic patterns unlike those associated with benign processes, they often give us the earliest warning signs of breast cancer, visible years before we would detect a palpable mass. Those screening mammograms universally recommended for women over age 50 do not turn up all that many occult tumors. What they turn up most often are tiny clusters of suspicious calcifications.

We should perhaps explain that the cells of the mammary gland are naturally oriented toward the processing and secretion of calcium, since this mineral is a principal ingredient of milk and absolutely essential for an infant's bone formation. Should some of these mammary cells undergo malignant transformation, that inherent potential for calcium processing will be reawakened as the cells become abnormally active. This time the calcium is not secreted as a vital foodstuff in solution, but simply dumped outside the cells as minuscule flakes of irregular shape and size which serve no biological purpose. Back in the 1970s studies with an electron microscope revealed that human breast cancer cells grown in culture typically excrete fine particles of calcium. Our pioneer mammographer Robert L. Egan assures us that "calcifications can be demonstrated by light microscopy in almost all duct carcinomas."[21] While mammography cannot aspire to capture the details seen on tissue sections examined under a microscope, it can demonstrate calcifications in a large majority of breast cancers. Calcium deposits fulfill the great desideratum of X-ray imaging—they are radio-opaque and show up marvelously on film. With the aid of a magnifying glass, calcifications as small as one-tenth or even one-twentieth of a millimeter can be seen—a particle in this size range is considerably smaller than the period at the end of

this sentence. The largest calcifications, of perhaps two or three millimeters in diameter, appear as white blots on film and are readily visible to the naked eye.

Radiologists are constantly writing books and articles on ways to distinguish the calcifications caused by breast cancer from the more commonplace benign presentations. The proposed criteria are not absolute, but very useful. We may safely assume that the larger, coarser calcifications—those "blots" and "streaks" on mammograms—are due to benign processes. The tried-and-true rule of bilaterality also remains valid: calcifications which are scattered throughout both breasts have nothing to do with cancer. In fact, the only calcifications which raise any suspicion of malignancy are tiny little ones which seem to be clustered in a particular locus on one breast. Such a "cluster" suggests a focal point of metabolic activity. Dr. Egan has formulated three simple criteria for malignant presentations, which are worth repeating as they reflect his unparalleled experience in breast radiology. He believes that calcifications resulting from malignancy will fulfill these conditions: first, "they must be relatively fine"—secondly, "they must be uncountable"—and thirdly, "they must be confined to a measurable area." For Dr. Egan a suspicious cluster would consist of five or more tiny calcifications in a space half a centimeter square. "The finer the calcifications, the more important." Egan observes that large calcifications may serve to draw the radiologist's attention to a particular spot on a breast film, "but it is the much finer interspersed ones that really elevate the suspicion of malignancy." If inspection with a magnifying glass "brings countless additional fine flecks into view," the spot in question is "probably cancer."[22] *An uncountable multitude of the tiniest white flecks*—yet another radiological red flag! Yet this scarlet banner is not quite as

Clustered Calcifications

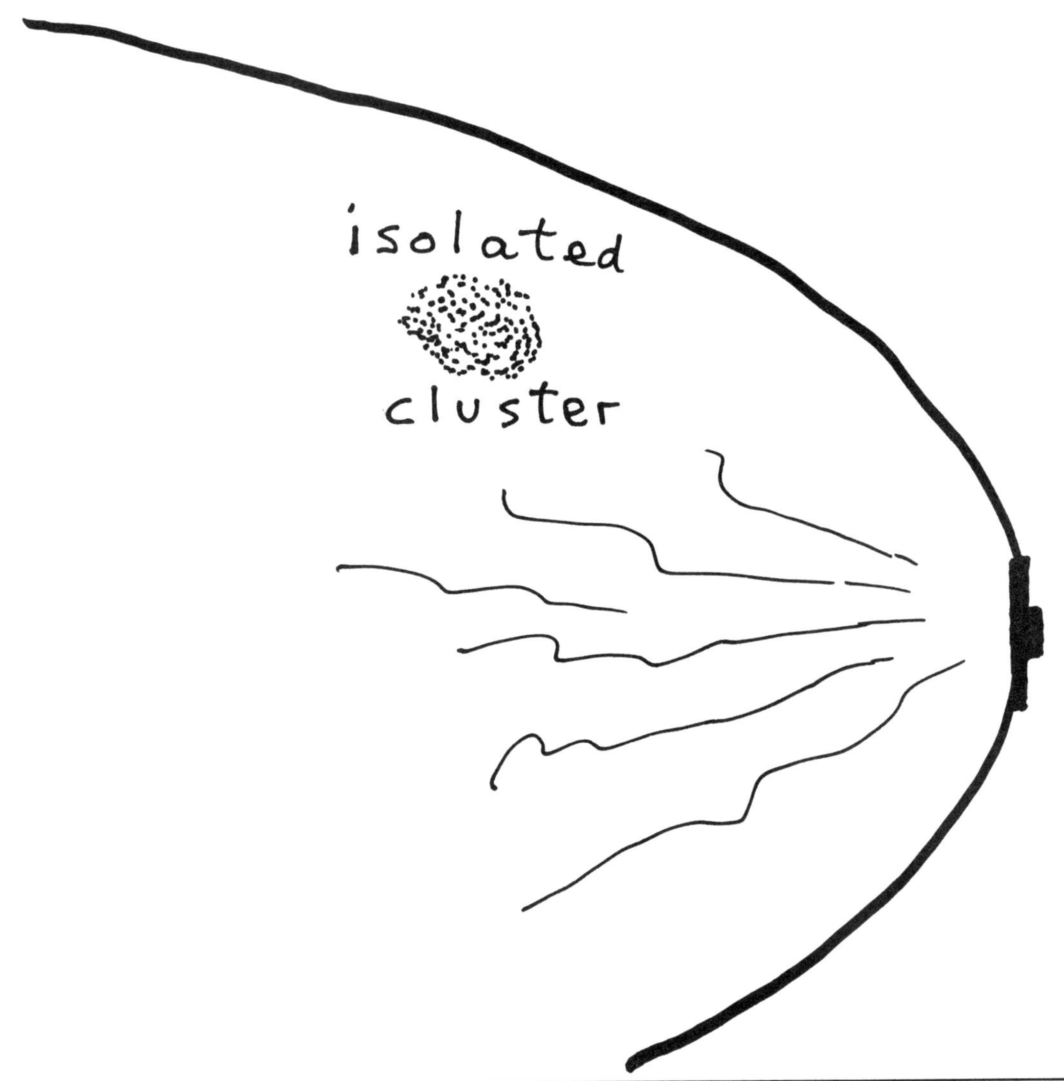

Numerous tiny calcifications confined to a small area on a mammogram may possibly be the result of malignant transformation. Additional measures to establish the nature of an isolated cluster of calcifications are warranted. Larger, coarser calcifications which are scattered throughout both breasts normally result from benign processes.

threatening as an irregular mass with spiculated borders, because this time its caption reads "EARLY BREAST CANCER."

Calcifications also prove useful in diagnosing benign disorders of the breast. Daniel B. Kopans, director of breast imaging at Boston's Massachusetts General Hospital, points out that the typical benign calcifications "are smooth, round, larger than one millimeter and have lucent centers."[23] Breast cancers rarely produce calcifications this large, most calcium deposits associated with malignancy being well under half a millimeter in diameter. Cysts frequently calcify— the crescent or ring-shaped calcification is characteristic, mineral deposition occurring at the cyst's wall and thus making its outline visible. Large coarse blots of calcification seen in a rounded well-defined mass are indicative of a mature fibroadenoma which has stopped growing. Sometimes such amorphous blots will be detected in the postmenopausal breast without any evidence of an existing mass or masses; Dr. Egan suspects that these calcifications are simply "the residual finding of old degenerated fibroadenomata."[24]

The milk ducts are prone to several types of mineralization. The duct walls themselves may calcify, in much the same way that blood vessels become hardened in arteriosclerosis. Moreover, any cellular debris or fluid secretions accumulating inside the ducts will eventually become calcified and radio-opaque. Finally, calcification may occur in the stroma surrounding the ducts, not uncommonly as a result of duct ectasia and periductal inflammation. Mammograms of aging breasts often contain broad white streaks which are either linear or branching in configuration, following the path of milk ducts. Dr. Kopans observes that these benign ductal calcifications are characteristically

either "solid and rod-shaped" or "lucent-centered and tubular."[25] When cancer cells proliferate inside the milk ducts, as they do in ductal carcinoma *in situ* (DCIS), they also produce calcifications in linear or branching configurations. But DCIS is not often confused with the aforementioned benign processes. In DCIS the calcifications are not dispersed throughout the breast, but are seemingly confined to a single duct or ductal network in a particular area. And DCIS calcium depositions are neither solid rods nor lucent tubes, but clusters of microcalcifications which just happen to suggest the outlines of a duct or ducts.

When Is Biopsy Necessary?

Even when highly suspicious, calcifications by themselves are no cause for undue alarm, though they certainly merit attention. Back in the 1970s we learned that those breast cancers which produce calcifications tend to be the slow-growing variety. The really aggressive tumors, those which can pop up terrifyingly in the intervals between annual mammograms, seem to be in too much of a hurry to leave calcium deposits.[26] A substantial majority of the cancers detected on the basis of calcifications alone, without any physical findings suggestive of malignancy, will prove to be "minimal"—either *in situ* (noninvasive) cancers or tiny invasive tumors which have hardly begun to infiltrate the surrounding tissues. But historically only 25% of the biopsies done for mammography-detected calcifications have resulted in a positive diagnosis. The Emory University series of 895 breast biopsies performed for "clustered calcifications not in a mass," as reported by Dr. Egan and his colleagues, yielded "one carcinoma for each four biopsies." A subsequent University of Virginia series of 325 biopsies produced comparable

Branching Calcifications

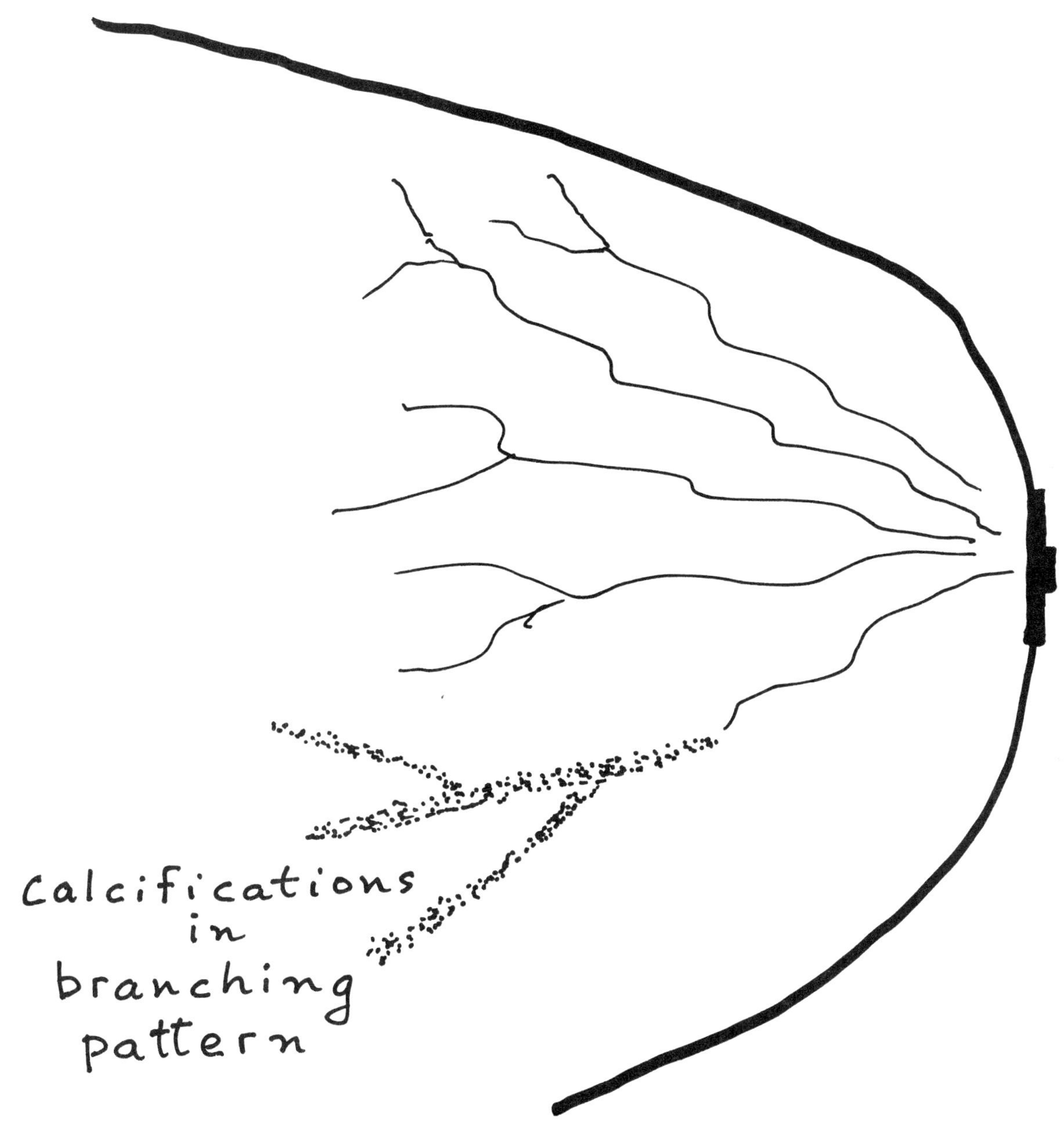

Tiny calcifications observed in linear or branching patterns suggest the outlines of the larger milk ducts. This radiological finding is often associated with ductal carcinoma *in situ*.

results: "About one-fourth of clustered or grouped microcalcifications are associated with malignant lesions."[27] This 25% rate, with most of the cancers discovered being low-risk or *in situ* lesions, should be contrasted with that almost overwhelming rate and risk demonstrated for palpable masses with spiculated margins—over 90% malignant, with almost all the cancers being invasive.

The majority of biopsies done for clustered calcifications (75% or so) will prove to be false alarms simply because this radiological sign is not limited to malignancies. Usually the calcifications in question are too suspicious to ignore, but only occasionally can they be said to be virtually diagnostic of breast cancer. In contrast, the firm spiculated mass is a highly specific sign for infiltrating ductal carcinomas—just a few benign conditions mimic it. With calcifications this situation is reversed—mimicry by benign conditions outweighs malignancy. The calcifications produced by "fibrocystic disease" are typically round and smooth, fairly uniform in shape, size, and density, and diffusely scattered throughout both breasts. But Dr. Egan cautions us that this benign species "often occurs in localized clumps that are indistinguishable from malignant calcifications."[28] That pesky and ubiquitous fibrocystic disease (every clinician's favorite breast diagnosis) would seem to be behind most of the false alarms, yet pathology reports frequently cite **epithelial hyperplasia** as the histological finding in these cases. Hyperplasia involves an excessive proliferation of cells and unwarranted metabolic activity. This diagnosis would explain why these cells might be secreting tiny calcium particles, but the cells themselves are not malignant and not necessarily on the road to malignancy. Other benign conditions which can lead to biopsy include **ductal papillomas,** which sometimes produce calcifications

suggestive of breast cancer, and that superb mime **sclerosing adenosis**, which usually does so.

Patients generally concede the necessity of biopsying persistent lumps, but not many women relish the thought of undergoing breast surgery solely because of a few white flecks seen on a mammogram. A woman who receives a biopsy recommendation for the latter reason should feel free to question her physicians about the nature of the visualized abnormality and about the technique of the proposed biopsy procedure. The main problem in examining clusters of microcalcifications lies not with the one-in-four rate of positive findings, but simply in the fact that a lot of surgery may be required to remove small and rather elusive tissue specimens. Traditionally, surgeons have relied on wire localization in these cases. A thin wire with a small hook at the end would be shoved down to the area of the calcifications, and a mammogram would be taken to confirm that the hooked end was adjacent to the lesion. The surgeon would now cut down to the end of the wire and remove the surrounding tissues, the specimen being X-rayed immediately to ensure that it contained the suspect calcifications. In recent years some breast specialists have begun to wonder whether fine-needle aspiration or a core-needle tissue sampling, if aided by mammographic guidance, might not establish the diagnosis almost as effectively as the old wire-localization technique.

For patients with mildly irregular patterns of calcification, observation by means of sequential mammograms might be adopted as the initial strategy. Myron Moskowitz and his colleagues at the University of Cincinnati have long followed a policy of attentive surveillance. After three months they take additional mammograms of the breast with the suspect calcifications: "If no change is seen, the assumption is made that the disease, if present, is not growing rapidly." Another series of mammograms would then be taken six months later: "If all remains stable, annual mammography is again advised. If the calcium has developed as an interval finding, performance of a biopsy is usually the most prudent course."[29] The San Francisco radiologist Edward A. Sickles believes that intensified mammographic surveillance, with exams every six months, stands to identify those lesions which are progressing toward malignancy, "and will do so while the tumors still have a favorable prognosis."[30] But observation is never a reasonable policy if the clustered calcifications are associated with a definite mass or an area of increased density. In these cases the likelihood of malignancy approaches 50%, and biopsy is always indicated. William L. Donegan reminds us that fine microcalcifications in a mass or density are "the most ominous finding," more than twice as likely to prove malignant as calcium deposits which are not associated with a mass or density.[31]

Some Specialized Techniques
And the Newer Imaging Modalities

In evaluating any breast abnormality, whether palpable or not, the radiologist can use specialized mammographic techniques to come closer to a diagnosis. One of these, **ductography**, has already been mentioned as a means of visualizing a nipple discharge. A fluid contrast medium is injected into the discharging duct, thus making the particular ductal network radio-opaque and allowing us to see any obstructions in it. Contrast mediums are not often used in mammography. In most cases the supplementary techniques involve no more than slight changes in positioning or the degree of breast compression.

The breast is pliable and easy to reposition. If the problem isn't seen on the first exposure, additional views taken from different angles may give us the information we need. A lead marker, paper-thin and self-adherent, can be placed on the breast surface above any suspected abnormality, so that the radiologist can be sure that the problem area has been captured on film.

Today's mammography machines have helpful features which allow for **spot compression** as well as **magnification views**. A higher degree of compression can be applied to that area of the breast regarded as suspicious, making for a better defined image on the film. The image can also be enlarged (magnified) to reveal its smaller details. Both focal compression and sectional magnification are essential for the radiologist who's struggling to form an opinion on a group of calcifications or to decide whether the borders of a mass are intact or just a little bit spiculated. Joseph T. Ennis, a contributor to Bland and Copeland's massive textbook, believes that "the optimal degree of magnification is 1.5 times life size."[32]

Mammography remains the fastest and cheapest imaging tool for breast disorders. For a few applications, however, breast radiologists and their patients may wish to consider those glamorous and elaborate technologies which provide cross-sectional images of the body. **Computerized axial tomography,** or **CAT** for short, came of age in the late 1970s. CAT relies on multiple X-rays made as a radiation source rotates slowly around a body part—these fractional images are processed by a computer to yield the desired cross section. CAT is much more expensive and time-consuming than plain X-rays, and it involves a much higher dose of radiation. Moreover, CAT scans of the breast typically require the administration of an intravenous contrast agent to produce meaningful images. The rationale is that since breast cancers and other proliferative lesions tend toward neovascularity (the generation of new blood vessels), they would absorb more of the radio-opaque contrast agent than normal tissues, and hence they would be "enhanced" (more visible) on the scan. In the early 1980s CAT showed promise in detecting small tumors in the dense glandular breasts of premenopausal women. The scans also permitted visualization of a broader area than that allowed by mammography, including the chest muscles underlying the mammary gland as well as the lymph nodes in the axilla (armpit) and beneath the sternum (breastbone).

By the late 1980s CAT imaging of the breast had become far less attractive, not so much because of its cost and complexity, but because it was being overshadowed by another computer-based modality. **Magnetic resonance imaging** (MRI) emerged as the latest innovation in diagnostic imaging. Unlike CAT or mammography. MRI did not use ionizing radiation—it relied on radio waves transmitted into the body in the presence of an extremely powerful magnetic field. Tissues of different composition and density respond differently to these radio waves, sending back "echoes" of varying strength. A computer converts these echoes into the detailed cross-sectional image.[34] MRI imaging of the breast, like that by CAT, requires an intravenous contrast agent; and it is expensive and time-consuming. During the 1990s, however, MRI found a modest niche in breast imaging; and manufacturers began to produce dedicated equipment—i.e., machines designed specifically to image this body part. For certain applications MRI often proved superior to mammography. In evaluating dense premenopausal breasts, the new modality could usually distinguish between the dominant masses caused by tumors and the pronounced nodularities due to age-related fibrosis. Malignant breast

tumors readily enhance (show up) on MRI due to their increased vascularity, while fibrocystic changes, fat necrosis, and old scar tissues typically fail to enhance. But MRI scans of the breast are not always unequivocal. Proliferative lesions like fibroadenomas and sclerosing adenosis, as well as epithelial hyperplasia, can give positive results, thus raising a needless suspicion of malignancy. Steven E. Harms and other researchers at Baylor University caution that premenopausal women should not undergo MRI "during the proliferative phase (last two weeks) of the menstrual cycle," because even normal glandular tissues could possibly be enhanced.[35] MRI performed shortly after a biopsy of, or trauma to, the breast will also give a false-positive result, since newly-healing tissues consistently enhance.

Neither CAT nor MRI has an established role in screening for the earliest stages of breast cancer, which are nonpalpable and otherwise asymptomatic. Neither modality can image tiny calcifications; and neither could consistently detect ductal carcinoma *in situ*, where the cancer cells remain confined within the milk ducts and have not yet produced increased vascularity in the surrounding tissues. CAT imaging of the breast now seems a bit irrelevant, but at present there are three indications for MRI scans. The first is to look for a tumor in a premenopausal patient who complains of a "lump" but whose breasts are too densely glandular to permit informative mammography. The second is to rule out the possibility of undiscovered smaller tumors in a breast cancer patient who has chosen lumpectomy as a treatment rather than mastectomy. The presence of one or more additional tumors in the affected breast would be, of course, a counterindication to its preservation. A third application is to assess the integrity of a silicone-gel breast implant. We have discovered that MRI is

Ductography

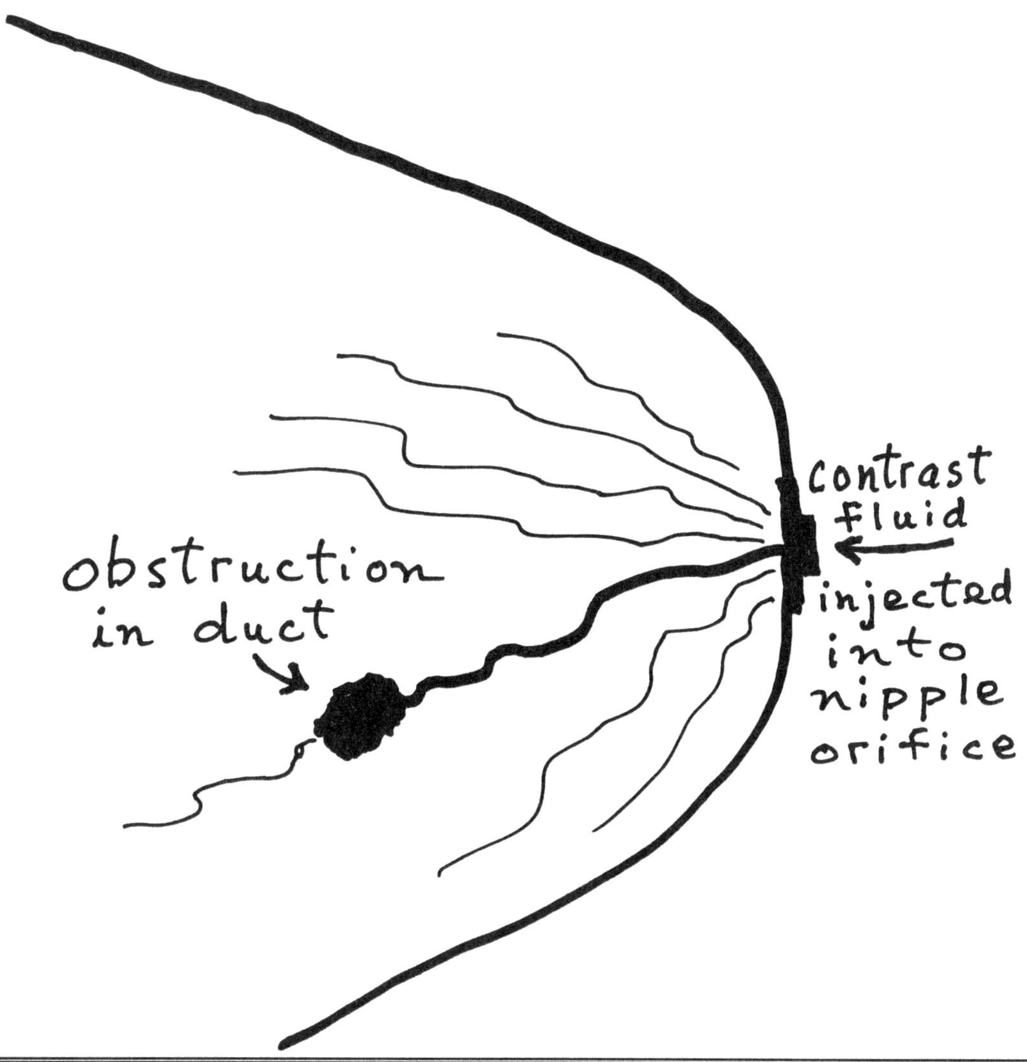

Ductography is a mammographic technique used to locate the source of a nipple discharge. An opaque contrast fluid is first injected into the orifice of the discharging duct. The outline of the involved duct as well as any obstructions in it will then be visible on the ensuing mammogram. Most nipple discharges result from papillomas or from duct ectasias rather than from malignant transformation.

the best modality for visualizing implants and for detecting silicone leaks from them.[36]

While readily available in most American communities, MRI scans of the breast have at best supplemented film-screen mammography; they are not appropriate for routine imaging. In recent years our efforts to develop a better all-purpose tool have been focused on **digital mammography**, which promises to bring the power of computer graphics to traditional radiology.[37] In digital mammography the information gathered from breast X-rays is digitized and processed by a computer. The resulting images can then be displayed on a high-resolution video monitor or on film. This emerging technology would allow the mammographer to manipulate the breast image, heightening its contrast or enlarging specific areas of it. The contrast enhancement would help to overcome the perennial difficulty of visualizing structures in dense glandular breasts. Digital systems have had problems in imaging the entire breast—that is, in **full-field mammography**—but once these are overcome, they stand to offer several practical advantages. One is speed, because there are no films to develop. Another would be easy distribution of the image, which could be electronically transmitted to the referring physician or to a consultant in a distant city. Some researchers hope to reduce the inevitable errors and oversights due to human frailty through computer-aided diagnosis, in which a software program would serve as a consulting radiologist and provide a second opinion on breast images.[38] Ideally a program could be developed which would recognize irregular densities or suspicious calcifications, and point them out to the radiologist. At the moment, however, the effective interpretation of breast images continues to remain dependent on sharp eyes and individual experience.

FALSE NEGATIVES
Why Cancer Can Be Overlooked

If we consider that pathologists often struggle to make a diagnosis when looking at a cellular specimen under high magnification, we will not be surprised that radiologists looking at X-rays can miss malignancy altogether, even when a palpable mass is present. Numerical estimates vary for **false negatives**, those clean bills of health mistakenly given for breast cancer. In the early days of mammography, the rate of error was appallingly high. One analysis of 499 patients with palpable malignant tumors who were mammogramed between 1976 and 1985 provided some eye-opening statistics.[39] Overall, 22% of these patients received false-negative reports—but the error rate for women under age 50 was a shocking 44%! Never foolproof, X-ray mammography is considerably more error-prone when aimed at premenopausal breasts or at the breasts of postmenopausal women who have been taking hormone replacement therapy. But negative mammographic findings should never be used as an excuse to postpone tissue sampling in a woman of any age who has a clinical symptom suggestive of malignancy—e.g., an unidentified dominant mass, an unexplained nipple discharge, or a unilateral change of contour. Experienced radiologists readily concede the possibility of error. David G. Bragg of the University of Utah School of Medicine emphasizes that "it should be clearly understood that mammography will fail to recognize some 10% to 15% of cancers for a variety of reasons." Another radiologist, R. James Brenner of the Cedars-Sinai Medical Center in Los Angeles, offers a more guarded estimate: "Even in the best of hands about 7% to 10% of tumors are missed on mammography."[40]

How can mammography possibly fail to detect a solid lump which both the patient and her physician can unquestionably feel? The answer boils down to a lack of contrast. A mammary gland which is under constant hormonal stimulation tends to be composed primarily of fibrous and glandular tissues, with minimal interspersed fat. Radiologists describe a breast like this as "radiographically dense"; its tissues are said to attenuate (impede) the passage of X-rays. Daniel B. Kopans of the Massachusetts General Hospital reminds us that breast cancers are "almost always high in X-ray attenuation" due to their increased cellularity and the fibrotic stromal reaction they usually induce. "Small breast cancers that are surrounded by fat are easily seen," Dr. Kopans explains, "because of the contrast between the high X-ray attenuation of the cancer and the relatively low attenuation of the fat." The difficulty in visualizing malignant tumors in some premenopausal breasts arises from the fact that the entire mammary gland is comparatively high in X-ray attenuation. Dr. Kopans observes: "If two abutting, but different, tissue types produce similar X-ray attenuation, then they will appear as a continuous tissue structure without visible separation." In other words, if the surrounding normal tissues are just as "radiodense" as the malignant tumor, then that tumor will be indistinguishable; it's mammographically invisible even if it's as palpable as a plum! Dr. Kopans has found that spot compression sometimes aids tumor visualization "by displacing the confusing, overlapping structures."[41] Another option to be considered in cases of palpable masses but negative mammograms is MRI. This modality's detection of breast cancers doesn't depend on differences in X-ray attenuation, but upon the differential absorption of a contrast agent, which would be greater in well-vascularized proliferative lesions. A mammographically invisible tumor may show up clearly on MRI.

While radiographically dense breasts are the most obvious cause of misleading or uninformative mammograms, there are many lesser pitfalls. Mammography has yet to become an automated, self-correcting procedure; it is adversely affected by less than optimal techniques. And the breast remains a tricky object to image. The complete visualization of the mammary gland is not always accomplished—the glandular tissues wrap around the curved chest, stretching out elusively toward the axilla. Positioning and breast compression have to be painstakingly individualized for each patient, and successful imaging ultimately depends on the skills of the personnel working in the radiologist's office. In 1992 the United States Congress passed an important law entitled the **Mammography Quality Standards Act**, which mandated professional certification for all radiologists and their assisting technicians as well as the annual inspection of all mammographic equipment.[42] The advice routinely given to women in the 1980s, to have mammograms taken only at "accredited centers," has become less pertinent. Henceforth all the centers and personnel will have accreditation, but this hardly removes the possibility of error. Good mammography remains a complex and time-consuming undertaking which requires close attention to numerous small details.

Chapter Eleven

Biopsy Becomes a Friend

In most cases a breast lesion cannot be conclusively diagnosed without submitting a tissue sample for pathological analysis. The generic term for such tissue sampling is **biopsy**. When applied to the breast, this word has been known to evoke almost as much uneasiness as the dreaded *CANCER*-word itself. For the first three quarters of the twentieth century, breast biopsies were almost always performed under total anesthesia in hospital operating rooms. Patients undergoing these procedures feared a loss of control over their bodies and possible mutilation, and these fears were not without reason. Today breast biopsies and needle tissue samplings are usually performed on an outpatient basis, with only local anesthesia and mild sedation. Patients are informed and consulted at every step in the process.

The traditional procedure under total anesthesia came to be called the **one-step biopsy**, because it could conveniently combine the sampling of tissue (biopsy) with the surgical therapy for breast malignancies (mastectomy) in a single operation. The one-step biopsy grew out of a fixed belief in the mechanical dissemination of cancer cells. That is to say, a tumor in the breast or elsewhere was viewed as a self-contained hive of contagion—by cutting into it, the surgeon would release the agents of disease (cancer cells), spreading them throughout the operative field with his scalpel and freeing them to migrate to other parts of the body. We now know that the potential of cancer cells to migrate and establish metastases is determined by genetic changes occurring within the cells themselves, and that any mechanical dissemination during surgery has little or no effect on the matter. But in the early decades of the twentieth century, this simplistic idea was accepted as an article of faith. Cutting into a tumor seemed like cutting open a hornets' nest—if you did so, you had to be prepared to remove and destroy that nest and any surrounding tissues which might harbor some of its swarming occupants. Thus a biopsy which revealed cancer had to be followed immediately by a definitive surgical therapy. In the case of breast malignancies, treatment always consisted of that surgical mutilation known as the **radical mastectomy**.

The traditional combination of biopsy and mastectomy depended upon getting a pathology report intraoperatively, within a few minutes after the tissue specimen was removed. This immediate diagnosis became possible through the **frozen section**, a time-honored pathological technique developed in the 1870s. In this assay, a small portion of the tumor specimen is flash-frozen, so that it will be firm enough to be sliced into the extremely thin sections necessary for microscopic examination. A frozen section, once stained with dyes which make the cells and their nuclei visible, can usually tell us in an instant whether a tissue sample is benign or malignant. Prior to the late 1970s breast biopsies done in the United States were characterized by a ritual lull in activity—the surgeon and operating room nurses had to stand idle while the excised specimen was rushed off to the hospital pathology department for a frozen section. Ten or fifteen minutes later, the pathologist's voice would come creakily over the intercom to announce the verdict. If the specimen proved to be benign, the surgeon would simply close the incision. If malignancy was established, the operative team would resume purposeful activity. The affected breast, the muscles beneath it, and all the lymph nodes in the axilla had to be promptly removed—there was no time to waste! That hornet's nest had been opened, the malignant cells had been stirred up and spread about, and the patient's life depended upon *getting them all out!*

This exercise was well-intended and entirely rational, being based on cancer biology as it was then understood. But four generations of American patients suffered mightily from that erroneous concept of mechanical dissemination and the inflexible biopsy procedure it inspired. To begin with, women undergoing breast biopsies were not consulted about treatment options in the event that malignancy should be discovered. Their surgeons, masculine in gender and paternalistic in attitude, assumed the easy posture of omniscience and provided the honeyed words of reassurance: "Don't worry—it's probably nothing." Why mention an unsettling topic like mastectomy? For breast cancer patients the shock of recognition came only in the recovery room, when they awakened to find themselves pierced by drainage tubes and wrapped about

with sterile dressings. A hovering nurse typically whispered the standard explanation: "Dear, it was malignant; they had to remove your breast . . . etc., etc." One patient who experienced such a problematic awakening was Terese Lasser, who underwent a breast biopsy in 1952 expecting "to be out of the hospital the next morning," and instead found herself "tight-wrapped as a mummy in surgical gauze." Mrs. Lasser later started **Reach to Recovery**, the American Cancer Society program which sends trained volunteers on hospital visits to women who have just undergone surgery for breast cancer.[1]

The Two-Step Biopsy

With our present knowledge we may find it difficult to understand why surgeons of the 1950s and 1960s adhered so passionately to the one-step biopsy. At the time the most eminent specialists in cancer medicine, dripping with credentials and prestige, wrote articles and textbooks explaining that a breast cancer patient's chances of survival would be seriously diminished by even a short delay between the performance of a biopsy and the definitive surgical therapy. These gentlemen also emphasized that the one-step procedure was far more convenient for both patient and practitioner, since it required but a single hospitalization for both diagnosis and putative cure. A *third* reason, never stated in print, was probably as important as the publicly announced arguments. One-step biopsies allowed surgeons to sidestep meaningful consultations with patients about eventual treatment—these could only be difficult and unpleasant, given the fact that a sweeping amputation was standard practice in all cases of mammary carcinoma. Best do the deed first, afterwards whisper the C-word, and let the patient come to her own terms with a *fait accompli*.

By the early 1970s, however, those arguments for the one-step biopsy began to look less convincing. George Crile, Jr., and other progressive surgeons had reached the conclusion that the modified radical mastectomy, which sacrificed the breast but preserved the underlying chest muscles, was every bit as effective as the mutilative radical mastectomy which had held sway since the 1890s. More innovative practitioners wondered whether some cases of breast cancer could not be satisfactorily treated by lumpectomy, the mere removal of the tumor with an encircling margin of normal tissue. There were even a few heretics who thought that the customary axillary dissection might be minimized or omitted altogether. Gradually the reformers gained ground; before long clinical trials were underway pitting their heretical propositions against the prevailing surgical orthodoxy. Suddenly there were alternative treatments being loudly promoted by highly regarded physicians—and the very existence of alternatives tended to promote consultation between surgeon and patient about the choice of the most appropriate therapy. But most American surgeons wanted irrefutable evidence before abandoning the one-step biopsy and the radical mastectomy. In late 1974 Rose Kushner visited nineteen surgeons in the Washington, D.C., area before she found one willing to do a "two-step operation"—that is, a biopsy performed for diagnosis only, with intervening consultations before any decision on the extent of the definitive cancer surgery. Some of these gentlemen she queried about biopsying her breast lump reacted in a less-than-genteel fashion. "No patient is going to tell me how to do my surgery," said one abruptly. Another told her: "You're absolutely ridiculous! If the diagnosis is positive on frozen section, the breast must come off immediately."[2]

The most powerful impetus toward the two-step biopsy came not from scientific data, but from legislative action. Concerned laypersons and sympathetic medical professionals began to lobby state legislatures to pass laws requiring that physicians disclose all available treatment options to breast cancer patients. In 1979 Massachusetts became the first state to enact this legislation, followed by California a year later. By 1989 twelve additional states had also passed informed consent laws.[3] While the wording and content of the pertinent legislation varied from state to state, the national impact was clear enough. It had become illegal to perform mastectomy on an anesthetized patient who had consented to nothing more than a diagnostic biopsy.

By the mid-1980s the old beliefs that surgical biopsy would dangerously disseminate tumor cells and that any delay afterward would imperil a patient's chances of survival had lost credibility. An authoritative clinical trial conducted by Bernard Fisher and his co-workers found no difference in the ten-year survival rates between those breast cancer patients who underwent the one-step procedure (simultaneous biopsy and mastectomy) and those who had the two-step procedure, with the definitive surgery coming about two weeks after the biopsy.[4] Another study done at Italy's National Tumor Institute in Milan yielded comparable results—there was no difference in the survival rates between those patients having immediate surgery and those who had surgery as late as thirty days after the biopsy.[5] As screening mammography became more prevalent during the 1970s, pathologists began to voice doubts about the accuracy of frozen sections in diagnosing small nonpalpable cancers detected by calcifications. More and more of these early-stage lesions were showing up on mammograms; and they could be confidently diagnosed only on **permanent sections**, which required a day or two to prepare. In this technique, the excised tissue specimens are not frozen but embedded in paraffin, which must be allowed to dry before being sliced into thin sections and stained with dyes. In 1979 a Consensus Development Conference on breast cancer held at the National Institutes of Health gave its sanction to the two-step biopsy and consultation before surgery. "A diagnostic biopsy," advised the Conference panelists, "should be studied by permanent histologic sections before definitive therapeutic alternatives are discussed with the patient."[6]

In the ten years between 1975 and 1985, a tremendous revolution in breast biopsy procedures was quietly effected. The standard practice became outpatient biopsy, with a delay of a week or two before any decision on the advisability of additional surgery. This delay allows the pathologist time to evaluate the permanent sections and to compose a detailed report on the lesion. For her part the patient has time to confer with both the pathologist and the surgeon, as well as to obtain second opinions on the specimen slides and on alternative therapies. These days nothing can be done without the patient's consent to the proposed treatment and without her full understanding of its probable side effects. The old one-step procedure combining biopsy under total anesthesia, immediate frozen-section diagnosis, and contingent mastectomy is still available. It remains a reasonable option for patients who probably have breast cancer as indicated by a spiculated mass detected on a mammogram or by positive cytological findings after fine-needle aspiration, and who would prefer removal of the breast to its preservation.

Undergoing Outpatient Biopsy

If surgical breast biopsies are no longer the momentous and threatening experiences they once were, they are still too complicated to be casually performed in a doctor's office. Biopsy typically takes place in a hospital operating room designed for "day surgery" or other minor procedures. The hospital setting offers several advantages—a sterile environment reducing the risk of postoperative infection, as well as a wide range of support services. The pathology lab is usually in the same building; thus the possibility that a tissue specimen will be lost in transit or otherwise mishandled is minimal. But not all hospitals are equal. If the patient and her personal physician are wise, the day surgery will be scheduled at a facility where breast biopsies and the pathological analysis of mammary specimens are commonplace. The choice of a surgeon is equally important. John Laszlo of the American Cancer Society worries about the quality of biopsies performed by gynecologists "who may operate on women with lumps in the breast no more than once or twice a year." He refers his patients to surgeons "who are making such decisions and doing such operations frequently."[7] The surgeon's level of expertise can be a crucial factor if the lesion biopsied should prove malignant. For a patient who desires to preserve her breast, the "biopsy" now tends to constitute the definitive surgical procedure—it becomes that lumpectomy which is intended to remove all the tumor with a thin rim of surrounding normal tissue. Getting a clean margin around a tumor, that safety zone free of cancer cells, is a difficult task even for experienced breast surgeons.

Most biopsies can be performed in an hour or less, and do not require an overnight stay in the hospital. But a woman undergoing biopsy would be prudent to enlist a friend or relative to drive her to and from the hospital. On the one hand, breast biopsies are emotionally stressful; on the other, fairly powerful sedatives may be given intravenously to alleviate anxiety during the procedure. Both the stress and the sedation can have lingering effects and impair one's ability to operate an auto. Once the patient has changed into a hospital-issued gown and arrived in the operating room, the mandatory preparations can begin. The first step is to coat the affected breast with an antiseptic solution; the second is to inject a local anesthetic around the spot where the incision will be made. If the patient feels any pain during surgery, additional anesthetic can be injected as needed. But most patients will feel little beyond sensations of pressure or tugging— the sort of thing you experience when a dentist drills and fills your tooth after giving you a shot of Novocaine. Unless heavily sedated, the patient will be very much awake during the biopsy and can hear everything. Seeing is another matter. The patient's observation of the operative field is effectively discouraged, either by hanging a thin drape between her head and the breast being incised, or simply by asking her to turn her head away.[8] The surgeon's incision is carefully considered so that it leaves only a thin scar which heals rapidly and eventually becomes almost imperceptible. The best incisions for these purposes are slightly curved and parallel the outline of the areola; hence they are called **circumareolar**. Radical incisions, made at right angles to the areolar edge, are usually avoided because they interrupt the lines of cutaneous tension in the breast and may leave larger scars.

Breast biopsies can be either **excisional** (removing the entire lesion) or **incisional** (removing only a tissue sample from the lesion). An excision is preferred for dominant masses (definite lumps) of small to moderate size—say, up to three centimeters

in diameter (about an inch and a quarter). A modest excisional biopsy usually does not produce a noticeable cosmetic defect (i.e., distort the breast's appearance); and for benign lesions it is often curative, getting rid of the problem altogether. In the case of malignant tumors, an excision provides a complete specimen from which the pathologist can gather much more information than from an incisional sampling. A "slice" taken from a tumor's center would not necessarily tell us whether there is malignant infiltration of nearby lymphatic vessels or of adjacent tissues on its periphery. But incisional biopsies almost always provide enough material for the positive identification of lesions as benign or malignant; and they may be deemed appropriate for large masses (over an inch or two) and for ill-defined areas of increased density. A biopsy specimen, whether consisting of the entire lesion or merely a slice from it, needs to be placed on ice and promptly transported to the pathology department. These days the specimen is not merely sectioned for microscopic examination. If it's malignant, portions of it will be subjected to various tests designed to tell us how aggressive the tumor might be, and to estimate the likelihood of metastatic spread. The best known of these assays attempt to determine whether the cancer cells are still hormonally responsive—that is, estrogen and progesterone receptor-positive—and whether they overexpress the accelerative oncogene HER-2/*neu*. A frozen section may still be made from a large biopsy specimen, simply with a view to relieving the patient's anxiety by providing a diagnosis before she leaves the hospital.

As with other surgical procedures, **hemostasis** (the control of bleeding) is of paramount importance in breast biopsies. Today most surgeons rely on electrocautery to stop bleeding from the smaller blood vessels—a slight touch from a red-hot wire will immediately staunch the flow. Larger vessels can be sealed in the old-fashioned way, by tying the open ends with absorbable sutures. The defect left by the removal of a breast mass may—or may not—be sutured, depending on the surgeon's individual judgment. William L. Donegan advises against suturing the defect, "because it can reconstitute itself in a more natural way than the surgeon can contrive."[9] Wiley W. Souba and Kirby I. Bland observe that "closure of the breast tissue defect is not mandatory," but they recommend doing so.[10] The subcutaneous fat and the skin incision are closed with fine absorbable sutures—the stitching should not be so tight that it promotes contracture or scarring. Drainage tubes to remove any postoperative fluid accumulation are not often used; but then if the tissue defect is unusually large, a thin flexible tube may be left in place for a day or two. In general, the defects produced by the removal of well-defined or encapsulated benign lesions will be smaller than those produced by the excision of malignant tumors, which requires an accompanying margin of normal tissue on all sides. It is these larger defects associated with cancer which are most likely to need suture closure and postop drainage.

Of course, a patient undergoing biopsy does not notice the fine details of suturing. When the operation is over, all she sees is the light sterile dressing which has been placed on the wound. In most cases this amounts to no more than a large band-aid. Some pain is likely once the anesthetic has worn off; the patient typically receives a prescription for a mild narcotic painkiller like codeine. But an over-the-counter analgesic like Tylenol (a brand name for acetaminophen) may do the trick. Any consumption of aspirin should be limited for several days, because sizable doses of this painkiller can hamper the blood's ability to clot. The wound should be kept dry until it heals, and during this period vigorous exercise should probably be avoided. The recommendation to wear a "firm support bra" after a breast biopsy is universal. One European surgeon goes so far as to suggest wearing a bra "night and day for some months, since it would seem to diminish traction on the scar."[11]

The Needle Samplings

As discussed in Chapter Nine, **fine-needle aspiration** (FNA) is a routine office procedure which can often diagnose malignant and benign disorders of the breast. But FNA cannot be properly termed "a biopsy," since it provides no tissue sample, only an aspirate of loose cells and accompanying cellular debris. And FNA is not a substitute for biopsy, though it may sometimes make tissue sampling unnecessary by positively identifying a benign condition. These days FNA often serves as a prelude to biopsy. If the cytological analysis of a needle aspirate yields equivocal results, we would naturally want to obtain a tissue sample so as to be sure of the diagnosis. If the analysis should indicate malignancy, we would need an excisional biopsy (lumpectomy) for both therapeutic and diagnostic purposes. A few aspirated cancer cells can't tell us whether the tumor is invasive or not, and they hold few clues to its histological subtype and its degree of aggressiveness.

Fine-needle aspiration may be performed on suspicious breast masses which we already plan to remove, because there are advantages to be had from knowing whether cancer is present *before* *the* *actual* *biopsy*. An early warning of malignancy allows us to ponder the therapeutic options ahead of time. Additional views of the breast with magnification mammography or with magnetic resonance imaging (MRI) could be taken, both to estimate the extent of the malignant lesion and to reveal any other abnormalities in the affected breast or in the contralateral (opposite) breast.[12] The positive FNA results and the radiographic images would determine the course of the biopsy. Surgeons operate in different ways depending upon whether a breast lesion is regarded as benign or as malignant. When removing a presumably benign lesion, the surgeon will try to minimize the defect left by its excision—and will purposely remove as little of the adjacent tissue as possible. When faced with a verified malignancy, the surgeon will be concerned not only to remove the entire tumor, but also to obtain an adequate margin (safety zone) of nonmalignant tissue on all sides. Lumpectomy patients usually tolerate the larger defect, knowing that the risk of cancer recurring in the affected breast has thereby been reduced.

Skinny needles aren't the only ones around. Fine-needle aspiration must be distinguished from the **core-needle biopsy**. Both procedures involve needle penetration of a breast lesion and the removal of a specimen for laboratory analysis. They differ in the size (diameter) of the needle used and in the type of specimen extracted. The core needle, sometimes referred to as a "wide needle" or "cutting needle," is much broader than the more familiar fine needles. It has a hollow bore specifically designed to extract a thin sliver of tissue. Since a core needle provides a tissue cross section rather than just an aspirate of cells, it accomplishes a minimal incisional biopsy. A handheld core needle resembles a slender pen or pencil—it has a solid pointed tip followed by a hollow "specimen notch" covered with a retractable sleeve. During a core-needle biopsy, a tiny incision is first made in the skin overlying a breast mass; the needle is then advanced through the incision into the mass. Now the retractable sleeve is pulled back to expose

the specimen notch, and then pushed forward again, thus entrapping the thinnest strip (or core) of tissue in the notch.[13] The needle is withdrawn from the breast, the tissue specimen retrieved and sent to the pathology lab, and compression is applied to the puncture wound to stop the bleeding.

A core-needle biopsy can be done as an office procedure. It's quick and inexpensive, requires only a dab of local anesthetic and a band-aid afterwards, and leaves no defect or scar to speak of. But it has substantial limitations. A handheld core needle cannot accurately sample small, deep-set, or otherwise elusive masses, and it has no role in sampling those nonpalpable lesions detected on mammograms. This technique is suitable mainly for large palpable masses right at the surface of the breast, where a mass can be immobilized with one hand at same time a core needle is advanced with the other. While the pathologist is more likely to reach a definite diagnosis from a core-needle specimen than from a cellular aspirate, a negative finding would not eliminate the need for the surgical excision of a mass which had clinical or mammographic features suggestive of malignancy. With needles, whether wide or thin, the possibility of sampling error always exists. If the needle is placed in the wrong spot, or if a specimen is too small, malignancy may be overlooked.

In the 1990s improved radiographic visualization began to expand the indications for needle sampling of breast abnormalities, by giving us more reliable ways of targeting small or deep-set lesions. Ultrasound offered the simplest and least expensive guidance for needle probes; the technique in question came to be dubbed **freehand interventional sonography**. Here a transducer (scanner) is held against the breast, while a needle (either fine or wide) is moved toward the solid mass or fluid-filled cyst. Flickering images appear

Handheld Core Needle

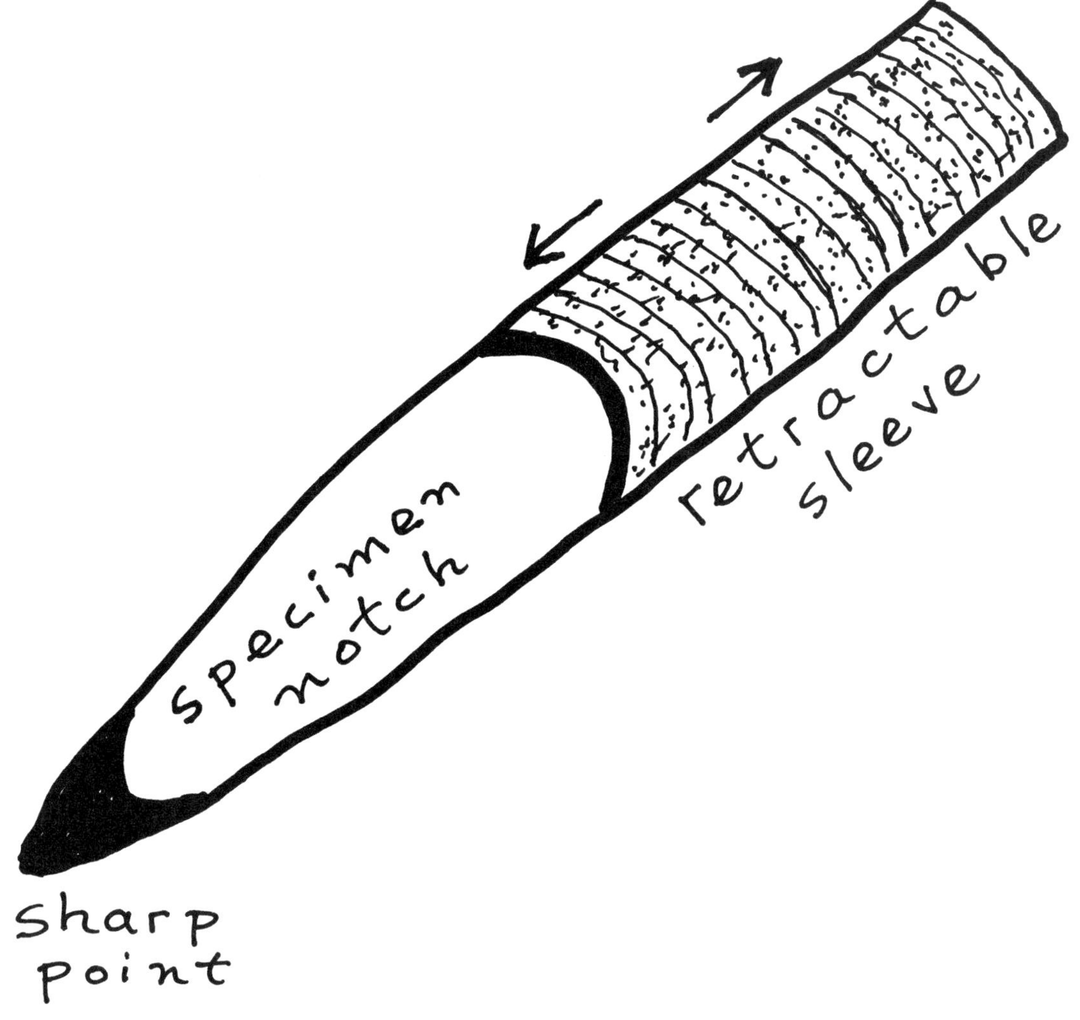

A handheld core needle offers an uncomplicated and inexpensive way to biopsy a palpable mass located near the breast's surface. After the needle point is advanced into the mass, the retractable sleeve is pulled back and then pushed forward. A thin sliver of tissue is thus entrapped in the specimen notch.

on a video monitor—the picture is fuzzy, but it's usually sufficient to show us the spatial relationship between the advancing needle and the lesion we wish to aspirate or biopsy. This type of guidance can be accomplished with standard ultrasound equipment, and it requires minimal training on the operator's part. One recipe for schooling freehand sonographers called for an uncooked turkey breast stuffed with pimento-filled olives. The poultry item was found to simulate breast tissue better than a synthetic product, and the olives gave a reasonable approximation of breast masses.[14] Just a trip to the supermarket, and any ultrasound technician could become proficient at guiding needle probes of breast lesions—and have leftovers for sandwiches!

Stuart S. Kaplan and other radiologists at the University of California in Los Angeles have pioneered a sophisticated ultrasound technique which is particularly suited for core-needle biopsies. They use two needles. The first is a hollow "introducer needle" of 12-gauge diameter, large enough to be easily visualized with ultrasound technology. After this introducer needle is advanced up against the breast mass, a core-biopsy needle of 14-gauge diameter (slightly narrower) is threaded through it to sample the mass. The advantage here is that the introducer needle can be left in place, while the narrower core-biopsy needle can be moved in and out at will, taking multiple tissue samples. Damage to the surrounding normal tissues is minimized, and the odds of getting adequate pathological specimens greatly improved.[15] Even with such innovations, however, ultrasound-guided needle samplings are suitable only for solid or cystic masses of one centimeter or more in diameter (upwards of half an inch or so). Ultrasound cannot visualize clusters of microcalcifications or ill-defined areas of increased density.

Nonpalpable Lesions

An unhappy truism of breast biopsies is: **"The smaller the lesion, the more difficulty in sampling it."** This principle can sometimes hold true for small palpable masses right beneath the skin, which may seem to slip away—indeed, to disappear—as soon as the surgeon makes an incision. But the truism is always applicable to nonpalpable lesions—that is, to those suspicious calcifications or atypical densities which we can detect only by mammography. The most reliable method of sampling such lesions has long been **wire localization and excisional biopsy**. Unfortunately, this technique is neither simple nor innocuous. Years ago, if a nonpalpable lesion happened to lie deep in a large breast, the surgery needed for an effective biopsy was often extensive enough to require total anesthesia and overnight hospitalization. More recently, these procedures have been done on an outpatient basis, but for many women they still meant a very bad day in the hospital. First, a patient had to visit the radiology department, where the biopsy-bound breast was mammogramed several times. A hollow introducer needle was stuck in the breast, and then a thin wire with a hooked end threaded through the needle. The needle came out—the wire being left in place to guide the surgeon to the elusive calcifications or area of density. At some hospitals a little bit of colored dye might be injected at the lesion's site as a safety measure. If the locator wire should be pulled out of position, the dye would surely mark the spot, being colored (so that the surgeon could see it) as well as radio-opaque (so that it would show up on mammograms). Patients were typically wide-awake during the localization procedure (anesthesia being reserved for the surgical biopsy itself); and some of them could experience considerable discomfort, especially if the needles and wires had to be re-inserted or otherwise maneuvered so as to be in just the right spot. The writer Gayle Feldman has recalled her reactions during a difficult localization for tiny calcifications: "I felt nauseated and faint. I gripped the mammography machine as the radiologist threaded the hook and wire through. My God, I hadn't expected the localization to hurt like this."[16]

Once wire localization was completed, the patient would be shuttled off to the operating room for the biopsy. The surgeon would simply follow the wire down to the nonpalpable lesion, taking pains to excise a broad tissue section around the wire's hooked end. As soon as the specimen was removed, it would be rushed off to the hospital's radiology department. An X-ray of the specimen had to be compared with the patient's preoperative mammograms. Did the excised tissues really contain the suspicious calcifications or density which had prompted the biopsy? Only when both surgeon and radiologist were satisfied of the lesion's removal, could the biopsy incision be closed, and the patient dismissed from the hospital.

Stereotactic Needle Biopsies

Wire localization and an ample excision continue to be the gold standard for diagnosing and treating nonpalpable lesions, but nobody wants to perform this procedure. Localization is time-consuming and expensive. The subsequent surgery may leave a largish defect in the breast; and the scar tissue which forms as the defect heals can appear as a star-shaped mass on future mammograms, looking just like an infiltrating ductal carcinoma and making radiological interpretations more difficult. Patients would gladly suffer these many drawbacks if wire localization biopsies really saved lives; but as we've seen in Chapter Ten, most

biopsies done for calcifications or asymmetrical densities result in verdicts of "epithelial hyperplasia" or "fibrocystic change." All that anxiety, expense, and scarring—and all done simply to identify harmless benign processes!

It would be far better if we could use fine-needle aspirations or core-needle biopsies, those relatively cheap and painless procedures, to sort out the benign lesions—and thus reserve wire localization and excisional biopsy for the early-stage cancers. A core-needle tissue sampling would almost always give us a reliable diagnosis of nonpalpable lesions if we could position the needle and its specimen notch properly. Unfortunately, in the 1980s we simply did not have the technology to achieve that optimal positioning. Just try sampling a deep-set nonpalpable lesion with a handheld needle! And imagine that you have no good way of seeing either the tiny lesion or the needle point during the procedure—and that you have moreover no good way of immobilizing the relentlessly heaving breast or your tremulous hand! Could it be done? The upsurge in the number of nonpalpable lesions being recommended for biopsy provided equipment manufacturers with an incentive to work on these formidable obstacles. By the early 1990s Yankee ingenuity had triumphed, and we had some elaborate devices which enabled us to perform **stereotactic needle biopsies**. The new machines used digital mammography to achieve immediate radiographic guidance, that essential visualization of both lesion and needle during the sampling procedure. Stabilization was also provided for. A specially designed biopsy table held the breast motionless, while an automated biopsy gun replaced the physician's tremulous hand. Needle sampling of any and all abnormalities in the breast had become feasible.

The idea of stereotactic breast biopsies originated in Sweden. As early as 1976 the Karolinska Hospital in Stockholm introduced a crude stereotactic system for nonpalpable lesions. Mammograms of the affected breast were taken from two different angles. The lesion's spatial location was then carefully coordinated (mapped) from these "two stereoradiographs," and through the use of a calibrated grid, a handheld needle was aimed with passable accuracy.[17] American radiologists did not become excited about the technique until the late 1980s, when it became clear that a high degree of automation and precision could be obtained. **Steve H. Parker**, director of a Denver breast imaging clinic appropriately called the **Swedish Medical Center**, emerged as the leading American proponent of the new technology. Other radiologists soon came to refer to the "Parker approach" for stereotactic needle biopsies of the breast. The equipment used was *dedicated* (designed for the purpose intended)—Fischer Imaging of Denver produced the *Mammotest* unit, while Lorad Medical Systems (Danbury, Connecticut) manufactured the competing *StereoGuide*. Both units featured a biopsy table, upon which a patient would lie prone and suspend her breasts into the compression paddles beneath. The elaborate apparatus underneath the table surpassed the fantasies of Rube Goldberg. A digital mammography system flashed images of the affected breast on a video monitor. Admittedly, the visual field was narrow (five centimeters or so), and the resolution much less than that in film-screen mammography, but both the nonpalpable lesion and the biopsy needle could be seen. A computer figured out the lesion's coordinates and plotted the best trajectory to it, while simultaneously aiming a biopsy gun. The most popular of these automated sampling devices was the **Biopty gun** distributed by Bard Urological (Covington, Georgia),

but a **Pro-Mag** from Manan Medical Products (Northbrook, Illinois) accomplished the job equally well. Both guns "fired" a core-biopsy needle in an unwaveringly straight line for a distance of up to two-and-a-quarter centimeters (about an inch).

In 1990 Steve H. Parker and other avant-garde radiologists published the results of a small clinical trial conducted in the Denver area. Parker et al had enrolled 103 patients with nonpalpable breast lesions, who had first undergone stereotactic needle biopsies, and then subsequently had the traditional wire locations and excisional biopsies. The pathology reports from the needle biopsies were compared with those from the elaborate surgical biopsies. Dr. Parker and his colleagues enthusiastically announced that the stereotactic biopsies gave the correct diagnosis 97% of the time, and they sung the praises of the Mammotest table and the Bard Biopty gun. This biopsy procedure caused little discomfort, left no noticeable defect or scar, and cost only half as much as a wire-localization biopsy. *It was all so simple!* Just get the patient on the Mammotest table, then take a few digital mammograms and feed them into the computer, which will calculate exact coordinates for the lesion. Now inject a bit of local anesthetic; make a small nick in the skin, and advance the needle through it to the precalculated depth. "The Biopty gun is aligned automatically on the proper trajectory," observed Parker et al, "but stereo views are obtained again to confirm that the needle is poised over the lesion." The needle is now backed up for a fraction of an inch ("at least two millimeters"); and then it's fired, instantly springing forward to entrap a slender strip of tissue in its specimen notch. "The needle is removed, and the core tissue obtained is placed in formalin." Parker et al recommended that this sampling procedure be repeated three or four times, the needle's position being constantly monitored by digital mammography to ensure that the lesion is "canvassed anteriorly to posteriorly in measured increments." All the "biopsy passes" are made through the single nick in the skin; when they are completed, the patient usually needs nothing more than temporary compression and a band-aid to stop the bleeding. The risk of complications is minuscule, being limited to an occasional hematoma (blood accumulation) or a very infrequent infection at the biopsy site.[18]

A Better Mousetrap?

Somebody certainly seemed to have come up with a better way to diagnose nonpalpable lesions. During the 1990s the most up-to-date hospitals and breast imaging clinics rushed to acquire their Mammotest or their StereoGuide. These devices were expensive, costing about $125,000 apiece.[19] And there was also the question of training—how much did one need to operate the new machines, and could equally accurate biopsies be performed by operators less experienced than Steve Parker and his associates. The inevitable turf wars broke out. Should stereotactic needle biopsies be regarded primarily as mammographic investigations, and hence done by radiologists?—or were they really operative procedures best accomplished by a surgeon? In 1994 a correspondent to the *American Surgery News* offered an optimistic opinion: "A surgeon can learn his technique in one day." Crash courses in stereotactic breast biopsy sprang up in idyllic locales, and many radiologists and surgeons heard the same advice from their colleagues: "Go to Bermuda for the weekend. Get trained."[20]

In the meantime research-oriented physicians at the large cancer hospitals were undertaking studies designed to verify the reliability of stereotactic needle biopsies. Was this technique more effective for some types of breast lesion than for others? Were there any pitfalls? Laura Liberman and her colleagues at the Memorial Sloan-Kettering Cancer Center in New York City emphasized that when core-needle biopsies are performed for suspicious microcalcifications, the tiny specimens still need to be X-rayed immediately to ensure the presence of the calcifications in question. At Sloan-Kettering the pathologists were able to reach a definite diagnosis in 81% of the cases where the core specimens contained the suspicious calcifications, but only in 38% of those cases where they did not.[21] How many core specimens are necessary? The Sloan-Kettering experience, as reported by Liberman et al, suggests that a single specimen will suffice for a definite diagnosis in some 70% of stereotactic biopsies; yet the likelihood of diagnosis improves as more specimens are taken. With five core specimens, the Sloan-Kettering pathologists were able to diagnose 99% of the solid masses sampled and 87% of the nonpalpable lesions discovered by mammographic calcifications. Taking six specimens upped the diagnostic yield from those nonpalpable lesions to 92%.[22] Radiologist Liberman and her colleagues point out that stereotactic core biopsies, unlike fine-needle aspirations, can distinguish between ductal carcinoma *in situ* (DCIS) and infiltrating ductal carcinomas. The problem they see is that this technique cannot rule out the possibility of a hidden focus of invasive cancer somewhere in a DCIS lesion.[23] With core-needle biopsies, of course, the entire lesion isn't submitted for pathological analysis— only tiny specimens taken from different areas of the lesion.

In 1994 Roger J. Jackman and other radiologists at the Stanford University Medical Center reported that stereotactic needle sampling had replaced wire localization and excisional biopsy "as the preferred method for histological diagnosis in all our patients with nonpalpable lesions." But Jackman et al acknowledged that the core specimens did not always provide sufficient material to distinguish **atypical ductal hyperplasia** (ADH) from ductal carcinoma *in situ*: "We recommend excision of all ADH lesions diagnosed with large-core needle biopsy."[24] But the diagnostic accuracy of stereotactic samplings was generally conceded. Steve H. Parker and his colleagues did an analysis of 4,744 core-needle biopsies performed at twenty institutions across the United States. Only twelve of these biopsies, 0.25%, proved to be false-negatives—that is, gave a clean bill of health when cancer was present.[25]

A Biopsy for All Lesions

We have made remarkable progress in the accurate pathological diagnosis of breast abnormalities. In the early 1970s we had but a single tissue-sampling procedure, the old one-step biopsy, which was universally agreed upon and invariably adopted whenever there was the slightest chance that a malignancy might be discovered. In those unenlightened days breast symptoms were often ignored—and palpable lumps allowed to double in size—because physicians and patients alike knew that a proper diagnosis involved hospitalization, open surgery, total anesthesia, a lasting scar for benign conditions, and an irrevocable amputation for even the tiniest focus of cancer. These days we have a variety of procedures which can accomplish tissue sampling of suspicious lesions, and naturally there is some uncertainty about the best way to sample this or that type of lesion. Confusing? Yes, but that's the price you pay for progress! With the proper forethought, we can minimize the anxiety, discomfort, expense, and scarring

which have long been associated with breast biopsies. All abnormalities can now be sampled by needle penetration done on an outpatient basis and with only a local anesthetic. Given the combination of adequate preliminary mammograms and skillful needle placement, we can arrive at the proper diagnosis over 90% of the time without resort to surgery. Palpable masses of at least one centimeter (half an inch) in diameter can usually be sampled with a handheld needle. The use of a core needle mandates a few antiseptic precautions, but it is more likely to lead to a conclusive diagnosis than fine-needle aspiration. The new stereotactic needle biopsies are more expensive, but then they permit the accurate needle sampling of nonpalpable lesions anywhere in the breast. Steve Parker and his colleagues sometimes have conveyed the impression that stereotactic biopsy with a Mammotest table and Biopty gun ought to be the diagnostic procedure of choice for almost every breast problem. It is certainly welcome as an option; but in many cases the freehand techniques would suffice to arrive at a diagnosis, and in others an excisional biopsy would be the most logical choice. Unlike any of the needle sampling procedures, the excisional biopsy can accomplish a therapeutic purpose as well as a diagnostic one.

The cost-effectiveness of a preliminary stereotactic biopsy is open to question in those cases where malignancy is strongly suspected and an excisional biopsy anticipated. For example, a core-needle sampling which revealed ductal carcinoma *in situ* would probably need to be followed by wire localization and a surgical excision which would now be termed "lumpectomy." A full excision would be necessary both to treat the DCIS by removing it, and to verify that the lesion contained no foci of occult infiltration. In this case the cost of the therapeutic excision would be added to that of the diagnostic stereotactic biopsy—would it not therefore be cheaper just to do the excision in the first place? The answer isn't as clear as you might think. A cost-benefit analysis done in Saint Louis at the Barnes Hospital and the Washington University School of Medicine reported an average price of $549 for a stereotactic needle biopsy and $1,570 for the traditional wire-localization biopsy. The study's authors recommended preliminary stereotactic samplings for all nonpalpable lesions. Even if cancer should be discovered and open surgery later required, they argued that an initial stereotactic diagnosis might save time and money in the long run: "There was a significant improvement in the surgical margins achieved when the diagnosis of breast cancer was known before operation, and the need for re-excision as a part of breast conservation was eliminated."[26]

The clearest indication for stereotactic needle biopsies still remains low-risk lesions, those mammographically discovered calcifications or asymmetrical densities which have perhaps one chance in five or in ten of turning up malignant. The University of Chicago Hospital has recorded its experience with 246 patients with low-risk lesions who underwent stereotactic needle samplings. A full 85% of these patients were found to have harmless benign conditions and were thus spared surgical biopsy. In this instance a stereotactic procedure costing $1,100 to $1,300 saved each patient with a benign condition over $2,000, because wire-localization biopsies in the Chicago-area hospitals then cost anywhere from $3,500 to $5,000 or more.[27] Those Chicago prices tower like skyscrapers over the estimates Steve Parker and his associates reported for the Denver area— $675 for a stereotactic needle sampling and $1,217 for an outpatient surgical biopsy.[28] Stereotactic biopsy tables and automated tissue-sampling guns are not presently available in small-town America, but hopefully these wondrous devices will soon be found in every sizable city and hospital. Sometimes they can save your money as well as your breast.

Chapter Twelve

PATHOLOGY REPORT
Understanding the Varieties of Breast Cancer

In cancer medicine the pathologist is king. The verdict coming from the pathology lab after a biopsy determines whether a patient will be liberated from anxiety, or rather involuntarily consigned to a protracted round of consultation and therapy. Pathologists are physicians who specialize in disease processes. They do not generally examine or treat patients, but rather provide precise diagnoses based upon the examination of tissue specimens under a microscope. In pathology a good bedside manner accounts for very little—knowledge is everything, and a meticulous attention to small details the hallmark of the true professional.

In the past breast cancer patients rarely had occasion to see a pathologist in the flesh. The pathologist's role seemed to be limited to a momentary appearance as a disembodied voice, which came over the operating room intercom to report on a frozen section. Things have changed considerably, because we now recognize that "breast cancer" is not a single disease, but rather a broad spectrum of disorders which require different therapeutic approaches. Since the treatment must be tailored to suit the individual case, we must look to the pathologist for more explicit guidance. Will surgical excision alone cure this particular type of mammary cancer? Can

the breast be preserved, or does extensive tumor spread make mastectomy a more rational alternative? Is postoperative radiotherapy advisable? Is chemotherapy indicated, and if so, what kind? Often a skilled pathologist can give authoritative answers to these questions simply by looking at the biopsy specimen. Of course, pathologists do not treat patients or decree therapy, but their advice on these matters should be valued for precisely that reason. They are more likely to be impartial, having neither an inflexible commitment to this or that therapy nor any financial incentive to recommend one treatment over another.

The interpretation of breast biopsies is not always straightforward. In spite of its relatively simple anatomy, the breast can give rise to a bewildering assortment of benign and malignant lesions. Not all pathologists are equally conversant with its mysteries. A pathology lab which mainly analyzed Pap smears for gynecologists would no doubt be stymied by the conundrums posed by the mammary gland. A biopsy specimen which has been processed by one lab cannot be processed again by another— but fortunately the permanent sections from the specimen (those glass slides which are kept indefinitely by the hospital) can be readily transported for a second opinion or even a third. Pathologists rarely overlook frank malignancy; but the degree of malignancy may occasionally be overstated or understated, with the result that either excessive or insufficient treatments will be adopted by the referring physicians.

This chapter is intended to acquaint the reader with the complex work that pathologists do, and to introduce and define some terms which are commonly used on breast pathology reports. Insofar as a patient diagnosed with "breast cancer" might wish to participate in treatment decisions, she should know enough to grasp the general drift and implications of her pathology report—and, if necessary, to ask meaningful questions of her pathologist. This chapter also describes the principal varieties of mammary malignancy and assesses the degree of aggressiveness associated with each. The benign conditions covered in Chapter Eight are not discussed here, for the simple reason that a benign diagnosis on a pathology report prompts us only to a sigh of relief. On the other hand, a report indicating malignancy ought to encourage us to further study. That report may have to be "translated" for us, but it should be thoroughly understood before treatment options are pondered.

SPECIMEN PREPARATION
Fixation, Embedding, Staining

Fresh biopsy specimens are raw blobs of tissue, by themselves relatively uninformative. To interpret them, we have to see the shape and configuration of their constituent cells. The visualization of cells in solid mammalian tissues was first accomplished in the late 1870s—the basic techniques have not changed much. The most important tool remains the microscope with compound lenses, first introduced around 1830. It is called a **light microscope**, because visualization depends upon the waves of light which pass through the extremely thin specimens. A magnification of about 1,000 times the original size can be obtained. The **electron microscope** offers far greater magnifications, up to 50,000 or more, enabling us to see the tiny structures in a cell's cytoplasm. Visualization depends upon waves of electrons, which are aimed at incredibly thin specimens in a vacuum chamber. Electron microscopy is far too expensive and complicated for routine specimen analysis. When we speak of "the microscope," we therefore mean the light microscope, which can reveal the general size and condition of cellular nuclei and cytoplasms, but not any smaller structures.

As mentioned in Chapter Eleven, the frozen-section technique offers immediate specimen preparation; its drawbacks are that the tissue used cannot be preserved and that cellular details cannot be seen with the greatest clarity. Permanent sections are preferred, but their preparation takes a day or two. The entire biopsy specimen must first be immersed in chemicals such as formalin (a formaldehyde solution) which act to arrest the rapid process of decay—this step is called **fixation**. Subsequently the specimen is rinsed and dehydrated by passing it through a series of alcohol solutions. **Embedding** comes next, the specimen being placed in warm liquefied paraffin. After the paraffin has infiltrated the tissues and been allowed to harden, the specimen can be sectioned. A precision instrument called a **microtome** divides it into thin slices called **sections**, which are just a few microns thick (about one-hundredth of a millimeter).

These slivers are still not ready to be placed under a microscope, because they are colorless and essentially invisible. **Staining** is a necessary final step—the coloring dyes are differentially absorbed by the various cellular structures, thus enabling us to distinguish them. Nuclei absorb the lion's share of these chemicals. The enlarged nuclei of cancer cells appear vividly hyperchromatic, leaping up to the observing eye as the bright warning signs of malignancy. Over the decades many stains have been introduced; some are better than others for visualizing this or that particular cellular structure. But the most useful stain remains the first one developed, the combination of **hematoxylin and eosin** which has been around since the 1870s. Pathologists employ the initials **H&E** to designate this combination, which stains nuclei dark blue and gives cytoplasms a pink-to-reddish hue.

After fixation, dehydration, embedding, sectioning, and staining, all the preparations can be said to be complete. The slices of processed tissue, mounted between little panes of glass, are called **permanent sections** because they are wonderfully enduring. They will last indefinitely, and you can examine them as often as you like. Alas, the cells and tissues so enshrined are dead and dry—archival relics which tell us as much about the metabolic processes of a growing malignancy as a mummy from ancient Egypt tells us about the living Pharaoh. The magnifications obtained with light microscopy, hundreds of times larger than the original, may sound impressive to the layperson; but they are puny for the task at hand. The cells are, as it were, seen from afar. Looking down at a tissue cross section with a light microscope is like looking down at a housing subdivision while flying in an airplane at an altitude of 5,000 feet. You might perceive an orderly arrangement of houses, trees, and streets in the subdivision while being oblivious to any particular details—the type of street paving, the species of tree, the use of brick or wood for home construction. But if you happened to fly over that subdivision

shortly after it had been destroyed by a violent tornado or a large earthquake, you would know that some catastrophic event had taken place. Houses would be flattened, trees uprooted, streets jolted asunder. Similarly, a pathologist looking at a permanent section can appreciate the orderly arrangement of normal tissues—the expected regularity of cells resting on a basement membrane, and the gentle branching of blood vessels. A cataclysmic transformation is equally obvious in the malignant specimen. There would be haphazard variations in the size, structure, and arrangement of cells—as well as a disappearing basement membrane and swollen blood vessels wandering out of their usual courses. With light microscopy, as during air travel one mile up, we can recognize the effects of a massive natural disaster on the landscape beneath us.

TUMOR EXAMINATION
The Gross Specimen

Tumor analysis always begins with a visual inspection of the "gross specimen"—that is, the unprocessed tissue sample removed by the biopsy. The pathology department's record-keeping should also begin here, as the pathologist takes a minute or two to measure the specimen and record its size and general appearance. Such measurements can be deceptive, for the overall specimen size usually does not correlate with the dimensions of the malignant tumor. The specimen may in fact consist largely of nonmalignant tissue, because tumors rarely grow in a regular fashion and because the surgeon will have purposely included an encircling margin of healthy flesh. The cancer itself could be much smaller. The pathologist can often get a better idea of its actual size and probable aggressiveness by cutting the specimen in two, and then inspecting the interior surfaces of these halves with a magnifying glass. The border of the tumor—the line where it impinges on the surrounding tissues—provides the first clue of prognostic import. If the tumor border appears well-defined and seems to "push" the normal tissues outward in an "expansile" growth pattern, the patient's long-term prognosis is usually good. On the other hand, if the border is indistinct and tendrils of tumor appear to be infiltrating the surrounding tissues, any judgment on the patient's prognosis should be reserved. Malignant infiltration visible to the naked eye is always a danger signal, and it becomes increasingly ominous after a tumor reaches a diameter of about one centimeter.

To a greater or lesser degree, invasive breast cancers tend to induce a fibrotic reaction in the stroma (bed of connective tissue) surrounding the mammary gland's ducts and lobules. This reaction can often be observed on the gross (visual) inspection of a halved specimen; and its extent should be duly noted on the pathology report, where it might be termed **desmoplasia** (Greek for an abnormal proliferation of fibrous tissue). A strong desmoplastic reaction is regarded as a favorable indicator in medullary breast cancers, but as an unhappy finding in those rock-hard tumors sometimes called "scirrhous carcinomas." **Necrosis** (the death of tissues) is actually a marker of tumor aggressiveness. It is apparent to the naked eye as a white chalky area at the tumor's center, consisting of dead cells, cellular debris, and calcifications. You might perhaps suspect that dead or dying cancer cells would be a good thing; but it's important to remember the reason why these cells died. These cells perished because they could not obtain an adequate blood supply; and in all probability this happened because the tumor grew too fast, with the rapidly multiplying cancer cells on the periphery absorbing most of the blood-borne nutrients

while the interior cells were left to famish. Thus an area of visible necrosis usually serves to indicate a fast-growing, highly invasive breast tumor. Thanks to an authoritative clinical trial with long-term follow-up, we know that such necrosis identifies a subgroup of node-negative patients who are especially likely to experience recurrence.[1] The combination of an **infiltrative border** and **central necrosis** bodes ill in a breast tumor of any size; conversely, the absence of these two characteristics is a positive omen.

What are we to make of those inflammatory reactions which can sometimes be detected around the edges of tumors? Under the microscope we might see large numbers of infection-fighting white cells, principally lymphocytes of the T-cell variety, intermingling with the cancer cells. Back in the 1970s some pathologists thought that such a **lymphocytic reaction** indicated a strong immune response to the cancer and thus pointed toward a better prognosis.[2] Sadly, our clinical trials have demonstrated that the presence of lymphocytes—like an area of necrosis—is usually associated with the more aggressive breast tumors and therefore more likely to foreshadow a poorer prognosis. Paul Peter Rosen of New York's Memorial Sloan-Kettering observes that "duct carcinomas with a prominent lymphocytic reaction tend to be poorly differentiated" and "almost always estrogen and progesterone receptor-negative."[3] The biochemical changes produced by malignant infiltration of the surrounding tissues probably are responsible for summoning all the white cells. But upon arriving at the scene, the T-cells seem to remain mere bystanders, doing nothing to impede the tumor's growth. Neither dying cancer cells nor onrushing white cells can offer us any reason for optimism—but there is safety in a non-infiltrative border.

MICROSCOPIC ANALYSIS
Histological and Nuclear Grading

Specimen inspection with the naked eye is likely to be informative only in the case of the larger breast tumors. For small lesions, especially nonpalpable ones, we have to await the completion of microscopic studies before drawing any conclusions. When malignancy is considered even a remote possibility, the biopsy specimen should be thoroughly studied on permanent sections. The principal goal of microscopic analysis can be briefly stated—to determine a specimen's degree of **differentiation**. This word, first introduced in Chapter One, designates the functional adulthood of cells as they are encountered in particular glands and specialized tissues. A variation of the term will be found on a cancer pathology report, used in an attempt to evaluate how closely the cells in a malignant tumor resemble those in the normal tissue from which it arose. Thus the cellular structure of a "well-differentiated" breast tumor closely resembles the normal organization of the mammary gland. A tumor might also be described as "moderately differentiated"—as "poorly differentiated" (having little resemblance to the cells and tissues from which it arose)—or as "undifferentiated" (having no resemblance). Loss of differentiation is a progressive biological catastrophe; it has the most profound implications for a tumor's growth rate and metastatic potential. John Laszlo of the American Cancer Society reminds us that well-differentiated malignancies "are generally slow-growing," while poorly differentiated ones "are generally more rapidly growing."[4] An undifferentiated tumor might also be described as **anaplastic**—from the Greek *an*, "without," and *plasis*, "a molding." These terms can be used interchangeably to label the presumably dangerous tumor.

Since the 1920s pathologists interested in breast malignancies have been trying to develop a uniform, reproducible method of **tumor grading**—that is, a way of objectively measuring a tumor's degree of differentiation and of predicting its behavior. The most widely used system is **histological**: pathologists try to assign an evaluative grade based on a tumor's overall organization (from the Greek *histos*, "web" or "tissue"). Jean F. Simpson and David L. Page of Vanderbilt University observe that the histological grading of breast cancers "consists of assessment of three features: tubular formation, nuclei, and mitoses."[5] An arrangement into small duct-like structures, or tubules, constitutes a very favorable sign, because this is the normal architecture of the mammary gland. The nuclei of malignant cells reveal wide variations in size and shape, from the small and regular to the enormous and bizarre. Nuclei which look bad are typically described as **pleomorphic** and **hyperchromatic**. The former term indicates a variety of different shapes; the latter simply means that the nuclei are brightly colored, having absorbed excessive amounts of staining dye because they contain excessive quantities of DNA. Mitosis occurs when a cell physically divides in two—this reproductive event is clearly visible under the microscope. And the more mitoses a pathologist can count on a permanent section, the faster a tumor is likely to grow. Most systems for histological grading use a numerical scale of one to three, with "one" representing well-differentiated breast cancers and "three" the poorly differentiated tumors. Simpson and Page remind us that low-grade breast carcinomas (prognosticly favorable) have "very regular nuclei, lack of mitoses, prominent tubular formation." But high-grade tumors (prognosticly unfavorable) reveal "pleomorphic nuclei, frequent mitoses, and lack of tubule formation."[6]

While the basic techniques of specimen preparation and light microscopy have not changed much in the past century, pathology is as dynamic and progressive a medical discipline as any other. Back in the 1970s Maurice M. Black, a famous pathologist in New York City, started a small revolution by developing the concept of **nuclear grading**, which he touted as superior to the traditional histological grading.[7] Black and his colleagues argued that a breast tumor's behavior could be predicted better by looking at the nuclei of its individual cancer cells rather than by assessing its histological (structural) features. Of course, all malignancies result from malfunctions in the genetic material (DNA) stored in the nucleus. Black's idea was perfectly logical, but how practical was it for routine laboratory analysis? We can't see malfunctioning genes even with an electron microscope, so what could we discover about the complicated nuclear machinery with a light microscope? Not a great deal; but if we turn up the magnification to 400 or more, we can discern a few significant clues. Nuclear grading evaluates the tiny structures and tissues within the nucleus, namely the **nucleoli** and the **chromatin**. Nucleoli are small round bodies involved in the production of RNA (ribonucleic acid), which carries coded instructions for protein manufacture to the workshops (ribosomes) in the cytoplasm. Each human cell has at least one nucleolus in its nucleus, sometimes as many as four; but nucleoli usually remain invisible, even at high magnifications. They become prominent only in rapidly multiplying cells, such as we find in an embryo or a malignant tumor. The more nucleoli visible in breast cancer cells, the more aggressive the tumor is likely to be. The tissue evaluated in nuclear grading is chromatin, the combination of DNA and adhesive proteins which forms the chromosomes and genes. In well-differentiated breast cancer cells, the chromatin appears fine in texture, stains lightly, and is evenly distributed throughout the nucleus. But in undifferentiated breast cancer cells, the chromatin has a coarse texture—and it piles up in heavily staining "clumps" or *vesiculae* (blisters) which are erratically positioned.

Nuclear grading gives us additional guidance in selecting the optimal therapy, but American pathologists have been slow to embrace this microscopic assay, most of them having been trained to do only histological grading. To make matters worse, the assay's proponents had difficulty in agreeing on a uniform system of grading. Dr. Black and his colleagues used a numerical scale from one to three; but wishing to distinguish nuclear grading from histological grading, they reversed the order of evaluations, assigning a grade of "one" to nuclei in bad shape and "three" to those that seemed almost normal. In the 1980s Edwin R. Fisher, head pathologist of the influential **National Surgical Adjuvant Breast and Bowel Project** (NSABP), took up the cause of nuclear grade. Fisher and his NSABP co-workers also used a numerical scale, but they called well-differentiated nuclei "grade one" and poorly differentiated nuclei "grade three," thereby bringing nuclear grading into line with the traditional histological evaluations.[8]

As of late our pathologists have tended to accept the NSABP practice for grading nuclei; but to avoid any possible confusion, future references in this book will be to "good," "moderate," or "poor" nuclear grade. K. Kendall Pierson and Edward J. Wilkinson of the University of Florida have published some general criteria for these three grades, which are worth quoting. **Good nuclear grade** "is characterized by small, relatively uniform, rounded nuclei with few nucleoli and rare mitoses." A breast tumor with **moderate nuclear grade** reveals "increased nuclear size, pleomorphism, and chromatin/DNA variability." In breast malignancies with **poor nuclear grade**, we can expect to see markedly enlarged, highly pleomorphic nuclei "with vesicular and variable chromatin patterns, prominent nucleoli, and conspicuous, often atypical, mitotic figures."[9]

During the 1990s the importance of nuclear grading became widely recognized as a steady stream of NSABP reports linked poor nuclear grade to an increased risk of tumor recurrence and early death. The Saint Louis pathologist John S. Meyer and his colleagues demonstrated that the proliferation rate of breast cancer cells "increases impressively with progression of the nuclear grade from one [good] to three [poor]."[10] Unlike histological analysis, nuclear grading can be done on isolated cancer cells obtained by fine-needle aspiration, thus giving us clues to a tumor's biological aggressiveness even before its excision. At the Consensus Development Conference on breast cancer therapies held in 1990, Edwin R. Fisher proclaimed that "there is a power in nuclear grade." Dr. Fisher explained that if he knew the histological variety of a patient's tumor and the nuclear grade of its constituent cells, he could make all treatment decisions simply on the basis of these two facts. Suitably impressed, the Conference panelists recommended that nuclear grading be included in "the routine pathologic review of breast cancer specimens."[11]

Lymphatic Invasion

Plausible evidence of a mammary tumor's ability to spread throughout the body is obtained when we find breast cancer cells outside the breast. In looking for proof of tumor dissemination, physicians have traditionally begun by examining the regional lymph nodes in the axilla (armpit). Yet a close microscopic analysis of the primary tumor (i.e., biopsy specimen) may produce evidence of dissemination which is almost as compelling as positive axillary nodes— sometimes we can see cancer cells invading the lymphatic channels adjacent to the tumor. Such **lymphatic invasion** is an acknowledged risk factor for local recurrence in the breast and for eventual metastasis to other organs. Paul Peter Rosen of Memorial Sloan-Kettering observes that malignant invasion of the breast lymphatics can be detected in "approximately 25% of invasive duct carcinomas." He advises pathologists to look carefully for cancer cells in the lymphatic channels "adjacent to, or well beyond, the invasive tumor margin." The long-term effects of lymphatic invasion are evident from a study Rosen and his colleagues did of 378 breast cancer patients with negative axillary nodes (usually a favorable prognostic indicator). Of those patients who had no evidence of lymphatic invasion near the primary tumor, only 10% died from breast cancer during the ten years following their diagnosis—but 33% of the patients with lymphatic invasion died during this time period. Dr. Rosen reports that recurrences in node-negative patients with lymphatic invasion "tend to occur more than five years after diagnosis," and are "almost always systemic."[12] Like tumor necrosis and poor nuclear grade, evidence of lymphatic invasion would seem to be especially useful in identifying those node-negative patients who stand to benefit from chemotherapy. This finding would be merely incidental in node-positive patients, because in these cases we already know that regional tumor dissemination has occurred.

Malignant invasion of the small blood vessels near the primary tumor is not detected as easily as lymphatic invasion, nor has its prognostic significance been clearly defined. There have been two reasons for our lack of knowledge. The first is that the tiny capillaries and veins are extremely difficult to distinguish with conventional H&E (hematoxylin and eosin) staining. To see them we must use special reagents which selectively stain the elastic fibers in the vessel walls.[13] A second reason is that we really do not know how often breast tumor cells escape into the nearby blood vessels and how this invasion might affect disease progression. However, several NSABP reports have linked vascular invasion with other unfavorable indicators. It is usually found in conjunction with four or more positive axillary nodes, or with poor nuclear grade, or with tumor necrosis.[14]

Looking at Angiogenesis

Angiogenesis, the spontaneous generation of new blood vessels, is essential to the growth of breast carcinomas and other solid tumors; and it is unquestionably fraught with prognostic import. But as recently as the 1980s our pathologists lacked a practical assay for assessing the degree of angiogenesis in tumor specimens. Understandably, an article published in the *New England Journal of Medicine* in 1991 attracted much attention because it seemed to offer a remedy for this methodological deficiency. The Harvard pathologist Noel Weidner and his co-workers had used a "standard immunoperoxidase technique" to stain the tiny blood vessels in the paraffin-embedded specimens (permanent sections) taken from 49 patients with invasive breast cancer. Weidner et al announced that they were able to assess the degree of angiogenesis simply by counting the number of stained vessels in each specimen, and moreover, that the number and density of these highlighted microvessels identified those patients whose tumors eventually metastasized. "There was a clear distinction," Dr. Weidner and his colleagues discovered, "between a stage without neovascularization, which correlated with a paucity of metastases, and a stage in which increasing neovascularization correlated with a rising rate of metastasis."[15] The following year Dr. Weidner, the angiogenesis authority Judah Folkman, and six other researchers published a more detailed report in the *Journal of the National Cancer Institute*, based on the examination of permanent sections from 165 breast cancer patients. Color illustrations revealed how immunoperoxidase staining makes tumor-associated microvessels stand out as dark brown streaks against the pinkish background achieved by previous H&E staining. Weidner and his colleagues explained that they first scan the specimen slides at low-power magnification (50 or 100 times the original size) to find "hotspots," areas of apparent angiogenetic vascularization. They then switch to high-power magnification (200 times the original size) and start counting. The density of microvessels per 200X microscopic field is the key factor they wish to ascertain, and their results are "expressed as the highest number of microvessels identified within any single 200X field." Weidner et al had no doubt that tumor angiogenesis measured in this way is "an independent and highly significant prognostic indicator" in early-stage breast cancer: "All patients having more than 100 microvessels per 200X field experienced tumor recurrence within 33 months of diagnosis, compared with less than 5% of the patients having 33 or fewer microvessels per 200X field."[16]

Other groups of cancer researchers now rushed to study angiogenetic microvessel density. An Italian team monitored 254 patients with node-negative breast cancer "for a median of 62 months," finding that angiogenesis measured in this way was "significantly predictive" of recurrence. The more microvessels per 200X field, the greater the odds of early relapse.[17] The Weidner technique was soon applied to other human tumors, with comparable results—an increase in microvessel density also seemed to fore-shadow treatment failures in bladder, colon, lung, and prostate cancers. In the case of breast cancers, this innovative technique was sure to be—well, *controversial!* Karen Axelsson and other skeptical pathologists published a study based on paraffin specimens taken from 220 breast cancer patients treated at Boston's Massachusetts General Hospital. Dr. Axelsson's team found that microvessel counting had "an intrinsic variability that was unacceptably high." No two pathologists working independently were likely to achieve the same result, because of "the inescapable heterogeneity of vascularization within any tumor as well as the subjective processes of selection and counting required to score the tumor." In this study the scores recorded for microvessel density did not accurately predict either the rate of tumor recurrence or the probability of long-term survival: "Nodal status was the most powerful criterion." Axelsson et al argued that microvessel counting is "not yet a suitable assay for general application."[18]

We should no doubt anticipate further debates about this intriguing assay. No one would question either that the visual grading of tumor specimens tends to be somewhat subjective, with inevitable variations between individual pathologists, or that the proliferation of new blood vessels near a malignant tumor is an inauspicious finding.

Too Many Prognosticators?

Breast cancer pathology has come a long way. Back in the 1950s and 1960s all that patients and their physicians really expected from the pathology lab was a simplistic announcement stating whether "cancer" was present. These days we expect the lab to determine the histological subtype of breast cancer and, more importantly, to tell us how aggressive the particular tumor is likely to be. Our pathologists have made remarkable strides in distinguishing between the breast tumor which is merely a localized proliferation of abnormal cells, presumably curable by a modest excision, and the tumor which is rapidly becoming a deadly systemic malignancy. Substantial harm can be done to patients if this distinction is not made. We should therefore welcome any and all tests and assays designed to evaluate the metastatic potential of breast cancers. The problem is that, all of a sudden, there seem to be too many assays—as well as too many differences of opinion about their utility. In 1994 the *Journal of the National Cancer Institute* reported that no fewer than 58 prognostic assays were under investigation in breast malignancies.[19] Our cancer specialists face a daunting task just trying *to stay abreast* (pardon the pun!) of a burgeoning literature, and to evaluate the conflicting claims and counterclaims. Controversies flourish about which new indicator is truly "independent" (providing prognostic information not obtainable with more established assays), and about which new test gives the most "reproducible" results. The researchers involved naturally show exceptional enthusiasm for the assay upon which they happen to be working.

The tremendous ongoing research on prognostic indicators is commendable, but it has presented the author of this book with a small dilemma. Although all the new assays are performed in the pathology lab, any attempt to discuss them in Chapter Twelve would overload it with details. This chapter is intended only as a short introduction to the nuts and bolts of pathology—that is, to such basic matters as specimen preparation, microscopic analysis, and the classification of breast cancers by type. These newer assays are therefore being shifted to Chapter

Fourteen on "Staging," where there will be more room to discuss them comfortably. While **staging** reflects the results of tumor analysis, it has traditionally been used as a shorthand measurement of anatomical spread—Stage One signifying localized cancer, Stage Two regional (axillary spread), Stage Three advanced, and Stage Four metastatic (systemic). These old anatomical stages are still used, but nowadays they tend to get mentioned in the same breath with the results from the newest prognostic assays. That's another reason to combine staging and the new predictive factors in Chapter Fourteen; but since some of these assays are likely to be mentioned on a pathology report, they need to be briefly listed here.

The assays best established as independent and reproducible are those which test for the presence of **estrogen and progesterone receptors**. Breast cancer cells having large quantities of these hormone receptor proteins tend to be well-differentiated and slow-growing; they will usually respond to therapy with oral drugs (e.g., tamoxifen) which gently block the proliferative stimulus provided by the sex hormones. An assay intended to measure a tumor's growth rate can be profitably included on any pathology report. The results may be expressed as an **S-phase fraction**—that is, as the percentage of cells synthesizing DNA in preparation for mitosis. The higher the S-phase, the faster the tumor grows; this is a well-established prognostic factor. The relationship of **ploidy** to prognosis is less clearly defined. The term refers to the amount of DNA present in the cellular nuclei, with **diploid tumors** (normal or near-normal DNA quantities) being seen as less threatening than **aneuploid tumors** (excessive quantities of DNA). **Flow cytometry**, a computer-based assay which became popular in the 1980s, can yield measurements of both S-phase and ploidy.

Since the early 1990s pathology labs have been increasingly relying on immunohistochemical methods to perform all sorts of assays. As previously mentioned, "immunostaining" uses monoclonal antibodies which bind to proteins or other antigens in cells, thus giving us visible evidence of their presence. The reagent *Ki-67*, which stains a nuclear molecule involved in cell division, provides another way of estimating a tumor's growth rate. Immunohistochemical assays have also been useful in evaluating **gene activity**. We are particularly concerned to detect aberrant behavior by the tumor suppressor genes *p53* and *nm23*, and by the breast cancer oncogene HER-2/*neu*. The utility of gene assays remains under investigation. We are on firmer ground with the traditional indicators—viz., histological grade, nuclear morphology, and nodal status. The division of breast tumors into well-described histological subtypes also conveys an impression of solidity and long tradition. That enterprise began over a century ago, and it continues today.

DUCTAL CARCINOMAS
<u>Commonplace</u> <u>and</u> <u>Dangerous</u>

The most common type of breast malignancy is responsible for most of the morbidity and mortality. The designation **infiltrating ductal carcinoma** usefully summarizes both its origin and its behavior. It arises from the thin layer of epithelial cells which line the mammary gland's ductal system, and sooner or later it will infiltrate (invade) the surrounding tissues and lymphatic vessels. In the days before widespread mammography screening, perhaps 80% of all breast cancers diagnosed in American women were infiltrating ductal carcinomas, the remaining 20% being mostly lobular carcinomas or the better-prognosis variants of ductal cancer. Mammography has changed these percentages. In recent years perhaps 35% of diagnosed breast cancers have been **ductal carcinoma *in situ***, where the transformed cells are completely confined within the ducts. These lesions are not invasive and not immediately threatening, but they are regarded as the presumptive forerunners of all types of invasive ductal cancers. Ductal cells are much more prone to malignant transformation than lobular cells. While infiltrating ductal carcinomas can occur anywhere in the breast's ductal system, pathologists believe that most of these tumors arise from the **terminal ductal lobular unit**—that is, from the small ducts which drain the lobules.[20]

The term **adenocarcinoma** is sometimes used on pathology reports instead of "infiltrating ductal carcinoma." This word is not especially informative, since that prefix *adeno* simply denotes a glandular origin (from the Greek *aden*, "gland"). Pathologists use these two terms interchangeably; but when they wish to specify the garden variety of infiltrating ductal carcinoma, they will always append the initials **NOS** or **NST** to the diagnosis. The first abbreviation stands for **<u>Not</u> <u>Otherwise</u> <u>Specified</u>**, the second for **<u>No</u> <u>Special</u> <u>Type</u>**. These abbreviations are used to verify that the tumor in question cannot be classified as one of the better-prognosis variants of ductal cancer—which are the tubular, medullary, mucinous, and papillary carcinomas. We know from long experience that these histologically favorable subtypes generally begin with expansile growth patterns; they "push" the surrounding tissues outward rather than infiltrating them, and they are less prone to invade the lymphatic channels and spread throughout the body. In contrast, even small infiltrating ductal carcinomas, NOS or NST, must be regarded as potentially metastatic. This species is also quite familiar. Clinically, it

typically presents as that "hard painless lump" described in all those handout brochures from the American Cancer Society. A fibrotic reaction in the connective tissues (stroma) surrounding the tumor is so common and so anticipated that the pathology report may not even mention it, except for the addition of the three words "with productive fibrosis" right after the NOS or NST. If the tumor has been growing for some time, and the surrounding stroma has become so mineralized that it feels like a gritty, coarsely-textured rock, the term **scirrhous carcinoma** may be used (from the Greek *skirrhos*, "hard"). The mammographic image of a NOS tumor is similarly characteristic—it appears as that "stellate" or "spiculated" mass which sets off the alarm bells in the radiologist's office. Upon excisional biopsy, a largish tumor belonging to this species can often be recognized by "gross inspection"— that is, with the naked eye. The pathologists K. Kendall Pierson and Edward J. Wilkinson describe the visual appearance of a large specimen which has been cut into two halves: "The cut surface of the mass reveals the central radiating stellate tumor with chalky white or yellow streaks extending into the surrounding breast tissues. The tumor characteristically has a poorly defined visible border."[21] The self-evident infiltration and necrosis in this advanced tumor bespeak a poor prognosis. In all probability, a tumor like this has already metastasized; but we should not assume that all infiltrating ductal carcinomas are equal. They can exhibit a wide range of clinical presentations and subsequent behaviors; and of course, in their earliest stages they can be cured by adequate surgical excision.

The Better-Prognosis Variants

As invasive ductal carcinomas go, the best kind to have is a histological subtype known as **tubular carcinoma** or (as it is sometimes called) **well-differentiated carcinoma**. Historically, tubular carcinoma has been an infrequent diagnosis, representing only about two percent of breast cancer cases; but the reported incidence has been rising due to the tumor's detection by calcifications seen on mammograms. The distinctive feature of this subtype is its orderly architecture, easily discernible with low-power magnification. It forms tubules or duct-like structures which resemble those in the normal mammary gland, except that they seem haphazardly arranged or jumbled together. The tumor's constituent cells look almost normal—the nuclei are relatively small and regular, with only an occasional mitotic figure. As pathologists Pierson and Wilkinson point out, only "the absence of well-defined basement membranes" reliably distinguishes tubular carcinomas from benign proliferative disorders like sclerosing adenosis.[22]

Tubular cancers tend to be small, usually about one centimeter or so in diameter; and their clinical presentations and mammographic appearances are noticeably different from those we associate with infiltrating ductal carcinomas. R. Robinson Baker, a breast surgeon at the Johns Hopkins University Hospital, observes that "the majority of tubular cancers present as a well-circumscribed mass." Neither palpation nor mammography is likely to yield any findings suggestive of infiltration into the surrounding tissues. Dr. Baker adds that tubular cancers do not pull on the breast's ligaments: "Skin and nipple retraction are never seen." This subtype cannot be reliably diagnosed by fine-needle aspiration or core-needle biopsy, or on a frozen section. Any aspirated cells would probably seem deceptively benign; the distinction between this low-grade cancer and sclerosing adenosis is difficult to make using a core-needle specimen or on a frozen section. Dr. Baker assures us that "pure" tubular carcinomas are unlikely to metastasize and may be safely treated by wide excision (lumpectomy) alone, without any need for an axillary dissection, breast irradiation, or chemotherapy.[23] The problem is that tubular carcinomas do not always occur in their pure form. If a particular tumor contains a small infiltrative element, its behavior may actually be dictated by that minority element. A study of fifty patients with tubular carcinoma treated at Houston's M. D. Anderson Cancer Center suggests that while this variant may not represent an aggressive malignancy, it does have some potential for lymphatic dissemination. Fully 20% of the M. D. Anderson patients had evidence of axillary involvement, though no more than one or two nodes were positive in any individual.[24] Probably we would be wise to assume that the larger a tubular carcinoma grows, the more likely it is to develop infiltrative features and to invade the lymphatics.

Medullary cancers offer a study in contrasts, combining unfavorable cellular characteristics with an expansile growth pattern. About five percent of diagnosed breast cancers can be classified as medullary; patients with this variant tend to be younger than average, often in their late forties or early fifties. These tumors are relatively fast-growing and may become quite large; but unlike infiltrating ductal carcinomas, they are well-circumscribed. A medullary cancer will be quickly encapsulated by a layer of fibrotic overgrowth, just like a benign fibroadenoma. While the cancer tends to be a little softer and slightly less mobile than a fibroadenoma, these two lesions can be easily confused, both on palpation and on mammography. Microscopic analysis makes the distinction:

medullary cancers reveal a loss of structural organization as well as constituent cells whose nuclei are enlarged, hyperchromatic, and pleomorphic. The pathologist often detects numerous mitoses, indicative of a rapid rate of cellular division. Edwin R. Fisher and his NSABP colleagues caution that this variant has the potential to develop into an aggressive malignancy, citing unpropitious findings including "its high [poor] nuclear and histologic grades, frequent lack of estrogen and progesterone receptors, and tumor necrosis."[25] The redeeming feature of "pure" or typical medullary tumors is their well-defined, non-infiltrative border. Those subtle genetic alterations which allow cancer cells to readily infiltrate adjacent tissues and lymphatic vessels have not yet occurred, and therefore the odds of positive axillary nodes are considerably lower than with infiltrating ductal carcinomas. But a medullary tumor whose border reveals areas of infiltration would be termed "atypical," and it could conceivably behave like an infiltrating ductal carcinoma. Medullary breast cancers cannot be adequately diagnosed by fine-needle aspiration or by core-needle biopsy; any specimen produced by an excisional biopsy needs to be thoroughly reviewed on permanent sections. In a few instances, a second opinion on the slides may be helpful. In her book *My Breast* Joyce Wadler provides an enlightening account of a medullary tumor whose classification was debated by half-a-dozen pathologists in New York City. A year after Ms. Wadler's diagnosis, the verdict on her medullary tumor was changed from "typical" to "atypical," with an accompanying recommendation for some much-delayed chemotherapy.[26] Anyone who thinks that breast cancer pathology is always an exact science should read Ms. Wadler's memoir for an eye-opener.

Mucinous carcinomas, also known as "colloid" or "gelatinous" carcinomas, are slow-growing tumors which mainly afflict elderly women and represent about three percent of breast cancer cases. The several names reflect the fact that the individual cancer cells secrete large quantities of mucin, giving this subtype a glistening or gelatinous appearance both grossly and microscopically. These tumors tend to present as large well-circumscribed masses which feel soft to the touch. Unlike tubular and medullary cancers, the mucinous variant can be diagnosed with fine-needle aspiration—the abundant mucin in and around the aspirated cells is a give-away.[27] According to pathologist Carlos M. Perez-Mesa of the Roswell Park Cancer Institute in Buffalo, "the tumor cells are uniform and hyperchromatic, with regular nuclei but rare nucleoli. The interface between tumor and neighboring tissue is characteristically sharp." The combination of good nuclear grade and a pushing, sharply defined border bespeaks a good prognosis. Additional assays typically reveal that the tumor cells are estrogen receptor-positive and diploid (with normal or near-normal levels of DNA). Dr. Perez-Mesa observes that no more than 15% of those patients with "pure" mucinous carcinomas will be found to have positive axillary nodes, and that even in node-positive cases distant metastases may not occur for a decade or two, owing to this tumor's sluggish growth rate.[28] Those patients with disseminated tumors, usually ranging in age from 60 to 80 at diagnosis, are probably more likely to die from causes other than cancer.

As with the other better-prognosis variants, the outlook for mucinous tumors changes considerably when they are not pure or typical, but have histological features reminiscent of infiltrating ductal carcinomas. The larger the infiltrative element, the more questionable the prognosis. "When reporting mucinous carcinomas," Perez-Mesa cautions, "pathologists are obliged to state the proportion of pure and mixed types because of the different behavior of the two." Previous studies have found positive axillary nodes in 33% to 46% of the mixed or atypical tumors.[29] This rate of axillary involvement is not appreciably different from that which we would expect with infiltrating ductal carcinomas.

Papillary carcinomas also occur principally in older postmenopausal women, mostly after age 60. At least some of these tumors may result from the malignant transformation of benign papillomas, those slender fingerlike projections of epithelial cells which often arise in the milk ducts. In any event, it is clear that papillary carcinomas begin as tiny stalks of malignant cells growing from the sides of ducts or (less frequently) from the walls of cysts. These tumors may remain confined to the involved ducts or cysts for a long time. Once they invade the surrounding tissues, they typically display an expansile growth pattern like the medullary and mucinous variants. Paul Peter Rosen of Memorial Sloan-Kettering observes that "the majority of papillary carcinomas are estrogen receptor-rich, and they generally have a low growth rate." Even when invasive, these tumors "have a relatively low frequency of axillary nodal metastases."[30]

The pathologist may need to take pains to distinguish a papillary carcinoma from the commonplace papilloma. Both lesions often develop in the large ducts beneath the nipple, and both may present with a bloody or bloodstained nipple discharge. But a papillary carcinoma is far more likely to produce a palpable mass, especially as it progresses beyond the confines of the duct. Neither mammography nor fine-needle aspiration is consistently useful in distinguishing between benign and malignant papillary lesions;

microscopic examination of a biopsy specimen (permanent section) establishes the diagnosis. Papillary carcinomas constitute about one or two percent of the breast cancers currently being diagnosed. When discovered early, they can be treated by local excision.

Two Unusual Presentations

Textbook writers often convey the erroneous impression that Paget's disease and inflammatory carcinoma are distinct histological subtypes of breast cancer. Both these conditions are more accurately described as unusual presentations of the garden variety (infiltrating ductal carcinoma NOS). With both a breast malignancy will first manifest itself not by that familiar lump, but by what seems to be no more than a superficial irritation or inflammation of the nipple or skin. And with both the diagnosis of cancer is almost inevitably delayed, because the presenting symptoms are clinically indistinguishable from those of a commonplace nipple eczema or of a mastitis (inflammation) caused by bacterial infection.

The term **Paget's disease** does not refer to a specific histological diagnosis. It's simply a cover-all expression for any breast malignancy which presents on the nipple-areola complex, echoing an 1874 description by James Paget. This versatile English doctor observed that certain superficial changes on or around the nipple were apt to be followed a year or two later by an obvious malignant tumor in the underlying breast. Paget's disease typically begins with eczema-like alterations affecting the nipple—these may be either dry and scaly, or moist, raw, and reddish. The affected area soon grows larger, spreading outward to involve the entire areola and then the surrounding skin. Eventually the nipple will become ulcerated, or it will begin to flatten out. Either circumstance tends to alert the patient that her condition is no ordinary skin disorder. Paget's disease is relatively uncommon. A survey of 9,000 breast cancer cases in Philadelphia found that only 1.5% had the characteristic nipple-areola presentation. Paget's may also be seen in men, at roughly the same percentage rate. A survey of 138 men with breast cancer turned up two cases (a 1.45% rate) with Pagetoid symptoms.[31]

On rare occasions a breast malignancy might actually originate in the nipple-areola complex. But we now know that the overwhelming majority of Paget's cases are caused by cancers which develop in the underlying ductal system, and then spread upward through one or more nipple orifices. Diagnosis is easy. Under a microscope a skin biopsy specimen would reveal the cells typical of Paget's—pale-staining cells with abundant cytoplasms, enlarged nuclei, and prominent nucleoli.[32] The patient's long-term prognosis has less to do with the extent of the skin erosion than with the aggressiveness of the underlying malignancy. Patients whose cutaneous symptoms are accompanied by a palpable subareolar mass generally face a more problematic outlook. Biopsy of such a mass usually detects an infiltrating ductal carcinoma; but when both palpation and mammograms have failed to locate an underlying mass, breast biopsies will reveal ductal carcinoma *in situ* in two cases out of three. Of course, purely *in situ* breast cancers can always be cured by adequate surgery. Robert T. Osteen, a surgeon at the Harvard Medical School, gives us some pertinent statistics based on a follow-up of 890 women diagnosed with Paget's disease. In this group 54% of the patients presented with a palpable mass, and 46% without a mass. Those patients with a mass had a five-year survival rate of only 38%, while those without achieved an 88% rate.[33]

Inflammatory carcinomas may also present in the nipple area, as well as anywhere else on the surface of the breast; but these cases are not likely to be confused with Paget's disease, which mimics a persistent eczema and spreads slowly over a period of months or years. The inflammatory designation is reserved for those cases which mimic fairly acute infections and develop over a period of a few weeks. Every textbook on breast cancer lists the principal clinical symptoms—erythema (redness), sensations of localized warmth, and subcutaneous edema (fluid retention) which eventually gives the overlying skin a pitted appearance like an orange—the so-called *peau d'orange sign*. The affected breast may also change in size and texture, growing smaller and firmer, or (more frequently) larger and tenderer. These symptoms may vary from case to case; only microscopic analysis can establish the diagnosis. A full-thickness skin biopsy will lead to the startling finding which both identifies and characterizes inflammatory breast cancer—the lymphatic vessels in the dermis (the inner layer of the skin) are clogged up with poorly differentiated cancer cells which have impeded fluid drainage and have thus produced the symptoms of erythema, warmth, and edema. This is lymphatic invasion with a vengeance! Unfortunately, by the time the dermal lymphatics have been so thoroughly invaded, malignant cells will have inevitably spread throughout the affected breast as well as to the axillary lymph nodes and to other anatomical locations. Sandra M. Swain and Marc E. Lippman, oncologists at the Georgetown University Medical Center, remind us that "inflammatory breast carcinoma is a systemic disease at diagnosis." The malignancy responsible for the striking skin alterations almost always proves to be a ductal carcinoma NOS, which is (needless to say) extremely infiltrative. Additional diagnostic assays are hardly necessary—they would be sure to reveal that the tumor cells have poor nuclear grade and a high S-phase fraction, and are estrogen and progesterone receptor-negative. Inflammatory presentations occur only in about one percent of the breast cancer cases diagnosed in the United States. Unfortunately, the women afflicted tend to be younger than other patients, and thus stand to have their lives shortened by several decades. According to Swain and Lippman, surveys of these patients have reported "mean ages ranging from 45 to 54 years."[34]

An underlying mass may—or may not—be detected in cases of inflammatory breast cancer. Neither excision of a mass nor amputation of the breast has been shown to extend patient survival. The initial treatment consists of rigorous intravenous chemotherapy; this often induces prolonged remissions, because the rapidly multiplying tumor cells tend to be susceptible to cytotoxic drugs. Mastectomy or radiation therapy might be performed afterwards, either to prevent local recurrences in the breast or to treat those which have already occurred.

In cases of Paget's disease, mastectomy is usually the surgical treatment of choice. The nipple and the areola almost always need to be removed for tumor control, creating such a large cosmetic defect that breast preservation becomes a less attractive option. Dr. Osteen recommends mastectomy for Paget's patients with "diffuse *in situ* or invasive cancer" in the affected breast. But he believes that an attempt at breast preservation—excision only of the nipple-areola complex and the affected underlying ducts—might be considered for "patients with a small subareolar cancer and with an otherwise negative mammogram and physical examination."[35]

Infiltrating Lobular Carcinomas

About five to ten percent of invasive breast cancers are classified as **infiltrating lobular carcinomas**; they arise from the epithelial cells lining the lobules rather than from those which line the milk ducts. Like other breast cancers, lobular carcinomas are most frequently diagnosed in postmenopausal women in their late fifties or early sixties. But these tumors are subtly different from infiltrating ductal carcinomas both in their initial symptoms and in their subsequent biological behavior. Malignant lobular cells are easy to recognize under the microscope. Small round cells with prominent but relatively uniform nuclei constitute the hallmark of lobular carcinogenesis—the telltale nuclei are decidedly hyperchromatic but only mildly pleomorphic, with infrequent mitoses.[36] Invasive lobular carcinomas are assumed to have developed from lobular carcinoma *in situ*, a jumbled proliferation of cells which is not exactly cancer, but certainly an atypical hyperplasia indicative of genetic instability and a significantly increased risk of malignant transformation. The abnormal cells look alike in both infiltrating and *in situ* lobular lesions.

When lobular tumors invade the surrounding stroma, they tend to reveal characteristic patterns of infiltration which are remarkably orderly. Paul Peter Rosen of Memorial Sloan-Kettering describes the two principal patterns as "Indian-file" and "targetoid." In the first those distinctive malignant cells seem to march into the surrounding tissues in straight columns, one cell behind another, Indian-file. In the second the invading cells seem to grow in concentric circles around the nearby ducts and lobules. These curving columns of cells are so pronounced and so regular that they resemble those dark lines which circle the bull's-eyes on archery and marksmanship targets. But Dr. Rosen cautions us that lobular tumors sometimes follow other, less regular patterns of infiltration.[37]

The clinical presentations of infiltrating lobular carcinomas are less obvious than the symptoms we associate with infiltrating ductal carcinomas. As a consequence, these tumors often grow to considerable sizes before they are detected and diagnosed. Lobular carcinomas do not normally present as dominant masses with irregular borders— that is, as those hard lumps which give us the stellate or spiculated images on mammograms. Just as their infiltration of surrounding tissues tends to be subtle and diffuse, so is the stromal reaction they elicit similarly subtle and diffuse. Palpation of an affected breast typically discovers an area of vague induration (thickening) or nodularity—in short, the sort of thing that might lead one to suspect fibrocystic lumpiness rather than cancer. Mammography is also less effective in detecting lobular carcinomas. Dr. Perez-Mesa points out that these tumors usually lack discernible margination and that "calcifications frequently are not present."[38] Ductal symptoms like nipple discharge or Paget's disease do not occur with lobular carcinogenesis. These tumors are also less likely to produce dimpling (retraction of breast contour) or discoloration on the overlying skin. Even the gross specimens of lobular carcinomas can look very different from those of other tumor types. Dr. Rosen observes that "the tumor tissue may not be visibly abnormal.[39]

Our knowledge of the behavior of lobular carcinomas has been inferred from miscellaneous studies lacking in rigorous methodology. We do know that lobular tumors are about twice as likely as ductal carcinomas to eventually prove **multifocal** (with several malignant foci appearing in the same breast) as well as **bilateral** (with cancer also arising in the opposite breast).[40] The larger size of lobular carcinomas at diagnosis, and their greater tendency to be multifocal and bilateral, makes presurgical screening and counseling highly advisable for those patients desiring breast preservation (lumpectomy). A study done at the H. Lee Moffitt Cancer Center of the University of South Florida (Tampa) found that lumpectomies planned for lobular patients sometimes had to be converted into mastectomies once the surgery was underway. In these cases the preoperative mammograms did not reveal the full extent of tumor involvement; and the surgical team discovered intraoperatively that they could not obtain tumor-free margins, or that they would need to remove so much tissue that the cosmetic outcome would be unacceptable.[41]

As with other epithelial breast cancers, the long-term prognosis with infiltrating lobular carcinomas depends largely on the degree of lymphatic tumor dissemination, which is best demonstrated by the number of positive axillary nodes. But disseminated lobular tumors usually behave less aggressively than comparable ductal carcinomas which have also spread beyond the confines of the breast. The favorable short-term prognosis for most lobular carcinomas is no doubt due to the good prognostic features of their constituent cells. These cells have lower mitotic rates than those seen in ductal carcinomas, reveal good nuclear grade, and are much more likely to be positive for estrogen and progesterone receptors. According to Perez-Mesa, "estrogen receptor positivity has been noted in as many as 92% of infiltrating lobular carcinomas."[42] Jean F. Simpson and David L. Page observe that "women with the pure, classical type of invasive lobular carcinoma have an excellent short-term prognosis, with about 90% surviving for ten years, almost without regard to stage." For node-positive patients, however, "treatment failure is frequent after that time."[43]

Metastases from systemic lobular carcinomas may sometimes spring up in organs which are left untouched by systemic ductal carcinomas. The lobular species frequently metastasizes to the stomach and other locations in the gastrointestinal tract; ductal carcinomas almost never do so.[44]

Rare Invasive Cancers

May the author take a moment to review the preceding paragraphs and place them in perspective? So far we have covered the principal varieties of invasive breast cancer—namely, infiltrating ductal carcinomas NOS and the four better-prognosis ductal carcinomas (tubular, medullary, mucinous, papillary), as well as infiltrating lobular carcinomas. Probably 99% of invasive breast cancers with the potential to metastasize can ultimately be placed in one of these six categories. However, attentive readers of Chapter One should recall a broad statement (page 10) that there are "about thirty types" of pathologically distinguishable breast malignancies, and they will allow that the author needs to account for about two dozen additional varieties to avoid being caught in an apparent inconsistency. Well, naming two dozen additional types is not a problem; but taking the time to discuss them would be, sorely overloading readers with information that even breast specialists need to look up. All the remaining types are *great rarities*, which taken together amount to less than one percent of diagnosed breast malignancies. Physicians at large research-oriented cancer centers like Memorial Sloan-Kettering or Houston's M. D. Anderson sometimes write articles describing a few cases of this or that rare species, gathered from institutional records going back thirty or forty years. Like the six common varieties we've already discussed, most of these rarer breast cancers

arise from epithelial cells; and their names reflect this fact—for example, adenoid cystic carcinoma, apocrine carcinoma, endocrine carcinoma, metaplastic carcinoma, secretory carcinoma, and squamous cell carcinoma. These names are dropped into the text primarily to emphasize **Lesson One** ("breast cancer" is not a single entity but a broad spectrum of different processes), and to reinforce **Lesson Two** (a wise patient will confer with several specialists to discover what that vague diagnostic pronouncement really means in her case).

Not all breast cancers are carcinomas arising from the mammary gland. A tiny minority will turn out to be **sarcomas** arising from connective tissues. Pathologists have identified eight different types of sarcoma which can originate in the breast; but since all of them together account for considerably less than one-half of one percent of breast malignancies, readers wishing information on such rarities as liposarcomas or leiomyosarcomas must be referred to the big textbooks and large cancer centers. We should merely point out that breast sarcomas behave differently from the commonplace epithelial tumors and require different treatment strategies. Perhaps the most striking difference is that breast sarcomas spread hematogenously (through the bloodstream) rather than through the lymphatic system. Those time-honored surgical procedures intended to sample or remove the axillary lymph nodes serve little purpose in diagnosing and treating these malignancies, and they are usually omitted.

The only sarcoma encountered with any degree of frequency is **cystosarcoma phyllodes**, which poses a diagnostic enigma for breast cancer pathologists. This term should be reserved for phyllodes tumors with malignant characteristics. As mentioned in Chapter Eight, phyllodes tumors are first cousins to fibroadenomas—both species of neoplasm involve abnormal proliferation of the lobular epithelial cells and of the surrounding stromal (connective) cells. But phyllodes tumors are far more troublesome. Unlike fibroadenomas, they are not rigorously encased in a fibrous shell, and their growth is not self-limited. Even when clearly benign, these tumors can grow so large that they deform the breast; and if not fully excised, they are likely to recur. Malignant transformation is the greatest danger: the stromal component in a phyllodes tumor may occasionally evolve into an aggressive sarcoma. Consequently, all phyllodes tumors need to be carefully evaluated to assess their malignant potential. But predicting an individual patient's cancer risk is not easy. Neither a phyllodes tumor's size nor its growth rate is a reliable indicator of malignancy; the pathologist looks instead for signs of excessive cellularity and mitotic activity in the stromal component. If the stroma contains numerous atypical cells with hyperchromatic and pleomorphic nuclei, and if the tumor's border is infiltrative rather than expansile, then prudence would demand that a phyllodes tumor be regarded as malignant.[45]

Another species of sarcoma which can present in the breast is the **angiosarcoma**. Sometimes called a "hemangiosarcoma," this vascular tumor arises from the endothelial cells lining blood vessel walls. Breast angiosarcomas are extremely rare. Jeanne A. Petrek, a breast surgeon at Memorial Sloan-Kettering, observes that "about one hundred cases have been reported in the medical literature," including "two probable cases in men."[46] Yet angiosarcomas have attracted a lot of attention because of their unusual clinical course and their sometimes spectacular aggressiveness. In their worst form they can kill within several months after diagnosis, surpassing even inflammatory breast carcinomas in rapid lethality. A few angiosarcomas have a better prognosis. As with other malignancies, the histological features and cellular characteristics of the particular tumor dictate the probable outcome. Breast angiosarcomas typically present as a painless mass, but that is perhaps the only significant behavior they share with the commonplace mammary carcinomas.

The breast can also harbor various and sundry cancers which have nothing to do with the mammary gland and its surrounding connective tissues. **Skin cancers** can present on the breast's surface, both the ubiquitous basal cell carcinomas (pesky but curable) as well as the potentially lethal melanomas. **Metastatic tumors** deriving from malignancies in other organs can produce masses in the breast; occasionally these tumors will be discovered there before they are detected at their point of origin. Lung cancers are responsible for most of these extraneous metastases in the breast, although ovarian, renal (kidney), and stomach tumors have been implicated in a few cases. Metastatic tumors tend to present as small superficially-located lumps, mostly in the upper outer quadrant near the axilla. While microscopic analysis cannot always identify their point of origin, metastases are usually recognizable as such, because the malignant cells will be located outside the breast's ducts and lobules (the cells in these mammary structures being normal).

Lymphomas, principally of the non-Hodgkin's varieties, may cause symptoms in the breast. While these malignant proliferations of lymphocytes (white blood cells) cannot be classified as "solid tumors," they can form distinct masses anywhere in the lymphatic system (usually in the form of enlarged lymph nodes) and occasionally at other anatomical sites. Presentations in the breast are normally secondary manifestations of systemic lymphomas. Once in a blue moon, however, a non-Hodgkin's lymphoma will present solely as a rapidly growing breast mass, with no evidence of disease discernable elsewhere in the body. These rare cases are called **primary lymphomas of the breast**. In the years from 1949 to 1984, Memorial Sloan-Kettering treated only 53 patients with primary lymphoma of the breast; and M. D. Anderson recorded a mere ten cases in the years from 1944 to 1990. While treatment always begins with the surgical excision of the breast mass, it consists mainly of intravenous chemotherapy intended to combat occult systemic disease.[47]

The Dilemma of _In Situ_ Cancer

It is unrealistic to believe that normal cells can suddenly be transformed into malignant ones. We know that the solid tumors afflicting adults are typically many years, perhaps even several decades, in the making. Cells must divide, then divide again and again, dozens of times, before they have accumulated all those genetic errors which constitute malignancy. Our efforts to understand this process have focused largely on cervical and colonic cancers, because with these tumors we can see the step-by-step carcinogenetic changes as they occur. The surface of the uterine cervix is readily inspected with an instrument called a **colposcope** (from the Greek word for vagina, _kolpos_). And the lining of the sigmoid colon (the S-shaped lower portion) can be observed with a flexible **sigmoidoscope**. Tissue sampling both of the cervix and of the sigmoid colon is easy and precise. In the matter of cervical cancer, we can demonstrate how the abnormal cells we might detect on a Pap smear may eventually give rise to a superficial tumor, which would tend to become increasingly invasive. For colon cancer we have not only learned

how benign polyps can sometimes develop into infiltrating tumors, but we know the gene malfunctions which occur at each step in the carcinogenetic process. This knowledge has saved many lives. With both cervical and colonic malignancies, a timely surgical intervention can nip an emergent tumor in the bud, curing the disease without appreciably harming the patient.

In the case of breast cancers, we can postulate a step-by-step transformation more readily than we can demonstrate it. We have no "mammoscope" which would enable us to look inside the minuscule ducts and lobules of the mammary gland. And the accurate tissue sampling of breast lesions is usually far more difficult than the sampling of cervical or colonic abnormalities. Our imperfect knowledge of mammary carcinogenesis derives largely from the pathological analysis of nonpalpable _in situ_ cancers, which have in the past been discovered fortuitously, mostly as incidental findings after exploratory biopsies for symptomatic benign lesions or after mastectomies for invasive tumors. The Latin term _in situ_ means "in place." As used in breast cancer pathology reports, it signifies that the transformed cells remain confined within the ducts or lobules, and that the basement membranes separating them from the surrounding tissues (stroma) are still intact. These _in situ_ cells may exhibit considerable powers of proliferation, expanding the girth of ducts or lobules with their growing numbers, or spreading sideways to fill up several interconnected groups of ducts or lobules. But they usually do not form palpable masses, because the particular genetic mutations which impart an ability to dissolve the basement membranes and create havoc in the stroma have yet to occur.

Pathologists have long assumed that _in situ_ breast cancers give rise to the infiltrating ductal and lobular carcinomas. Microscopic examinations of invasive tumors often reveal foci of *in situ* cells right alongside the infiltrative portions—presumably, the malignant cells invading the stroma began as *in situ* cells, but later acquired an invasive potential through an additional mutation or two. Prior to the 1980s, however, nobody really knew anything about the natural history of *in situ* breast cancers. How frequently did these lesions occur? Did they always progress to become invasive tumors, and if so, how long did this process take? Back in the 1950s and 1960s, when an occult *in situ* cancer chanced to be discovered during a biopsy performed for a benign condition, the patient was subjected to radical mastectomy, that sweeping amputation removing the breast, the chest muscles, and all the lymph nodes in the axilla. Of course, this treatment deprived physicians of any opportunity to observe and record the progression of *in situ* lesions. It was also barbaric and unenlightened, sort of like amputating your foot to cure an ingrown toenail. Today we know that purely *in situ* breast cancers never involve the chest muscles or spread to the axillary lymph nodes. Even an *in situ* cancer involving large areas of the mammary gland can be treated by simple mastectomy (removal of the breast alone), with a virtual certainty of cure. Unless we suspect that a sizable *in situ* lesion could contain foci of occult infiltration, there is no need to sample any axillary nodes.

In recent years *in situ* breast cancers have come under scrutiny because of the growing numbers of them being discovered by screening mammography and because of the uncertainty regarding their optimal treatment. Given the fact that many invasive cancers are currently treated with breast-conserving surgery (lumpectomy), it seems unreasonable to recommend mastectomy for small noninvasive cancers. But there remain unresolved issues about our strategies for breast preservation. What are the recurrence rates after local excision of *in situ* cancers?

Are some types of *in situ* cancer more prone to recur than others? How wide a margin of normal tissue should be excised? Should the involved breast be irradiated after surgery? As *in situ* breast cancer became a routine diagnosis instead of an occasional finding, these issues seemed likely to affect the health and financial security of more and more women. In 1996 the San Francisco pathologist Michael D. Lagios estimated that ductal carcinoma *in situ* accounted for 35% of the breast cancers being diagnosed by "institutions effectively using mammography."[48] Fortunately, we now recognize that some types of *in situ* breast cancer are more dangerous than others and thus may warrant more aggressive therapies. A fundamental distinction has been made between ductal carcinoma *in situ* and lobular carcinoma *in situ*. The two species are separate entities and behave differently. *In situ* ductal cells may spill into the lobules, and *in situ* lobular cells can spread into the ducts; but pathologists have no trouble in telling the two species apart, regardless of where they might be found.

Ductal Carcinoma *In Situ*

David L. Page and William D. Dupont of Vanderbilt University have observed that "ductal carcinoma *in situ* should be considered an intrinsically precancerous lesion because of its regular association with recurrence at the site of its initial diagnosis."[49] Whenever we do an excisional biopsy for a focus of ductal carcinoma *in situ* (DCIS), and then years later discover an infiltrating ductal carcinoma in the affected breast, we usually find that the invasive cancer has developed right at the spot of the original biopsy, or very close to it. We may therefore reasonably conclude that DCIS tends to begin as a focal lesion—at a single spot in the breast rather than at multiple locations—and that it tends to progress toward invasive cancer. Any recurrence after an initial excision, whether of DCIS or of infiltrating carcinoma, would probably be due to DCIS cells which were inadvertently left behind.

Ductal carcinoma *in situ* represents a much bigger problem than lobular carcinoma *in situ*. The former species is encountered far more often, being regularly discovered through the tiny calcifications which show up on mammograms. In contrast, the lobular species seldom generates calcifications. We assume that DCIS gives rise to a large majority of invasive breast cancers, but not all cases of DCIS are equally risky. Pathologists now distinguish between several subtypes of DCIS, each of which carries a different level of risk for infiltrative progression. Our DCIS classifications are made principally on the patterns of cellular growth seen in the ducts upon microscopic examination. Most pathologists cite four subtypes. The most prognosticly favorable is called **cribriform**. In cribriform DCIS the transformed cells are relatively uniform in size, and arranged in a so-called "sievelike pattern." They fill the duct involved, except that there are lots of "holes" (unoccupied spaces), just like a sieve. Stuart J. Schnitt, a pathologist at the Harvard Medical School, points out that "the cells composing this type are generally small to medium sized, and the nuclei are uniformly hyperchromatic. Mitoses are relatively infrequent."[50] Good nuclear grade and low proliferative rates characterize this well-differentiated DCIS subtype. The variant called **micropapillary** also reveals smallish, more or less uniform cells, but this time they will be found growing in fingerlike or frondlike projections from the duct walls. Carlos M. Perez-Mesa observes that the cribriform and micropapillary patterns are frequently found mixed together in DCIS specimens. This circumstance and the fact

that both represent low-grade, well-differentiated lesions have led some authors to consider them as a single entity. Paul Peter Rosen believes that tubular carcinoma, the most differentiated of the invasive ductal malignancies, "invariably arises from an orderly micropapillary or cribriform intraductal carcinoma."[51]

The DCIS variant called **solid** has an easily recognizable growth pattern, but its cellular features are not always auspicious. In this subtype the malignant cells fill the entire duct; there are no sievelike holes (gaps) or tiny papillary projections. Sometimes these cells may be relatively small and uniform, with rounded nuclei of good grade. At other times they can be, as Perez-Mesa states, "pleomorphic cells with atypical nuclei (prominent nucleoli) and abnormal mitoses." Dr. Rosen points out that aggressive infiltrating carcinomas may evolve from unpropitious cases of solid DCIS.[52] But the real villain among DCIS lesions is called **comedo**. As used on pathology reports, this Latinate term indicates that the involved duct contains an area of central necrosis, which resembles a comedo (blackhead) when viewed under the microscope. We have already seen that central necrosis is an ominous sign for invasive tumors; with DCIS it indicates a strong likelihood of infiltrative progression. The intraductal necrosis may be so pronounced that it becomes grossly apparent (visible to the naked eye upon clinical examination). According to Dr. Schnitt, "cords of pasty material" may occasionally be "expressed from the involved ducts."[53] The individual cells in comedo DCIS tend to be large and pleomorphic, with irregular nuclei and frequent mitoses. Recent molecular analyses have suggested that comedo cells are far more prone than other DCIS cells to lack the metastasis suppressor gene *nm23* and to express the accelerative oncogene HER-2/*neu*. Writing in the *Journal of the*

"Cribriform"
Ductal Carcinoma *in situ*

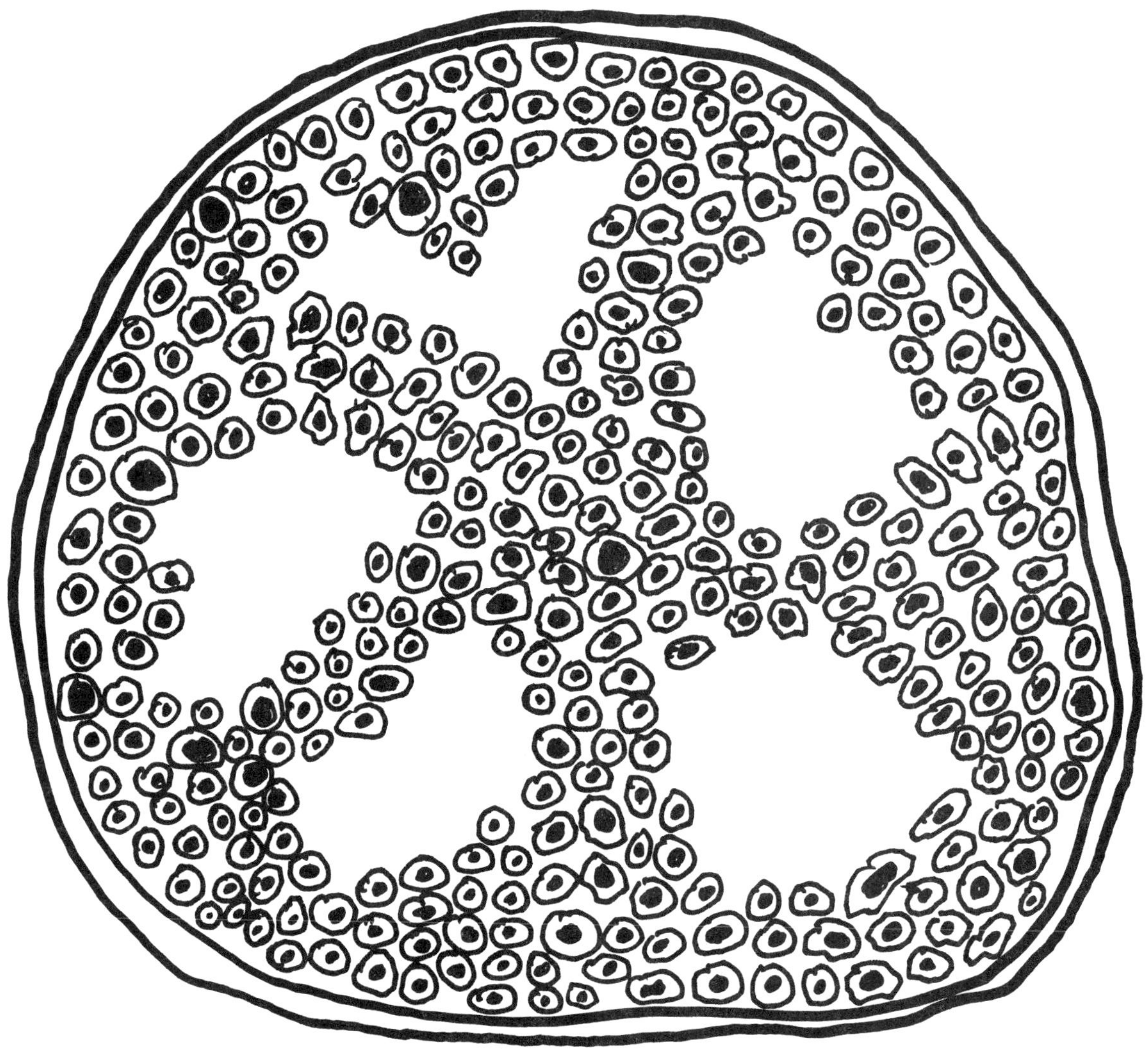

The cribriform or "sievelike" pattern of DCIS has been associated with a low risk of local recurrence after lumpectomy. In this variant the transformed cells are relatively uniform in size and reveal good nuclear grade. These cells do not completely fill the ductal lumen (passageway), which contains several sievelike "holes."

"Micropapillary"
Ductal Carcinoma *in situ*

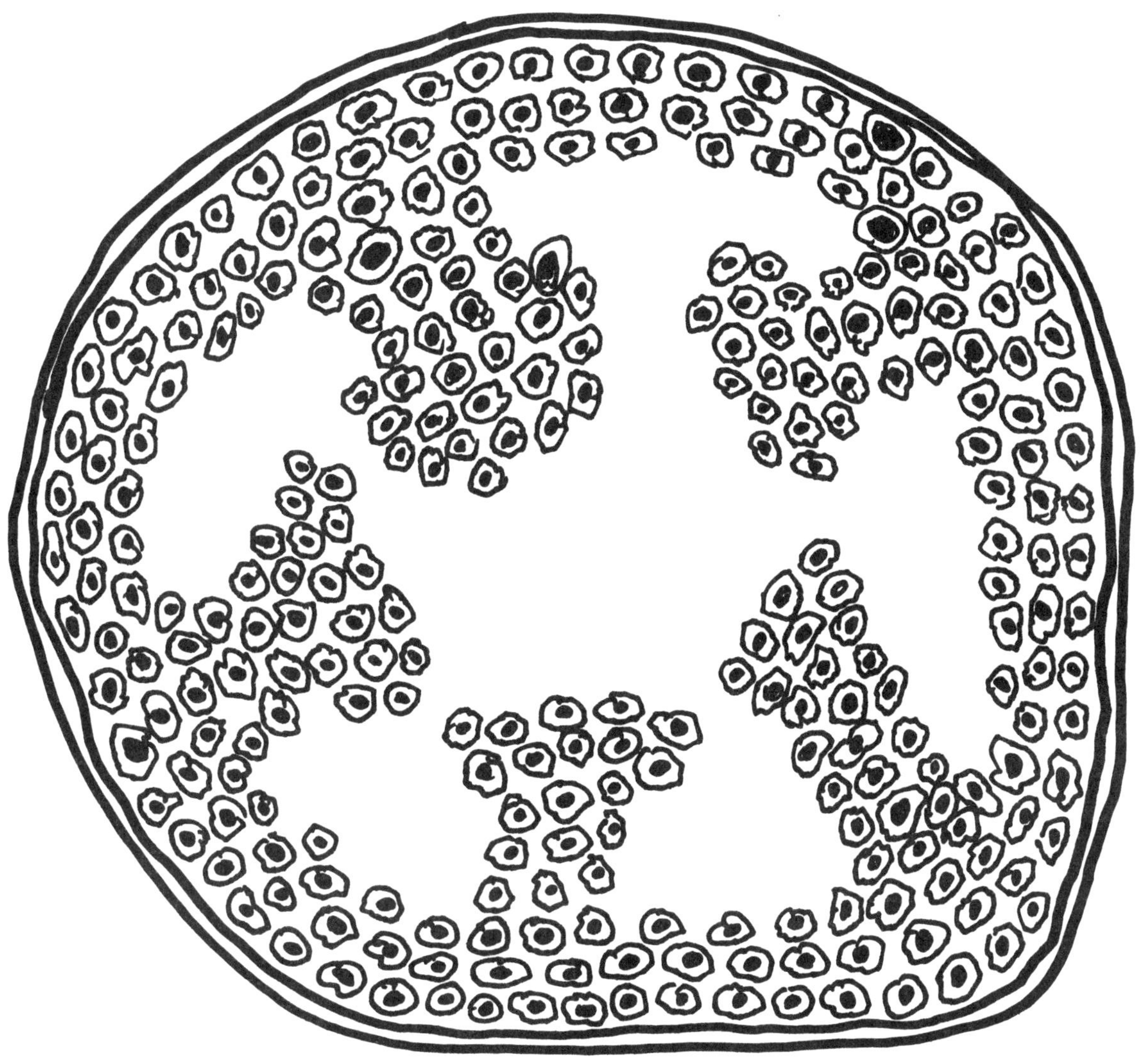

The micropapillary growth pattern tends to occur in the larger milk ducts. The fingerlike or frondlike projections from the ductal walls are composed of small to medium-sized cells with good nuclear grade. This DCIS variant is associated with a low risk for local recurrence after lumpectomy.

American Medical Association, the Chicago breast surgeon Monica Morrow observed that comedo DCIS lesions frequently have "high proliferative rates, absent estrogen receptors, abnormal DNA content, and abnormalities of oncogenes, as well as the ability to produce angiogenesis in the surrounding stroma."[54] Comedo DCIS would seem to be the direct predecessor of most infiltrating ductal carcinomas NOS. About the only good thing we can say about this variant is that it can be detected early by mammography and cured by adequate excision. The necrotic cores of comedo lesions typically contain calcifications which show up clearly on mammograms.

These four subtypes of DCIS should not be viewed as absolutes. Often two or more variants will be found in the same biopsy specimen, rendering a precise classification impossible. What is important is that we now recognize a crucial distinction among DCIS lesions. On the one hand, there are orderly formations of relatively uniform cells with low-grade (good-featured) nuclei; on the other, pleomorphic cells with bizarre nuclei may be jumbled together in the duct or huddled around a central necrotic core. Comedo-type necrosis is the most ominous feature. Many pathologists classify DCIS specimens simply as "comedo" or "noncomedo," an oversimplification which nonetheless serves to separate most of the gentle sheep (typically noncomedo) from the problematic goats.

Learning How to Treat DCIS

For decades proponents of mastectomy were accustomed to cite ductal carcinoma *in situ* as proof that breast cancer can be cured by surgery. This proposition is certainly true with DCIS—but is mastectomy necessary?

Since DCIS typically begins at a single spot, why not just excise that locus and leave the rest of the breast alone? These questions were first raised in the late 1970s, as the arguments for lumpectomy became louder, and as the clinical trials of mammographic screening began to turn up numerous DCIS cases. Unfortunately, nobody had any data upon which plausible answers might be based. In 1978 a group of pathologists at Memorial Sloan-Kettering dug deeply into that institution's voluminous records and retrieved a grand total of ten (10) cases of low-grade noncomedo DCIS which had been mistakenly diagnosed as "hyperplasia" or some other benign condition, and thus treated with excisional biopsy instead of mastectomy. The ten cases were ancient (from the years between 1945 and 1950), and neither the treatments nor the follow-up on patient outcomes possessed any degree of uniformity. This retrospective study was so lacking in methodology that it could not begin to address our questions, much less answer them; but the fact that it was featured in the *Journal of the American Medical Association* can serve to illustrate the state of medical knowledge at that time.[55]

Women with diagnosed DCIS who wish to keep their breasts owe a debt of gratitude to Michael D. Lagios and his colleagues in San Francisco (at the Children's Hospital and the University of California), who began to produce more convincing data in the early 1980s. Dr. Lagios and his team initially analyzed 53 mastectomy specimens, all the breasts having been amputated solely because of DCIS. Lagios et al sought to determine how frequently these lesions were multifocal (present at several different locations in the breast), and how often they were accompanied by foci of occult infiltration. Their findings strongly suggested that DCIS lesions ought to be treated while they are still small. None of the 29 lesions smaller than

"Solid"
Ductal Carcinoma *in situ*

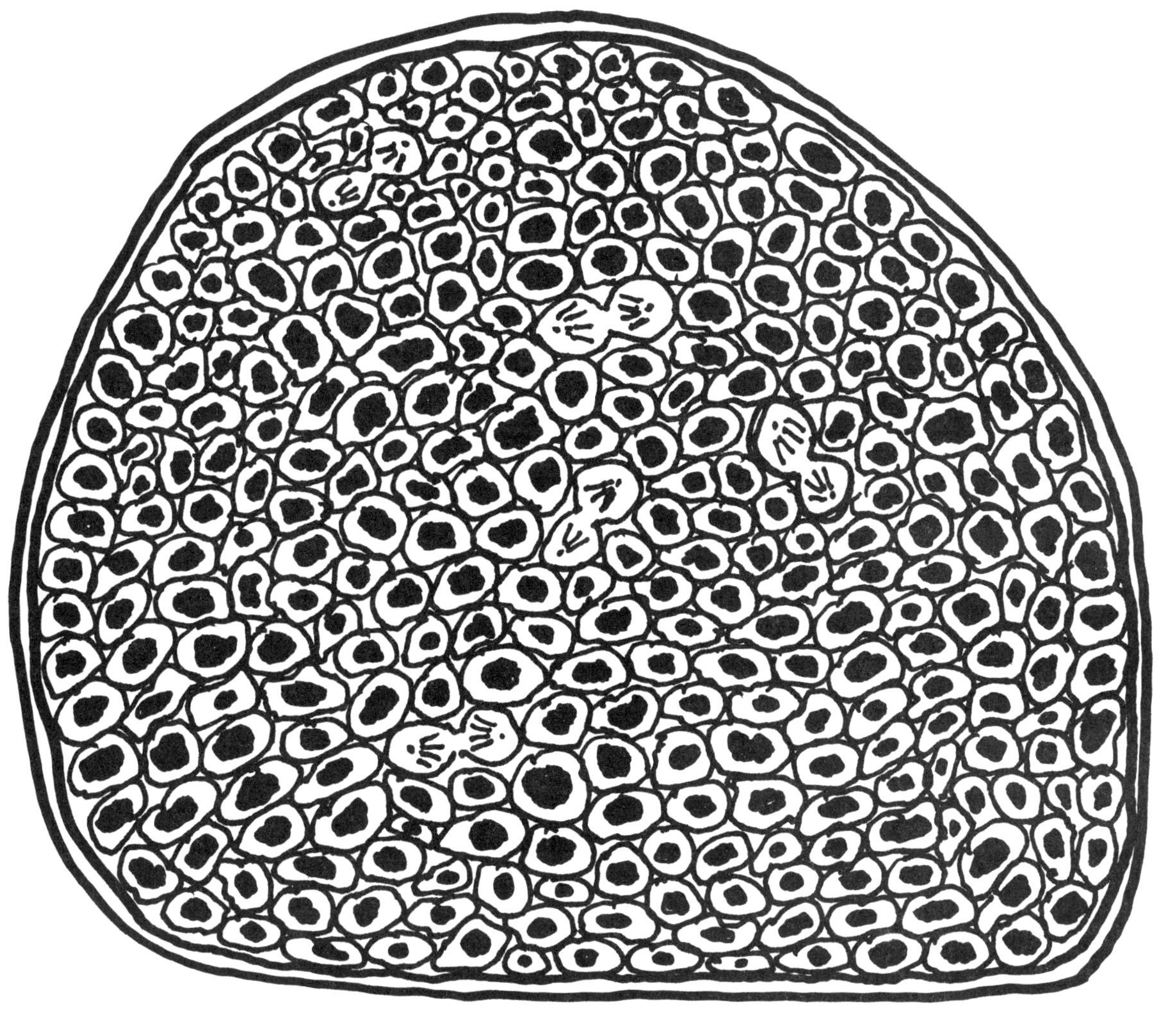

In the solid growth pattern of DCIS, the transformed cells completely obliterate the ductal lumen. The risk of local recurrence after lumpectomy will vary according to the characteristics of these cells. The above illustration depicts cells with **poor nuclear grade** (suggested by the large irregular nuclei) and a **high growth rate** (suggested by the "mitotic figures," cells in the process of division).

25 millimeters in extent (2.5 centimeters, about an inch and one-eighth) revealed any evidence of occult infiltration, and only four proved multifocal. But of the 24 lesions larger than 25 mm in extent, eleven showed "occult foci of invasion." Thirteen patients with these larger lesions had DCIS at other spots in the affected breast (multifocal disease), and six had nipple involvement. Most of the DCIS lesions over 25 mm were really large, 60 mm or more (about two and a half inches or more).[56]

For their next study Dr. Lagios and his colleagues selected 25 mm (2.5 cm) as an arbitrary boundary for conservative therapy: 79 patients with DCIS "of histologically confirmed extents of 25 mm or less" were treated by lumpectomy "without irradiation or axillary dissection." Lagios, a pathologist, worked closely with the collaborating surgeons and radiologists to ensure "adequacy of excision" (cancer-free margins) in all patients. After a follow-up averaging about four years, the San Francisco team reported that "eight patients (10.1%) have recurred locally in the immediate vicinity of the biopsy site." Four of the recurrences were just DCIS again, but the remaining four were small invasive cancers. When publishing their results in 1989, Lagios et al took pains to identify the type of DCIS lesion which was prone to recur after surgical excision. Seven of the eight patients experiencing local recurrence had DCIS lesions characterized by "high-grade nuclear morphology [poor nuclear grade] and comedo-type necrosis." Only one patient judged to have had "intermediate grade DCIS" experienced local recurrence, and then only at seven years after her lumpectomy. "None of the 33 patients with DCIS of micropapillary/non-necrotic cribriform type and low-grade nuclear morphology developed local recurrence."[57]

The ground-breaking studies of Lagios et al demonstrated the difficulty of verifying cancer-free margins with DCIS—the tumor borders are hard to see either with the naked eye or with a microscope. But these same studies provided reassuring evidence that only lesions with comedo features or poor nuclear grade were especially prone to early recurrence after lumpectomy. Several groups of East Coast researchers hastened to provide corroboration. Writing in the *New England Journal of Medicine*, Stuart J. Schnitt and other Harvard-affiliated physicians argued that breast preservation should be the initial strategy in DCIS treatment. Even if the tumor recurred locally after excision, there would still be "an excellent chance for salvage" (i.e., a strong probability that the cancer could still be cured with salvage therapy).[58] In the early 1990s two teams headed respectively by Gordon F. Schwartz of Philadelphia's Jefferson Medical College and by Lawrence J. Solin of the University of Pennsylvania published the results from small trials of breast preservation strategies for DCIS. Schwartz et al treated 70 women having nonpalpable DCIS lesions no larger than 25 mm with local excision alone. After a follow-up averaging four years, ten patients had experienced a recurrence "at the same site as the primary lesion." Nine of these recurring patients had "the comedo type of DCIS as the initial lesion."[59] Solin et al treated 172 women with small DCIS lesions by excision (lumpectomy) and "definitive breast irradiation." The addition of radiation therapy resulted in a lower rate of local recurrences than those reported by the Lagios and Schwartz teams, but it did not prevent them altogether. After a median follow-up of seven years, Solin et al had counted 16 local recurrences at or near the site of the original diagnosis. They concluded that a combination of comedo features and "nuclear grade three" (poor nuclear grade) strongly indicated those patients who were most likely to experience treatment failure. The projected

"Comedo"
Ductal Carcinoma *in situ*

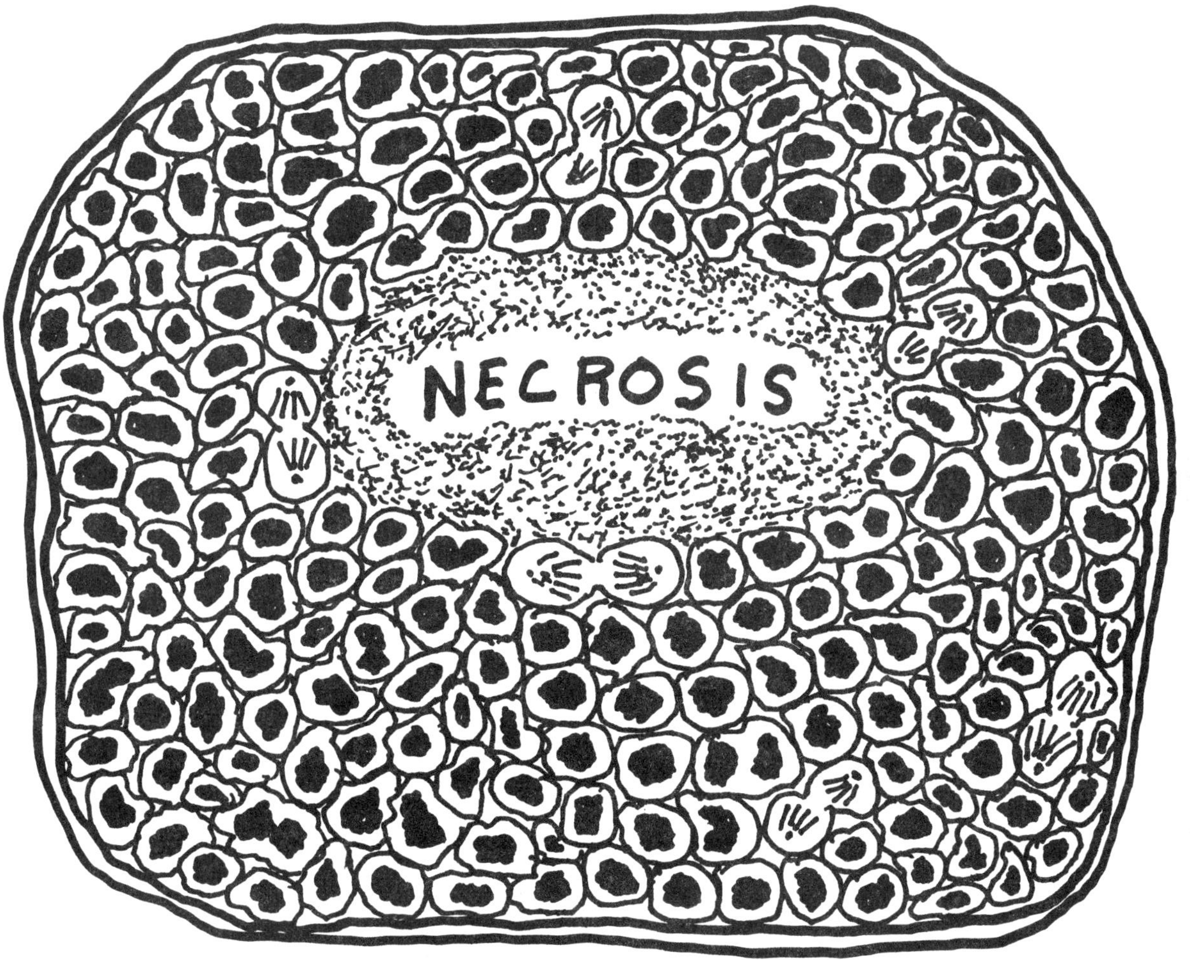

The comedo subtype of DCIS may evolve from poorly differentiated cases of solid DCIS. It is recognizable by an area of **central necrotic material**, suggestive of a high growth rate. Comedo cells are frequently enlarged and irregular, with poor nuclear grade. Tumor excision with wide disease-free margins and subsequent whole-breast irradiation help to lower the elevated risk both of local recurrence and of progression to invasive cancer.

rate of local recurrence at eight years was 20% for patients with this combination, but only 5% for those without it.[60]

The clinical trial whose results were most eagerly awaited by DCIS researchers was **Protocol B-17** conducted by the **National Surgical Adjuvant Breast and Bowel Project**. Begun in 1985, this NSABP trial randomly assigned 790 women with limited DCIS to undergo lumpectomy alone, or lumpectomy followed by five weeks of daily radiation therapy to the involved breast. The initial results of B-17, appearing as the lead article in the *New England Journal of Medicine* on June 3, 1993, received substantial coverage in American newspapers and TV newscasts. The five-year rate of recurrence in the involved breast was 16.4% in the 391 patients treated by lumpectomy alone, but only 7% in the 399 patients who had both lumpectomy and subsequent irradiation. The NSABP team concluded: "Breast irradiation after lumpectomy is more appropriate than lumpectomy alone for localized ductal carcinoma *in situ*."[61] Two years later Edwin R. Fisher, the NSABP's lead pathologist, and his colleagues published a more detailed analysis of the B-17 findings. They reported that two factors, "moderate/marked comedo necrosis" and "uncertain/involved lumpectomy margins," were "the only statistically significant independent predictors" of recurrence in the affected breast, both for those patients who were irradiated and for those who were not. But Fisher et al sang the praises of radiotherapy, suggesting that "gross margin assessment may be sufficient for local control if irradiation is administered."[62]

Unfortunately, a consensus about the need for adjuvant irradiation after DCIS lumpectomies was not to be had. David L. Page and Michael D. Lagios published a blistering critique of B-17, complaining that the trial did not adequately stratify DCIS lesions by subtype pattern, by nuclear grade, or by size, and implying that the NSABP did not do an optimal job of obtaining cancer-free margins. Page and Lagios argued "that the pathologic data collection and analysis in B-17 were focused insufficiently to identify cases that probably may be cured by planned excision without radiation." They observed that the results from earlier clinical trials indicate that "small, low-grade DCIS (determined by lack of comedo pattern necrosis and low nuclear grade primarily) is highly unlikely to recur within four-to-eight years of follow-up, even without radiation therapy." Edwin R. Fisher and his NSABP co-workers were not at all happy with this critique, which they described as "laced with a surfeit of academic prolix and nonsequiturs."[63]

Dr. Lagios has continued to promote minimal treatment for minimal lesions. In 1996 he pointed out that the size of DCIS lesions at diagnosis had dropped "from an average approximate 60 mm in those few detected by palpation to 10 mm or less in those detected mammographically." But Lagios and his San Francisco team will accept DCIS lesions larger than 25 mm for breast conservation surgery, assuming that both cancer-free margins and an acceptable cosmetic result can be obtained. Dr. Lagios cautions that an unaided visual inspection of margins is never appropriate: "Involvement of a margin in DCIS is like the disease— invisible and nonpalpable." The entire specimen should therefore be studied on permanent sections to rule out marginal involvement: "We recommend minimum margins of 5 mm as well as a careful review of preoperative and postoperative film mammograms and specimen radiograms." Lagios does not believe that breast irradiation is advisable for the smallest lesions: "It may be more appropriate to reserve radiation therapy for invasive recurrences, should they occur."[64]

Lobular Carcinoma *In Situ*

Unlike DCIS, lobular carcinoma *in situ* (LCIS) has largely remained an incidental finding—it's encountered by chance in a biopsy specimen obtained for some other reason. LCIS never presents as a palpable mass which we might detect during a physical examination, and only occasionally will it produce calcifications which might raise our suspicions on mammograms. This condition was first described in 1941 by two pathologists at Memorial Sloan-Kettering, Frank W. Foote, Jr., and Fred W. Stewart, who had observed a curious proliferation of lobular cells in several biopsy specimens. Their original description is still valid: "The compact, orderly arrangement of the epithelium of the normal lobule gives place to a decided looseness, a loss of cohesion. Layers do not multiply as layers, but cells are progressively displaced toward the lumina [centers] in a disorderly fashion, eventually obliterating the space."[65] No breast pathologist today is likely to mistake lobular carcinoma *in situ*: the lobules are jammed full of cells which, while definitely abnormal, display a monotonous regularity. In 1991, fifty years after Foote and Stewart, the Harvard pathologist Stuart J. Schnitt wrote that LCIS is characterized by "a solid proliferation of relatively small monomorphic cells," which distend and obliterate "the acinar units" (the milk-producing indentations). The nuclei of LCIS cells are slightly enlarged and mildly hyperchromatic, but not at all pleomorphic. As Dr. Schnitt points out, the nuclei tend to be uniform in size and "round-to-oval" in their shape.[66]

Is lobular carcinoma *in situ* really a form of preinvasive breast cancer? Foote

and Stewart both thought so, describing LCIS as "an extreme hazard" and recommending prompt mastectomy as "essential." Back in the 1950s the breast specialist C. D. Haagensen concluded that the striking regularity of LCIS cells and their nuclei argued against malignancy. He proposed that this condition be called **lobular neoplasia**, a term which would signify an abnormal "new growth" without specifying whether it might be benign or malignant. Haagensen did not perform mastectomies on his LCIS patients; he merely kept them under close observation. We now know that Haagensen was pretty much right—but neither the name he chose nor his watch-and-wait policy found many adherents. Carcinoma meant cancer, and there was only one thing to do for breast cancer. In 1969 a retrospective study of a few cases from Memorial Sloan-Kettering urged that LCIS "be treated by modified radical mastectomy."[67]

In recent decades we have learned much more about lobular carcinoma *in situ* and the ways in which it differs from ductal carcinoma *in situ*. LCIS is typically diagnosed in premenopausal women. According to Carlos M. Perez-Mesa, "80% to 89% of patients are younger than 55 years."[68] The fact that we find this lesion in younger women but not in older ones suggests that, in most cases, it regresses of its own accord with the postmenopausal involution of the lobules. Therefore the old assumption that LCIS necessarily evolves into invasive cancer is not warranted. LCIS also differs from DCIS in its pattern of occurrence in the breast. DCIS usually begins as a focal lesion—that is, as a single area of malignant transformation which has a greater or lesser potential for infiltrative progression. If we find DCIS at several different spots in the breast, we tend to assume that the malignant cells have spread through the ductal system from an initial focus. No one believes that

Lobular Carcinoma *in situ*

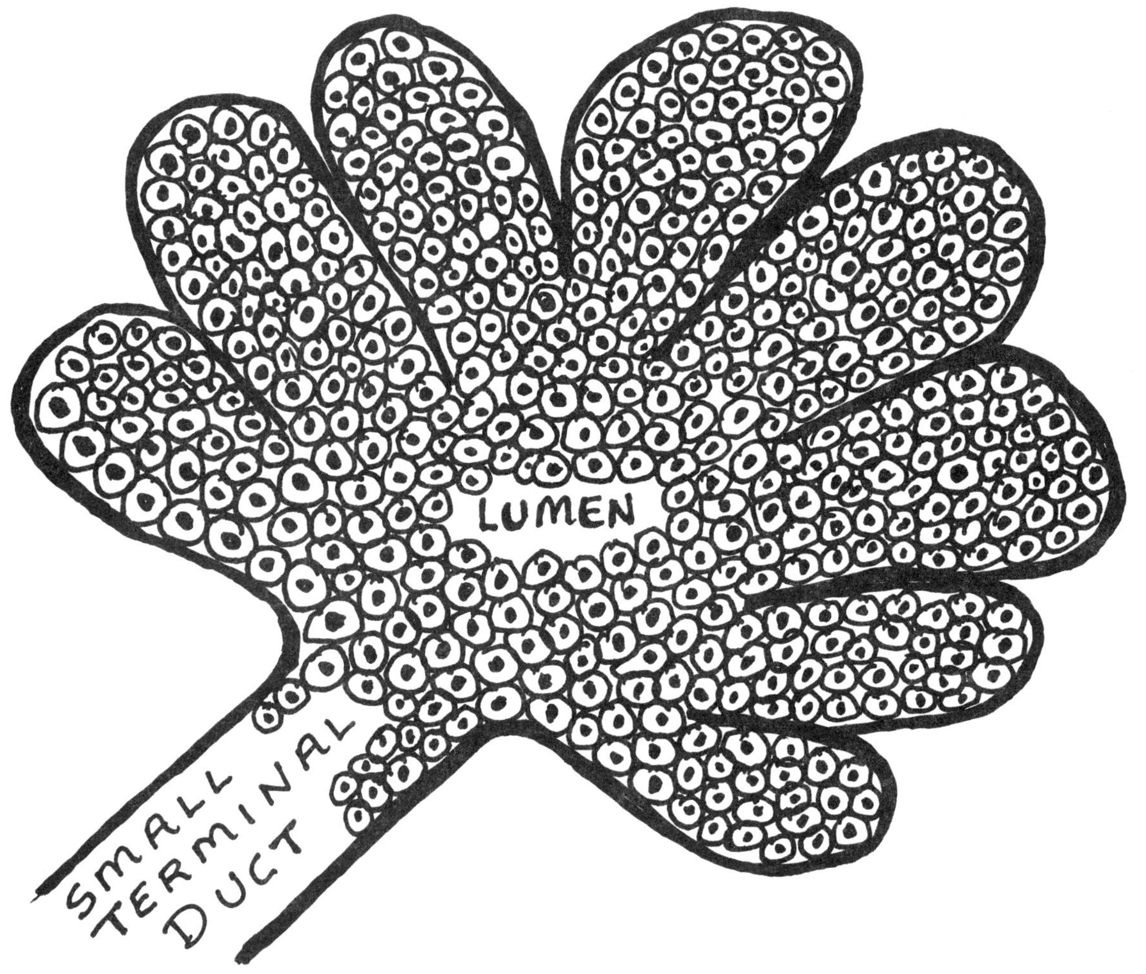

In lobular carcinoma *in situ* (LCIS), relatively uniform epithelial cells with slightly enlarged nuclei fill the affected lobules. This condition is **neoplastic**—that is, an abnormal proliferation of cells—without being malignant. While LCIS cells are not the immediate forerunner of invasive cancer, their presence is indicative of genetic instability affecting the entire mammary gland. Patients diagnosed with LCIS have an elevated risk for subsequent carcinogenesis, which could occur in either breast.

DCIS is inherently **multicentric**, a descriptive term we should reserve for those tumors which arise independently and more or less simultaneously in several different quadrants of an affected breast. In contrast, LCIS tends not only to be multicentric, but also to be bilateral (affecting both breasts). Nobody can claim to have exact figures, but the ballpark statistics cited in recent textbooks estimate that about 70% to 80% of LCIS cases are multicentric, and about 30% to 40% are bilateral.[69] The incidence of bilaterality could be much higher, since it's impossible to rule out LCIS bilaterality without amputating an apparently normal breast and then examining the whole of it microscopically.

Notwithstanding the fuzziness of our data, the multicentric and bilateral nature of LCIS has been generally acknowledged. It's clearly indicated not only by tissue analyses, but also by the way in which invasive cancers occur in the decades following this diagnosis. When a focus of LCIS is discovered in one breast and then years later the patient develops an infiltrating carcinoma, we typically find that the invasive tumor has developed *somewhere else than at the site of the original LCIS diagnosis.* Moreover, about half the time we will find that the tumor has developed *in the opposite breast.* The best data we have comes from C. D. Haagensen and his co-workers, who kept tabs on 295 LCIS patients for a mean follow-up period of 16.3 years. A total of 63 patients (21.4%) developed invasive cancers during follow-up, half of the tumors arising in the breast originally biopsied, and half arising in the opposite breast. Surprisingly, only 25% of the tumors in Haagensen's series proved to be infiltrating lobular carcinomas, the histological species we would

expect to arise from LCIS. The majority of these invasive cancers were infiltrating ductal carcinomas, which could not have arisen from the transformed lobular cells.[70]

If the neoplastic cells are not themselves the forerunners of invasive cancer, what is the significance of lobular carcinoma *in situ*? The best answer we have is that LCIS indicates genetic instability in the mammary gland generally, which may result in either ductal or lobular carcinogenesis, in either breast. Frank E. Gump of Columbia University's Breast Service points out that "the cells in and of themselves are not the danger," but they constitute "a powerful marker of increased risk" which is "bilateral."[71] This new understanding of LCIS biology has presented us with a treatment dilemma. Lumpectomy, now the most frequent treatment for DCIS lesions, has no role in LCIS therapy, since the disease must be assumed to be multicentric. But mastectomy of the breast in which LCIS was discovered would also be a half measure, since the disease must also be assumed to be bilateral. Thus we have only two logical management options—prolonged surveillance featuring frequent mammography and physical exams, or bilateral mastectomy. David W. Kinne, a breast surgeon at Memorial Sloan-Kettering, observes that many physicians consider bilateral mastectomy "excessively drastic given the level of risk."[72] But that risk is not negligible. Jean F. Simpson and David L. Page of Vanderbilt University estimate that the breast cancer risk for LCIS patients "approaches ten times that of comparable women in the general population," and that "20% to 25% will develop invasive cancer within about fifteen years after the discovery biopsy."[73]

Chapter Thirteen

Dealing with a Cancer Diagnosis

Telling a patient that he or she has cancer would seem to be one of the most difficult things that a physician may be called upon to do. The oncology journals are full of articles purporting to identify the best way of delivering this verdict. But the message is neither appropriate nor appreciated, regardless of how thoughtfully it may be conveyed. The physician may mention the diagnosis casually during a telephone conversation ("Yes, it's cancer alright"), or place an intimate arm around the patient's shoulder while saying "We'll get through this together!" These strategies are of little avail. Physicians shouldering this burden tend to feel like those fabled messengers of antiquity who trembled when they approached certain despotic kings in Asia Minor, knowing full well that these monarchs routinely killed any bearer of bad news.

Who can predict how a layperson will react to a cancer diagnosis? Some patients want complete disclosure of the facts; others would prefer to know as little as possible. A few adopt denial as a coping mechanism, pretending that the diagnosis must be in error. Others accept the diagnosis but get angry about it, pointlessly venting resentments toward their blameless physicians. Breast cancer patients would seem to have a fairly standardized reaction to the initial diagnosis. If we can draw a conclusion from all those personal memoirs of breast cancer struggles, it would be that these patients typically burst into tears at the very instant the horrid C-word is mentioned. If not obligatory, this reaction is quite common. Hester Hill Schnipper, an oncology social worker who herself developed breast cancer, has recorded a memorable instance: "After telling me that I had cancer, my surgeon wept. Then we wept together. And then she promised me that she would not cry into the incision at the next surgery."[1] Tears, whether coming conventionally from the patient or most unconventionally from the physician, no doubt serve a valuable cleansing function. They also act as a safety valve for pent-up emotions and escalating fears whose intensity can hardly be imagined by persons in excellent health. Tears are a perfectly normal response; but there's no point in carrying on a prolonged crying spell, for the simple reason that tears do not solve problems or make treatment decisions.

For many patients, weeping will prove to be an overwrought reaction. As we've seen in the preceding chapter, the term "breast cancer" always needs clarification before it really means anything. It is heterogeneously applied to cellular proliferations which do not necessarily require treatment (e.g., lobular carcinoma *in situ*), to low-grade malignancies which are curable with a wide excision, and to terribly aggressive tumors which are already disseminated at diagnosis. Every patient has the right to know what her diagnosis might mean or not mean, and to decide which of the several treatment strategies she will accept. A breast cancer diagnosis does not represent a medical emergency like a heart attack or a gunshot wound. In most cases the tumor will have been slowly growing for years before it becomes radiographically or clinically apparent. Postponing treatment for a few days or several weeks is unlikely to affect the outcome; there is no reason why any patient should feel rushed or pressured into accepting this or that therapy. But while breast cancer patients may have time to gather information about their individual cases, the quality of the information they receive depends heavily upon both the knowledgeability and the honesty of their physicians. One sophisticated patient in New York City has formulated a Golden Rule for these information transfers, which is worth repeating and keeping ever in mind: **"Be sure your doctors are absolutely straight with you."**[2]

Unfortunately, straight talk about a cancer diagnosis and an impartial judgment on prospective treatments remain desiderata which are more easily hypothesized than actually obtained. Back in the 1950s and 1960s a few American doctors felt it prudent to withhold all news of malignant findings from their patients. Even today some Japanese physicians refrain from divulging a cancer diagnosis, arguing that the patient should not be "burdened" with worries about the disease or with the dilemma of choosing between the different treatments. In the United States the only patients who are presently likely to encounter such a wall of stone-faced silence are children under the age of ten (they somehow manage to grasp the true state of affairs). But it is not unusual for adult patients to receive subtly evasive answers or euphemistic descriptions which have the effect of misrepresenting both the disease and the prognosis. Instead of answering a patient's legitimate query, the doctor might just gaze out the window—or give a confident reply which has no bearing on the question asked. Why do physicians intentionally convey disinformation in this fashion? Much of the blame has to be placed on the patients themselves, who are perceived as being woefully ignorant of oncology and prone to inappropriate emotional reactions. Physicians do not relish those weeping bouts or flare-ups of temper, which they regard (rightly so) as nonproductive, time-consuming, and psychologically draining. They are apt to be much more "straight" with those few patients who obviously know something about breast anatomy and cancer medicine. The best advice the author of this book has to offer is that during post-diagnosis consultations the patient should assume the posture of an attentive medical student. That is, she should appear as someone who is intellectually curious rather than as someone who is emotionally distraught. It would not hurt to reveal a basic knowledge of cancer biology and to display a fair amount of respect—but not awe—for the involved physicians and their respective medical specialties.

SECOND OPINIONS
A Lesson from Lumpectomy Rates

These days the diagnosis of breast cancer typically requires three medical specialists— a diagnostic radiologist, a surgeon, and a pathologist. The number of specialists called upon to *treat* breast cancer, especially if breast reconstruction is desired or complex chemotherapy regimens needed, may seem to increase exponentially. Diagnosis can be difficult enough, but the majority of the ongoing controversies and turf wars have always centered around proposed treatments. Doctors, like judges and politicians, readily fall into the habit of appearing self-confident and knowledgeable. Unfortunately, knowledge about breast cancer is relative, often with a large element of uncertainty. In most cases newly diagnosed patients thus stand to benefit from independent second opinions. It's not just that individual physicians can possess only incomplete knowledge, but that the treatment recommendations they make are likely to reflect the particular training they have received and to embody the particular procedures they customarily perform. Now that strong bias toward one's own medical specialty and therapeutic procedures is entirely understandable—it's powerfully reinforced by personal pride as well as by economic self-interest. But a problem arises when the treatment the doctor prefers and recommends is not the treatment that is most appropriate for the patient's type of breast cancer and for her personal situation. And this happens a lot more often than you might think.

There are oodles of controversies about the systemic therapies for breast cancer— whether this or that chemo regimen is most effective for this or that stage of disease, whether node-negative patients should take chemo at all, whether node-positive post-menopausal patients do better on chemo or on tamoxifen. But the most obvious and inevitable controversy concerns the primary surgical therapy. Should a breast tumor be initially treated by wide excision (lumpec-tomy) or by removal of the entire organ (mastectomy)? It is instructive to consider the varying percentages of American patients who have been treated by lumpectomy, because the relevant statistics show us how the therapies adopted may be determined by

specialty bias or by local custom rather than by any medical necessity. Historically, surgeons have favored the exclusively surgi-cal remedy (mastectomy), while radiation oncologists have worked hard to prove that lumpectomy followed by conscientious irradiation of the affected breast is equally effective. There are advantages and disad-vantages inherent in each approach, as well as indications and counterindications which may make one or the other far more suitable for select groups of patients. These matters will be covered more fully in subsequent chapters; for the present we're concerned simply with the unscientific bias which may creep into treatment recommendations. Over the decades there has been a mighty turf war centering on the primary surgical therapy. Financial reward is never mentioned by the combatants, but any nonpartisan observer cannot fail to notice this aspect. A mastec-tomy patient is entirely the surgeon's patient, but a woman who opts for lumpectomy and subsequent irradiation quickly becomes the radiotherapist's patient.

By the mid-1980s the results from large clinical trials comparing mastectomy and lumpectomy revealed that the long-term survival rates were equivalent for these two procedures. Lumpectomy patients were not at increased risk of dying from breast cancer. Therefore the main therapeutic advantage of mastectomy is that it removes the risk of a local recurrence within the affected breast (this is something lumpectomy patients always need to watch out for). In 1990 the Consensus Development Conference spon-sored by the National Institutes of Health (NIH) concluded that "breast conservation treatment is an appropriate method of pri-mary therapy for the majority of women with Stage I and II breast cancer and is prefer-able."[3] You might think that the highly publicized clinical trials and an NIH recom-mendation would have made mastectomy almost obsolete, especially in view of the fact that perhaps 90% or more of the tumors currently being diagnosed might be deemed suitable for "conservative therapy" (i.e., breast preservation). But a nationwide lumpectomy revolution did not occur; what we found instead were the most astonishing variations in the percentage of patients treated by conservative therapy. Lumpectomy triumphed convincingly only in the New England states; a victory in this region could have been anticipated, since the most influential studies of breast preservation techniques had been done at Boston's Joint Center for Radiation Therapy. Mastectomy remained the most common treatment in the South and Midwest, while in California and the other Pacific Coast states the two therapies received roughly equal billing. A study based on data collected by the American College of Surgeons reported that 53.1% of the Stage One patients in New England received lumpectomies, but only 15.3% of comparable patients in the states of Alabama, Kentucky, Mississippi, and Tennessee. The rate was 34.5% in the Pacific Coast states, Alaska, and Hawaii.[4] A study published in 1996 found that the overall lumpectomy rate in North Carolina rose from 7.3% in 1988 to 14.3% in 1993; but the hospital of the University of North Carolina at Chapel Hill reported a rate of 46% for the year 1994, more than three times the state average.[5]

What are we to conclude from these statistical vagaries? First of all, that the percentage of patients treated with breast-conserving surgery and subsequent radiotherapy will be significantly higher in those communities with numbers of well-qualified radiation oncologists. The type of hospital at which the surgery is performed may also matter a great deal. The North Carolina study found that the smallest hospitals—those with one hundred or fewer beds—had a lumpectomy rate of only 4.9%. Patients wanting breast preservation usually fare better at the larger hospitals in sizable cities, at university hospitals, or at the major cancer centers. The hospital of the University of Vermont in Burlington recorded a lumpectomy rate of 73% "for invasive breast cancer of all stages," well above the regional average for New England.[6] With breast cancer the treatment recommendations will vary, depending not only upon which door in the hospital a patient might open, but upon where that hospital happens to be located.

Some breast cancer activists have raised a hue and cry about gender bias, hinting that male surgeons urge mastectomy more often than female ones. Perhaps there's some truth in this idea, but it should be remembered that many of the radiotherapists who preach lumpectomy are male. The North Carolina study found no evidence of gender bias among the state's surgeons, but it did find that surgeons who graduated from medical school before 1980 were slightly more prone to perform mastectomies. The difference might be due to training received in an era when mastectomy was emphasized as the only reasonable therapy, or it might be that these older surgeons attract older patients who may be wary of radiation treatments or less interested in breast preservation. In North Carolina patients over age 70 were much more likely to be treated with mastectomy than with lumpectomy and irradiation; so were patients who lacked private health insurance. Adjuvant radiotherapy for breast preservation represents an added expense; and it requires that the patient spend six weeks or so in the close vicinity of a radiation facility. Financially secure, well-educated women living in urban centers or university towns are in a better position to know about breast conservation—and to follow this option if they choose. Women living in rural areas are presently at a disadvantage. But the assumption that everybody would prefer lumpectomy and irradiation is no more warranted than the old assumption that mastectomy was universally appropriate. Blake Cady, a professor of surgery at the Harvard Medical School, offers an anecdote which challenges our preconceptions about gender bias and the power of physician recommendations: "I met a young woman surgeon in a Midwestern farming community who told me that she could not talk her farmers' wives into even considering breast conservation and radiation therapy. It was too complicated, too prolonged apparently, to satisfy their pragmatic and practical approach to life."[7]

No Patient Stands Alone

Newly diagnosed cancer patients often feel awfully alone, as though they were suddenly isolated from the rest of the healthy workaday world. But the fact is that they have lots of company. About one-third of present-day Americans will be diagnosed with a serious malignancy at some time in their lives; few families and certainly no neighborhoods will remain untouched. Fortunately, numerous support organizations stand ready to give information and advice to this mass of suffering humanity. And there are more support groups specifically devoted to breast cancer than to any other type of malignancy. Most sizable hospitals sponsor instructional seminars and social gatherings designed to assist the breast cancer patients who have passed through their doors. And in most cities these patients have also formed their own independent groups, whose functions could range from recreational trips to health care activism. The sort of assistance needed by breast cancer patients will be as varied as the disease. Minimally, those patients diagnosed with invasive tumors stand to need advice on selecting a prosthesis to replace a missing breast, or on caring for the skin of a breast that is being irradiated. Those patients who must undergo several months of chemotherapy will need counseling on how to cope with the treatment side effects and to maintain an attractive physical appearance in spite of them. Any patient, regardless of whether the prognosis is good or problematic, will find her life changed by a breast cancer diagnosis. But help is never more than a phone call away. Any local chapter of the American Cancer Society can usually direct a patient to an appropriate support group or to a physician competent to provide a second opinion. And these days a "mouse click" on the Internet can open vast storehouses of information, available free of charge.

memento mori

While cancer represents a public health problem of major dimensions, each individual diagnosis might be better described as a crisis in someone's private life. Suddenly a formerly independent person is consigned to the complex world of doctors and nurses, becoming largely dependent on the expertise and good will of professionals who are strangers. The patient's journey will be at best an expensive nuisance, at worst a protracted ordeal. But whether or not a tumor is curable, the diagnosis itself serves as a forceful *memento mori*—a reminder that life is fragile and brief, and that all biological organisms must decay and die. Most of us have been so busy, so preoccupied, with trivial but necessary matters that we are positively shocked to find ourselves face to face with this overwhelming reality. The gospel of dissolution is written with the hand of God in every cell's genetic material—it is correct and irrefutable. But the divine message is grudgingly received in a secular society given over to problem-solving and mass marketing—a land where advertisements sell the illusion of enduring youth, and where the news media are always reporting apparent therapeutic breakthroughs. Cancer patients learn to heed this gospel; once they have gotten over the shock of diagnosis and the dilemma of treatment choices, they often achieve a tranquility that is denied to others. Many report a sense of wonder at the natural world, marveling at occurrences they seem never to have properly observed prior to their diagnosis. Roger C. Bone, a physician with metastatic renal cancer, describes such an awakening: "Death has opened my eyes to life—literally. Since learning that I have a terminal illness, I believe my mind has expanded and its appetite has become insatiable. My evenings now have not one but three remarkable sunsets, each changing as my perspective of the sun changes."[8] Bonnie Marona, a breast cancer patient in California, recalls that she learned to take pleasure in small things: "Having cancer has robbed me of that blissful ignorance that I once had; believing that tomorrow stretched forever. In exchange, I am granted the vision to see each day as precious; a gift to be used wisely and richly."[9]

More Pussycats than Tigers

Notwithstanding the efficient way in which a cancer diagnosis awakens intimations of mortality, we should not overlook the salient fact that most breast cancer patients do not die from breast cancer. These days no more than one patient in every five actually succumbs because of this particular diagnosis, an estimate which is borne out by national statistics. In a recent year the American Cancer Society projected a nationwide total of 217,440 new cases of breast cancer, but only 40,580 deaths.[10] The low mortality rate is not due to any amazing breakthroughs in treatment—it's simply that the majority of breast tumors are biological pussycats rather than tigers. Many tend to remain localized in the affected breast, and those which do metastasize often behave indolently. We can't exactly say that a patient is "lucky" to have developed a mammary carcinoma; but compared to patients with other common malignancies, breast cancer patients are fortunate. A diagnosis of lung or pancreatic cancer has usually been equivalent to a somber tolling of the funereal bell—about 90% of these patients die within five years, regardless of the treatment strategies adopted. Most ovarian and hepatic (liver) tumors will eventually prove resistant to the standard therapies. These cancers are discovered too late for adequate surgical excision; any curative dose of radiation therapy would destroy the adjacent tissues, and chemotherapy has been of limited value. Compared to the aforementioned malignancies, breast cancers are wonderfully treatable, with proven roles for each of the three main modalities. Even in cases of metastatic disease, a strategy to relieve symptoms and prolong survival can usually be developed.

Breast malignancies would be much more deadly if the breast were—like the pancreas and liver—a vital organ in close proximity to other vital organs. Consisting mainly of that subtle mammary gland and a mass of surrounding fat, the breast is not at all vital. Moreover, it's separated from the closest vital organs by the pectoral muscles, the rib cage, and the sternum. This muscular and skeletal barrier retards any local extension of breast tumors into the chest cavity. The surgical treatment alone—either mastectomy or lumpectomy—stands to cure about 75% of apparent Stage One (node-negative) tumors. And these days a patient who loses a breast to cancer can have a lifelike replacement through the now sophisticated techniques for breast reconstruction. However distressing a breast cancer diagnosis may be when it is received, the majority of present-day patients will not suffer a noticeably shortened lifespan. Nor will their appearance and their ability to function in society be noticeably impaired. Years later most of them will recall their diagnosis and treatment as a big nuisance rather than as a life-and-death struggle. Merle O'Rourke Thompson, a breast cancer survivor, discovered that she "could live on a higher plane, not noticing daily annoyances." For six months after finishing chemotherapy she lived "somewhat mystically" with her husband: "But one day I walked into the bedroom, stopped dead, and yelled at Ed, _'Pick up those socks!'_ He kissed me, saying, 'Welcome back.'"[11] Breast cancer patients should anticipate a bothersome year of consultation with medical professionals, but most will eventually be "welcomed back" to their former lives.

Job Security and Insurance

Recovering cancer patients, particularly those under age 65, often worry about losing their job or their health insurance, or both. Susan J. Mellette, a physician dealing with cancer rehabilitation at the Medical College of Virginia, observes that many horror stories about job discrimination "date back to the 1970s, a time when there was less public knowledge of cancer and fewer prominent people discussed their cancer experience openly."[12] Back in those benighted days some cancer patients took pains to conceal their illness from their employers, as well as from their relatives and friends. This tactic now seems excessive. While the C-word can still provoke unreasonable responses, cancer patients and other persons perceived as handicapped acquired significant employment protection in 1991 when Congress passed the **Americans with Disabilities Act**.

Briefly stated, this national legislation prohibits any employer with fifteen or more employees from engaging in discriminatory hiring and promotional practices directed against persons with medical disabilities. The only stipulation is that a handicapped person seeking employment must be able to perform the job for which he or she would be hired. _Fair enough!_ But as we've seen, the majority of breast cancer patients currently being diagnosed are not going to be disabled; they will in fact be _cured_—and their risk of eventually dying from some form of cancer will be only slightly higher than that of persons with no history of cancer. Job discrimination against such patients is irrational as well as illegal. The best policy to govern relationships between cancer patients and their employers should be one of openness, whereby the ramifications of a medical diagnosis are honestly discussed and impassively evaluated. Physicians need to get involved, if only momentarily, to explain what the diagnosis might mean and to confirm the patient's ability to continue working. Properly informed, most employers are willing to allow time off for radiation treatments or chemotherapy sessions, both because they are sympathetic to their employees' problems and because they realize that these problems will be temporary. Other problems employees can have—absenteeism, domestic difficulties, drug dependency, migraine headaches—may be less terrifying, but then they are far more likely to be prolonged and to cause considerable disruption in the workplace.

Unlike the right to fair employment practices, any right to modestly priced health insurance remains a thorny and unresolved issue, both for cancer patients and for persons with numerous other medical conditions. The United States lacks a uniform national system of health care services. For persons ineligible for Medicare or Medicaid, health insurance is provided by private companies which must earn a profit to stay in business. Understandably, these companies are no more enthusiastic about insuring individuals likely to need fabulously expensive treatments than they are about providing collision insurance for drunk drivers or flood insurance for houses built on riverbanks. In the 1980s the triumph of medical innovation left the health insurance industry in turmoil. Hospital bills of $100,000 or more became commonplace as certain experimental procedures became standard practice—open-heart bypass surgery, organ transplantation, and for cancer patients, those elaborate inpatient chemotherapy regimens loosely called "bone marrow transplantation." American patients demanded the very best care; and what's more, they sued when they did not get it. Juries awarded enormous sums in malpractice cases. Many doctors felt themselves caught in a financial bind between judicial extortion and skyrocketing premiums for malpractice insurance; defensively, they doubled or tripled their fees. Hospitals also upped their charges. This unhappy situation wrought by superlative technology and whiny litigation almost makes us yearn for those simpler days of medieval yore, when unlettered barbers performed surgery without anesthesia for a shilling or two. Some insurance companies ceased to underwrite medical policies; those which continued to do so wanted to look more carefully at the patients they insured and the procedures they covered.

Health insurance premiums seem to rise each year, even for persons thought to be in good health. But cancer patients have been singled out. The *Journal of the National Cancer Institute* has reported that these patients "are often faced with premiums that rise 500% once they are diagnosed."[13] Policies can be surreptitiously revised so that

they not only require higher premiums but offer substantially reduced coverage. Cancer patients who do not have Medicare or Medicaid must seek their own individual solutions, which will vary from case to case. Patients covered by group insurance at their place of employment usually try to hold onto their job even if they're unhappy with it, fearing that seeking another position would entail a loss of coverage. The resulting career stasis has been aptly dubbed "job-lock." Patricia A. Ganz, an oncologist at the University of California in Los Angeles, points out that some states have established "high-risk insurance pools" to aid individuals whom private insurers are reluctant to cover. Other alternatives mentioned by Dr. Ganz include "obtaining dependent coverage under the spouse's insurance plan" or "joining a health maintenance organization during open enrollment."[14] Full disclosure would seem to be a reasonable approach for those increasing numbers of women diagnosed with ductal carcinoma *in situ* or with tiny low-grade infiltrating tumors. That is, the diagnosis could be communicated in detail to the patient's insurance company, along with a clear statement that she has little risk of developing metastatic disease. The administrative personnel at large insurance companies typically possess a fair amount of medical sophistication (a few may even have prior credentials as nurses or physicians); and most of them will readily appreciate that localized breast carcinoma is a more propitious diagnosis than, say, diabetes or poorly controlled hypertension.

Personal Relationships

While a cancer diagnosis may change the way an individual is regarded by employers and insurance companies, legislative action has helped to remedy the most flagrant injustices. Unfortunately, there is nothing that Congress, state legislatures, or support groups can do about those subtle alterations in personal relationships which follow on the heels of diagnosis. Friends and relatives may suddenly become rather distant, feeling awkward about the whole thing and not knowing what to say. On the other hand, friends and relatives may rush in with untold quantities of uninformed advice. Patients have been bombarded with books on positive thinking (inspirational enough but scientifically dubious), and urged to devour large servings of dietary items rumored to "fight cancer" (asparagus, broccoli, carrots, garlic, grapes). A breast cancer patient's relationship with her husband or other intimate partner will be changed, either for better or for worse.

Much has been written specifically about the preservation of physical attractiveness and sexual functioning after a breast cancer diagnosis. In this matter as in all others, the effects of diagnosis and treatment are going to vary from case to case. Cytotoxic chemotherapy has adverse effects both on fertility and on sexual activity. Premenopausal women over the age of 40 often do not recover ovarian function, and virtually all patients will experience a temporary loss of libido. But breast surgery by itself, whether mastectomy or lumpectomy, cannot be said to have permanent physiological effects on sexual functioning. The *psychological* effects are another matter: these may be profound. For many women the breast is part and parcel of what it means to be female, the outward badge of gender and desirability. And any thought that a breast may be mutilated or removed looms as a barbarous castration and desexing. This focus on the breast, while understandable, is nonetheless excessive. Physical beauty is in the eye of the beholder, but in any case it involves the entire body—arms, hands, legs, skin, hair, and face. The loss of any body part may detract from the whole; but the loss of a breast to cancer is a minor inconvenience compared to the loss of an arm or a leg due to a traffic accident or industrial mishap.

We hesitate to predict how any individual man will react to a breast cancer diagnosis in a wife or girlfriend. Boys in junior high school take an intense interest in the profound changes occurring in their own bodies—deepening of voice, increased height and musculature, growth of facial hair. Naturally they're also very curious about the physical changes which sexual maturity brings to their female classmates, most visibly embodied in breast development. In adolescent males these nascent curiosities usually find expression in silly locker-room snickerings about girls who are "well-endowed." For adult men, at least for those who are not retarded, the novelty of breasts will have long since worn off; and gratifying sexual experiences will have less to do with anatomical equipment than with intellectual communication and spiritual union. These latter commodities cannot be quantified with a tape measure; however, we may safely conclude that a smile or a kind word is likely to be a better aphrodisiac than an exposed breast.

Any "intimate relationship" which becomes less intimate because of a cancer diagnosis was never very intimate to begin with. Of course, relationships in which the partners have no intent of commitment are by their nature self-serving and temporary—but then so are many marriages. Couples often agree to a wedding ceremony for reasons which have nothing to do with the holiness of the heart's affections. Some people get married simply to comply with social convention; others may be motivated by thoughts of economic security or social advantage. Marriages like these are at best *polished glass*, an abundant commodity which only looks like the far rarer diamond. One problem with glass marriages is that they shatter under pressure, such as might be occasioned by a serious illness or the death of a child. Is that sparkling relationship really diamond or just the glass look-alike? A cancer diagnosis is a test which usually separates the fake from the genuine article. One husband of a breast cancer patient had this to say about his wife's illness: "My greatest concern is to keep her in my life. As far as the loss of the breast, loss of the hair and chemotherapy goes, they're insignificant compared to having her."[15] These sentiments reveal the *unyielding diamond.*

The Rest of this Book

This chapter marks a turning point. Previous chapters have dealt largely with subjects which should be of concern to any woman—breast anatomy, risk factors, symptoms, and diagnostic procedures. The rest of this book deals largely with the current modalities for treating breast malignancies, and should be of especial interest to persons who must live with a prior diagnosis. It is not easy to com-prehend the merits and limitations of the existing therapeutic strategies, or to make informed decisions about them. Even the most sophisticated laypersons can have trouble. Sandra Day O'Connor, the first woman appointed to the Supreme Court, has recalled her reactions to the breast cancer diagnosis given her in 1988: "The big C. The word cancer, it overwhelms the psyche, just the word. I couldn't believe it. I was unprepared for the enormous emotional jolt that I received from the diagnosis." Judge O'Connor, although one of the nation's best legal minds, found herself ill-equipped for the extensive research she needed to perform. And she was baffled by the conflicting rec-ommendations from different specialists: "Moving from doctor to doctor with separate appointments and separate approaches and one doctor not hearing what the other said increased the uncertainty and increased the trauma."[16]

Hopefully the ensuing chapters of this book will assist patients like Judge O'Connor, those bright laypersons who wish to understand the disease and to participate in treatment decisions, but who need a synopsis of research and an unbiased appraisal of the "separate approaches."

Chapter Fourteen

Staging—The Evolving Art of Prognosis

The word *stage* is one which cancer patients are likely to hear frequently, whatever type of malignancy they may have been diagnosed with. Unfortunately, in this context that word has nothing to do with the Broadway theaters or the acting profession. Cancer staging is simply a method of estimating and describing disease progression. A "stage" also serves as a convenient abbreviation to put in a patient's medical records—it indicates the seriousness of the situation, at least in the doctor's opinion. Our existing systems for staging malignancies tend to be elaborate and complicated; they also vary considerably from one type of cancer to the next. But the broad outlines of breast cancer staging are easy to comprehend. Most textbooks use roman numerals for these stages; for convenience we'll spell them out in plain English. The designation **Stage Zero** or **Null** (0) usually refers to an *in situ* (noninvasive) tumor. **Stage One** (I) identifies a small infiltrating tumor which gives no sign of having spread to the axillary lymph nodes; patients so staged are called "node-negative." The designation **Stage Two** (II) is used for invasive tumors whose malignant cells have spread to one or more axillary lymph nodes. The designation **Stage Three** (III) is reserved for patients with a really big breast tumor (several inches in diameter), or with extensive axillary spread

(palpable nodes), or with both conditions. Any patient with a demonstrable metastasis in some other part of the body is said to be in **Stage Four** (IV).

Breast cancer treatments correlate fairly well with this staging system, and they can be profitably summarized stage-wise. A large majority of patients with *in situ* or Stage One tumors will be cured by local therapy alone, either by surgery or by surgery followed by radiotherapy. Many patients with Stage Two disease also have a good prognosis; but almost all of them will be urged to take some form of adjuvant systemic therapy, either oral tamoxifen (an antiestrogenic drug) or intravenous chemotherapy, or both. Stage Three tumors are difficult to treat; many of these patients will eventually develop distant metastases. Stage Four breast cancer, metastatic disease, has not been curable with the existing therapies, but often it can be effectively managed. Although Stage Four patients are likely to die from cancer, their individual life expectancies may vary greatly.

Of course, it is premature to talk about stage or treatment before the entire tumor has been surgically excised and pathologically examined. Historically, the excision and examination of a dozen or more axillary lymph nodes has also been considered a prerequisite for staging; but just before the year 2000 this standard practice underwent a sea change. Such extensive axillary dissections are no longer likely to be performed unless the first node filtering the breast's lymph fluid, the so-called **sentinel node**, proves to contain cancer cells. But any patient scheduled for breast surgery (lumpectomy or mastectomy) is still required to submit to the conventional battery of preoperative assays, with a view to ruling out occult (subclinical) metastases as well as any coexisting nonmalignant diseases. Before surgery both breasts must be studiously mammogramed, and both axillae searchingly palpated for hints of nodal enlargement. Then come the chest X-rays to be sure the lungs are clear. Blood samples are taken to measure the level of serum electrolytes and to verify proper hepatic (liver) function. The "CBC" (complete blood count) would alert us to any imbalance between the red and white cells. And the inevitable urinalysis is included to be sure the kidneys are doing their job. These standard tests (chest X-rays, blood, urine) are relatively inexpensive, as well as fast and painless. When performed on a patient with early-stage breast cancer (Stages Zero, One, or Two), they usually do not detect a single abnormality. These tests are done principally for documentation—that is, to have proof that they were in fact *done* and that nothing abnormal was detected. If an abnormality should be recorded, or if the patient complains of bone pain, dyspnea (breathing difficulty), headaches or other neurological symptoms, the surgeon or the referring physician may order more elaborate tests to search for possible metastatic disease. These could include a "bone scan" of the body with radioactive isotopes, as well as CAT or MRI scans of symptomatic areas. Bone scans, CAT, and MRI do not often play a role in the breast cancer patient's initial workup; they are expensive and rarely yield positive findings.

Dr. Haagensen's *Grave Signs*

Efforts to develop a useful system of staging breast cancers—and therefore of predicting their course and eventual outcome—began almost a century ago. The pioneering breast surgeon William Stewart Halsted observed that his extremely thorough operation (the radical mastectomy) hardly benefited some of his patients. In these cases, nodules of recurrent tumor promptly sprouted along the surgical scar, soon followed by the symptoms of metastatic disease. There was really no point in operating upon such patients, but how could a surgeon distinguish them from those other patients for whom mastectomy provided years or even decades of disease-free survival? Nobody knew. In the 1930s Halsted's most illustrious follower, C. D. Haagensen of Columbia University, tried to catalogue "certain clinical features" which would consistently indicate "far advanced and incurable disease." Dr. Haagensen called these features **grave signs**. They were also "gross signs," meaning that an experienced physician could readily perceive them by visual inspection or by palpation. In 1943 Haagensen and his colleague Arthur Purdy Stout published a landmark paper in which they argued "that patients with these clinical features should not be operated upon." The grave signs Haagensen and Stout identified were "edema of the skin over the breast, satellite nodules in it, solid fixation of the tumor to the chest wall, axillary lymph nodes 2.5 centimeters or more in diameter, fixation of axillary nodes to the overlying skin or the underlying chest wall, supraclavicular metastases, and inflammatory carcinoma."[1] These days, of course, we would regard tumor fixation to the chest wall or overlying skin, or massive axillary nodes, simply as evidence of a locally advanced breast cancer (Stage Three), one that has been allowed to grow—and grow—and grow—before the patient came in for treatment. Haagensen saw numerous cases like this, but the conclusion he drew from them is not universally applicable. Locally advanced cases are quite operable and not always incurable. If the malignant cells are not too aggressive, these patients may even enjoy long-term survival. On the other hand, "inflammatory" signs and "edema" typically characterize those terribly aggressive carcinomas which mimic severe infections in their presentation. Dr. Haagensen was right on target in this instance—inflammatory breast cancer is systemic (Stage Four) at diagnosis, and surgery by itself does nothing to prolong the patient's survival.

The TNM Classification

Haagensen's system of clinical features led physicians to ponder a single momentous question: "Can *the operation* be performed?" If this question seems simple-minded today, we should remember that in Haagensen's era "the operation" (radical mastectomy) was about all that could be done for breast cancer patients. By the early 1950s, however, breast specialists began to recognize that Haagensen's criteria were not only a bit idiosyncratic, but that they could not adequately account for (or "stage") all the disease presentations seen in breast malignancies. In 1954 an international committee proposed a more comprehensive and uniform system for staging breast cancers, the **TNM classification.** This new system quickly won wide acceptance; in its revised and expanded editions it remains the basis for our current staging. The capital letters **TNM** refer to three things the physician is asked to evaluate as separate entities—the primary **TUMOR** in the breast, any involvement of the axillary lymph **NODES**, and any possible **METASTASIS**. Numbers and small letters

are placed after the capital letters, enabling us to express what is known about the tumor and nodes in an abbreviated fashion. For example, **T1** would indicate a primary tumor no larger than two centimeters (about an inch) in its greatest dimension. The addition of a lower case letter allows for more precision. Thus **T1a** identifies a primary tumor 0.5 cm or smaller, while **T1b** designates a tumor larger than 0.5 cm but not over 1.0 cm, and **T1c** refers to a tumor larger than 1.0 cm but not over 2.0 cm. Assuming the lymph nodes are negative and distant metastases not apparent, T1 tumors will be classified as Stage One breast cancer. Adjuvant systemic therapy for T1a tumors is probably unwarranted, but almost all American oncologists would recommend it for T1c tumors with unfavorable histologic features or poor nuclear grade.

Really large breast tumors are regarded as Stage Two disease in the TNM classification even if the axillary lymph nodes seem to be negative (cancer-free). A **T2** rating, designating a primary tumor larger than two centimeters, or a **T3** rating (tumor over 5.0 cm), would be sufficient to raise the suspicion of metastatic potential and merit a Stage Two billing. The **T4** rating does not specify a lesion's size, but denotes its fixation to the overlying skin or underlying chest wall—one of Dr. Haagensen's grave signs. T4 tumors are always regarded as Stage Three disease, whatever condition the regional lymph nodes might be in.

The best nodal status is always **N0**—that is, **node-negative**. The **N1** rating indicates that one to four axillary lymph nodes have tested positive for breast cancer cells. But the addition of letters improves this picture slightly—**N1a** means that these nodes contain only small "micrometastases" (no tumor deposits larger than 0.2 cm), and **N1b** limits the number of involved nodes to three. Breast tumors rated T1 or T2 with N1, N1a, or N1b nodes are classified as Stage Two disease. But any **N2** rating warrants a Stage Three diagnosis, regardless of the primary tumor's size. N2 indicates considerable nodal involvement—either five or more axillary nodes found to be positive, or at least one positive node which is greatly enlarged (over 3.0 cm in diameter), or at least one positive node discovered in the internal mammary chain beneath the sternum (breast-bone).

The **M** of the TNM classification is the easiest element to remember. It refers to any established colony of breast cancer cells found elsewhere in the body—that is, away from the breast with the primary tumor and the ipsilateral (same side) lymph nodes. Such colonies are called **distant metastases**. The designation **M0** indicates that no distant metastasis has been found; in this case the patient's stage is determined by the tumor characteristics (T) and the nodal status (N). **M1** indicates that at least one distant metastasis is known to be present; and any patient with this finding is said to have Stage Four breast cancer, regardless of the condition of the primary tumor and the ipsilateral nodes. In the TNM classification breast cancer cells discovered in either the supraclavicular nodes (those over the collarbone) or in the cervical nodes (those in the neck) are regarded as distant metastases; and they would warrant an M1 rating.[2]

What TNM Doesn't Tell Us

The TNM classification is a model of schematic ingenuity which allows for the annotation and cataloguing of all breast cancers. After the appropriate numbers and lower-case letters are jotted down, the physician can consult a staging manual and then confidently pronounce *The Stage* to satisfy the patient's naive curiosity. We should accord

TNM staging a certain degree of respect—it has its uses—but we ought not to take it as a definitive prognostication. Cancer staging systems grew out of our human need for tidiness and our understandable desire to impose a sense of order upon baffling and unpredictable malignancies. Unfortunately, none of these staging schemata fully correlate with the unwieldy biological phenomena they're supposed to pigeonhole. The main drawbacks of TNM staging are that it is merely anatomical in its measurements, and that it conveys the impression that tumor growth and dissemination proceed in a neat step-by-step fashion. Breast cancers often fail to follow this stepwise scenario. A few tumors designated Stage One will nonetheless rapidly give rise to metastatic disease, while some Stage Three tumors will be cured by local therapy alone. Patients with a single limited metastasis sometimes can remain fully functional for many years.

The question which TNM staging seeks to answer is not irrelevant, yet it is that simplistic query which occurs to even the most uninformed patient: "How far has that tumor spread?" TNM staging does not address a subtler but ultimately more important issue—**the metastatic potential of the individual cancer cells**. Back in the 1970s an accurate TNM assessment seemed to provide sufficient information to make treatment decisions; but since the 1980s the most up-to-date specialists have wanted to see much more data coming from the pathology lab. As explained in Chapter Twelve, a pathology report ought to identify the type of breast cancer, describe the tumor's degree of differentiation and its histological and nuclear grades, and call attention to any evidence of lymphatic invasion or angiogenesis. Assays to estimate the cancer cells' hormonal responsiveness (measurements of estrogen and progesterone receptor protein), and to gauge their rate of proliferation (S-phase), should be performed on all but the most minuscule tumors. We'll have more to say about the aforementioned assays later in this chapter; but for the moment we must point out that physicians dealing with breast cancer, surgeons and oncologists alike, still rely heavily on tumor size and nodal status in making treatment decisions. It is prudent that they do so. Surveys of hospital records and clinical trials have established that for most patients tumor size and nodal status at the time of diagnosis will be significant indicators of the eventual outcome.

Tumor Size and Prognosis

With malignant breast tumors, bigger is _not_ better. There will be occasional exceptions to this rule. It is better to have a large tumor with little metastatic potential than a small tumor capable of rapid dissemination. But in most cases the larger the primary tumor is, the poorer the patient's chances of long-term survival. Breast preservation also becomes much more difficult.

Since tumor size may well dictate the type of surgery required (mastectomy or lumpectomy), and provide an indication for chemotherapy, it should be meticulously measured in the pathology lab and prominently entered in the patient's records. Presurgical estimations of tumor size, whether done by palpation or by mammography, are notoriously prone to error; and even laboratory measurements of excised specimens are not as simple as you might think. The pathologist Edwin R. Fisher cautions that "breast tumors don't grow like a solid cherry."[3] There may be intervening normal tissue between the tendrils of tumor, and the malignant portions themselves may be quite heterogeneous. Some specimens pronounced "invasive" may consist largely of _in situ_ cells; others may have little or no _in situ_

component. The proportion of infiltrating tumor relative to normal tissue or to any _in situ_ component has prognostic import, perhaps even more than overall size; and it should be clearly stated in the pathology report along with the lesion's general dimensions.

When thinking about tumor size as a prognostic indicator, we would do well to remember that the volume or "capacity" of a two-centimeter tumor is not simply twice that of a one-centimeter tumor, but about four times as great. Thus the 2.0 cm tumor presumably contains many more cancer cells than the 1.0 cm tumor, and typically these cells have been multiplying and mutating for a longer period than those in the smaller tumor. During this time they will have had a better opportunity to acquire those genetic changes needed for lymphatic invasion and metastatic colonization. The TNM criterion which automatically categorizes any tumor over 2.0 cm as Stage Two may be arbitrary, but it is not illogical. The larger breast tumors grow, the more likely they are to spread to the axillary lymph nodes. William L. Donegan has given us some ballpark estimates which are worth repeating. According to Dr. Donegan, only 26% of patients with tumors "1.0 cm or less in diameter" will be found to be node-positive; but 78% of patients with tumors over 10 cm will have axillary involvement.[4]

Nodal status remains the most convincing prognostic indicator for breast cancers; but when that status has not been determined, or when a patient is node-negative or has just one or two positive nodes, tumor size can suddenly become extremely important. Christine L. Carter and her colleagues at the National Cancer Institute have analyzed the five-year survival data on 24,740 American patients diagnosed with primary breast cancer. Their results suggest that "tumor diameter and lymph node status act as independent but additive prognostic indicators. As tumor size increases, survival decreases regardless of lymph node status; and as lymph node involvement increases, survival also decreases regardless of tumor size." The statistics from this large cohort reveal extensive nodal involvement as the most ominous signpost pointing toward premature death, but tumor size had an obvious effect both on nodal status and on survival. For example, of the 7,282 patients having tumors between 2.0 cm and 2.9 cm in diameter (about an inch or so), a solid majority (4,010 patients) proved to be node-negative. And the short-term survival rates for these middling-sized tumors were good—92.3% of the node-negative patients survived the first five years after their diagnosis, as did 83.4% of the patients with one to three positive nodes and 63.4% of those with four or more positive nodes. The statistics were quite different for those 2,698 patients having tumors of 5.0 cm (two inches) or more in diameter. Over two-thirds of this subgroup—1,889 patients—proved to be node-positive; and two-thirds of these node-positive patients—1,259—had extensive axillary involvement (four or more nodes affected). The five-year survival rates dropped noticeably for these largest tumors—82.2% of the node-negative patients passed that milestone, as did 73.0% of those with one to three positive nodes. But only 45.5% of those with four or more positive nodes were alive five years after their diagnosis. The combination of large tumor size and extensive nodal involvement thus identifies a patient population with an especially poor prognosis. It's worth emphasizing that some node-positive patients (one to three nodes) with the middling-sized tumors (2.0 to 2.9 cm) actually had a better five-year survival rate (83.4%) than did the node-negative patients with the larger tumors (82.2%). Dr. Carter sand her NCI colleagues observe "that the metastatic potential evolves as the tumor grows, and that nodal status simply reflects the ability of the tumor to spread. However, the evolution of this metastatic potential is not the same in all tumors."[5]

We must vigorously applaud Carter et al for their solid data and plausible conclusions. The main weakness of this NCI study was its lack of long-term follow-up. Fortunately, the pathologist Paul Peter Rosen and his colleagues at the Memorial Sloan-Kettering Cancer Center have shown us how tumor size at diagnosis affects the likelihood of developing metastatic disease over a time period of two decades. Rosen et al looked at the ongoing medical records of 767 patients treated at Sloan-Kettering for node-negative breast cancer between 1964 and 1970. All these women received mastectomies and axillary dissections—none had any form of adjuvant systemic therapy like chemotherapy or tamoxifen. Their case histories thus give us a good idea of the curative potential of surgery alone in Stage One disease. By the time Dr. Rosen and his colleagues published their analysis in 1993 (over twenty years later), 193 of these node-negative patients—25% of the group—had developed distant metastases. Rosen et al found that the odds of remaining healthy were strongly related both to tumor size and to histological subtype. Those 219 patients who had infiltrating ductal or lobular carcinomas 1.0 cm or smaller in diameter, or who had "special tumor types" (tubular, medullary, mucinous, papillary) 3.0 cm or smaller in diameter, had a good long-term prognosis. At ten years after treatment, 91% were disease-free; and 87% were still healthy twenty years afterward. But the outcome was less certain for those 548 patients having infiltrating ductal or lobular carcinomas over 1.0 cm, or special tumor types over 3.0 cm—only 73% of these patients remained disease-free at ten years, and only 68% at twenty years.[6]

We may draw several useful conclusions from this well-documented Sloan-Kettering study. The first is that as a rule of thumb, about 75% of node-negative tumors will not have evolved metastatic potential before diagnosis and hence may be cured by surgery alone. A second is that most node-negative tumors which are going to recur will do so within ten years after their diagnosis, the recurrence rate dropping off sharply thereafter. A third conclusion has important implications for the use of systemic therapies in node-negative cases. Those invasive ductal or lobular carcinomas larger than one centimeter are about three times more likely to give rise to distant metastases than comparable tumors whose maximum diameter does not exceed one centimeter. Dr. Rosen and his colleagues argued that the routine use of chemotherapy for these smaller tumors (1.0 cm or less) is not warranted, "unless new forms of treatment prove to be less toxic and/or more effective in enhancing relapse-free survival."[7]

NODAL STATUS
The Weightiest Prognosticator

In recent years the investigation of prognostic indicators in breast cancer has focused on molecular biology—on oncogenes running out of control, on nonfunctional tumor suppressors, and on elusive cellular proteins thought to fuel angiogenesis and metastasis. But we should not lose sight of the fact that no indicator carries more weight with practicing physicians than nodal status. Rightly or wrongly, the presence of a few malignant cells in a single axillary lymph node tends to be accepted as presumptive evidence that localized breast cancer is rapidly becoming systemic disease. This is not always the case. There are ascending degrees of nodal involvement, which correlate impressively (but not absolutely) with descending odds for long-term disease-free survival.

As explained in Chapter Four, lymph fluid draining from the breast and arm is filtered through some thirty or so nodes located in the axilla. Under normal conditions these nodes are not palpable—we can't feel them, and we are not even aware of their presence. But in advanced breast cancer these nodes can become terribly apparent, individually swelling up to a centimeter or more in size, and then collectively sticking together so that the axilla becomes a rubbery mass of unsightly tumor. A century ago William Stewart Halsted frequently encountered such matted masses of axillary nodes in his patients. For Halsted and his successors, a thorough axillary dissection—that is, the surgical excision of all axillary nodes and the surrounding fatty tissues—was a therapeutic imperative. It represented a matter of life and death, every bit as important as the removal of the diseased breast.

Today, of course, surgeons initially remove only the leading sentinel node which receives the most direct drainage from the tumor area. If the sentinel node is positive, a limited axillary dissection may be performed both to gauge the extent of nodal involvement and to prevent subsequent recurrences in the axilla. But any excision of axillary nodes is done mainly for prognostic purposes rather than for therapeutic advantage—this surgery has little or no effect on patient survival. For our understanding of the prognostic significance of positive nodes, we are indebted to the large clinical trials conducted by the **National Surgical Adjuvant Breast and Bowel Project**. From the late 1960s through the early 1980s, the NSABP investigators were especially curious to determine how increasing numbers of positive nodes affected patient outcome. Did a patient with cancer cells in just one axillary node have a better chance at long-term survival than a patient with a dozen involved nodes? And if so, how much better? By 1972 Bernard Fisher, the NSABP's chief administrator, was able to report preliminary findings from a group of 297 node-positive patients who had been treated by radical mastectomy. Of those patients who had one to three positive nodes, 53% developed metastatic disease within five years after their surgery. But 80% of those patients who had four or more positive nodes developed metastases within five years.[8] This early NSABP study highlighted two general rules about node-positive breast cancer—first, the more nodes positive, the greater the likelihood of subsequent systemic disease; and second, if metastases are going to occur, most of them will become apparent within five years after diagnosis and treatment.

From the mid-1970s onward, physicians who treated breast malignancies took the NSABP hint and divided their node-positive patients into two groups—those having one to three involved nodes (guarded prognosis assumed) and those having four or more (bad prognosis assumed). But the NSABP researchers decided to modify this arbitrary dividing line after they reviewed the data from **Protocol B-04**, that celebrated clinical trial which proved that radical mastectomy was no more effective than less mutilative procedures. Patients enrolled in NSABP's Protocol B-04 were recruited and treated between 1971 and 1974; all received an axillary dissection, none had postsurgical chemotherapy. The trial thus constitutes a unique source of information on the "natural history" of node-positive breast cancer, because the patients' nodal status was carefully determined, and the evolution of disease not influenced by adjuvant drug therapies. In 1985 the NSABP's pathologist Edwin R. Fisher presented the ten-year

results on 614 patients from Protocol B-04. Ten years after surgery only 20% of 279 node-negative patients had developed distant metastases, but 47% of the 160 patients with one to three involved nodes had done so. Overall, 71% of those 175 patients having four or more positive nodes experienced systemic recurrence; but Dr. Fisher further subdivided this group, emphasizing the large variations within it. For patients with four to six involved nodes, the recurrence rate was 59%; with seven to twelve nodes, 69%; and with thirteen or more nodes, a whopping 87%.[9]

Henceforth the NSABP would campaign against the practice of lumping all "four-or-more" patients into a single high-risk group. Other researchers heeded this basic message, while shying away from the NSABP's proposed four-step stratification. After the mid-1980s patients with node-positive breast cancer were typically stratified into three groups—(1) those with one to three involved nodes, assumed to be at some risk of metastatic disease; (2) those with four to nine involved nodes, assumed to be at high risk; and (3) those with ten or more involved nodes, assumed to be at extremely high risk. Writing in the *Journal of the National Cancer Institute*, the Italian oncologists Gianni Bonadonna and Pinuccia Valagussa observed that this three-subset stratification of node-positive patients "allows a more accurate prediction of treatment outcome." They then offered some ballpark probabilities for systemic (metastatic) recurrence among patients who have been treated for local control of the breast tumor, but who have not yet received chemotherapy. According to Bonadonna and Valagussa, "65% to 67%" of those patients with one to three positive nodes could be expected to relapse within ten years after their surgery. The estimated rate cited for the four-to-nine subset was "75% to 77%," and "in excess of 90%" for the ten-or-more group of patients.[10] The attentive reader will have noticed that these ten-year relapse rates are just a trifle higher than those Edwin R. Fisher announced as the B-04 findings in 1985—especially in that "one-to-three" subset! A small caveat is therefore in order. Women diagnosed with node-positive breast cancer are likely to be quoted some very glib statistics about node counts and the probability of recurrence, with professional oncologists having a tendency to regard even a single positive node as an indication for rigorous chemotherapy. You should be aware that these statistics are not sacrosanct. The recurrence rates reported for nodal subsets vary from study to study, being affected by the characteristics of the patients recruited, by the type of surgery performed for local control, and by the thoroughness of follow-up monitoring.

Unfortunately, we're unlikely to have any statistics more plausible than those provided by NSABP Protocol B-04; after the mid-1970s almost all American patients with positive nodes were urged to take adjuvant drug therapy. There would be no more clinical trials demonstrating the "natural history" of node-positive breast cancer as it evolves without chemotherapeutic interventions. In 1996, however, Coral A. Quiet and other researchers published retrospective data on node-positive patients treated at the University of Chicago back in the pre-chemotherapy era, from the 1930s until the 1970s. These patients did not receive systemic therapy, yet their recurrence rates were considerably lower than those cited by Bonadonna and Valagussa. The Chicago series included 127 patients with a single positive node, whose risk of developing metastases proved to be significantly related to tumor size. For example, all 15 patients in this category with small primary tumors (one centimeter or less) remained disease-free at twenty years after surgery—but only 73% of

of the 35 patients with middling-size tumors (1.1 cm to 2.0 cm) and 62% of the 77 patients with larger tumors (over 2.0 cm). These low relapse rates for a single-node subset are not too different from those we associate with node-negative breast cancer. The most surprising finding from the Chicago study concerned the highest-risk subset, those patients with ten or more positive nodes. An astonishing 29% of the 26 patients in this subset survived twenty years without recurrence, a rate that is more than twice as good as the 13% disease-free survival at ten years reported for the NSABP's highest-risk nodal subset.[11]

What can we conclude from the well-documented NSABP and Chicago findings? First of all, that while the discovery of one or more positive lymph nodes should always be viewed with concern, it does not by itself provide conclusive evidence that a patient is going to develop metastatic disease. In a few cases even patients with ten or more positive nodes have enjoyed long-term survival without detectable recurrences, apparently having been cured by surgery alone. There are several hypotheses which might be cited to explain these anomalous cases. The old Halstedian surgeons would have argued that the axillary nodes acted as "a barrier" and temporarily arrested the migration of cancer cells; and that when the nodes were excised, the patients were cured of their tumors—just in the nick of time! Today's physicians would prefer a more "molecular" explanation. Perhaps the cancer cells had acquired genetic changes enabling them to invade the lymphatic channels and travel to the regional nodes, but still lacked those mutations which facilitate metastatic engraftment in distant anatomical sites.

The Axillary Dissection

There are only mild controversies about the relapse rates to be expected in node-positive breast cancer, understandably tinged with specialty bias. Surgeons have tended to cite lower rates (thus subtly emphasizing the curative power of adequate surgery); oncologists have tended to up the percentages (thus subtly emphasizing the advisability of chemotherapy or other systemic drugs). But everybody accepts the general position—the more nodal involvement, the greater the probability of eventual metastatic disease. What nobody has quite agreed upon is that pesky axillary dissection—a prerequisite for accurate nodal staging, since it supplies the nodes to be examined. In what particular types of breast cancer must the axilla be operated upon, and how many nodes should be removed? Do thorough axillary dissections improve survival rates? Not a few surgeons still harbor the traditional belief that this procedure serves a double therapeutic function, not only preventing regional recurrences in the axilla, but probably reducing the incidence of distant metastases as well. Unfortunately, the results from the NSABP trials did not support the second proposition. Bernard Fisher and his NSABP colleagues have emphatically stated the B-04 findings: "Treatment failure and mortality five years following operation was unaffected by the number of axillary nodes removed and examined. There is no evidence that the removal of more nodes, positive or negative, improves the survival rate." According to Fisher et al, positive nodes are not themselves "instigators of distant disease," but merely "indicators reflecting an interrelation that permits the development of metastases."[12]

While the NSABP investigators saw no therapeutic benefit to be had from a thorough dissection removing 25 or 30 nodes, they vigorously advocated a limited dissection for diagnostic purposes. But they were worried that samplings removing fewer than ten nodes could result in staging errors—for example, some patients actually having four or more positive nodes might get mistakenly classified with the "one-to-three" patients, a more prognosticly favorable group.[13] Inadequate sampling of the axilla is only one of several causes for incorrect nodal staging. Another is inadequate examination of the nodal specimens. During the 1990s it became clear that the axillary nodes can contain "occult micrometastases," little clusters of cancer cells which are likely to be missed with the standard H&E staining techniques, but which may be detected with the more sophisticated immunostaining procedures. A European study of nodal specimens from 921 breast cancer patients found 83 cases (a 9% rate) revealing these occult cancer cells; other studies have yielded different results, but most suggest that from 15% to 25% of sampled axillary nodes that would be deemed negative with the standard H&E staining actually contain hidden foci of tumor cells.[14] We may surmise that many breast cancers historically judged node-negative were in fact surreptitiously node-positive. This hypothesis helps to explain the 25% rate of treatment failure commonly reported for node-negative patients.

Sentinel Node Sampling

The major drawback to axillary dissections has always been the danger of permanent side effects. The more complete the dissection, the more accurate will be the determination of nodal status, and the lower the risk of tumor recurrence in the axilla. But then we run the risk of seriously impeding lymphatic drainage, causing the patient's arm to retain lymph fluid and swell up painfully to twice its normal size. In the 1990s the wisdom of excising axillary nodes began to be debated as never before. A retrospective analysis of 283 cases of invasive breast cancer treated at the Johns Hopkins Hospital found that only 46% of these patients could be said to have benefited from their axillary dissections. The Hopkins researchers assumed that those few patients with palpable "clinically involved" nodes—15% of the study group—received a "therapeutic benefit" from the procedure. And they believed that 31% of the group received a "diagnostic benefit," because in these cases the discovery of positive nodes provided the principal indication for chemo-therapy. But the remaining 54% did not benefit.[15]

Of course, no breast cancer patient who proves node-negative—i.e., no tumor dissemination to the axilla—can be said to have profited from axillary surgery. And the majority of patients currently being diagnosed are going to be node-negative. The likelihood of diagnostic or therapeutic benefits has been steadily decreasing in the era of public awareness and mammography screening. Was there any way to obtain accurate information on nodal status without resorting to extensive dissections? In the 1990s breast cancer specialists in California and Florida developed the technique of **sentinel node dissection**, which quickly found wide acceptance among American surgeons. The idea here is to identify the first (or sentinel) node which would be reached by the lymph fluid draining from a breast tumor. Once we are sure that the sentinel node has been identified, it is excised and subjected to a thorough pathological examination using both H&E and immunostaining. If the sentinel node proves negative for cancer cells, the patient is assumed to be node-negative and spared the traditional axillary dissection. If the node proves positive, a more extensive dissection may be done, both to provide information on

the number of involved lymph nodes and to reduce the risk of axillary recurrences. The main drawback to sentinel node sampling is that it requires considerable training and practice to identify the first node filtering lymph fluid from the tumor area. The California team relied on a blue dye which was injected into the tumor area and allowed to drain into the axilla, thereby adding a touch of color to the lymphatic channels and nodes for visual identification. The Florida team combined a radionuclide tracer with the colored dye. By using a small handheld "Geiger counter," the surgeon could identify radioactive "hot spots" as the suspect axillary nodes before making an incision.

We'll have more to say about the pros and cons of sentinel node sampling in Chapter Seventeen. For the moment we need to alert the reader that traditional axillary dissections with their lingering side effects are no longer necessary in many breast malignancies. No patient with ductal carcinoma *in situ* needs any type of axillary exploration, and probably only a very few patients with small invasive tumors (those of one centimeter or less) would benefit from a traditional dissection. Patients having larger tumors with unfavorable histological characteristics (e. g., infiltrating ductal carcinomas of 2.0 cm or more) are likely to receive a recommendation for adjuvant systemic therapy regardless of their nodal status. Hence the potential diagnostic benefit to be had from an axillary dissection in such cases seems less obvious than it did in previous decades. Thanks to the NSABP trials, we know that this procedure is not likely to affect the long-term survival rates for any subgroup of breast cancer patients.

Toward a Cellular Staging:
Separating Tigers from Pussycats

By the 1970s the TNM model of breast cancer staging was widely used by American physicians; but the heterogeneity of breast tumors, which did not altogether escape the notice of old-time surgeons like Halsted and Haagensen, now began to represent a major dilemma. Public awareness campaigns and mammography screening meant that more and more "cases" were being diagnosed—yet most of them turned out to be biological pussycats rather than the grisly tigers the Halstedians had to deal with. In an oft-cited article published in 1979, the biologist Maurice S. Fox of the Massachusetts Institute of Technology worried that "the aggressive search for early or minimal disease" would lead to the diagnosis "of increasing numbers of women with lesions exhibiting histological characteristics of cancer but with relatively benign biological properties." In other words, you're going to detect a lot of pussycats! In support of his thesis Fox observed that although the number of reported cases had jumped 50% between 1965 and 1975, "breast cancer mortality has remained unchanged for at least the past forty years." While a minority of patients will have "fatal outcome," the majority "exhibit a relative mortality only modestly different from that of women of similar ages without evidence of disease." And the traditional pathological workups are not especially efficient in distinguishing between the lethal and nonlethal varieties. "Histological examination," Fox asserted, "does not permit a prediction of the likelihood that a lesion will follow the sequential steps believed to characterize the natural history of breast cancer. Some lesions may rarely, or never, make the transition to metastatic disease."[16]

From the late 1970s onward, advances in chemotherapy provided us with an urgent reason to find better ways of identifying those particular early-stage tumors destined to produce metastases. We now had new multidrug regimens which were somewhat effective in holding the metastatic tigers at bay, but which were too toxic and too unpredictable to use against presumably localized pussycats. When do you call for the chemo? Anatomical staging along the TNM lines could not always give us a precise answer to this query. We needed a cellular staging focusing on the malignant potential of the individual cancer cells. Ultimately, it is the characteristics of the individual cells which determine the outcome.

Hormonal Responsiveness
The Role of Estrogen Receptors

The first cellular assays to be widely used sought to measure the responsiveness of breast cancer cells to the steroid sex hormones. Estrogen is the most important of these hormones; it stimulates breast development at puberty, and thereafter keeps the cells lining the mammary gland's ducts and lobules in constant activity. Prior to the 1970s, however, very little was known about the mechanisms through which estrogen exerts its effects. In the 1960s mice and rats had been injected with radioactive estrogenic compounds, thereby demonstrating that heavy uptake of this hormone occurs only in certain target tissues such as the endometrium (uterine lining) or the mammary gland. Researchers postulated that the cells of these tissues expressed specific estrogen-binding components, variously referred to as "estrophiles" or "estrogen receptors." By 1970 Elwood V. Jensen and his co-workers at the University of Chicago had shown us that the binding component was a protein bounteously present in the cytoplasms of the target cells. A molecule of estrogen binds to the receptor protein; the complex thus formed travels to the cellular nucleus, where it activates the transcription of genes. Jensen et al devised methods of measuring the quantity of this protein in tumor samples; and they established that those breast cancer cells containing the protein responded to estrogen, but that those without it rarely did so.[17]

Physicians took immediate notice of the Jensen group's methodology, because it offered a way of predicting which patients would respond to hormonal therapies. At the time there were no standard chemotherapy regimens for breast cancer; but cases of metastatic disease sometimes responded dramatically to manipulations of the body's hormone levels. These treatments could be either **ablative** (e.g., shutting off the flow of estrogen by surgical excision of the ovaries) or **additive** (e.g., giving so much synthetic estrogen that the cancer cells become saturated with it and cease to proliferate). Either strategy could shrink tumor metastases, even cause them to disappear for long periods of time. The problem was that in any sizable group of Stage Four patients, only about one-third had significant responses to such manipulations; the majority did not benefit. Measurements of the estrogen receptor protein changed things. For the first time physicians had a tool—a cellular assay—which could distinguish reasonably well between those patients likely to respond and those patients who almost certainly would not.

During the 1970s and 1980s numerous laboratory experiments and clinical trials were conducted to further define the role of estrogen receptor (ER) measurements in breast cancer medicine. We can summarize a voluminous literature by saying that ER assays not only help us in selecting appropriate systemic therapies, but they give us some inkling of the course that individual tumors

may be inclined to follow. **ER status is an independent prognostic indicator, second in importance only to nodal status and tumor size.** A positive reading, indicating the presence of receptor protein in the cancer cells, tends to be associated with the pussycat variety of breast malignancy. Normal cells in the mammary epithelium are rich in ER protein, and their growth is estrogen dependent. When we find this protein in transformed tumor cells, we can assume that they retain at least some of the functional attributes of the healthy differentiated cells from which they arose. The pathologist Edwin R. Fisher has aptly described "high estrogen receptor content" as "a biochemical reflection of tumor differentiation."[18] The quantity of receptor protein in the cancer cells usually correlates with a tumor's size and its stage. As a rule nonpalpable *in situ* lesions have more of the protein than palpable invasive tumors, while distant metastases have least of all. Breast cancer cells presumably begin as ER-positive and subsequently evolve into an ER-negative phenotype. Estrogen receptor positivity is often (but not always) found in conjunction with other tumor characteristics known to be prognosticly favorable—good nuclear grade, well-differentiated histology, and low S-phase (slow proliferation rates).[19]

We do not know exactly what happens when breast cancer cells lose their cytoplasmic ER protein; in some cases this transformation may be due to nuclear malfunctions affecting the recently located gene (long arm of chromosome six) which directs the manufacture of this protein.[20] While the cause may be open to question, nobody thinks that the loss of ER protein is an auspicious event. A negative finding on an ER assay indicates that the tumor cells are sufficiently deregulated that they can multiply without the customary hormonal stimulation. ER negativity does not by itself identify any tumor as a metastatic tiger, yet physicians suspect that as a group these cases are going to behave more aggressively. Some clinical trials have revealed a significantly poorer outcome for ER-negative patients. The Italian National Cancer Institute in Milan kept tabs on 464 women who had been treated for Stage One (node-negative) breast cancer. Four years after surgery only 11.6% of the ER-positive premenopausal patients had experienced disease recurrence; in contrast, 41.3% of the ER-negative premenopausal patients suffered a relapse.[21] Striking statistics like these explain why physicians want to look closely at ER status in early breast cancer, Stages One and Two. Node-negative patients with middling-sized tumors and negative ER readings are often advised to take chemotherapy, especially if they are premenopausal.

We should emphasize that ER expression is no more an absolute indicator of prognosis than nodal status or tumor size. High levels of receptor protein provide no assurance that distant metastases will not occur. But clinical experience has consistently demonstrated that ER-positive patients tend to enjoy longer disease-free intervals than comparable patients who are ER-negative, and that those metastases which do develop in the former group are more likely to be sluggish osseous (bone) lesions rather than fast-moving visceral growths which could take root in the liver or lungs.

Measuring Cellular ER Levels

Estrogen receptor positivity is not an all-or-nothing proposition. There are ascending degrees of ER expression in breast tumors, which correlate fairly well with increasing response to hormonal therapies and increasing odds of long-term survival. From the early 1970s to the mid-1980s, the standard method of measuring cellular concentrations of ER protein was a biochemical test called a **ligand-binding assay**. A sizable portion of the tumor specimen, about 500 milligrams or so, would be chemically treated and then centrifuged, leaving a homogeneous fluid. Radiolabeled estradiol (the ligand) would be added to this homogenate; and the mildly radioactive hormone would bind to any unoccupied estrogen receptors in the cytosol, producing a sedimentation reaction whose extent could be measured. This simple assay has one major drawback—it requires a largish quantity of tumor that has been either just removed from the patient (i.e., fresh) or immediately frozen after surgery. The ER protein is heat labile; at room temperatures it rapidly loses its ability to interact with estrogen molecules.

The major advantage of this assay is that it gives a quantitative reading of the ER present in the specimen, conveniently expressed in **femtomoles (fmol) of estradiol binding per milligram of cytosol protein**. Any reading of less than 3 fmol/mg is interpreted as decidedly ER-negative; no appreciable amount of the receptor protein can be detected. Readings of 3 to 9 fmol/mg are marginal: the likelihood of response to hormonal therapy is uncertain. A reading of 10 fmol/mg or more indicates clinically significant ER positivity, with a good chance of response to hormonal therapy. The higher the reading, the better the odds of response and of long-term survival. Donegan and Spratt's weighty textbook contains a table correlating ER assay results with the observed response rates to endocrine therapies. Here are some ballpark figures taken from this source—only 9% of breast cancer patients having 0 to 9 fmol/mg respond to hormonal manipulations, but 50% of those patients having 10 to 50 fmol/mg respond, as do 83% of the patients having 100 fmol/mg.[22]

Patients with ER readings below 10

fmol/mg are dubious candidates for the estrogen-blocking drug tamoxifen. If they were deemed at risk of metastatic disease, they would probably receive a recommendation for cytotoxic chemotherapy. Back in 1978 the *New England Journal of Medicine* published a "retrospective study" by Marc E. Lippman and his co-workers at the National Cancer Institute, who sought to correlate assayed levels of ER protein with the observed response rates to chemotherapy in 69 women with Stage Four (metastatic) breast cancer. The NCI team found that only 3 of 25 patients having positive ER readings (10 fmol/mg or better) responded to chemotherapy, but that 34 of 45 patients with negative ER assays registered objective responses.[23] Almost everybody now accepts the general proposition—viz., chemo is indicated for ER-negative patients having, or deemed to be at risk of, metastatic disease. But we need to stress that subsequent clinical trials have not confirmed this early finding that ER-positive patients are intrinsically unresponsive to chemo. The rate of tumor cell proliferation (S-phase) is a much better indicator of chemo responsiveness than ER status; but as we've seen, ER-positive patients tend to have lower proliferation rates and may fail to respond for that reason.

ER assays principally tell us about the probable response to *hormonal* therapies. But quantitative measurements of ER protein have also helped to explain the clinical observation that premenopausal breast cancers tend to behave more aggressively than comparable postmenopausal tumors. Besides having an intrinsically high proliferation rate, breast cancer cells from premenopausal women are frequently ER-negative. In contrast, most cancer cells from postmenopausal women will prove to be ER-positive. Gary M. Clark, C. Kent Osborne, and William L. McGuire, those dedicated steroid researchers at the University of Texas in San Antonio, looked at the ER concentrations in 2,777 breast malignancies. The tumors taken from 625 premenopausal women revealed a median ER reading of 8 fmol/mg—the tumors from 2,152 postmenopausal women, a median reading of 46 fmol/mg![24] When we consider that most breast cancer patients are postmenopausal, and that most postmenopausal tumors are decidedly ER-positive, we will not be surprised that tamoxifen has long been the most widely used adjuvant drug.

Immunostaining for ER Protein

By the late 1980s, just when oncologists had become accustomed to ER readings in femtomoles, avant-garde pathologists began to beat the drums for **immunohistochemical assays** of the receptor protein. As explained in Chapter Three, "immunostaining" relies on the old-fashioned visualization of cells placed under the microscope, as enhanced by newfangled reagents (monoclonal antibodies) which impart a bright coloration to hitherto invisible cellular components. The pathologist can actually see the evidence of ER accumulation in a cell's cytoplasm and nucleus, thus verifying the protein's presence and its presumptive activity. Immunostaining is very different from the standard biochemical assay that gave us our present knowledge about the role that ER protein plays in breast malignancies. Not everybody is ready to abandon the older assay, but the newer methodology offers several advantages. For example, the biochemical assay can be subject to sampling errors. In it a large tumor specimen is transformed into a fluid homogenate, then a ligand (estradiol) introduced whose binding activity may be measured. But the ER reading reported for the breast cancer cells will be too low (a false-negative result) if the specimen contains too many stromal (connective) cells—

or fatty cells—or inflammatory (white) cells. While these healthy cells are found in close association with the malignant mammary cells, they are not estrogen-dependent, do not produce estrogen receptors, and would be assayed as negative. False-positive readings can also occur. Let's suppose that some of the breast cancer cells in a specimen express a lot of ER, but that the majority of them actually have low levels. In this case the pathology lab might report ER positivity, while the tumor's subsequent behavior would accord with the ER-negative phenotype. Properly performed immunohistochemical assays eliminate the aforementioned sources of error. The pathologist would make a visual distinction between the malignant cells with ER protein and the adjacent nonmammary cells without it, or he would notice that while some of the malignant cells might be ER-rich, most of them are ER-deficient.

Clive Roy Taylor and Richard J. Cote, pathologists at the University of Southern California, sing the praises of this new methodology in their impressive book entitled *Immunomicroscopy*, while adding an appropriate caveat: "Immunohistochemical assays for hormone receptor content are technically demanding to perform and interpret." But the biggest obstacle is that immunostaining reports are perceived as being vaguely qualitative rather than precisely quantitative. Oncologists love that aura of scientific precision conveyed by numerical statements of femtomoles per milligram! Alas, the immunostainers have yet to agree on a rating system which would possess a comparable aura. Taylor and Cote observe that two factors, "the proportion of positive cells" and "the intensity of stain," must serve as the basis for any system that might be devised in the future.[25] For the time being, we can enthusiastically recommend ER immunostaining for tumor samples which can't be evaluated with the older biochemical assay. An *in situ*

breast cancer should never be reduced to a homogenate—the entire specimen must be embedded in paraffin, sectioned, and studied under the microscope, because it is far more important to rule out any possibility of malignant infiltration (i.e., an invasive portion) than it is to establish the ER status. Fortunately, the newest antibody reagents will react to traces of inert receptor protein found in paraffin-embedded tumor slides. Thus immunostaining can usually give us ER status reports on recently processed *in situ* specimens, or on archival slides taken from tumor specimens processed many years before. Large quantities of tissue are not needed. Immunostaining works well on individual cells obtained by fine-needle aspiration and on those tiny slivers extracted with core-needle biopsies. The technique's applicability to any and all specimens is a strong selling point in an era when the breast cancers being diagnosed are getting smaller and smaller.

Progesterone Receptors Too?

Some breast cancer researchers, especially the San Antonio group, have postulated that the cellular levels of progesterone receptor (PgR) protein would give us better clues to prognosis and hormonal responsiveness than ER levels. The reasoning behind this hypothesis was simple. Mammary cells synthesize the PgR protein only after they have been stimulated (or primed) by estrogen; hence if we find PgR in a breast cancer cell, we might conclude that both its estrogen and progesterone pathways are functional, and that it is truly hormonally responsive. In 1983 Gary M. Clark and his San Antonio colleagues published a preliminary study in the *New England Journal of Medicine*: the data they had gathered from 189 Stage Two patients suggested that PgR positivity was a better indicator of "extended disease-free survival" than ER positivity. "Progesterone-receptor levels," Clark et al argued, "should be routinely measured."[26] Clark and William L. McGuire examined retrospective data from 638 breast cancer patients treated with various endocrine therapies, correlating ER and PgR status with the reported response rates. Of those patients positive for both ER and PgR, fully 71% were listed as responders. In contrast, only 32% of the patients who were ER-positive but PgR-negative appeared on the responders' list. According to Clark and McGuire, ER status by itself was not always sufficient to predict responsiveness to hormonal manipulations; one needed a PgR reading as well.[27]

The studies of PgR status had as yet been too small or too poorly designed to generate convincing statistical power. Other groups of researchers questioned whether PgR levels really helped to predict the hormonal responsiveness of breast cancer cells. By 1992 we had some plausible answers from a clinical trial conducted by the Southwest Oncology Group (SWOG), who had monitored 342 patients with Stage Four (metastatic) breast cancer being treated with tamoxifen. Those patients assayed as being both ER-positive and PgR-positive had the highest response rates, but patients who were ER-positive and PgR-negative also had respectable rates. For example, patients seen as decidedly ER-positive (50 or more fmol/mg) achieved a 53% response rate even when they had the lowest PgR levels (less than 10 fmol/mg). Comparable ER-positive patients who were also decidedly PgR-positive (100 or more fmol/mg) registered a 66% response rate—i.e., somewhat better than those assayed ER-positive and PgR-negative, but not overwhelmingly better. The SWOG researchers modestly concluded "that knowledge of PgR levels can improve the pretreatment assessment of ER-positive breast cancer patients"; but they observed that "no groups of ER-positive patients had such a low response rate as to preclude consideration for the use of tamoxifen."[28]

ER assays still remain our principal indicator for the hormonal differentiation of breast cancer cells—ER status should always be considered when treatment strategies are pondered. As with ER, the levels of cellular PgR protein can be measured by ligand-binding assay or by immunostaining. While there is less agreement about the significance of progesterone receptors, it is clear that tumors which are strongly positive for both ER and PgR stand the best chance of responding to hormonal therapies.

Measuring Growth Rates:
S-phase, Flow Cytometry, Ki-67

Cellular proliferation rates vary tremendously among the different types of human malignancy. Some cancerous cells, notably those born in prostate and thyroid tumors, may have metastatic potential, but they usually multiply so slowly that most patients die from old age rather than from their malignancies. At the other extreme, the cells found in acute leukemias and rare angiosarcomas can proliferate with such explosive rapidity that most patients would die within a few weeks after diagnosis if they were not promptly treated with chemotherapy. That broad spectrum of disease we call "breast cancer" contains both extremes. A slow rate of cellular proliferation characterizes the pussycat variety; this is generally found in association with other prognosticly favorable features—histological differentiation, good nuclear grade, and ER and PgR positivity. A rapid growth rate suggests the metastatic tiger, especially when it's detected in a tumor with other prognosticly unfavorable features.

There are several assays which we can use to measure the proliferation rates of breast cancer cells. The traditional method, dating back to the 1950s and 1960s, is called **mitotic indexing**. Any pathology lab can do it—no special equipment is required, just the permanent sections (glass slides) from the tumor in question. Mitosis, the division of one cell into two, is clearly visible under the microscope. The pathologist simply adds up the number of mitoses seen on the slides to arrive at the "mitotic index," which is the ratio of these "mitotic figures" to the total number of cells present. While simple enough, this technique represents an enormous expenditure of time and eyestrain because mitosis is a relatively rare event in solid mammalian tissues. John S. Meyer, a pioneering researcher of cellular proliferation rates, observes that in some breast carcinomas "more than 10,000 cells must be counted to find five or more mitotic figures."[29]

A more practical way of distinguishing between rapid and slow cellular proliferation in solid tumors is by calculating the percentage of cells in **S-phase**. This abbreviation refers to the "synthesis phase," that period in which an individual cell duplicates its chromosomal DNA in preparation for its division into two daughter cells. In any tissue specimen, many more cells will be found in S-phase than can be detected undergoing mitosis. The final process of one cell becoming two takes only a few minutes, but S-phase can occupy a full day or more. Dr. Meyer has cited a ballpark average of "near 19 hours" for the S-phase of breast cancer cells, concluding that "the number of S-phase cells is clearly approximately 20 times the number of M-phase cells (those undergoing mitosis) at any given time."[30] Counting S-phase cells would not be like looking for needles in haystacks, but this cellular synthetic activity is not normally visible under the microscope. Visualization first became possible through the technique of **thymidine labeling**, which was perfected in the 1970s. Thymidine, a chemical base, is one of the necessary components (or building blocks) of DNA. As such, it is readily absorbed by cells duplicating their DNA—that is, by cells in S-phase—but not by cells in other phases of the cell cycle. Thymidine is "labeled" (made traceable) by combining it with the radioactive isotope tritium. In this assay small pieces of a tumor, each about one cubic millimeter in size, are incubated with the radiolabeled thymidine in an oxygen-rich atmosphere (oxygen being a prerequisite for DNA synthesis). Subsequently the tiny specimens are embedded in paraffin, sectioned, and photographed by autoradiography. The nuclei of cells in S-phase would appear black on the developed autoradiographs, because they would have taken up the radiolabeled thymidine. As with mitotic indexing, the pathologist's job now becomes one of close visual inspection and accurate enumeration. The **thymidine labeling index** (TLI) is expressed as the ratio of S-phase cells (those with thymidine-labeled nuclei) to the total number of cells counted.

During the 1980s the prognostic significance of S-phase in breast malignancies, as measured by thymidine labeling, became much clearer. John S. Meyer demonstrated that S-phase readings can vary several-fold among different histological subtypes. The better-prognosis variants of infiltrating carcinoma (tubular, mucinous, papillary) usually reveal low S-phase readings. But the unpropitious comedo form of ductal carcinoma *in situ* typically has a high S-phase reading or TLI, about three times as great as the favorable cribriform and micropapillary varieties of DCIS. According to Dr. Meyer's analysis, S-phase expressed by TLI correlates neatly with nuclear grade. The TLI of invasive breast tumors exhibiting poor nuclear grade

(224 specimens studied) proved to be about four times that of comparable tumors with good nuclear grade (207 specimens studied).[31] These broad differences in S-phase activity are associated with marked variations in disease recurrence and overall survival. Rosella Silvestrini and her colleagues at Milan's Cancer Institute followed 258 node-negative patients treated by mastectomy between 1972 and 1981. Of those patients judged to have low S-phase (low TLI), 80.5% remained disease-free six years after surgery; but only 59.6% of those patients with high S-phase (high TLI) avoided a relapse. Silvestrini et al concluded that high S-phase is "a marker of risk in patients with node-negative tumors." The danger would seem to be especially pronounced for premenopausal women, whose mammary cells have higher proliferation rates even before any malignant transformation. In this study only 9.8% of the premenopausal patients with low S-phase readings died of recurrent breast cancer during the six-year follow-up, but 30.1% of those with high readings succumbed.[32]

Dr. Silvestrini and her team subsequently performed thymidine labeling assays on the tumors taken from 523 node-positive patients treated in Milan. After a five-year follow-up, 34% of the patients with "slowly proliferating tumors" (low S-phase or TLI) had experienced recurrence, as had 50% of the patients with "rapidly proliferating tumors." At five years 85% of the patients with low S-phase were still alive, as were 73% of those with high S-phase. Silvestrini et al concluded that high S-phase (high TLI) identifies those node-positive patients "at high risk for early relapse"; however, they cautioned that a low reading offers no guarantee that metastases will not eventually occur.[33]

By the 1990s oncologists recognized that S-phase was an important prognostic factor in early-stage breast cancer, one that ought to be considered along with nodal status, tumor size, and ER content before making those difficult decisions about the advisability of chemotherapy. But thymidine labeling never became popular because it is too time-consuming. The process of thymidine incubation and autoradiography can take about two weeks, and afterwards the pathologist faces the arduous task of counting the labeled cells. Breast cancer specialists were understandably enthusiastic when a new automated assay called **flow cytometry** promised to deliver speedy evaluations of the S-phase of tumor specimens. Flow cytometry was originally developed back in the 1960s under the name "spectrophotometry," simply as a tinkertoy for research biologists. The technique works best with fresh tissue specimens, but frozen or paraffin-embedded samples can also be used. First, however, a tumor specimen has to be "disaggregated" (broken down) into its individual cells; this may be accomplished either by digestive enzymes or by mechanical means. The resulting suspension of cells is then incubated with a fluorescent dye which binds to the DNA in the cellular nuclei. A machine called a "cytometer" does the rest. The dissociated cells flow single-file under a powerful light beam, hundreds of cells per second. Each individual nucleus emits a pulse of fluorescence, whose intensity depends upon the quantity of DNA present. The more DNA in a cell's nucleus, the more fluorescent dye absorbed, and the stronger the emission. All these pulses of light, one for each of the thousands and thousands of cells, are recorded by a photosensitive device in the cytometer, being simultaneously transmitted as electric signals to a computer. The computer's software program performs a rapid analysis of these multitudinous pulses, yielding a printout reading of the specimen's **S-phase fraction**—that is, the percentage of its cells in S-phase.[34]

Since the early 1990s pathologists have also had immunohistochemical assays to use in estimating tumor growth rates. The **monoclonal antibody Ki-67** binds to an elusive protein which is expressed in the nuclei of actively replicating cells (those in S-phase or undergoing mitosis), but not in the nuclei of resting cells. All the pathologist has to do is to treat a specimen slide with the Ki-67 reagent, and then total up the number of positive (stained) nuclei to arrive at a "labeling index" (estimate of the growth rate). We soon discovered that the proliferation estimates obtained by Ki-67 immunostaining correlate quite well with those obtained by mitotic indexing and DNA flow cytometry. But one noticeable drawback to the technique is that Ki-67 will react only with fresh or frozen tissue specimens. Fortunately, a newer monoclonal antibody called **MIB-1** can detect the telltale nuclear protein in paraffin-embedded specimens (permanent sections).[35]

Like other immunostaining assays, tests with Ki-67 or MIB-1 are relatively inexpensive and quick; and they require just the smallest sliver of tumor. Sampling errors do not occur, because the pathologist can see whether the positive (stained) cells are actually breast cancer cells. The usual complaints can be lodged—viz., that the evaluation of staining intensities tends to be subjective, and that the expression of results (grading) is not precisely quantitative. In 1994, however, a team of Italian researchers reported that they had developed a "computer-assisted image analysis system" for breast cancer specimens stained with Ki-67 or MIB-1. While the new system needs a few manual interventions, the computer program "allows automatic nuclear counting, detects positive nuclei, and measures their staining intensity."[36] In the future, standardized grading by an automated system could make immunostaining reports more acceptable to practicing oncologists. At the moment, neither flow cytometry nor immunostaining can lay claim to perfect accuracy. But given the unquestionable importance of proliferation rates in breast cancer prognosis, all invasive tumors ought to be tested by at least one of these useful assays.

PLOIDY:
Quantifying a Cell's DNA

Flow cytometry can also give us an estimate of a tumor specimen's **ploidy**. This term refers to the chromosomal composition of the individual cells—**diploid cells** having the expected number of chromosomes for the species in question, and **aneuploid cells** having an abnormal number (usually too many). Cytometric readings for both ploidy and the S-phase fraction are based on the quantity of DNA present in cellular nuclei, but they are not the same thing. S-phase cells contain more DNA because they are duplicating their chromosomes in preparation for mitosis; thus an S-phase fraction is a measurement of the tumor's growth rate. Aneuploid cells contain more DNA because they have duplicated their chromosomes without a subsequent mitosis; thus ploidy is a measure of cellular functionality. Aneuploid nuclei, swollen and distorted by superfluous sets of chromosomes, are frequently encountered in advanced malignancies.

Ploidy and the S-phase fraction possess prognostic import for every type of cancer. Flow cytometry has proven especially suitable for the analysis of leukemias and lymphomas, because these tumor specimens (white blood cells) are disaggregated at the outset. The technique's potential in evaluating breast cancers has been championed by the late William L. McGuire and his colleagues at the University of Texas in San Antonio. In 1985 Dr. McGuire and Lynn G. Dressler announced in the *Journal of the National Cancer Institute* that "the determination of S-phase fraction and aneuploidy can now be implemented in the clinical setting. After a preparation of a single cell suspension, the DNA content of 100,000 cells can be measured by flow cytometry in a few minutes."[37] In 1989 Gary M. Clark, Dressler, McGuire, and other San Antonio researchers called attention to flow cytometry with an article in the *New England Journal of Medicine*. They reported that they had performed flow cytometric measurements of ploidy and S-phase "on 395 specimens of node-negative breast cancer from our bank of frozen tumors." Ploidy proved to be the most significant indicator of prognosis in this group. About 88% of the patients with diploid tumors remained disease-free five years after treatment, but only 74% of those patients with aneuploid tumors stayed healthy. Clark et al found that S-phase fractions were especially helpful in predicting the likelihood of relapse among node-negative patients with diploid tumors: "The risk of recurrence among such patients with high S-phase was 4.0 times that among those with low S-phase." But node-negative patients "with diploid low S-phase tumors" were found to have "a particularly good prognosis." Clark and his colleagues suggested that "for such patients the risks and costs of adjuvant systemic therapy may outweigh the benefits."[38]

Not everybody shared the San Antonio team's confidence in flow cytometric analysis. Michael J. Kornstein of the Medical College of Virginia was one of many physicians who worried about the lack of uniformity among laboratories using flow cytometry. Kornstein wrote the *New England Journal of Medicine*: "The percentage of cells in S-phase in solid tumors is difficult to measure

meaningfully. The numbers obtained by Clark et al cannot be used to evaluate results obtained by other laboratories, particularly if those laboratories used different computer software."[39] Flow cytometry is also subject to sampling errors. The assay results will be misleading if the suspension of cells flowing through the machine contains too many nonmalignant cells—for example, too many of those fibroblasts (connective cells) and lymphocytes (white cells) which are usually found adjacent to breast tumors.

Ploidy is easier to determine by flow cytometry than S-phase, but then the value of ploidy in predicting recurrence and survival among breast cancer patients has been more controversial than S-phase. Researchers at the University of Leiden in Holland performed flow cytometry on 690 breast tumors, reaching different conclusions from those drawn by Clark and his colleagues. The Dutch team found that aneuploidy did not affect the outcome among 349 node-negative patients, although it had an adverse effect on both recurrence and survival in 341 node-positive patients. "Aneuploidy," surmised the Hollanders, "has predominantly a positive effect on the growth rate of occult distant metastases rather than on metastatic capacity."[40] While the prognostic implications of aneuploidy in breast malignancies may need further clarification, no one has ever suggested that this finding is auspicious.

EXPERIMENTAL ASSAYS
The Case of *Cathepsin D*

All sorts of esoterica are under investigation as prognostic markers in early-stage breast cancer. Much research has been focused on **growth factors** which stimulate cellular proliferation or on the **receptors** for them. The **epidermal growth factor receptor** is frequently mentioned in this regard. Then there are those minuscule quantities of rare proteins which have been implicated in angiogenesis or metastasis—would an assay for these proteins tell us whether an apparently localized breast tumor is actually spreading throughout the body? From time to time a scientific publication on one of these esoterica gets blazoned in the popular media (newspapers and television) as a great breakthrough in breast cancer prognostication. These reports typically prove to be overstated. There is no microscope which lets us observe the molecular alterations occurring in a malignant cell, but our problem in studying them is not simply a lack of visualization. The alterations are manifold; they will vary from cell to cell, and they are terribly difficult to measure with demonstrable accuracy. The results obtained by different laboratories using different assays can reveal appalling inconsistencies.

The case of **cathepsin D** illustrates how glowing initial reports of a breakthrough may be dimmed by subsequent investigations. Cathepsin D is a proteolytic enzyme which is present in small quantities in normal cells, and in larger quantities in malignant ones. In the late 1980s some researchers suspected that this surfeit of cathepsin D enabled malignant cells to perform those mysterious dissolutions of basement membranes and the extracellular matrix which are a prerequisite for tumor dissemination. If this were true, then a reading of a tumor's cathepsin D levels ought to give us a good clue to its metastatic potential. In 1989 the British medical journal *Lancet* published a study by a team of French researchers who had assayed cathepsin D concentrations in the tumors from 122 breast cancer patients. Of those 94 patients judged to have low levels of this enzyme, only 20 (about 21.3%) developed metastases during a median follow-up of 4.6 years. In contrast, 20 of the 28

patients judged to have high levels—about 71.4%—developed metastases during follow-up. Given the study's small size, we may doubt its statistical power; but the authors were emphatic in describing its implications. "Cathepsin D," they asserted, "is unique in its association with breast cancer which has a high risk of metastasis. Cathepsin D concentration can be used to identify patients who may benefit from adjuvant therapy."[41]

In the United States the breast cancer team at the University of Texas did much to bring cathepsin D to the public's attention. The San Antonio researchers ran to their iceboxes and retrieved frozen tumor specimens taken from 397 patients. Enzyme concentrations were compared with the relevant patient histories. On February 1, 1990, the *New England Journal of Medicine* published the study's findings. High levels of cathepsin D did not seem predictive of outcome for the 198 node-positive patients, but looked quite ominous for the 199 node-negative patients. After a median follow-up of 64 months, the node-negative patients with high cathepsin D levels revealed 2.6 times the risk of recurrence and 3.9 times the risk of death compared to comparable node-negative patients with low levels of this enzyme. Like the French scientists, the Texans were adamant about the implications: "In multivariate analyses, a high level of cathepsin D was the most important independent factor in predicting shorter disease-free and overall survival in patients with node-negative disease."[42]

Patients and physicians rushed to embrace the new prognostic marker. At the Consensus Development Conference on breast cancer treatments held in June 1990, the panel chairman William C. Wood observed that various commercial laboratories were already offering cathepsin D assays and that "patients are coming in clutching assay reports."[43] But the cathepsin D euphoria proved to be short-lived. Some subsequent studies tended to confirm the findings from France and Texas; but others found no association, and at least one found that high levels of cathepsin D were associated with an improved prognosis. The San Antonio team planned a more elaborate study which would hopefully corroborate their first publication and resolve the growing controversy. This time they retrieved 927 frozen specimens from their tumor bank, all taken from node-negative patients; and they painstakingly measured the levels of cathepsin D expression, using both the traditional Western blot assay and an improved monoclonal antibody for immunostaining. When the Texans published their new results in 1994, they had to make a surprising admission: "We were unable to demonstrate that cathepsin D expression correlates with disease-free survival or overall survival." They speculated that subtle differences in assay methodology might be responsible for the tremendous discrepancy between their two studies: "Our results show the danger of extrapolating the value of a prognostic marker between studies where the marker is evaluated by different assay methods."[44] The second San Antonio report was not acclaimed in the newspapers or on TV, but word of the Texans' about-face spread quickly among cancer researchers. The *Journal of the National Cancer Institute* observed that "the use of cathepsin D is fraught with problems."[45]

Bone Marrow Sampling

The fate of cathepsin D suggests why it may be a long time before any assay measuring cellular proteins will appear on that pedestal where generations of surgeons and pathologists have placed nodal status. But one experimental assay which might have the potential to rival the time-honored sampling

of axillary nodes would seem to be **bone marrow sampling**. Both these "samplings" rest upon the same basic assumption. Viz., when we find breast cancer cells outside the affected breast, we have solid evidence that malignant dissemination has already taken place, and we should conclude that there is a possibility that destructive metastases will eventually appear in other organs. With the newer assay, we're simply checking a different extramammary site—one which is entirely plausible and easily accessible. Metastatic breast cancers almost invariably spread to the bone marrow. Osseous metastases predominate with sluggish postmenopausal tumors; but even in those cases where death results from rapidly progressive metastases to the lungs, liver, or brain, postmortem examinations often turn up evidence of subclinical marrow involvement.

In adults the active bone marrow is concentrated in the porous latticelike interiors of the sternum (breastbone), ribs, vertebrae, and ilia (hip bones). Marrow is a soft jellylike substance teaming with cellular life—it's the birthplace and nursery of all the millions of blood cells, both red and white, that must be generated daily if the body is to survive. Unfortunately, malignant cells shed by solid tumors into the lymphatic channels or blood vessels are likely to be carried to the marrow, where they can easily come to rest. Pathologists Taylor and Cote observe: "The bone marrow vasculature consists of a unique sinusoidal system that may simply act as a filter that traps or concentrates malignant cells."[46] Not every tumor cell which might journey to the marrow will form a metastatic lesion there, but visiting breast cancer cells always merit concern. We may surmise that most breast cancer cells reaching the marrow have first traveled through the lymphatic channels and nodes located in the axilla, prior to entering the subclavian blood veins. But taking a routine blood sample to look for circulating cancer cells in early-stage disease would be a needle-in-the-haystack quest— the chances of finding any are remote. Until recently the likelihood of identifying tumor cells arrested in the bone marrow was also very small. Extracting a marrow sample has always been easy enough; a large-bore needle inserted into the sternum or iliac crest (top of the hip bone) will provide an aspirated specimen which can be smeared on the pathologist's glass slides. But the customary staining procedures are not especially helpful in distinguishing between all those multitudinous blood cells which properly inhabit the marrow and the occasional tumor cell which has no business being there. The development of monoclonal antibodies provided a solution: since the early 1980s we have had reagents which would react with particular antigens expressed on the surface membranes or in the cytoplasms of epithelial cells. Henceforth a pathologist looking at a marrow smear under a microscope could easily detect any extraneous tumor cells—(these would be epithelial cells)—because they would be brightly stained by the colored reagent used. The blood cells native to the marrow would not be stained because they do not express the particular antigens that the reagents bind to.[47]

British physicians affiliated with the Ludwig Institute for Cancer Research (London branch) were the first to demonstrate that these immunostaining techniques could effectively identify breast cancer "micrometastases" in the bone marrow. In the *Lancet* for December 3, 1983, they reported that 28 of 110 patients undergoing an initial surgery for early-stage breast cancer had tested positive: "The number of tumor cells detected ranged from one to more than 500; none were detected in conventionally stained specimens."[48] Naturally everybody wanted to know whether positive marrow assays at the time of diagnosis possessed long-term

prognostic significance. In New York City pathologists at Memorial Sloan-Kettering tested 51 patients undergoing surgery, correlating the results with nodal status. Breast cancer cells were detected in the marrow of 27% of the node-negatives (6 of 22 patients) and 41% of the node-positives (12 of 29 patients). Not only did more node-positive patients test positive on the new assay, but those who did typically had more cancer cells detectable in their bone marrow than the node-negatives who tested positive.[49]

In 1985 the Ludwig Institute group in London reported that the women in their expanding study who had tested positive were more prone to recurrence than those who had tested negative. The number of cells found in the marrow seemed to have prognostic import: "Patients with fewer than 20 cancer cells present are relapsing faster than those with no cancer cells but slower than those with 20 or more."[50] Two years later the Ludwig researchers announced that positive assay results at diagnosis indicated an elevated risk for subsequent osseous involvement: "Ten out of 19 patients (53%) who developed bone metastases at first relapse had micrometastases at presentation."[51] But the London team's study took an unexpected turn; in 1989 they reported a finding that they had not anticipated. They retested some of the patients originally judged marrow positive "at a median time of 18 months after surgery." Surprisingly, only two of the 21 patients retested still had detectable cancer cells in their bone marrow. In the others the cancer cells seemed to have vanished—at least from the marrow! The London team hypothesized that while the breast tumors of these 19 patients had indeed been shedding malignant cells, the surgery had effectively removed the source of the circulating cells. And those cells already present in the marrow before surgery might just have died out.[52] This novel finding should remind us that although one or two positive axillary nodes or a few cancer cells in the bone marrow do give incontrovertible evidence of tumor dissemination, they may not always identify a tumor as a metastatic tiger. Not every malignant cell arriving in systemic circulation is going to have the potential for metastatic evolution—probably most of them will never acquire that capacity. Tumor cells found lingering in the marrow a year or two after surgery may be a more valid indicator of impending metastasis than cells detected at the time of the original diagnosis. The Ludwig Institute researchers concluded that the tumor cells they had found in patients undergoing surgery were simply "circulating" rather than "aspirated from an actual deposit."[53]

But breast cancer cells in the bone marrow are hardly a propitious sign. The Memorial Sloan-Kettering pathologists kept tabs on the 51 patients they had assayed: "The estimated two-year recurrence rate for patients with no bone marrow micrometastases (BMM) was 3%; in patients with BMM, the two-year recurrence rate was 33%. Bone marrow tumor burden was related to early recurrence. Among patients with BMM, those who did not recur had on average fewer extrinsic cells in their marrow than those who recurred (15 versus 43 cells, respectively)."[54] For a larger study with longer follow-up, we are indebted to Ingo J. Diel and other German physicians at the Women's Hospital of the University of Heidelberg, who have been taking bone marrow samples from breast cancer patients undergoing an initial surgery since 1985. In the *Journal of the National Cancer Institute* for November 20, 1996, Dr. Diel and his colleagues analyzed data gathered from 727 patients. Cancer cells were detected in the marrow of 112 of 360 node-negative patients (a 31% rate), and of 203 of 367 node-positive patients

(a 55% rate). At a median follow-up of 36 months, 143 patients had developed distant metastases; and of these patients, 109—or 76%—had recorded positive marrow assays at the time of surgery. Those patients who assayed positive proved to be at higher risk of metastases not only in the skeletal framework, but elsewhere in the body. Marrow positivity was intimately associated with increasing nodal involvement, with larger tumor size, and with higher (poorer) histological grade. This German study by Diel et al differed from the American and British investigations in firmly asserting that marrow positivity is "an independent prognostic indicator" both for disease-free survival and for overall survival, and that it is "superior" to nodal status in this regard. For those breast tumors smaller than two centimeters in diameter, Diel and his colleagues found the presence of cancer cells in the marrow to be "the most powerful predictor of outcome."[55]

None of the aforementioned studies was a randomized clinical trial which might definitively establish the prognostic superiority of bone marrow sampling over axillary node dissections. The patients in these studies underwent both types of assay. If some future trial should prove that marrow sampling consistently provides better prognostic information than that obtained by axillary dissection, we might be able to dispense with the latter examination in many cases. Marrow sampling has become a safe outpatient procedure which can usually be completed in less than an hour. Serious complications are unlikely.[56] Patients experience a sore hip or breastbone, but these symptoms resolve within a week. The body quickly replaces the aspirated marrow, and there are no long-term side effects.

GENETIC ANALYSIS
Looking at *p53* and HER-2/*neu*

Malignancies originate in genetic defects. Those discrete lengths of DNA which code for cellular proteins, popularly known as "genes," can malfunction in many different ways, producing diverse disease manifestations. In theory, the genetic analysis of tumor cells ought to give us our essential staging factors, which would carry far more prognostic import than the traditional gross assessments of tumor size and nodal status. In practice, genetic analysis has become crucial in staging the leukemias and lymphomas, and in selecting the best therapies for them. For breast malignancies and the other solid tumors, however, genetic analysis might be described as a promising area of research rather than as a mature science. Breast cancer researchers have tended to focus their investigations on two highly-publicized genes, *p53* and HER-2/*neu*. The first of these had been implicated in so many different malignancies that it began to look like a universal cancer gene. *Newsweek* ran a cover story featuring *p53* as "THE CANCER KILLER," thus bringing a bit of molecular biology to popular attention.[57]

As discussed in Chapter Three, *p53* is a tumor suppressor gene located on the short arm of chromosome 17. When it is functioning properly, it acts as a regulator of the cell cycle, keeping a cell from needlessly entering S-phase and hastening toward mitosis. When *p53* is damaged by a point mutation, it may encode an abnormal, nonfunctional protein, allowing a cell to remain constantly in the reproductive mode. References to the "overexpression" of *p53* protein refer exclusively to abnormal versions of this protein, which typically have extended half-lives and accumulate as ineffectual deposits in cellular

nuclei. Most studies of *p53* in cancer prognosis have not attempted to identify the point mutations in the DNA, but have simply tried to determine whether the nuclei of the cancer cells contained the abnormal protein. This determination is much easier. Immunostaining with a monoclonal antibody directed against the protein imparts a bright colorization to the nuclei so treated. The normal *p53* protein has a short half-life and does not accumulate in the cell's nuclei. Positive nuclear staining thus indicates a problem with the gene and its product.

Most *p53* malfunctions have been detected in advanced malignancies. But breast cancer specialists are also interested in them as pivotal events in early-stage disease. The molecular clarification of the Li-Fraumeni syndrome has established that germline (hereditary) mutations of *p53* can strongly predispose women to early-onset breast cancer.[58] Did sporadic (nonhereditary) mutations in this gene likewise chart a course toward tumorigenesis? More importantly, could they tell us which seemingly localized breast tumors were actually prone to metastasize? In search of answers, those dedicated researchers at the University of Texas in San Antonio delved into their famous iceboxes and retrieved frozen tumor specimens from 700 node-negative patients. Expression of mutant *p53* protein was then evaluated by immunostaining. The Texans soon reported that *p53* overexpression as indicated by positive immunostaining was directly correlated with a high proliferation rate (high S-phase). "Both factors were independently associated with poor prognosis, suggesting that *p53* may have other biological functions in addition to cell-cycle regulation." Five years after treatment, 80% of the 388 patients judged "negative" for the mutant protein remained disease-free (no apparent recurrences); and 72% of 263 patients judged "low-positive" for the protein were similarly healthy. But only 58% of those 99 patients deemed "high-positive" for *p53* overexpression were free of recurrent cancer. The five-year survival statistics were analogous—88% for the negatives, 84% for the low-positives, and 74% for the high-positives.[59]

Rosella Silvestrini and her colleagues at Italy's National Cancer Institute in Milan also reported that *p53* overexpression "is an independent marker for shortened relapse-free and overall survival in node-negative breast patients." The Milan group had tested 256 paraffin-embedded specimens, passing a verdict of overexpression whenever more than 5% of the nuclei stained positive. "The hazard of relapse was consistently three times higher for patients with *p53*-overexpressing tumors, up to the fourth year from mastectomy."[60]

Mutant *p53* protein is also an inauspicious marker in node-positive breast cancer. A study of node-positive tumors done at the Mayo Clinic in Rochester, Minnesota, found perceptible nuclear staining for *p53* to be "associated with negative estrogen receptor (ER) status, high (poor) nuclear grade, and high (poor) histologic grade."[61] Dr. Silvestrini and her Milan colleagues reported comparable findings based upon the immunostaining of tumor specimens from 240 postmenopausal patients: "Relapse-free and distant metastasis-free survival at five years were significantly lower for patients with tumors that highly expressed *p53*." According to Silvestrini et al, *p53* overexpression in node-positive breast cancer "provided prognostic information independent of tumor size, axillary node involvement, steroid receptors, and thymidine labeling index."[62]

No one could doubt that a malfunctioning *p53* gene was a bad omen in any breast malignancy; but since this finding tended to be closely associated with so many other negative factors, some researchers wondered whether it provided significant additional information. Do we really need a *p53* assay if we already know tumor size, nuclear and histological grades, nodal status, ER, PgR, and S-phase? Foremost among the skeptics were Paul Peter Rosen and his colleagues at Memorial Sloan-Kettering, who used immunostaining to assay "formaldehyde-fixed, paraffin-embedded primary invasive carcinomas from 440 node-negative patients." Rosen et al found that *p53* overexpression occurred most often in the commonplace ductal carcinomas NOS and in fast-growing medullary carcinomas, and that it tended to be associated with poor nuclear grade and with ER-negativity. Mutant *p53* protein was rarely detected in the better-prognosis tumor subspecies, namely the "tubular, papillary, pure lobular, or duct carcinoma with lobular features." When the Sloan-Kettering team correlated the assay results with the patients' case histories (median follow-up of 119 months), they found nothing to hoot about. "The presence or absence of *p53* expression alone," Rosen and his colleagues concluded, "cannot be considered a reliable prognostic indicator independently in node-negative breast carcinoma."[63]

The discrepancies between the various studies of *p53* in breast malignancies may be partially attributed to the limitations of immunohistochemical techniques. The protein's antigen intensity—that is, its reactivity with reagents—quickly diminishes in paraffin slides stored at room temperature, creating a possibility of false-negative results. Immunoreactivity is retained better in tumor specimens which are either frozen or kept in paraffin blocks.[64] Other factors can also influence assay findings, including the type of fixative used to preserve the specimen and the particular reagent applied to it. The biggest shortcoming is the lack of a uniform system for grading *p53* overexpression. No two research groups seem to have used precisely the same criterion for declaring tumors negative or positive, making comparisons of the different studies problematic. Citing "insufficient data," the American Society of Clinical Oncology has declined to recommend the routine use of *p53* assays in breast cancer staging.[65]

*   *   *

The HER-2/*neu* oncogene, also known as *erb*B-2, is located on the same chromosome (number 17) as *p53*, but it illustrates a different mechanism of tumorigenesis. As we've seen in Chapter Three, HER-2 acts as an accelerator of cellular proliferation—it encodes a growth factor receptor for the cell's outer membrane. Problems with this gene do not occur because its protein is mutant and nonfunctional (as in the case of *p53*). They come about whenever the normal protein is present in excessive quantities, a condition which by itself promotes undue mitotic activity. DNA analysis typically reveals the cause of the protein surfeit to be **amplification** (i.e., too many copies of the gene encoding for the protein). But most studies correlating breast cancer prognosis with excessive HER-2 protein have relied on the simpler immunohistochemical methodology rather than on DNA analysis. The more pronounced the immunostaining of the cancer cells' outer membranes, the more protein we may assume to be present.

The groundbreaking publications by Dennis J. Slamon and his UCLA co-workers in 1987 and 1989 stimulated international interest in HER-2/*neu*. An early Japanese study found that amplification of this gene was "a prognostic factor independent of tumor size and nodal status," and that an increasing number of gene copies strongly correlated "with both degree of nuclear

atypia and number of mitotic figures." Yet HER-2 amplification does not play a role in most breast cancers. The Tokyo team found evidence of it only in 28 of the 176 specimens they tested, a 15.9% rate, and these cases were all infiltrating ductal carcinomas.[66] Researchers in London used immunostaining to compare the rates of HER-2 overexpression in the different types of breast cancer, and they reported "the almost consistent absence of immunostaining in the uncommon histological varieties." None of the 33 lobular carcinomas they assayed revealed excessive HER-2 expression; the better-prognosis variants of ductal carcinoma (tubular, medullary, mucinous, papillary) also proved negative. And only 14 of the 63 ductal carcinomas NOS (22%) were positive. The London team concluded that overexpression of the HER-2 receptor protein "is mainly seen in a subgroup of ductal tumors, and that almost all other histological types, especially those associated with good prognosis, lack this expression."[67] The genetic malfunction may well be an early event in this subgroup, occurring before the tumors become invasive. Researchers at the Netherlands Cancer Institute consistently detected HER-2 overexpression in the unpropitious comedo variety of ductal carcinoma *in situ*—all 19 specimens the Amsterdam team examined tested positive. In contrast, none of the favorable DCIS variants assayed—16 specimens of "small-cell, papillary, or cribriform growth type"—revealed positive membrane staining.[68]

Most studies of HER-2/*neu* and breast cancer prognosis have supported the original conclusion of Slamon's UCLA team—viz., that protein overexpression points toward early recurrence and shortened survival in node-positive patients, but does not seem to be especially predictive in node-negative patients. In 1992, however, the San Antonio group published a notable study dissenting from this majority opinion. The Texans had first stratified 613 node-negative tumor specimens "into low-risk and high-risk groups on the basis of tumor size and estrogen-receptor (ER) status." An independent prognostic value for HER-2 immunostaining became apparent only in a subset analysis performed on 179 patients judged "low-risk," all of whom had ER-positive invasive tumors smaller than three centimeters in diameter. After a median follow-up of 5.1 years, over 80% of the 165 low-risk patients whose tumors did not overexpress the HER-2 protein remained free of disease (no detectable recurrences). In contrast, only 43% of the 14 low-risk patients with positive membrane staining were still disease-free. The San Antonio team surmised that HER-2 overexpression might thus identify a small subset of node-negative patients with good-risk features (e.g., small tumor size and ER-positivity) who are actually at considerable risk of developing metastatic disease.[69]

Another intriguing finding which emerged from the San Antonio study concerned the relationship between HER-2 overexpression and tumor responsiveness to chemotherapy. The Texans looked closely at 75 node-negative patients classified "high-risk," with tumors which were ER-negative and/or over three centimeters in size. All these patients had tested positive for HER-2 overexpression—40 of them got chemotherapy after surgery, 35 of them did not. But a subset analysis performed after a five-year follow-up revealed no difference in the recurrence rates between those who received the chemo and those who didn't. While conceding that the number of patients was too small to draw definite conclusions, the San Antonio team wondered whether HER-2 overexpression was responsible for the lack of benefit from adjuvant therapy: "An involvement of this oncogene in drug resistance

might also partially explain why most studies of node-positive disease find an association between HER-2/*neu* and poor clinical outcome, as these patients routinely receive adjuvant chemotherapy."[70] Any mechanisms by which HER-2 might promote drug resistance have yet to be deciphered, but several subsequent analyses of patient outcome have reached the same conclusion. Canadian researchers tracking 888 node-positive patients on a long-term basis (2.5 to 10.5 years of follow-up) reported that HER-2 overexpression proved to be "an independent prognostic factor," but was "useful in predicting survival time only in patients receiving adjuvant chemotherapy, thus suggesting that it may be a marker of drug resistance."[71] On May 5, 1994, the *New England Journal of Medicine* published the results from an American clinical trial relating the effectiveness of different doses of chemotherapy to different levels of HER-2 expression. For this study 442 women with node-positive breast cancer (Stage Two) had been randomly assigned to receive "high, moderate, or low" doses of CAF, a standard regimen using cyclophosphamide, Adriamycin (brand name for doxorubicin), and fluorouracil. There was "no clear evidence of a dose-response effect" in those patients with little or no positive immunostaining. But those patients whose tumors noticeably overexpressed the HER-2 protein had "significantly longer disease-free and overall survival" if they received the highest dose of CAF. The trial investigators suggested that HER-2 overexpression "may indeed be a marker of relative resistance to chemotherapy, but an escalation of the dose may overcome that resistance."[72]

By the mid-1990s everybody knew that HER-2/*neu* overexpression was often associated with nasty ductal carcinomas, those metastatic tigers which are responsible for the lion's share of breast cancer mortality. But not a few researchers wondered how "independent" this indicator really was, since HER-2 overexpression typically occurs in a context of other ominous findings. The aforementioned Canadian study discovered that "positive membrane staining was correlated with more involved lymph nodes, aneuploidy, poor nuclear and histologic grades, absence of estrogen and progesterone receptor content, and cathepsin D expression." The aforementioned American trial found a correlation between HER-2 overexpression and high S-phase. Unfortunately, the immunostaining assays being used to evaluate the oncogene's status had not been standardized. And as the literature on HER-2 increased, so did the number of conflicting judgments on its prognostic utility.[73] We may safely assert that the gene's role in mammary cells, both normal and malignant, needs further clarification. Why is HER-2 overexpressed much more often in ductal carcinomas than in lobular ones? How can this gene be deemed responsible for drug resistance, when conventional wisdom holds that undifferentiated, rapidly proliferating tumors are more responsive to chemo? Given our present uncertainties, the results from any HER-2 assay done for staging purposes must be interpreted with caution.

A Quiz for Readers

To those readers who have found this chapter overly long and technical, the author has only to say—"Just try reading all those articles cited in my notes to know the true meaning of the words <u>LONG</u> and <u>TECHNICAL</u>." This chapter simply presents the highlights from a humongous body of research attempting to identify reliable methods of distinguishing between those early-stage breast cancers which are going to metastasize, and

those which have little chance of doing so. No single prognostic indicator, nor all of them together, can offer us complete certainty in making this crucial distinction. Nobody can infallibly predict whether any given breast tumor is—or is not—going to metastasize. But patients and physicians who know and ponder their indicators have at least a rational basis for making treatment decisions.

Back in the "old days"—before 1975—breast cancer staging tended to be an academic exercise, just something for the medical records. The treatment was essentially one and the same (radical mastectomy), whatever the prognosis might be. These days we know a lot more about the diverse natural histories of the different types of breast malignancy; and the correct staging—that is, the plausible forecasting of a given tumor's evolution—ought to affect the choice of treatment. Our prognostic indicators must lead us toward a reasonable answer to a therapeutic riddle of urgent import. **Is systemic therapy advisable, and if so, what kind?** The available options range from high-dose cytotoxic regimens to gentle anti-estrogenic drugs like tamoxifen. Cytotoxic chemotherapy and tamoxifen have been proven to extend survival for many patients, but there is presently no adjuvant therapy which we could describe as "routinely and predictably curative." Systemic therapy, even with tamoxifen, may involve considerable expense and unwanted side effects; therefore it should be reserved for patients with unfavorable prognostic indicators. In some cases the indicators are so uniformly ominous that everyone, surgeons and oncologists alike, would agree on the advisability of chemotherapy. But in many other cases the indicators leave ample room for divergent interpretations, and the recommendation a patient will receive may well depend upon which door in the hospital she happens to open. In all cases of *in situ* breast cancer and in most cases of small Stage One tumors, there is no indication for cytotoxic therapy—the odds are that these patients would be harmed more by the chemo than by their cancers. Such presumably localized tumors have been presumably arrested by surgery, either with or without irradiation of the affected breast. The use of tamoxifen as a prophylactic in these localized cases—that is, solely as preventive measure against the development of new primary tumors either in the affected breast or in the contralateral one—can be rationally advocated only when we know that the original lesion was estrogen receptor-positive.

Treatment decisions in breast malignancies have necessarily become much more complex, because the number of prognostic indicators and therapeutic alternatives has increased dramatically since the early 1970s. Needless to say, only an informed patient can meaningfully participate in treatment decisions, or know when to seek another opinion. Are you adequately prepared to talk with an oncologist? The following **two-part** **quiz** should test whether you, the reader, have retained sufficient information from our chapters on pathology and staging. All you need to do is to decide whether cytotoxic chemotherapy would be indicated for the two cases described below.

CASE NUMBER ONE is drawn from life. A patient went to I. Craig Henderson, one of the nation's mostly highly respected oncologists, "for a consultation regarding her adjuvant therapy." As Dr. Henderson recalled in the *New England Journal of Medicine*, this patient had "a small diploid tumor with a very low S-phase fraction, a high estrogen-receptor level, and a very high progesterone-receptor level." In the way of treatment she had already received "six months of intensive adjuvant chemotherapy,

and her physician had recommended that she continue taking tamoxifen for life."[74] *What's wrong with this picture?* Why would Dr. Henderson be editorializing about it in the *Journal*, and wondering "how frequently such things happen"? If you do not immediately recognize that the tumor in question would seem to be a localized pussycat, and that the type of systemic therapy being given ought to be reserved for metastatic tigers, then you need to re-read Chapter Fourteen! That's a stiff penalty, but perhaps not so stiff as being on the receiving end of unnecessary chemotherapy.

CASE NUMBER TWO is a beast of a different stripe, entirely hypothetical but not at all mythological. The patient's pathology report begins with this brief synopsis: "Poorly differentiated ductal carcinoma NOS, 3 cm in diameter, with infiltrative border, central necrosis, and adjacent lymphatic invasion. Pleomorphic cells, enlarged nuclei with visible nucleoli, occasional mitotic figures." If you do not immediately recognize that any breast tumor fitting this description must be assumed to be a metastatic tiger, please re-read Chapter Twelve, our little introduction to pathological analysis. The surgical excision of this particular tumor has probably failed to arrest the disease, and the aforementioned "six months of intensive adjuvant chemotherapy" (wrongly prescribed for Case Number One) might be considered an appropriate option.

It is noteworthy that in this second case we reached a reasonable conclusion without any knowledge of ER status, S-phase, ploidy, *p53* mutations, or any other of those newfangled prognostic indicators that began to be emphasized in the 1980s. Old-fashioned pathology work—i.e., attentive microscopy of H&E-stained permanent sections—told us what we needed to know. The **tumor size** of three centimeters should by itself set off alarm bells when the malignant species is a ductal carcinoma NOS (not otherwise specified). While we did not know the patient's nodal status, the determination of adjacent **lymphatic invasion** provides strong evidence that malignant cells have already begun to spread away from a primary tumor. **Central necrosis** and the observation of **mitotic figures** were both indicative of a high rate of cellular proliferation, and we could therefore assume a **high S-phase** even without doing flow cytometry. "Visible nucleoli" in "enlarged nuclei" warranted our assumption of **poor nuclear grade**.

Our quiz is finished. Please keep in mind that the two cases cited were rather obvious examples of the pussycat and the tiger. In less obvious cases physicians still place the most reliance on nodal status in making that crucial distinction between these species. But because axillary dissection can produce lasting side effects as well as prognostic information, this procedure is never indicated with purely *in situ* tumors, and its value in small invasive tumors with good features might be questioned. Any patient facing axillary surgery should earnestly inquire about the extent of the procedure and the reasons for it. **Sentinel node dissection** is a less invasive technique which can determine the likelihood of axillary involvement.

Historically, about 75% of Stage One (node-negative) patients have been cured by local therapy alone. Tumor size has been the major factor in deciding which subgroup of node-negative patients should receive chemo. The Consensus Development Conference held in 1990 concluded that "node-negative patients with tumors 1 cm or less have an excellent prognosis and do not require adju-

vant systemic therapy outside of clinical trials."[75] In deciding whether a node-negative patient might be at higher risk of recurrence, wise physicians also take into consideration her age and her family history. Youthful age (premenopausal) and a positive family history (mother or sister previously diagnosed) may tend to slant the balance toward chemotherapy.[76] The molecular indicators carrying the most weight in this matter are a negative ER status and a high S-phase; both point toward a fast-moving tumor which could metastasize but which would probably respond to cytotoxic therapy. However, since most node-negative patients with small tumors do not need systemic therapy, any patient in this category who receives a recommendation for chemotherapy should require some very convincing explanations from her physicians.

* * *

Our next chapter touches on the history of breast cancer treatments in the United States. This story is essentially one of progress, albeit *slow* progress. As we'll see, patients have long been subjected to deplorable *over*-treatments or *under*-treatments, or both. From 1900 to 1975 the customary surgical procedure used to obtain local control (radical mastectomy) represented needless overtreatment for almost all patients. At the same time patients at risk of metastatic disease were always undertreated, because we had only crude systemic therapies. Even today the specters of overtreatment or undertreatment remain frightening, especially with regard to chemotherapy. A misstep in either direction can do irreparable harm, and missteps are sure to occur if the pertinent staging assays are not conscientiously performed and interpreted.

Chapter Fifteen

BREAST CANCER SURGERY
From Antiquity to the NSABP

There is nothing new about breast cancers. They were the first malignancies mentioned in recorded history, for the obvious reason that the other commonplace tumors remain inside the body and hence out of sight. Physicians in ancient Egypt or Babylon would note the puzzling symptoms and recognize the gravity of these illnesses, but they usually had no clue to the underlying causes. They could not see the actual tumors. Malignancies of the stomach and pancreas were understood simply as relentless gnawing aches in the belly. Colon cancers were just bloody stools and difficulty in defecation—bladder and kidney tumors, just blood in the urine—cervical and endometrial cancers, just unexplained vaginal bleeding—and hepatic (liver) tumors, just a curious yellowing of the skin (jaundice). With most malignancies the doctors of antiquity saw only the secondary effects. But breast cancers represented a notable exception. Here the cause was all too appallingly visible—that hard lump which slowly grew and grew until it transformed the entire breast into an odorous and painful mass of necrotic tissue. The anguish and mortification of women with these locally advanced tumors can hardly be imagined. In ancient times there was no chance of prompt relief, for the

cancers were not immediately lethal (patients might survive for years), and the doctors had no effective palliation. The earliest known reference to breast cancer occurs in an Egyptian papyrus written about 3000 BC. The hieroglyphics tell us that there is "no treatment" for "bulging tumors of the breast" which are "cool to the touch" and "do not generate secretions of fluid."[1]

No doubt the physicians of Egypt and Babylon had frequent recourse to placebos, recommending the application of soothing oils or balms to give their patients a momentary glimpse of illusory hope. The Greeks and Romans also had to deal with mammary carcinomas; their remedies were not much better. Hippocrates mentioned breast tumors twice, without saying how they should be treated. Some five centuries later Galen, the great anatomist of Roman times, looked closely at developing breast tumors and then coined a name which remains current. He called them *cancer*—the Latin word for "crab"—because the hard tumor with tendrils radiating outward reminded him of a crab in its shell with outstretched claws. Galen also formulated a treatment strategy which is still fundamental. "Cut out the whole tumor," he advised, "so as not to leave a single root."[2] Unfortunately, breast surgery in the later

Roman Empire was only slightly less torturous than the crucifixions imposed upon criminals. Mastectomy involved a protracted round of incision and cautery, without benefit of anesthesia. The surgeon would cut a bit and then apply a red hot iron to staunch the bleeding—the process was repeated again and again, until the breast finally came off. No one kept statistics on the number of patients who were cured of their cancers or, indeed, even survived their operations. But the fact that women willingly submitted to these procedures should remind us of what a terrible affliction locally advanced breast cancer can be. Most physicians today will never have an opportunity to see a truly advanced tumor, unless they undertake missionary work in a very remote region of the globe.

From the Roman era to the late nineteenth century, progress in breast cancer surgery was almost imperceptible. During the seventeenth and eighteenth centuries, European surgeons tried to operate as rapidly as possible, thus minimizing the time that wide-awake patients would have to spend undergoing excruciating procedures. An ingenious German surgeon named Johann Schultes ("Scultetus" in Latin) recommended that leather thongs be sutured through the base of the affected breast prior to mastectomy. Once the operation was under way, an assistant would pull vigorously on the thongs while the surgeon hastily wielded his scalpel. The breast came off in a flash, but hemostasis (control of bleeding) was as primitive as ever, a hot iron being pressed against the surgical wound to achieve this end.[3]

Two innovations essential to effective surgery were made in the mid-nineteenth century—namely, the introduction of anesthesia in the 1840s and of antiseptic precautions in the 1860s. But several decades had to pass before surgeons fully grasped the importance of these discoveries. Most of them continued to operate as before, rapidly and with scant regard for the possibility of bacterial wound contamination. Mastectomy remained dangerous and ineffective, with much surgical morbidity as well as subsequent tumor recurrence in the operative field. A series of 170 mastectomies performed in Vienna between 1867 and 1876 yielded a depressing statistic—only eight patients were still alive three years after their operations. In 1891 the American writer Alice James— sister to the novelist Henry James and the philosopher William James—learned that the painful lump in her breast was malignant. "Nothing can be done but to alleviate the pain," said her doctor.[4] Alice died in 1892; if her breast tumor had presented a few years later, she might have had better prospects. During the 1890s mastectomy became not only a safe operation but also an effective way to stop a breast tumor's local progression. This unprecedented achievement was largely due to the efforts of a single American surgeon, whose life and legacy we need to examine in some detail.

Halsted's Radical Mastectomy

William Stewart Halsted (1852-1922) can be justly described as "the father of modern American surgery." Any American who has undergone a surgical procedure and survived it is greatly in his debt.[5] Halsted was born into a well-to-do family in New York City. In 1870 he entered Yale College, where he seems to have spent more time playing football and baseball than studying in the library. During his senior year at Yale, however, he developed an intense interest in medicine; and when he returned to New York, he enrolled in the College of Physicians and Surgeons. After he received his M.D. degree in 1877, he spent two years in Europe, studying the techniques and instruments being used by avant-garde surgeons in Germany and Austria. By the early 1880s he was a busy practitioner in New York, professionally respected and socially active. But this conventional career—that of a successful clinician—came to an abrupt end in 1886. Halsted had experimented with cocaine ("a remarkable new drug") and become addicted to it. Emotionally shattered and physically debilitated, he underwent a seven-month hospitalization for rehabilitation. These experiences changed his life in fundamental ways; thereafter he shied away from social activities, devoting himself to laboratory research and the solution of hitherto intractable surgical problems. The year 1889 proved fortuitous both for Halsted and for American surgery—he received an appointment to the new Johns Hopkins Hospital in Baltimore, a unique institution which specifically sought to encourage experimental medicine.

Halsted remained at Hopkins until his death in 1922, his growing reputation being inseparably interwoven with that of his institution. Some of the innovations that Halsted introduced at Hopkins seem so obvious to us today that we can hardly imagine that medicine was ever practiced without them. Those **hospital charts** at the foot of patients' beds recording variations in temperature and pulse rate, and those **rubber gloves** worn by surgeons and their helpers during operations, both had their origins in Halsted's brainstorms. But his most valuable contribution came not in the realm of medical supplies, but of operative methodology. Unlike his predecessors and most of his contemporaries, Halsted paid close attention to antiseptic precautions; and he took full advantage of the artificial sleep induced by anesthesia. The operations he performed became prolonged affairs; his movements were always deliberate and gentle, reflecting a profound knowledge of anatomy and an extreme desire to avoid unnecessary injury to delicate tissues.

At every step he took pains to maintain hemostasis, sealing off leaky blood vessels with sutures of fine silk rather than with the coarser catgut then in common use. And when closing the wound he sought to achieve a thorough reapproximation of the incised tissues. Halsted's contemporaries scoffed at the length of time he devoted to surgery—one of his mastectomies typically required five hours or more—but the fact is that his patients survived their operations. Moreover, they did not later succumb to postoperative infections or hemorrhages, those terrible sequelae of operating-room carelessness.

The list of operative procedures associated with Halsted's name is formidable. He was the first surgeon to devise an operation curing inguinal hernias, and he performed one of the earliest cholecystectomies (removal of stones from the gallbladder). He pioneered the use of implanted screws to stabilize fractures of the long bones, and his refined suturing techniques made surgery of the gastrointestinal tract feasible. But Halsted is most often remembered for the **radical mastectomy** that he frequently performed at Johns Hopkins. What was "radical" about the procedure is that it was not limited to the removal of the breast, nipple, and all glandular tissues—(today we would call this a "total" or "simple" mastectomy)—but that it also removed the underlying chest muscles (pectoralis major and minor) as well as the axillary lymph nodes. Why did Halsted advocate routine removal of the chest muscles? Some of the contemporary European surgeons, particularly the Germans, had observed that advanced breast carcinomas can spread to the **fascia** (fibrous membrane) overlying these muscles; but fear of fascial involvement was not the reason Halsted gave in an 1894 account of his procedure. It was necessary to remove the chest muscles, he explained, so as to do an *en bloc* resection of the entire breast, "lest the wound become infected by the division of tissue."[6] The outdated idea implicit in Halsted's choice of words ("infected") holds that cancer cells are like some bacterial contamination which could easily be spread about by the surgeon's scalpel. The possibility of mechanical dissemination, while not entirely discounted, is taken much less seriously today. In this instance Halsted's admirable traits of thoroughness and asepsis led to a pernicious overtreatment being established as standard practice. The chest muscles are not involved in early breast cancer (Stages One and Two); and their removal causes problems for the patient since they are needed to give the chest its normal rounded contour and to control arm movements.

Halsted's *en bloc* resection also included the contents of the axilla. A single incision encircling the breast was extended diagonally toward the shoulder so that the surgeon could remove all the axillary nodes. For Halsted and untold numbers of later American surgeons, the lymphatic dissemination of breast cancer cells was the main obstacle to overcome if patients were to be cured. The Halstedians thought they understood this matter perfectly. Malignancies beginning in the breast were assumed to spread in a predictable fashion—the cancer cells traveled first to the axillary lymph nodes, <u>which</u> <u>acted</u> <u>as</u> <u>barriers</u> <u>and</u> <u>temporarily</u> <u>prevented</u> <u>further</u> <u>dissemination</u>. After a while, however, the nodes were so thoroughly overrun by multiplying cancer cells that they ceased to function as barriers. They became instead sources of further dissemination, as the cancer cells escaped from their confines and began to establish metastatic colonies elsewhere. By excising all the nodes and the fatty tissues surrounding them, the surgeon would hopefully interrupt this process and thereby cure the patient. Today, of course, we regard these ideas as overly

simplistic—and we know that the regional lymph nodes are not effective as barriers, even on a temporary basis. But Halsted was emphatic about the need "to clean out the axilla," stressing it in his lectures and writings.

Subsequent generations of American surgeons tinkered with the placement of the mastectomy incision—but otherwise tended to accept Halsted's dictates without question. Radical mastectomy remained the operative procedure of choice for the next eight decades. We cannot blame Dr. Halsted for this appalling intellectual stasis—he was himself an innovator. He could proudly point out that 34 of the 76 breast cancer patients he treated at Johns Hopkins between 1889 and 1894 were alive and seemingly healthy three years after their surgery.[7] This 45% "cure rate" would be unimpressive if contrasted with present-day survival rates—but then it should be contrasted with the previously mentioned Vienna mastectomy series done between 1867 and 1876, which reported a paltry 4.7% "cure rate" (only eight of 170 patients alive at three years). Halsted's survival figures were the best that any surgeon had achieved up to that time. While the effectiveness of extensive local surgery in reducing distant metastases is questionable, no one can doubt that Halsted's operation did a good job of preventing recurrences on the chest wall and in the axilla. By and large he achieved local control. The rate of local recurrence he reported in 1894 was 6%, yet by current definitions about 18% of his patients would be deemed to have suffered a recurrence at or near the tumor site.[8] This second estimate will still impress us if we consider the sort of breast tumors Halsted had to deal with. He did not see the raisin-sized lesions that might be detected by modern mammography, or the cherry-sized lumps that might be discovered by manual breast examinations. The tumors he encountered were as large as plums or oranges, sometimes even grapefruits. In that era of false modesty and of general ignorance about bodily functions, women were unlikely to pay much attention to small breast lumps and sought medical treatment only for those larger ones which had become a source of embarrassment or pain. Like the surgeons of the Roman Empire, Halsted dealt exclusively with advanced disease—the sort of cases we would classify as Stage Three or Four.

It is difficult to understand Halsted's persistent influence on breast cancer surgery in the United States without remembering that he was a superb teacher as well as an anatomical technician. From 1892 until his death he held the post of Professor of Surgery at a medical school whose program for training surgical residents was a model of its kind. And the young surgeons who passed under Halsted's tutelage often became heads of surgical departments at other hospitals and universities. The Halsted-Hopkins alumni were more likely to teach future surgeons and to write textbooks than to become small-town practitioners. In this way Halsted's doctrines and methodology were powerfully transmitted as gospel truth to the entire surgical profession. Overall Halsted's legacy had positive effects on American surgical practice; but in the matter of breast carcinomas, it tended to discourage further scientific investigations. Here innovation was replaced by orthodoxy. Experimentation yielded to a veneration of the Halstedian tradition and an unquestioning adherence to its dogmas.

Some Surgical Heretics

By the 1920s inflexible procedures for diagnosing and treating breast cancers prevailed throughout the United States—viz., biopsy under general anesthesia, frozen section for instantaneous diagnosis, and an immediate *en bloc* mastectomy in response to any positive verdict, whereby the breast, chest muscles, and axillary nodes were removed with a single incision. Every effort was made to prevent even a single cancer cell from escaping the operative field. But in the 1920s the breast cancer cases encountered by surgeons were beginning to be different from those Halsted saw back in the 1890s. If tumors were still plum-sized at diagnosis, at least the plums were getting smaller. Public awareness of malignant disease was growing, thanks to a fledgling organization founded in 1913 under the name "American Society for the Control of Cancer"; it was later to be rechristened the **American Cancer Society**. The Society's unchanging leitmotif became apparent shortly after its birth—viz., cancer is a most terrible disease, but can be cured if detected early. "Any lump, especially in the breast," warned a Society poster circulated in 1919, is a "danger signal" which "should take you to a competent doctor for a thorough examination."[9]

The fact that some breast cancers were now being diagnosed earlier did not prompt American surgeons to consider the possibility of less radical mastectomies. Any significant departure from the Halsted procedure would have been viewed as rank heresy. Nonetheless, a few heretics did exist—the most prominent American dissenter was **George W. Crile** (1864-1943), a surgeon in Cleveland, Ohio. In 1921 Crile and several of his colleagues had founded the city's famous Cleveland Clinic; he served as this hospital's president from its inauguration to 1940. The Clinic has consistently reflected Crile's interest in finding less mutilative ways to treat breast tumors. "Halsted," said Dr. Crile, "was a putterer who took all day to do an operation which shouldn't be done at all."[10] Crile also performed mastectomies on his breast cancer patients, but unlike Halsted he never removed the underlying chest muscles. He believed that if these muscles revealed malignant infiltration, the tumor was so far advanced as to be already disseminated, and hence incurable by any degree of local surgery.

Crile's departure from Halstedian orthodoxy was mild and judicious. A more pronounced heresy soon began to flourish across the Canadian border. **Vera Peters** (1911-1993), a radiotherapist at Toronto's Princess Margaret Hospital, reached the conclusion that breast carcinomas could be effectively treated without mastectomy. As a young M.D. in the mid-1930s, Peters originally thought that mastectomy was the only rational treatment. But then some of the breast cancer patients at Princess Margaret simply refused to consent to mastectomy; their tumors were small, and they wanted to keep their breasts. These patients received no treatment except for excisional biopsies— and the subsequent breast irradiation supplied by Dr. Peters and her colleagues. The hospital kept track of the handful of recalcitrant patients. Surprisingly, at five and ten years after diagnosis their survival rates were just as good as those of the patients who received radical mastectomies. Princess Margaret soon became the first institution in North America to offer conservative surgery (lumpectomy) and radiation therapy as a standard treatment option for breast carcinomas. "The patients who refused mastectomy were the true pioneers," Dr. Peters recalled in 1984. "Our apprehension about their outlook soon changed to interest, and later to conviction on observing that the majority were free of disease ten to twenty years later."[11]

Some physicians who ventured to treat breast tumors by excisional biopsy and irradiation cannot properly be described as heretics from Halstedian orthodoxy, because they were English or French, and hence not so thoroughly imbued with the American dogmas. The surgeon **Geoffrey Keynes** (1887-1982) was the most prominent innovator in England. During the First World War Keynes had served with the Royal Army Medical Corps in France. In 1921 he joined the staff of Saint Bartholomew's Hospital in London, where he began to specialize in breast diseases and to investigate the value of radium therapy in managing breast cancers. Keynes later recalled that in the 1920s the best way to deliver a therapeutic dose of radiation to the breast and axilla was "by using hollow platinum needles filled with radium chloride." The first patients he treated had "disease so advanced that it was regarded as inoperable. The needles were inserted in a careful pattern so that the tumor and its related lymph nodes in the axilla were fully irradiated." Keynes and his colleagues were impressed by the resulting tumor shrinkage and delay in local progression. At the time Keynes was still performing radical mastectomies on operable patients; in 1925 he inadvertently removed the breast of a patient whose "carcinoma" turned out to be fat necrosis, an altogether benign condition. He was, in his words, "filled with shame at having been guilty of performing so mutilating an operation when in fact a small local removal would have sufficed." Thereafter he completely abandoned radical surgery. With the approval of his colleagues, he began to treat all his breast cancer patients with conservative surgery and radium needle implants. In the late 1920s and early 1930s Keynes became a crusader, arguing in articles and lectures that breast tumors could be adequately managed by excision and irradiation. He hinted that the survival rates might even be better than with radical surgery, because patients would come in sooner for diagnosis and treatment: "It was apparent that many women knew enough of the horrors of radical mastectomy to create a dread of what would follow a visit to their doctor." Keynes' crusade had little or no effect on surgical practices, either in England or in the United States. He found that his views were "clearly unpalatable to most surgeons and almost universally ignored by other writers on cancer of the breast."[12]

France, the country where Marie Curie had discovered radium in 1902, proved more receptive to the idea of treating breast tumors by irradiating them. Between 1936 and 1942 Francois Baclesse and other physicians at the Curie Institute in Paris treated 145 breast cancer patients with radiation therapy. These patients were a heterogeneous group—some had advanced tumors classified as inoperable, while others received adjuvant radiotherapy after their mastectomies. Only ten patients were what we would now call "lumpectomy patients"—that is, their treatment consisted of excisional biopsy for tumor removal and ensuing irradiation to destroy any residual cancer cells in the breast. But Baclesse and his colleagues marveled at how well this subgroup fared; nine out of ten (90%) were still alive five years later. Encouraged, the Curie Institute physicians tried to determine the appropriate dose of radiation for lumpectomy patients. They discovered that the larger the primary tumor was, the higher the dose that would typically be needed to prevent local recurrences in the breast. By the 1950s breast-conserving surgery and radiotherapy were routinely used to treat small breast tumors seen at the Curie Institute.[13]

Debating Radical Surgery

The small group of far-flung innovators— Crile in Cleveland, Peters in Toronto, Keynes in London, and the Curie Institute radiotherapists in Paris—could not begin to stem the flood tide of radical mastectomies. In the 1950s the trend toward extensive ablative surgery for solid tumors actually became more pronounced. At the time radiotherapy remained crude and imprecise; and chemotherapy was being used only experimentally, against a few leukemias and lymphomas. By default, so to speak, surgeons were the sole cancer doctors. Their specialty then epitomized the best in modern medicine—all eyes were turned toward the drama of the operating room, just as in the Rock Hudson movie "Magnificent Obsession" (1954), a box office hit which mingled mushy romance with brain surgery. The American dread of *cancer* was as excessive as the American dread of *communism*—both words denoted horrible, insidious, unspeakable things which had to be contained at all costs. The mere mention of either word elicited an emotional over-reaction. By now the American Cancer Society had grown into a most powerful advocate. Its public service messages had certainly taught Americans not to ignore persistent lumps and other unexplained symptoms; but because of their brevity and simplicity, these communications could not instill a sophisticated understanding of the diverse types of human malignancy. Alas, the practical result of the Society's campaigns was not discretion, but **cancerphobia**.

These two trends in American popular culture—the apotheosis of heroic surgeons and a pervasive anxiety about cancer— combined to produce appalling operative excesses. Ablative surgery reached its high water mark. Solid tumors were deemed curable by "adequate surgery"—if a patient had a bad outcome, perhaps the resection had not been extensive enough! Surgeons rose to the challenge by devising operations which demonstrated extraordinary technical proficiency. But all too often if a life was preserved, the quality of that life seemed to have been seriously compromised. In the 1950s many cancer survivors could not hide their operative scars. There were teenage osteosarcoma victims whose legs had been amputated at the hip socket, and middle-aged victims of laryngeal cancer (usually heavy smokers) whose voice boxes had been removed, and elderly victims of colon or rectal carcinomas who wore bulky colostomy bags under their clothing. Then as now, the tumor species with the most long-term survivors was breast cancer. Former patients wore cumbersome breast prostheses to conceal their chest concavities; yet their arms, often swollen and painful as a result of vigorous axillary evacuations, tended to reveal the history of mastectomy that they would have preferred to hide.

The Halstedian tradition of breast cancer surgery was stronger than ever. From the 1950s through the 1980s, the tradition found an articulate defender in **Jerome A. Urban**, a breast surgeon at New York's Memorial Sloan-Kettering Cancer Center. Dr. Urban always emphasized that mammary carcinomas originate as local phenomena in the breast and that adequate surgery can cure them in many instances. This fact is self-evident; but as we'll see, controversies were soon to erupt over exactly how extensive a resection must be to qualify as "adequate." Urban consistently promoted mastectomy as the best treatment—when in doubt he preferred to err on the side of too much surgery rather than too little, fearing that the opportunity for cure might be irretrievably lost. Naturally he tailored his resections to suit the particular pathological diagnosis. He performed total (simple) mastectomies for *in situ* breast cancers, but opted for more radical procedures whenever there was a possibility of malignant dissemination. Urban firmly believed that any lymph nodes which might harbor cancer cells should be removed; to leave them behind, he argued, was to endanger the patient's life.[14] Lest some readers too casually dismiss this philosophy, we should point out that Urban, like Halsted and C. D. Haagensen before him, frequently encountered advanced cases with grossly involved lymph nodes. Those troublesome Stage Three patients that other surgeons hesitated to treat were often referred to Sloan-Kettering's famous practitioner. Urban commanded the most sophisticated techniques for ensuring local control of advanced breast tumors. In the early 1950s he had won accolades by developing the **extended radical mastectomy**, during which the sternum (breastbone) is resected to allow surgical excision of the internal mammary nodes beneath. The **"Urban procedure"** (as this operation was sometimes called) went a step beyond Halsted, ensuring that the *en bloc* mastectomy really removed all the nodes involved in the breast's lymphatic drainage (axillary nodes, Rotter's nodes between the chest muscles, and the internal mammary chain). In lesser hands, sternal resection can be accompanied by dangerous complications, but the patients Urban operated upon usually enjoyed uneventful recoveries. The Urban procedure was reserved for those few patients with suspected involvement of the internal mammary nodes; it did reduce the number of sternum-area recurrences in this group. Dr. Urban could cite several studies reporting that it improved the survival rates among these patients, but this effect is much less certain.[15]

Not everybody applauded the development of ever more radical surgical procedures. The innovators who believed that even the standard radical mastectomy was an excessive treatment for early-stage breast cancer found an extraordinarily able spokesman in **George Crile, Jr.** A surgeon at the Cleveland Clinic, he was the son of George W. Crile, who modified the Halstedian mastectomy to preserve the chest muscles back in the 1920s. The younger Crile had graduated from the Harvard Medical School in 1933, joining the staff of the Cleveland Clinic the following year. At first he accepted the prevalent surgical doctrines and performed radical mastectomies on all his breast cancer patients. He was, as he later recalled, horrified at the more conservative operations his father did, with their "thick skin flaps and no disturbance of muscles."[16] But by the early 1950s he had begun to suspect that the survival rates achieved by radical mastectomy were no better than those achieved by simple mastectomies or even by the breast-preserving operations of Geoffrey Keynes. After 1954 George Crile, Jr., never performed another radical mastectomy. His conversion involved much more than the abandonment of a particular procedure—he had come to believe that the fear of cancer was worse than the disease itself. It was this fear he argued, that led patients to agree to horribly mutilating operations in the hope of being cancer-free.

Besides being a competent surgeon, Crile was also a prolific writer; in a stream of articles and books he campaigned against cancerphobia and overtreatment, two evils that went hand-in-hand. An article he contributed to *Life* magazine in 1955, headed "A Plea Against Blind Fear of Cancer," reveals his characteristic themes. He pooh-poohed the recent achievements in ablative surgery— "the frontier is no longer surgery, it is basic research"—as well as the intense efforts aimed at early discovery. "Even if a person had X-rays of the chest, stomach and intestinal track every four months, the possible development of fatal cancer could not be forestalled." While Crile observed that surgery can routinely cure some malignancies, he felt that "many of the modern ultra radical operations can be a cruel waste." And he advised his readers not to be too hasty in consenting to cancer operations. "There is no clear evidence," he wrote, "that

immediate treatment is any more effective than treatment given a little later." Crile's text in *Life* was accompanied by statements of protest from several officers of the American Cancer Society and the American College of Surgeons, all of whom affirmed the value of early detection and prompt treatment.[17]

During the 1960s and early 1970s, Crile's crusade against surgical overtreatments focused specifically on the radical mastectomy. Experiences in his private life probably played a role in bringing him to the battlements of the mastectomy controversy. His beloved wife Jane had been diagnosed with a small but aggressive breast cancer in 1958; she died five years later from brain metastases. Now a bereaved survivor, Crile provided the reading public with graphic descriptions of the aftereffects of radical mastectomy—that ugly scar which was so difficult to hide, the paper-thin flaps of skin stretched tautly over the bare rib cage, the ipsilateral arm swollen by irremediable lymphedema. Like his father before him, Crile had now concluded that the breast's underlying muscles and most of its overlying skin should be preserved. But he also took a position that even his father might have viewed as heretical. He proposed that routine axillary dissections should be abandoned, arguing that the regional lymph nodes, instead of being potential sources of metastatic dissemination, were actually involved with the body's "immunologic resistance" to the breast tumor. Removing them might even hurt a patient's chances for survival; certainly it seemed to do no good.[18]

TALK ABOUT CONTROVERSY!!
The learned Doctors Urban and Crile sure gave us a big one back in the 1950s and 1960s! The former wrote mainly in textbooks and medical journals, addressing an

audience of physicians and assuring them that radical mastectomy was necessary so as to be sure of removing all those dangerous lymph nodes. The latter broke from the ranks of the secretive surgical fraternity and took his arguments to the general public, depicting radical mastectomy as senseless mutilation and hinting that those lymph nodes were really allies in the patient's struggle against disease. Needless to say, Crile did not endear himself to the majority of American surgeons. In a book entitled *What Women Should Know About the Breast Cancer Controversy* (1973), he pointedly advised prospective patients to refuse treatment by any surgeon who insisted upon radical mastectomy.[19] One of the readers who took his advice to heart was the writer Rose Kushner. Of course, all Crile's propagandizing had not altered the Halstedian tradition, as Kushner learned to her chagrin from the nineteen surgeons she fruitlessly consulted in 1974.[20] The one-step biopsy and *en bloc* radical mastectomy remained standard practice. Any surgeon who performed a more conservative operation ran the risk of being sued for malpractice if the patient should have a bad outcome. George Crile, Jr., did not have sufficiently convincing data to overturn the existing state of affairs. But by going public with the technicalities of breast cancer surgery, he created a climate of controversy in which many people began to perceive the need for a large clinical trial to resolve the issues being so hotly debated.

The Advent of Clinical Trials:
Bernard Fisher and the NSABP

Today we all agree that the best way to determine the relative effectiveness of two different treatments is by conducting a large trial. Thousands of patients would be recruited at hospitals across the country; then they would be randomly assigned to receive treatment "A" or treatment "B." After an appropriate follow-up time, the patient outcomes would be compared and—*presto!*—we'd know that the treatment "A" works better than "B," or vice versa. The problem is that this process is much more complicated than it sounds. The planning and execution of a convincing clinical trial requires astronomical quantities of time and money. Considerable intellectual acumen must be exercised to remove the possible sources of bias; then those numerous patients must be carefully monitored, so as to generate the statistical power which would indicate that the trial's results are not due to mere chance. Properly done, a clinical trial can provide persuasive data and forever alter the treatment strategy for a particular disease. We learned this much from those prototypical trials of the late 1940s and early 1950s, which decisively proved that the antibiotic combination of streptomycin and isoniazid could cure tuberculosis, and that the Salk vaccine could prevent polio. Unfortunately, for breast malignancies there had been no clinical trials. In the 1960s therapy was still based on the essentially untested hypotheses and pronouncements of famous specialists like C. D. Haagensen and Jerome A. Urban. The studies of patient outcome being cited to support therapeutic decisions involved small numbers of patients treated by the very same physicians who naturally hoped to demonstrate the effectiveness of their particular approaches. We should always be suspicious of studies like this.

Fortunately, a bright new day began to dawn in 1957, when officials at the National Cancer Institute formulated plans for a clinical trials organization to be called the **National Surgical Adjuvant Breast Project**.

As the name implies, the NSABP was originally conceived as a means of testing the value of postsurgical adjuvants—that is, chemotherapy and irradiation—in breast cancer medicine. Over the years the organization expanded its scope to include trials of chemotherapy for colorectal cancer; it was thus rechristened the "Breast and Bowel Project," while retaining the same initials (NSABP) that everybody had become familiar with. The NSABP is of the greatest importance: it conducts large clinical trials specifically designed to resolve those disputed issues which are always popping up in breast cancer therapeutics. And the NSABP is very big. Starting out with a few dozen participating hospitals in the 1960s, it had over 200 American and Canadian institutions participating in its trials by the 1990s.

We cannot discuss the NSABP without mentioning its longtime chairman **Bernard Fisher**. A 1943 graduate of the University of Pittsburgh Medical School, Fisher was a surgeon who abandoned the scalpel for the science of statistics. As he recalled, he had initially "no interest in chemotherapy, clinical trials, or breast cancer." But his career changed direction in the spring of 1958, when he attended an NSABP meeting on these topics at the National Institutes of Health in Bethesda, Maryland.[21] Within several years Fisher became the NSABP's prime mover and transferred its headquarters from Bethesda to the campus of the University of Pittsburgh. Yet the NSABP always remained closely associated with the National Cancer Institute, which provided the funds for its numerous trials as well as suggestions on how they should be conducted. The NSABP/NCI alliance packed a lot of clout. During the 1960s and 1970s breast cancer specialists learned to read the articles bylined "Bernard Fisher et al" with especial care. After all, the NSABP trials had been sanctioned by the NCI, and they sought to answer the most urgent questions regarding patient care. Readers could be sure that considerable efforts had been made to eliminate those subtle biases and confounding factors which are forever creeping into scientific studies, and that the number of patients recruited was large enough that the reported results possessed a strong statistical likelihood of being true. Not infrequently NSABP communications tended to overturn biological hypotheses and clinical practices whose validity had previously seemed self-evident.

The NSABP Looks at Nodes

"Breast cancer," Bernard Fisher liked to say, "is a field of *hard opinions and soft data*." As we've seen, nowhere were the opinions harder and the data softer than in the matter of the regional lymph nodes. Should radical surgery be performed to ensure the removal of all these nodes, or was it better to leave them alone? Were the long-term survival rates adversely affected if nodes containing cancer cells should be left behind? Back in the 1960s the only answers we had were based on soft data. The NSABP got busy to produce some hard facts. Bernard Fisher and his younger brother Edwin R. Fisher (the NSABP's chief pathologist) went to their laboratory in Pittsburgh and performed a groundbreaking experiment. They injected malignant cells into the foot pads of anesthetized rabbits; then an hour or two later they removed the animals' popliteal lymph nodes (those behind the knee joint) as well as the lymphatic vessels leading into and away from these nodes. When the Fisher brothers examined the excised tissues under a microscope, they observed a phenomenon contrary to the accepted theory of nodal function. Yes, most of the injected cancer cells had been temporarily arrested in the nodes; but in every case a few malignant cells were found in the *efferent* lymph vessels—those leading away from the nodes. In 1966 the brothers published an account of their little experiment in *Science*, commenting briefly on its significance: "This finding indicates that lymph nodes are not the effective barrier to dissemination of tumor cells they had previously been assumed to be. While tumor cells *may* be sequestrated in the lymph nodes, they also traverse that structure."[22]

That the regional lymph nodes are ineffective at stopping tumor cell dissemination should come as no surprise to readers of the preceding chapter. We now know that wandering breast cancer cells can sometimes be detected in the bone marrow of ostensibly node-negative patients.[23] But the Fisher brothers' hypothesis was not obvious in the 1960s and 1970s, nor was it likely to be welcomed by orthodox surgeons, for it cast doubt on the rationale behind radical mastectomy in early-stage disease. If the nodes are not barriers and if the cancer cells can easily slip through them, why perform an *en bloc* resection of the regional lymphatics? The operation has severe side effects, and in most cases it would be just like closing the corral gate after the horses have already escaped.

The NSABP team began to build a case against radical mastectomy. By 1969 Bernard Fisher and his colleagues had a bit of indirect evidence from an early clinical trial suggesting that nodal resections did not improve the odds of survival. American surgeons had long believed that invasive tumors arising in the inner quadrants of the breast tended to have a poorer prognosis, because they could shed cancer cells into the internal mammary nodes (those beneath the sternum). Being difficult to access, these nodes were not routinely dissected; and presumably they might serve as stepping stones for metastatic dissemination. But the NSABP discovered that inner-quadrant tumors with unresected substernal nodes had exactly the same prognosis as outer-quadrant tumors. The location of a breast tumor did not constitute a prognostic factor insofar as survival was concerned.[24] During the 1970s, when data from the famous Protocol B-04 trial began to roll in, the NSABP reached an even more revolutionary conclusion. The axillary dissection, said Fisher et al, has no effect on survival rates. It makes no difference how many axillary nodes are removed, or whether any at all are removed—the patient's chances of surviving her disease remain unchanged.[25] The main value the NSABP saw in axillary dissection was diagnostic—increasing numbers of positive nodes give us an indication of a tumor's metastatic potential as well as an approximate measurement of the tumor cell dissemination which has occurred before surgery. In the NSABP trials subsequent to B-04, whenever patients underwent axillary dissection, the number of nodes removed and examined averaged around 15. With the NSABP this time-honored procedure became a modest sampling for diagnostic purposes rather than a full-fledged evacuation (30 or more nodes excised) done as a last-ditch effort to halt metastasis.[26]

The NSABP's investigation of the regional lymph nodes has broad implications for our understanding of tumor biology and our choice of surgical procedures. The NSABP results strongly suggest that those breast tumors which are destined to give rise to metastatic disease will become systemic much earlier than American surgeons had previously believed. Therefore while extensive local surgery might free the patient from distressing local recurrences, it cannot usually prevent the eventual appearance of distant metastases in these unpropitious cases. According to the NSABP hypothesis, positive nodes should be viewed neither as barriers nor as stepping-off places for systemic dissemination, but as "indicators of a host-tumor relationship which permits the development of metastases."[27] In 1980 Bernard Fisher delivered the Karnofsky Memorial Lecture before the American Society of Clinical Oncology. He told his audience that the Halstedian hypothesis postulating an orderly and predictable tumor spread via the regional lymphatics had become untenable. The malignant cells shed by breast tumors manage to go through or around the lymph nodes, getting into the bloodstream almost immediately: "The two vascular systems are so interrelated that it is impractical to consider them as independent routes of neoplastic dissemination." He explained that the likelihood of metastatic disease is "not solely dictated by anatomical considerations," but is "influenced by intrinsic factors in tumor cells and in the organs to which they gain access."[28] Today we would recognize **genetic mutations** as the most important of Dr. Fisher's "intrinsic factors." While we now have assays for a few genes whose mutations cause lots of trouble (e.g., *p53*), our data on the aforementioned "host-tumor relationship" remains quite soft.

Overtreatment by Radiation

In addition to excessive surgery, the cancerphobia of the 1950s and 1960s also led to indiscriminate applications of radiation therapy. Breast cancer patients suffered more than others. At many hospitals it was routine practice to irradiate the chest wall and axilla after radical mastectomy. If a few cancer cells had somehow managed to escape the surgeon's *en bloc* resection, the postoperative irradiation would surely kill them! Every weapon in the hospital's armamentarium had to be used whenever the terrible C-word was mentioned! Of course, nobody had

any hard data proving that postmastectomy irradiation of the operative field actually improved survival rates. But the side effects were clear enough and permanent—large patches of necrotic skin and increased lymphedema (fluid retention) in the ipsilateral arm. Today we would not tolerate these side effects; but in the 1950s and 1960s they were an inevitable consequence of poorly trained personnel and old-fashioned X-ray machines. Typically the individual who administered postmastectomy irradiation was not a board-certified radiation oncologist (the specialty hardly existed then), but a radiologist whose expertise was largely limited to diagnostic X-rays. The "orthovoltage" (low-voltage) machines then being used delivered the heaviest dose of radiation to the skin (it always got burned), while the underlying tissues were inadequately treated.

The NSABP was quick to examine the value of this surgical adjuvant. In 1961 Bernard Fisher and his co-workers initiated a prospective clinical trial which eventually involved 1,103 breast cancer patients treated at 25 institutions. All these patients received the standard radical mastectomies and full axillary dissections. Thereafter they were divided into two groups, one which served as a control and one which received "parasternal, axillary, and supraclavicular irradiation." In 1970 Fisher et al reported the trial's five-year results. The irradiated patients proved to have fewer recurrences in the areas treated, but there were no significant differences between the two groups either in the development of distant metastases or in the overall survival rate.[29] The attempts to improve long-term survival by irradiating the chest wall and the areas of lymph node concentrations were not working. In some cases they might even shorten life expectancies, by inflicting additional anguish and morbidity on patients already burdened with the aftereffects of radical mastectomy.

During the 1970s the practice of post-mastectomy irradiation was gradually abandoned, as physicians across the country realized the implications of the NSABP trial. Viz., radiotherapy can prevent or control recurrences at or near the site of a breast tumor, but it usually cannot forestall distant metastases. Insofar as systemic disease is concerned, regional radiotherapy—like regional ablative surgery—tends to shut the door after an escape has occurred. Today the only patients who are irradiated after mastectomy have advanced tumors (Stage Three) with a high probability of local recurrence. Some indications for prophylactic irradiation of the chest wall and axilla include tumor fixation to the overlying skin or to the fascia covering the chest muscles, or very considerable nodal involvement (e.g., palpable nodes). The main advantage gained by giving radiation before the local recurrences become apparent rather than after they do, is that lower doses will suffice to obtain control.[30] These days any suspected involvement of the internal mammary nodes, which Dr. Urban proposed to treat by surgery back in the 1950s and 1960s, is likely to be handled by radiotherapy.

NSABP PROTOCOL B-04
Twilight of the Radical Mastectomy

During the 1970s a revolution occurred in the primary surgical treatment of breast cancers in the United States. At the beginning of the decade, the *en bloc* radical mastectomy held sway; it was supported not only by long-standing tradition but also by a vast body of published literature. At the end of the decade, this procedure was being used only for a few patients with locally advanced tumors. The instrument used to overturn the

the Halstedian tradition was an NSABP clinical trial known as **Protocol B-04**. This trial had been in the planning stages since the early 1960s—Bernard Fisher and his colleagues had long pondered the details of a "protocol" (i.e., strict rules governing patient enrollment, eligibility, and follow-up) which would make the trial's findings unimpeachable. The first patient for NSABP Protocol B-04 was enrolled on July 22, 1971; the last patient, on September 6, 1974. Altogether the trial evaluated the outcomes of 1,665 breast cancer patients who had been treated at 34 institutions. These patients were randomly assigned to receive one of three surgical treatments—(1) radical mastectomy removing the breast, chest muscles, and axillary nodes *en bloc*—or (2) total (simple) mastectomy removing the breast but leaving the chest muscles and axillary nodes untouched—or (3) total (simple) mastectomy followed within six weeks by 25 fractions (treatment days) of radiation therapy "encompassing the ipsilateral chest wall, axilla, supraclavicular and internal mammary node regions."[31]

In June 1977 the NSABP published its first report of the trial's results. After an average follow-up of 36 months, there had been no significant differences in outcome between the three treatment arms. About 15% of the patients who received only a total mastectomy (no irradiation given) did develop local recurrences in the axilla; they then underwent axillary dissections for tumor control. But Bernard Fisher and his colleagues were heartened by their discovery that the positive nodes left behind had not as yet resulted in a higher incidence of distant metastases—as they expressed the matter, these nodes proved to be only "a manifestation" of tumor cell dissemination rather than "a predecessor" of disease in other organs.[32] Fisher et al gave a more detailed analysis of the trial's findings and implications in 1985, when they published the ten-year results in the *New England Journal of Medicine*. They had found "no significant differences" among the three treatment arms either with regard to the development of metastatic disease or to overall survival. "The variations of local and regional treatment used in this study," they concluded, "are not important in determining survival of patients with breast cancer." After ten years 18% of the patients who received just a total mastectomy had developed "detectable nodes" in the axilla, but the overall survival rate of this treatment arm was not affected: "The need for a delayed dissection in these patients (the 18 percent) was the only discernible disadvantage of not routinely performing an axillary dissection."[33]

Protocol B-04 did not address the question of breast preservation; all patients received mastectomies. This trial was conducted to determine whether the treatment of the regional lymph nodes in early-stage breast cancer affects the eventual outcome. Are the survival rates improved when these nodes are excised or irradiated? The answer that B-04 gave us was unequivocal, and it destroyed the rationale supporting both the radical mastectomy and the practice of post-mastectomy irradiation.

The NIH Consensus of 1979

Radical mastectomy was in eclipse even before a **Consensus Development Conference** (CDC) convened at the National Institutes of Health (NIH) in June 1979. Fully half of the breast cancer operations performed in 1972 were Halsted-type radical mastectomies; but in 1976 only 28% were, and in 1981 just a mere 3%.[34] No doubt the big NIH conference played a role in hastening the Halsted's demise. In their official

"Consensus Statement" the CDC panel noted that about 85% of the breast cancers being diagnosed in the United States were in Stages One or Two: "The presenting size of the primary tumor has also diminished notably and now averages about two centimeters." In view of these facts and of the emerging data from the NSABP's Protocol B-04, the panel concluded "that total mastectomy with axillary dissection is the current treatment standard." The surgical excision of axillary nodes was deemed "necessary for staging purposes" because the new chemotherapy regimens would be "indicated only with pathological confirmation of tumor involvement in one or more nodes."[35]

If the 1979 Consensus Statement seems fairly restrained today, we should remember that it contained much that was anathema to surgeons imbued with the first principle of Halstedian resection—viz., *all* lymph nodes that might be involved with tumor cells must be removed for urgent therapeutic reasons. The eleven-member panel had consisted mainly of reformers who wanted to see less mutilative breast surgery, including such familiar figures as Bernard Fisher, Rose Kushner, the Harvard radiotherapist Samuel Hellman, and the Italian surgeon Umberto Veronesi. But the panel did contain one prominent Halstedian, none other than Jerome A. Urban, who issued a "Minority Report" dissenting from the majority opinion. Urban wrote that total mastectomy could be hazardous because it compromised the surgeon's ability to do a thorough axillary dissection. He endorsed the modified radical mastectomy, in which the smaller chest muscle (pectoralis minor) is resected so as to allow better access to the axilla. And if the breast tumor was too close to the pectoralis major muscle, why then a radical mastectomy would be necessary—only with this procedure, Dr. Urban explained, could one be sure of removing those elusive Rotter's nodes which lie between the two chest muscles.[36]

Urban's views were shared by most American surgeons of the time, and he could cite various and sundry studies reporting improvements in disease-free and overall survival achieved by thorough nodal evacuations. But the CDC majority was more impressed by the far harder data coming from Protocol B-04. The era of radical breast surgery had ended. Precise observation and statistical power had won out over a venerated tradition and the clinical impressions of three generations of practitioners. First the Fisher brothers' laboratory experiments had demonstrated that the regional lymph nodes could not stop tumor cell dissemination; and then the NSABP's randomized clinical trial had proven that neither the surgical excision of these nodes nor their irradiation significantly improved the survival rates in early-stage breast cancer. And the practice of medicine began to change. It was a great victory for the scientific method.

The Lumpectomy Debate:
Are Tumors <u>Focal</u> or <u>Multifocal</u>?

Privately, most American surgeons were happy to get rid of the radical mastectomy— that's the main reason this procedure vanished almost overnight, once the NSABP's clinical trial had shown that it was no better than lesser operations. The Halsted was relatively easy to perform; but surgeons had a difficult time in postop consultations, having to face patients who had first been terrified by that dreaded C-word, and who were now either angry or depressed about that terrible amputation. As a group the surgical fraternity could live with total (simple) mastectomy; and at least one branch of the guild— the reconstructive (plastic) surgeons—found

themselves delighted with the operative standard endorsed by the Consensus Development Conference of 1979. The preservation of the chest muscles and a bit more overlying skin allowed sophisticated breast reconstructions, which had been impossible in the radical mastectomy era. From a strictly "business" point of view, one could say that a whole new market had suddenly opened up, with a potential of 100,000 or more breast reconstructions every year in the United States. Of course, the "product" being offered was greatly improved. Both providers and consumers stood to benefit from it, the former professionally and economically, the latter cosmetically and spiritually.

Breast preservation was an entirely different matter. For business reasons, as well as because of ingrained professional training, American surgeons did not like the idea of lumpectomy as a primary surgical therapy for breast cancer. It was not simply that a woman who opted for breast preservation and radiation therapy quickly ceased to be the surgeon's patient and became instead the radiotherapist's patient. Surgeons truly believed that the survival rates following lumpectomy could not possibly be as good as those following mastectomy. Writing in a 1977 textbook, the breast surgeon R. Robinson Baker of Johns Hopkins grudgingly conceded that a "more conservative procedure" had to be offered to a patient who refused mastectomy, while adding the customary scary caveat: "The patient should be aware that the procedure may not be associated with the same chance of survival."[37] At the time nobody had any hard data on this matter.

The debate over lumpectomy in the 1970s and 1980s, like the preceding debate over radical mastectomy, ultimately boiled down to a single issue in biology. Here the

the unresolved question was not the supposed barrier function of the regional lymph nodes, but the very nature of primary breast tumors. Are they essentially **<u>focal</u>** or **<u>multifocal</u>**? If a tumor's origination is focal—i.e., if it begins only at a single spot (or focus)—then we should be able to cure it by excising that spot with a modest margin of normal healthy tissue. On the other hand, if a tumor is actually multifocal—i.e., if the single lump or lesion we initially detect signifies that all the breast's glandular tissue will soon undergo malignant transformation—then a lumpectomy would merely postpone the day of reckoning. Another clinically apparently cancer was sure to pop up somewhere else in the affected breast, necessitating a belated "salvage" mastectomy—and maybe even costing the patient her chance for long-term survival.

Some writers on this issue use the term <u>multicentric</u> instead of "multifocal." Others speak of lesions simultaneously existing in different quadrants. All these usages—multifocal, multicentric, and "different quadrants"—convey more or less the same idea. That is, cancer would be seen as a disseminated process within the affected breast and therefore unlikely to be controlled by focal excision (lumpectomy). The term <u>bilateral</u> takes the idea of tumor dissemination a step further—that is, cancer would be seen as originating at multiple foci in *both breasts*, and hence unlikely to be arrested by any procedure short of double mastectomy.

Back in the 1960s and 1970s some meticulous surgeons felt the need to rule out the possibility of bilaterality by performing a **contralateral breast biopsy**. During the mastectomy of the breast with a primary tumor, they would take a tissue sample from the other (contralateral) breast, usually at the quadrant location corresponding to (or "mirroring") the site of the ipsilateral cancer. The

perceived advantage was that if malignancy should be discovered in the contralateral breast, the surgeon could proceed to do the second mastectomy while the patient remained under anesthesia, thus saving her a second trip to the operating room. The contralateral biopsy came to public attention in the fall of 1974, after Jerome A. Urban biopsied the right breast of "Happy" Rockefeller (wife of Vice-President Nelson Rockefeller) while performing a radical mastectomy for the infiltrating tumor in her left breast. Unfortunately, the intraoperative frozen section was inconclusive—two pinhead-sized clusters of *in situ* cancer cells were later detected on the permanent (paraffin) sections. And the next month Mrs. Rockefeller had to return to Sloan-Kettering for a total (simple) mastectomy of her right breast.[38]

These days the intraoperative contralateral biopsy has fallen into disfavor. The yield (percentage of positive findings) is extremely low, and no one wants to perform an unannounced second mastectomy on an anesthetized patient. But you may well imagine that Dr. Urban and other surgeons who routinely biopsied the contralateral breast to look for bilateral disease would not be overly receptive to the arguments for lumpectomy, which are based on the premise that early-stage breast cancer usually begins at a discrete unilateral focus. Today we know that a few breast cancers can be both multifocal and bilateral—indeed, this is often true of hereditary (familial) syndromes, because here all the cells of the mammary gland are carrying one or more germline mutations predisposing them to malignant transformation. In these cases the eventual appearance of a new primary tumor in a different quadrant or in the contralateral breast almost seems like a foregone conclusion. In sporadic (nonhereditary) cases, however, there is no reason to assume either multifocal or bilateral disease unless we have evidence to that effect. What percentage of sporadic breast cancers will prove to be multifocal at inception? In the 1970s the estimates being bandied about were as soft as cotton candy, having been spun out by cancer researchers who just might have prejudged the issue. The technique used to document the presence of multifocal disease has been the "simulated lumpectomy"—that is, the primary tumor is first removed with a wide excision, and then the pathologist examines the mastectomy specimen *sans* tumor for evidence of residual cancer cells. In 1974 Harold J. Wanebo, a senior surgical resident at Sloan-Kettering, and Andrew G. Huvos of the hospital's pathology department, reported on their examination of 162 breasts removed by Dr. Urban for diverse malignant conditions: "Residual cancer was found in 52% of the mastectomy specimens after generous excisional biopsies."[39] The following year Edwin R. Fisher and his NSABP colleagues reported a 13.4% incidence of residual cancer when they published findings derived from Protocol B-04: "Microscopic foci of multicentric cancer were detected in 121 of 904 breasts surgically removed for a clinically overt invasive cancer."[40] *Wow!* The rate of multifocal involvement reported by Urban's associates was almost four times that reported by the NSABP team—52% versus 13.4%! We cannot help but suspect a degree of political bias in these two studies, Dr. Urban being so publicly committed to the concept of mastectomy, and the NSABP now beginning to embrace the proposition that lumpectomies would suffice for most patients. Perhaps the NSABP's estimate is a little low; but the one based on Dr. Urban's mastectomy series is clearly much too high, because almost one-third of these patients (49 of the 162) had lobular carcinoma *in situ* (LCIS). As attentive readers of our pathology chapter will recall, LCIS is usually multifocal and often bilateral, *but not really*

cancer. Of course, back in the mid-1970s nobody recognized these facts, not even the breast specialists at Sloan-Kettering.

While the multifocal dissemination of primary breast tumors may never be quantified in percentages, several studies appearing after those by Urban's associates and the NSABP gave us estimates which seem more plausible. The Sloan-Kettering pathologist Paul Peter Rosen examined 203 mastectomy specimens after simulated lumpectomies, finding that the risk of residual cancer elsewhere in the breast was related to the size of the primary tumor. Of 100 patients with tumors less than two centimeters in diameter, 26% had subclinical malignant foci elsewhere. But the rate was 38% for those 103 patients with tumors over two centimeters. Patients whose primary tumors were subareolar—i.e., located right beneath the nipple and hence in a position to infiltrate the milk ducts converging there—proved more than twice as likely to have disseminated foci as those patients "with lesions less centrally placed."[41]

In 1986 the breast surgeon Frank E. Gump and other researchers at Columbia University published a highly informative study based on 657 patients with Stage One or Two disease who had undergone mastectomies at the Columbia-Presbyterian Medical Center. Overall, 179 of the 657 patients (27%) "were found to have separate foci"; but Gump et al discovered that the incidence of residual cancer elsewhere in the breast varied by histological type. The infiltrating ductal carcinomas, by far the most frequent histology (496 of the 657 cases), had the lowest rate of distant foci—19%—and this percentage rose or fell according to tumor size. Of those 298 patients with ductal carcinomas over two centimeters in diameter, 69—or 23%—had subclinical foci beyond the tumor border. But only 12% of those patients with ductal malignancies smaller than two centimeters (24 of 198 cases) revealed such foci. From their cross-sectional analysis of mastectomy specimens, Gump et al concluded that infiltrating ductal carcinomas typically originate at a single focus and that any distant deposits of tumor cells usually result from an outward spreading through the ductal system. They pointed out that the term multicentric is less appropriate for this histological type, since it tends to suggest multiple tumor foci arising independently in different quadrants. This had not occurred with the ductal carcinomas they examined. "Ninety percent of the secondary foci were found in close proximity to the primary, suggesting spread rather than multicentricity." In contrast, the secondary foci from the 92 infiltrating lobular carcinomas they examined tended to represent apparent multicentricity "as opposed to spread of cancer from the primary." Fully half of these primary lobular carcinomas (46 of the 92 cases) were accompanied by subclinical malignant foci well beyond the tumor border and often in other quadrants. The Columbia-Presbyterian series also included 42 mastectomies performed for clinically detectable (palpable) cases of ductal carcinoma *in situ* (DCIS). As we've seen in our pathology chapter, DCIS does not usually produce palpable masses. Those few cases which do so are probably far advanced, with considerable spread through the ductal system. The findings of Gump et al corroborated this assumption—81% of these DCIS cases (34 of the 42) had malignant foci at some distance from the main lesion.[42]

The debate over the multifocal nature of some breast tumors did not—and could not—end with a simple "yes-or-no" answer. What we have learned through painstaking research is that some breast tumors are much more likely than others to be accompanied by residual cancer elsewhere in the breast, and hence much less suitable for attempts at breast preservation. Increasing tumor size not only poses difficulties with regard to the cosmetic outcome (final appearance of the preserved breast), but it also increases the probability of distant foci. Those tumors located under the nipple can be a problem on both counts—*cosmesis* cannot always be obtained because the nipple cannot always be preserved, and *multifocal disease* easily results from spread through the ductal network.

We now know that infiltrating lobular carcinomas are often multicentric and sometimes bilateral. Even when small, these tumors may be poor candidates for breast preservation (lumpectomy). In contrast, the vast majority of the commonplace ductal carcinomas, both invasive and *in situ*, have focal inception. If detected when small, these tumors are quite suitable for lumpectomy. Complete excision becomes more difficult with the larger ductal cancers—the bigger they get, the more likely they are to have spread through the ductal system.

A Recipe for Preservation:
The "Joint Center" Radiotherapists

The possibility of residual cancer remaining in the breast after lumpectomy, whether due to incomplete tumor removal or to independent malignant foci in other quadrants, did not deter the proponents of breast preservation. Indeed, one group of physicians—the radiation oncologists—actually welcomed the challenge posed by multifocal residual disease, seeing an opportunity for the frequent application of their emerging specialty. Radiotherapy, they argued, was precisely the modality that should be used to sterilize the few remaining cancer cells. Why remove the entire breast when only a small portion was grossly involved with tumor? For reasons which we will explain in Chapter Nineteen, it is not practical to eliminate large tumor masses with irradiation. This modality serves principally as a "mopping up operation," destroying any cancer cells left behind after surgery. The appropriate dosage for this purpose can vary greatly from one type of cancer to another, but it must be precisely determined in all cases. Too little radiation, and the residual cancer cells survive to produce recurrences—too much radiation, and the side effects become irreversible. What was needed was a standard recipe for breast preservation, just the right dose to eliminate residual cancer cells without sacrificing long-term cosmesis. By convention radiotherapy regimens are stated in units of the **radiation absorbed dose** (or "rads"), delivered in so many daily treatment increments (called **fractions**), to certain well-delineated areas of the body (called **fields**). The dose may also be expressed in **grays**, a term which recalls the British radiologist Louis Harold Gray. One gray (Gy) is equivalent to 100 rads or to 100 centigrays (cGy).

Those early pioneers of radiotherapy for breast preservation, Geoffrey Keynes and Vera Peters, may have ventured into unexplored territory, but they did not leave us an established regimen which could serve as a road map to the goal. Keynes and Peters were mavericks whose treatments and success rates look more than a little anecdotal. We have no convincing data on the doses, fractions, and fields they used, nor on the cosmetic results they obtained. But thanks to Dr. Keynes, a few English hospitals kept tinkering with limited surgery (lumpectomy) and radiotherapy in the 1950s. In 1961 Guy's Hospital in London began a primitive clinical trial to test the therapeutic value of

these breast preservation strategies. Within the next decade 372 breast cancer patients at Guy's were randomly assigned to receive either the standard radical mastectomy with axillary dissection, or wide excision of the tumor (lumpectomy) followed by irradiation of the breast and axilla. The radiation course consisted of "30 Gy (3,000 rads) over two weeks." The results published in 1972 indicated that the lumpectomy and radiotherapy group had significantly more local recurrences than the mastectomy group—and their survival rate also seemed to be slightly poorer.[43] The dose used in the Guy's trial was obviously too low, and given in too few fractions.

In the United States there had been no notable studies of lumpectomy and irradiation for breast preservation. True, even in the mastectomy-minded 1950s and 1960s, George Crile, Jr., and his colleagues at the Cleveland Clinic, and the radiotherapist Eleanor D. Montague at Houston's M. D. Anderson Hospital had been treating breast cancer patients with these strategies—but at the time breast preservation was always a second-line therapy, offered only to those few patients who were either too ill to undergo mastectomy, or who refused to submit to it in spite of their physicians' entreaties.[44] No hard data on cosmesis, recurrence rates, or overall survival could be generated from motley patient populations like these. By the end of the 1960s, however, new "supervoltage" machines delivering more precise doses of radiation were becoming widely available; and radiation oncology was becoming a distinct medical specialty. And one American institution now started to offer lumpectomy and irradiation as a first-line treatment to those patients who might prefer it over mastectomy. That institution was Boston's **Joint Center for Radiation Therapy**, staffed by members of Harvard's Department of Radiation Oncology and serving hospitals in the surrounding New England area. Henceforth the leading proponents of breast preservation were no longer solitary physicians resisting the currents of mainstream theory and practice; they would be instead the rising young radiotherapists at the Harvard Medical School, including such future luminaries as Samuel Hellman and Jay R. Harris.

The Joint Center packed a lot of clout. Soon that heretical therapy began to acquire respectability. For the first time patients were being carefully screened before treatment to ensure that they were suitable candidates for breast preservation, with a strong probability of tumor control and good cosmetic outcome. Early on the Joint Center physicians decided not to irradiate the axilla of breast cancer patients, as had been done in the Guy's Hospital trial. They wanted to give the maximum tolerable dose to the affected breast—if a comparable dose were delivered to the axilla, there would be undesirable "matchline" fibrosis (hardening of tissues) where the breast and axillary fields overlapped. To prevent tumor recurrence in the axilla and to obtain staging information, the Joint Center regimen required a limited dissection of the lower and middle portions of the axilla. After a patient had recovered from the initial surgery (lumpectomy and axillary dissection), the business of irradiation could begin—180 to 200 rads every workday for five weeks (25 fractions), resulting in an accumulative whole-breast dosage of 4,500 to 5,000 rads. An extra bit of irradiation called **a boost** was given to the **tumor bed** (location where the tumor had been), so that this area received a total of 6,000 rads or more. In the 1970s the boost to the tumor bed was typically delivered by radioactive iridium "seeds" (pellets) which were temporarily implanted in the breast; the patient had to remain isolated in a hospital room for two or three days. By the 1980s

boosts were given on an outpatient basis, using external electron-beam radiation. The additional fractions aimed at the tumor bed (200 rads daily) added another week to the treatment time.[45]

The goal of breast irradiation at the Joint Center was twofold—first, to destroy any cancer cells persisting at or near the tumor site, and secondly, to sterilize any multicentric foci of tumor which might be secretly developing in other quadrants. The Center's regimen had almost twice the overall dose and over twice as many fractions as the disappointing regimen used in the Guy's Hospital trial. It represented about all the radiation that could be given safely if cosmesis was to be maintained. With accumulative whole-breast doses exceeding 5,000 rads, the incidence of fibrosis (thickening of breast and skin) and retraction (breast shrinkage) increased significantly. Was the regimen powerful enough to obtain local tumor control? In 1988 Abram Recht and other Joint Center radiotherapists reported the recurrence rates observed in 607 patients with Stage One or Stage Two breast cancer whom they had treated between 1968 and 1981. Altogether 67 patients (11%) had suffered a recurrence in the irradiated breast; the majority of these relapses (48 of the 67, or 72%) occurred at or near the site of the primary tumor. The chances of relapse in the treated breast were greatest from two to five years after therapy, falling off sharply thereafter.[46]

The preceding results suggest that long-term preservation of the breast was being accomplished for most patients given the regimen (no local recurrence in 540 of the 607). But control of residual cancer at or near the tumor site was less than optimal. Until 1981 the Joint Center required only the "gross excision" of malignant breast tumors; reflecting a belief that radiotherapy could sterilize any traces of the primary cancer left behind. This expectation was not fulfilled in a noticeable minority—48 (or 7.9%) of the 607 cases. Beginning in 1982 the rules were strengthened to require that the tumor margins be "microscopically negative"—i.e., no cancer cells at all on the borders of the excision, as verified by pathological examination. The original Joint Center regimen seems to have been reasonably effective in controlling occult malignant foci in other breast quadrants. A ten-year follow-up on 783 lumpectomy patients given this regimen revealed that while 12% of them developed a new primary tumor in the opposite (untreated) breast, only 4% developed a new primary tumor somewhere else in the ipsilateral (treated) breast.[47]

Whole-breast irradiation clearly tended to forestall the development of independent tumors in other quadrants. Recurrence of the original tumor was the more troublesome problem. During the 1980s the Joint Center radiotherapists took pains to identify the risk factors for recurrence in the treated breast. One factor was implicated much more often than others—the presence of a large area of ductal carcinoma *in situ* (DCIS) in or near the primary tumor. The Joint Center publications always referred to this condition as an **extensive intraductal component** (EIC).[48] The finding is hardly surprising. Readers of our pathology chapter will recall that DCIS is difficult to detect by unaided visual inspection, sometimes even on pathological examination, and that it can spread surreptitiously throughout the milk ducts without causing clinical symptoms. According to Jay R. Harris and Abram Recht, the Joint Center patients with an EIC had "a 27% crude incidence of local recurrence," whereas those without an EIC had only an 8% incidence.[49] We must emphasize that an EIC does not elevate the risk of developing distant metastases. An EIC does indicate a much higher likelihood of recurrence at or near the site of the primary tumor, but only if some of the

DCIS cells happen to be left behind. By 1994 researchers from the Joint Center and other Boston-area hospitals were able to report that EIC-positive patients did not have an elevated risk of local recurrence <u>if the tumor margins were microscopically negative</u>. The Joint Center subsequently regarded "all patients with uninvolved margins" as possible candidates for breast preservation, regardless of whether they were EIC-positive or EIC-negative.[50]

NSABP Protocol B-06
Lumpectomy Becomes Orthodoxy

The Joint Center for Radiation Therapy gave us detailed information on the factors governing the cosmetic outcome and the risk of local recurrence after lumpectomy and irradiation. But since the Joint Center was not a clinical trials organization, it could not address the single question paramount in the minds of both patients and physicians. Are the survival rates as good with breast preservation as with mastectomy? By the mid-1970s the NSABP was planning a big clinical trial to resolve this issue. Enrollment in **Protocol B-06**, as the trial came to be called, began in April 1976 and ended in January 1984. Eligible patients had invasive breast cancer (Stages One or Two), with primary tumors less than four centimeters (about an inch and a half) in diameter. These patients were randomly assigned to one of three treatment arms—(1) total (simple) mastectomy, or (2) lumpectomy followed by breast irradiation, or (3) lumpectomy alone (no further local treatment given). Although the protocol description infelicitously used the term "segmental mastectomy" instead of "lumpectomy," the surgery in the breast preservation arms amounted to no more than a meticulous excision. "The operation," said

Bernard Fisher and his NSABP colleagues, "removes only sufficient tissue to ensure that margins of resected specimens are free of tumor." Removal of the skin overlying the breast tumor was not required and was generally avoided, but tumor-free margins were an absolute prerequisite for breast preservation. If the pathologist "noted tumor at the specimen margin upon completing the microscopical examination," any patient placed in one of the lumpectomy arms would be given a total mastectomy and then reassigned to the mastectomy arm. Patients in all arms received a limited dissection of the lower and middle axilla: "The mean number of nodes removed was 15." And all node-positive patients received adjuvant chemotherapy, regardless of treatment arm. Those lumpectomy patients assigned to irradiation received a minimum of 5,000 rads to the entire breast, delivered over five weeks ("200 rads per day, five days per week"). The radiotherapy regimen in Protocol B-06 differed from the Joint Center's in that no boost was given to the tumor bed.[51]

By 1984 the NSABP was ready to release its initial results from Protocol B-06, based on a five-year follow-up of 1,843 patients treated at 89 different institutions. But the *New England Journal of Medicine* seems to have been hesitant about publishing findings which were so contrary to the prevalent notions of breast cancer biology. As Bernard Fisher later recalled, "our manuscript was in limbo for almost a year."[52] Eventually the *Journal* made amends to Fisher et al by prominently featuring two NSABP reports in its issue for March 14, 1985—the five-year results from Protocol B-06 and the ten-year results from Protocol B-04. To those surgeons who believed that thorough mastectomies must surely improve survival rates, the B-06 findings cannot have been comforting. The NSABP reported "no significant differences" between the three treatment arms, either with regard to the development of distant metastases or to overall survival. However, the incidence of local recurrence in the breast varied markedly between the two lumpectomy arms. Those lumpectomy patients who received irradiation had a 7.7% rate of breast recurrence; for those who did not, the rate was 27.9%, more than three-and-a-half times as great. Bernard Fisher and his numerous colleagues concluded that lumpectomy followed by irradiation is "suitable for the initial treatment of breast tumors that are no larger than 4 cm." The only stipulations they offered were that the local excision be "achieved with tumor-free specimen margins," and that node-positive patients "also receive adjuvant chemotherapy."[53]

This issue of the *Journal* with detailed results from Protocols B-04 and B-06 constituted a landmark event in our research on breast carcinomas. Both these clinical trials pointed toward the same general conclusion—viz., the variations in surgery and radiotherapy may affect the local and regional control of breast malignancies, but they do not significantly affect the development of distant metastases or the long-term survival rates. Therefore it would be humane and reasonable to select the least disfiguring surgical procedure, assuming it gave adequate local and regional control. The type of breast tumor a patient has, not the extent of surgery, determines the chances of survival. Either mastectomy or wide excision can manage those essentially localized "pussycats"; neither operation suffices to tame metastatic "tigers." Writing in a *Journal* editorial accompanying the two NSABP reports, C. Barber Mueller of the McMaster University Medical Centre (Hamilton, Ontario) aptly summarized their implications: "These data strongly suggest that patients who are going to die of breast cancer after surgical treatment and local irradiation already have micrometastases at the time of treatment, which foreordain the outcome."[54]

NSABP Protocol B-06 proved a bitter pill for surgeons of the Halstedian school, who continued to believe that variations in local and regional therapy do indeed affect a patient's chances of survival. Donald J. Ferguson of the University of Chicago wrote the *Journal* to challenge Fisher et al: "Their negation of rational surgery and their preliminary conclusions should be critically evaluated before they are applied to patients." Dr. Ferguson, an advocate of the extended radical mastectomy for inner-quadrant tumors, seemed oblivious of the NSABP findings regarding the regional lymph nodes. He faulted Protocol B-06 because its axillary dissections averaged only 15 nodes per procedure: "The fact suggests that none of them approached surgical completeness in the axilla."[55] Jerome A. Urban was not tardy in raising his objections to the NSABP's new doctrines. He appeared on the ABC television show "Nightline" the day before the B-06 findings were published. "The results and conclusions from this study," he informed viewers, "are premature. You really need ten-year follow-up." According to Dr. Urban, the incidence of local recurrence is "much higher" with lumpectomy than with mastectomy: "The survival rate is much worse."[56]

The NSABP was not perturbed by the protests from traditionalist surgeons. Bernard Fisher and his co-workers were confident that they possessed the hardest data available on the issues being disputed. Moreover, they had the backing of the National Cancer Institute and the *New England Journal of Medicine*. On March 30, 1989, the *Journal* published the eight-year results from Protocol B-06. Even with the more extended follow-up, the overall survival rates were "remarkably similar" for the three

therapeutic variations—about 71% of the patients in each arm remained alive. But the gap in the local recurrence rates between the two lumpectomy arms had widened. Only 10.4% of the patients assigned to irradiation were reported to have experienced a recurrence in the affected breast (a modest 2.7% increase since the five-year analysis). In contrast, 39.4% of the patients assigned to lumpectomy alone (no irradiation given) experienced recurrences (an 11.5% increase since the first analysis). There were no significant differences between the three treatment arms in the development of distant metastases—a fact which demonstrates that the metastatic potential of the primary tumor is more important in determining outcome than any local or regional recurrence.[57] While a recurrence in the treated breast may pose no threat to life expectancy, it is understandably distressing to the patient and a big thorn in the side of breast preservation (most local recurrences are followed by mastectomy). Protocol B-06 clearly indicated that tumor excision by itself, even when the margins are free of cancer cells, will be insufficient to prevent breast recurrences in a substantial minority of lumpectomy patients. In most cases of invasive breast cancer, irradiation improves the odds of success.

When the NSABP published the twelve-year results from Protocol B-06 in 1995, Bernard Fisher and his colleagues had to do a lot of tedious explaining. In 1990 staff workers at the NSABP headquarters in Pittsburgh discovered that some of the data submitted by one of the participating institutions was fraudulent. The ensuing investigation soon snowballed into a terrible controversy, with accusations and innuendoes being bandied about as several government organizations scrutinized every aspect of the NSABP's procedures. Dr. Fisher had done nothing wrong. The problem originated with the responsible physician at the Saint Luc Hospital in Montreal, Dr. Roger Poisson, who decided to fudge on the strict admission criteria of Protocol B-06. As he later explained, he acted so that six of his breast cancer patients who were ineligible for this trial could nonetheless be admitted to it and receive "the best therapy and follow-up treatment."[58] Thus did Dr. Poisson's good intentions lead to a bit of minor scientific misconduct which thoroughly disrupted the NSABP's operations and almost paved the road back to radical mastectomy!

The upshot was that Dr. Fisher and his NSABP colleagues had to prepare a detailed reanalysis of the Protocol B-06 results, excluding "all St. Luc patients with falsified data" as well as a few patients treated at other institutions who did not precisely meet the trial's criteria. The amended twelve-year results, published in the *New England Journal of Medicine* on November 30, 1995, were based on a close follow-up of 1,851 eligible patients. As in the five-year and eight-year analyses, the NSABP again found "no significant differences" between the three treatment arms, either with regard to the appearance of distant metastases or to the survival rates. Local recurrence in the breast, seen only in the two lumpectomy arms, had no noticeable effect on survival. Fisher et al discovered that node-positive patients assigned to lumpectomy alone had a higher rate of breast recurrence than did the node-negative patients in the same treatment arm. But those node-positive patients receiving whole-breast irradiation after lumpectomy had a very low rate, "only five percent at twelve years," indicating that the combination of radiotherapy and chemotherapy can be highly effective in maintaining local control. "This low incidence," Fisher et al argued, "precludes one from considering positive axillary nodes as a contraindication to breast-conserving surgery."[59]

The NSABP's twelve-year results from Protocol B-06 were accompanied by a "Special Article" written by researchers at the National Cancer Institute, who had audited the medical records of 1,554 patients in this trial. The NCI team reported that "discrepancies between the NSABP data and the audit results were uncommon"; and they confirmed "the adequacy of the data" upon which the twelve-year analysis had been based.[60] While Protocol B-06 remains our most convincing study comparing lumpectomy and mastectomy, other clinical trials have reached the same conclusion. Jeffrey Abrams and his colleagues in the NCI's Division of Cancer Treatment prepared a "meta-analysis," pooling the survival data from the NCI's own little trial of lumpectomy (237 patients) and four larger European trials. Altogether these five trials involved 2,854 patients—1,447 had been randomized to breast preservation and irradiation, and 1,407 had been randomized to mastectomy. The mortality figures proved to be essentially identical—302 deaths (or 20.9%) in the breast preservation arms, and 285 deaths (or 20.3%) in the mastectomy arms. Citing a "tight confidence interval" (a great virtue in statistics), Abrams et al found it "unlikely that meaningful survival differences exist between breast-sparing procedures and mastectomy."[61]

The NIH Consensus of 1990

A **Consensus Development Conference** on early-stage breast cancer, sponsored by the National Institutes of Health, was held on the NIH campus in Bethesda, Maryland, in June 1990. This conference did not begin a revolution in breast cancer treatments; its function was simply to give an official NIH sanction and some high-profile publicity to a revolution which had been in progress for over a decade. The "consensus" can be briefly stated—viz., lumpectomy and whole-breast irradiation for the local control of small invasive tumors, followed by adjuvant systemic therapy (chemotherapy or tamoxifen or both) in those cases at risk of developing metastatic disease. The microphones in the spacious NIH auditorium were held by the leading proponents of these therapeutic strategies, notably Bernard Fisher of the NSABP, Jay R. Harris from the Joint Center, and the famed Italian oncologist Gianni Bonadonna. Nobody extolled the virtues of mastectomy, or even mentioned that procedure save to disparage it as a surgical anachronism. The Halstedians had not been invited. Given these circumstances, it is hardly surprising that the CDC panel unanimously recommended "breast conservation treatment" as "preferable" for "the majority of women with stage I and II breast cancer."[62]

As we've seen in Chapter Thirteen, mastectomy continued to be the prevalent surgical treatment in some regions of the United States, demonstrating that the NIH cannot always dictate the policies of individual physicians and hospitals, nor alter patient preferences.[63] The Consensus Development Conference of 1990 did not end the debate over the relative merits of lumpectomy and mastectomy; however, it does provide a convenient milestone to end our historical review of breast cancer surgery. We've covered a full century of American efforts to understand and combat this disease, from 1889 when William Stewart Halsted went to Johns Hopkins, to 1990 when the NIH conference applied its imprimatur to breast preservation. This century that began with Halsted and radical mastectomy ended with Bernard Fisher, the NSABP trials, and the science of statistical probabilities. It was a remarkable century. For the first 5,000 years of recorded history, from ancient Egypt circa

3,000 BC to about 1890, there was no effective treatment of any kind for breast malignancies. Attempts at mastectomy for local control amounted to barbarous tortures which were ineffectual and sometimes fatal. Halsted achieved local control with minimal morbidity; he successfully removed large tumors from the chest wall. But his assumption that such local control significantly affects systemic outcome (survival) led subsequent surgeons to perform operations that were appallingly excessive for small tumors. The rationale behind radical surgery for breast carcinomas may be summarized in a single word—*nodes!* The Halstedians had no desire to mutilate healthy tissues gratuitously; they removed the chest muscles, evacuated the axilla, and resected the sternum because these measures were necessary to be certain of removing all the regional lymph nodes. In the 1960s and 1970s the NSABP convincingly demonstrated, first in laboratory experiments and then in clinical trials, that these nodes are not effective barriers to tumor cell dissemination. Hence radical surgery to remove them is unlikely to improve a patient's chances of survival. Another inference to be drawn from the NSABP trials is that what we call *early* breast cancer is often *late*—viz., an invasive tumor can surreptitiously shed millions of cancer cells into systemic circulation before it's detected with our present diagnostic tools. In this situation any local and regional therapies, regardless of their comprehensiveness, would ultimately prove ineffectual. Outcome would be determined by the metastatic potential of the previously disseminated cancer cells—only systemic drug therapies might stand a chance of altering the disease's natural history.

American mortality from breast cancer remained fairly constant throughout eight decades of radical mastectomy. Bigger operations did not save more lives. As a result the therapeutic pendulum has moved in the opposite direction. Today's standard is minimal surgery—adequate to completely remove the tumor, but leaving the surrounding tissues untouched. Of course, the judgment as to what constitutes "adequate" surgery varies from practitioner to practitioner; a few still operate on subtly Halstedian principles. As a necessary corrective, we will simply cite the widely publicized guidelines of the NSABP and the Joint Center for Radiation Therapy—both organizations favor the excision of a primary tumor with narrow but altogether cancer-free margins, followed by whole-breast irradiation. The general prescription is no different from that proposed by Galen in the second century— ("remove the entire tumor leaving no root behind")—but the methods of accomplishing it have finally become sophisticated. Breast preservation tends to require more work than mastectomy. Bernard Fisher and Carol Redmond of the NSABP give us a chastening admonition: "The retreat from Halsted principles of cancer surgery does not imply that careless surgery is acceptable. We recommend that surgeons and pathologists make the effort to ensure that resected specimen margins are free of tumor and that radiation therapy of the breast be administered by those with expertise."[64] Neither the NSABP nor the Joint Center for Radiation Therapy had discovered any miracle cure or wonder drug, but their collective message was the best news that breast cancer patients have ever heard. Viz., *Come in early for diagnosis and treatment—your breast can be saved, and your chance of survival will not be compromised.*

Chapter Sixteen

MAKING A DECISION
Lumpectomy or Mastectomy?

About the only uncontroversial matter in breast cancer medicine is the doctrine that the primary tumor must be surgically removed. The prospect of breast surgery is not pleasant, but readers of the last chapter should have a profound appreciation of the progress that has been made in this area. The next chapter will describe the current surgical procedures—readers may be surprised to learn how easy and uneventful breast operations have become. Recovery is swift, without those lingering debilitations that were common a few decades ago. The present chapter is about decision making, for ultimately it is the patient alone who must make that difficult but necessary choice of procedure. At the moment there are **three surgical options** for early-stage breast cancers. The first two—simple (total) mastectomy and lumpectomy followed by whole-breast irradiation—are now standard therapies, having been authorized by the NIH conferences of 1979 and 1990. A third option—lumpectomy *without irradiation*—remains controversial; nonetheless, some breast cancer specialists with impeccable credentials have argued that it should be the initial strategy for the smallest tumors.

The advice patients receive from practicing physicians almost inevitably contains an element of specialty bias. Understandably, doctors tend to recommend the procedures they themselves perform and believe in. Judicious impartiality is often very hard to come by. By way of aiding any reader who might be facing a decision about breast cancer surgery, let's briefly review the indications and counterindications for each of the three surgical options. Please be assured that these indications are common knowledge, and that they are discussed without the slightest hint of specialty bias.

The Mastectomy Option

Mastectomy is the only available option for really large tumors, those usually rated Stage Three. In this instance the breast cannot be preserved. But mastectomy offers several advantages for smaller lesions, those which might be deemed suitable for lumpectomy. Surgical ablation (removal) of the mammary gland remains the gold standard of local control. There are no worries about recurrence in the treated breast, and the follow-up examinations after surgery are greatly simplified. Mastectomy is likely to be somewhat cheaper and much faster than the standard breast preservation regimens, which call for five or six weeks of daily radiation therapy after lumpectomy. If local tumor control, freedom from anxiety, and speedy cost-effective treatment are the principal concerns, then mastectomy could well be the logical choice for many patients.

On the other hand, a woman who is appalled at the prospect of losing a breast should consult with board-certified radiation oncologists about her suitability for lumpectomy and irradiation. These specialists have a positive incentive to find ways in which a breast may be preserved. Not all physicians are sympathetic to the concept of breast preservation. James Owen Drife, a bearded OB/GYN at the University of Leeds in England, goes so far as to advocate prophylactic mastectomy "to abolish breast cancer." For women past childbearing age, he argues, "the breast has no function apart from its psychological one." It is just "a redundant gland and a pad of fat." Defending himself against potential brickbats, Dr. Drife explains his position: "I have seen relatives, friends, and colleagues killed painfully by glands they didn't need. I refer questioners to my own secondary sexual characteristics and point out that if my beard had a 6% chance of turning malignant I would shave it off."[1]

The decision to forfeit a breast is much more agonizing than getting a clean shave, but Drife's premises are biologically correct. The loss of a breast is not quite comparable to the loss of a voice box to laryngeal cancer or the loss of a leg to osteosarcoma. These days there are excellent appliances (prostheses) to enable laryngeal patients to talk again and osteosarcoma patients to walk again; but patients whose voice boxes or legs have been amputated always need training before they're actually able to walk or talk. In contrast, today's mastectomy patients have no problems with communication, mobility, or other essential functions; and they do not require training in the use of prosthetic appliances. A realistic silicone prosthesis (breast form) can be worn within a few days after surgery, and a skillful breast reconstruction can usually be completed within a few months. Women who freely and knowingly choose mastectomy, with or without subsequent reconstruction, tend to be content with their decision. Nancy Reagan, diagnosed with a small breast cancer in October 1987, decided to have a mastectomy because she could not fit radiation treatments into her busy schedule as First Lady. Two years later Mrs. Reagan wrote: "I have never felt better. My activities have not changed in any way. I feel wonderful and my husband tells me every day that he loves me more than the day we were married."[2]

The Lumpectomy Option:
Indications and Counterindications

One essential prerequisite for lumpectomy and irradiation is not physiological—it has to do with the individual patient's attitude. Breast preservation means more work. A woman must be sufficiently motivated to undergo five or six weeks of radiotherapy, with its consequent side effects. She must also be psychologically prepared for a lifetime of watchful follow-up, because there is no certain way of predicting whether cancer will recur in the treated breast. Assuming the patient has these personal characteristics, lumpectomy and irradiation should generally be encouraged as the initial strategy for early-stage breast cancer. Looking at the results published by the Joint Center for Radiation Therapy and the NSABP, we might hazard a ballpark estimate that about 90% of patients with tumors two centimeters or less in diameter are suitable candidates for this strategy, and furthermore that about 90% of the presumed candidates can achieve successful long-term preservation. As we've seen in the preceding chapter, ductal carcinomas limited to a single focus in the breast are especially suitable for lumpectomy and irradiation. The cosmetic results after radiotherapy are often described as "good" or "excellent"; this is usually the case when the tumor is small and located in an outer quadrant.

Unfortunately, there are several definite **counterindications to lumpectomy**. When they are present, it could be foolish to subject patients to the expense and discomfort of radiation therapy, because there is a highly elevated risk of local recurrence in the treated breast and a consequent need for salvage mastectomy. In the event of recurrence, we would have to admit that not only has irradiation failed to sterilize the residual cancer cells in the breast, but that it has made any breast reconstruction more difficult by reducing the elasticity of the overlying skin. Cosmetically and psychologically, those lumpectomy patients who suffer such treatment failures would have been better off had they opted for mastectomy and reconstruction in the first place.

The most obvious counterindication to breast preservation is the presence of **a second tumor elsewhere in the affected breast**. When we discover one or more foci of cancer at some distance from the initial primary tumor—for example, in other breast quadrants—we tend to assume that the malignant process is multifocal, possibly affecting large areas of the breast, and that the local excision of one or two foci may not arrest it. For this reason, conscientious radiotherapists (like those at the Joint Center) want to study several mammograms of the affected breast before accepting a patient for treatment. In the case of a radiographically

"dense" premenopausal breast, supplemental examination with MRI (magnetic resonance imaging) should be considered. MRI can sometimes detect tumors missed by mammography.[3] Most American breast specialists regard multiple tumor foci as an absolute counterindication to preservation; but by way of presenting other points of view, we should point out that radiotherapists at the Marseille Cancer Institute (France) have treated patients like these with conservative surgery and irradiation. After a follow-up of 71 months, the Institute's patients with multiple foci had a local recurrence rate of 25% (15 of 61 patients recurring in the treated breast), more than twice as high as that of patients with single tumors (11% rate, 56 of 525 patients recurring).[4] While it is not impossible to perform multiple lumpectomies for multiple lesions, the risk of recurrence is decidedly elevated, and the cosmetic outcome quite problematic.

Even if no secondary malignant foci can be detected on mammograms or MRI, the characteristics of the primary tumor may give us pause when thinking about breast preservation. We now know that lobular tumors (as opposed to ductal ones) are often more widespread than is apparent on preoperative mammograms. The reader is referred to the previous discussions of **lobular histology** in Chapters Twelve and Fifteen. Many textbooks also cite **"diffuse microcalcifications"** visible on mammograms of the affected breast as a relative counterindication. This is a very tricky criterion which requires an expert radiologist like Robert L. Egan or Daniel B. Kopans for an informed interpretation. Most calcifications, even if disseminated throughout the breast, result from benign processes. Only a few patterns of calcification are suggestive of malignancy and thus likely to pose an obstacle to preservation.[5]

Genetic inheritance may represent a

major stumbling block, and it should always be considered whenever there is a family history of breast cancer. However, the fact that one or more close relatives of a patient also received a breast cancer diagnosis does not necessarily mean that she is suffering from a hereditary syndrome in which all the cells of the mammary gland carry a genetic defect predisposing them to malignancy. The age at which these relatives developed cancer is an important clue—hereditary breast tumors typically have early onset (usually before age 50), and they tend to be bilateral (both breasts are eventually affected). A history of early-onset bilateral tumors in first-degree relatives (mother or sisters) would thus seem to be a strong counterindication, unless we could isolate the genetic defect behind the syndrome and verify that the patient has *not* inherited it. Fortunately, our ability to isolate these defects and to identify the family members carrying them has been growing rapidly. Most non-carriers would be suitable candidates for breast preservation; at present the logical strategy for carriers already diagnosed with breast cancer would appear to be bilateral (double) mastectomy. Several studies have reported that prophylactic bilateral mastectomies effectively prevent future breast tumors among women carrying mutations of the *BRCA1* or *BRCA2* genes.[6]

Most laypersons imagine that **advanced age** would be a counterindication to lumpectomy. The converse is true. As a group, lumpectomy patients over age 50 have fewer recurrences in the treated breast. With older women there are also fewer worries about the possible long-term side effects of high-dose radiation. Quite a few textbooks cite "age under 40 years" as a relative counterindication to breast preservation; but this too is an oversimplification. A higher percentage of premenopausal patients have had recurrences in the treated breast, because a higher percentage of these patients have had tumors with unfavorable characteristics (estrogen receptor negativity, high S-phase, poor nuclear grade). The tumor characteristics, not chronological age, are what we should be principally concerned about. But as we've seen in the last chapter, the combination of irradiation and chemotherapy can usually forestall recurrences in the treated breast, even among node-positive patients with aggressive tumors.

Large tumor size can be a counterindication, but then we have no firm guidelines as to what size is actually "too large." The size limits bandied about in the literature (two centimeters, four centimeters, etc.) have varied from one clinical trial to the next. The smaller the tumor, the more suitable it's likely to be for lumpectomy; but size *per se* is not the most meaningful criterion. The necessary criteria are cancer-free margins on the excised specimen (i.e., presumed local control) and a cosmetic result acceptable to the patient. A large tumor might be removed from a large breast with an acceptable cosmetic result. If the same size tumor were removed from a small breast, the cosmetic result might be unacceptable.

A prospective lumpectomy patient should discuss the issue of cosmesis (final appearance of the treated breast) with those physicians who would be treating her. While nobody can infallibly predict the cosmetic outcome, experienced surgeons and radiotherapists have the best judgment in this matter. Factors associated with inferior results may—or may not—be counterindications to preservation, depending upon how badly the patient wants to keep her breast and on what outcome she would regard as satisfactory. The **tumor's location** can be as important to cosmesis as its dimensions. Locations in close proximity to the nipple pose a cosmetic dilemma because the nipple and its surrounding areola may have to be removed for tumor control. Locations in the inner and lower quadrants are sometimes associated with inferior results, especially in the case of large lesions. A patient's overall physique should also be factored into the cosmetic equation. Obese women and women with large pendulous breasts may have poorer results because their body configurations make it difficult to deliver uniform doses of radiation to the affected breast.

Radiotherapy's Limitations

Like other cancer therapies, whole-breast irradiation has its limitations. Laypersons usually assume that radiotherapy helps to prevent systemic disease and thereby works to extend survival; but the NSABP clinical trials have demonstrated that any survival advantage afforded by breast irradiation is likely to be insignificant. The principal advantage is tumor control in the areas treated. Irradiation greatly reduces the possibility of breast recurrences, both near the tumor site and in other quadrants.

The side effects of breast radiotherapy are not exactly pleasant, but they are tolerable. During therapy they are limited to a general sense of fatigue and an uncomfortable reddening of the skin; both symptoms quickly resolve after the treatments are completed. Over the next year the irradiated breast may reveal a slight degree of contraction (shrinkage), and it will become firmer. The skin of the breast will become thicker, and it may take on a slightly darker coloration. By two or three years after therapy, however, these progressive changes will have ceased. In various subtle ways the breast exposed to high-dose radiation will always be different from the untreated breast; but it is now stable, and under clothing it usually cannot be distinguished from the untreated breast.

The worst side effect that might occur after radiotherapy is the induction of a second malignancy entirely unrelated to the primary breast tumor. Ionizing radiation easily disrupts the unstable, malfunctioning DNA of cancer cells, thus causing them to die. Unfortunately, it also has the potential to cause genetic mutations in *normal* cells, which may result in the development of a treatment-related malignancy years or even decades later. Such induced cancers are extremely rare after breast radiotherapy; we cannot honestly say that the risk is nonexistent, but it is certainly minimal. We know from long-term follow-up on atomic bomb survivors and on women given radiotherapy for Hodgkin's disease that the adult breast can tolerate very high doses of radiation without incurring an elevated risk of mammary carcinomas.[7] Moreover, the contralateral (untreated) breast is shielded during the treatments given to the affected breast, so that it receives only a small amount of scatter radiation. Second breast cancers attributable to post-lumpectomy radiotherapy must therefore be viewed as remote hypothetical possibilities rather than as noteworthy dangers. The risk of sarcomas developing in the irradiated bone or other connective tissues is also infinitesimal. Leukemias, those malignant proliferations of white blood cells, pose a greater concern because whole-breast irradiation necessarily falls upon cells circulating in the blood and upon the bone marrow in the sternum. But here again the potential hazard posed by radiation treatments alone is extremely small, any elevation in risk being much less than one percent. Only when radiotherapy is combined with chemotherapy does the incidence of post-treatment leukemias begin to rise noticeably—and in this case the principal culprit is not radiation, but alkylating agents such as the commonplace drug cyclophosphamide. With current techniques the bone marrow receives very little exposure during whole-breast irradiation.[8]

The main drawback of breast radiotherapy is neither the side effects (which tend to resolve with time) nor the risk of carcinogenesis (which is remote), but the fact that **this treatment cannot be repeated**. Radiation exposure is cumulative. With a fractionated dose of 5,000 to 6,000 rads, we are approaching the maximum lifetime tolerance of the affected breast. If we were to irradiate the breast again, we would produce so much contraction and tissue necrosis that the cosmetic result would be worse than mastectomy. That's the reason why tumor recurrences in the breast after lumpectomy and irradiation are usually followed by mastectomy—a second course of radiotherapy is not an option. Considering this limitation, some breast specialists have proposed that the smallest tumors ought to be treated by lumpectomy alone, saving the whole-breast irradiation for use against possible recurrences. Of course, this proposition is still rank heresy, yet it has been advocated with increasing frequency.

LUMPECTOMY ALONE
Can Radiotherapy Be Omitted?

As we've seen in Chapter Fifteen, the results from NSABP Protocol B-06 suggested that long-term local control of *some* breast cancers could be achieved by lumpectomy alone. But neither the NSABP nor the National Cancer Institute has been anxious to propose guidelines for the omission of radiotherapy. The official statement from the Consensus Development Conference of 1990 advised that "no subgroups have been identified in which radiation therapy can be avoided."[9] In the same year the eminent radiotherapist Samuel Hellman argued that "it's too soon to know" whether whole-breast irradiation can ever be omitted after lumpectomy. Understandably, Dr. Hellman and his colleagues have been no more enthusiastic about a departure from radiotherapy than American surgeons were about the departure from mastectomy.

This new heresy first began to flourish in the usual places—viz., the Cleveland Clinic and the Princess Margaret Hospital in Toronto, the very same institutions which had deviated from the doctrines of radical mastectomy back in the 1920s and 1930s. In 1993 the surgeon Robert E. Hermann of the Cleveland Clinic observed that not only has radiation therapy after lumpectomy "not improved survival," but that "it increases the time of treatment, triples its cost, causes some early and late morbidity, and makes small recurrences in the breast more difficult to identify both mammographically and by clinical exam."[11] As early as 1975 Hermann and his colleagues began to offer selected patients breast-preserving operations without subsequent irradiation. Naturally the Cleveland Clinic team tailored their surgery to fit the individual patient and the particular tumor. Modified radical mastectomies were sometimes used for clinically apparent Stage Two disease ("tumor larger than 2.0 cm or involved axillary lymph nodes"). But almost all patients who wished to keep their breasts were given lumpectomies, the advisability of postoperative irradiation being determined on a case-by-case basis. If the resected tumor was "2.0 to 4.0 cm in size" or "showed tumor near the margins," radiation therapy was recommended. Lumpectomy without irradiation was reserved for "small tumors (less than 2.0 cm) located in the periphery of the breast."[12] From 1975 through 1988 the Cleveland Clinic physicians treated 620 patients with lumpectomy alone. According to Dr. Hermann, "local recurrence in these selected patients at five and ten years was not in the range suggested by the NSABP studies (i.e., 30% to 40%), but was only 11% at five years and 14% at ten years."[13] By way of accounting for this big discrepancy in recurrence rates, we should remind the reader that NSABP Protocol B-06 accepted invasive cancers up to four centimeters (4.0 cm) in diameter for its arm featuring lumpectomy without irradiation. Not only was the Cleveland Clinic's size limitation for this strategy set at two centimeters, but Dr. Hermann and his colleagues required much wider negative margins on the excised tumor specimens (1.0 to 2.0 cm cancer-free).

Across the Canadian border in Toronto, Roy M. Clark and other physicians at the Princess Margaret Hospital began a clinical trial in 1984, randomly assigning 837 node-negative patients to receive lumpectomy with subsequent whole-breast irradiation or to receive lumpectomy alone. In 1992, after a median follow-up of 43 months, Clark et al reported the rate of local recurrence in the treated breast—it was only 5.5% in the irradiated patients, but 25.7% in those who received no further treatment after lumpectomy. The Princess Margaret team concluded that tumor size over two centimeters, age under 40, and poor nuclear grade were all "important predictors for breast relapse." In contrast, patients over age 50 with tumors smaller than two centimeters had only a 13.5% rate of breast relapse even when radiotherapy was omitted.[14] In 1996 Clark and his colleagues published an updated report on the Princess Margaret trial. Like NSABP Protocol B-06, it revealed no significant difference in survival rates between those lumpectomy patients who received whole-breast irradiation and those who did not.[15]

Are there any indications for the omission of breast irradiation? The answer to this question has to be *YES!*—but we must observe that surgeons and pathologists seem more interested in discovering these indications than radiotherapists are. At a National Cancer Institute workshop on breast preservation, Jay R. Harris of the Joint Center advocated irradiation of all lumpectomy patients because "assessing negative margins is not an exact science." Roy M. Clark (also a radiation oncologist) explained his reason for favoring breast radiotherapy: "Patients are profoundly distressed when they are told they have a recurrence. You can't just say 'we can deal with this' and move on."[16] Perhaps some patients might be more distressed by the prospect of radiation exposure than by the possibility of a purely local recurrence in the breast. And all patients should be free to form their own opinions on the value of any proposed treatment strategy. At the moment, however, the most logical candidates for lumpectomy without irradiation would seem to be those patients with nonpalpable lesions, those tiny malignancies which are only detected by mammography and which physicians have been just a trifle embarrassed to treat. Whether invasive or *in situ*, these lesions tend to be so small that there is little chance of spread to the axillary lymph nodes. Frankly, we have no good way of predicting when—or if—these neoplasms will progress to become clinically apparent tumors. Back in the 1970s some pathologists coined the term **minimal breast cancer** for such lesions, which were then being detected in significant numbers by the early trials of screening mammography.[17] Cases like this are not so "minimal" that we would risk leaving them untreated, yet mastectomy would clearly be overtreatment, and giving irradiation after a lumpectomy would deprive us of any opportunity to use this modality again. A practical solution might be to use wide excision (lumpectomy) alone, naturally with much attention paid to getting cancer-free margins on the specimen, and naturally with intensive follow-up on any patients so treated. One suggestion has been that lumpectomy patients who are not irradiated should have mammograms every six months for the first three years after treatment.[18] *Theoretically*, any recurrence near the original site or elsewhere in the breast would be detected while still small enough for a second lumpectomy to be feasible, with the option to use irradiation at that time.

We should emphasize that the "heretics" proposing lumpectomy without irradiation are not advocating any wholesale abandonment of breast cancer radiotherapy, only suggesting that in selected cases the benefit of this modality for tumor control is problematic and thus likely to be outweighed by its inevitable disadvantages (e.g., side effects and expense). As recounted in Chapter Twelve, the pathologist Michael D. Lagios has vigorously argued that lumpectomy alone should be the initial treatment for all those small foci of ductal carcinoma *in situ* (DCIS) now being detected by mammography. Some surgeons have hinted that lumpectomy alone might also suffice for palpable invasive tumors; the size limit most frequently bandied about has been one centimeter. Richard G. Margolese of Montreal's Jewish General Hospital, a longtime participant in the NSABP trials, points out that when the tumor diameter was one centimeter or less, Protocol B-06 failed to find a significant difference in the local (breast) recurrence rates between those lumpectomy patients who were irradiated and those who were not.[19] Surgeons Blake Cady and Michael D. Stone of the Harvard Medical School predict that breast-preserving surgery without subsequent irradiation will soon be "a relatively common mode of therapy," both for DCIS and for "small primary invasive cancers."[20]

Chapter Seventeen

UNDERGOING SURGERY
And Recovering from It

Bernard Fisher has said that if there were one word he could eliminate from the medical vocabulary, that word would be *biopsy*.[1]   While Dr. Fisher may be overstating the case for vocabulary reform, his grievance is valid. Breast preservation efforts get into trouble whenever the distinction between an **excisional biopsy** and a **lumpectomy** is not made sharply enough. These terms denote surgical procedures which are identical in basic technique, but have different end points.   A biopsy is a **diagnostic procedure** which we perform to identify a breast lesion assumed to be benign. A lumpectomy is a **therapeutic operation** performed to control a tumor known or assumed to be malignant. With lumpectomy it is imperative that the entire tumor be removed as a single intact specimen with sufficiently   wide   negative   (cancer-free) margins on all sides.   And the attending pathologist must be able to verify the complete removal of the tumor and the presence of negative margins.   A previous surgical biopsy of the tumor, whether incisional or excisional, always complicates the pathologist's job. Richard G. Margolese and other surgeons who participated in NSABP Protocol B-06 point out that "lumpectomy as a second procedure" is problematic, because

"the bloody infiltration that causes induration and discoloration of tissues surrounding a cavity makes it difficult to define the borders for further resection. The chance for good tumor control is lessened, and cosmesis may be compromised."[2]

Any lumpectomy should be carefully planned in advance, regardless of the tumor's size or location. Ideally we would confirm the diagnosis of malignancy before surgery through fine-needle aspiration or core-needle biopsy, those minimally invasive procedures we discussed in Chapters Nine and Eleven. The amount of information a pathologist can gather from a cellular aspirate or core-needle specimen is limited, but properly done these procedures can identify malignant lesions as such about 90% of the time. In the case of a breast lesion which seems suspicious on clinical examination (palpation) or on mammograms, but whose nature could not be established by the initial aspiration or core sampling, Dr. Margolese and his NSABP colleagues urge that "the surgical biopsy should be performed as if it were a lumpectomy, with full attention given to margins."[3] Almost all breast biopsies require at least a loose collaboration between a surgeon, a pathologist, and a radiologist (mammographer). In contrast, a satisfactory lumpectomy requires the *intimate* collaboration of these three specialists—they must work together as a team. The NSABP lumpectomy guidelines emphasize that an experienced pathologist should be present in the operating room to inspect the tumor specimen as soon as the surgeon removes it.[4] Although the radiologist may not need to be physically present in the OR, the preoperative mammograms should be prominently displayed there on illuminated viewing boxes.

A patient with a known or suspected malignancy should remember that exploratory biopsies are counterindicated if breast preservation is desired. But if she has chosen her physicians and hospital wisely, her personal experience of undergoing lumpectomy for breast cancer should not be noticeably different from that of a patient undergoing the standard excisional biopsy, as described in Chapter Eleven. Overnight hospitalization is not often necessary. Most patients can walk in the hospital that morning and then walk out that afternoon, but being under sedation they should not attempt to drive a car or operate machinery before the following day.

Lumpectomy requires a single incision, which is placed so as to heal with the smallest possible scar. Most incisions will be slightly curved, paralleling the curved outlines of the areola. Cosmesis-conscious surgeons may want to put the incision in the areola itself, where the scar would be least visible; but Dr. Margolese and his NSABP colleagues caution that an areola incision is not advisable if the surgeon has to "tunnel" through breast tissue to reach the tumor. "The incision is best made directly over the mass." The NSABP guidelines call for the removal of an overlying skin segment only when the tumor is "superficial" (near the breast's surface), simply "as a method of obtaining an adequate margin." With tumors at other locations, the surgeon may wish to

leave a "narrow ellipse of skin" (less than five millimeters wide) at "the center of the specimen to orient the pathologist and to allow histologic examination of the dermal lymphatics."[5]

Most textbooks on breast cancer surgery recommend that a lumpectomy incision be placed so as to encompass—and ensure the removal of—any "needle tracks" which may have resulted from a preoperative fine-needle aspiration or core-needle biopsy. The old fear that cancer cells might be mechanically disseminated by a scalpel or a probing needle is remarkably persistent. A needle-track excision seems relatively harmless compared to the *en bloc* radical mastectomy, but surgeon William C. Wood of Emory University reminds us that the value of this recommendation is "untested." Needle-track excisions are probably less important "in breasts that will be irradiated as part of breast conservation treatment."[6]

Getting a Cancer-free Margin

Everybody agrees that a negative margin surrounding the tumor specimen—i.e., a strip of tissue entirely free of cancer cells—is the foremost desideratum in breast preservation surgery; but there is no agreement on how wide that margin should be. The widest margins are produced by **quadrantectomy**, a procedure which has been frequently used by the surgeon Umberto Veronesi and his colleagues at Italy's National Cancer Institute in Milan. As the name suggests, a quadrantectomy removes the entire breast quadrant in which the tumor is located, along with a sizable segment of overlying skin. The rate of local recurrence in the breast tends to be very low; the cosmetic outcome is less certain. Boston's Joint Center for Radiation Therapy represents the other extreme on this question—the Center's radiotherapists regard a margin as "negative" if no cancer cells are found within one millimeter of the specimen's border. That's a truly microscopic safety zone, less than one-twentieth of an inch. It is acceptable to the Center's radiotherapists because they require whole-breast irradiation with an additional boost, so that the tumor bed receives a total of 6,000 rads or more.[7] The margins required by those institutions which have offered lumpectomy without irradiation have been much more substantial. The Cleveland Clinic guidelines for this strategy specify a negative margin of one to two centimeters. The Princess Margaret clinical trial, which had a fairly high recurrence rate among its non-irradiated participants, required negative margins of one-half to one centimeter.[8] Unless a patient has very large breasts, a negative margin of two centimeters (about three-quarters inch) on all sides of the tumor may result in a noticeable cosmetic defect. The Consensus Development Conference of 1990 tried to reach a happy medium, recommending "a normal tissue margin of approximately one centimeter."[9]

Margins are a difficult tightrope to walk. If they're too narrow, the recurrence rate rises; if they're too wide, cosmesis suffers. While the issue of margins should be pondered before surgery, an informed decision on their adequacy cannot be made until after the pathologist looks at the tumor specimen. With lumpectomy as with the old-fashioned one-step biopsy, we need answers while the operation is still in progress. Is the tumor specimen surrounded by cancer-free margins, and is it now safe to close the incision? A second operation to obtain clean margins, while feasible, would be detrimental both to cosmesis and to the patient's state of mind. Fortunately, the pathologist will be right there in the OR to inspect the operative cavity (surgical field), process the specimen,

and advise the surgeon. Usually the surgeon will first tag the excised specimen with one or two sutures for orientation, thereby distinguishing its top from its bottom. Then the pathologist will lightly coat the specimen's surface with India ink, which serves as a permanent marker. If under microscopic examination cancer cells are seen near the inked surface, the margins would be rated "close." If the cancer cells are actually detected in the ink, the margins would be deemed "involved," and further excision would be indicated. While in the OR the pathologist will cut the tumor specimen in two and examine its exposed interior with a magnifying glass. If there is any question of marginal involvement, microscopic examination of a frozen section taken from the suspect area should be done immediately, so as to determine whether more tissue must be removed from the operative cavity. In the case of a nonpalpable lesion discovered by mammography, the excised specimen should be immediately radiographed (X-rayed) to verify that it contains the calcifications or other abnormality which prompted the breast surgery.

The preceding techniques for the intraoperative assessment of margins represent common sense and standard practice. If rigorously adhered to, they will usually eliminate the unpleasant possibility that a second lumpectomy might have to be done on the heels of the first, because the permanent sections revealed involved margins or because postoperative mammograms discovered the suspicious calcifications still lodged in the breast. These precautions cannot be said to eliminate the long-term problem posed by tumor recurrences cropping up near the lumpectomy site a few years later. An innovative hypothesis which helps to explain such local failures rests upon the concept of **molecular margins**. Joseph A. Brennan and his colleagues at Johns Hopkins suggest that these recurrences may not be due to any obviously malignant cells left behind at surgery, but rather to cells near the tumor which seem normal enough yet carry genetic mutations leading to malignant evolution. Brennan et al used an assay based on the polymerase chain reaction (PCR) to look for carcinogenetic mutations of the *p53* gene in tumor margins declared "negative" after routine microscopic examinations. What they found was that adjacent "normal-appearing tissue" can sometimes harbor the same *p53* mutations as the excised tumor, and that these "positive molecular margins" foreshadow "a substantially increased risk of local recurrence."[10] Assays to evaluate the DNA mutations of apparently normal cells near a malignant tumor remain experimental; if they should become standard, they might give us a better idea of how wide a margin must be to be truly cancer-free.

That Pesky Axillary Dissection

Surgery to remove the regional lymph nodes in the axilla (armpit) has been one of the holiest icons in breast cancer medicine. It has been unconditionally venerated by traditionalist surgeons, and even the breast preservationists of the NSABP and the Joint Center for Radiation Therapy have been known to genuflect before it. But these days any indiscriminate application of this procedure starts to look like mindless ritualism. Patients with *in situ* or node-negative tumors derive no benefit from axillary surgery, and they now constitute a majority of American patients diagnosed with breast cancer. Node-positive patients typically receive very good protection against tumor recurrence in the axilla as well as improved staging (prognostic assessment). Yet we know from the NSABP trials that there is little or no survival

benefit to be had, even for patients with numerous positive nodes. By the year 2000 the **sentinel node biopsy** performed during lumpectomy or mastectomy was increasingly being used for patients with small breast tumors, and most American surgeons saw no reason to remove additional nodes if the sentinel node proved free of cancer cells.[11]

The traditional axillary dissection does not automatically go in tandem with lumpectomy, because it requires general anesthesia rather than sedation, and thus it would convert an outpatient procedure into an inpatient one. Moreover, while lumpectomy and axillary dissection can be performed on the same occasion, they constitute two different operations which ideally require two separate incisions. Richard G. Margolese and his NSABP colleagues stress that "a separate incision for the axillary dissection is always better." When the primary tumor is located in the upper outer quadrant (near the axilla), some surgeons may try to accomplish both procedures with one incision, extending the lumpectomy incision made over the tumor diagonally up into the axilla. This technique is possibly easier and faster for the surgeon; but as Dr. Margolese and his colleagues point out, it involves "a long suture line" which interrupts "the skin's normal lines of tension" and leads to "poor cosmesis."[12] In the worst cases this extension of the lumpectomy incision can result in a noticeable scar and a distorted breast contour. Lumpectomy patients who must undergo axillary dissection are better served by a separate incision discretely placed under the arm, where the scar will be naturally concealed.

Unlike the outpatient lumpectomy, almost any type of mastectomy can conveniently accommodate axillary dissection as an accompanying procedure. During mastectomy the patient is already under general anesthesia; and since cosmesis of the pre-served breast is not an issue, extending the incision toward the axilla poses no problem. The controversies here have centered around the number and location of the nodes to be removed; as usual in breast cancer matters, consensus is lacking. However, surgeons have agreed to discuss the axillary nodes as though they were divided into three distinct levels, using the pectoralis minor muscle as an anatomical reference point. The level I nodes are found in the fatty tissue lateral to (alongside of) the pectoralis minor—the level II nodes, beneath it—and the level III nodes, above it. These three levels are also referred to as "low" (level I), as "middle" (level II), and as "high" or "apex" (level III). When a breast tumor sheds cancer cells into the lymphatic system, the lower axillary nodes (level I) are usually the first to be involved. But a surgeon performing an axillary dissec-tion for staging (diagnostic) purposes may want to remove the middle nodes under the pectoralis minor muscle (level II) as well as the lower nodes, because occasionally posi-tive nodes will be found in level II while level I proves negative. We refer to this phenomenon as "nodal skip metastases"; it happens just often enough to make us slightly suspicious of the diagnostic reliabil-ity of samplings limited to the lower axillary nodes. The highest or apex nodes (level III), located well up in the axilla, are almost never involved with breast cancer dissemination if the lower and middle nodes (levels I and II) prove negative.[13]

The lower axillary nodes (level I) are the easiest to access, and in the case of small breast tumors some surgeons have been content simply to take a few nodes from that level. But Blake Cady and Michael D. Stone of the Harvard Medical School condemn any "blind, non-anatomic removal in the low axilla," pointing out that not only is the staging information less reliable, but that

"without a formal controlled exposure of the pertinent nerves (long thoracic and thora-codorsal), they are at risk of injury."[14] Axil-lary surgery is a tricky business, more diffi-cult than mastectomy, because the axilla contains lots of delicate nerves and small blood vessels essential to the healthy func-tioning of the arm and shoulder. The nerves in particular must be spared at all costs. An injury to the long thoracic nerve can paralyze the serratus anterior muscle, causing that uncontrollable protrusion of the shoulder blade, the so-called "winged scapula," which used to be an often encountered reminder of exuberant axillary dissections. If the thora-codorsal nerve is cut, the latissimus dorsi muscle will be paralyzed, making it difficult for the patient to rotate her arm. Stripping the fatty tissue from around the axillary artery will not capture many breast cancer cells, but does invite lymphedema—the nodes and lymphatic vessels found there are involved with the drainage of the arm, not the mammary gland.[15]

These days the worst side effects of axillary dissections—edematous arms swol-len with fluid, atrophied muscles, winged scapulas—are rarely encountered. Not only do surgeons proceed more cautiously and knowledgeably than their predecessors, but in current American practice the apex of the axilla is not dissected in early-stage breast cancer. Historically, those efforts to remove the highest nodes (level III) have caused the most serious disruptions of nerves and lym-phatics. With this fact in mind, the NSABP guidelines for axillary dissections would limit the intervention to the lower and middle axilla, removing "all level I and II nodes." Dr. Margolese and his colleagues assure us that this sampling "will provide a highly accurate staging of axillary nodes." The median number of nodes examined in the NSABP trials has been 15, a figure which has been "strikingly constant" for both

The Three Levels of Axillary Nodes

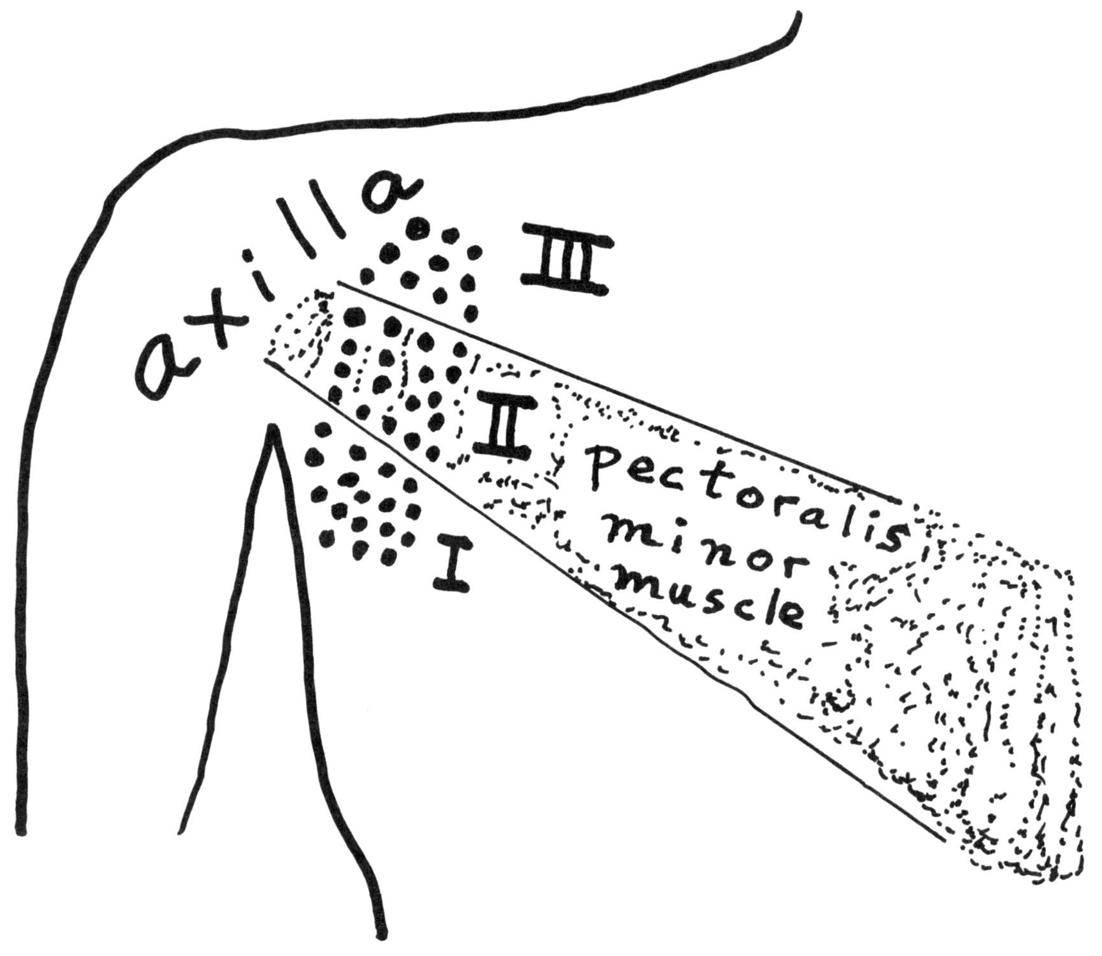

The **axillary dissections** performed during the radical mastectomy era removed all three levels of nodes, compromising the arm's lymphatic drainage and leading to severe lymphedema. The **"high" or "apex" nodes (level III)** are no longer dissected in early-stage breast cancer. For most node-positive patients, removal of the **lower (level I) and middle (level II) nodes** will provide adequate protection against axillary recurrences. The **pectoralis minor muscle** must be temporarily retracted to access the underlying level II nodes, but its function should not be impaired. **Sentinel node mapping** usually identifies a single node in the lower axilla (level I), which can be biopsied without causing any significant side effects.

lumpectomies and mastectomies.[16] Cady and Stone suggest that surgeons "obtain at least 10 lymph nodes for analysis." All this is a far cry from the total evacuations practiced by Halstedians like C. D. Haagensen, who once reported that he got "an average of 50.3 lymph nodes out of the axillary portion of radical mastectomy specimens."[17]

The Sentinel Node Biopsy

Even the most careful dissection of the lower and middle axilla will necessarily impair the arm's lymphatic drainage to some extent. Henceforth the affected arm will always be more prone to fluid accumulation (lymphedema) and infections than the contralateral arm, and as a result it will be subject to a long list of restrictions. The patient will be cautioned that injections and blood pressure monitoring should be performed on the other arm—that she should try to avoid injuring the involved hand or arm (even small cuts and burns can lead to unpleasant consequences)—and that she should not hamper the arm's circulation by wearing tight clothing or rings. These lingering side effects— and the fact that the therapeutic value of an axillary dissection is no longer as apparent as it once was—have led some breast specialists to ponder whether this time-honored procedure might often be replaced for staging purposes by the **sentinel node biopsy**. This newer technique is purely diagnostic in intent; it would not prevent tumor recurrences in the axilla, and therefore it would be most suitable for patients who are unlikely to have positive axillary nodes. The most plausible candidates would be patients with ductal carcinoma *in situ* or small invasive tumors less than one centimeter in diameter. About 90% of these cases are going to be node-negative; for that large majority it's a terrible waste to undergo axillary surgery just to prove the anticipated absence of axillary involvement. At the other extreme, most patients with large invasive tumors (say, over two centimeters) or with palpable nodes stand to benefit from a careful axillary dissection, because that's the best way of preventing the probable axillary recurrences.

The technique of sentinel node biopsy already plays a role in the staging of melanomas, the most threatening variety of skin cancer. The principal advocates of its use in breast malignancies have been Armando E. Giuliano and his colleagues at the John Wayne Cancer Institute in Santa Monica, California, and John J. Albertini and his coworkers at the H. Lee Moffitt Cancer Center at the University of South Florida in Tampa. A sentinel node biopsy must be done right before the scheduled lumpectomy or mastectomy. As Dr. Giuliano and his colleagues explain, they first inject a little bit of "blue vital dye" (about five milliliters) into the tumor and the surrounding area; then they wait "approximately five minutes, the time required for dye to reach the axillary drainage basin." An incision is now made in the axilla "just below the hair-bearing region," and the surgeon carefully probes about to find either a "blue-stained node" or a bluish lymphatic vessel which would lead to such a node. That blue node is assumed to be **the sentinel node**, the first one which filters the lymphatic fluid draining from the tumor area. It's excised and subjected to intense pathological examination, using not only the traditional hematoxylin and eosin (H&E) staining but also the newer and more expensive immunostaining.[18] "While that does increase the cost of looking at that lymph node," Giuliano observes, "it diminishes the cost of caring for that patient because the technique would be an outpatient procedure under local anesthesia."[19]

Between 1991 and 1994 the Giuliano

team tested sentinel node mapping and sampling on 172 breast cancer patients undergoing surgery at the John Wayne Cancer Institute. All these patients had traditional axillary dissections (removal of level I and II nodes "and at least some level III") after the sentinel node biopsy was finished. Giuliano and his colleagues discovered that there is a pronounced "learning curve" for surgeons trying to identify and excise sentinel nodes. Early attempts were often unsuccessful, but "in the last 50 cases the rate of detection was 78.0%." Once a sentinel node had been located, it proved to be a remarkably accurate predictor of the axillary status (positive or negative) as later determined by the axillary dissection. "The sentinel node," reported Giuliano et al, "accurately identified axillary nodal status in 109 of 114 cases (95.6%)."[20]

At the University of South Florida in Tampa, John J. Albertini and his co-workers improved the odds of successful lymphatic mapping by adding a radioactive marker ("technetium-labeled sulfur colloid") to the blue dye. Before making an incision, the surgeon used "a handheld gamma-detection probe" to "identify the area of greatest activity in the axilla." The miniature Geiger counter came into play again once a blue node had been exposed, being "used to confirm that the node contained a significantly higher level of radioactivity than background tissue or neighboring, non-sentinel lymph nodes." Albertini et al tested their two-marker technique (dye plus radioisotope) on 62 breast cancer patients treated at the Moffitt Cancer Center; they reported a 92% success rate in detecting a sentinel node (57 out of the 62 cases).[21]

One serendipitous benefit from sentinel node mapping has been a better understanding of the breast's lymphatic drainage—we now know that it can vary considerably from individual to individual. Most of the sentinel nodes identified by the Giuliano team were in the lower axilla (level I); but as they pointed out, "23.3% of our most recent dissections yielded a sentinel node in level II alone."[22] This surprising finding does much to explain the phenomenon of nodal skip metastases which had puzzled breast cancer specialists for many years. Intense examination of one sentinel node with immunostaining may actually be a more sensitive indicator of subtle axillary involvement than the routine H&E studies of a dozen or more nodes which have been randomly excised. The effectiveness of this new technique means that future surgery for small breast tumors will be conducted on an outpatient basis, with lower costs and fewer side effects. Mammography and fine-needle aspiration would give us a preliminary diagnosis—the sentinel node biopsy and the lumpectomy could then be done together. In 1997 the breast surgeon Umberto Veronesi and his colleagues in Milan, Italy, reported their satisfaction with preoperative nodal mapping, concluding that "patients without clinical involvement of the axilla should undergo sentinel node biopsy routinely, and may be spared complete axillary dissection when the sentinel node is disease-free."[23] The Milan team's endorsement is especially significant because it represents an about-face. Hitherto Veronesi et al had been sticklers for total axillary evacuations.

The Moffitt Cancer Center of the University of South Florida has made an effort to re-educate surgeons trained to do traditional axillary dissections, offering a brief course on the sentinel node biopsy featuring "intraoperative sessions on melanoma and breast cancer patients."[24] However, Dr. Giuliano stresses that mastery of the proper technique requires considerable practice: "I caution surgeons not to abandon routine axillary dissection until they have achieved a consistently high rate of sentinel node identification."[25] The shortage of proficient surgeons is not the only obstacle to the universal adoption of sentinel node biopsy; another is the fact that oncologists have long been accustomed to plan adjuvant therapy based on the total number of positive nodes detected. Patients with ten or more positive nodes have been regarded as candidates for exceptionally rigorous chemotherapy. Sentinel node biopsy is therefore most practical when the indicator node conveniently proves negative. Walter Lawrence, Jr., a surgeon in Richmond, Virginia, has considered the other possibility: "If one obtains a positive report from the sentinel node biopsy, what should one do? Should one go ahead and perform a node dissection? Or should we now say that we have enough information and proceed with the adjuvant therapy?" In these cases Armando E. Giuliano's approach would be entirely traditional. "I think patients with positive nodes should have an axillary dissection," Dr. Giuliano advises. "There are therapeutic advantages. There is regional control, and there may be survival advantages. We cannot conclude that leaving residual cancer in the axilla is good."[26]

The Types of Mastectomy:
Making Sense of Nomenclature

Laypersons readily grasp the concept of lumpectomy; but mastectomy nomenclature tends to be all Greek to them, a difficulty compounded by the fact that different surgeons may use different names for the same procedure. It may be easy to suspect that a "modified radical" mastectomy removes less flesh than the more forbidding-sounding "total" mastectomy—but the converse is true, as readers of Chapter Fifteen will remember.

What the different types of mastectomy have in common is an intent to remove the mammary gland in its entirety. This normally means excision of the nipple and areola, all the ducts and lobules, and the subcutaneous fat which makes up the bulk of the breast. There are considerable variations in the amount of skin removed, in the size and placement of the incision, and in the completeness of any axillary dissection that might accompany the procedure. The prevalent nomenclature reflects these variations, but does not do so as precisely as we might like. Unfortunately, no mastectomy technique can offer a 100% guarantee that all glandular tissues will be removed. The mammary gland is not a well-defined capsulated organ like the pancreas or the prostate; it consists largely of subtly disseminated tissues which are not distinguishable by the naked eye. Grant W. Carlson, a surgeon at Emory University, reminds us that residual glandular tissue can sometimes adhere to the skin. To be sure of its complete removal, Dr. Carlson adds, "you would almost have to come so close to the skin to either slough the skin, or you would have to remove a large portion of skin."[27]

The **radical mastectomy** remains the biggest hammer in the surgical armamentarium. This procedure removes the breast, the underlying muscles, most of the skin, and all the axillary lymph nodes, leaving the patient with a perfectly flat chest and a tendency to arm lymphedema. These days only Stage Three tumors involving the skin or chest muscles might be thought to warrant a true radical operation. The term **modified radical mastectomy** is bandied about much more frequently, being used to cover a multitude of surgical variations rather than to define a particular operative plan. But the mere mention of the word "radical" should alert you that an axillary dissection is intended.

Back in the 1930s the London surgeon D. H. Patey discovered that he could leave the large pectoralis major muscle in place and still do a thorough axillary dissection provided he removed the pectoralis minor. This smaller muscle must be excised or at least divided to gain full access to the lymph nodes in the apex of the axilla (the level III nodes). The so-called **Patey-type mastectomy** offers local tumor control comparable to that obtained by radical mastectomy, yet with better cosmesis and improved arm function. The concave appearance of the chest is avoided. One drawback is that by removing or cutting the pectoralis minor muscle, the surgeon will usually destroy the lateral pectoral nerve, thereby causing the lower third of the pectoralis major muscle to atrophy and consequently producing some stiffness of shoulder movements.[28] This disability is mild compared to those left by radical mastectomy; in the 1970s Patey's modification won general acceptance in the United States. When American breast surgeons spoke of a "modified radical mastectomy" in that decade, they almost always meant the Patey procedure. For Jerome A. Urban and David W. Kinne at New York's Sloan-Kettering Cancer Center, or for Francis E. Rosato at Philadelphia's Jefferson Medical College, it was the procedure of choice for small to moderate-sized invasive tumors.

By the 1980s, however, surgeons taking their cue from Bernard Fisher and the NSABP came to regard Patey-type mastectomies as excessive. Even before the NSABP's clinical trials, the surgeon Hugh Auchincloss of New York City had concluded that there was no necessity to dissect the apex of the axilla. He plausibly reasoned that the apical (level III) nodes are not often involved in early-stage breast cancer, and that if they are, the patient is probably going to develop metastatic disease regardless of the thoroughness of the axillary dissection.

Auchincloss developed and promoted a modified radical mastectomy in which both chest muscles (pectoralis major and minor) are preserved with full innervation and vascular supply. The two muscles are merely retracted—temporarily pulled out of the way—so as to allow the surgeon to remove the lower and middle axillary nodes (levels I and II). This procedure does not cause the pectoralis major atrophy and the resulting arm and shoulder disabilities which can sometimes accompany the Patey modification. The **Auchincloss-type mastectomy** has been modified so much that it is no longer "radical" in a proper Halstedian sense. Nonetheless it also is referred to as a "modified radical mastectomy." And it may also be called an **Auchincloss-Madden-type mastectomy**, picking up the surname of breast surgeon John L. Madden, who similarly advocated the preservation of both chest muscles.[29]

Dr. Auchincloss, who publicized his procedure in the early 1960s, was simply ahead of his time. Careful retraction of the chest muscles to allow a restricted axillary dissection (levels I and II only) now constitutes the standard modification, endorsed by the Consensus Development Conference of 1979 and by the NSABP surgeons.[30] Nonetheless, whenever that imprecise term "modified radical mastectomy" is dropped into a preoperative consultation, the wise patient will inquire about the extent of the axillary surgery being planned and the reasons for it. Only patients with extensive nodal involvement would seem to be appropriate candidates for Patey-type operations.

The terms **simple mastectomy** and **total mastectomy** are equivalent. Neither usage implies axillary dissection; both denote a complete removal of the mammary gland. The most obvious indications for this basic mastectomy are widespread *in situ* cancer or a genetic predisposition to carcinogenesis as seen in familial breast cancer syndromes. In these two instances, we have ample reason to believe that the entire breast—and possibly the patient's life—may be at considerable risk; but we have as yet no evidence which would suggest malignant dissemination to the axilla. Therefore any lumpectomy would be insufficient, and any excision of regional lymph nodes would be unwarranted. The chest muscles are preserved in total (simple) mastectomies. The Consensus Development Conference of 1979 recommended "total mastectomy with axillary dissection" by way of emphasizing that while axillary staging was desirable in early-stage breast cancer, the chest muscles should be left intact. The procedure intended was an Auchincloss-type mastectomy; presumably the CDC panel did not wish to sow confusion by citing a "modified radical mastectomy," that term being traditionally associated with Patey and pectoralis minor excision.

Two specialized mastectomy procedures have been developed for patients who are anxious to get rid of cancer-prone or otherwise troublesome glands while holding onto cosmetically pleasing breast contours. The combination of **subcutaneous mastectomy and silicone implant** elicited a great deal of enthusiasm back in the 1970s. In this procedure an easily concealable incision is first made in the inframammary fold—that crease at the bottom of the breast where it rests on the lower chest wall. Then the surgeon tunnels under the skin to remove the breast's fatty and glandular tissues, afterwards inserting a silicone implant in their place.[31] The procedure thus promises much—preservation of the nipple-areola complex and all the skin, removal of that dangerous gland and a lifelike reconstruction, all done in just one trip to the operating room. Unfortunately, this procedure is technically demanding. It sometimes involves

appreciable blood loss, and it carries a higher risk of complications (skin slough and infections) than purely ablative mastectomies. A meticulous subcutaneous mastectomy might remove as much as 90% of the mammary gland; but remnants of the ductal system necessarily remain in the nipple-areola complex, and traces of glandular tissue may be left on the underside of the skin. William C. Wood of Emory University speculates that prophylactic subcutaneous mastectomies could reduce the likelihood of breast cancer in high-risk women almost as effectively as total mastectomies: "Some women want to have a marked reduction in risk but are not convinced that giving up a nipple will significantly affect that risk reduction. There are no convincing trials to suggest that it will."[32] In the 1990s, however, the subcutaneous mastectomy and silicone implant fell into disrepute, not so much because of the perennial worries about residual mammary tissues, but because of the torrents of bad publicity unleashed on silicone implants.

Dr. Wood, Grant W. Carlson, the reconstructive surgeon John Bostwick III, and other physicians at the Emory Hospital in Atlanta have promoted another innovative procedure called the **skin-sparing mastectomy**. First used in 1991, this term denotes a mastectomy which attempts to remove the entire mammary gland while preserving most of the breast's skin so as to facilitate simultaneous reconstruction. The technique can be used either for prophylaxis (cancer prevention) or for the treatment of small invasive cancers with no significant skin involvement. The main difference between the skin-sparing mastectomy and more traditional procedures has to do with the size and placement of the incision. Instead of a broad elliptical incision encompassing most of the breast's skin, the surgeon typically makes an oval incision around the outline of the nipple and areola. All the glandular tissue is then removed through that small opening. If a breast cancer is located at some distance from the areola, the surgeon may either extend the circumareolar incision to the tumor area or make a separate lumpectomy-type incision directly over the tumor. Once the oncologic surgeon has finished, the reconstructive (plastic) surgeon can immediately re-create the breast mound either with the patient's own tissue (flap transfer) or with an expander (inflatable shell). The Emory team points out that "skin-sparing mastectomy facilitates reconstruction by reducing remedial surgery. Preservation of the inframammary fold and native skin envelope allows breast symmetry to be achieved without altering the opposite breast. The periareolar incisions are more inconspicuous."[33] This particular procedure of simultaneous mastectomy and breast reconstruction requires considerable finesse from both the oncologic and the reconstructive surgeon; it is not available at all hospitals.

Undergoing Mastectomy

Mastectomy is a safe operation, not at all life-threatening, yet it remains major surgery which has normally required general anesthesia and hospitalization. Patients typically check into the hospital the day before so as to undergo a battery of tests—chest X-rays, electrocardiograms, and laboratory workups of blood samples. The surgery itself may take several hours; an accompanying axillary dissection increases the operating time. The amount of blood lost during mastectomy is highly variable; transfusion may be necessary in some cases, but surgeons now do everything they can to avoid that contingency. While the mandatory testing of donated blood has greatly reduced the risk of infection with a virus causing hepatitis or AIDS, there are several other reasons to be leery of

transfusions. William L. Donegan and John S. Spratt observe that blood transfusions have "well-documented immunosuppressive effects" which might possibly retard wound healing. Banking of the patient's own blood (autologous blood) before surgery is the safest option if a substantial blood loss is anticipated. During mastectomy the anesthesiologist will continually monitor the volume of the patient's blood, its pressure, and its oxygen-carrying capacity. Transfusion or other supportive measures are indicated whenever the intravascular volume falls so low that the patient's blood pressure cannot be maintained, or when hemoglobin depletion signals that the cells are not getting enough oxygen. Donegan and Spratt observe that the infusion of electrolyte solutions during surgery helps to maintain a steady intravascular volume: "Postoperatively, administration of oral iron supplements helps to reconstitute normal levels of hemoglobin."[34]

Dr. Halsted's basic lessons of careful dissection and constant hemostasis remain as important as they ever were, but his old-fashioned incision encircling the breast has gone by the board. The modern mastectomy incision is elliptical. It encompasses the tumor site, the "track" of any previous surgical biopsy or needle sampling procedure, and the nipple-areola complex. Depending on the tumor's location and the breast's configuration, the ellipse may lie horizontally, vertically, or diagonally. Kirby I. Bland and Edward M. Copeland of the University of Florida recommend that "the incision incorporate skin at least three centimeters from the periphery of the tumor in three dimensions. Less skin is excised when lesions are located deep within the breast and are small in transverse diameter."[35] Three centimeters (about an inch and a quarter) may sound like a lot, but present-day incisions are narrow compared to those prevalent in the era of radical

Elliptical Mastectomy Incision

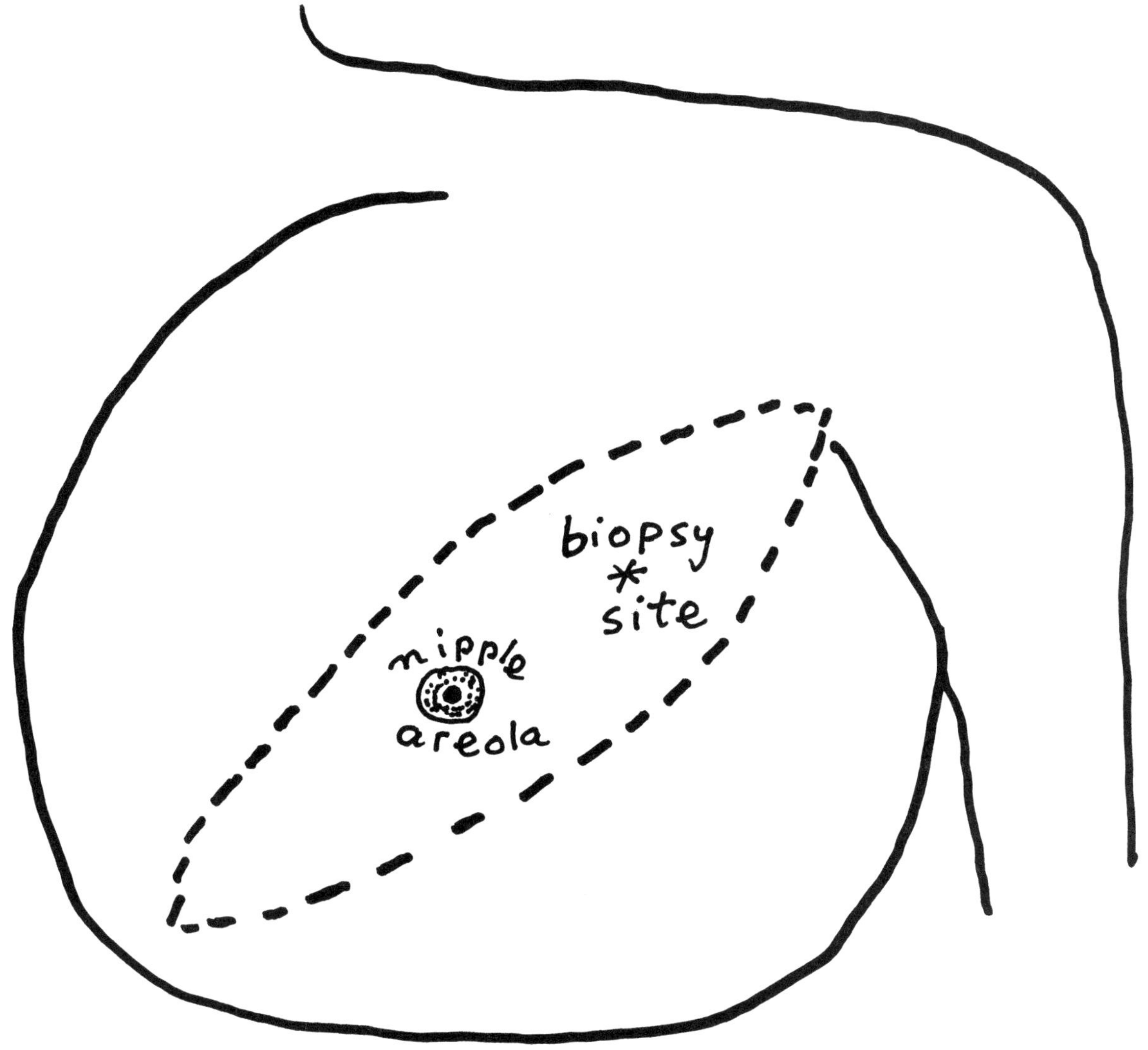

Today's mastectomy incisions are not nearly as wide or as long as those used in the era of radical surgery. Nonetheless, with a view to removing the entire mammary gland, they normally encompass **the nipple-areola complex**. And with a nod to the old worries about a possible mechanical dissemination of tumor cells, they will also encompass **the site of any previous biopsy or needle-sampling procedure**.

mastectomy. Skin grafts are rarely needed to close the wound. If the patient desires reconstruction with an implant, an inflatable **tissue expander** is usually put in place before wound closure. Later it is gradually enlarged to accomplish the regrowth of the skin envelope—that is, the replacement of the skin excised during mastectomy.

An <u>Outpatient</u> Mastectomy?

The most cost-saving innovation in breast surgery has been the development of regional anesthesia techniques which allow almost all procedures to be performed on an outpatient basis. As recently as the 1980s mastectomies, axillary dissections, and breast reconstructions typically required hospitalization for the better part of a week. The main obstacle preventing mastectomy patients from walking out of the hospital on the same day they entered has always been the necessity for general anesthesia, with its ensuing postoperative grogginess and often frequent nausea. By the 1990s, however, avant-garde anesthesiologists discovered that mastectomies and axillary dissections could be safely performed without general anesthesia if only the spinal nerves relaying sensations from the breast and axilla could be temporarily "blocked" (deadened). Eileen P. Lynch and other anesthesiologists at Boston's famed Brigham and Women's Hospital began to use **thoracic epidural anesthesia** in 1993 for selected patients undergoing mastectomies or other extensive breast operations. In this technique the patient is first given intravenous sedation; then a needle with an attached catheter is inserted in the upper spine, "in one of the spaces between the second and sixth thoracic vertebrae." According to Dr. Lynch and her colleagues, the combination of lidocaine and epinephrine is administered through the catheter until "the lateral and medial pectoral nerves are blocked," producing "adequate sensory anesthesia of the anterior chest wall." The goal is to bathe the spinal cord with anesthetic solution—but the tough membrane (dura mater) surrounding the cord should not be penetrated. As the anesthetic rapidly disseminates beyond the epidural space, additional doses have to be given "every 20 to 40 minutes" while the operation is in progress. The collaborating surgeon at Brigham and Women's Hospital, Dr. Timothy J. Eberlein, has been free to discharge patients given epidural anesthesia once he verified the absence of surgical complications and obtained postoperative pain control. In practice, however, most patients undergoing mastectomy or axillary dissection were kept in the hospital overnight, being released on the second day.[36]

A breast cancer team at the Duke University Medical Center, headed by surgeons Christina F. Weltz and H. Kim Lyerly and the anesthesiologist Roy A. Greengrass, has adhered more strictly to the concept of outpatient mastectomy. Operative pain control at this North Carolina institution is obtained by **paravertebral block**. With this technique a long-lasting local anesthetic is injected into the "thoracic paravertebral space" to block (deaden) the relevant nerves as they emerge from the spinal column. Dr. Weltz and her colleagues assure us that paravertebral block, unlike epidural anesthesia, carries no risk of injury to the spinal cord and can provide "pain control for up to 20 hours after operation." The Duke mastectomy patients who seemed suitable for immediate release were kept in the recovery room for two or three hours (the average stay was 169 minutes). They were then given instructions on how to care for the incision and the indwelling drains, provided with tablets for pain (acetaminophen and codeine), and allowed to go home.[37]

The advent of outpatient mastectomy, with same-day or day-after discharge, has elicited both loud applause and cries of apprehension. Insurance companies paying for mastectomies and subsequent reconstructions are understandably enthusiastic about an innovation which could lower the typical hospital bill by several thousand dollars. From the patients' point of view, the principal advantages to having breast surgery done under spinal anesthesia rather than general anesthesia are an expedited recovery and a reduced incidence of postoperative nausea. Naturally there are a few drawbacks. Not all anesthesiologists are sufficiently proficient in the necessary techniques. And some surgeons may be uncomfortable about removing a breast or maneuvering around the axilla while the patient is conscious enough to be aware of these events. Activist groups have been quick to point out that mastectomy is often a severe psychological and physiological shock to patients, who may feel much more comfortable and secure if they can remain in the hospital for the first two or three days after surgery. Dr. Weltz and her colleagues at Duke caution that candidates for outpatient mastectomy should be carefully screened. These patients must be knowledgeable enough to recognize postoperative complications like subcutaneous bleeding or wound infection, and able to go back to the hospital at the first sign of trouble. All the Duke mastectomy patients given a same-day discharge were "seen at the outpatient breast clinic within ten days and thereafter as needed for wound examination, drain removal, and consultation." According to Dr. Weltz and her colleagues, "the ability to avoid hospitalization softens the impact of a cancer diagnosis and encourages early return to normal activity."[38]

Recovering from Surgery

Back in the days of radical mastectomy, recovery from breast surgery often amounted to a protracted ordeal—six months of rehabilitative exercises might be necessary to restore the basic functions of arm and shoulder. These days recovery is likely to be swift and complete, regardless of whether the patient has spent a week in the hospital or just a few hours. Lumpectomy patients are sent home with a light dressing over the incision; they are advised to wear supportive bras and to avoid overly vigorous activities. As the lumpectomy incision heals, the patient may notice a gradual hardening at the tumor site. This is a normal occurrence resulting from tissue reconstitution, not a sign of resurgent malignancy.

The tiny lymphatic vessels which are inevitably cut during breast surgery will continue to drain lymphatic fluid into the operative field; it usually takes two or three days before these vessels begin to close of their own accord. In the meantime, fluid accumulation is a problem which must be dealt with. Fine-needle aspiration can always be used to remove fluid accumulations under the skin—these are called **seromas**—but it is better to prevent their formation. Surgeons try to do this by leaving flexible soft-plastic drains in place. These drains are sometimes attached to a gentle suction device, much like those devices which dentists put in your mouth while drilling on your teeth. The purpose is to evacuate the serous fluid and to encourage early closure of the severed lymphatics. Modified radical mastectomies have typically required two drains—one being placed under the skin flaps on the chest wall, and the other being left in the axilla.[39] In the 1980s mastectomy patients were expected to stay in the hospital until the fluid output from each drain had slowed down to a trickle (30 milliliters or less per day). The tubes were then taken out, and the patients discharged. Current practice at some institutions allows patients to go home with the drains in place, and then return as outpatients several days later to have them removed. Lumpectomy usually does not require drainage tubes at the tumor site; but when this procedure is done in conjunction with axillary dissection, a tube should be placed in the axilla. The intact breast goes on secreting lymphatic fluid into the axilla, so much so that the risk of seroma formation there with lumpectomy and axillary dissection may actually be greater than with modified radical mastectomy.[40]

The effects of anesthesia and blood loss are understandably felt more by patients who have had mastectomies than by those who have had lumpectomies. Nonetheless mastectomy patients are expected to be ambulatory—up and walking about—the day after surgery. Typically the wound has been covered with a light dressing, loosely attached so as not to unduly restrict arm and shoulder movements, or to retard fluid collection with the drainage tubes. There are differences of opinion on how soon the affected arm and shoulder should be used after mastectomy and axillary dissection. Vigorous exercise right after surgery would have the effect of increasing lymphatic flow into the operative field, preventing severed lymphatics from closing. For this reason Kirby I. Bland and his colleagues have advocated that the shoulder and upper arm be kept relatively immobile for several days, "while mobility is permitted below the elbow in the forearm and hand." Other surgeons encourage patients to use the arm normally but carefully from the very first day. Age and physical condition are factors which dictate the speed of recovery. Bland et al observe that "young women usually regain full arm and shoulder range of motion before leaving the hospital."[41]

Older patients are more prone to **neuropraxia** of the ipsilateral arm or shoulder, transient paralysis which occurs because the pertinent nerves have been manipulated (pulled out of position) during axillary dissection, and have therefore temporarily lost their ability to activate muscles. Such commonplace postmastectomy symptoms as numbness or tingling affecting the arm and shoulder may also be chalked up to this bruising of the axillary nerves. Any patient who experiences muscular weakness stands to benefit from a structured exercise program, which should be begun as soon as the lymphatic flow subsides. The "spider walk" has long been recommended as an initial exercise—the patient slowly walks her fingers up a wall like a spider, going a little bit higher with each passing day. Later, a week or two after surgery, she may be encouraged to raise her arm over her head, again going higher on each subsequent day. It should be emphasized that no one who has had an axillary dissection should attempt to raise her arm over her head before being advised to do so by her surgeon or by a physical therapist trained in postmastectomy rehabilitation. Moderation remains the best policy for exercises in the immediate postoperative period. Whether they are recovering in the hospital or at home, breast surgery patients need rest more than they need activity.

Long-term Adjustments

Either mastectomy by itself or lumpectomy with axillary dissection will bring some permanent changes to the patient's life. Regaining full mobility of the affected arm and shoulder is but the first obstacle which must be overcome. For mastectomy patients, the loss of a breast will have created an imbalance—one side of the chest still carries its customary weight, while the other is suddenly disburdened. If the remaining breast is large and heavy, this imbalance can rapidly lead to nagging aches of the back, neck, and shoulder. Almost all mastectomy patients will eventually seek a permanent solution to this problem, either by acquiring and wearing a weighted silicone prosthesis (breast form), or by undergoing breast reconstruction. In the meantime there is the matter of leaving the hospital in the same clothes one wore when entering it. Since the 1950s this fashion dilemma has usually been solved by a volunteer from the American Cancer Society's **"Reach to Recovery"** program, who would appear in the patient's hospital room a day or two after surgery bringing words of consolation, lots of ACS brochures, and a temporary prosthesis made of Dacron or another lightweight material.

For most patients that hospital visit from an ACS representative or some other volunteer worker has marked their first experience with a cancer support group. Not everybody is thrilled to discover that they have been automatically and involuntarily "grouped" with cancer patients. This is an affiliation that nobody would consciously seek to acquire, and some patients may want nothing to do with organizations which are perceived as being based solely on mutual illness. The degree of participation in a cancer support group—a little, a lot, or none at all—is left to the individual; but there are often decided advantages to be had from active involvement. Physicians and nurses simply do not have time to discuss all the personal problems which ensue upon cancer diagnosis and treatment. And they are not likely to welcome phone calls at odd hours to chat about these problems. In contrast, the members of a support group generally find the time to talk. While not medical professionals, they do have firsthand experience of coping with cancer treatments. Of course, as we've seen, breast cancers are extremely

heterogeneous and require very different treatments. The Reach to Recovery program has never tried to match its volunteers with new patients on the basis of pathological diagnoses and projected adjuvant therapies. It does attempt to match them on the basis of age, marital status, and initial surgical therapy. Thus a married woman in her seventies who had a mastectomy ten years previously would not normally be asked to visit a single woman in her thirties who has just had a lumpectomy and is scheduled for whole-breast irradiation two weeks hence. But if the first volunteer who comes has no first-hand experience with a projected treatment like radiotherapy or chemo, the odds are very good that she can provide the name and telephone number of another person in the local support group who has "been there." Names, telephone numbers, and Internet addresses are what cancer support is all about. The patient needs to be connected with people who know how to help. Often lasting friendships and new opportunities are unexpected but highly gratifying byproducts of participation in a support group.

Each mastectomy patient must make her own private adjustments to the loss of a breast. Some patients may find it emotionally painful to look at the mastectomy incision, which may be half a foot in length and stretch from the sternum to the axilla. For purely practical reasons, however, the incision needs to be looked at and looked after. It should be kept dry; and while it ought to be ventilated, it should also be cushioned against blows and chafing clothing. A week or two after surgery, the patient must return to the surgeon's office for inspection of the incision and suture removal. But she should contact her surgeon immediately if undue redness or swelling develops near the incision—this could well indicate an infection.

As soon as the incision is fully healed, a weighted prosthesis can be worn. Breast replacement forms come in various sizes and shapes, ranging in price from under $100 to over $1,000. Pliable prostheses filled with silicone gel best simulate the weight and feel of a natural breast; they can be obtained with or without a nipple replica. In larger cities a glance at the Yellow Pages of the phone book will suffice to identify a surgical supply company or specialty shop which carries breast prostheses. The relevant listings are typically given under headings like "prosthetic devices" or "brassieres." Patients living in small towns or rural areas can order breast prostheses from mail order catalogs or over the Internet, yet they might find it worthwhile to travel to a big-city specialty shop for an opportunity to try on various prostheses and to benefit from an experienced salesperson's advice. The task of finding a suitable prosthesis is, of course, left to the individual patient. A doctor's prescription is necessary only if Medicare or an insurance company is being asked to foot the bill, or if the cost is to be deducted as a medical expense on an income tax return.

As we've seen, the inadvertent destruction of nerves during an axillary dissection can lead to the irreversible atrophy of muscles involved in arm and shoulder function. Fortunately, these major problems are not nearly as common as they once were; but all mastectomy patients still have to cope with an annoying **postoperative numbness** of the skin on the chest wall. In order to remove the breast tissue, the tiny nerves relaying sensations from the overlying skin are necessarily severed. If the mastectomy has been accompanied by axillary dissection, the area of skin insensitivity will include the axilla and possibly the inner side of the upper arm. Patients experiencing axillary numbness may

want to shave off underarm hair with an electric razor instead of a razor blade, thereby minimizing the risk of nicks and cuts. William L. Donegan and John S. Spratt assure us that these areas of skin anesthesia gradually become smaller over the course of a year, "because of regeneration of sensory nerves."[42] Other postmastectomy symptoms due to severed nerves include a feeling of tightness across the chest and tingling or itching sensations in the skin—these also subside with the passage of time. A few patients are temporarily troubled by the so-called "phantom breast syndrome," in which they perceive sensations coming from the amputated breast. In this case the nerves which had led to the breast are simply continuing to send their accustomed messages to the brain. The phantom breast phenomenon does not occur as frequently as those phantom arm or leg sensations after the amputation of these limbs, nor is it as severe when it does occur.

The **lymphatic drainage of the arm** is necessarily disrupted by any axillary dissection, even a limited one. With time the drainage may improve due to the development of collateral lymph vessels bypassing the severed ones. But if any axillary surgery has been done, it is always wise to assume that the arm's ability to remove lymph fluid and to fight infections has been compromised, and to take appropriate precautions. This advice is applicable to both lumpectomy and mastectomy patients. We cannot surely predict which patients are going to develop lymphedema, that generalized swelling of the arm and hand due to fluid retention. The obvious risk factors are an increasing thoroughness of the axillary dissection (especially if the level III nodes are removed), as well as obesity and advanced age. The customary treatments for persistent lymphedema have included compression of the arm with elastic sleeves, elevation of the arm to foster drainage, antibiotics for any local infections, and (as a last resort) surgery to remove the edematous tissues. None of these measures is consistently effective; therefore a patient who has had axillary surgery should always keep prevention in mind. The affected arm and hand should be protected from injury (cuts, scrapes, burns, bruises) as well as from undue constriction brought about by overly tight clothing and rings or by blood pressure monitoring.

BREAST RECONSTRUCTION

Virtually all mastectomy patients are suitable candidates for breast reconstruction, which is now regarded as necessary rehabilitation and therefore covered by Medicare and by private insurance plans. The breast mound (the overall shape) can be reproduced by an implanted prosthesis, by a transfer of tissue from another site, or by a combination of both techniques. Reduction or augmentation mammoplasty (surgery) may sometimes have to be performed on the opposite breast to achieve symmetry. In recent years many plastic surgeons have advocated immediate reconstruction of the breast mound, reasoning that implant placement or tissue transfer could be accomplished most advantageously during the same operation in which the affected breast is removed. A lifelike simulation of the nipple and areola can be achieved through several minor procedures, which are usually done in the surgeon's office some three to six months after reconstruction of the breast mound.

The important thing to remember about breast reconstruction is that **every case is different**. Each presents a unique challenge to the plastic surgeon. For her part the patient has to choose from among various options. Immediate reconstruction during the mastectomy operation or reconstruction at some later date? Implant or tissue transfer?

Each alternative has different advantages, disadvantages, and risks. Ideally the patient would make her choices without anxiety or stress, but with a basic understanding of the issues involved. Breast reconstruction has its limitations. Upon its completion the patient's appearance in street clothes may actually be improved, as previously ptotic (drooping) breasts now appear uplifted. But a reconstructed breast has no sensation to speak of, cannot secrete milk or respond to erotic stimuli, and usually bears a perceptible scar. We must be realistic about this matter. Yet if we survey the history of attempts at breast reconstruction, we will appreciate the advances that have been made.

The Role of Silicone Implants

Back in the days of radical mastectomy, plastic surgeons shied away from breast reconstruction. The defects produced by mastectomy seemed to doom any attempt to failure—there were no pectoral muscles left behind which could cover an implant or anchor a tissue transplant, and usually there was barely sufficient skin to close the gaping surgical wound, much less to enclose a new breast mound. But the biggest obstacle to reconstructive efforts was the absence of an implantable material which would be soft and cushiony enough to feel like a natural breast, yet durable enough to retain its shape indefinitely. In the 1940s plastic surgeons used paraffin to simulate breast mounds; at least this crude substance was soft. The 1950s saw the introduction of the polyvinyl alcohol sponge—the so-called "Ivalon" sponge. Being both cushiony and durable, these first synthetic implants were greeted with much enthusiasm; but it soon became obvious that Ivalon was not biologically inert. The human body reacts to foreign materials by surrounding them with a fibrous shell consisting of collagen. With the passage of time that shell tends to become harder and tighter, compressing any foreign object into the smallest possible volume— that is, into a sphere. This is exactly what happened with the Ivalon implants. After a few years those implanted breasts which had originally been so soft and pliable began to resemble baseballs stuck under the skin— they became hard painful spheres which were not only cosmetically unattractive, but quite difficult to live with. Of course, the implants themselves had not changed; they had simply been compressed, or "walled off," by the body's defense mechanisms. When the fibrous capsule surrounding an implant becomes so firm that it distorts the shape of the breast, plastic surgeons will speak of **contracture**. The word aptly describes the most common long-term complication after reconstruction or augmentation with breast implants.[1]

By the early 1960s researchers were looking for another material which would be considerably less reactive than Ivalon. They focused their attention on **silicone**, a versatile synthetic plastic derived from a pervasive natural element. Silicone, first produced in the 1930s, had a longstanding reputation for chemical inertness; moreover, it could be manufactured in three distinct forms—a liquid, a soft gel, and a flexible solid called **elastomer**. Silicone has found so many commercial and industrial applications that it is practically unavoidable in modern society. It's used as a lubricant and as insulating material, and it's a featured ingredient in dozens of household products. Silicone was also to prove useful in medicine. Back in the 1940s and 1950s plastic surgeons smoothed out the wrinkles of movie stars with subcutaneous injections of liquid silicone. All sorts of prostheses have been made from the solid elastomer—cardiac pacemakers, heart valves, artificial joints, erectile penile implants, and contact lenses. *And as for the gel?* Why, it seemed the very thing to reproduce the soft cushiony feel of the human breast. The Dow Corning Corporation introduced the first **silicone gel implant** in 1962; this device consisted of an outer envelope (or shell) made of thin elastomer which was filled with the softer gel.[2]

Silicone gel implants represented a big improvement over paraffin and Ivalon. They were more durable, and unlike earlier prostheses they did not always provoke that relentless fibrotic reaction from the host. To be sure, the body will form a capsule around a silicone breast implant, but normally the process stops short of contracture. Ross Rudolph, a plastic surgeon at the University of California in San Diego, explains that the resulting capsule tends to be "a smooth nonreactive bursa which, while containing the implant, allows it mobility."[3] Surgeons also learned that contracture was less likely to occur if the implant was placed under the pectoralis major muscle rather than above it, and if extreme care was taken to avoid introducing bacteria into the operative field. Satisfactory long-term results were finally being achieved; breasts reconstructed or augmented with the new silicone implants stayed soft and pliable year after year.

By the late 1970s, with the transition to modified mastectomy procedures which preserved the pectoral muscles and much more skin, breast reconstruction was fast becoming an integral part of every plastic surgeon's repertoire. Robert M. Goldwyn of the Harvard Medical School points out that the number of breast reconstructions done in the United States jumped from 20,000 in 1981 to 98,000 in 1984—almost a fivefold increase in just four years![4] The silicone implant was largely responsible for this amazing statistic. By making duplication of the breast mound easy and predictable, it gave a powerful stimulus to reconstructive endeavors, not only with implants but with tissue transfers and nipple-areola simulations as well. Plastic surgeons now became adept at duplicating the breast mound with tissue borrowed from the back (the latissimus dorsi flap) or from the lower abdomen (the TRAM flap). The lion's share of breast reconstructions continued to be done with silicone implants, because the necessary procedure amounted to little more than a sophisticated insertion. Compared to tissue reconstructions, the implant method was considerably cheaper and faster; and it carried fewer risks of postoperative complications.

Dow Corning and other manufacturers responded to the growing demand by bringing out improved implant prostheses, in a variety of sizes. The silicone gel implant remained a standard item, but several other types were introduced in an effort to further reduce the risk of contracture or to remove the possibility of silicone gel escaping into the surrounding tissues. The **saline implant** also had an elastomer outer envelope; but instead of silicone gel, it contained sterile salt water. Some plastic surgeons believed that saline implants were less likely to induce contracture. A few patients complained that the saline fill felt less natural than the silicone gel; but the biggest drawback to saline

implants, especially the early models, was their tendency to rupture. Any leak in the outer envelope meant prompt deflation—the reconstructed breast suddenly went flat. Fortunately, mishaps of this kind constituted social embarrassments rather than medical emergencies; the escaping fluid was harmless, and it was quickly reabsorbed by the body. Later models of the saline implant featured thicker and stronger envelopes, greatly reducing the risk of rupture.

To many plastic surgeons in the 1980s, the **double-lumen implant** was the best choice. This more expensive model featured two envelopes (or shells) and therefore two lumens (or fillable spaces). The inner lumen contained silicone gel; the outer, saline. This double-lumen construction greatly reduced the possibility of silicone gel leaking from the implant—the gel was now enclosed within two elastomer shells as well as the intervening layer of saline. The outer lumen (the one holding just saline) could be filled with antibiotics, which would slowly be released into the surrounding tissues. The antibiotics were designed to combat any bacterial contamination occurring during the implant insertion, since subclinical (undetected) infection had long been suspected as a contributory factor in cases of contracture. Plastic surgeons knew that occasionally a patient who had silicone implants in both breasts would develop contracture in one breast, while the other breast remained soft and pliable. The observation suggested a bacterial etiology—if a genetic predisposition toward contracture or an immune system response to silicone had been at fault, both breasts would have been affected.[5]

It was anticipated that **implants coated with polyurethane foam** would also reduce the incidence of contracture; their irregular, somewhat porous surfaces were thought to be more acceptable to the body—that is, less likely to provoke an immune response—than the smooth surfaces of other implants.[6] Alas, the foam-covered implants were vigorously touted in the 1980s only to be double-damned in the 1990s! Researchers discovered that not only did the foam coating tend to deteriorate after a few years, but that in so deteriorating it released chemical byproducts (toluene diisocyanate diamines or TDAs) known to cause cancer in mice and rats. The risk of human carcinogenesis from the minuscule TDA quantities involved seems to have been negligible, perhaps one in a million; but some 200,000 American women who received implants with polyurethane foam coatings were terrified by the alarming reports which appeared in newspapers and magazines and on TV. These implants were withdrawn from the market by the early 1990s.[7] Yet the idea that irregular outer surfaces are less likely to provoke fibrotic reactions is very much alive. Many implants currently being used, both saline and silicone gel, feature a so-called **textured surface**. As the roughened surface in these models is simply wrinkled elastomer, the issue of carcinogenetic byproducts has not been raised.

The Great Implant War
(The Story Behind It)

If silicone gel implants had been used exclusively for the reconstruction of breasts lost to mastectomy, they probably would have remained as uncontroversial as artificial legs and false teeth. However, only about one-fourth of the implants manufactured in the United States went to breast cancer patients.[8] It would appear that American plastic surgeons immediately realized that the largest market for these devices was not represented by cancer victims, most of whom were over age fifty, but by healthy young women in their twenties and thirties who perceived their breasts as being too small. We must loudly applaud the wonderful work plastic surgeons do in repairing birth defects like cleft lips or in reconstructing the facial features of accident or burn victims. But unlike other surgeons they principally perform operations done for cosmetic enhancement rather than for therapeutic necessity. Often this surgery enables patients to feel better about themselves and to function more gracefully in society. Plastic surgeons are truly the artists of the surgical profession, moving tissue to re-create faces, noses, eyelids, and abdomens—simultaneously displaying the anatomical knowledge of Michelangelo and the aesthetic sensibilities of da Vinci. But a caveat is in order. These specialists are also salesmen, for they must sell the benefits of expensive procedures (face lifts, nose jobs, tummy tucks) which are not medically indicated, all the while assuring patients and their family members that a speedy recovery and a good outcome may be assumed. In the 1980s our plastic surgeons were not shy about selling cosmetic breast enlargements by means of the silicone gel implant. Some of them went on national TV shows, talking enthusiastically about augmentation mammoplasty while holding sample implants for camera close-ups. Many others gave discreet presentations in their home communities, addressing small groups of women while flashing color slides of before-and-after appearances. In one way or another the word got out that bust enlargement was really quite safe and a reasonable thing to do.

Inserting a breast implant for cosmetic purposes was indeed easy. The patient was first given local anesthesia and sedation. The plastic surgeon would then make a small incision at a spot where the resulting scar would be thoroughly concealed, most often in the inframammary fold (the crease at the bottom of the breast), but sometimes in the areola or in the axilla. The implant was usually placed under the large pectoralis major muscle, which helped to hold it in position. In the case of athletic women who vigorously flexed their pectoral muscles—for example, weight lifters or tennis players—a subglandular placement (i.e., above the pectoralis major) might be preferred. After surgery the patient had to restrict her physical activities for a few days, but subsequently she could resume her usual routine with significantly enlarged breasts which looked and felt "normal." At least most men had no clue to the surgical secret. Implanted breasts did tend to feel a little firmer than nonimplanted ones; but unless a man was an OB/GYN by profession, or otherwise in the habit of palpating dozens of breasts on a daily basis, he would not notice the difference.

No one knows exactly how many American women have received silicone gel implants for cosmetic breast enhancement. A ballpark figure frequently bandied about sets their number at two million. Most of these women received a tremendous psychological boost from their surgery. The implants freed them from the burden of being small-breasted in a society hooked on the Hollywood notion that large breasts are somehow more feminine or more sexy. But not every implant recipient had a good outcome. Complications could arise from flaws either in the surgical technique or in the prosthesis. A lingering postoperative infection might force the surgeon to remove an implant and to drain the festering wound. Implants could rupture, they could slip out of position, they might even protrude through the skin. Contracture still caused problems for a few implant recipients—that old devil had never been completely explained, much less banished. We did know that surgical sloppiness leading to bacterial contamination or inadequate hemostasis (poor control of bleeding) invited both infection and contracture. Some plastic surgeons may have been guilty of faulty technique because they were working too hastily. Implant insertions could be done on an assembly-line basis, one case right after another, two or three a day. A practice of this sort may have been lucrative for the surgeon, but was it conducive to the best results? We have no reliable national statistics on the number of bad outcomes following implant surgery. Neither the implant manufacturers nor the individual surgeons seem to have been anxious to collect and publicize this data. However, considering that several million American women have received breast implants, we may plausibly speculate that tens of thousands of recipients have had problematic outcomes, due either to postoperative infections or to progressive contracture or to prosthesis failure. Perhaps most mastectomy patients would have faced a setback after implant reconstruction with a degree of stoicism; after all, they had a dread disease, and they had already lost a breast. In contrast, the young women who simply opted for cosmetic breast enlargement had been healthy to begin with; and most of them had been led to believe that a satisfactory outcome was a near certainty. If their implants had to be removed because of complications, they were worse off than they had been before. While some of these unfortunate patients may have been disappointed, those who suspected that they had been the victims of misrepresentation perpetrated by their physicians or by the implant manufacturers were apt to be extremely angry. The upshot was that the Food and Drug Administration received more complaints about breast implants than about any other medical device. If the breast implant was the most widely used silicone prosthesis, it was also the one that generated the most worries. In the late 1980s a growing mountain of complaints in the FDA offices foreshadowed a great battle.

The FDA Opens Fire!

In the early 1960s, when silicone gel breast implants first went on the market, the Food and Drug Administration did not have specific authority from Congress to regulate medical devices. As a result of this legislative oversight, any safety testing that these implants received was performed exclusively by the manufacturers, not by impartial government scientists. In 1976 Congress finally gave the FDA authority to supervise new medical devices, adding a proviso that the agency could also require evidence that the devices marketed before this time were safe. The FDA took no immediate steps to investigate breast implants—these devices had long been on the market, were considered "grandfathered," and were presumed to be safe. Only in the late 1980s, as the defects in the polyurethane-foam models began to generate negative publicity, did the FDA urge implant manufacturers to prove that their products were safe. The agency was not satisfied with the answers it received. On January 6, 1992, it took dramatic action, declaring a moratorium on the sale of silicone gel implants.[9] In February an FDA advisory panel convened in Bethesda, Maryland, held a three-day public hearing on breast implants. The panel heard graphic tales of leaking implants, of ruptured ones, and of silicone gel which was not cohesive like jelly but almost as fluid as water. Several physicians testified that there could be a link between silicone implants and immune system disorders. The most disturbing evidence came from internal documents provided by Dow Corning, the largest manufacturer of implants. These documents established that company employees had long been aware of various product failures and were concerned that not enough research had been done on silicone and its components. On February 20 the panel members unanimously announced their recommendations.

They had concluded that there was insufficient evidence to convict silicone gel implants of causing systemic disease or to recommend that women with these implants have them removed. However, the panel urged that their use be sharply restricted, pointing out that we really did not know how often the implants ruptured or about what side effects any escaping gel could cause in the human body. Henceforth women who wanted silicone gel implants simply for cosmetic breast enhancement would be required to participate in clinical trials, which would keep track of any complications or illnesses following implantation. On April 16, 1992, the FDA accepted the panel's recommendations—in effect, the agency had begun a national prohibition on the casual use of silicone gel implants for breast augmentation. David A. Kessler, commissioner of the FDA, was quick to emphasize that the agency's decision did not mean that gel implants were hazardous, only that their safety and durability had not been properly established. Dr. Kessler added that saline implants, those whose elastomer shell was filled with harmless saline, would remain readily available to all women. And breast cancer patients, "whose need is greatest," would still have access to gel implants for reconstruction after mastectomy.[10]

Alas, the public perception of breast implants had been altered by all those scary stories in the news media. Those supposedly harmless bust enhancers were starting to look like the medical devices from Hell! In 1991 the polyurethane-foam models had been mercilessly pounded in news reports; when the FDA announced a moratorium on all silicone gel implants the following January, many implant recipients took it as an official confirmation of their worst fears. Were they carrying time bombs in their breasts? The FDA's public hearing held in February 1992 generated a week of front-page revelations for newspapers across the country—the headlines tended toward the sensational, and the stories beneath were terribly disquieting. An implant recipient in New Mexico was so upset by what she read and heard that she removed her two implants by herself, using Valium tablets for sedation and a razor blade for a scalpel.[11]

America's plastic surgeons were livid at what the FDA and the health reporters had wrought. Although besieged by anxious patients, they leaped on the barricades, firing off letters to newspaper editors, then bashing the FDA on the TV talk shows! Breast implants, said the doctors, had brought joy to their patients and were no more dangerous than all the other medical devices made of silicone. One implant defender argued that silicon (the natural element) is "essential for plants and probably essential for mammals, including humans." This element is present in human bodily fluids, "including serum, urine, cerebrospinal fluid, and bile." Why, you were likely to ingest more silicon compounds by drinking ordinary tap water than you would get from a leaking gel implant![12]

Other physicians soon joined the plastic surgeons' counterattack. Marcia Angell, executive editor of the *New England Journal of Medicine*, found that the FDA's restrictions on silicone gel implants smacked of paternalism. All drugs and medical devices, Dr. Angell observed, have possible risks and side effects: "Greater risks are permitted for greater benefits. In the case of breast implants, the benefit has to do with personal judgments about the quality of life, which are subjective and unique to each woman." Why shouldn't women decide for themselves in this matter? "People are regularly permitted to take risks that are probably much greater than the likely risk from breast implants; they do so when they smoke cigarettes, for example, or drink alcohol to excess."[13] In 1993

the American Medical Association joined the fray. The AMA's Council on Scientific Affairs released its own report, concluding that there was no clinical data to prove that silicone gel implants caused any form of cancer or any immune disorder, and that "the considerable public anxiety is not warranted based on current scientific evidence." The AMA's House of Delegates went on record as supporting "the position that women have the right to choose silicone gel-filled or saline-filled breast implants for both augmentation and reconstruction."[14]

For their part David A. Kessler and his FDA co-workers fiercely defended the federal position, blasting the AMA conclusions with barbed retorts: "For thirty years, physicians implanted silicone gel implants in women without having adequate information on what risks they might pose. Such practice represents an abrogation of responsibility on the part of physicians."[15]

Silicone and Systemic Disease

The principal issue which led to the Great Implant War was not the risk of local complications like infections or contracture—everybody admitted this risk—but an unresolved scientific question of broad import. Did silicone exposure ever induce systemic disease in the body? The FDA was not greatly concerned about saline implants, because the only silicone used in their construction was the elastomer outer envelope. The elastomer (solid) form of silicone tends to be molecularly stable; it does not regularly shed particles. In contrast, the traditional gel implants might contain a pound or more of silicone in a molecularly loose form. A leak or rupture in one of these implants was tantamount to getting a large injection of gelatinous silicone right in the breast. And not all the escaping gel necessarily remained at the site of its release. Nodular silicone deposits might be recovered from lymph nodes in the axilla, groin, and elsewhere. But even when the outer shell of a gel implant stayed intact, tiny microscopic particles of silicone would often be shed by a well-known phenomenon called **gel bleed**. The number of silicone particles which can bleed (seep) through an elastomer outer shell is affected by the thickness and strength of that shell. The thicker and stronger the envelope, the less gel bleed; but then with a thicker envelope the reconstructed or augmented breast begins to feel unnaturally starchy. Plastic surgeons naturally favored gel implants with thinner envelopes, because they resulted in softer, more pliable breasts. They also shed lots of minuscule silicone particles.

Was silicone really that perfectly nonreactive substance that it had been portrayed as, or could constant exposure to it provoke undesirable reactions among certain individuals? By the early 1990s researchers had discovered that silicone in its gel form could readily induce antibody formation (an immune response) in laboratory rats. The elastomer form was found to be less reactive; but a team at the University of Texas in Galveston described two patients who experienced intense inflammatory reactions to implanted elastomer tubing. Some rheumatologists postulated that women with gel implants might even be subject to "a new and unique rheumatic syndrome" caused by silicone exposure.[16] But the most curiosity was aroused by three puzzling, chronic, and debilitating diseases which had been recognized long before the advent of silicone breast implants—rheumatoid arthritis, lupus, and scleroderma. These three maladies are called **autoimmune diseases** because they occur when the immune system wrongly attacks the body's own tissues. They are also referred to as **connective-tissue diseases**,

since they painfully affect the joints (hands, wrists, knees). The etiologies (causes) of rheumatoid arthritis, lupus, and scleroderma have not been precisely defined. Genetic inheritance seems to play a role in these diseases, as might also environmental agents like chemicals and viruses. A basic epidemiological observation probably foreordained that silicone particles from leaky breast implants would come under suspicion. These three diseases afflict women much more often than they afflict men, and they typically present (become clinically apparent) between the ages of 20 and 50. Needless to say, young premenopausal women in this age bracket were the very people who were receiving all the silicone gel implants. But compared to the general population, this particular gender and age subset has an elevated risk for these diseases even without factoring breast implants into the equation. The medical writer Nancy Bruning has given a thought-provoking statistic. If we assume that the incidence rate of rheumatoid arthritis among young women ranges from 1% to 2%, and that about two million young women have received silicone gel implants, then we could expect that "20,000 to 40,000 women with implants have it by chance."[17] The incidence rates are considerably lower for lupus (which is rare) and lower still for scleroderma (which is extremely rare). Yet with our present knowledge, if we were confronted with a young implant recipient diagnosed with one of these three diseases or with some vaguer rheumatic syndrome, we could not say to a certainty whether silicone exposure did—or did not—contribute to the illness. Attentive readers of Chapter Five will recall that well-designed epidemiological studies could at least demonstrate a probable cause-and-effect relationship (or the probable absence of such a relationship), by showing that gel implant recipients as a group have—or do not have—elevated rates of connective-tissue diseases. But in the late 1980s we had no good epidemiological studies of this matter—what we had instead were scattered reports from rheumatologists who had observed multiple cases of early-onset scleroderma among implant recipients and who suspected silicone exposure as the probable cause. Before the epidemiologists could properly begin their work, the whole issue was taken into the nation's courtrooms, a forum where glib talking and appealing theatrics all too often carry the day over tedious disquisitions about scientific probabilities.

Lawyers to the Front—
Manufacturers in Full Retreat!

The implant war had been begun in a most gentlemanly fashion by FDA commissioner David A. Kessler, a dedicated physician and public servant who could not have possibly foreseen the destruction that was to follow. Certain storm troopers of the legal profession were to launch ferocious frontal assaults against the implant manufacturers—and no quarter would be given! In October and November 1991 product liability lawyers throughout the United States were closely observing a celebrated case being tried in a federal courtroom in San Francisco. Mariann Hopkins, a college secretary, had sued the Dow Corning Corporation for damages. She claimed that silicone gel exposure from ruptured breast implants had caused her progressive rheumatic disease, which presented with severe joint pains, fatigue, and weight loss. Mrs. Hopkins' physician testified that her symptoms had begun *before she received the implants.* Notwithstanding this fact, the jury found that the implants were defectively designed and that Dow Corning has not warned Mrs. Hopkins of their possible dangers. On December 13, 1991, it awarded a record sum of 7.34 million dollars to the plaintiff.[18] This case clearly demonstrated that implant liability lawsuits could be won without definite proof that silicone exposure had actually caused a plaintiff's illness. Some three weeks later, when the FDA announced a moratorium on silicone gel implants, the legal bombardment commenced in earnest.

If the liability lawyers had hoped to avoid simulating a shark feeding frenzy, they did not succeed. Shamelessly seductive advertisements suddenly appeared in newspapers and magazines throughout the country, warning implant recipients of the "time bombs" in their breasts and providing the telephone numbers of legal firms. An advertisement which ran in the April 1992 *Vogue* read like a typo-prone rheumatology textbook: "SILICONE BREAST IMPLANT SUFFERERS . . . You may possibly have a legal claim for damages if you have been diagnosed with: Human Adjuvant Disease, Connective Tissue Disease (Lupus, Chronic Arthritis and Scleroderma), Carpal-Tunnel and Raynauds Syndrome, Polio-myositis [*sic*], Morphea, Hepatitis, Fibromyalgia, Sjogren's Syndrome and Thyroiditis."[19]

Dow Corning bore the brunt of the assault. Some 10,000 implant-related law suits were filed against this corporation in 1992, and another 10,000 in 1993.[20] Any case against Dow Corning or other manufacturers that actually went to trial immediately became a battle of the doctors, with a few rheumatologists testifying for the plaintiffs while some plastic surgeons spoke up for the defendants. Juries composed of laypersons were being asked to decide on complex scientific hypotheses which had not as yet been sufficiently tested. Which set of expert witnesses should be believed? Astronomical sums were sometimes awarded to plaintiffs who truthfully and tearfully testified that their health problems began around the time they received their implants. Fearing financial annihilation, Dow Corning and eight other manufacturers capitulated in April 1994; they agreed to establish a fund of 4.25 *billion* dollars to pay for any existing or future claims arising from breast implants.[21] This was the largest product liability settlement in history—but it was not enough! Spurred on by sensational publicity and pettifogger advertising, some 440,000 implant recipients registered to participate in the fabulously rich settlement, sharply reducing the value of any payments to individual sufferers.[22] The litigation seemed likely to drag on for years, with nobody getting paid on a regular basis except lawyers and judges.

American manufacturers had already retreated from the field of breast prostheses. Dow Corning stopped producing silicone gel implants in March 1992; in May 1995 the company filed for bankruptcy protection. Other manufacturers wondered whether they should relocate to foreign countries, where product liability claims might be less likely. Marcia Angell of the *New England Journal of Medicine* was appalled at the litigious excesses of the implant war; she wrote a book about them entitled *Science on Trial*, in which she called for reform of the tort system. Dr. Angell worried that the fate of Dow Corning might generally discourage pharmaceutical and prosthetic research in the United States: "This controversy sent a clear message to the medical device industry that a company can be brought to its knees in the utter absence of scientific evidence."[23]

How Dangerous Are Implants?

One positive result from the implant war was that epidemiologists finally tried to quantify the level of risk posed by silicone implants.

Researchers at the Mayo Clinic in Rochester, Minnesota, dug deeply into that institution's well-preserved records and identified 749 women who had received one or more breast implants there between 1964 and 1991. The Mayo Clinic team then selected a control group consisting of 1,498 women from the surrounding community who had never received an implant. When these two groups were compared, the relative risk of connective-tissue disease in the implant recipients proved to be 1.06—this minor elevation in risk (up 6%) was "not statistically significant." The Mayo Clinic study appeared in the *New England Journal of Medicine* on June 16, 1994—it was hailed by the implant manufacturers and the plastic surgeons, but damned by those who felt that silicone implants could be dangerous. The usual complaints were made (e.g., inadequate sample size, faulty design, abbreviated follow-up). One group of skeptics raised a fundamental objection to any study which simply compares the medical histories of implant recipients to those of nonrecipients: "Clinical data from the population of women who are exposed to free silicone gel, from either ruptured implants or free injection, need to be compared with data from a control population before a conclusion can be reached about an association between breast implants and disease."[24]

On June 22, 1995, the *Journal* published a contribution from the Nurses' Health Study, a venerable epidemiological engine still chugging along after two decades. The Harvard team had compared the self-reported incidence of connective-tissue disease in 1,183 nurses with silicone implants and 86,318 nurses without them. Their findings were reassuring: "We did not find an increased risk of any connective-tissue disease among women with any breast implant or with specific types of breast implants."[25] Presumably, if silicone gel implants had posed as big a risk for rheumatoid arthritis and other autoimmune diseases as cigarette smoking poses for lung cancer, the Mayo Clinic and Nurses' Health surveys would have recorded strong positive associations. FDA commissioner David A. Kessler had also come to believe that the risk posed by implants was rather small, but he was not willing to dismiss it altogether. Testifying before a Congressional committee, Kessler had to defend his agency's 1992 decision to ban silicone gel implants for cosmetic breast augmentation. He explained that "certain women, perhaps as many as ten thousand," might be "particularly vulnerable" to silicone exposure, and thus at increased risk of auto-immune diseases if their implants were to rupture. Unfortunately, the FDA did not have adequate data either to say how often breast implants might fail or to identify any women who might be at increased risk.[26]

Dr. Kessler's position soon received considerable buttressing from a study con-ducted by the epidemiologist Charles H. Hennekens and his colleagues at the Harvard Medical School. This team of researchers went over 395,543 four-page questionnaires which had been voluntarily completed by 395,543 female health care professionals (nurses, dental hygienists, pharmacists). On its third page the questionnaire had asked whether the respondent had ever been diag-nosed with rheumatoid arthritis, lupus, scleroderma, or any other connective-tissue disease. And on the fourth page it inquired whether the respondent had ever had a breast implant. No information was obtained as to the type of implant (silicone gel, saline, or double lumen) or as to whether the implant had ever ruptured, leaked, or otherwise caused problems. In spite of the fact that the questionnaire was not specifically designed to elicit data on a possible relationship be-tween breast implants and connective-tissue

diseases, some provocative findings emerged when the 395,543 responses were fed into the computer. The incidence of rheumatoid arthritis proved to be 18% higher in the implant recipients, who also had a 15% higher rate of lupus and an 84% higher rate of scleroderma. The overall risk of any connective-tissue disease was 1.24 (up 24%) in the implant group. Hennekens et al con-cluded that their results "do suggest small increased risks of connective-tissue diseases among women with breast implants. The very large sample size makes chance an unlikely explanation for the results, but bias due to differential overreporting of connec-tive-tissue diseases or selective participation by affected women with breast implants remains a plausible alternative explana-tion."[27]

Breast implants, whether filled with silicone gel or with saline, are hardly a health hazard to be compared with smoking ciga-rettes or being obese. But the fact that sili-cone is chemically inert does not necessarily mean that it is biologically inert. At the moment we do not know whether silicone exposure might occasionally provoke an inappropriate immune response in certain individuals, possibly even leading to auto-immune diseases like lupus or scleroderma. One dread disease which has not been plau-sibly associated with breast implants is can-cer. The available evidence suggests that silicone is not carcinogenic, does not damage the DNA in the surrounding cells, and plays no role in the origin of breast malignancies or other solid tumors.[28] On the other hand, cosmetic breast implants do tend to reduce the effectiveness of mammography. Silicone gel is very radio-opaque; and a gel implant, particularly if placed above the pectoralis major muscle, can obscure sizable areas of glandular tissue. Marie A. Ganott and other radiologists at the University of Pittsburgh assure us that "saline implants are less radio-opaque, allowing partial visibility of tissue detail through the implant."[29] But both silicone gel and saline implants make it more difficult to achieve the degree of compression necessary for good mammography. One study found that while breasts without implants could be compressed to an average thickness of 4.5 centimeters, breasts with implants could be compressed only to 7.0 centimeters. If contracture should develop around the implant, both visualization and compression will be especially difficult.[30]

The issue of post-implant mammography usually does not arise in the case of a reconstructed breast, since the glandular tissue has presumably been removed by the mastectomy. However, this issue should be discussed with young women who want implants simply to increase the size of their breasts. In the past both the plastic surgeons and their patients have approached augmentation mammoplasty much too casually. The potential risks also need to be taken into account. Prospective augmentation patients may also wish to consider that men who are principally excited by frontal protrusions on the chest wall may not be as intelligent as those who are aroused by smiles, kind words, and acts of compassion (romantic stimuli that can be accomplished without incurring a $5,000 surgical bill).

But implants can be enthusiastically recommended for the vast majority of mastectomy patients who want breast reconstruction. Implants are usually the cheapest, fastest, and safest way to accomplish this task. They also lend themselves to immediate reconstruction—that is, to the replacement of the breast mound during the mastectomy operation. For those patients who are worried about the still undefined risks of silicone gel exposure, saline-filled implants would be a better choice.

Immediate Reconstruction: The Role of Tissue Expanders

Back in the 1970s the idea of immediate breast reconstruction was peremptorily dismissed. The cancer surgeons claimed to be worried that breast reconstructions performed too early would hinder the detection of local recurrences—you had to be sure that "the cancer was cured" before even thinking about reconstruction. With solemn faces and the accustomed posture of superior knowledge, surgeons advised their mastectomy patients to wait at least two years. The plastic surgeons of that era cited patient psychology as the principal reason for delaying reconstruction. A breast cancer patient was deemed to be "under too much stress" at the time of her mastectomy operation to make intelligent decisions about this matter. Moreover (so the patronizing reasoning went) the patient should "experience the loss of a breast" for a year or two, in order that she would "appreciate" an inevitably imperfect reconstruction!

By the mid-1980s, however, delayed breast reconstructions began to look as outdated as the one-step biopsy and the radical mastectomy. All these surgical dogmas had their roots in practitioner traditions and untested biological hypotheses rather than in any medical necessity. As early as 1977 R. Barrett Noone of the University of Pennsylvania and other plastic surgeons in the Philadelphia area began to offer immediate reconstruction to their mastectomy patients, most of whom responded favorably to this option. Within a few years it became clear that immediate reconstructions of the breast mound were aesthetically equal to those performed on a delayed basis, and that they had no adverse effect on tumor behavior.[31] Implants placed under the pectoralis major muscle during mastectomy operations did not lead to a noticeably higher incidence of postoperative complications; they did not retard wound healing, nor did they delay any scheduled administration of chemotherapy. At worst, prosthesis insertion might extend the mastectomy operation by about an hour; but compared to delayed reconstruction, this method was remarkably cost-effective. It saved both time and money. According to Dr. Noone, plastic surgeons are pleased "to coordinate planning and proper incisions with the general surgeons," and they especially welcome "the opportunity to work with unscarred, fresh muscle and skin."[32]

The re-creation of the breast mound by means of an implant cannot always be achieved in one easy step. Implant insertions are most effective when the patient's opposite breast is small and upright, and when the skin deficit produced by mastectomy is not too great. When the opposite breast is large, a larger implant would have to be used to obtain symmetry; but then mastectomy wounds usually cannot be closed over larger implants, because of the amount of skin removed. Plastic surgeons have increasingly relied on **tissue expanders** to solve this problem. These devices are simply inflatable saline implants; each is equipped with a tiny tube leading to a little port (valve), through which fluid can be added or removed. Expanders are easy to use and highly effective. During the mastectomy operation, as soon as the cancer surgeon is finished, the plastic surgeon will insert a partially inflated tissue expander beneath the pectoralis major muscle, leaving the fill tube and its port outside the muscle margin but beneath the skin. Ten days or two weeks later, after the mastectomy scar has begun to heal, the patient must return to the plastic surgeon's office. Using a thin hypodermic needle, the surgeon now accesses the subcutaneous port and adds more saline fluid. The idea is to gradually increase the tissue expander volume so that a gentle pressure is put on the overlying skin, thereby stimulating expansion of the skin envelope—just like in pregnancy! A week or two later the patient returns again, and still more fluid is added to the expander. The process is repeated again and again, the number and timing of office visits being determined by the rate of skin regrowth. Eventually the breast being reconstructed with the tissue expander is about the same size as the opposite breast. At this time the expander is overinflated by 25% or 30%, and then left alone for three or four months. The protracted overinflation ensures that the "pocket" created for the implant will be ample and that the reconstructed breast mound will have a more natural "hang" to it. In the past, when the period of overinflation was finished, the plastic surgeon would perform a second operation (usually on an outpatient basis) to remove the expander and to insert a permanent implant (usually silicone gel) in its place. These days manufacturers are producing more durable expanders which can be left in place indefinitely. With these newer models all the surgeon need do is to withdraw the excess fluid used in the overinflation phase. The tissue expander then functions as a permanent saline implant; and the reconstructed breast, now partially deflated, hangs down slightly just like the other breast.[33]

Tissue expanders offer several prominent advantages. With the expander method there's no need for a skin graft to close the mastectomy wound over a large implant. And the reconstructed breast will look better, because the new skin has the same coloration and texture as the skin removed by the mastectomy. The drawbacks to this method are that it typically takes six months or more to complete and that it is mildly uncomfortable. A mastectomy patient who chooses it should count on a dozen visits to her plastic surgeon's office. Every time saline is added to the expander, she will experience an awkward feeling of tightness across the chest. During the overinflation phase there's a cosmetic imbalance as well—the reconstructed breast is larger than the opposite breast and sits higher on the chest wall. Yet such difficulties are minor compared to those which have sometimes occurred with skin grafts or tissue transfers, and in most cases the expander method is likely to yield better cosmetic results than grafts or transfers.

The Logistics of Consultation

Currently the main obstacle to immediate reconstruction of the breast mound is posed by the logistics of consultation. Combining reconstruction with mastectomy requires that two different surgical teams be present in the operating room—the first to remove the tumor and the troublesome mammary gland, the second to reconstruct the missing breast. A phone call usually suffices to arrange a collaboration between the general (cancer) surgeon and the reconstructive (plastic) surgeon. Adequate consultation with the patient is more difficult. These days we may anticipate an interval of a week or two between the discovery of malignant cells in a biopsy specimen or fine-needle aspirate, and the scheduling of surgery. That is not much time for the patient, who's naturally upset and feeling harried, to learn about reconstructive options. Fortunately, plastic surgeons understand the dilemma faced by breast cancer patients and will give them consultations on short notice.

A preoperative consultation does not confer an obligation on the patient. Breast reconstruction can be done at any time after mastectomy, even years or decades later. If a patient is uncertain or uneasy about this matter, she would be wise to postpone it. The consultation with a plastic surgeon is likely to be informative and pleasant, and therefore worthwhile regardless of whether a reconstructive procedure ensues in the near future. Unlike general surgeons whose task is often to remove diseased organs, plastic surgeons are always building something or sculpting something into more pleasing proportions. And like other artists they will talk enthusiastically about their work and proudly display samples of it. No consultation would be complete without color photos (or slides) of mastectomy scars—(so that the patient can "experience the loss of a breast")—and then of the impressive results obtained by various reconstructive procedures. No one procedure is suitable for everybody. Patients are different—some are thin, some heavy; some are large-breasted, some small-breasted; some are young and healthy, others older with diverse medical problems. It is usually intriguing to hear a plastic surgeon's opinion on how he or she would handle your particular case. And with the aid of a video camera and a computer, today's surgeons can give you simulated results in an instant, showing you how you might look after reconstruction. Of course, as a patient you may have your own ideas and requirements. Women with large ptotic (drooping) breasts might seize the opportunity to have smaller uplifted ones, knowing that breast cancer reconstructions are covered by insurance plans which would never pay for purely cosmetic surgery. At the other extreme, a patient with small breasts can emerge from the reconstructive process with two larger breasts, both finely proportioned. Not all attempts at breast reconstruction are unequivocally successful, but these days there are more successes than failures.

Achieving Symmetry

Good breast reconstructions typically involve three distinct steps—(1) re-creating the breast mound, (2) achieving symmetry between the new mound and the other breast, and (3) simulating the nipple-areola complex. The first and third steps are relatively straight-forward; the second step can be tricky, financially as well as surgically, for it often raises the eyebrows of philistine insurance adjusters who may regard procedures promoting symmetry as bill padding. But implant reconstructions by themselves, even if preceded by tissue expansion techniques, are likely to achieve a cosmetically pleasing degree of symmetry only with patients who begin with small to moderate-sized breasts sitting relatively high on the chest wall. If the opposite breast is fairly large or quite large, or if it reveals a significant degree of ptosis (downward hang), just putting a subpectoral implant on the mastectomy side will not suffice. In such cases the achievement of symmetry between the two breast mounds will require an operation on the opposite breast. This operation would be called **reduction mammoplasty** if smaller size is the principal goal, or **mastopexy** if the main object is breast elevation (i.e., correction of an existing ptosis). An uplifting mastopexy can some-times be accomplished by removing a little skin and thereby tightening the skin enve-lope; reduction mammoplasty tends to be considerably more involved.[34] But neither procedure should prevent the immediate reconstruction of a breast lost to mastectomy

It may be cost-effective to do the mas-tectomy, the implant or tissue expander insertion, and the symmetry procedure on the opposite breast during a single trip to the operating room. But this surgical trio neces-sarily increases operating time, blood loss, and the recovery period—not everybody is

enticed by it. Some plastic surgeons would prefer to see the finished implant reconstruc-tion, after the new breast mound has had time to heal and settle into position, before at-tempting any modification on the opposite breast. Some patients may object to an operation which would leave a scar on their remaining healthy breast and which may possibly alter the nipple's sensitivity. When a patient with a large or ptotic opposite breast declines any contralateral surgery, a tissue transfer reconstruction on the mastectomy side is the only way to achieve symmetry. Unlike implants, tissue transfers can be used to duplicate the dimensions of oversized or ptotic breasts. These reconstructions require far more time in the operating room than implant insertions, yet they too can be ac-complished on an immediate basis, as a lengthy coda to mastectomy.

Tissue Transfers

John B. McCraw and other plastic surgeons at the Eastern Virginia Medical School in Norfolk assure us that "the most natural results, as far as softness and symmetry, are achieved with autogenous tissue." When successful, tissue reconstructions of the breast mound are also the most durable—they stay soft and warm, and they are not subject to distortions caused by contracture or implant displacement. "The real ques-tion," according to Dr. McCraw and his colleagues, "is whether the results are worth the risk and expense of a very sophisticated procedure."[35] Prominent among the risks are the possibilities of postoperative infection or of tissue necrosis due to an inadequate blood supply. Either of these complications can lead to the total loss of the transferred tissue, which is a most distressing outcome. With tissue transfers, cosmesis is never perfect. The scars on the reconstructed breast mound may be more noticeable than with an implant reconstruction. There will also be a scar at the donor site, the spot from which the borrowed tissue was taken.

Tissue reconstructions are indicated for mastectomy patients who are poor candidates for implants. The patient whose previous implant (or implants) had to be removed because of severe contracture probably should not chance a repeat episode of fibrosis. Another plausible candidate for a tissue transfer would be a patient whose pectoralis major muscle is either very small or has atrophied due to nerve damage suffered during axillary dissection. In either case the muscle would not be able to hold an implant securely in place. A third class of tissue transfer candidate is represented by the breast cancer patient who chose lumpectomy and irradiation as the initial treatment, but then years later had to undergo a "salvage" mastectomy because of tumor recurrence in the preserved breast. Unfortunately, salvage mastectomies usually result in large skin deficits because the cancer surgeons now want to eliminate the possibility of future local recurrences. And the skin left behind at mastectomy is not suitable for tissue expander methods. Previously irradiated skin is not elastic, and it does not expand well.

The ideal candidate for tissue transfer reconstruction would be an otherwise healthy patient who, while not obese, has a little excess flesh on the lower abdomen, on the back of the shoulder, and on the buttocks. But successful tissue reconstructions can also be accomplished with very thin patients, though the defect left at the donor site may be more noticeable. The unconditional prerequisite is not body size or configuration, but the continuous circulation of well-oxygenated blood throughout the transferred tissue. Any underlying conditions which adversely affect the circulation or the small blood vessels represent a decided obstacle to

tissue reconstructions, as they would predispose any transferred tissue to necrosis. J. Brien Murphy of the University of Pennsylvania School of Medicine identifies four conditions as major counterindications to tissue transfer techniques: "chronic obstructive pulmonary disease, severe cardiovascular disease, uncontrolled hypertension, and insulin-dependent diabetes." For Dr. Murphy, obesity and smoking would be classified as minor counterindications. He points out that "complication rates approaching 40 percent" have been reported in obese patients undergoing tissue reconstructions. Since the nicotine obtained from tobacco products acts to constrict the small blood vessels, smokers are well-advised to abstain from their habit both before and after any reconstructive breast surgery, whether with implants or with tissue transfers.

The Pedicle Flaps

The tissue transferred in a reconstructive procedure is called **a flap**. It consists of an adequate segment of skin together with the fatty tissue beneath and a strip of the underlying muscle. A fuller name would therefore be **musculocutaneous flap**—but the term **myocutaneous flap** is also current (from the Greek *mys*, "muscle," and the Latin *cutis*, "skin"). The strip of muscle must be included to obtain the blood vessels which nourish the skin and fatty tissues; these vessels pass through the muscle prior to branching out as tiny capillaries in the subcutaneous area. The flaps used most often in breast mound reconstructions are **the pedicle flaps**—that is, the transferred tissue is not completely excised from its donor site, but is rotated on a pedicle (the strip of muscle) into its new position on the chest wall. With pedicle flaps most of the original blood supply to the tissue is maintained; the vessels passing through the muscle are not severed, simply moved in a new direction.

The first pedicle flap that plastic surgeons learned to use was the **latissimus dorsi flap**, based on a wide flat muscle (latissimus dorsi) from the upper back which helps with arm and shoulder movements. This flap had actually been used as early as 1896, but simply to provide skin to close the gaping mastectomy wounds of that era. Only in the late 1970s did plastic surgeons begin to appreciate its wonderful utility in breast reconstructions. A segment of latissimus dorsi, rotated to the front of the body, could simulate a missing or atrophic pectoralis major muscle and provide the necessary cover for an implant. At first latissimus dorsi flaps were used mainly in conjunction with implants, often for patients who had undergone radical mastectomies. Later surgeons discovered that if a little more fat and skin were included on the carrying strip of muscle, they would have sufficient bulk to reconstruct a small or moderate-sized breast even without an implant.

Latissimus dorsi reconstructions of the breast mound are relatively easy to perform. Dr. McCraw and his colleagues observe that "an immediate reconstruction adds approximately one hour and thirty minutes to the time of a mastectomy and should not necessitate additional transfusion."[37] The risk of necrosis is low, even among regular smokers, because this flap has an excellent blood supply. The scar at the donor site can be concealed under clothing, but the partial excision of the latissimus dorsi cannot be remedied. Women who are active in sports requiring vigorous arm movements, such as swimming or tennis, may notice a difference in their performance after this procedure. If a patient has been a frequent sunbather, the skin transferred from the back may be darker than that found in the breast area, so that the reconstructed mound would initially have a patchwork appearance. This contrast in coloration could be expected to fade with time.

The second pedicle flap used in breast reconstruction is the **TRAM flap**, based on a *transverse* section of abdominal skin and fat carried on the **rectus abdominis muscle** (as the initials TRAM suggest). This technique was pioneered in the early 1980s by Carl R. Hartrampf, Jr., and other plastic surgeons at the Emory University School of Medicine; by the end of the decade it had surpassed latissimus dorsi reconstructions in popularity.[38] The TRAM flap offers several advantages. Usually enough tissue is made available to reconstruct the largest breast without any need for an implant or for reductive surgery on the opposite breast. Since the procedure removes excess flesh from the lower abdomen, it conveniently doubles as a "tummy tuck"; the patient's postoperative appearance will be slimmer. TRAM flap reconstructions are often performed in conjunction with mastectomy, adding to the operating time. Timothy J. Eberlein and his colleagues at the Harvard Medical School report that "a typical TRAM flap reconstruction takes an additional two-and-a-half to three hours after the mastectomy."[39] The procedure greatly increases both the recovery time and the hospital bill.

During a TRAM flap reconstruction the plastic surgeon will excise a generous ellipse of abdominal skin and fat, going from one hip to the other. Most of the tissue comes from beneath the navel. According to Dr. Hartrampf and his Emory colleague L. Franklyn Elliott, "the ellipse generally extends vertically from one fingerbreadth above the umbilicus to one fingerbreadth above the pubis."[40] The flap-carrying rectus abdominis is a broad flat muscle which descends from the rib cage to the pubic bone; it serves to hold the intestines in place and to help flex the spinal column. Fortuitously, this muscle comes in pairs, one on each side of the abdominal midline. The pedicle—that is, the partially dissected strip of carrier muscle with its constituent blood vessels—is normally taken from the ipsilateral muscle (i.e., the muscle on the same side of the body as the mastectomy wound). Having harvested the necessary flap and pedicle, the surgeon will next "tunnel" beneath the skin of the upper abdomen to reach the mastectomy wound. The flap is then vertically oriented and pulled through the subcutaneous tunnel to the wound area, where it will be shaped and trimmed so as to match the opposite breast. It is then sutured in place to complete the reconstruction of the breast mound. A fair amount of abdominal skin and fat is usually discarded during a TRAM flap reconstruction; the blood loss can also be considerable. Doctors Hartrampf and Elliott report that in their expert hands "only a rare patient needs blood transfusions"—but they recommend that a prospective patient be given the option to set aside units of blood specifically for her operation, either "autologous (self-donated) blood" or "blood from a close friend or family member."[41]

Most TRAM flap candidates have an excess inch or two of flesh in the midsection, but the procedure can also give satisfactory results in women who are not noticeably overweight. A history of prior abdominal surgery may—or many not—disqualify a patient; a previous TRAM flap procedure normally constitutes a strong counterindication. The distribution of blood in harvested TRAM flaps is less predictable than with latissimus dorsi flaps; smoking thus tends to invite areas of necrosis. Hartrampf and Elliott recommend that patients who smoke should quit the habit "three months before surgery," but if this is not possible, then at least "two to three weeks before."[42]

The breast mound produced by TRAM flap reconstruction is wondrously soft and soon comes to feel quite natural. Abdominal cosmesis is less satisfactory. The operation will leave a scar in the lower abdomen running from hip to hip; the navel is preserved, but its postoperative appearance will be different. The defect created in the rectus abdominis muscle is usually well tolerated if the surgeon has carefully obtained abdominal closure. In most cases the disability will be limited to a reduction in the number of sit-ups a patient can perform, but certain individuals may be prone to develop aesthetically unpleasant abdominal bulging or even true hernias protruding through the weakened abdominal wall. Patients noticeably at risk for bulging or hernias include those who are obese as well as those who have had two TRAM flap reconstructions to replace both breasts. To forestall bulging or herniation in these cases, the surgeon may suture a lightweight synthetic mesh over the abdominal donor sites before wound closure. The mesh can provide considerable support.

The Free Flaps

When plastic surgeons speak of **free flaps**, they are referring to musculocutaneous flaps which have been completely excised from the donor sites. There are no pedicles (or stalks) which would maintain the original blood supply to these tissue transplants—all the blood vessels nourishing them have been severed. How then do these flaps manage to survive? We can answer that question with a single Greek word which is prominent in every surgeon's vocabulary but which few laypersons know—**anastomosis**. Surgically speaking, the term refers to the suturing together of two open tubular structures—for example, the severed ends of two blood vessels. Prior to the 1970s an anastomosis of small blood vessels was an impossible task; but after the introduction of the **operating**

microscope, it became a routine one. Albeit somewhat bulky, this device has enabled surgeons to perform feats of virtuosity that we take for granted, but which were unheard of only a few decades ago—for example, the reattachment of the severed limbs of accident victims. The utilization of free flaps in breast reconstruction also derives from those microsurgical techniques which permit tiny vascular anastomoses. Unfortunately, not every plastic surgeon is sufficiently proficient in microsurgery, nor are free flaps at all "free" by dollar-and-cents reckonings. In 1992 the free-flap pioneer William W. Shaw of the UCLA School of Medicine gave us some revealing ballpark statistics: "The surgical procedure takes approximately four hours for one breast and seven hours for two breasts, and costs between \$35,000 and \$50,000."[43] Free-flap reconstruction of the breast mound, not available everywhere, is the most expensive and time-consuming way to do it. Still, the results can be very good, and free-flap reconstruction can become an attractive option when simpler methods are counterindicated.

By far the most popular free flap used in breast reconstruction is the **TRAM free flap**, which offers several advantages over the traditional (pedicled) TRAM flap. As there is no need for a pedicle, the section of rectus abdominis muscle cut away is much smaller, reducing the risk of postoperative bulging or herniation. Once the severed blood vessels in the muscular strip are anastomosed to the thoracodorsal vessels in the axilla, the TRAM free flap will have a good blood supply throughout, better in fact than can be obtained with the traditional pedicle. These advantages mean that a TRAM free flap might be considered for patients who are poor candidates for the pedicled TRAM—for example, those who are obese or who have had prior abdominal surgery (both these groups stand to suffer from any rectus

abdominis deficiency), as well as those who are regular smokers (this group is prone to flap necrosis because nicotine constricts the small blood vessels).

TRAM free-flap reconstructions can be advantageously performed on an immediate basis, since mastectomy tends to expose the axillary blood vessels which must be anastomosed to the vessels in the flap. The procedure also lends itself to bilateral reconstructions. Many patients have enough abdominal excess that one elliptical TRAM flap would suffice to reconstruct both breasts—the flap could be simply divided in two. The main obstacle to reconstructing both breasts with the traditional TRAM technique is that two largish pedicles would be required, one from the rectus abdominis muscle on each side, and that consequently the entire abdominal wall would be greatly weakened. With the free-flap TRAM technique, the two strips which would be taken from the rectus abdominis muscles are much smaller. Roger K. Khouri of Washington University in Saint Louis and his colleagues suggest that bilateral TRAM free-flap reconstructions could be a boon to women having bilateral prophylactic mastectomies because of inherited *BRCA1* or *BRCA2* mutations. Khouri et al analyzed the results of 120 bilateral free-flap TRAMs: the average operating time was 8.6 hours, and the average stay in the hospital 7.6 days. Most patients needed supplemental blood during their operation, either autologous (their own) blood or from a donor. "Over the course of this series," Khouri et al point out, "operative times and the requirement for blood transfusion decreased markedly."[44]

The other free-flap reconstructions require even more anatomical inventiveness and microsurgical expertise. The **gluteal free flap** draws on the skin and fatty tissue covering the buttocks, with a section of the underlying gluteus maximus muscle being used as a carrier. Depending on whether the tissue transfer is taken from the top or the bottom of the buttocks, it would be termed a **superior gluteal flap** (top) or an **inferior gluteal flap** (bottom). Both the tissue harvest and the blood vessel anastomoses are technically demanding. A gluteal flap can be anastomosed to the axillary vessels, but it usually will be better positioned on the chest wall if the anastomoses are made to the internal mammary vessels beneath the sternum. The nature of the tissue obtained from a gluteal donor site may dictate the type of breast mound which can be reconstructed. William W. Shaw and his UCLA colleague Christina Y. Ahn observe that "a gluteal free flap is most suitable for reconstructing a firm, conical breast, whereas a free TRAM flap is ideal for reconstructing a soft, slightly ptotic breast."[45] A gluteal free flap is most likely to be considered when a patient strongly objects to a TRAM reconstruction for personal reasons. Some women do not want a long scar running across the lower abdomen. Those who are active athletes may wish to avoid the slight functional disability which harvest of the rectus abdominis or latissimus dorsi muscles invariably entails.

Any donor site in the body could conceivably provide tissue for a free-flap breast reconstruction. Other sites which have occasionally been used include the front of the thigh (the **tensor fascia lata flap**) and the roll of flesh at the top of the hipbone (the so-called **Ruben's flap**). With free-flap techniques, virtually all mastectomy patients without prohibitive pathological conditions have been suitable candidates for tissue-transfer reconstruction.

The Nipple-Areola Complex

The final step in breast reconstruction is the simulation of a nipple-areola complex. Usually this is not done until three months or so after the completion of the breast mound reconstruction. Before turning their attention to the nipple and areola, plastic surgeons want to be certain that any new breast mound created by tissue transfer is fully healed and has adequate circulation throughout, and that any new mound created by implant or tissue expander has settled into its permanent position on the chest wall. Hence they will preach the unpleasant gospel of delay in all cases. The good news is that the various procedures used in nipple-areola simulations are done on an outpatient basis (typically in the surgeon's office) and require no more than a dab of local anesthetic.

The foremost issue to be considered in planning a new nipple and areola is symmetry. The simulation must be a reasonable match for the nipple and areola on the other breast, not only in size and shape but in position and coloration. Even minor discrepancies between the two nipple-areola complexes will be obvious to the observer. Historically, plastic surgeons have succeeded fairly well with short-term simulations, though the long-term results were less satisfactory. Over a period of months or years, the coloration of simulated areolas tended to fade, and simulated nipples tended to lose projection. Areola coloration and nipple projection continue to represent major challenges.

Back in the late 1970s and early 1980s plastic surgeons relied mainly on tissue grafts to simulate nipple-areola complexes. If the nipple and the areola on the opposite breast were large enough, "sharing" was the preferred method. One half of the existing nipple and areola would be carefully excised and then sutured in place on the new breast mound, resulting in two complexes which initially looked identical. The technique's drawbacks included perceptible scarring on the donor nipple and reduced sensitivity in the donor nipple. Moreover, in their new location the transferred areola might lose pigmentation, and the transferred nipple might suffer a loss of projection. Plastic surgeons therefore experimented with other donor sites. Skin grafts from the upper inner thigh or from the genital area (usually from the labia minora) were frequently used in areola reconstructions. The coloration looked good at first; but as Thomas J. Krizek of the University of Chicago recalls, "groin skin became darker, and labial tissue became very pigmented and unnatural looking."[46] The ear had the greatest utility for some practitioners. A post-auricular graft (skin from behind the ear) could be used for the areola simulation, while a segment of ear lobe or conchal cartilage would do nicely for a nipple simulation. Tiny bits of ear cartilage could also be placed under the new areola to simulate Montgomery's glands, those tiny bumps which enlarge during pregnancy and lactation. The ear-derived nipples kept their projection better than nipples re-created from labial tissue or from toe pads, but the post-auricular skin used for the areolas soon faded to pale or pink colorations.[47]

By the 1990s tissue grafting had largely given way to simpler methods of nipple-areola reconstruction. Nipples were most often simulated with "local flap" techniques—little strips of skin were partially excised from the breast mound, lifted up, and then sutured together to create a nipple-like prominence. John William Little of Georgetown University assures us that "virtually any opposite nipple can be matched with local flap techniques," and that with an adequate blood supply to the flaps, nipple projection will be "reliable and lasting." Intradermal tattooing with durable pigments has become the preferred method of areola simulation. Some plastic surgeons will tattoo the areola simulation as soon as nipple reconstruction is finished. But Dr. Little counsels delay, explaining that tattooing can also serve as "the ultimate fine-tooling tool" to disguise any small discrepancies in nipple position. "Such subtle distinctions," he argues, "cannot be made until the two breast mounds are in a stable state, with the postsurgical phase essentially resolved."[48] Areola tattoos are not prone to early loss of coloration, because the pigments are embedded deep in the dermis. When a tattoo eventually begins to fade, a brief visit to the surgeon's office will suffice to restore the original tints. Touch-up tattooing is easy.

Chapter Nineteen

Radiation Therapy after Lumpectomy

By itself mastectomy is a cheaper and faster treatment than lumpectomy and subsequent whole-breast irradiation; but as we've seen in the preceding chapter, mastectomy combined with subsequent breast reconstruction can sometimes be considerably more expensive and time-consuming. Since the survival rates achieved by these therapeutic options are equivalent, lumpectomy and irradiation may well be the most advantageous initial strategy for the patient who wishes to retain a breast. Radiotherapy has become very safe and effective, with tolerable side effects which quickly resolve in most cases. Breast irradiation is given to destroy any cancer cells left behind after lumpectomy, thereby lowering the risk of recurrence in the treated breast. Most lumpectomy patients readily understand that this therapy will help with breast preservation, while failing to fully comprehend its two main limitations. Firstly, breast irradiation does not seem to have any effect on survival rates. Secondly, it cannot be repeated without producing unacceptable cosmetic changes.

The old horror stories about patients who were "burned for life" by radiation treatments are no longer appropriate. Back in the 1950s and 1960s, however, these tales had a factual basis. The low-energy orthovoltage machines then being used delivered the maximum dose to the patient's skin.

Attempts to eradicate any cancer cells left behind in the breast usually left the overlying skin looking like charcoal. During the 1970s and 1980s those radiotherapeutic model T's were gradually replaced with versatile high-energy machines called **linear accelerators**, which can produce well-defined beams of irradiation to deliver the maximum dose at a predetermined depth. **Proton beams** are used for deep penetration—in whole-breast radiotherapy they provide a relatively homogeneous dose throughout the organ, while sparing the overlying skin. **Electron beams** are used when limited penetration is desired; for example, they would be called upon to irradiate skin cancers or superficial tumor recurrences, or to deliver a boost (extra dose) to a tumor bed (site) located just a centimeter or two beneath the skin. Today's radiotherapists can control the dose and the field (irradiated area) with great precision. By changing the proportion of electrons and protons, or by adjusting the size or direction of the invisible beams, they can treat virtually any site in the body.

Radiation Kills Cancer Cells

Around the year 1900 physicians in Europe and the United States began to take note of a seemingly miraculous phenomenon. When tiny quantities of the newly discovered element **radium** were applied to superficial malignancies, these tumors inexplicably shrank, or even faded away altogether, while the surrounding normal tissues appeared to be unharmed. Cancer radiotherapy had been born, although at the time no one understood the biological mechanisms involved. How did radiation which fell equally on both malignant and nonmalignant cells manage to select only the former for destruction? The answer lies in the unstable nature of the cancer cells themselves. These cells have a decided growth advantage over normal cells, but that advantage is their undoing as far as radiotherapy is concerned. The streams of subatomic particles (protons or electrons) preferentially damage cells which are either preparing to divide (in S-phase) or are actually engaged in the process of division (mitosis). Cells which are at rest, as most normal cells would be, are relatively insensitive to radiation. But the faster cancer cells multiply, the more vulnerable they become. A direct hit on a strand of chromosomal DNA can kill a cancer cell outright; more often radiotherapy just inflicts sublethal damage on cancer cells, which fortunately cannot repair themselves as well as normal cells. While the damage is immediate, death usually ensues only when a maimed cancer cell enters the cell cycle and attempts to divide. This delayed reaction explains why irradiated tumors will continue to shrink long after therapy has been completed.[1]

The word **hypoxia** denotes a condition which is the foremost obstacle to radiotherapeutic success. It refers to the inadequate oxygenation of an irradiated malignancy (from *hypo*, Greek for "beneath," and *oxygen*). Without oxygen, the cancer cells will not divide or even prepare to divide; they thus become much more resistant to irradiation. In solid tumors the cells around the periphery are typically well-oxygenated and rapidly multiplying, and therefore vulnerable to radiotherapy. In contrast, the cancer cells near the tumor's center tend to be oxygen-deprived and therefore necessarily at rest—and highly radio-resistant. The disorderly growth patterns of malignant tumors dictate that hypoxia will be a constant in cancer biology. Even with tumors as small as a millimeter or two in diameter, the peripheral cancer cells receive noticeably more oxygen than those in the interior. Hypoxia explains why radiotherapy comes into play principally as a "mopping up" procedure, being used after a surgeon has excised all visible traces of tumor. If we were to attempt to eradicate a solid tumor with irradiation alone, the dose required to sterilize those hypoxic interior cells would be so high that it would destroy the surrounding normal tissues. Conceivably, we might irradiate large breast tumors as an initial procedure—that is, before surgery—but only with a view to shrinking them a bit so that lumpectomy or mastectomy would be feasible. Surgical excision remains necessarily in all breast carcinomas.

The Rationale of Fractionation

When performed for palliation (pain relief), radiotherapy may be performed at a single sitting. One exposure will often suffice to relieve the pain from bone metastases or to shrink metastatic tumors pressing upon nerves or obstructing airways. However, when performed with a view to eliminating all cancer cells, radiotherapy has to be given **in fractions**—that is, in numerous treatment sessions. Fractionation is simultaneously the lumpectomy patient's worst aggravation and greatest ally. Irradiation given in fractions has a better chance of catching (sooner or later) the cancer cells when they are preparing to divide or actually dividing—and thus of inflicting damage on their DNA which would eventually prove lethal. Moreover, the time interval between fractions affords the irradiated normal cells a better opportunity to repair any damage they might have suffered. Thus with fractionation we can deliver a much larger cumulative dose of radiation than we could administer at a single sitting. The dose which would exceed the tolerance of the irradiated tissues if delivered all at once can be safely given in small increments, with far superior results both with regard to tumor control and to cosmesis.

The only drawback to fractionation is that it sorely tests a cancer patient's patience; this is especially true of the standard breast-preservation regimens. Normally radiotherapy is not scheduled until a week or two after lumpectomy, to allow for wound healing. Thereafter the patient has to visit the radiation oncology office on a daily basis, five days a week, for at least one month and quite possibly longer. The treatment usually has two distinct phases. The first involves **whole-breast irradiation with proton beams**. As we've seen in Chapter Fifteen, the influential regimen developed by Boston's Joint Center for Radiotherapy calls for a dose of 4,500 to 5,000 rads (45 to 50 grays) to the entire breast, delivered in fractions of 180 to 200 rads each, over some 25 workdays.[2] After whole-breast irradiation the patient may be given time off, a week or two to recover from the first phase of treatment, prior to beginning the second phase. This consists of **boost irradiation to the tumor bed**. The "boost," an extra dose aimed at the site where the tumor had been, would seem to be especially indicated for infiltrating (invasive) cancers excised with relatively narrow margins. In these cases we must allow for the possibility that a few cancer cells may persist in the surrounding tissues, and moreover that these cells may have become somewhat hypoxic because their blood supply has been disrupted by the tumor

surgery. Back in the 1970s boosts were often delivered by implanting radioactive iridium "seeds" (pellets) in the breast for several days, a practice which ensured a high dose to the tumor bed but which did not always result in the best cosmesis. By the 1990s most institutions relied on external beam irradiation for this purpose—the penetration of the electron beams can be adjusted so that the maximum dose occurs right at the tumor bed depth. The boost may consist of an additional 1,000 to 2,000 rads (10 to 20 grays), given in fractions no greater than 200 rads per day. Carl M. Mansfield and other radiotherapists at Philadelphia's Thomas Jefferson University Hospital assure us that "a small area of the breast can be given a higher dose without undue fibrosis and loss in cosmesis."[3]

Treatment Planning Session:
Marking Out the Fields

The first visit to the radiotherapist's office is always the longest, being devoted to a lengthy treatment planning session. These preparatory activities are also known as **simulation**—they are necessary because radiation treatments must be individualized to suit each patient's body configuration. The **fields**—that is, the areas of the body to be irradiated—must be determined with the utmost care and then marked out in a highly visible fashion. Immobilization is an absolute prerequisite. A patient receiving irradiation must remain motionless, just like a patient who receives a mammogram or a chest X-ray. The problem is that the breast radiotherapy patient must remain motionless not for a few seconds but for minutes at a time, and furthermore, that she must be immobilized in exactly the same position for each treatment session, from the first fraction to the last. If she were to slip out of position by only a half inch or so, then the beam of radiation would begin to fall on tissues which should not be treated. Radiotherapists rely on a combination of body casts, wedges, and adhesive tape to achieve the essential immobility. Nancy Price Mendenhall of the University of Florida describes her institution's procedures: "At simulation, the chest wall is leveled by placing the patient on a prefabricated wedge. To increase reproducibility of the position each day, a customized polyurethane upper torso mold, which fits over the wedge, is then fashioned for each patient."[4] The arm on the affected side is abducted (drawn up and away from the body); during treatment it may be taped or otherwise secured so as to keep it well above the irradiated area.

Whole-breast irradiation is accomplished with **tangential fields**. That is, the proton beam will be angled so that it can encompass the entire breast while hardly touching the ribs, lungs, or esophagus. The adult breast can tolerate considerable radiation, but this is not true of the delicate structures contained in the thorax (chest cavity). For example, if the lungs or esophagus were to be significantly included in the breast fields, these organs would soon suffer from pronounced inflammation and fibrosis. Carl M. Mansfield and his colleagues observe that with well-planned tangential fields the unwanted radiation exposure will be limited to "a thin margin of the lung and a portion of four or six ribs."[5] Normally this small exposure does not result in subsequent clinical symptoms. To achieve homogeneous dosage throughout, tangential irradiation is administered from both sides of the affected breast. For the **lateral field** the machine's head lies by the patient's side, releasing a beam which enters at the side of the breast and exits at the sternum. For the **medial field** the machine's head is placed above the patient's body; the beam enters at the sternum and exits from the side of the breast.

Boost irradiation to the tumor bed is usually accomplished with a **small perpendicular field**. The machine's head hovers over the breast's surface so as to aim a concentrated electron beam down the surgical tract (lumpectomy incision) to the spot where the tumor had been. The maximum dose must fall on the tumor bed, not on the overlying scar or on the underlying lungs. The depth of penetration is controlled by modulating the energy of the beam. Jay R. Harris and Abram Recht of Boston's Joint Center for Radiotherapy observe that the electron energy selected can be "based on the thickness of the breast tissue from the skin surface to the anterior chest wall, which is determined by ultrasonography."[6] Currently radiation oncologists at many institutions also make use of CAT scans and computer dosimetry to plan the most advantageous fields and the proper beam energies.

Preparing a personalized body cast for the patient and calculating the precise dosage and fields with the help of ultrasound, CAT, and computers can prove quite time-consuming. But the increasingly restless patient cannot be dismissed from the treatment planning session until the fields have been marked out in the old-fashioned way. Radiotherapists have traditionally marked the field borders on their patients' skin with brightly colored ink—the visible lines serving as a safeguard against mistakes due to carelessness or haste. The ink used is permanent in that it resists being washed off; over a period of several months the markings will fade away as the skin gradually renews itself. At New York's Memorial Sloan-Kettering and some other institutions, the field borders are also indicated by tiny bluish dots tattooed in the skin. The supplementary tattoos are almost too small to see—the sole

A Tangential Field
for Breast Irradiation

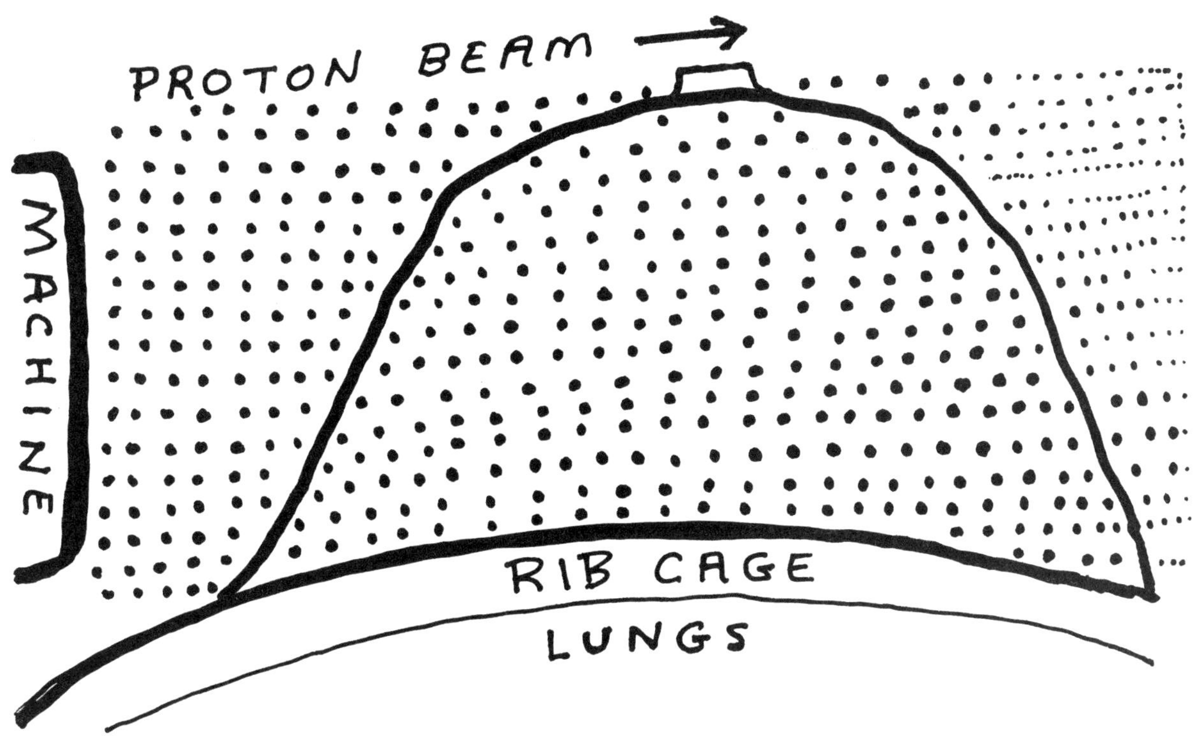

The patient normally rests on her back, with the head of the machine (linear accelerator) by her side. The energy of the proton beam is controlled so that it will deeply penetrate the affected breast, but then dissipate at a distance of some 20 centimeters (about 8 inches) from the machine's head. **Tangential fields are sharply angled so as to minimize the amount of radiation falling on the rib cage and on the underlying lungs.**

advantage in adding them is that they provide a permanent record of the initial radiotherapy. Should the patient suffer a recurrence some years later, either in the treated breast or near it (e.g., in the axilla), any radiotherapist treating her at that time would not only be aware of the prior irradiation, but would know what fields had been used. Since previously irradiated tissues often cannot tolerate significant additional exposures, a tattooed record of the initial fields can be helpful in planning the management of local recurrences.

SPECIAL CIRCUMSTANCES
Large Breasts? Suspect Nodes?

Radiotherapy is usually a routine undertaking when administered to patients who are prime candidates for breast preservation, both in regard to tumor staging and body configuration. The hypothetical "ideal candidate" would have small to moderate-sized breasts, with a small ductal carcinoma (Stage Null or One) which gives no indication of dissemination to the regional lymph nodes. The radiotherapist's task becomes more complicated when a patient has large or pendulous breasts, or when the regional lymph nodes must be irradiated because of known or suspected tumor involvement. Nancy Price Mendenhall stresses that large or pendulous breasts are not a counterindication to preservation, although they are "technically more difficult to irradiate, and dose homogeneity within the breast is more difficult to achieve." For whole-breast radiotherapy in these cases, she recommends using proton beams with "higher energies," thereby obtaining deeper penetration. "The dose to the entire breast is often limited to 4,500 centigrays (rads) at 180 centigrays per treatment, because of dose inhomogeneities and acute

skin reactions." Carl M. Mansfield and his colleagues in Philadelphia argue that "extra large breasts should be an indication for conservative management. When one breast is removed, these patients have major problems with cosmesis, asymmetry, and even balance." But Mansfield et al emphasize that careful treatment planning is necessary to avoid severe skin reactions and subsequent breast retraction: "Our results have been very good, and the majority of our patients have had no major complications."[7]

When whole-breast irradiation must be combined with irradiation of regional lymph nodes, even the most skilled radiotherapists will be hard pressed to avoid overlapping fields. "Hot spots" (areas of excessive radiation exposure) are a natural consequence of overlapping fields. As we've seen in Chapter Fifteen, the Joint Center for Radiotherapy long ago abandoned routine axillary irradiation because of cosmetic concerns. Severe skin reactions and fibrotic contracture can develop in the outer upper quadrant of the breast, where the whole-breast and axillary fields would necessarily overlap. To prevent tumor recurrences in the axilla, the Joint Center physicians favor a limited axillary dissection (removal of the lower and middle nodes—levels I and II). We may be sure that most lumpectomy patients with probable axillary involvement would be better served by surgery than by irradiation—*the Joint Center says so!* But even at the Joint Center the occasional patient with extensive axillary involvement (lots of positive nodes) may sometimes be given irradiation to the apical nodes (level III) and the neighboring supraclavicular nodes.[8] In general, however, we want to avoid irradiating the axilla.

With the internal mammary nodes located under the sternum (breastbone), the situation is reversed—surgical dissection here tends to produce more morbidity than radiotherapy. If a patient has a large invasive tumor in an inner breast quadrant, the internal mammary nodes may be given external beam radiation to forestall possible parasternal recurrences (i.e., recurrences on either side of the sternum). In some individuals these nodes can be adequately irradiated simply by lowering the angle of the tangential proton beams used in the whole-breast treatment. In other individuals it may be better to use a perpendicular electron beam directed through the sternum. Both these procedures are tricky. A supplementary perpendicular beam would tend to overlap with the tangential whole-breast fields, creating hot spots in the center of the chest. A lowered tangential beam avoids the problem of sternal overlapping, but it necessarily increases the volume of lung tissue irradiated. Before attempting to treat the internal mammary nodes, radiotherapists usually want to study a CAT scan of the patient's thorax to determine the precise location of these nodes and their spatial relationship to the lungs and heart. Both the fields and the dosage must be precisely calculated to avoid serious complications.[9]

Side Effects during Treatment

The actual administration of breast irradiation takes only a few seconds, and it is completely painless. Far more time is devoted to setup—for each and every session the patient must be snugly fitted in her personalized body cast, and the machine precisely aligned with the markings (field border indications) drawn on her body. Setup being completed, the patient is then left alone in the treatment room. The radiotherapy personnel must retreat to the adjoining room, which is shielded against radiation exposure. They remain in constant communication with the patient by means of the intercom and the closed-circuit television. The radiotherapy machine makes a little whirring or buzzing sound while emitting the invisible beams. When it stops, the session is over—the personnel return, and the patient can get dressed and leave.

The only generalized symptom produced by breast radiotherapy is **fatigue**. Almost all patients will begin to feel tired or run-down before the end of the course. Carrie F. Dunne-Daly, a radiation oncology nurse at Chicago's Saint Joseph Hospital, suggests that this fatigue may be "related to the presence of excess toxic metabolites and waste products during cell destruction."[10] In any event, the body's energies must now be devoted to repairing the damage caused by radiation exposure, leaving little energy for nonessential tasks. We might add that breast radiotherapy regimens are inherently fatiguing because of their unavoidable monotony: the same setup routine has to be repeated in precisely the same way on every weekday for five weeks or more. Even before beginning the course, most patients are likely to feel themselves somewhat "drained" by the prolonged anxieties which accompany any cancer diagnosis. During treatment all patients thus stand to benefit from a reduced activity level and extra rest, and from the enthusiastic support of family members, friends, and medical professionals.

The amount of instruction needed by radiotherapy patients varies from individual to individual. A few naive patients may have to be assured that they will not be made radioactive and that they cannot transmit radioactivity to those around them. Detailed dietary instruction is not necessary. Although patients may notice changes in their appetite, they can eat pretty much what they like and what agrees with them. Unlike chemotherapy, breast radiotherapy does not affect the taste buds or the gastrointestinal tract. Patients do not experience nausea or vomiting—at least none which can be specifically attributed to irradiation. **Localized skin reactions** affecting the treated breast are another matter: they are inevitable, and all patients need to be informed about them.

Within the first week or two of treatment, the irradiated breast will show signs of **erythema**—a gradual reddening of the skin caused by dilation of the underlying capillaries. The skin soon becomes quite red; it will feel warm to the touch, and it may appear slightly edematous (puffy) because of fluid retention. After three or four weeks of treatment, erythema is succeeded by a condition known as **dry desquamation** (from the Latin *desquamare*, "to scale off"). As nurse Dunne-Daly explains, the skin now becomes "dry, flaky, scaly, and itchy," because of "the decreased ability of the basal cells of the epidermis to replace the surface layer cells, and the decreased ability of the sweat and sebaceous glands to produce sweat."[11] Dry desquamation is distressing to the patient, but usually it can be relieved by simple remedies. More importantly, it does not require interruption of radiotherapy. **Wet desquamation** is cause for greater concern; in this condition the skin takes on an angry red coloration, and it becomes extremely tender and moist. It has been so damaged by excessive radiation that it can no longer retain lymphatic fluid, which oozes upward in the affected areas. Fortunately, wet desquamation is not common during breast radiotherapy; but patients with large or pendulous breasts sometimes reveal traces of this problem along the inframammary fold, that crease at the bottom of the breast which is susceptible to local irritations and which often tends to receive a larger dose of radiation. Areas affected by wet desquamation may have to be covered with a sterile dressing; occasionally, the treatment course will have to be suspended for several weeks while waiting for healing to occur.

Skin Care at Home

The task of caring for the breast's dry irritated skin is left largely to the patient. The Golden Rule is that she should pay close attention to any instructions, oral or printed, which she may be given by the radiotherapist or by nursing personnel. Drugstores and supermarkets carry numerous lotions and creams which claim to moisturize dry skin; but the patient should use only those products recommended by her radiotherapy professionals, because some of these commercial products contain ingredients likely to do more harm than good. Dunne-Daly cautions that "ointments and creams that contain zinc" should not be used in the treatment fields. The prohibition also includes scented powders, perfumes, deodorants, and the like—in general, cosmetics should not be applied to the irritated skin. Kathleen L. McGowan, a longtime radiation oncology nurse, recommends instead "a light coating of pure aloe vera" to relieve dryness—this natural product is "available in gel form from health food stores and pharmacies." Brand-name moisturizers like Eucerin or Lubriderm may also be recommended. When the symptoms of dry desquamation begin, the patient should resist that urge to scratch the itchy flaking skin. A dusting of ordinary cornstarch will usually relieve itching. But nurse McGowan cautions that cornstarch should not be used as an underarm deodorant or otherwise applied to moist areas, lest it promote a fungal infection: "Moisture and cornstarch generate glucose, a prime medium for fungal growth."[12] If desquamative itching persists after the cornstarch remedy has been tried, the radiation oncologist can prescribe a steroidal cream or lotion to provide relief.

Most skin care during and after radiotherapy is simply a matter of avoiding things likely to cause further irritation. A breast being irradiated should not be exposed to direct sunlight—you must postpone that trip to the beach if it involves sunbathing with no more protection than a scant bikini top! Temperature extremes also need to be avoided. Don't apply a heating pad or an electric blanket to the treated breast—and don't sit in front of a window air conditioner or an open refrigerator. While bathing and showering are not forbidden, they should be kept within certain limits. Those pleasant showers with streams of hot water beating down on the body are no longer a good idea—ditto for sitting in a hot tub! Water exposure should be minimized as far as the treated breast is concerned. Use lukewarm water, briefly and sparingly. Choose a soap which is gentle enough for a baby's tender skin, and keep the suds to a minimum! Loose blouses and soft fabrics are the preferred apparel—constrictive bras and other tight upper-body clothing should not be worn.

The temporary skin reactions do not stop on the last day of treatment. In fact, they may not actually peak until a week or two later, because the cells in the skin's basal layer are still continuing to die. Thereafter the acute reactions will slowly begin to resolve. Complete healing normally requires between three and six months—but the breast's skin will never again be as resilient as it was before irradiation. Commonsense precautions against excessive exposure to sunlight, hot water, and harsh soaps should be observed for a lifetime.

The Lingering Sequelae

The best news regarding long-term side effects is that breast irradiation does not affect the patient's general health. It does not increase the incidence of cardiovascular disease, hypertension, arthritis, diabetes, osteoporosis, and all those other degenerative disorders which afflict aging *Homo sapiens*. Moreover the small dose of radiation which falls on the sternum's bone marrow is not likely to induce a second cancer (e.g., a treatment-related leukemia or lymphoma). Back in the 1960s and 1970s, before the advent of linear accelerators, the imprecise dosage and poorly defined fields characteristic of the old orthovoltage machines could indeed lead to distressing side effects. Sometimes the patient's ability to function could be significantly impaired. The ribs, given a trifle too much irradiation, could eventually become pressure-sensitive, making it painful to hug a child or to carry a bag of groceries. In a few cases rib fractures might ensue from gentle contact. The underlying lungs responded to inadvertent overdosage with fibrosis and inflammation—some months after the excessive irradiation, an affected patient might present with a nonproductive cough and a vague dyspnea (difficulty in breathing). Radiation-induced osteitis and pneumonitis were always *late* effects. Any overdose did not become apparent during treatment, because bone and lung cells divide far less often than the skin's basal cells and therefore would not die off in large numbers until long after any sublethal radiation damage. These cells might die months or years later, when they finally attempted to reproduce themselves. Fortunately, debilitating sequelae affecting the ribs and lungs are quite rare in contemporary radiotherapy done for breast preservation. With CAT scans and computer-assisted dosimetry we know in advance how much radiation the lungs and ribs are going to receive.

Although the final cosmetic results of lumpectomy and radiation therapy are usually described as "good" or "excellent," all patients should be informed about—and psychologically prepared for—long-term changes affecting the treated breast. These changes may not be readily apparent to the casual observer, but they are an inevitable consequence of treatment. Irradiated skin is affected in subtle ways—the inert outer layer which you see becomes thicker, while the living basal layer beneath becomes thinner. Irradiated skin also tends toward hyperpigmentation—it can become darker. This effect may be more noticeable in fair-skinned individuals who sunburn easily, and it would naturally be more pronounced at the site given the boost (the extra dose to the tumor bed). A very few patients will develop a condition known as **telangiectasia**. The formidable Greek term simply means that the tiny blood vessels supplying the skin have become abnormally visible because they are permanently dilated. In other patients the skin's pores may appear to become larger. There are no easy remedies for such superficial changes should they occur; they may become less noticeable with the passage of time.

The breast's overall size and configuration can also be altered as a result of irradiation. Unfortunately, these changes cannot be predicted before therapy; they typically develop slowly over a period of several years. In the first six months following radiotherapy, the treated breast may actually be somewhat larger and softer than the contralateral breast because of edema (fluid retention). When this swelling resolves, the treated breast will tend to become firmer than its opposite because its fatty tissues are now being replaced by collagen, that fibrous protein which the body calls upon to repair injuries. If the fibrosis is too pronounced, the treated breast will gradually shrink, becoming smaller than its opposite and sitting noticeably higher on the chest wall. Radiotherapists use the term **retraction** to describe this late sequela. Large pendulous breasts with a high fat content are slightly more prone to retraction, both because dose inhomogeneities during treatment can create hot spots predisposed to fibrosis, and because more of the breast's volume will be replaced by collagen. Patients beginning with small tumors in small to moderate-sized breasts naturally fare better in this regard. The lumpectomy removes less tissue, and the irradiated breast is far less prone to retraction.

Any lumpectomy patient choosing subsequent irradiation should prepare herself for the possibility that the treated breast will eventually be somewhat smaller than its opposite; but severe, cosmetically unacceptable retraction is seldom seen. Mary Ann Rose, Jay R. Harris, and other Boston-area radiotherapists and surgeons have evaluated the long-term cosmetic outcomes of 593 lumpectomy patients treated at the Joint Center. They found that "breast retraction generally occurred in the first three years and remained stable thereafter." According to their grading system, half of the patients studied had "no retraction" at three years— and "35% had slight retraction, 13% had moderate, and 2% had severe." Dr. Rose and her colleagues believe that three years after therapy is the earliest date when the cosmetic outcome of lumpectomy and breast irradiation can be definitively evaluated. They are encouraged that satisfactory results seen at that time have been shown to remain relatively stable: "No patient with either an excellent or good score at three years who was re-evaluated at seven years had results which deteriorated to poor."[13]

Follow-up after Radiotherapy

The lumpectomy patient who receives breast irradiation can count on making regular visits to her radiotherapist's office long after the completion of treatment. Follow-up is more complicated than after mastectomy because it has two special objectives—firstly, documentation of the progressive changes occurring in the treated breast, and secondly, surveillance of the treated breast for any recurrence of cancer. Abram Recht of the Joint Center and his Boston-area colleagues observe that "the optimal intervals" for follow-up examinations have not been determined: "During the first two to three years after treatment, we usually perform physical examinations every two to three months. The gradual changes attributable to radiotherapy may be distinguished more easily from those of a recurrence in this manner." Dr. Recht and his co-workers believe that mammograms of both breasts should be taken at "approximately six months after the completion of radiotherapy," and that a second set of bilateral mammograms taken "six months later" (at one year) "may be helpful in documenting the resolution of radiotherapy-induced changes." Thereafter patients should have "annual mammography for life."[14]

Mammograms taken of irradiated breasts require special attentiveness and expertise for their proper interpretation. The progressive changes wrought by radiotherapy in the treated breast—skin thickening, collagen fibrosis, and the sudden appearance of calcifications in areas of increased density—tend to resemble the warning signs for breast carcinoma that every radiologist knows. The tumor bed, having been troubled first by invasive surgery and later by a boost dose of radiation, typically responds with localized fibrosis and fat necrosis. This reaction often produces an induration (hardening) at the site, which can be felt during physical exams. On mammograms the site sometimes looks like a star-shaped or spiculated mass, in close mimicry of the radiographic signature of an infiltrating ductal carcinoma.[15]

The distinction between radiation-induced alteration and cancer recurrence is not always easy to make. Surgical biopsy would give us a conclusive answer; but we naturally wish to avoid biopsying an irradiated breast, because it is disturbing to the patient and because it would cause additional scarring, making subsequent mammography even more difficult. Nancy Price Mendenhall observes that at the University of Florida continued surveillance is usually preferred to biopsy: "For patients with equivocal or suspicious findings, the mammograms are repeated at three and six-month intervals." Abram Recht and his colleagues have a lower tolerance level for suspicious lesions seen on mammograms: "A modest-sized open biopsy does not appear to create complications or worsen the cosmetic results. If necessary, core-needle biopsies can be done repeatedly with little patient discomfort in the surgeon's office. Biopsies may be helpful in reducing patient and physician uncertainty."[16]

Fortunately, the perceived need for biopsies has greatly diminished in recent years as radiologists have become more familiar with the mammographic appearance of irradiated breasts. The important thing to remember is that the breast changes occurring during the first year or two after lumpectomy and radiotherapy are much more likely to be due to the treatment than to a cancer recurrence. Kathleen M. Harris and other radiologists at the University of Pittsburgh School of Medicine point out that "the natural course of the postoperative and post-irradiation changes is regression or stability over time." The radiographic changes are "maximum at one year"; thereafter they will resolve or remain stable. "Any increase in the changes or development of a new density or new microcalcifications should alert the radiologist to possible recurrence of carcinoma."[17]

The Scheduling Dilemmas:
Chemotherapy and Pregnancy

While breast irradiation is relatively uncomplicated for most lumpectomy patients, it can become a tricky balancing act when administered to node-positive patients who need prompt chemotherapy to combat presumably imminent metastases, or to pregnant patients who want to deliver healthy babies. These situations pose scheduling dilemmas. In the case of patients needing both chemotherapy and radiotherapy, which should come first—the chemo or the radiation? Can you ever give the two treatments concurrently—i.e., at the same time—without producing intolerable side effects, or without having to reduce the dose levels of one or both? In the case of pregnant patients, how can you treat the breast without exposing the fetus to radiation?

As we've seen in Chapter Fifteen, NSABP Protocol B-06 demonstrated that positive nodes were not a counterindication to lumpectomy, because the combination of localized radiotherapy and systemic chemotherapy is highly effective in preventing tumor recurrences in the breast. The chemo normally takes precedence over irradiation, because it is more important to forestall distant metastases which can kill the patient than it is to prevent purely local recurrences in the breast. In Protocol B-06 all the node-positive patients assigned to the lumpectomy and radiotherapy arm received one course of chemotherapy before being given their whole-breast irradiation.[18] The physicians at Boston's Joint Center for Radiotherapy have long looked askance at the concurrent (simultaneous) administration of irradiation and chemotherapy, fearing that it might detract from the cosmetic outcome. Abram Recht and his colleagues published the results of a little clinical trial done at the Joint Center—244 lumpectomy patients deemed "at substantial risk for distant metastases" had been "randomly assigned to receive a 12-week course of chemotherapy either before or after radiation therapy." According to Recht et al, the patients who received the chemo first had a better survival rate; but the patients who received the radiotherapy first had fewer recurrences in the breast.[19] This is pretty much what we would expect.

As a group, node-positive lumpectomy patients are at noticeably higher risk both for local recurrences in the breast and for the development of metastatic disease. Obviously, it is not advantageous to delay either the breast irradiation or the systemic chemotherapy. The problem is that giving these treatments concurrently constitutes a "double whammy" as far as side effects are concerned; the patient's physical and psychological resources would be taxed to their limits. But there is no biological reason why irradiation and chemotherapy could not be given concurrently, because the dose-limiting effects of each modality are different. As we've seen, the administration of radiation to the breast tends to be limited by skin reactions, notably by moist desquamation. It does not cause significant bone marrow suppression (i.e., a dangerous reduction in the number of red and white blood cells), nor does it lead to a distressing gastrointestinal symptoms like nausea and vomiting. In contrast, the administration of chemotherapy is principally limited by bone marrow suppression. It often produces acute gastrointestinal symptoms, but it usually does not cause skin reactions like desquamation. Therefore lumpectomy patients who do not have underlying medical problems can receive irradiation and chemotherapy concurrently, or very nearly so, without a forced reduction in the dose levels of either treatment. Therapeutic effectiveness of both modalities would thus be maintained.

There have never been hard-and-fast rules for the sequencing of chemotherapy and whole-breast irradiation. But we may cite three general possibilities—(1) sequential administration, typically with the chemo preceding the irradiation; or (2) alternating administration, usually with one course of chemo before the irradiation and the remaining courses after it; or (3) concurrent administration. If the patient is otherwise healthy, her wishes should be the paramount factor in making scheduling decisions. Some patients may want to complete their postsurgical treatments as soon as possible, and might elect concurrent administration for that reason. Still others might lean toward this option if they believe that it offers the best chance to preserve their breasts and to avoid metastatic disease. But the type of chemotherapy being considered can sometimes dictate scheduling. Concurrent administration with CMF does not cause insurmountable difficulties—this standard regimen developed in the 1970s uses the drugs cyclophosphamide, methotrexate, and fluorouracil. Nancy Price Mendenhall observes that her group at the University of Florida routinely delivers breast irradiation concurrently with CMF chemotherapy, "the only noticeable effect being a slight increase in the rate of pneumonitis."[20] Yet the concurrent administration of CAF or FAC, standard breast cancer regimens featuring the potent drug Adriamycin (brand name for doxorubicin), usually involves an unacceptable level of side effects. Adriamycin by itself will cause severe bone marrow suppression, total alopecia (hair loss), and the usual gastrointestinal symptoms. Moreover, the drug tends to aggravate the skin symptoms produced by radiotherapy. Dr. Mendenhall and her colleagues report that this pharmaceutical straw

breaks the camel's back: "In our experience it has not been possible to use a doxorubicin-containing regimen concurrently with irradiation."[21]

Some cancer centers and oncology groups have embraced Adriamycin-based chemotherapy with more enthusiasm than others. Houston's M. D. Anderson Cancer Center has long been almost synonymous with the FAC regimen for breast cancer. At M. D. Anderson lumpectomy patients with four or more positive nodes were typically given three cycles of FAC before beginning breast radiotherapy. But those lumpectomy patients considered to be at lower risk for distant metastases were given their irradiation first, then allowed a recovery period (three to six weeks off) prior to beginning their FAC cycles.[22]

Nothing seems to complicate attempts at breast preservation so much as **pregnancy**. Back in the 1950s and 1960s breast cancer specialists did not often encounter a patient who was pregnant. When they did, they usually recommended abortion, fearing that continuation of the pregnancy might contribute to aggressive tumor behavior and jeopardize the patient's chances of survival. In recent decades, breast cancer diagnoses during pregnancy have become almost commonplace, as more and more women have been delaying motherhood until their thirties or forties, age brackets in which the disease incidence starts to rise. While unfortunate, the conjunction of breast cancer and pregnancy is no longer viewed ominously. We've learned that by itself pregnancy does not always indicate an aggressive tumor, nor does the continuation of pregnancy necessarily make cancer cells behave more aggressively. Abortion remains an option for the patient who does not wish to cope with both motherhood and cancer treatments, but it is no longer seen as an essential therapeutic measure.   Herbert C. Hoover, Jr., of the Harvard Medical School goes so far as to state that "termination of pregnancy has no role in the management of stage I and II breast cancer patients."[23]

Today's physicians are becoming increasingly adept at a balancing act whereby the breast tumor is treated with one hand while a baby is delivered with the other. If mastectomy is the only therapy intended, the balancing act is easy—the surgery can be performed at any time during pregnancy, with no particular danger to the mother or the fetus. Adjuvant chemotherapy after lumpectomy or mastectomy is another matter. Cytotoxic drugs cannot be given during the first trimester of pregnancy, a time when the embryo's organs are in the process of forming. The likely result would be miscarriage or birth defects. We now know that chemotherapy can be administered during the second and third trimesters without causing fetal organ malformations. However, when breast cancer is diagnosed near the end of pregnancy, most physicians would prefer to wait until after delivery before beginning chemotherapy. Drug exposure during the second and third trimesters may possibly contribute to low birth weights or to an increased incidence of complications during childbirth. The babies being born to mothers who have received breast cancer chemotherapy during pregnancy seem healthy enough, but at present we do not know whether these children will subsequently face a higher risk of leukemia or other malignancies as a result of their *in utero* exposure to cytotoxic drugs.[24]

Radiotherapy for breast preservation during pregnancy remains *terra incognita.* As we've seen, the adult breast can tolerate large doses of radiation; but this is not true of the developing fetus, which would be irrevocably damaged by far smaller doses. Of course, we could protect the fetus from 98% or 99% of the radiation directed at the breast by such simple measures as shielding the abdomen with lead or by angling the beam away from the abdomen. But the radiotherapist Allen S. Lichter and the oncologist Marc E. Lippman point out that no amount of shielding can completely eliminate that "internal scatter" radiation which would be deflected from the mother's ribs and chest cavity. They estimate that during early pregnancy, when the uterus is confined to the pelvis, the internal scatter dose to the new embryo might be "10 to 20 rads." In late pregnancy, when the top of the uterus approaches the sternum, the scatter dose to the fetus might be "100 rads or more."[25] These exposure levels are tiny compared to the 5,000 rads or more that the breast would typically receive, but they are nonetheless cause for concern. Jeanne A. Petrek, a breast surgeon at New York's Memorial Sloan-Kettering, observes that "in the pregnant women of Hiroshima and Nagasaki, an air dose of one to nine centigrays (rads) during weeks six to eleven of pregnancy resulted in an 11% incidence of microcephaly and mental retardation in children." Citing "the atomic bomb experience and animal experimentation," Dr. Petrek concludes that "five centigrays (rads) is the dose level for early pregnancy at which radiation-induced anomalies become meaningful. After some thirty weeks of gestation, radiation-induced congenital defects are extremely rare."[26]

While sympathetic to breast preservation, Lichter and Lippman believe that the standard irradiation regimens pose too much danger during pregnancy. They suggest that the surgical excision of the tumor (lumpectomy) could be performed upon diagnosis and the radiotherapy postponed until after childbirth. "Alternatively," advise Lichter and Lippman, "one could conceivably excise the breast mass and irradiate the tumor bed with an electron beam, using a small boost field to a dose of 2,000 to 2,5000 rads.

After delivery the whole-breast irradiation with proton beams could be performed. Such a strategy would deliver less than two rads to the fetus."[27] These approaches sound reasonable; unfortunately, there have been no large-scale studies evaluating their effectiveness either with regard to cosmesis or to local tumor control. Dr. Petrek points out that our knowledge of radiotherapy for breast preservation has been derived from nonpregnant women. She worries that the established techniques may not be altogether appropriate for pregnant or postpartum women: "The pregnant woman's breast, with the large inter-anastomosing ducts and sizable lymph/blood vessels, is not anatomically and physiologically similar to the less active breast."[28]

Chapter Twenty

The Threat of Recurrence

Most breast cancer patients being diagnosed today, especially those with *in situ* or Stage One (node-negative) tumors, are not going to experience a recurrence. But all patients must face the possibility of recurrence, being at greater or lesser risk for that eventuality. Therefore all patients would do well to know a little bit about the different types of recurrence, about their presenting symptoms, and about the treatment strategies for them. Unfortunately, honest information on these complex and largely unpalatable matters is hard to come by. Physicians usually shy away from the topic of recurrence; and if they do speak, their comments are often so brief or so reassuring as to be evasive. Appropriate printed materials for laypersons have also been scanty. Back in the 1980s Rose Kushner complained that "in the reams of expensive brochures, pamphlets, leaflets, and booklets published by the American Cancer Society, there is not a single line addressed to patients to warn them about a second cancer."[1] While obviously nobody wants to talk about treatment failures or new malignant tumors, any educational program which neglects to do so is seriously incomplete.

The term *recurrence*, like the term *breast cancer*, is a vague "catch-all" usage covering many heterogeneous events. Some of these events are not much more than a nuisance, being adequately handled by simple interventions. Other events amount to a death knell, since they signal the onset of relentless metastatic disease. Broadly speaking, we can divide recurrences into two main categories. The first is **the reappearance of the original tumor**, which may also be called "treatment failure." The second is **the development of a new primary tumor**—that is, another tumor arising *de novo* (Latin for "anew" and independently) in the opposite breast or in a different location in the treated (preserved) breast. The risk levels for these events vary wildly among the diverse patient subgroups. Patients with *in situ* or small Stage One tumors, if treated by mastectomy, are at such low risk for the reappearance of their original lesions that we may confidently speak of their "being cured." But like any patients previously diagnosed with breast cancer, their risk of developing a *de novo* tumor in the opposite breast is substantially higher than the risk faced by members of the general population. At the other end of the spectrum, some Stage Two or Three patients with unfavorable tumor characteristics (e.g., poorly differentiated histology, poor nuclear grade, high S-phase, estrogen-receptor negativity) are at such terribly high risk for a recurrence of their original cancers that we don't give much thought to *de novo* malignancies.

When confronted with a reappearance of the original tumor, breast cancer specialists apply two commonsense yardsticks to judge the seriousness of the event. The first is the **disease-free interval** or **DFI**—that is, the length of time which has passed between the completion of treatment and the discovery of the recurrence. The second is the **extent of the recurrent disease**. A long DFI is seen as propitious, a short one as ominous. The interpretation of "disease extent" is even more self-evident. Thus a small focus of recurrent tumor discovered in a preserved breast many months after lumpectomy, or a solitary malignant nodule found at the mastectomy site some years after surgery, would usually be interpreted as a manageable event. At the other extreme, scattered tumor foci appearing in a preserved breast soon after radiotherapy, or numerous tumor nodules cropping up in the skin flaps soon after mastectomy, could only be described as tragic treatment failures. All too often recurrences like these are quickly succeeded by distant metastases.

The Basics of Follow-up

An exact prescription for follow-up examinations after a breast cancer diagnosis and treatment has never been written down on stone tablets. But since we know that with invasive tumors, especially those graded Stage Two or Three, treatment failures are most likely to become apparent in the first two years after therapy, follow-up has traditionally been more intense during that period. After five years the number of recurrences being detected diminishes markedly, with a corresponding decrease in the frequency of doctor appointments. Back in the 1980s the National Cancer Institute went so far as to issue guidelines for breast cancer follow-up, calling for physician examinations every three months during the first two years, then at least every six months during the third to fifth years, with annual examinations thereafter.[2] Regardless of whether a patient has had a lumpectomy or a mastectomy, and regardless of how long ago the treatment took place, the physician must be alert to four areas of concern during any follow-up examination. These are: (1) **the opposite breast**, which might give rise to a new primary cancer; (2) **local recurrences**, which could occur either in the skin flaps after mastectomy or in the preserved breast after lumpectomy; (3) **regional recurrences**, by which is meant tumor cells growing in the regional lymph nodes; and finally (4) **distant metastases**. Recurrent cancer detected in a preserved breast, in skin flaps, or in the regional lymph nodes often indicates an elevated risk for metastatic disease. But we cannot make that final diagnosis until we find colonies of breast cancer cells flourishing in distant organs where they clearly do not belong—for example, in the skeletal framework (bones) or, more ominously, in the lungs or the liver or the brain.

Follow-up still relies heavily on the physician's visual and palpatory skills. At every office visit, the preserved breast or the mastectomy scar is closely inspected and carefully palpated, as is the opposite breast. The axillae and the supraclavicular regions, both ipsilateral and contralateral, are felt for signs of enlarging lymph nodes. The abdomen is palpated to detect possible abnormalities of the liver or the spleen. The conventional blood work, done at least once a year, includes a complete blood count (CBC) as well as an alkaline phosphatase assay to monitor liver function. The conventional radiographic studies, mammography and a chest X-ray, might be done at six months post-treatment and then again at one year, thereafter being repeated at annual intervals.

Physicians must use their discretion in deciding what laboratory tests might be indicated and how often mammograms should be taken.

Any symptom or assay result suggestive of recurrent cancer typically leads to more elaborate tests. A bone scan can usually highlight those skeletal sites which might possibly be involved with metastatic disease. CAT scans, particularly if performed with radionuclide contrast agents, can give us helpful cross-sectional images of the abdomen and liver, the thorax (chest cavity), and the axillary lymph nodes. These days magnetic resonance imaging (MRI) is the modality of choice for evaluating suspect lesions in the brain or spine. Any cancer discovered, be it local or regional recurrence, *de novo* primary tumor, or distant metastasis, needs to be resected (surgically excised) insofar as possible. Then the new tumor specimen must be subjected to a full pathology workup, just like the original tumor. We need to know the specimen's histological subtype, its degree of differentiation, its nuclear grade, and its S-phase (rate of proliferation). Is this specimen exactly identical to the original tumor, or is it less differentiated and more aggressive? Is it a new primary? A metastasis? Skilled pathologists can answer these questions, which are not simply academic, but have a direct bearing on treatment strategies. Recurrence often brings a recommendation for systemic therapy. In this regard it is imperative that we know whether the newly discovered cancer cells are estrogen and progesterone receptor-positive, and thus likely to respond to hormonal drugs like tamoxifen. The fact that an original tumor was slow-growing and hormone receptor-positive is no guarantee that a recurrence will be. Any cancer cell populations flourishing in the regional lymph nodes or in metastatic deposits may well have evolved to become receptor-negative and

highly proliferative; in this case, cytotoxic chemotherapy would be the logical systemic treatment.

With some solid tumors those patients who have gone five years without a recurrence are regarded as cancer-free, and they can be confidently dismissed from follow-up. Passing the five-year milestone is also a celebratory occasion for breast cancer patients, but it does not necessarily provide an assurance that the original tumor will not return. C. D. Haagensen, the influential breast surgeon who practiced from the 1930s through the 1970s, recalled that some of his patients developed recurrences after being seemingly disease-free for ten, twenty, or even thirty years. The biology of breast carcinomas has not changed since Haagensen's day. Most patients who are fated to develop local recurrences or distant metastases will do so in the first five years after the initial diagnosis and treatment. But with other patients tiny congregations of disseminated tumor cells can survive unnoticed in the body, multiplying so slowly that a decade or two will elapse before they produce symptoms. Dr. Haagensen's dusty statistics are still worth quoting, because he maintained an exceptionally long follow-up on a large patient population. He records that 74% of bone metastases, "the most frequent type," developed "within five years after operation, but 10% became apparent after more than ten years." Of the lung metastases he encountered, 65% appeared within five years, "and 11% after ten years."[3] Taking our cue from Dr. Haagensen, we can only conclude that follow-up for breast cancer patients should be a lifelong proposition—the number of office visits might be reduced after five years, but vigilance can never be altogether relaxed.

The _Other_ Breast

Most malignancies detected in the other (contralateral) breast can be only loosely described as "recurrences." Usually they are new primaries—viz., *de novo* cancers arising independently of, and with no necessary relation to, the previously diagnosed tumor in the ipsilateral breast. Sometimes a new primary will resemble the first tumor, but this is not always true. The new primary might be *in situ* while the first tumor was invasive, or vice versa. The new primary might reveal better—or worse—prognostic features. With most newly discovered lesions in the opposite breast, we therefore have to repeat the diagnostic and therapeutic procedures which have been described in previous chapters. The initial detection by mammography or palpation is followed by diagnostic sampling (fine-needle aspiration or core-needle biopsy), by lumpectomy or mastectomy, by a full pathological workup, and (for invasive tumors) by a determination of axillary nodal status. If the patient chooses lumpectomy, breast irradiation is usually indicated. The advisability of adjuvant chemotherapy or of hormonal drugs would be decided on a case-by-case basis, depending on the axillary status and on other prognostic features.

The thought of a new cancer arising in the previously unaffected breast is understandably depressing. The good news is that for most patients the risk is relatively low, and that if a contralateral primary should develop, it will probably be detected early. Even such sticklers for radical surgery as C. D. Haagensen and Jerome A. Urban never advocated prophylactic mastectomy of the contralateral breast. But surveillance is certainly warranted. A ballpark estimate bandied about in many textbooks is that a woman previously diagnosed with breast cancer has "five times the risk of the general population" for *de novo* malignancy in the other breast.[4] The National Surgical Adjuvant Breast and Bowel Project attempted to quantify the risk more precisely by looking at the contralateral malignancies "encountered over a ten-year period in 1,578 women with invasive breast cancer enrolled in Protocol B-04." According to the pathologist Edwin F. Fisher and his NSABP colleagues, "the annual incidence was constant and less than 1%," with the exception of "a peak of 1.75% in the second postoperative year."[5] Paul Peter Rosen and his colleagues published a "Twenty-Year Follow-up" on 610 breast cancer patients (Stage One and Two) treated at New York's Memorial Sloan-Kettering Cancer Center. "Subsequent contralateral breast carcinomas," reported Rosen et al, "were detected in 57 of 610 women (9%). The average annual hazard rate was 8 per 1,000 patients per year, without significant fluctuations throughout the twenty years of follow-up."[6] Both the NSABP and the Sloan-Kettering results suggest that by and large the risk of *de novo* carcinogenesis in the contralateral breast stays steady at a little less than 1% per year. Thus younger patients would naturally face a greater lifetime risk because of their greater life expectancies. Using the Sloan-Kettering hazard rate and assuming an average life expectancy of eighty years, we can calculate that in a hypothetical group of 1,000 breast cancer patients diagnosed at age 40, about a third of them (320) would eventually develop a tumor in the opposite breast. If our hypothetical group of 1,000 patients were all age 60 at diagnosis, only about a sixth of them (160) could be expected to develop a contralateral tumor.

The aforementioned incidence rate—less than 1% per year—may be fairly accurate for breast cancer patients in general, but certain subgroups have rates which are substantially higher or lower. Dr. Fisher and his NSABP colleagues cite several pathological characteristics of ipsilateral tumors which are strongly associated with subsequent contralateral carcinogenesis. In Protocol B-04, if the first breast cancer was multicentric (present in several quadrants), or accompanied by "proliferative fibrocystic disease," or of infiltrating lobular histology with adjacent areas of lobular carcinoma *in situ*, then the risk to the contralateral breast proved to be significantly elevated. This is exactly what we would expect, because any of these findings would be suggestive of genetic instability and abnormal proliferation throughout the entire mammary gland (i.e., both breasts).[7] The very highest risk would be found in patients carrying genetic mutations predisposing them to bilateral breast cancer. In recent years we have made great progress in understanding how certain mutations in the *p53* tumor suppressor gene or in the breast cancer genes *BRCA1* and *BRCA2* will almost inevitably translate into clinically apparent malignancies.[8] A patient who is curious about the level of risk posed by her opposite breast should consult an appropriately qualified specialist for more information. And a pathologist, rather than a surgeon or a radiotherapist, might be the best judge of those ipsilateral tumor characteristics which could indicate a high probability of subsequent contralateral malignancy. Only a counselor thoroughly schooled in hereditary cancer syndromes and in molecular biology would be competent to assess the risk level posed by a particular mutation in *p53*, *BRCA1*, or *BRCA2*.

On rare occasions a cancer detected in the contralateral breast will not be a new primary, but a metastasis coming from the original ipsilateral tumor. The distinction between *de novo* carcinogenesis and metastatic spread is not always easy to make, but we need to make it because it affects our treatment strategies. We always approach new primary tumors with a view to curing them by surgical excision if at all possible. With metastatic disease, surgery is a preliminary measure which can help only with local control—we must employ systemic therapy in the hope of preventing further dissemination. Fortunately, pathologists can usually identify metastases as such. Location is an important clue: metastatic deposits are not often found in the mammary gland proper, but rather in fatty tissues at the breast's periphery—e.g., near the sternal midline or in the axillary tail. Metastases to the contralateral breast also do not reveal the growth patterns characteristic of primary tumors. The surgeon Kirby I. Bland and his colleagues point out that "metastases tend to be multiple and show expansile growth rather than an infiltrative stellate pattern."[9] Primary invasive breast cancers are often found adjacent to areas of *in situ* cancer; this finding would be extremely unlikely with metastatic disease.

Recurrence after Lumpectomy

No breast preservation strategy offers the same degree of protection against local recurrences as a meticulous mastectomy. As we learned from NSABP Protocol B-06, when lumpectomy is not followed by irradiation, the risk of recurrent disease in the preserved breast can sometimes be substantial.[10] But radiotherapy gives no absolute guarantee of local control. Recurrences in the preserved breast may be either regrowths of the original tumor (presumably due to incomplete excision), or new primary tumors arising in previously unaffected tissues (*de novo* carcinogenesis). Physicians tend to assume that a recurrence found near the tumor bed (site of the original tumor) probably represents a regrowth (treatment failure), and that a recurrence found several centimeters away from the tumor bed or in another breast quadrant probably represents a new primary. The disease-free interval is also factored into these diagnostic assumptions. Most recurrences detected within the first few years after the initial treatment are found at or near the site of the original tumor. Presumably, a few cancer cells have managed to survive in the surrounding tissues, eluding both scalpel and irradiation, and have caused the regrowth. Most recurrences detected in later years are new primaries which have developed in other breast quadrants. Abram Recht and his knowledgeable colleagues give us a useful rule of thumb from the Joint Center for Radiotherapy: "Recurrences in or near the tumor bed are uncommon later than eight years after treatment, whereas tumor development in other parts of the breast is rare earlier than five years after the end of therapy."[11] Thus the threat of regrowth from residual tumor cells diminishes with the passage of time, while the possibility of *de novo* malignant transformation increases.

For plausible estimates of the risk of local recurrence, we are especially indebted to the long-term follow-up conducted by the Marseille Cancer Institute in France, which began to treat numerous patients with breast-conserving surgery and modern megavoltage radiotherapy in the early 1960s, several years ahead of any American institution. The radiotherapist John M. Kurtz and his colleagues kept track of 1,593 lumpectomy patients treated at the Institute between 1963 and 1982, recording 178 local recurrences (11% of the group) by the end of 1987. "The actuarial freedom from mammary recurrence," Kurtz et al observe, "was 93% at five years, 86% at ten years, and 80% at twenty years." The Marseille results are tidy enough, indicating an ongoing risk over a period of two decades which neatly averages out to 1% per year. The lion's share of the recorded recurrences (79%) occurred "in the

vicinity of the tumor bed" and were therefore "considered true recurrences" (i.e., regrowths). But after ten years the majority of recurrences being detected (64%) "were located elsewhere in the breast." Dr. Kurtz and his Marseille colleagues conclude that "after fifteen years the risk appears to be small."[12]

What's the best way to treat a local recurrence in a previously irradiated breast? The answer a concerned patient receives to this perplexing question may well depend upon which radiation oncologist she happens to ask. As stated in Chapters Sixteen and Nineteen, a second course of whole-breast radiotherapy is not an option, because the cumulative exposure would exceed the breast's tolerance.[13] The American reaction to treatment failure after lumpectomy and irradiation has usually been salvage mastectomy, but this option can only be terribly distressing to patients who have endured protracted therapy for the purpose of breast preservation. Moreover, it seems unlikely that salvage mastectomy significantly affects the subsequent survival rates in these patients, especially in the case of recurrences detected near the tumor bed. Dr. Kurtz and his colleagues at the Marseille Cancer Institute have been actively promoting "wide excision" as an initial strategy for "small, well-localized recurrences." The salvage lumpectomies performed at the Institute were not as effective as salvage mastectomies in maintaining local tumor control, but they seemed to suffice for many patients. "Survival after recurrence," Kurtz et al assure us, "did not depend upon the type of salvage operation. Locoregional control was 88% at five years after salvage mastectomy, and 64% after breast-conserving salvage procedures."[14] In the United States Carl M. Mansfield and his colleagues at Philadelphia's Thomas Jefferson University Hospital will treat "solitary recurrences" in the breast, either near the tumor bed or in a new area, by local excision; they then give additional boost irradiation to the recurrence site "using an implant or an electron beam."[15] But Abram Recht and his Joint Center colleagues worry that patients given second lumpectomies for initial local recurrences will be prone to further local or regional treatment failures. "After careful clinical and radiological evaluation to rule out multifocal disease," the Joint Center radiotherapists advise, "selected patients might be treated with wide local excision. However, we currently feel that mastectomy, with or without immediate reconstruction, is the treatment of choice."[16]

The only encouraging aspect of local recurrence after lumpectomy is that the vast majority of these events are strictly local both in their nature and in their import—they do not necessarily foreshadow the simultaneous or subsequent development of metastatic disease. Of course, there are exceptions to this rule. If the local recurrence becomes apparent soon after treatment and involves large areas of the breast or the overlying skin, the patient's prospects are much more questionable. The aforementioned presentations bespeak a fast-growing, highly infiltrative tumor whose cells are widely disseminated throughout the glandular tissues or the dermal (skin) lymphatic vessels. We would naturally be apprehensive that other parts of the body could have been invaded as well. Under these circumstances the breast cannot be preserved; salvage mastectomy is indicated, and systemic chemotherapy should be considered.[17]

Recurrence after Mastectomy

Local recurrences after mastectomy are rare in early-stage breast cancer (Stages One and Two). But the risk is appreciably higher in Stage Three patients, those with numerous positive nodes or with large original tumors. A recurrence typically presents as one or more small nodules (tiny painless lumps) arising in the surgical field, usually at the mastectomy scar or on the adjacent skin flaps. Sometimes gradual discoloration is the only clue—patches of skin may take on reddish or purplish hues. The relevant symptoms can be subtle—by themselves they are not necessarily indicative of malignancy—but they should not be ignored. Once established, local recurrences in the skin flaps can be difficult to control; naturally we'd like to detect them early, so as to give prophylactic irradiation to the affected areas. Yet in many cases the biopsy report will suffice to relieve our anxieties, by demonstrating that a suspect nodule is nothing more than a little fibrotic cyst, or that a skin discoloration has been produced by an infiltration of inflammatory (white) cells. Inflammation and fibrosis, commonplace sequelae of invasive surgery, frequently mimic recurrent malignancy, but they are in no way related to it and have nothing to do with its causation.

Local recurrences in the skin flaps after mastectomy have traditionally been considered more ominous than local recurrences in the breast after lumpectomy. The reason for this is simple—*the post-mastectomy lesions should not be there*. Lumpectomy leaves behind the bulk of the mammary tissues as well as an obvious possibility of recurrence in them. With mastectomy we tend to assume that surgery has removed all these tissues as well as the possibility of local recurrence. Therefore something must have gone wrong if a local recurrence is detected.

Of the three explanations which come to mind, only the first one is reassuring—perhaps the prior mastectomy did not remove all the tumor, and the remaining cancer cells continued to grow until they produced a clinical symptom. This scenario would not necessarily indicate an elevated risk for metastatic disease; we would be dealing with a mere "regrowth" (local treatment failure) comparable to those typically seen in lumpectomy patients. Occasionally an alert pathologist can confirm this less threatening hypothesis by identifying residual glandular tissue in the excised specimen, thus demonstrating that the mastectomy was not complete. But in most cases of local recurrence after mastectomy, physicians will cite two other possibilities by way of explanation. Perhaps cancer cells circulating in the bloodstream have found their way back to the surgical field, where they would naturally tend to implant and start growing to form nodules. If the responsible cancer cells did not come from systemic circulation, then perhaps they had invaded the nearby dermal lymphatics prior to mastectomy and were thus already implanted in the skin. Either of these explanations points toward a greatly elevated risk for metastatic disease. Malignant infiltration of the skin has been recognized as a "grave sign" since Haagensen's day. The prognostic significance of cancer cells which can survive an arduous journey in the bloodstream and thereafter implant and flourish should be self-evident.

Breast cancer specialists have long known that the majority of mastectomy patients who develop cutaneous (skin) recurrences will eventually present with distant metastases, although these may not become symptomatic until some years later. Accordingly, confirmation of a local recurrence usually brings a recommendation for systemic therapy. Frederick C. Ames and Charles M. Balch of the M. D. Anderson Cancer Center in Houston regard even "solitary recurrences" as indicative of malignant dissemination: "In all patients there remains a high risk of subsequent systemic failure. For healthy patients we currently recommend an aggressive regimen using fluorouracil, doxorubicin, and cyclophosphamide [FAC chemotherapy]. In elderly (over 75 years) or infirm patients whose disease is estrogen receptor-positive, tamoxifen is given."[18] For many specialists the length of the disease-free interval (DFI) and the extent of the recurrence will strongly influence deliberations about the advisability of chemotherapy. A solitary nodule of locally recurrent cancer detected years after mastectomy may not foreshadow imminent metastatic disease or a shortened life expectancy. True, cancer cells could be present in the bloodstream or in the dermal lymphatics; but obviously they are not particularly aggressive or fast-growing, as evidenced by the long DFI and by the limited nature of the recurrence. At the other extreme, numerous malignant nodules arising in the skin shortly after mastectomy almost certainly indicate a highly aggressive tumor as well as an urgent need for powerful systemic therapy.

Regardless of the threat of metastatic disease, the physician's first objective will be to obtain local control—that is, to remove any nodules of recurrent tumor and to prevent new nodules from forming. In the case of a small solitary nodule which arises years after mastectomy, surgical excision alone might provide satisfactory control. But in the vast majority of cases, the excision of any palpable nodules is quickly followed by an extended course of radiation therapy. Irradiation is given not only to the obvious areas of recurrence, but to the entire surgical field and to the regional lymph nodes in the axilla and beneath the sternum. Nancy Price Mendenhall of the University of Florida and her colleagues explain: "Irradiation is the mainstay of management if the initial treatment did not include irradiation. All areas at risk for subclinical involvement are given 5,000 centigrays (rads) in five weeks at 200 centigrays (rads) per fraction." Mendenhall et al would also give a boost dose—another 1,000 rads in five fractions of 200 rads each—to "areas around surgical incisions," as well as an even larger boost (1,500 to 2,000 rads in fractions of 200 to 250 each) to "areas of gross involvement."[19] Readers of Chapter Nineteen will recognize that this regimen for local cutaneous recurrences is quite as intense as the typical radiotherapy regimens for breast preservation, perhaps even more so if boosts are given to the mastectomy scar or to areas grossly involved with resurgent cancer. The side effects would be similar to those encountered with whole-breast radiotherapy after lumpectomy. However, the fields and the type of irradiation may be different. In this instance radiotherapists would rely more on perpendicular fields and electron beams, so as to give a large dose to the skin flaps while limiting exposure to the heart and lungs. Temporarily implanted radioactive needles or seeds (pellets) have historically been used to deliver large boosts to grossly involved areas—these implants expose the surrounding tissues to steady high-dose irradiation, which diminishes after a distance of a centimeter or two.

Local recurrences in the skin after mastectomy are profoundly distressing to physician and patient alike. In most cases, however, a fractionated course of radiotherapy will be effective in achieving and maintaining local control. If the cytotoxic or hormonal drugs given for systemic control also prove effective, the patient can anticipate long-term disease-free survival, yet this optimistic scenario does not always come to pass. If recurrences arise in skin which has

been previously irradiated—for example, during a failed attempt at breast preservation—our ability to combat them with additional radiotherapy will be limited. Dr. Mendenhall and her colleagues caution that in these cases "retreatment with irradiation is not likely to be successful" and "may result in severe complications."[20] Some radiotherapy can usually be given as a boost dose to small areas of local recurrence; but if we were to again expose large areas of the skin to 5,000 rads or so, we would be inviting widespread skin necrosis. The lungs, the ribs, and the sternum would also begin to receive cumulative doses exceeding their respective tolerances. For local recurrences in previously irradiated skin, we are therefore forced to rely principally on wide excision. With repeated recurrences the surgical defects will become progressively larger, and their healing ever more problematic. A plastic surgeon must therefore be enlisted to perform skin grafts or a tissue transfer in an attempt to remedy the damage. These strategies are less likely to achieve permanent control.

Uncontrolled cutaneous recurrences at or near the mastectomy site are an occasional complication of terminal breast cancer. Of course, the patient is not going to die from the local recurrences, but rather from the distant metastases which are simultaneously present. However, these local manifestations of disease can cause untold discomfort and embarrassment; the multiple sores tend to become painful as well as unsightly, and they may ooze fluid. Historically, all that physicians were able to do in these cases was to change the dressings, since the main therapeutic strategies (surgery and irradiation) had already been applied to their limits. More recently, researchers have explored other techniques for regaining local control in patients with persistent cutaneous recurrences. **Hyperthermia** may well be a useful adjunct to traditional radiotherapy—the temperature of superficial lesions could be elevated by microwave equipment before treatment, thereby enabling us to use lower doses of radiation.[21] **Photodynamic therapy** promises to destroy tumors without recourse to irradiation. In this technique patients with skin cancers or with tumors in accessible cavernous organs (e.g., bladder, esophagus, or lungs) are first given a light-sensitizing drug like Photofrin (brand name for porfimer sodium). The unstable cancer cells absorb more of the drug than normal cells. Thus when a powerful light source (laser beam) is aimed at the lesions, it will preferentially induce destructive biochemical reactions in the sensitized cancer cells, bringing about their death. The adjacent normal cells are relatively unharmed. Clinical trials designed to evaluate photodynamic therapy have been begun at the Mayo Clinic in Rochester, Minnesota, and at the Roswell Park Cancer Institute in Buffalo, New York.[22]

The Regional Lymph Nodes

Like recurrences in the skin flaps after mastectomy, nodal recurrences are interpreted as evidence of tumor cell dissemination and as an indication for systemic therapy. This holds true for both lumpectomy and mastectomy patients. The length of the disease-free interval and the extent of the recurrence may give us hints as to whether aggressive chemotherapy or gentler hormonal drugs would be more appropriately employed. However, the first task is to regain control of the affected nodal areas. Uncontrolled recurrences in the regional lymph nodes will bring pain and disability in their wake—that's one reason why the Halstedian surgeons were such sticklers for removing these nodes prophylactically.

Recurrence in the axilla is extremely improbable after adequate treatment for *in situ* breast cancers. It is also unlikely with early-stage invasive tumors if the previous treatment included an axillary dissection removing at least the lower and middle nodes (levels I and II). But monthly palpation of the axillae should be done by all patients: it is the most practical strategy for the timely detection of axillary involvement. Recurrences typically present as one or more enlarged, palpable nodes detectable during a manual examination. Other symptoms affecting the axilla, the arm, or the shoulder also merit prompt diagnostic investigations. William L. Donegan cautions that "pain in the arm and shoulder" or "increasing loss of motor and sensory sensation in the arm and hand" could be due to an unnoticed axillary recurrence. Left untreated, recurrences in the individual axillary nodes tend to grow until they coalesce into a solid mass of tumor. The resulting compression of the brachial plexus (the nerve network in the axilla) soon renders the arm and hand painful and nonfunctional. Dr. Donegan observes that CAT scans or magnetic resonance imaging (MRI) "can be helpful in evaluating the axillary nodes," but "in the absence of obvious recurrence, exploration of the brachial plexus may be necessary for diagnosis."[23] The initial treatment for any recurrence is surgery—an axillary dissection if one has not been performed previously, or if one has, excision of the recurrent tumor insofar as possible. Radiotherapy would be indicated in those cases where we anticipate that cancer cells may be lingering behind in the remaining axillary tissues. A fractionated course of irradiation is sometimes given to the apical nodes (level III) and the neighboring supraclavicular nodes following a dissection of the lower and middle axilla. But irradiation of the entire axilla may be deemed prudent in cases of extensive axillary recurrence.

A recurrence in the internal

mammary nodes, those located beneath the sternum, is relatively uncommon; but it can occur if the primary tumor was invasive and found in an inner breast quadrant. The typical presentation is a parasternal mass—that is, a little lump right between the sternum and the breast. Physical examination alone may be insufficient to determine whether that parasternal mass is strictly a cutaneous (skin) recurrence or whether it represents an extension of a nodal involvement originating beneath the sternum. A chest X-ray can sometimes give us the answer; but if it doesn't, a CAT scan of the thorax (chest cavity) should be performed. We need to identify recurrences in the internal mammary nodes promptly. Untreated, nodal recurrences here can progress until they begin to painfully destroy the sternum and the ribs. Even more ominously, the tumor cells will often leap from involved substernal nodes to the pleura, the membrane covering the lungs—in this instance, breathing difficulties would soon ensue. While surgery is our most effective weapon against substernal nodal recurrences, irradiation is usually tried first, because resection (removal) of the sternum is a difficult and risky procedure. External electron-beam therapy can be aimed down at the internal mammary nodes. An alternative technique would be to thread an iridium or cobalt wire through the internal mammary artery, a large blood vessel which passes within a centimeter or so of these nodes. The radioactive wire implant can deliver a dose as high as 9,000 rads to the nodal chain without causing significant complications in the surrounding tissues.[24] But if the nodal involvement is extensive to begin with, or if irradiation fails to arrest the recurrence, our recourse must be to surgery. Patricia M. McCormack and other thoracic surgeons at New York's Memorial Sloan-Kettering Cancer Center are adept at treating those advanced cases where the sternum and

ribs have been invaded by tumor. Dr. McCormack and her colleagues resect the sternum and the affected portions of the ribs; they then cover the large surgical defect with a polyethylene template mesh, spreading a pliable synthetic composite over the mesh to simulate the natural contours of the chest wall. Subsequent plastic surgery may be necessary to replace the missing skin or to reconstruct a missing breast. As McCormack et al point out, the long-term prognosis of these patients "depends on whether they have evidence of disease elsewhere."[25]

Recurrence in the supraclavicular nodes, those located above the collarbone, has been viewed ominously since Halsted's day. Breast cancer specialists have long interpreted any recurrence here as a harbinger of metastatic disease. As we've seen in Chapter Fourteen, the standard TNM staging automatically categorizes patients with involved supraclavicular nodes as Stage Four. The lymphatic vessels of the breast do not drain directly into these nodes—a recurrence in them typically follows involvement of the apical (level III) axillary nodes, and it suggests pervasive tumor dissemination throughout the regional lymphatics. The presenting symptom is usually one or more palpable nodes above the collarbone. Untreated, these nodes may grow to golf-ball size; the timely combination of surgical excision and irradiation can prevent this development, but the eventual outcome remains problematic. One study of patients who were treated for supraclavicular involvement found that 80% of them developed overt metastases within four years.[26] Only rigorous systemic therapy would seem to stand a chance of slowing or stopping disease progression in these cases.

Looking for Metastatic Disease

Distant metastases represent the worst type of recurrence. In this eventuality the cancer cells do not merely recur in the breast or in the neighboring lymph nodes, but they demonstrate a much greater malignant potential by establishing parasitic colonizations in one or more distant organs. With rare exceptions we have not been able to reverse the metastatic process once it has become established. However, in many cases we can effectively manage symptoms and avert complications, thereby keeping patients functional and independent for a longer time than they would otherwise be. The management of metastatic breast cancer is a complicated topic whose discussion we must postpone until Chapter Twenty-six. For the moment we need to consider the tools which are used to search for metastatic disease, and which may be employed during follow-up. Any hint of recurrence, even a purely local event, almost invariably leads to a battery of tests intended to rule out—or to detect—distant metastases. In early-stage breast cancer, most patients will consistently test negative; even with those fated to develop metastatic disease, several years usually elapse between the diagnosis of the original tumor and the appearance of distant lesions large enough to set off the alarm bells on our current tests.

The old-fashioned **chest X-ray** remains the most frequently used tool. It's cheap, it's fast, and it does a fairly good job of detecting metastatic tumors in the lungs. The **CAT scan**, diagnostic offspring of a marriage between a revolving X-ray apparatus and the computer, gets called upon whenever chest X-rays fail to remove our suspicions or to satisfy our curiosity. CAT can give us cross-sectional images of the lungs and other thoracic organs—if not exactly cheap, it is quite fast and entirely painless, and it is readily available in American hospitals. The level of radiation exposure, while more than that of conventional X-rays, is relatively low and does not raise concerns about side effects.

With breast cancers the most frequent site of metastatic disease is the skeletal framework. We are especially concerned about possible metastases in important weight-bearing structures like the hip, the femur (thighbone), or the spinal vertebrae—in any of these bones either a sudden fracture or a gradual disintegration would cause considerable pain and lasting disability. Node-positive patients and those with any type of recurrence are routinely asked to undergo a skeletal radiograph, popularly known as a **bone scan**. This test is as painless as an X-ray but far more time-consuming. The patient must first visit her hospital's "Department of Nuclear Medicine," where she receives an intravenous injection of a mildly radioactive substance which would tend to concentrate in bone (e.g., radiolabeled phosphate or strontium). Two or three hours later the patient returns for the bone scan—she must now lie motionless for thirty minutes or so while the scanning device passes slowly over her body. The end result is a large radiographic image of the entire skeleton. Areas of abnormal activity, such as might be caused by osseous (bone) metastases, will show up as "hot spots" because they have absorbed more of the radioisotope. The advantages of a bone scan are that it images the skeletal framework at one sitting and that it can detect metastatic lesions before they would cause symptoms or be noticeable on standard X-rays. About 50% of a bone's mass has to be lost before an X-ray will detect any abnormality. The disadvantages of bone scanning are that benign processes like arthritis also show up as hot spots, and that the "yield" (percentage of true positive findings) is extremely low in asymptomatic patients. The NSABP tallied the yield from 7,984 bone scans done on patients with early-stage disease enrolled in its clinical trials: only 52 scans (less than 1%) actually detected osseous metastases.[27]

Back in the 1970s the **liver scan** was touted for the early detection of hepatic metastases. Taking this test is much like undergoing a bone scan. The patient first receives an intravenous injection of a mildly radioactive substance which would be preferentially taken up by the liver (e.g., radio-labeled colloidal sulfur). Later she must lie still under a scanner for thirty minutes or so while the organ is imaged. A noticeable difference from the bone scan is that any metastases would show up as "cold spots," areas of the liver which had failed to absorb the radioisotope. Unfortunately, liver scans are prone to false positives because cirrhosis, hepatitis, and other nonmalignant conditions will also produce cold spots on the radiograph. In the 1980s breast cancer specialists learned that CAT scans of the liver done with intravenous contrast agents tended to be more accurate than radioisotope scanning. Dr. Donegan observes that in patients with liver involvement, CAT "provides optimum sensitivity but still detects fewer than 50% of the metastases detected at laparotomy [surgical exploration]."[28] Normally neither a radioisotope scan nor a CAT scan would be done on an asymptomatic patient unless a rising level of alkaline phosphatase in the blood had previously suggested abnormal liver function. The inexpensive test for this enzyme is a routine part of follow-up.

Magnetic resonance imaging, the newest technology for looking at cross sections of the body, is not significantly better than CAT for viewing the abdominal and thoracic cavities. Moreover, MRI exams have hitherto been more expensive and more time-consuming than CAT, factors which have predisposed physicians toward the older system. But MRI has become the system of choice for evaluating suspected metastatic lesions in the brain or the spinal vertebrae. This tool is not employed in routine follow-up. MRI of the brain would be done only if the patient were to experience neurological symptoms like persistent headaches or unexplained dizziness. An exam focusing on the vertebrae would be indicated only if the patient were to experience localized back pain or if a bone scan had previously suggested osteolytic activity (destruction of bone) in the spinal column.[29]

Serum Tumor Markers

The Holy Grail of cancer detection strategies, whether we are looking for new tumors or for recurrences, is a simple blood test which would conclusively tell us if malignant cells are active in the body. The development of such a test rests upon the assumption that cancer cells must produce one or more substances which are not produced by normal cells. Thus, if we should detect one of these telltale substances in the blood, we would have an indication of malignancy long before the formation of a tumor large enough to be detected on an X-ray, a mammogram, or a CAT scan. Oncology textbooks sometimes refer to these substances as **biomarkers**— they are also called **serum tumor markers**, "serum" being the fluid portion of the blood (as distinguished from its cellular portion). One of these markers, **prostate-specific antigen** (PSA), has already found wide acceptance as a screening tool. Elevated levels of PSA usually (but not always) give us a clue to an initial malignant transformation taking place in the male prostate. PSA also comes in handy after the treatment of prostate cancer. Low levels of the PSA protein are suggestive of tumor control, while rising levels suggest recurrent disease. While the utility of PSA readings has often been debated, PSA nonetheless represents a major success story among biomarkers. For the other solid tumors the quest has been less rewarding.[30]

The measurement of **carcinoembryonic antigen** (CEA) in breast and colon cancers has been advocated for many years. **CEA** is a protein which is secreted by certain tissues in developing fetuses, but which is not normally present in adults. In the 1960s researchers learned that many colon cancers and some breast cancers also secrete tiny quantities of CEA. Shortly thereafter monitoring of CEA levels in the blood became routine in the follow-up of diagnosed colon cancers. This inexpensive assay is generally done for breast cancers as well, but very little weight can be placed on the results. While some breast tumors produce CEA in measurable amounts, others do not. Moreover, CEA levels can also be elevated in various benign conditions. In the mid-1980s Centocor, a pharmaceutical company, started to market a monoclonal antibody assay called **CA 15-3**, which reacts with an elusive protein shed by breast cancer cells into the bloodstream. This biomarker is more specific than CEA; in most studies rising levels of CA 15-3 have been shown to correlate with disease progression. According to guidelines published by the American Society of Clinical Oncology, "9% of women with Stage One and 19% of women with Stage Two breast cancer have elevated CA 15-3 levels. The incidence of abnormal values increases to 38% and 75% for patients with Stage Three and Stage Four, respectively." The Society cautions its members that "low CA 15-3 levels do not exclude metastases, and a given CA 15-3 level cannot be used to determine the stage of disease."[31]

Since neither CEA nor CA 15-3 is an altogether reliable indicator, most breast cancer specialists have wanted both assays to be performed. Elevated readings during follow-up, especially if the readings right

after surgery were low, are suggestive of metastatic progression. Unfortunately, these assays do not tell us the anatomical location of the metastatic colonies, nor do they give us any clues as to how we might eliminate them.

Is Follow-up Really Needed?

In the matter of follow-up after an initial breast cancer diagnosis and treatment, we find ourselves between a rock and a hard place. How many of those follow-up office visits and diagnostic tests might justly be described as "prudent and reasonable"? And how many are merely "encyclopedic and habitual," accomplishing nothing to speak of beyond an elevation of patient anxieties and the perpetual ringing of practitioner cash registers? Perhaps we can agree that an attitude of vigilance, by patient and physician alike, is always prudent. Furthermore, there is substantial agreement among physicians that annual physical examinations and annual mammograms constitute a reasonable strategy—viz., a strategy which is unlikely to overtax a patient's patience or her pocketbook. But additional consensus is lacking. In spite of all those doctor-ordered assays, most recurrences and most new primary tumors are discovered by the patients themselves, who typically perform breast examinations with a thoroughness surpassing even the American Cancer Society's recommendations. While our current assays for metastatic disease can often detect distant lesions before they cause symptoms, it is not at all certain that discovering these lesions while they are asymptomatic will produce a survival benefit. The *Journal of the American Medical Association* has published the results of two Italian clinical trials which together had randomly assigned 2,563 breast cancer patients to receive either an intensive follow-up with regular bone scans and chest X-rays, or to receive a minimal follow-up limited to annual physical examinations and annual mammograms. In neither trial did the group of patients receiving regular bone scans and chest X-rays reveal any survival advantage over the group who just received the physical examinations and the mammograms.[32]

The surgeon John S. Spratt, co-editor with Dr. Donegan of a standard textbook, has been a vocal proponent of the minimalist philosophy which holds that expensive diagnostic tests should be done only on those breast cancer patients with symptoms suggestive of recurrent disease. Dr. Spratt is concerned that "as much as a billion dollars per year could be spent on follow-up testing with no survival benefit. Those patients whose cases are followed simply by self-surveillance and prompt evaluation of symptoms do just as well."[33] Of course, other breast cancer specialists will argue that the patients' interests are best served by intensive follow-up. The reason why Dr. Spratt and his fellow minimalists are probably right about the absence of a demonstrable survival benefit is that our current tests for metastatic disease are not nearly sensitive enough. Those marvelous high-tech scans, CAT and MRI, have been extremely helpful in evaluating symptoms; but they cannot begin to detect micrometastases, tiny pinpoint clusters of disseminated cancer cells which are just beginning to take root in other organs, and which cause no symptoms whatsoever. The smallest lesions we can predictably see on CAT or MRI scans are likely to be upwards of a centimeter in diameter. Clinically speaking, a tumor in this size range (0.5 to 1.0 cm) is "small"; but from a molecular view point it's enormous, being composed of millions and millions of cancer cells. Bone scans have comparable limitations. The osseous metastases they will predictably

detect represent advanced disease. Detection is "early" only by comparison to conventional X-rays or to a clinical presentation (e.g., a patient in pain). When we encounter a positive finding on any of these scans, we are not looking toward the beginning of the metastatic process, but rather toward its end. By this time systemic disease tends to be so firmly established in the body that even rigorous chemotherapy cannot eliminate it. The only current assay which would seem to show us *early* metastatic disease is **bone marrow sampling with subsequent immunostaining**—that is, with a pathology workup to detect isolated cancer cells in the marrow aspirate. We've already discussed this new technique in Chapter Fourteen; unfortunately, any role it might play in the routine follow-up of breast cancer patients has not as yet been defined.

Patients need to be sophisticated consumers who can judge for themselves the value of the particular follow-up strategies being recommended. The vast majority of patients who have been adequately treated for *in situ* or small Stage One tumors are not going to benefit from tests designed to detect metastatic disease, since they are not at risk for it. On the other hand, all these patients would stand to benefit from the early detection of new primary tumors, which could arise either in the other (contralateral) breast or in a treated (preserved) breast. All lumpectomy patients are also at greater or lesser risk for local recurrences in the preserved breast, and they merit regular physical examinations and mammograms simply on that account. Node-positive patients and those node-negative patients with larger tumors or discouraging pathology reports are at risk for metastatic disease; they may well benefit from a more intensive follow-up. Disregarding the slippery issue of survival benefit, we can safely say that the early detection and treatment of distant metastases is prudent, because it often enables us to avoid complications. The lung metastasis detected as a spot on an X-ray film and effectively managed by surgical excision or by chemotherapy does not grow until it afflicts the patient with coughing fits and respiratory distress. Metastatic foci detected on a bone scan can often be ameliorated with irradiation before they begin to cause painful symptoms. Impending fractures of vertebrae, hips, or thighbones can often be averted by inserting surgical pins. From an afflicted patient's point of view, the trouble and expense caused by one fracture could be greater than that occasioned by a hundred bone scans. The surgeon Michael D. Wertheimer reminds us that follow-up may also be psychologically beneficial: "Patients with cancer rarely miss follow-up appointments, and need and deserve the intense link that their post-treatment surveillance program provides. There are many tangible and intangible attributes of follow-up based on this long-term physician-patient relationship that cannot be measured."[34]

Chapter Twenty-one

ALTERNATIVE MEDICINE
Vitamins, Diet, and Positive Thinking

Orthodox cancer treatments remain profoundly frightening, and not without reason. They tend to be mutilative or toxic, and they do not always work. It is hardly surprising that many patients are powerfully attracted to so-called **alternative therapies**, which hold out the promise of therapeutic effects obtainable without mutilation or toxicity, and at minimal expense. In this case the "alternatives" usually involve no more than slight changes in lifestyle. ***Can a modification in diet or some positive thinking enhance the body's resistance to tumor cells and stave off the appearance of distant metastases?*** Obviously, we'd all like to think so—but the fact that we desperately want to believe in these strategies is perhaps the very reason why we should insist on the most stringent scientific evidence of effectiveness before recommending them. Unfortunately, the task of designing experiments which would properly measure the effects that diet and mindset might have on disease progression is not easy. Laypersons often embrace dietary or mindset strategies uncritically and much too passionately—on the other hand, physicians often dismiss these approaches a little too peremptorily.

The Vitamin Revolution:
Miracles or Marketing?

The first "miracle cures" were not wrought by pharmaceutical companies but by grocers. In the eighteenth century we began to understand that certain terrible illnesses could be cured by incredibly minor modifications in diet. English sailors, confined for months at a time in ships sailing to the far-flung outposts of the British Empire, often developed a mysterious and devastating disorder called **scurvy**. Afflicted sailors would lose weight, their gums would bleed, and their teeth would fall out; many of them eventually died. The culprit behind this strange epidemic was not an infectious agent but a nutritional omission. The sailors' diet of salted beef and hardtack was rich enough in macronutrients (carbohydrates, fats, and proteins); but it lacked a micronutrient essential for the formation of collagen, that fibrous constructive material which holds the body together and prevents blood vessels from leaking. Scurvy is an example of a **vitamin-deficiency disease**—it results from the absence of vitamin C (ascorbic acid), which is supplied by fresh fruits and vegetables. In the eighteen and nineteenth centuries, no-body knew anything about vitamins, those elusive organic substances found in food-stuffs which are necessary only in the tiniest trace amounts. But the observation was made that if citrus fruits like limes or lemons were added to the nautical diet, scurvy did not occur. English sailors soon acquired the nickname *limeys* because they spent a lot of time sucking on lemons or limes.

These days clinically apparent vitamin deficiencies are extremely rare in American society; this was not always the case. At the beginning of the twentieth century, children growing up in the gloomy tenement slums of Northern cities often suffered from a syndrome called **rickets**. Their leg and arm bones were soft and spindly due to insufficient vitamin D, a micronutrient which the body produces by itself when exposed to sunlight. Poor people in the rural South, a sunnier locale, weren't troubled by rickets; but since their diet consisted largely of corn bread and blackstrap molasses, they were prone to develop **pellagra**. Physicians at first suspected that some subtle infectious agent lay behind pellagra's characteristic symptoms—viz., red and crusty skin, diarrhea, eventual dementia. The cause proved to be an absence of the B vitamin niacin. Rickets and pellagra disappeared from the American scene at about the time the super-market arrived. Fish liver oil and fortified milk vanquished the former disease; niacin-rich brewer's yeast took care of the latter.[1]

The aforementioned diseases (scurvy, rickets, pellagra) arise only in cases of those extraordinary dietary deprivations which are associated with extreme poverty or appalling ignorance. Do well-educated, middle-class Americans need to constantly consume supplements of synthetic vitamins to pre-serve their health? This issue remains debatable, but there is no question that for decades American pharmaceutical companies have been slyly portraying universal vitamin supplementation as an urgent public health measure. The medical historian Rima D. Apple has chronicled these marketing excesses in a book entitled *Vitamania*. "Throughout the 1920s and 1930s," she points out, "researchers isolated and even synthesized many of these rare micronutri-ents, thereby laying the foundation for a lucrative industry." In 1921 only three vitamins (A, B, C) were officially recognized; by 1940 the list included over twenty vitamins.[2] Marketing began innocuously back in the 1920s, with cod liver oil—mothers were urged to give their children a teaspoon or two each day during the gloomy winter months, thereby supplying the fat-soluble vitamin D (the so-called "sunshine vitamin") and pro-moting "sturdy bones and teeth." The 1930s saw the introduction of irradiated (and there-fore vitamin D fortified) milk, bread, and cereals. When multivitamin pills became available in the 1940s, manufacturers em-barked on more extensive campaigns to educate the public. The message conveyed was simple—even if you did not have an overt deficiency disease, you could still suffer from all sorts of maladies if you did not get enough vitamins. Advertisements from Miles Laboratories, manufacturer of the popular "One-a-day" brand of multivitamin pills, warned consumers that pernicious subclinical deficiencies were difficult to diagnose; but might be manifested by "low resistance to colds, irritability, fatigue, loss of vitality, weakness, nervousness, indigestion, gas, certain skin troubles, sleepless-ness." The list of symptoms, Dr. Apple observes, was "very long and nonspecific." The Kroger supermarket chain took a differ-ent tack—its advertising flyers emphasized the benefits to be had from vitamins, which included "bright eyes," "lustrous hair," and "buoyant vitality."[3] Daily supplements were deemed necessary because the American diet was terribly vitamin-deficient, or so it seemed! Canned foods weren't a good source of these micronutrients because modern processing methods diminished their vitamin content. And as for fresh fruits and vegetables, they weren't fresh enough! Why, if the vitamins in these foodstuffs did not decay during that long journey from the farm to the market, they would almost certainly be lost during cooking! Thus did the American public learn about vitamins, and thus did the daily multivitamin pill come to be regarded as an insurance policy against a wide range of subtle deficiencies and their resulting manifold symptoms. You had to be absolutely sure that you got your vitamins!

In the last half of the twentieth century, vitamin supplementation became a multi-billion-dollar industry in the United States. Our pharmaceutical companies love vitamins because these products are so cheap to manufacture and (being relatively free of side effects) open few doors to liability litigation. In most cases any excess consumption is simply eliminated through the body's normal excretory functions. Since vitamins are food elements rather than drugs, they have avoided rigorous regulation by the Food and Drug Administration. The FDA does not allow vitamin manufacturers to claim specific medicinal effects in their advertising; but—as we've seen—any number of benefits can be *implied*. American consumers also love vitamins. These products are "natural," yet they come packaged in little bottles just like "real medicine" and are similarly invested with "scientific authority." Moreover, the consumer can self-prescribe at will. A vast array of supplements is displayed in every drug store and supermarket. These pills are cheaper than prescription drugs, and reports of their wondrous efficacies are appearing daily in the newspapers and on TV.

Antioxidants Get <u>Over</u>hyped

In the 1980s nutrition-oriented researchers began to advance claims for vitamins that made the old-fashioned hype about radiant hair and vibrant energy look modest and restrained. Numerous studies seemed to suggest that vitamins might play a role in preventing cancer and cardiovascular disease. Most of this research was done on those vitamins with **antioxidant properties**. Oxidation, the combination of oxygen with other elements and the resulting release of energy, is essential to life as we know it. This process is constantly occurring in individual cells throughout the body. Oxidation *per se* would not seem to promote either cancer or atherosclerosis (the narrowing of blood vessels due to fatty deposits in them); but certain unstable molecules released as byproducts of intracellular chemical reactions have been implicated in both diseases. These molecules are called **free radicals**: they can damage nuclear DNA, possibly causing carcinogenic mutations. They can also damage the membranes of the endothelial cells lining the blood vessels, possibly predisposing the coronary arteries to atherosclerotic obstructions. The vitamins referred to as "antioxidants"—**vitamins C, E, and beta carotene** (a precursor of vitamin A)—are believed to neutralize free radicals and thereby to help minimize oxidative damage.

Unfortunately, the evidence that antioxidant vitamins can prevent cancer and cardiovascular disease in humans is far from being conclusive. There have been oodles of laboratory experiments involving "nude" (immunodeficient) mice or using individual cells grown in Petri dishes. Marcia Will and Joseph A. Fontana of the University of Maryland Cancer Center in Baltimore remind us that vitamin A and its precursors can delay breast tumor formation in rats and mice exposed to mammary carcinogens, and that vitamin C inhibits the growth of cultured breast cancer cells.[4]   Notwithstanding these experimental results, anybody at all familiar with cancer research knows that just about everything seems to induce malignancy in nude mice and that just about anything seems to cure it.   We had better not place too much weight on these tiny beasties—ditto for cancer cells artificially kept alive in Petri dishes, whose growth can be stymied by all sorts of compounds.   The *human* studies have been almost entirely epidemiological in nature, attempting to correlate a higher or lower consumption of antioxidant vitamins with higher or lower rates of cancer and cardiovascular disease.   Many of these studies have reported protective effects, but others have failed to find an association. Epidemiological studies of diet and disease are especially prone to bias and confounding, methodological pitfalls which we discussed in Chapter Five.   You can't control human consumption of foodstuffs in the same way that you can control the diet of laboratory animals.   Moreover, when you do find an apparent protective effect, it is hard to identify the nutritional component responsible because human diets are so varied.

In the 1990s the most plausible epidemiological studies of antioxidant vitamins were those postulating a role for vitamin E in the prevention of cardiovascular disease.   On May 20, 1993, the *New England Journal of Medicine* published the results of two studies performed by Meir J. Stampfer, Eric B. Rimm, Walter C. Willett, and other epidemiologists at Harvard University.   The Nurses' Health Study had polled 87,245 female nurses—those in the top fifth for vitamin E consumption had "a relative risk of major coronary disease of 0.66" (a 34% reduction) compared to those in the lowest fifth.[5]   In the Health Professionals Follow-up Study 33,910 men were polled—those who took vitamin E supplements ("at least 100 IU per day for at

least two years") had "a multivariate relative risk of coronary disease of 0.63" (a 37% reduction) compared to those who did not.[6] In an editorial accompanying the two articles, Daniel Steinberg of the University of California at San Diego worried about confounding factors ("the men in the upper fifth in terms of vitamin E intake did exercise more"), as well as the possible long-term side effects: "Are we really sure that 500 or 1,000 IU of vitamin E daily carries no risk over a five-year period?   A twenty-year period?" Dr. Steinberg urged that "large double-blind clinical trials" be performed before any universal recommendation for vitamin E supplementation.[7]

Other people were more disposed to interpret the tentative Harvard findings as mighty pillars of scientific fact.   The pharmaceutical firm Hoffmann-La Roche (a manufacturer of vitamin pills) ran advertisements touting antioxidants for cardiovascular health in *Time* and the *Journal of the American Medical Association*.   An advertisement in the latter weekly warned physicians that "more than 90%" of the American population have "a shortfall for essential nutrients, including an 'antioxidant gap.'   Thus, where appropriate, consider recommending fortified foods and/or dietary supplements containing vitamins C and E and beta carotene."[8]   The Hoffmann-La Roche advertisements were thoughtfully composed and presented in the form of public service messages.   They did not specifically recommend the firm's vitamin pills, and they stopped just short of saying that antioxidant vitamins actually prevent heart attacks.   Notwithstanding the tactfulness of Hoffmann-La Roche's educational campaign, it was enough to elicit a vigorous response from Victor Herbert, a researcher affiliated with the Mount Sinai Medical Center in New York City.   Dr. Herbert, who had long been critical of the exaggerated benefits claimed for vitamin supplementation, fired off salvos of protest to the editors of the *Journal of the American Medical Association* and other scientific organs. "No supplement is a pure antioxidant," he explained. "This is a myth. Vitamins C, E, and beta carotene are mischaracterized by describing them solely as 'antioxidants' (fighters against harmful free radicals). They in fact are redox agents, antioxidant in some circumstances (often so in the physiologic quantities found in food), and pro-oxidant (producing billions of harmful free radicals) in other circumstances (often so in the pharmacologic quantities found in supplements)." Dr. Herbert argued that vitamin E's protective effects against heart attacks could be largely mediated by "the prohemorrhagic action of megadoses of vitamin E," which might also "promote excessive bleeding."[9]

Citations soon flew fast and furiously in the *Journal*'s correspondence columns as Dr. Herbert engaged Wolfgang Schalch of Hoffmann-La Roche in epistolary joust over the vitamin RDAs (Recommended Dietary Allowances). The former cited studies which "reported harms from above-RDA amounts of 'antioxidant' vitamins, including promotion of heart disease, cancer, and liver and kidney disease." The latter cited studies confirming "the safety of long-term use of higher than RDA levels."[10] The hard-fought stalemate between Doctors Herbert and Schalch should remind us that the voluminous literature on antioxidant vitamins is hardly consistent. There would seem to be substantial evidence that the RDA amounts of vitamin C, E, and beta carotene play an important role in maintaining health. Do supplements containing many times these amounts make one even healthier? Dr. Herbert, forever skeptical, sees no overall benefit: "Supplements help some, harm some, and do nothing for most, so the bottom line is a wash."[11]

Can Vitamins Cure Cancer?

The idea that foodstuffs, vitamins in particular, can influence the course (natural history) of human malignancies has never been taken very seriously by American physicians or by orthodox organizations like the American Cancer Society and the National Cancer Institute. For decades dietary "therapies" were advocated only by a few unorthodox physicians who tended to practice in certain clinics in Mexico, beyond the reach of the Food and Drug Administration and aggressive malpractice lawyers. In the 1970s and 1980s the notion that vitamins might slow or even reverse metastatic disease moved a bit closer to mainstream American medicine. If orthodox physicians and researchers still did not accept it, at least they became more willing to test it in clinical trials involving actual patients. The notion acquired a spokesman with august scientific credentials in the person of **Linus Pauling**, who had won two Nobel Prizes, one in chemistry and one peace award for social activism.[12] In the late 1960s Pauling turned his energies toward the interrelated fields of public health and nutrition, arguing that many diseases, even mental illnesses, could be prevented by the proper diet. He praised **vitamin C** (ascorbic acid) as a particularly versatile magic bullet. Pauling's book *Vitamin C and the Common Cold* became a best seller in the 1970s—its hypothesis that doses of vitamin C far in excess of the RDA can prevent most colds came to be accepted as an article of faith by millions of Americans. The ensuing clinical trials gave inconsistent results, not exactly proving the hypothesis but then not disproving it either.

Pauling also wrote a book entitled *Cancer and Vitamin C*, in collaboration with the Scottish physician Ewan Cameron who had dosed cancer patients with ten grams of vitamin C per day. Cameron claimed that those patients who received this megadose of vitamin C (about 167 times the RDA) fared better than comparable patients who had not. Researchers at the Linus Pauling Institute in California now performed the customary animal experimentation. Hairless mice were exposed to ultraviolet radiation, which typically induced squamous cell carcinomas of the skin. However, when the irradiated mice were fed a diet loaded with vitamin C, they often stayed tumor-free.[13] Cancer patients anxiously anticipated the therapeutic wonders hinted at by Pauling and Cameron. Cancer specialists were less impressed: Cameron's results seemed anecdotal—and mouse experiments usually have no more than marginal significance for human malignancies.

The highly respected oncologist Charles G. Moertel and his colleagues at the Mayo Clinic hoped to settle this issue with an impartial clinical trial. They randomly assigned one hundred patients with advanced colon cancer to receive either ten grams of daily vitamin C or a placebo. The results from this little trial did much to dispel any expectations that vitamin C would be a panacea for malignancy. Not only did the patients taking the supplements not have an improved outcome, they actually fared worse. "For patients taking vitamin C," Moertel et al reported in 1985, "the median survival was 2.9 months, and for placebo-treated patients it was 4.1 months."[14]

Pauling and other proponents of vitamin C were quick to point out the main limitation of the Mayo Clinic trial—only a few patients with terminal cancer had been enrolled. Would the added vitamin C have demonstrated therapeutic benefits if more patients with early-stage tumors had taken part? Does extra vitamin C possibly have prophylactic effects, helping to ward off the development of initial primary tumors? Many serious researchers continue to believe

that vitamin C could confer both prophylactic and therapeutic benefits, but nobody has hard data on the true effectiveness of such supplementation in humans, or on the appropriate dose levels for it. At a symposium on vitamin C and cancer hosted by the National Institutes of Health, most speakers told highly technical tales of effects observed in laboratory animals or in cultured cancer cells. But Gladys Block of the National Cancer Institute summarized the results of 46 epidemiological studies, pointing out that "33 described significant protective effects on cancer mortality and incidence."[15] Perhaps we should take our epidemiological findings with a grain of salt, but should we also consume a gram of daily vitamin C? Probably we should not take any more than that. Arthur Robinson, a researcher closely allied with Linus Pauling, came to believe that the daily ten-gram doses (10,000 mg) recommended by Ewan Cameron might actually tend to promote cancer.[16] Pauling's wife Ava Helen, who went on a ten-gram regiment in 1970, was diagnosed with a fatal stomach cancer in 1975. Pauling himself died of prostate cancer in August 1993, though at the ripe old age of 93.

By the late 1980s, as the prospects for vitamin C therapy seemed dimmer, most cancer researchers were pinning their hopes on **beta carotene**. This antioxidant precursor of vitamin A is found abundantly in carrots (as the name suggests) and in many other green or yellow vegetables (e.g., sweet potatoes, broccoli, spinach, and squash). A growing number of epidemiological studies had reported correlations between a low intake of beta carotene and an increased incidence of malignancy, especially of those cancers known to be induced by smoking (e.g., lung and esophageal cancers).[17] A natural compound derived from plants, beta carotene looked like an ideal chemopreventive agent. There would be little risk of toxic overdoses, since the body converts only the beta carotene it needs to vitamin A. The fat-soluble **vitamin A** also excited researchers, as did various related compounds known as **retinoids**. In Petri-dish experiments vitamin A and its retinoid forerunners were often able to induce differentiation in malignant cells. Writing in the *Journal of the American Medical Association* in 1991, Samuel Broder of the National Cancer Institute and his colleague Judith E. Karp enthusiastically reported that "the ability of vitamin A-related compounds to suppress the formation of new tumors" added "a new dimension to our anticancer strategies."[18]

Such enthusiasm proved contagious. Cancer patients were soon drinking freshly squeezed carrot juice at breakfast, to be sure of getting uncontaminated beta carotene straight from Mother Nature. And vitamin pill bottles now carried labels which boldly proclaimed **"Added Beta Carotene."** Does beta carotene supplementation really help to prevent cancer? Can retinoids reverse established malignancies? The emerging results from several large-scale clinical trials did not support these hypotheses. In 1994 an American trial found that high-dose vitamin A did not improve the survival rates of melanoma patients, and a large trial done in Finland yielded the surprising finding that cigarette smokers who took beta carotene supplements were more prone to develop lung cancer than smokers who did not.[19] The year 1996 brought a thorough debunking of beta carotene supplementation. On May 2, 1996, the *New England Journal of Medicine* published the findings from two major American trials. The Physicians' Health Study had enrolled 22,071 male physicians—half of them took beta carotene supplements ("50 mg on alternate days"), and half received a placebo. After an average follow-up of twelve years,

the Harvard epidemiologists conducting this study reported that "beta carotene produced neither benefit nor harm in terms of the incidence of malignant neoplasms, cardiovascular disease, or death from all causes."[20] The CARET trial (that's short for the "Beta Carotene and Retinol Efficacy Trial") was frankly interventional in its design. It had enrolled 18,314 men and women deemed to be at high risk of developing lung cancer and cardiovascular disease (e.g., smokers and former smokers, as well as persons exposed to asbestos). After only four years of follow-up, the CARET trial was abruptly halted— the participants receiving the proposed intervention (supplementary beta carotene and vitamin A) had a significantly *higher* incidence of disease. Their risk of death from any cause was up 17% compared to the control (placebo) group. Specifically, the risk of death from lung cancer proved to be up 46% in the intervention group, and the risk of death from cardiovascular disease was 26% higher.[21]

No one would question the very consistent epidemiological finding that persons consuming diets rich in fruits and vegetables have lower rates of cancer and cardiovascular disease than persons consuming diets noticeably deficient in these foodstuffs. But the assumption that we can precisely identify the nutritional component (or components) responsible for these protective effects, and then put that component (or components) into an efficacious prophylactic pill, has not been demonstrated. This assumption has less to do with scientific progress than with smug presumption and shameless marketing. Any positive identification of the protective component in fruits and vegetables remains problematic—diets rich in beta carotene are also likely to be rich in vitamin C and various other vitamins and minerals, as well as low in fat. Which particular component or combination of components does the trick? Are there dietary components we haven't identified yet? The participants enrolled in epidemiological studies of diet and disease represent still another source of possible confounding. Conceivably those reporting a higher intake of fruits and vegetables, or of particular vitamins, were generally more careful of their health than those reporting a lower intake.

Advertising for manufactured supplements usually plays on the theme that vitamins are "natural"—and by implication, proper and beneficial. We know this for a fact only when these micronutrients are supplied in micro-quantities. What happens when massive doses are consumed is less certain. Toxic overdoses easily occur with the fat soluble vitamins A and D, because these vitamins are stored by—and therefore accumulate in—the body. Hypervitaminosis A or D can lead to all sorts of strange symptoms, none of which are pleasant or trivial. The American Medical Association's Council on Scientific Affairs reminds us that "severe illness has resulted from the excessive use of vitamin A, and death has occurred after massive oral doses of vitamin D."[22] It is much harder to overdose on vitamin C because this water-soluble vitamin is not stored in the body—any excess quantities are simply excreted in the urine. But a massive consumption of vitamin C is not without risk. Victor Herbert cautions that "large doses of vitamin C can promote kidney stones," and that in those persons genetically predisposed to "high body iron," vitamin C is not antioxidant but "violently pro-oxidant." While Dr. Herbert concedes the fact that vitamin E increases activity among the body's immune (white) cells, he worries that large doses of it could "promote progression of autoimmune diseases" such as "asthma, food allergy,

diabetes, rheumatoid arthritis, multiple sclerosis, and lupus."[23] In pharmacologic quantities vitamins can also produce undesirable interactions with drugs or with other vitamins. Excessive vitamin C may interfere with the action of methotrexate, a drug widely used in breast cancer chemotherapy. A clinical trial conducted with human subjects found that long-term supplementation with beta carotene lowered the level of vitamin E in the blood. Conversely, animal studies have suggested that vitamin E supplementation may lower beta carotene levels. It would appear that you cannot greatly elevate the level of the one without simultaneously depressing the other.[24]

Uninformed laypersons usually jump to the conclusion that because small quantities of vitamins are beneficial and necessary, a "whole lot" of them must be wonderful. This simplistic notion could be dangerous. Those big trials of beta carotene supplementation ought to make us suspect that synthetic vitamins taken in pharmacologic doses will have different effects from the vitamins present as trace amounts in foodstuffs. There would seem to be little harm—and possibly some good—in taking a daily multivitamin pill as an insurance policy against surreptitious vitamin deficiencies. On the other hand, cancer patients should be cautioned against gobbling down massive supplements of this or that vitamin because of something they read in a newspaper or heard on TV. Like the vitamin manufacturers, the popular media somehow manage to inflate even the flimsiest experiment with nude mice into an imminent therapy for humans. Unfortunately, we have no established vitamin regimens for the commonplace tumors. Those retinoids whose potential was lauded by Doctors Broder and Karp continue to be tested for the prevention and treatment of skin and cervical cancers.[25] One retinoid actually became an accepted therapy.

Tretinoin (all-*trans*-retinoic acid) has been used to induce remission in acute promyelocytic leukemia. This relatively uncommon malignancy involves a translocation of the gene for the retinoic acid receptor—oral doses of tretinoin remedy the problem and stimulate the leukemic cells to differentiate.[26] With this particular leukemia we know for a fact that "vitamin therapy" really works, and we have at least a general idea of why it works.

A Practical Dietary Strategy:
Lower the Fat and Up the Fiber

Notwithstanding the ongoing hoopla over micronutrients (vitamins and minerals), the proposals for a nutritional intervention in breast malignancies have tended to center around that terribly suspect macronutrient, **dietary fat**. Would a low-fat diet improve the survival rates? To be sure, it certainly would—at least in the inevitable animal model! Researchers at the American Health Foundation in Valhalla, New York, randomized "58 female nude mice" to receive either a high-fat diet or a low-fat diet. Seven days after the diets were commenced, all these immunodeficient mice were injected with human breast cancer cells. Close observation revealed that tumors tended to appear earlier in the mice receiving the high-fat diet than in those receiving the low-fat diet. Fifteen weeks after the cancer cell inoculation, the mice were killed and autopsied. Eighteen mice on the high-fat diet proved to have "macroscopic lung metastases"; in contrast, only eight mice on the low-fat diet had lung metastases.[27]

The assumption that a high-fat diet might similarly promote the development of distant metastases in humans seems plausible enough. Breast cancer specialists have long entertained a strong clinical impression that the course of disease is more aggressive in overweight patients. Epidemiologists at Canada's National Cancer Institute in Toronto studied the "premorbid diet" of 678 breast cancer patients. They discovered that those patients who had consumed a high-fat diet before their diagnosis were far more likely to develop metastatic disease: "For every 5% increase in energy from saturated fat, the risk of dying of breast cancer increased by 50%."[28] Researchers at Stockholm's Karolinska Hospital also tried to correlate dietary fat consumption and prognosis. This team looked at tumor recurrences in 240 breast cancer patients between the ages of 50 and 65. "Total fat and saturated fatty acids," the Swedish researchers concluded, "were the dietary parameters most strongly associated with risk for treatment failure." But the study's finding held true only for patients with estrogen receptor-positive tumors; for those with estrogen receptor-negative tumors, dietary fat consumption had no effect on recurrence rates.[29] This is pretty much what we would expect, since dietary fat is the macronutrient most readily converted into the steroid sex hormones. In postmenopausal women a high-fat diet and excessive adipose tissue (body fat) correlate directly and impressively with the level of estrogen in the blood.

The hypothesis that a low-fat diet would improve tumor control and survival for many breast cancer patients needs to be verified in a large clinical trial. In the meantime, it does no harm to recommend calorie counting. Notwithstanding the advertising messages from vitamin manufacturers, there is no obvious epidemic of nutritional deficiencies among middle-class Americans. Over-nutrition is the main problem—most adults are overweight, and a hefty percentage of the population is frankly obese. **Dietary fiber** is one of the few things we ought to consume more of.   L. A. Cohen and his colleagues at the American Health Foundation suggest that increased fiber consumption might even offset the anticipated evils of a high-fat diet. "While the estimated fat intake in Finland is similar to that in the United States," Cohen et al point out, "the breast cancer incidence rate is considerably lower." They believe that "high dietary fiber intake by Finnish women, particularly in rural areas, modifies the otherwise adverse effect of a diet high in animal fat on breast cancer risk." There could be several mechanisms for fiber's protective effects: "High-fat diets enhance reabsorption of unconjugated estrogen; high-fiber diets exert the reverse effect. An additional factor that tends to decrease circulating estrogens is the binding of estrogens to fiber and their excretion in the feces." Dr. Cohen and his colleagues sing the praises of wheat bran for this purpose: "In human studies, when added to typical Western low-fiber diets, wheat fiber is among the most effective in increasing fecal weight and decreasing transit time."[30]

In recent decades the National Cancer Institute and the American Cancer Society, our principal agencies for public instruction, have confronted a baffling question. What dietary advice should be given to cancer patients who are concerned that what they eat may affect the course of their disease? As we have seen, vitamin supplementation remained much too controversial for these essentially conservative organizations. Neither the NCI nor the ACS wanted to go out on a limb (so to speak) with beta carotene, vitamins A, C, and D, the mineral selenium, or any other of the various micro-nutrients which have been put forth as having therapeutic effects. Yet neither organization could afford to ignore all those epidemiological studies suggesting that diet plays a significant role in breast, colon, and prostate

cancers. In the early 1990s the NCI began to publicize a dietary instructional program originally used by the California Department of Health Services—it was called **5-a-Day**. The admonition behind the headline motto is simple: we are called upon to eat five or more servings of fruits and vegetables every day, preferably fresh and not over-cooked. Ann Windham Wallace, the director of the Office of Consumer Affairs, hailed the NCI's new national campaign: "5-a-Day cuts through the confusion with a simple and actionable message. It vindicates the mothers of the world, who for years have been telling us to eat our vegetables." With support from the Produce Marketing Association of America, the NCI proposed to spend "over 90 million dollars" to "spread the word about fruits and vegetables and health."[31]

At least the American Cancer Society heard and heeded the 5-a-Day gospel. The Society's first dietary recommendation is— "*Eat five or more servings of fruits and vegetables each day.*" The ACS takes its cue from the fiber advocates at the American Health Foundation in making its second recommendation—namely, in urging that "grain products" be "included in every meal—whole grains in preference to processed (refined) grains." Other foods derived "from plant sources, such as breads, cereals, rice, pasta, or beans," also merit the Society's approval ("Eat several times a day"). But meat products get lambasted. "Choose beans as an alternative to meat," the ACS advises.[32] If this last prescription does not ignite blasts of flatulence, it will at least provoke every cattle rancher in Texas!

Some readers may be disappointed that the official revelations from our oracle organizations seem to amount to little more than a glorified "eat-your-vegetables" lecture, one that we've heard a thousand times before from our mothers and teachers. The large committees of physicians and scientists who cooked up the NCI's 5-a-Day campaign and the ACS guidelines were obviously trying to be innocuous rather than innovative. But as feasible recommendations for the general public, the NCI and ACS admonitions are right on target—they are unlikely to do harm if followed, and they reflect a broad consensus based on a vast body of biochemical and epidemiological research. The slew of fruits and vegetables would provide those antioxidant vitamins and essential minerals, without danger of overdose. Moreover, these foodstuffs are naturally high in fiber and low in fat, especially in that devilish saturated fat which comes from animal sources.

Implementation of 5-a-Day would seem to be easy enough. Thanks to advances in agriculture and transportation, American supermarkets now stock generous assortments of fresh fruits and vegetables all the year round. Understandably, this great variety poses the dilemma of choice. Which veggies will do the most to prevent cancer? Are rutabagas better than radishes? Are prunes preferable to apricots? Alas, the thin veneer of consensus starts to crumble when we get down to such specifics. Researchers doing work on the prophylactic qualities of this or that vegetable or fruit tend to be highly partial to it. Broccoli is frequently mentioned as a breast cancer preventive. Cruciferous vegetables (broccoli, cabbage, cauliflower, and Brussels sprouts) contain compounds known as **indoles** which can inhibit the growth of mammary tumors in mice and rats.[33] The low incidence of breast cancer among Japanese women might possibly be related to their high consumption of tofu—soy products contain compounds called **isoflavonoids** which have antioxidant and antiestrogenic qualities. One of these isoflavonoids, **genistein**, has excited considerable interest as a possible prophylactic for breast and prostate cancers. Genistein can

put the brakes on breast tumors growing in nude mice and on malignant prostatic cells growing in test tubes—nobody is altogether sure of the mechanism behind this phenomenon.[34]

The spectrum of fruits and vegetables being investigated by cancer researchers is truly astonishing. Garlic, long known to repel Hollywood vampires, has been loudly touted as a tumor repellent. Oranges and other citrus fruits have also been proposed for this purpose. At the University of Nebraska in Omaha, a few brave volunteers gulped down a mixture of garlic extract and orange juice in an attempt to test these novel notions.[35] If you find such cocktails unpalatable, you will be pleased to learn that a team of researchers at the University of Illinois in Chicago discovered that a compound in grapes called **resveratrol** effectively combats cancer in mice and in cell cultures. Yes, a daily glass of wine might do the trick! The Illinois researchers soberly report that "the concentration of resveratrol in red wine is in the range of 1.5 to 3.0 milligrams per liter. Appreciable amounts are also found in white and rosé wines."[36]

Those of us who still hunger and thirst for hamburgers and milk shakes can expect little solace from the **Designer Foods Program** initiated by the National Cancer Institute. This official NCI quest for cancer-fighting foodstuffs tends toward the vegetarian and (for lack of a better term) *the fruity*. Hugh D. Crone, an Australian chemist, looks askance at these overheated American enthusiasms for "the plant." He cautions that a total omission of meat and diary products from the diet would "rob the cancer victim of absorbable iron, calcium, and the most useful source of protein." Vegetables, fruits, and cereals "do not supply the missing requirements," Dr. Crone explains, "and may further compound the deficiencies. Thus a diet high in cereal and fiber may restrict the uptake from the gut of what little mineral content is in the diet."[37] Dr. Crone, we thank you for a different perspective—and an insight which suggests that in diet (as in other matters) *moderation is the best policy*.

The Mind-Body Connections

Cancer is not a psychosomatic disorder, any more than it is a vitamin-deficiency disease. But this is not to say that our state of mind and our dietary habits have no bearing on the development and progression of malignancies. They probably do—it's just that we cannot identify and measure psychological and dietary effects with the same precision that we can identify and measure, say, a chromosomal translocation or a mutation in the *p53* tumor suppressor gene.   Almost every serious researcher gives credence to the hypothesis that different dietary patterns help to explain why the incidence of breast, colon, and prostate cancers has been so high in some societies (e.g., the United States and western Europe) and so low in others (e.g., Japan). Unfortunately, there is no comparable consensus as to whether subtle states of mind or "personality types" can be cited to explain divergent incidence rates. From the 1920s through the 1950s various researchers who had been trained as psychologists or psychiatrists sought to create a profile of persons who would predictably develop cancer. Textbooks of psychology and psychiatry soon contained ponderous chapters on the so-called **cancer personality**. Persons of this mold were presumed to have had an unhappy childhood, suffering from a lack of closeness to their parents. As adults they remained inhibited, unable to express their emotions or to form intimate relationships with others. Regardless of their outward achievements, they were beset by feelings of unworthiness. In short, individuals with the aforesaid cancer personality were studies in frustration—many of them might commit suicide, but if they didn't, they would almost certainly develop a tumor! No doubt any individual fitting this psychological profile would be prone to multiple physical ailments, cancer being only one of them.

While the concept of a cancer personality sounded plausible enough, the actual diagnosis remained problematic and subjective.   The relevant traits are necessarily elusive and variable—we cannot demonstrate their influence on incidence rates with the same degree of certainty that we can for such obvious risk factors as advancing age, exposure to carcinogens, and inheritance of genetic defects. Cancer researchers trained in precisely quantitative or more experimentally verifiable sciences (e.g., cytology, pathology, or molecular biology) have long been inclined to pooh-pooh the ill-defined concepts put forward by psychological theorists. Writing in 1949, James Murphy of New York's Rockefeller Institute abruptly dismissed them. "Cancer occurs widely among animals and plants," he explained. "I find it hard to believe that mice or chickens suffer frustration in youth."[38] Dr. Murphy had a point, but his rejection was much too sweeping. Even if we do not believe that emotional deprivation and repressed desires are *per se* carcinogenic, we must admit that such frustrations typically lead human beings (who are not mice or chickens) into those destructive behavioral patterns associated with a high incidence of malignancy. Our hypothetical cancer personalities might smoke or engage in excessive drinking; they might not eat their vegetables or get enough exercise and sleep, and so forth. The psyche can often induce somatic disease—if not in one way, then in another.

Visualizing the Immune Cells

By the 1970s and 1980s a segment of the American public had accepted a seemingly logical extension of the cancer personality hypothesis—namely, if the mind can cause cancer, why then the mind must also be able to cure cancer! These notions gained in popularity, if not exactly in credibility, when several physicians with impressive credentials began to promote them. In the 1970s the radiation oncologist O. Carl Simonton and his wife Stephanie, a psychotherapist, developed a "mediation regimen" to serve as an adjunct to orthodox treatments like chemotherapy and irradiation. The Simontons opened counseling centers in Fort Worth and Dallas, where they instructed cancer patients to meditate several times a day and, more particularly, to "visualize" their immune (white) cells attacking and destroying their cancer cells. In articles, lectures, and a 1978 book entitled *Getting Well Again*, the Simontons claimed that persons who practiced these visualization techniques had better survival rates.[39] The meditation regimen itself did no harm, nor did it interfere with the administration of chemotherapy or radiotherapy. For many patients the regimen was psychologically comforting. But the Simontons' assertion of therapeutic benefits evoked some harsh criticisms from orthodox cancer specialists. John Laszlo of the American Cancer Society complained that "in a 246-page book," the Simontons "devote less than one page to the data that supposedly provide the scientific underpinning." Jimmie Holland of the Memorial Sloan-Kettering Cancer Center found the Simontons' enthusiastic reports to be a disservice: "I get distressed when I feel as if the public is being told you can heal your cancer with your thoughts."[40]

Rigorous clinical trials which might prove (or disprove) a therapeutic benefit have not been done. The cancer patients which the Simontons saw were probably healthier and wealthier than most, since they were able to travel to Fort Worth or Dallas for counseling sessions. Presumably, these patients were also predisposed to believe in the efficacy of visualization. Skeptics can thus raise objections of "selection bias" or "placebo effect" to explain away the Simontons' reported successes. In addition, we should emphasize that there is no known biological mechanism by which the mind can directly communicate with individual cancer cells or with individual immune cells, much less specifically instruct the latter to attack the former. Any benefits from the Simontons' regimen would therefore be achieved largely through stress reduction. It is very clear that stress or any other type of mental turmoil can depress the activity of the immune system. A study done at New York's Mount Sinai School of Medicine demonstrated that the responsiveness of circulating lymphocytes to antigenic challenges is significantly reduced in husbands whose wives have recently died.[41] We really don't need a scientific experiment to make this point—most of us know from personal experience that occasional anxiety and insomnia, whether resulting from the death of a loved one or from some other personal problem, make us much more prone to come down with a cold or the flu, those ubiquitous viral infections of the upper respiratory tract.[42] Stress reduction would almost certainly do much to lower the incidence of colds and the flu—would it likewise prevent distant metastases? Does the immune system routinely battle cancer cells with the same aggressiveness brought to bear against those rhinoviruses which make us sneeze? The Simontons' book might lead unwary laypersons to believe that the immune system does so, or at least can be made to do so. In fact, this issue has never been resolved.

The first and most essential lesson learned by our immune cells is to distinguish

"Self" (the body's own tissues) from "Not Self" (the highly antigenic foreign invaders). Except in cases of those regrettable autoimmune diseases, these cells do not attack the body's own tissues. Unfortunately, cancer cells are precisely that—Self, the body's own tissues—even if they now follow abnormal and unregulated growth patterns because of mutations in their nuclei. Malignant tumors as well as benign neoplasms (warts, moles, and freckles) are invisible insofar as the immune system is concerned. By way of illustration we might ponder the example of the most prevalent carcinomas, those pesky skin cancers which are the bane of middle-aged and elderly sunbathers. The body's immune system will tolerate dozens of basal cell carcinomas. There is no erythema (reddening) around these skin lesions, no systemic fever, no increase in the number of white cells in the blood, nor any other indication of an immunological response which we can readily measure. Yet the immune system almost always remains intact in the patient with basal cell carcinoma. If that patient were to receive a skin graft from any other person except an identical twin, the graft would be recognized as foreign (Not Self) and promptly rejected. The patient's immune cells are still there and quite potent—they just haven't been attacking the cancer cells in the same way that they would attack invading microorganisms (bacteria or viruses) or a tissue transplant from another person.

Cancer patients do indeed need to maintain proper nutrition and to control stress, for the explicit purpose of keeping their immune systems strong and of otherwise staying healthy. But it is irresponsible to convey the notion that the immune system by itself represents an effective defense against malignant progression. This posture oversimplifies an extremely complicated topic, and it goes counter to our customary experience. We all know that sarcomas and other extremely aggressive malignancies can occur in teenagers whose immune systems are presumably operating at peak efficiency. The breast and prostate cancers diagnosed in younger patients—say, those under age 50—often tend to behave more aggressively than comparably-staged tumors diagnosed in elderly patients, whose immune responses would be significantly weaker. With the leukemias and lymphomas, those vaunted immune cells have themselves turned malignant. Unfortunately, most of the experiments portraying a triumphant immune system vanquishing cancer have been done on mice or rats, and may have little or no relevance for human carcinogenesis. With humans we do have some intriguing hints that circulating lymphocytes, those B-cells and T-cells which effect the most sophisticated immunological responses, may sometimes be effective in slowing tumor progression. A Japanese study published in the *Journal of the National Cancer Institute* evaluated lymphocyte activity in 50 patients undergoing surgery for apparently localized lung cancer. These immune cells were isolated from each patient's blood, then mixed in a Petri dish with malignant cells freshly isolated from his tumor. Those patients whose lymphocytes killed their tumor cells *in vitro* had better outcomes than patients whose lymphocytes were ineffectual: "23 of the 27 patients with autologous tumor-killing activity remained tumor-free and survived more than five years after surgery, while all 23 who were negative for autologous tumor-killing activity relapsed by 18 months after surgery and died within 42 months after surgery."[43] William L. Donegan informs us that node-positive breast cancer patients who are still disease-free five years after surgery will tend to have "significantly higher pretreatment lymphocyte counts" than do comparable node-positive patients who experience recurrences.[44]

Findings like these suggest that the degree of immunocompetency may well influence the long-term prognosis; what they do not tell us is how we might induce sufficient immunocompetency in cancer patients who do not have it to begin with.

POSITIVE THINKING
Dr. Siegel's Best Seller

In the late 1980s Bernie S. Siegel brought the mind-over-matter hypothesis forcefully into the public consciousness with a best-selling book entitled *Love, Medicine & Miracles.* Dr. Siegel, a surgeon at Yale University, had come to the conclusion that a patient's mental attitude is as important to the success of an operation as is the proper surgical technique. His book, written in the heartwarming and inspirational vein, serves as a counterpoint to strictly physiological explanations of disease. Dr. Siegel reminds us that for most people intellectual and spiritual satisfactions have as much to do with staying healthy as any drugs that might be prescribed. Yet while *Love, Medicine & Miracles* brims with touching insights on human nature, it is too exasperatingly vague to use as a therapeutic manual. Anecdotal case follows anecdotal case, each describing a serious illness which disappeared as soon as the patient (in Dr. Siegel's words) "made some change toward a more loving and accepting attitude."[45] Cancer regressions abound—tumors just seem to melt away once a positive mindset is adopted!

The reception of Dr. Siegel's book was pretty much what you would expect. The public loved it, while orthodox cancer specialists saw red. John Laszlo of the American Cancer Society opined that "the book goes completely off the deep end because of a kind of religious fervor or conviction of the author concerning techniques of self-healing." Charles G. Moertel of the Mayo Clinic cited his long experience as a rejoinder to positive thinking. "I've been practicing medicine for 36 years and I've seen the most positive and optimistic patients die rapidly, and seen the most depressed and pessimistic patients live on and on."[46] We should give the nod to Dr. Moertel rather than Dr. Siegel, because the long-term prognosis in most malignancies still depends more on the particular pathological diagnosis (i.e., the type of cancer one has) than on the treatments applied or the mindset adopted. A breast cancer patient with cribriform ductal carcinoma *in situ* is not in any imminent danger, regardless of how depressed she might be. On the other hand, a breast cancer patient with a poorly differentiated infiltrating ductal carcinoma may need both chemotherapy and positive thinking, as well as considerable luck, to become a long-term survivor. We know for a fact that some pathological diagnoses have intrinsically good prognoses. A few tumors are rapidly fatal; and certain other tumors would be so, save for that surgical or medical intervention which often extends patients' life expectancies and sometimes accomplishes a cure.

Positive thinking should be universally recommended as an adjunct to surgical, radiological, and pharmaceutical interventions. But it cannot be regarded as an intervention, nor can we predict what effect it might have on outcome. "In the face of uncertainty," Dr. Siegel observes, "there is nothing wrong with hope."[47] The positive side of the Simontons' visualization exercises and of Siegel's love-equals-miracles prescription is that they provide spiritual comfort by giving patients a sense of combating their disease on their own initiative. Yet an overly credulous acceptance of such mindset philosophies can be as mistaken and as pernicious as the old-fashioned emphasis on radical surgery. By appearing to reduce malignant disease to an emotional imbalance, these doctrines tend to place the blame on the patient's own depressive thoughts if a tumor should develop or progress. This implication is no more true or charitable in the case of adult-onset cancers than it would be true or charitable in the case of early-onset genetic diseases like cystic fibrosis or muscular dystrophy. The writer Ruth Shereff recalls that after her diagnosis with ovarian cancer she was given three copies of *Love, Medicine & Miracles*—one from an aunt, one from an uncle, and one from a neighbor. "Whatever happened to science and the germ theory of disease?" Ms. Shereff asks. "The militant faith healers reminded me of religious fundamentalists who blame the victim for suffering. A hundred years ago, people might have said God was punishing me. Today my sin is that I do not handle stress properly."[48]

Getting a Handle on Stress

Stress, that terrible feeling of utter helplessness in the face of impending disaster or of overwhelming burdens, is as real a threat to health and well-being as any infectious agent. Yet because this syndrome is more insidious than an outbreak of cholera or the measles, its diagnosis can baffle physicians. We cannot measure "stress factors" in the same way that we might count the bacteria swimming in a urine sample. Nor can the diagnosis be made simply on the basis of a patient's outward circumstances. One individual in a lifeboat may be under tremendous stress, while the person in the next seat looks upon the storm and shipwreck only as an amusing lark. **Stress is not what happens to us—it has to do with the way our minds react to these events.** A few people can remain calm and cheerful during catastrophic natural disasters (e.g., earthquakes, hurricanes, or

tornadoes), but they are exceptions. Most of us would suffer extreme stress under these circumstances; and as a result some of us, while surviving the raging winds and tumbling buildings, would subsequently experience heart attacks, bouts of depression, suicidal impulses, and other psychological and somatic disorders. Survivors of natural or manmade disasters have good reason to be troubled—the point is that their post-traumatic symptoms usually do not originate in any physical injuries inflicted by the catastrophic events, but in the unbridled emotions generated by their own psyches.

Only those of us who die suddenly while still young and healthy are likely to escape the stress of a bad diagnosis. Sooner or later the rest of us will have to face a somber physician who explains that our medical problem is really quite serious and (given the current state of scientific knowledge) not easily fixed. The anticipated treatment stands to be costly, unpleasant, and prolonged—the outcome is doubtful. This particular "lifeboat" tends to be heavily populated with cancer patients, though it is not exactly reserved for them. Stress can only make things worse in this inherently disturbing situation of bodily peril and therapeutic uncertainty. Relatives and friends offer what assistance they can, rushing in with baskets of broccoli and multiple copies of Dr. Siegel's inspirational book. All this may—or may not—be helpful, depending upon how much one likes broccoli and upon how seriously one takes Dr. Siegel. For readers who want a more restrained assessment of the mind's ability to affect the course of somatic disease, Norman Cousins' *Head First: The Biology of Hope* is to be recommended. This book also abounds in anecdotes of seemingly miraculous recoveries, but Cousins goes beyond Siegel by trying to discover biological mechanisms which could explain the observed phenomena.[49]

In attempting to manage stress, we should be careful that the intervention we propose does not paradoxically have the effect of increasing stress. One recommendation which is unlikely to cause harm is to participate in a support group. This advice is customarily given to persons diagnosed with breast cancer. Because these patients are so numerous and (as a rule) so long-lived, there are support groups with relatively stable memberships in most American cities. Perhaps the most important benefit from such social support is a reduction of that stressful feeling of isolation. The aforementioned relatives and friends may not fully comprehend what a patient is going through—in contrast, the strangers in a support group tend to have a better comprehension of the mental anxieties and physical disabilities associated with the disease and its treatment. Does participation in a support group better the odds of survival? A randomized clinical trial conducted by researchers at Stanford University and the University of California, Berkeley, found that women with metastatic breast cancer who attended weekly discussion groups "lived significantly longer than did controls, by an average of nearly eighteen months."[50] This finding, published in the *Lancet* in 1989, spurred additional trials of social support interventions in advanced breast cancer. Not all of the subsequent trials detected a survival advantage.[51]

Norman Cousins' personal prescription for stress control is laughter.[52] In his book he goes so far as to list old slapstick movies featuring The Three Stooges or Laurel and Hardy as a therapeutic intervention of sorts. Any biological mechanisms by which laughter *per se* would prevent malignant progression remain to be identified. However, it is clear that anything which pleasantly distracts a patient and gets his or her mind off the topic of personal illness will reduce the level of stress. A certain attentiveness to one's physical condition is necessary for continued well-being; but a preoccupation with one's state of health tends to be unhealthy, because it raises an individual's stress levels and makes him or her into a bore. **Distraction**, whatever form it might take, is a better remedy for stress than any tranquilizers the doctors can prescribe. Laughing at old movies or corny jokes will provide momentary relief for many people—while bird watching, card playing, golfing, or going fishing might do the trick for others. Regardless of the medical verdicts we receive, our first task should be to enjoy life as much as we can, in whatever ways we choose. When we do not enjoy life, our immune responses as well as our social relationships are bound to suffer.

Meditation is a higher form of intellectual and spiritual distraction which may appeal to persons too intelligent to be significantly entertained by TV soap operas or by vintage slapstick. For many centuries the world's higher religions have encouraged meditative exercises as a pathway to enlightenment and salvation. Of late, the same techniques have been urged by psychotherapists who are careful to cite "science" rather than "religion" as the rationale. The Simontons' regimen of immune-cell visualization, for example, follows the format of traditional religious meditation. The cancer patient is advised to seek out a quiet room, free from noise and interruptions, so as to direct all mental energies toward a particular end—in this case, the activation of immune cells. Those readers who find this regimen somewhat naive may wish to consider that older and wiser meditation which aims to achieve closeness to God. In this instance, the meditative goal has nothing to do with prolonging our brief biological existence. It is rather to achieve an awakening to an undeniable but hardly demonstrable fact—namely, that there is a Power in the universe far beyond human understanding, and that this Power, although willing our death as well as our creation, is *infinitely benign.*

Chapter Twenty-two

HORMONAL THERAPY
The Triumph of Tamoxifen

With this chapter we begin to consider the pharmaceutical therapies for breast cancer. While systemic drugs can shrink primary breast tumors and forestall local recurrences, they are principally given with a view to preventing or controlling metastatic disease. A drug regimen which is commenced soon after the initial surgery for early-stage breast cancer will be referred to as **adjuvant therapy**. The drugs are intended as an "adjuvant" (supplement or aid) to the surgical treatment; they are given to combat the micrometastases (small clusters of disseminated cancer cells) which we cannot as yet detect with our current diagnostic tools, but which we fear may be lurking somewhere in the body. A drug regimen commenced after one or more distant metastases have been conclusively diagnosed is referred to as **salvage therapy**. Sensitive physicians may avoid mentioning that ominous word "salvage" in front of their patients, but the term is widely used.

So many drugs are now being used in breast cancer medicine that even professional oncologists can get a bit confused, and laypersons are apt to be totally perplexed. By way of simplification, we can group these varied medications into two broad categories: **hormonal drugs** and **cytotoxic chemotherapy**. The majority of breast and prostate tumors retain some degree of hormonal responsiveness. This means that the individual cancer cells, like the normal breast or prostate cells from which they arose, must be appropriately stimulated by a steroid sex hormone (estrogen or testosterone) before they can multiply. Pharmaceutical companies try to exploit this fact by developing **antiestrogens** or **antiandrogens**. Through one mechanism or another, these drugs will deprive malignant breast or prostate cells of hormonal stimuli; their action may be described as *cytostatic*—that is, they do not kill the cancer cells outright but simply stop them from reproducing. In contrast, our chemotherapy drugs are frankly *cytotoxic*—they kill cancer cells. Unfortunately, they also damage normal cells, causing temporary side effects like nausea and hair loss as well as permanent ones like diminished fertility and an elevated risk for hematologic malignancies (the various leukemias and lymphomas). The side effects produced by hormonal drugs are mild and usually do not greatly disturb a patient's lifestyle. More importantly, they tend to be reversible—they almost always fade away when the therapy is discontinued.

The most widely prescribed hormonal drug has long been **tamoxifen**, an antiestrogen taken orally which has proven useful not only in delaying the recurrence of previously diagnosed breast cancers but also in preventing new malignancies from developing in the contralateral (opposite) breast. We can point to this drug as one of the success stories in modern pharmacology; it was the prototype of a class of hormonal drugs now known as **Selective Estrogen Receptor Modulators** (SERMs). Tamoxifen is indicated in all cases of estrogen receptor-positive breast cancer which are at risk of metastatic dissemination. Of course, it is less certain whether this particular drug or some other hormonal drug should be prescribed for very small tumors which are presumably curable by local therapies, or given to healthy women who might simply be deemed at risk of breast cancer. In the 1980s and 1990s we witnessed a paradoxical situation in the United States. Because of mammography screening and increased public awareness, more and more breast tumors were being diagnosed in their earliest stages, when the possibility of metastatic dissemination would seem to be remote. At the same time adjuvant therapy was being urged for more and more subgroups of patients, so that even a tiny focus of ductal carcinoma *in situ* might conceivably elicit a recommendation for chemotherapy or long-term tamoxifen. We would have no problem with this trend toward universal adjuvant therapy if the drugs being used were 100% effective, caused no side effects, and carried no risks. This is not true of any of our current drugs. Moreover, only a minority of patients with small node-negative tumors (Stage One disease) have been shown to benefit from systemic therapies. Other patients in this good-prognosis subgroup would be treated unnecessarily. Fortunately, we have made considerable progress in determining which patients are actually in danger of metastatic dissemination and thus most likely to benefit from adjuvant therapy. Readers who are in doubt about their own status must be referred back to those weighty discussions touching on pathology reports (Chapter Twelve) and prognosis assessment (Chapter Fourteen).

The Surgical Ablations

Hormonal manipulations in breast cancer are not exactly new. The first successful maneuver was performed on June 15, 1895, by the Scottish surgeon George Thomas Beatson. He knew no more about hormones than anybody else in the 1890s, but he suspected that mammalian ovaries must secrete some elusive substance which controls lactation and other breast functions. One of his patients was a young woman of 33 who had undergone a mastectomy for breast cancer six months earlier; now she came to him in great distress because nodules of recurrent tumor were beginning to grow in the skin flaps surrounding the surgical scar. Perplexed, Dr. Beatson tried a desperate gambit: he did a **bilateral oophorectomy** (the removal of both ovaries). In the weeks and months following this operation, those tumor nodules grew smaller and smaller—then they seemed to vanish altogether! In 1896 Beatson did what many subsequent researchers have done: he rushed into print to announce his "cure" for breast cancer. The announcement was to prove premature; several years later the patient suffered a relapse, and this time the good doctor could do nothing to stymie the fatal progression of disease.[1]

Other surgeons took their cue from Beatson and began to perform oophorectomies on their breast cancer patients who suffered recurrences after mastectomy. It soon became apparent that the procedure had little or no effect on postmenopausal patients, and that only about a third of premenopausal patients could be expected to experience a dramatic remission like the one Beatson had described in 1896. The turn-of-the-century surgeons were thoroughly baffled by these results. Today, of course, we know that oophorectomy can be an effective ablation only in premenopausal patients—when you remove the ovaries, you are shutting down the principal source of estrogen in fertile women. Just a third of the younger patients responded satisfactorily, because only about a third of premenopausal breast cancers significantly express the estrogen receptor protein—**ER** for short—and are therefore dependent on estrogen for their growth. Postmenopausal breast cancers usually do express sufficient ER, but then oophorectomy would have little or no effect because postmenopausal ovaries have already ceased to secrete meaningful quantities of estrogen.[2] In postmenopausal women the adrenal glands situated atop the kidneys play a far more significant role in supplying the body's estrogen—they secrete androgens, which are then converted into estrogen in fatty tissues containing the enzyme aromatase.

Oophorectomy never won acceptance as an adjuvant—it was always a salvage procedure, to be tried as a last resort against metastatic disease in younger patients. No one could predict whether it would work with any given patient. Surgeons were also deterred by the prospect of morbidity. In the early decades of the twentieth century, an oophorectomy represented risky abdominal surgery. A mortality rate of over 6% was reported in a 1905 survey of breast cancer oophorectomies. In the 1920s irradiation of the ovaries became the ablative procedure of choice; it was far less traumatic for patients, and it did not involve the possibility of infection or death. True, the estrogen levels in the blood might fall more gradually, and any tumor regression take longer to occur; but

ultimately irradiation was just as effective as oophorectomy.[3] In the 1940s surgical castration again began to play a role in American cancer medicine—**orchiectomy** (the removal of the testicles) proved to be efficacious in the management of disseminated prostate cancer. Candidates for this procedure were usually elderly men troubled with gnawing pain from bone metastases; most readily consented to it when their physicians explained that the surgery was fast and safe, the response rate very impressive, and the side effects negligible.

The high-water mark for ablative hormonal manipulations came in the 1950s and 1960s, during the era of radical surgery. **Adrenalectomy** (removal of the adrenal glands) was promoted as a secondary procedure for relapsed breast or prostate cancer patients who had previously responded to castration (oophorectomy or orchiectomy). This surgical ablation often produced regressions in postmenopausal breast cancer. With premenopausal patients it might be done simultaneously with oophorectomy, thereby ensuring the immediate removal of the most important pathways for estrogen production. The drawbacks to adrenalectomy included the technical complexity of the operation, the possibility of postoperative complications, and the fact that adrenalectomized patients had to take cortisone for life. When adrenalectomy failed to stop disease progression, the radical surgeons had still another card up their sleeves—**hypophysectomy**, removal of the pituitary gland itself, a drastic measure which sometimes purchased a short reprieve for patients with advanced breast or prostatic malignancies at the cost of turning them into endocrine zombies. In retrospect, the tumor regressions achieved by the simple expedient of removing the hormone-producing glands look crude and barbaric. Oophorectomies were particularly unfortunate because they suddenly plunged young women into a menopausal state, necessitating a host of physiological and psychological adjustments. Today the only surgical ablation still performed with any frequency is orchiectomy.

ADDITIVE STRATEGIES
The Estrogen-Androgen Pendulum

While hormonal manipulations were first used to treat premenopausal patients, the most suitable candidates for this approach have always been postmenopausal patients, who are much more likely to have slow-growing, hormonally-dependent tumors. But prior to the 1940s we had no idea how these patients might be managed. The discovery of **diethylstilbestrol** in 1938 soon led to an effective postmenopausal strategy. We have encountered this drug before—it's that powerful synthetic estrogen **DES**, which those well-meaning obstetricians of the 1950s and 1960s so liberally dispensed in a vain attempt to prevent miscarriages.[4] However ill-conceived DES may have been for this particular purpose, it was to improve the survival rates of postmenopausal breast cancer patients by providing a convenient additive strategy. The earliest report of its effectiveness appeared in 1944; within a few years DES became the therapy of choice for postmenopausal women with recurrent breast cancer.[5]

You might logically pose the following question—if postmenopausal breast cancers are usually estrogen-dependent, would not an estrogenic compound like DES tend to accelerate tumor growth rather than retarding it? An up-to-date answer to this question would involve much gobbledygook about "hormone agonists" and the "down regulation of estrogen receptors." By way of simplification, we can say that, yes, estrogen does stimulate ER-positive breast tumors—but that any

abrupt change in the hormonal environment in which the cancer cells have been growing will often induce a temporary remission. We have long known that breast cancer cells maintained in laboratory Petri dishes will multiply continually if exposed to low doses of estrogen, but then stop growing when doused with much higher doses. Too much of a good thing breeds satiety. You might like chocolate ice cream, yet would quickly tire of that product if forced to eat it constantly, morning, noon, and night, seven days a week. Additive hormonal strategies work on much the same principle.

The postmenopausal DES regimen which held sway from the mid-1940s until the late 1970s was simple enough—take a pill (DES, 5 mg) three times a day. The breast cancer cells which had been growing in the low estrogen levels characteristic of the menopause were suddenly exposed to very high levels like those you find in well-advanced pregnancy. At first these cells would respond by multiplying furiously, causing malignant skin nodules to grow larger and bony metastases to become more painful. Physicians called this phenomenon ***"the flare."*** They would hasten to inform their anxious patients that a pronounced flare at the start of DES therapy was actually a good omen, because it indicated that the cancer cells were hormonally responsive and that a major remission could be expected to ensue. Sure enough, after a few days those estrogen-satiated breast cancer cells would stop multiplying—the skin nodules would shrink, and bony metastases become less painful. The patient was now in the first remission, which typically lasted for a year or two, occasionally longer. She continued to take daily diethylstilbestrol as maintenance therapy.

DES produced objective responses in a goodly majority of postmenopausal patients with metastatic breast cancer. The drug's drawback was that it also produced the physiological effects of estrogen excess—nausea and vomiting reminiscent of pregnancy's morning sickness, and that bloated feeling caused by fluid retention. Postmenopausal women taking DES may have been even more prone to thromboembolic events (blood clots in the legs, lungs, or coronary arteries) than the young women of the 1960s who took those early estrogen-rich oral contraceptives. As we explained in Chapter Seven, the added estrogen increases the liver's production of coagulation factors, predisposing susceptible individuals to thrombosis. Apart from the inevitable nauseous side effects and the possible thromboembolic complications, another problem with DES therapy was that it never cured the disease. Eventually the breast cancer cells which had regressed during the estrogen flood tide would become accustomed to their new hormonal environment and start to grow again. When tumor progression occurred, DES would be discontinued. However, in many cases the withdrawal of DES led to a second remission, which breast cancer specialists called *"a rebound."* The cancer cells which had learned to grow in the estrogen-rich environment were abruptly deprived of the copious synthetic hormone; and now they stopped growing because of its absence. Hormonal therapy for postmenopausal women with metastatic breast cancer thus swung back and forth like a pendulum—give the high-dose hormone to induce remission, then take it away upon disease progression to get a rebound, then give it again when the rebound started to fade. In this way physicians might produce two or three remissions; unfortunately, each successive response tended to be less complete and less durable than the one which preceded it.

DES therapy did not work very well in breast cancer patients who were either premenopausal or only very recently menopausal (within five years of the menopause). For these younger women, the additive strategy called for **synthetic androgens**, whose potential to induce remission in metastatic breast cancer had first been reported in 1939. The response rate was less impressive: a survey by the American Medical Association done in 1960 found that "androgens produced objective regression in 20% of premenopausal patients."[6] The side effects were not reminiscent of morning sickness, but of puberty in the male—growth of facial hair, deepening of voice, acne, and increased libido. In the 1940s high-dose androgens were occasionally used as a second-line therapy for postmenopausal patients who had relapsed while taking DES. After 1951 high-dose progestins (synthetic versions of progesterone) became the preferred second-line strategy for older women.

TAMOXIFEN:
Adjuvant Therapy Comes of Age

The surgical ablations and additive strategies used before the late 1970s shared a common failing. They were not suitable for use when they might do the most good—that is, as adjuvant therapy given before metastatic disease becomes so well-established that it is clinically apparent and presumably irreversible. We naturally anticipate that the maximum therapeutic benefit would result from a hormonal intervention performed while the patient's "tumor burden" is still small—i.e., limited to a few circulating cancer cells which have escaped from the primary breast tumor yet have not formed persistent colonies in other organs. But surgeons hesitated to perform oophorectomies on premenopausal patients with early-stage disease because the procedure was so mutilative and so psychologically disturbing, and no one could predict whether it would actually work. The odds that postmenopausal patients would respond to additive strategies were considerably better, but then DES with its nauseous side effects and thromboembolic dangers was not a drug to be casually prescribed. Fortunately, the 1970s brought two wonderful innovations in the hormonal therapy of breast cancers. Dedicated scientists in American and British laboratories not only discovered cellular assays which could predict whether tumors would respond to hormonal manipulation, but they came up with a drug called tamoxifen which was sufficiently nontoxic for routine adjuvant therapy and which worked for both premenopausal and post-menopausal patients.

As mentioned in Chapter Fourteen, Elwood V. Jensen and his colleagues at the University of Chicago were the first to demonstrate that an individual cell had to express the **estrogen receptor protein** (ER) before it could respond to that hormone. We are still learning about the way estrogen molecules, the ER protein, and appropriate genes in the cellular nucleus interact to alter a cell's behavior. The practical importance of the Chicago team's groundbreaking discovery was that it gave us a reasonably reliable means of determining whether the cancer cells originating from a particular breast tumor would respond to hormonal therapy. Subsequent American investigators emphasized that assays of **progesterone receptor protein** (PgR) were also needed to obtain the most accurate evaluation of a tumor's hormonal responsiveness. Today, of course, ER and PgR assays are standard; they should be performed on all malignant specimens, whether taken from a primary tumor in the breast or from a distant metastasis.[7]

While we are indebted to American scientists for our assays of hormonal responsiveness, the first convenient adjuvant drug came entirely from the "Mother Country." The British firm Imperial Chemical Industries, later known as ICI Pharma, developed an antiestrogenic compound (tamoxifen citrate) in the early 1960s, hoping that it could be marketed as an oral contraceptive. Tamoxifen did indeed prevent ovulation in rats and other laboratory animals; but when tested on humans, it was found to stimulate ovulation. Having no contraceptive application, the drug might have been shelved had not some of the firm's researchers had the foresight to test it on breast cancer cell lines. Tamoxifen stopped these malignant cells from multiplying. In the late 1960s the drug was given to patients with metastatic breast cancer by a team at the Christie Hospital in Manchester, England. The results published in 1971 were most encouraging—the patients taking tamoxifen achieved prolonged remissions, and they suffered virtually no side effects! In 1973 tamoxifen became an officially sanctioned treatment for recurrent breast cancer in the United Kingdom; on December 30, 1977, the Food and Drug Administration approved it for this purpose in the United States. Recognized as salvage therapy in the 1970s, tamoxifen was to win universal acceptance as an adjuvant in the following decade.[8]

No researcher has been more closely associated with tamoxifen than V. Craig Jordan, who began testing the drug on cell lines and laboratory animals while a graduate student at the University of Leeds. In 1980 Dr. Jordan received an appointment as a professor of oncology and pharmacology at the University of Wisconsin in Madison. He soon became tamoxifen's foremost advocate in the United States, publishing scores of articles and books explaining its merits. This drug has been <u>extensively</u> <u>studied</u>, not only in hundreds of laboratory experiments but in dozens of clinical trials involving human subjects. Dr. Jordan would seem to know the precise details of every test and every trial! Thus with an acknowledgment of indebtedness to his voluminous writings, what we know about tamoxifen can be *briefly* summarized.

The chemical structure of tamoxifen is very similar to that of the estrogens naturally produced by humans and by lower mammalian species. Insofar as this drug is acting as an antiestrogen, it does so by competitively binding to the ER protein. That is to say, tamoxifen (which is a lot like estrogen) occupies a cell's estrogen receptors, preventing the body's natural estrogen from binding to them. But unlike the customary estrogen-ER complex, the tamoxifen-ER complex tends to be inert—it does not stimulate those genes which force hormonally-responsive mammary cells to divide. Tamoxifen's mode of action is cytostatic; the drug does not directly kill breast cancer cells, though most of the affected cells will eventually die since their growth processes have been stymied. Tamoxifen can shrink ER-positive tumors both in human subjects and in laboratory animals, but understandably the response is not as rapid as one obtained by cytotoxic chemotherapy.

When we reflect that prior to the late 1970s all that American physicians could do in the way of hormonal therapy was to cut out the estrogen-producing glands or to flood the entire body with synthetic hormones, we will appreciate what a tremendous breakthrough tamoxifen represented. This drug unobtrusively blocks estrogen's action at the cellular level—the body's natural production of estrogen remains unchanged in postmenopausal women, and only slightly increased in premenopausal women. The many patients who were to take tamoxifen had relatively little to worry about, but they needed to remember two things. The first was to take the pills on time. Tamoxifen's effectiveness depends entirely upon keeping a constant level of the drug in the bloodstream. We know from laboratory experiments that tamoxifen can stop ER-positive breast cancer cells from multiplying even when these cells are exposed to estrogen. But when the drug level is reduced, the cancer cells quickly start growing again. A second thing patients needed to remember was that **tamoxifen is not a pure antiestrogen.** In some animal species and in some types of human tissue, this drug acts like estrogen and will promote cellular reproduction. Dr. Jordan reminds us that while tamoxifen is "an antiestrogen in the rat," it is estrogenic in mice: "No completely satisfactory subcellular mechanism for the species difference has yet been established."[9] In humans, tamoxifen has antiestrogenic, growth-retarding effects on cells derived from the mammary gland—but it has estrogenic, growth-promoting effects on the endometrial cells which line the interior of the uterus. A postmenopausal woman with an intact uterus who is taking tamoxifen should promptly report any vaginal bleeding to her physician. Like unopposed estrogen replacement therapy, this drug can promote endometrial hyperplasia and thereby increase the risk of endometrial cancer.

Tamoxifen's Side Effects

During the late 1980s ICI Pharma aggressively marketed tamoxifen in the United States under the brand name **Nolvadex**. A three-page advertisement appearing in the *New England Journal of Medicine* (May 25, 1989) challenged physicians to "*enter the era of molecular biology with Nolvadex.*" An accompanying illustration of a prescription pad reminded readers of the standard dosage: "10 mg b.i.d."—that is, a ten-milligram tablet twice a day. Some European trials had used 40 mg a day, but the higher dose did not seem any more effective. At either dosage tamoxifen was well-tolerated; in clinical trials comparing it to a placebo, the number of side effects reported for the drug was not much greater than those reported for the look-alike dummy tablets. Very few patients discontinued tamoxifen because they found the side effects intolerable. The only symptoms consistently reported more often for the drug than for placebos are related to its anti-estrogenic action. Postmenopausal women who experienced hot flashes during the menopause have about a 50% chance of experiencing hot flashes when they take tamoxifen.[10] Vaginal dryness and itching may also occur in postmenopausal patients. Estrogen creams quickly relieve this problem; but some physicians have been reluctant to prescribe them, fearing that they might increase the odds of recurrence. Richard R. Love, an oncologist at the University of Wisconsin in Madison, suggests that androgen creams could be tried for "severe vaginitis." Relief from hot flashes is less predictable. Dr. Love observes that "a phenobarbital preparation at bedtime and low-dose clonidine by mouth or given transdermally are helpful in some women."[11]

The side effects which may occur in premenopausal patients are quite different from those seen in postmenopausal patients. Tamoxifen increases the production of estradiol (the most active form of estrogen) by premenopausal ovaries; consequently, more estrogen will be circulating in the bloodstream of younger women taking the drug. This added estrogen does not seem to interfere with tamoxifen's inhibitory action on breast cancer cells, assuming a constant level of the drug is maintained.[12] But occasionally premenopausal patients will experience episodes of nausea and vomiting, the characteristic gastrointestinal reaction to excess estrogen. Tamoxifen has been associated with a higher incidence of irregular menses.

Since this drug does not prevent ovulation, premenopausal patients taking it can become pregnant and should use barrier methods of contraception to avoid this "complication." We do not know what effects tamoxifen might have on developing human embryos; the drug has been shown to induce birth defects in mice, rats, and guinea pigs. Breast feeding during therapy should also be avoided; the drug's possible effects on newborn infants are likewise unknown.[13]

When breast cancer patients with metastatic disease are started on tamoxifen, they typically experience "a flare" comparable to the flare traditionally encountered with the initiation of DES therapy. In this case, symptom exacerbation occurs because at low serum levels tamoxifen acts like estrogen on breast cancer cells. Once therapeutic levels of the drug are obtained in the bloodstream, the flare subsides.[14] Some patients taking tamoxifen have reported headaches and depression, but then patients taking placebos report these same symptoms. It seems most unlikely that tamoxifen induces neurological problems. A study done by Richard R. Love and his colleagues found that the incidence of headaches actually decreased in postmenopausal women taking the drug.[15]

The Clinical Trials:
How Effective Is Tamoxifen?

The value of adjuvant tamoxifen has been continually tested since the 1970s, by large clinical trials both in Europe and in the United States. Unfortunately, these trials have been quite heterogeneous, with variations in the patient populations studied, in the dose used and the length of treatment, and in record-keeping and follow-up. The reported results have naturally differed from trial to trial; but when all the trials are considered together, certain trends become apparent. We can confidently say that tamoxifen has been shown to extend **disease-free survival** (DFS) in estrogen receptor-positive breast cancer—in other words, it definitely tends to delay the reappearance of cancer, even in patients fated to eventually develop metastatic disease. The DFS advantage is most pronounced in postmenopausal patients with high levels of the ER protein, but it is also detectable in premenopausal patients who are comparably ER-positive. Most recent studies suggest that tamoxifen therapy also improves **overall survival** (OS) in ER-positive breast cancer. The evidence for a survival advantage is likewise clearer in postmenopausal populations. Younger patients at risk for recurrence have typically been given cytotoxic chemotherapy along with tamoxifen, leaving us a bit uncertain as to whether the chemo or the tamoxifen was principally responsible for the reported extension of life expectancy.

One of the earliest American trials of adjuvant tamoxifen was commenced by the National Surgical Adjuvant Breast and Bowel Project on January 1, 1977, some twelve months before the FDA approved the drug. The NSABP wanted to find out whether adding tamoxifen to a chemo regimen would help to extend DFS in node-positive breast cancer. While Protocol B-09 looks old-fashioned today, the trial had one extremely praiseworthy feature—the NSABP guidelines called for rigorously quantitative assays of tumor ER, and these were obtained for 1,414 trial participants. As stated in Chapter Fourteen, assay readings of at least 10 femtomoles of estradiol binding per milligram of cytosol protein (abbreviated as 10 fmol/mg) are regarded as positive, while lower readings are seen as borderline (3 to 9 fmol/mg) or negative (0 to 2 fmol/mg). The NSABP results published in the *New England Journal of Medicine* on July 2, 1981,

bore witness to the utility of ER testing. The trial did not detect any significant advantage from adding tamoxifen to chemotherapy in patients with negative or borderline readings, or in patients under age 50 (presumably premenopausal). For those trial participants over age 50 with positive ER readings, the NSABP team found that adding tamoxifen "reduced recurrence of disease at two years—by 51 percent in those with one to three positive nodes, and by 64 percent in those with four or more."[16]

We should always pay careful attention to the NSABP findings. In the 1980s reports from several clinical trials appeared to indicate that tamoxifen might delay recurrence or prolong survival in ER-*negative* breast cancer. To date, however, no biological mechanism by which the drug could predictably affect the course of ER-negative tumors has been established. The reports of its effectiveness in this subgroup may have been due to inaccurate ER assays (e.g., ER-positive specimens being labeled negative) or to confounding treatments (e.g., chemotherapy being given as well as tamoxifen). The European trials conducted during the 1970s and 1980s often went about ER determination in a haphazard fashion, yet some of these trials have been quite influential. The trial begun in England on November 1, 1977, by the Nolvadex Adjuvant Trial Organization (the so-called "NATO trial") did not feature a chemotherapy arm—the 1,285 breast cancer patients, mostly postmenopausal, were randomized to two years of adjuvant tamoxifen (10 mg twice daily) or to observation (control group). The six-year results published in 1985 revealed not only "a highly significant prolongation of the disease-free interval in the tamoxifen-treated group," but also "a highly significant reduction in the death rate, with 34% fewer deaths observed in the treated group than in the control group."[17] The "Scottish trial" begun in Edinburgh sought to determine whether a longer treatment period would be more effective: 1,312 breast cancer patients were randomly assigned to receive five years of adjuvant tamoxifen (20 mg daily) or simply to remain under observation, with tamoxifen therapy being commenced only after a recurrence had been detected. The *Lancet* for July 25, 1987, carried the Scottish researchers' enthusiastic report: "Recurrent disease developed in 157 patients in the adjuvant arm compared with 250 of those selected for tamoxifen therapy on relapse. The results indicate a pronounced advantage for immediate tamoxifen. Toxicity from tamoxifen given for five years is no greater than that found with a shorter course."[18] Neither trial paid the proper attention to tumor ER levels—just 46% of the NATO participants were assayed, and only 57% of the Scottish participants.

The long-running "Stockholm trial," begun in the Swedish capital in 1976, initially randomized 1,846 postmenopausal breast cancer patients to two years of adjuvant tamoxifen (40 mg daily, twice the standard American dose), or to an untreated control group. After two years the tamoxifen arm was further randomized, either to discontinue the drug or to take it for three additional years. The most remarkable findings from the Stockholm trial, as published in 1989, had to do with tamoxifen's potential to prevent or to induce second cancers. On the positive side, the drug seemed to prevent the development of *de novo* cancers in the contralateral (opposite) breast. The control group (915 patients) registered 32 contralateral tumors, the tamoxifen arm (931 patients) only 18. On the minus side, tamoxifen was associated with a higher incidence of endometrial cancer: there had been 13 cases in the treatment arm, only two in the control group. And this risk rose sharply with an increasing duration of treatment; it was greatest in those patients who took the drug for five years

instead of stopping at two.[19] In 1994 the Stockholm trial reported updated results—23 endometrial cancers detected in the 1,372 patients now getting tamoxifen, but only four detected in the 1,357 patients now in the control group. The FDA took prompt notice of this finding, requiring that a stronger warning accompany all tamoxifen bottles.[20] Of course, the fact that the drug was associated with endometrial carcinogenesis in postmenopausal women with intact uteri did not disqualify it for adjuvant breast cancer therapy. If detected early, endometrial cancers are easy to cure; this cannot be said of metastatic breast cancer.

By the late 1980s breast cancer specialists really needed some plausible estimates of the potential survival benefit, which could then be quoted to prospective tamoxifen patients. The **Early Breast Cancer Trialists' Collaborative Group**, composed of prominent European and American specialists, set about the task of **meta-analysis**— that is, the pooling of data from individual clinical trials to arrive at statistical "averages" which will hopefully be more convincing. Whether meta-analysis really gets us all that much closer to the truth is open to question, but at least it carries *the weight of numbers*. Thus the meta-analysis which the Trialists' Group published in the *New England Journal of Medicine* in 1988 attracted much attention. Analyzing 28 trials of tamoxifen involving 16,513 women, the Group found "a clear reduction in mortality only among women 50 or older." In this age bracket, tamoxifen therapy "reduced the annual odds of death during the first five years by about one fifth."[21] An updated meta-analysis published in 1992 was based on 42 tamoxifen trials involving 30,000 women. This time the Trialists' Group found that therapy reduced the annual odds of recurrence by about 12% in premenopausal women under age 50 and by about 28% or

29% in postmenopausal women aged 50 or older. The annual risk of death from breast cancer was reduced by about 6% for the premenopausal women and by about 17% to 21% for the postmenopausal women. The Trialists' Group pointed out that "tamoxifen also reduced the risk of contralateral breast cancer by 39%."[22] The 1998 update considered 55 tamoxifen trials involving 37,000 women, "comprising about 87% of the worldwide evidence." The Trialists' Group now sang the praises of long-term tamoxifen, citing "a highly significant trend towards greater effect with longer treatment." Two years of tamoxifen therapy reduced the recurrence rate by 29%, while five years reduced it by 47%. The overall reductions in mortality similarly revealed the benefits to be had from longer medication: the death rate was down 17% after two years on tamoxifen, and down 26% after five years.[23]

One noteworthy feature of the 1998 meta-analysis was that from the total of 37,000 trial participants, it identified 2,000 women whose breast tumors had assayed "ER-poor and PgR-poor," but who were nonetheless given tamoxifen. In this subgroup the drug "had no apparent effect on recurrence or mortality rates (1% reduction in both)." However, in an even smaller subgroup assayed ER-poor *but PgR-positive*, tamoxifen appeared to help—"the recurrence reduction was 23%, and the mortality reduction was 9%."[24] Although the small number of subjects in these two subgroups does not allow us to draw absolutely definitive conclusions, the meta-analysis results strongly underscore that necessity of assaying all tumor specimens for hormone receptors— PgR as well as ER—before considering any systemic therapy.

Do We Have <u>CONSENSUS</u>?

A consensus in any area of breast cancer medicine is as rare and elusive as a unicorn or the Abominable Snowman—at best we get only fleeting glimpses of the beast, and not everybody believes that it really exists. But the folks at the National Cancer Institute (NCI) are professional optimists, and they are in the business of promoting consensus in matters pertaining to diagnosis and treatment. A favored NCI instrument to achieve this end is the **Consensus Development Conference**, one of which was held in September 1985 to consider adjuvant therapies for early-stage breast cancer. Specialists from all over the world descended on the campus at Bethesda, Maryland, and pondered the implications of recent clinical trials. The conclusions which that CDC panel reached look simplistic today, but they are worth quoting because they give us a starting point for future deliberations. Briefly summarized, the NCI consensus of 1985 promulgated these self-evident truths: *"Adjuvant therapy delays recurrence and prolongs survival in node-positive breast cancer. Premenopausal patients should get cytotoxic chemotherapy; postmenopausal patients should get tamoxifen."*[25] Who could quibble with this? Our clinical trials have consistently found that *as a group* younger women benefit more from chemotherapy than older ones, and that *as a group* older women benefit more from tamoxifen than younger ones. Notwithstanding these facts, the CDC panel's distinctions between node-negative and node-positive disease, and between premenopausal and postmenopausal populations, were much too sharply drawn. The panel also sidestepped several pertinent questions which continue to demand our attention. What's the optimal treatment duration for tamoxifen? What subsets of node-negative patients might benefit from adjuvant therapy? Since we have two systemic modalities—i.e., cytotoxic chemotherapy and hormonal drugs like tamoxifen—can't we find ways to combine them so as to achieve greater therapeutic effectiveness?

While the Consensus Development Conference of 1985 did not settle a single unresolved question, it did serve to get the word out about tamoxifen, a drug which had hitherto been more widely used in Great Britain than in the United States. During the early 1980s the majority of American breast cancer patients were still being treated only by surgeons, most of whom seem to have been unaware of the impressive results emerging from the British tamoxifen trials. The NCI's own statistics are eye-opening. In 1984 only 17% of node-positive, ER-positive postmenopausal patients in the United States were receiving tamoxifen. By the end of 1985 about 50% of these patients were getting the drug.[26]

Tamoxifen *vs.* Oophorectomy

The possibility that tamoxifen or some other hormonal agent might play an important role in treating *premenopausal* breast cancer was sadly neglected by the Consensus Development Conference of 1985. The conferees went so far as to state that "adjuvant endocrine therapy appears to be of little, if any, benefit in women under age 50."[27] This blanket statement is a prime example of excessive revisionism—the value of hormonal manipulation was first demonstrated in a 33-year-old! Since 1896 physicians have known that oophorectomy can extend both the disease-free interval and overall survival for some younger patients, a fact reaffirmed in a 1996 meta-analysis.[28] Was tamoxifen as effective as oophorectomy in preventing the estrogenic stimulation of ER-positive premenopausal breast tumors? Convincing

statistics on this question have been hard to come by, since our tamoxifen trials have tended to focus on postmenopausal patients, and since oophorectomies are no longer routinely performed. A few small studies would seem to indicate that tamoxifen and oophorectomy are roughly equivalent in effectiveness. A trial done at the Christie Hospital in Manchester, England, randomized 354 premenopausal patients to adjuvant ovarian irradiation (oophorectomy equivalent) or to a year of adjuvant tamoxifen. A follow-up analysis at five years found "no significant difference in terms of survival, local recurrence, or distant metastases."[29] The Mayo Clinic in Rochester, Minnesota, did a little trial involving metastatic breast cancer, randomizing 26 patients to tamoxifen (10 mg twice daily) and 27 patients to surgical oophorectomy. Tamoxifen made bone metastases regress; but it was less effective on metastases elsewhere in the body, which proved more responsive to oophorectomy.[30]

American practice has leaned toward tamoxifen as an initial strategy. The drug is reversible—this cannot be said of surgical excision or of ovarian irradiation. If a premenopausal patient taking tamoxifen should develop progressive disease, then oophorectomy would be one of several secondary strategies which could be considered. ER-positive patients who experience recurrences during or after tamoxifen therapy often respond to oophorectomy, because these two manipulations rely on different mechanisms. The drug blocks estrogen action at the cellular level, while surgery or irradiation removes the glands which produce this hormone. Writing in the *New England Journal of Medicine* in 1998, the oncologist Gabriel N. Hortobagyi of Houston's M. D. Anderson Cancer Center suggested that tamoxifen alone could be tried as an initial adjuvant strategy in ER-positive patients "at low risk," regardless of their menopausal status. For all ER-positive patients "at moderate or high risk," whether premenopausal or postmenopausal, he recommended "the combination of chemotherapy and tamoxifen."[31]

Notwithstanding Hortobagyi's recommendations, tamoxifen prescriptions for premenopausal patients have been written more hesitatingly than for postmenopausal patients. In fertile women the drug stimulates the ovaries to churn out more estrogen. Even V. Craig Jordan and his colleagues at the University of Wisconsin wonder whether "increases in estrogen might be inappropriate for prolonged antitumor action."[32] Dr. Jordan and other authorities have suggested that when tamoxifen is given to premenopausal women, it could be combined with a **gonadotropin-releasing hormone agonist**—that is, with a drug which suppresses ovarian function. In theory, this hormonal combination would act synergistically, eliminating estrogen from the bloodstream and allowing the circulating tamoxifen molecules to bind to the cancer cells without competition. Thus the combination ought to be as effective in premenopausal patients as single-agent tamoxifen has been in postmenopausal patients with their naturally reduced estrogen levels. The stumbling blocks are that the proposed two-agent regimen has not been tested in large-scale clinical trials, and that the side effects (e.g., hot flashes and loss of bone mineralization) would be greater than with tamoxifen alone.

Adding Chemo to Tamoxifen

Cytotoxic chemotherapy continues to be the adjuvant therapy of choice for premenopausal patients who are node-positive or otherwise deemed at high risk for metastatic disease. Infiltrating breast malignancies in younger women tend to be ER-negative or ER-poor. In this instance nothing would be accomplished by incorporating tamoxifen or any other SERM in the adjuvant regimen. The NSABP's first trial of such combined therapy (Protocol B-09) found that patients under age 50 "with tumor ER and PgR levels under 10 fmol/mg" actually had "a poorer survival" when tamoxifen was given concurrently with chemo.[33] We cannot rule out the possibility that tamoxifen or some other antiestrogen could be effectively combined with cytotoxic chemotherapy to treat that subset of high-risk premenopausal tumors which are strongly ER-positive (say, 50 fmol/mg or more)—but as yet our clinical trials have not substantially documented this hypothesis. V. Craig Jordan reminds us that chemotherapy usually doubles as hormonal ablation in premenopausal women. Most regimens, especially those containing the alkylating agent cyclophosphamide, stop the ovaries from producing estrogen; and women over age 40 do not often recover ovarian function. "It is therefore possible," Dr. Jordan observes, "that the benefit to be gained from this form of endocrine therapy (i.e., chemical oophorectomy) is optimal, and tamoxifen can add little further benefit."[34]

The theoretical justifications for adding tamoxifen to premenopausal chemotherapy— or for adding chemotherapy to postmenopausal tamoxifen—rest on the known heterogeneity of breast malignancies and on the imperfection of our current ER and PgR assays. With mammary tumors we cannot assume that the cancer cells are clonal (exact duplicates of each other) or that the assay results perfectly represent their degree of hormonal responsiveness. We do know that over a period of time many ER-positive tumors tend to evolve toward a more aggressive ER-negative phenotype. Even when a tumor is assayed ER-positive, we have to wonder whether it might contain a few ER-negative cells whose growth is not dependent on the presence of estrogen. Thus if we assume tumor heterogeneity, we could logically give tamoxifen to stymie the slow-growing ER-positive cells, and chemotherapy to fight the faster-growing ER-negative cells. Everybody agrees with this general proposition—of course, there is no consensus as to which chemotherapy regimen might be preferable, or as to whether tamoxifen should be given *concurrently* (at the same time as the chemo) or *sequentially* (after the chemo). The oncologist C. Kent Osborne of the University of Texas at San Antonio has long entertained reservations about giving tamoxifen concurrently with certain chemo regimens. Back in the early 1980s Osborne and his colleagues studied the effect of tamoxifen on ER-positive breast cancer cells being grown in Petri dishes. What they discovered is that tamoxifen kept these cells in "gap one," the at-rest phase of the cell cycle. "Tamoxifen," they concluded, "might enhance the killing effect of drugs most active in G1 (gap one) cells, whereas the cytotoxic effect of drugs acting specifically during DNA synthesis (S phase) might be diminished."[35] Needless to say, most of our cytotoxic drugs work best on cells in S phase or cells undergoing mitosis, not on resting cells. Dr. Osborne later singled out cyclophosphamide and fluorouracil (5-FU), two drugs which are the "C" and "F" respectively of the breast cancer regimen CMF, as "potential candidates for an antagonistic net interaction when combined with tamoxifen." But laboratory experiments have suggested that giving tamoxifen concurrently with Adriamycin (doxorubicin), long the most potent drug in breast cancer chemotherapy, could be beneficial. The combination seems to pack more antitumor wallop than if the drugs were given separately. "On the basis of the preclinical data," Dr. Osborne writes, "one might predict a significant benefit by adding tamoxifen to doxorubicin alone. Predicting

the net effect of combining tamoxifen with regimens containing doxorubicin (Adriamycin) plus cyclophosphamide, with or without 5-FU, is more problematic."[36]

Thanks to the research of Dr. Osborne and other scientists, we can now be fairly sure that tamoxifen should not be administered concurrently with CMF. But nobody gave much thought to drug interactions in the late 1970s and early 1980s, when the first trials of tamoxifen plus chemotherapy for postmenopausal patients were designed. Beginning in July 1979 the Southwest Oncology Group (SWOG) randomized 892 postmenopausal women with node-positive, ER-positive breast cancer to receive tamoxifen by itself (10 mg twice daily), or to receive CMF chemotherapy by itself, or to receive concurrent CMF and tamoxifen. The SWOG results, eventually published in 1994, indicated that tamoxifen by itself performed as well as the chemo or the chemohormonal combination. The only thing gained by giving CMF-based chemo concurrently with tamoxifen seemed to be toxicity—61% of the patients getting the combination suffered troublesome side effects, while only 5% of those getting tamoxifen had problems.[37] Between 1984 and 1990 the National Cancer Institute of Canada, based in Toronto, randomly assigned 705 postmenopausal women with "node-positive, ER or PgR positive breast cancer" to two years of adjuvant tamoxifen (30 mg daily) or to concurrent tamoxifen and CMF. In 1996 the Canadian team released a preliminary report warning of thromboembolic complications—13.6% of the patients getting the combined therapy experienced blood clotting, while just 2.6% of those getting only tamoxifen did so.[38] The final verdict from this trial appeared in 1997: "The addition of concurrent CMF to tamoxifen adds no benefit and considerable toxicity."[39]

The SWOG and Canadian results did not exactly discourage oncologists from pondering chemohormonal regimens, but they sure prompted a rush to **tamoxifen maintenance**. That is to say—give a chemo regimen first if you think chemo is indicated, then put the patient on tamoxifen afterwards to help maintain the remission. With this scheduling there is no possibility of negative drug interactions (tamoxifen reducing the effectiveness of the chemo or vice versa). At the February 1992 international conference on breast cancer adjuvant therapy held in Saint Gallen, Switzerland, the pioneering Italian oncologist Gianni Bonadonna recommended this sequential approach, "with chemotherapy for six months, followed by tamoxifen for at least five years."[40] In matters related to breast cancer chemotherapy, American practice has typically followed in Dr. Bonadonna's wake; and it did so in this case. During the 1990s a short course of chemo (four to six months) and subsequent tamoxifen maintenance became a standard prescription, increasingly written for ER-positive patients with nodal involvement regardless of their menstrual status. The precise effect that these sequential regimens would have on recurrence and survival rates in different subgroups had not been determined; but the absence of data did not prevent broad acceptance of a scheduling strategy whose side effects were bearable and whose efficacy seemed assured, at least in theory.

Since the mid-1980s the National Surgical Adjuvant Breast and Bowel Project has worked hard to live up to that middle name—*adjuvant!* On various occasions the NSABP has reported that systemic therapies could benefit patients not previously thought to require them. For its part the National Cancer Institute has taken the NSABP findings with all possible seriousness, mailing out "*Clinical Alerts*" (official bulletins) so that American physicians could alter their practices accordingly. Alas, the upshot tended to be brickbats rather than consensus, because breast cancer specialists were no longer inclined to view the NSABP as a divine oracle, and because they resisted any governmental attempts to substitute treatment guidelines for the judgment of the individual physician.

NSABP Protocol B-16, begun in October 1984, eventually recruited 1,296 node-positive breast cancer patients over age 50. The most important question this trial asked was whether postmenopausal patients, usually given tamoxifen alone, would do better if they also received a short course of Adriamycin and cyclophosphamide (AC). Participants in NSABP Protocol B-16 were randomly assigned to receive five years of adjuvant tamoxifen (10 mg twice a day), or to receive ACT (i.e., the same tamoxifen with 63 days of AC given concurrently at the start of therapy). The NSABP published the results of a three-year follow-up in 1990. Disease-free survival (DFS) had been 84% for the ACT arm, but only 67% for the tamoxifen arm. Overall survival (OS) had been 93% for the trial participants taking ACT, but only 85% for those taking tamoxifen alone. Needless to say, the NSABP team recommended that chemo (the AC regimen) ought to be routinely added to tamoxifen for node-positive patients over age 50.[41] Saul E. Rivkin and other members of the Southwest Oncology Group (SWOG) took issue with this interpretation, complaining that the NSABP trial contained too many ER-poor participants—that is, too many patients who were not likely to benefit from tamoxifen, but who probably would have benefited from cytotoxic chemotherapy. About 20% of the women randomized in

Protocol B-16 had low or borderline ER and PgR assays (under 10 fmol/mg). Did this fact slant the trial's results in favor of ACT? Dr. Rivkin and his SWOG colleagues thought so: "When analyzed separately for ER-positive patients only, the ACT versus tamoxifen three-year survival benefit loses its significance."[42]

The extent to which the DFS and OS advantages found for ACT in Protocol B-16 could have been due to synergetic antitumor effects achieved by the concurrent administration of Adriamycin (doxorubicin) and tamoxifen remains to be seen. It is very clear, however, that this trial convinced NSABP chairman Bernard Fisher and his colleagues that there was nothing wrong with giving tamoxifen at the same time as chemotherapy. **NSABP Protocol B-20** asked whether ER-positive node-negative patients, traditionally considered a low-risk group, would benefit more from tamoxifen by itself or from chemo and tamoxifen. Between 1988 and 1993 the NSABP randomly assigned 2,306 eligible patients, both premenopausal and postmenopausal, to one of three adjuvant regimens—the standard five years of tamoxifen (10 mg twice a day), or MFT (methotrexate, fluorouracil, and concurrent tamoxifen), or CMFT (the prevalent CMF regimen and concurrent tamoxifen). The five-year results which the NSABP published in the *Journal of the National Cancer Institute* in 1997 revealed statistically significant advantages for the two chemohormonal arms, but the improvements in outcome were quite modest—no more than 5% in any category. For *disease-free survival* (freedom from all recurrence), the score was tamoxifen 85%, MFT 90%, and CMFT 89%. For *distant disease-free survival* (freedom from metastases), the score was tamoxifen 87%, MFT 92%, and CMFT 91%. *Overall survival* at five years was 94% for the tamoxifen arm,

97% for the MFT arm, and 96% for the CMFT arm. "No subgroup of patients," Bernard Fisher and his colleagues assure us, "failed to benefit from chemotherapy; however, the risk reduction was greatest in patients aged 49 years or less."[43]

NSABP Protocol B-20 demonstrates that even in a good-prognosis subgroup which has not always been given adjuvant therapy, a few patients—say, 3% to 5%—are going to benefit from the addition of cytotoxic chemotherapy to tamoxifen. What the trial does not tell us is how we might distinguish the few patients who will benefit from the majority who will not. That majority is really quite hefty—for example, it would be "about 95%" in the aforementioned DFS category if our basic calculations include the 10% or 11% of patients who experienced recurrence in the chemo arms and the 85% who stayed disease-free in the tamoxifen arm. That leaves us with about a 4% or 5% improvement in outcome achieved by the addition of chemotherapy. Is the smallish benefit worth the added toxicity? Since premenopausal patients at any risk of recurrence typically receive a recommendation for chemo, the question is most pertinent for ER-positive postmenopausal patients, that large subgroup which tends to do well with single agent tamoxifen.

Richard D. Gelber, a biostatistician at Boston's Dana-Farber Cancer Institute, collaborated with leading American and European breast specialists to produce a meta-analysis of nine clinical trials, in which tamoxifen plus chemotherapy had been administered to a total of 3,920 patients aged 50 or older with node-positive breast cancer. Dr. Gelber and his colleagues wanted to measure the survival benefit of these chemohormonal combinations not just in calendar months, but in terms of "quality-adjusted survival," whereby "time without symptoms or toxicity" would count as a plus, and any disease recurrence or treatment side effects would count as a minus. Using this yardstick, Gelber et al concluded that the nine trials had failed to demonstrate that "chemoendocrine therapy provides more quality-adjusted survival time than tamoxifen alone." By and large the time lost to chemo's toxicity seemed to cancel out the modest gains in life expectancy. Only when Gelber et al did a subgroup analysis based on ER-assay levels did they discern a benefit for the combined therapy. The 932 patients identified as having "less than 50 fmol/mg cytosol protein" appeared to gain an average 3.4 months of "quality time" (no symptoms or toxicity) from their added chemo. In contrast, the 1,898 strongly ER-positive patients having over 50 fmol/mg were deemed to have lost an average 6.6 months of quality time because of their added chemo.[44] Presumably many postmenopausal patients in this high-ER subgroup would be better off on tamoxifen alone until that future day when our chemotherapy regimens become less toxic or more effective.

Consensus (that fabulous beast) made a brief reappearance at the February 1998 international conference held in Saint Gallen, Switzerland. This time the consensus panel took pains to emphasize the importance of doing ER and PgR assays before prescribing tamoxifen or any combination of tamoxifen and chemotherapy. Menstrual status played a secondary role in the published Saint Gallen guidelines, which may be briefly summarized. All ER-negative and PgR-negative patients judged at risk of metastatic progression because of positive nodes or unfavorable tumor characteristics were identified as candidates for **chemotherapy**. Tamoxifen might be given afterwards in this subgroup when a tumor assay revealed "minimal/trace elements of either ER or PgR." The Saint Gallen consensus panel agreed that node-positive premenopausal patients who were either ER-positive and/or PgR-positive should receive both **chemotherapy and tamoxifen**. For node-positive postmenopausal patients who assayed ER-positive and/or PgR-positive, the panel recommended both **tamoxifen and chemotherapy**. The word order in the recommendation is telling, and moreover the consensus panelists left a very large and quite appropriate loophole. For this subgroup they advised, "considerations about a low relative risk of relapse, age, toxic effects, socioeconomic implications, and information on the patient's preference might justify the use of **tamoxifen alone**."[45]

LONG-TERM TAMOXIFEN:
Any Worms in the Apple?

How long should ER-positive patients stay on tamoxifen? In the earliest trials the drug was given for just a year or two, because we did not know much about its effectiveness or its side effects. During the 1980s we learned that two years of tamoxifen therapy were better than one—and during the 1990s, that five years were better than two. In 1996 a big Swedish trial involving 3,887 breast cancer patients released some pertinent survival statistics—80% of the ER-positive postmenopausal patients who had taken the drug for five years were still living at ten-year follow-up, as compared to only 74% of comparable patients who had taken the drug for two years.[46] If five years of tamoxifen therapy are so effective, would not ten years be even better? And what about tamoxifen for life? These tough questions sent that skittish filly *Consensus* packing for the hills! The National Cancer Institute took its cue from **NSABP Protocol B-14**, the big node-negative trial which failed to find a benefit from extending tamoxifen therapy beyond five years. On December 1, 1995, the NCI mailed out a "Clinical Announcement" to 22,000 cancer physicians, recommending that tamoxifen be "limited to five years" in node-negative patients.[47] But the issue of treatment duration has not exactly been laid to rest. The Eastern Cooperative Oncology Group (ECOG) conducted a trial of long-term tamoxifen maintenance given after chemotherapy for node-positive, ER-positive breast cancer. This study found an apparent advantage for those patients who continued to take tamoxifen after five years. "It appears to be reasonable," the ECOG team concluded, "to continue to evaluate the use of tamoxifen beyond five years in node-positive breast carcinoma."[48] The consensus panelists at the 1998 Saint Gallen Conference hedged their bets—they declared that "five years is the standard duration for node-negative breast cancer," while declining to set a time limit for node-positive patients.[49] V. Craig Jordan suggests that "long-term or indefinite therapy might be the best clinical strategy." He points out that although tamoxifen can efficiently suppress mammary tumors in laboratory rats, these lesions reappear when the drug is discontinued.[50]

Tamoxifen and Heart Disease

The fact that in the 1990s breast cancer specialists were debating whether tamoxifen should be taken for five years, for ten years, or for life, reflects favorably on those clinical trials which established that long-term administration of the drug usually did not entail adverse health consequences. The issue of sequelae did not arise during the first clinical trials, because here the drug was given simply as a palliative measure for patients with metastatic breast cancer, most of whom could be expected to die from the disease. But this issue assumes paramount importance when the drug is given as an adjuvant to patients with early-stage disease who may—*or may not*—develop metastatic disease in the future. but who have in any case an additional life expectancy of several decades. What would be the purpose of giving a drug which might delay death from breast cancer, while it hastened death from cardiovascular disease or from osteoporotic bone factures? As we've seen in Chapter Six, the natural reduction in estrogen levels which occurs during and after the menopause may dispose some women to atherosclerosis (formation of fatty deposits in blood vessels), and it is always associated with a loss of bone mineralization. Would the estrogen-blocking drug tamoxifen somehow accelerate these complicated processes?

The Wisconsin Tamoxifen Study did much to alleviate our fears. The oncologist Richard R. Love and his colleagues recruited 140 postmenopausal women previously diagnosed with node-negative breast cancer: half of them were given the standard dose of tamoxifen (10 mg twice daily), and half got placebo tablets. In 1990 the Wisconsin team reported that the women taking tamoxifen had considerably better "lipid profiles" than the control group. Their overall cholesterol levels declined during treatment, with a very noticeable decrease in low-density lipoprotein (the so-called "bad cholesterol" LDL), but only a modest reduction in high-density lipoprotein (the HDL cholesterol believed to protect against atherosclerosis). According to Dr. Love and his colleagues, the end result was that "the ratios of total cholesterol to HDL cholesterol and of LDL to HDL cholesterol changed favorably."[51]

Tamoxifen seemed to be acting like estrogen with regard to these cardiovascular risk factors, but how? Susan G. Nayfield and her colleagues at the National Cancer Institute suggested that "tamoxifen works as an estrogen agonist on the liver" and therefore alters lipid metabolism in a way "resembling estrogen-replacement therapy in postmenopausal women."[52] But nobody knew whether tamoxifen could really lower the incidence of cardiovascular disease—the findings from clinical trials touching upon this matter proved to be inconsistent. In 1991 the Scottish trial of long-term adjuvant tamoxifen (20 mg daily for five years) attracted a great deal of attention when it reported that women who took the drug suffered fewer than half as many fatal myocardial infarctions ("heart attacks") as the untreated control group.[53] In 1993 the Stockholm trial reported significantly fewer hospital admissions for "cardiac disease" among its postmenopausal participants assigned to tamoxifen than among its control group—the perceived benefit was more pronounced in those women who took the drug for five years instead of stopping at two.[54] But **NSABP Protocol P-1** (the gigantic "prevention trial" discussed in succeeding paragraphs) was unable to confirm any reduction in cardiovascular disease due to tamoxifen therapy. While the P-1 findings do assure us that tamoxifen is no cardiovascular ogre, they do not support the optimistic assumption that it is a wonder drug which might be casually prescribed to prevent heart attacks. Moreover, the NSABP's tamoxifen trials have consistently identified a small worm which occasionally infests the bright apple of tamoxifen therapy. Like exogenous estrogens, this drug slightly increases the likelihood of thrombosis (the formation of blood clots in the slow-moving venous circulation). Small clots in the superficial veins of the legs or arms may lead to localized irritation (thrombophlebitis)—but a larger clot in a deeper vein can prove lethal if it should be dislodged, enter the venous circulation, and eventually obstruct a significant blood vessel in the lungs (pulmonary embolism) or in the brain (occlusive stroke). NSABP Protocol B-14 found that "embolic phenomena, deep-vein thrombosis, and hospitalization occurred more often in the tamoxifen group (1.7%) than in the placebo group (0.4%)."[55] The risk involved is modest but undeniable. Therefore a woman taking tamoxifen is well advised to contact her physician if she should experience shortness of breath, painful swelling in the arms or legs, or a neurological complaint like headache or dizziness. While these symptoms are not necessarily related to deep-vein thrombosis, that possibility should always be considered in a woman who is taking tamoxifen or exogenous estrogens.

Tamoxifen and Bone Density

Tamoxifen researchers were especially anxious to determine whether long-term treatment with this drug would accelerate the postmenopausal loss of bone mineralization and thus promote early-onset osteoporosis. For many decades we knew that the menopausal decline in estrogen production was associated with a rapid decline in bone mass, but had no clue to the biological mechanism involved. Only in the late 1980s did American scientists discover that osteoblasts, the bone-building cells, express small quantities of the estrogen receptor protein (ER). Presumably the hormone must bind to the ER in these cells before they can do their work.[56] How did tamoxifen, that chameleon drug with varying estrogenic and antiestrogenic properties, act on osteoblasts? The Wisconsin Tamoxifen Study gave us a reassuring answer—the drug's effect on bone metabolism in postmenopausal women is decidedly estrogenic. For each of the trial's 140 participants, Richard R. Love and his colleagues measured "bone mineral density" at two skeletal locations: the lumbar (lower) spine, which consists mainly of the softer and more metabolically active trabecular bone, and the radius (the smaller of the two forearm bones), which consists mainly of the harder and less metabolically active cortical bone. The *New England Journal of Medicine* for March 26, 1992, published the results of the Wisconsin experiment: "In the women given tamoxifen, the mean bone mineral density of the lumbar spine increased by 0.61 percent per year, whereas in those given placebo it decreased by 1.00 percent per year." While the mineral density of the radius decreased by 0.88 percent per year in the women taking tamoxifen, it decreased even faster in the placebo-takers, going down by 1.29 percent per year. Tamoxifen seemed to be almost as effective as estrogen replacement therapy in preserving bone mass. The finding that the drug increased bone mass in the lumbar spine was deemed especially propitious. Dr. Love and his colleagues observed that "the decline in bone mass associated with the cessation of ovarian estrogen production involves mainly the trabecular bone found in the spine and to a lesser degree in the hips."[57]

The Wisconsin Tamoxifen Study followed its participants for two years. The Stockholm trial gave us a longer follow-up. The Swedish researchers measured the bone mineral density in the forearms of 75 postmenopausal breast cancer patients who had been previously randomized to two years of tamoxifen or to five years of tamoxifen or to a placebo. At seven years from randomization, there were no significant differences between these three groups: "The results thus did not indicate an accelerated postmenopausal bone loss with long-term adjuvant tamoxifen."[58] A little Danish trial also looked at the drug's effects on postmenopausal bone metabolism, randomizing 50 breast cancer patients to tamoxifen (30 mg daily for two years) or to a control group. The Copenhagen team found that bone mineral density of the lumbar spine "increased during the first year in women treated with tamoxifen and then stabilized, compared with decreased density in the control group. Bone mineral content at the forearms remained almost stable in tamoxifen-treated women compared with a decrease in the control group."[59] The Wisconsin, Stockholm, and Copenhagen experiments establish that tamoxifen does not accelerate the postmenopausal loss of bone mass; but because of their relatively short follow-ups, they do not tell us how effectively the drug would protect against bone fractures in the long run. Would a large group of 60-year-old women assigned today to lifelong tamoxifen therapy actually record fewer fractures some twenty or thirty years hence? At present we do not know.

An even broader gap in our knowledge concerns the drug's effect on premenopausal bone metabolism. What happens when you assign 40-year-olds to long-term tamoxifen therapy? What's the probable effect on their bone mineral density in future decades? Back in the 1980s laboratory experiments demonstrated that while the drug prevents the loss of bone mass in rats whose ovaries have been removed, it actually reduces bone density when given to rats with functioning ovaries. Trevor J. Powles of the Royal Marsden Hospital (Sutton, Surrcy) and other English researchers conducted a pertinent "chemoprevention" trial with human subjects. They randomly assigned 179 premenopausal women to tamoxifen (20 mg daily) or to a look-alike placebo. But the three-year results published in the *Journal of Clinical Oncology* in 1996 were not altogether reassuring. No loss of bone mineralization could be detected in the placebo group; but in the women taking tamoxifen, bone mineral density in the lumbar spine "decreased progressively and was significantly lower than pretreatment values at one, two, and three years." The women taking tamoxifen also experienced a slight loss of bone density in the hip, although this was not readily detected until the third year of therapy. "In the presence of premenopausal levels of estrogen," Powles et al concluded, "the net effects of tamoxifen are antiestrogenic with respect to skeletal metabolism." The bone loss is "more marked at sites of largely cancellous (trabecular) bone such as the spine compared with the hip, where the contribution of cortical bone is probably greater."[60]

We should emphasize that tamoxifen does not seem to be an osteoporotic ogre for premenopausal women. Dr. Powles and his colleagues hasten to assure us that "the loss of bone density was moderate and mostly in the first year of treatment." But they prudently urge further research on the drug's long-term effects in premenopausal women, because "even small differences in bone mineral density may have a significant effect on fracture risk."[61]

Risk of Endometrial Cancer

The nastiest worm that we might discover lurking in long-term tamoxifen therapy would be a potential to induce secondary malignancies. Laboratory experiments have repeatedly demonstrated that the drug can induce liver cancers in rats. Fortunately, our clinical trials involving tens of thousands of subjects have not indicated that hepatic carcinogenesis is a problem in humans. Bernard Fisher and his NSABP associates point out that the tamoxifen doses used to produce liver tumors in rats were twenty to a hundred times greater than the doses given to breast cancer patients: "Currently, this concern does not seem to be clinically or biochemically relevant."[62] Endometrial carcinomas are another matter. Tamoxifen's effect on the postmenopausal endometrium is strongly estrogenic, and long-term therapy

noticeably elevates the risk of malignant transformation. As in the case of estrogen replacement therapy, periodic administration of a progestin to induce endometrial shedding would reduce the risk; but this has not been a standard prescription, since we do not know how the progestin would affect tamoxifen's antitumor action. Some specialists have advocated annual endometrial evacuation (dilation and curettage) to reduce the risk, or regular endometrial biopsies to detect any transformation at an early stage. Either of these strategies ought to be effective; but as yet the only consensus we have is that postmenopausal patients with intact uteri should be informed of the risk and counseled to report any vaginal bleeding to their physician.

NSABP PROTOCOL B-14
The Big Node-Negative Trial

During the 1980s, as the evidence began to accumulate that tamoxifen not only combated hormonally responsive breast cancers but also lowered cholesterol levels and preserved bone mass in postmenopausal women, many researchers started to envision much broader indications for prescribing the drug. Why not give it to the low-risk patients (i.e., node-negative ones) or even to healthy women who might simply be deemed at higher risk of eventually developing breast cancer? The NSABP set out to test the value of these propositions in two clinical trials, **Protocols B-14 and P-1**, which were so large and so carefully monitored that their findings command our attention. Beginning in 1982, the NSABP randomly assigned 2,644 patients with node-negative breast cancer to five years of tamoxifen therapy (10 mg twice a day) or to a placebo. All the participants in B-14 were estrogen receptor-positive with assay readings of at least 10 fmol/mg—31% were under age 50 (presumably premenopausal), and 69% were age 50 or older (principally postmenopausal). The National Cancer Institute was so pleased with the trial's results that it could not wait for them to appear in print. In May 1988 the NCI mailed out unpublished B-14 data showing a tamoxifen advantage to 13,000 American oncologists. This premature news release, stamped ***CLINICAL ALERT—URGENT***, did not exactly endear the NCI to the editors of the *New England Journal of Medicine*, who did not publish the full NSABP report until the following February. Then breast cancer specialists finally had an opportunity to appreciate the design and statistical power of Protocol B-14, a trial which clearly demonstrated that premenopausal patients can benefit from adjuvant tamoxifen. At four years from randomization, 85% of the trial participants under age 50 who received tamoxifen remained free of disease (no recurrences detected)—but only 73% of comparably youthful participants who got the placebo tablets stayed disease-free. For the women aged 50 and older at randomization, the score at four years was 82% disease-free in the tamoxifen arm and 79% disease-free in the placebo arm.

NSABP Protocol B-14 did not detect a "statistically significant" survival advantage for tamoxifen, nor would it have been likely to do so, because very few node-negative patients die of metastatic disease within a few years of diagnosis. As with earlier clinical trials, the side effects that B-14 recorded were principally of the nuisance variety—hot flashes (57% of the participants taking tamoxifen were affected as compared to 40% in the placebo arm), vaginal discharge (23% tamoxifen, 12% placebo), and irregular menses (60% of the subjects under age 40 taking tamoxifen were affected as compared to 30% of the placebo takers in

the same age bracket). Bernard Fisher and his NSABP colleagues exercised a modicum of restraint when explaining the trial's implications for the *Journal*'s readers. They did not say that *all* ER-positive node-negative patients should take five years of tamoxifen; they simply said that they could not identify "any subsets" who failed to benefit. "Until there are better markers for more precisely identifying patients who require and will respond to tamoxifen," Fisher et al advised, "a physician's bias should not deny a patient the option to accept or reject the benefit that has been demonstrated. Although the benefit is moderate, it could have important public health consequences." The overall benefit as calculated for all B-14 participants was 6% in disease-free survival at four years—83% DFS in the tamoxifen arm as compared to 77% disease-free survival in the placebo arm.[63]

Not everybody was convinced by the NSABP's reasoning, and quite a few people were irritated by the NCI's decision to circulate snippets of B-14 data as the gospel truth before the scientific community had an opportunity to pass judgment on the published report. The radiotherapist Samuel Hellman complained that he first learned of the NCI's Clinical Alert by reading about it in a newspaper. Shortly afterwards he was swamped by "telephone messages from distraught patients who were concerned as to whether they had been mistreated or inadequately treated." K. C. Lee of Georgetown University's Lombardi Cancer Center pointed out that the NCI's hasty circulation of results amounted to "premature termination" of a trial still in the process of collecting data.[64] In an editorial accompanying the *Journal*'s publication of the B-14 results, William L. McGuire of the University of Texas at San Antonio emphasized that "the great majority (approximately 70 percent)" of patients who are node-negative can achieve long-term survival with adequate local therapy: "Most do not have distant micrometastases and therefore do not require systemic therapy." Dr. McGuire politely suggested that the B-14 findings did not warrant a policy of routine tamoxifen: "Relatively few patients benefited. The importance of this benefit in those few cannot be determined at present; no evidence of prolonged overall survival has yet been demonstrated." Before recommending systemic adjuvant therapy, physicians should use "the individual patient's risk factors (tumor size, steroid receptors, histopathology, proliferative rate, and ploidy) to weigh the probability of benefits." Having space to discuss only one of these factors, McGuire chose tumor size for his illustration: "Patients with node-negative tumors under 2 cm in diameter have an excellent prognosis, with an average five-year relapse rate of only 11%. As the tumor size increases beyond 2 cm in diameter, the relapse rate more than doubles."[65]

Indeed, tumor size happened to be the Achilles' heel in the B-14 data and consequently in any inflexible treatment guidelines which we might attempt to derive from that data. ER and PgR assays were required of all participants; these were performed with biochemical ligand-binding assays which typically give accurate quantitative readings (femtomoles per milligram), but require much more tumor tissue than immunostaining assays. The upshot was that really low-risk node-negative patients, those whose tumors were smaller than one centimeter in diameter, tended to be excluded from Protocol B-14 because the NSABP did not have ER and PgR readings for them.[66] Consequently, B-14 tells us nothing about those small infiltrating tumors (say, 0.5 to 1.0 cm in diameter) which might be detected by mammography or even by diligent breast self-examination. Patients with *in situ* breast cancers were never considered for this trial. Insofar as tumor size goes, Protocol B-14 was not so much a trial of low-risk node-negatives, but of *moderate to high-risk* node-negatives. The majority of participants had been diagnosed with tumors smaller than two centimeters in diameter; but 42% in the placebo arm and 43% in the tamoxifen arm had tumors larger than 2.0 cm, and thus would have been classified as Stage Two on the basis of tumor size alone.[67] The proposition that most Stage Two patients stand to benefit from adjuvant therapy has long since ceased to be controversial. What drove Dr. McGuire, Dr. Hellman, and other dedicated physicians to the barricades was the facile way in which the NCI and the news media managed to convey the impression that *all* node-negative patients urgently needed systemic therapy.

NSABP PROTOCOL P-1
Tamoxifen for Prevention?

While the NSABP and NCI had sown the seeds of dissension with Protocol B-14, these organizations did not reap a full harvest of brickbats until they proceeded with Protocol P-1, also known as the **Breast Cancer Prevention Trial**. It was one thing to give tamoxifen to women diagnosed with invasive breast cancer—everybody agreed on the drug's utility in ER-positive cases with nodal involvement. It was an entirely different matter to give a powerful pharmaceutical to healthy women who had not yet developed breast cancer. When we employ a therapeutic agent against lethal disease, we readily accept large risks and severe side effects in return for a small improvement in outcome. On the other hand, when we give a preventive agent to healthy persons, we require that the anticipated benefits far outweigh the ascertainable risks. Was the benefit-to-risk ratio for tamoxifen favorable enough to warrant its use as a breast cancer prophylactic? The NSABP and NCI thought so. In 1990 they began planning a clinical trial of truly monumental proportions to demonstrate the virtues of tamoxifen prophylaxis. This trial was scheduled to enroll 16,000 healthy women considered at risk for breast cancer, using 131 hospitals throughout the United States and Canada as recruitment centers. Half of the trial's participants would then receive five years of tamoxifen (20 mg daily), and half would get placebo tablets, in a "double-blinded fashion"—that is, neither the involved physicians nor the women participating would know who was actually getting the drug. The trial's cost was initially estimated at 68 million dollars. Bernard Fisher and his NSABP colleagues were sufficiently confident of success that in their protocol statement dated January 24, 1992, they projected a "net benefit" for the trial's treatment arm. Tamoxifen, calculated Fisher et al, ought to prevent 62 invasive breast cancers and 52 myocardial infarctions (heart attacks) for every 38 cases of endometrial cancer it induced.[68] Thus the final balance would be registered in the plus column—76 "events" prevented!

Nobody questioned the fact that tamoxifen could prevent—or at least greatly delay the presentation of—a significant number of breast cancers. Earlier clinical trials had consistently found a reduced incidence of contralateral tumors in patients given the drug. However, not a few physicians and breast cancer activists suspected that the NSABP's neat reckoning of anticipated benefits represented pie-in-the-sky optimism. Dr. Adriane Fugh-Berman of the Washington-based National Women's Health Network found that Protocol P-1 looked like "an experiment in disease substitution." The Harvard biologist Ruth Hubbard wondered

whether the big prevention trial was truly motivated by the spirit of disinterested scientific investigation: "A pharmaceutical firm could make huge profits if this drug were prescribed as a preventive treatment for healthy women."[69] Every side effect that had ever been associated with tamoxifen was now passionately rehashed by the trial's opponents, not just the acknowledged risks of endometrial cancer and thromboembolism, but problems like liver cancer and cataract formation which had been more convincingly demonstrated in rodents than in humans.[70] Writing in the *New England Journal of Medicine*, Adriane Fugh-Berman and Samuel Epstein complained that the consent form the NSABP asked trial participants to sign "misleadingly trivializes the risks while exaggerating potential benefits." Fugh-Berman and Epstein argued that the evidence that tamoxifen reduces the incidence of cardiovascular disease and osteoporosis was as yet "minimal and controversial." Only the Scottish trial had reported a decline in fatal heart attacks; other trials had not. "No study has demonstrated a decrease in fracture rates among tamoxifen users."[71]

The NSABP was unfazed by the frequent criticisms. In April 1992 it began to screen potential candidates for Protocol P-1; the trial started on the first of June. Criteria for admission were liberal—all women aged 60 or older were deemed eligible, as was any woman between 35 and 59 who had a family history of breast cancer (first-degree relatives affected) or a previous biopsy identifying a proliferative condition known to predispose to malignant transformation (e.g., atypical hyperplasia or lobular carcinoma *in situ*). Protocol P-1 did not want for candidates. In the year 1991 about 2,000 people signed up for the various clinical trials run by the NSABP; for 1993 the enrollment figure was 14,000—approximately 10,000 of whom accrued to the mammoth tamoxifen trial. According to later accounts, the NSABP operations office in Pittsburgh was "over-whelmed" by the influx of trial participants.[72] Was the NSABP overreaching itself? Quite possibly. Ensuing events illustrated the difficulty of running clinical trials which involve hundreds of physicians and thou-sands of patients scattered across the North American continent. Meticulous record-keeping and constant monitoring are neces-sary to avoid foul-ups of the most embarrass-ing kind.

The scandal which shook the NSABP and NCI in the spring of 1994 originated in a minor case of misconduct in Protocol B-06, the big lumpectomy trial. A well-meaning physician in Montreal had admitted ineligible patients to the trial and then submitted falsi-fied data to the NSABP headquarters.[73] Unfortunately, the revelation of wrongdoing triggered an avalanche of brickbats, most of which seemed to be personally aimed at the NSABP's chairman Bernard Fisher. At age 75 Dr. Fisher had long been the best known and most honored breast cancer specialist in the United States; now he found himself being grilled by a House of Representatives subcommittee headed by John Dingell of Michigan. Was it true that Zeneca Pharma-ceuticals, the manufacturer of tamoxifen, had paid for "lavish parties and receptions" held for NSABP-affiliated physicians? Citing the $80,000-plus expense recorded for a single NSABP function, Representative Dingell observed that the organization appeared to spend more money on social gatherings than on auditing clinical trials. He found it "not quite cricket" that Zeneca Pharmaceuticals had helped to fund an endowed professorship at Dr. Fisher's institution, the University of Pittsburgh. Was the academic quest for scientific truth being confused with a drug company's pursuit of profits?[74]

Dr. Fisher was eventually exonerated of any misconduct by the Department of Health and Human Services, and the NCI subsequently issued a statement acknowledg-ing his many contributions to breast cancer research during "the last forty years."[75] But the Congressional hearings of 1994 ought to serve as a perpetual caution. In this intensely controversial and competitive field, it is not enough for a researcher to be innocent of a conflict of interest—he or she must be above all suspicion! Insofar as the NSABP and Protocol P-1 were concerned, the scandal's upshot was delay, audits, reorganization, and a changing of the guard. Bernard Fisher relinquished the post of chairman with its heavy administrative duties; he now became the NSABP's "Scientific Director," still as visible as ever. Enrollment in Protocol P-1, which had been temporarily suspended in March 1994, resumed a year later; and it was completed on September 30, 1997.

Every six months NCI officials ana-lyzed the incoming data from Protocol P-1, looking for that solid evidence of benefit which would warrant ending the trial and disclosing its results. By March 1998 the reviewers were satisfied. On April 6 the NCI director Richard Klausner and his colleagues held a news conference to announce that, yes, tamoxifen did reduce the incidence of breast cancer by "40 to 50 percent among women at high risk." Klausner characterized the trial's results as "the first imperfect but very en-couraging step" in the search for drugs which can prevent cancer.[76] The popular news media, normally ready to interpret any suc-cessful experiment with laboratory mice as a harbinger of medical miracles, reacted coolly to the NCI announcement. *Time* magazine ran a two-page report on the trial's outcome under the heading "Beware this Break-through!" Tamoxifen, said the article, "comes with so many caveats that it won't help most women."[77] *Time* later made amends by publishing a letter from V. Craig Jordan, who assured the magazine's readers that they could take the drug at any time: "Tamoxifen does not wear out as a preventive after five years; in fact, it 'imprints' the breast and protects women for years after they stop taking it."[78]

Evaluating the P-1 Findings

For a more balanced account of the benefit-to-risk ratio of prophylactic tamoxifen, we are indebted—*as for so many things!*—to Bernard Fisher and his NSABP co-workers. The detailed report of the Protocol P-1 findings which they published in the *Journal of the National Cancer Institute* (September 16, 1998) is a model of scholarly discrimination, telling us honestly about the trial's failures as well as its successes. Their analysis was based on a conscientious follow-up of 13,175 women, fewer subjects than envisioned in the 1992 protocol, but far more than in any previous tamoxifen trial. The "mean time in the study" for all participants was four years (actually "47.7 months"), although a majority of participants (67.0%) "were followed for more than 48 months, and 36.8% had follow-up exceeding 60 months." The trial's two arms were evenly balanced (6,576 women on tamoxifen and 6,599 taking the placebo).

The analysis of the Protocol P-1 results positively drips with **statistical power**, that ability to tell us whether or not the recorded outcomes could have been due to chance alone. They were not—a strong tamoxifen advantage prevailed in all subgroups. There had been 175 cases of invasive breast cancer in the placebo arm, but only 89 in the tamoxifen arm; thus the NSABP researchers could claim "a 49% reduction in the overall risk." The drug also reduced the incidence of *in situ* (noninvasive) breast cancers by about 50%—there had been 69 cases detected in

the placebo arm, but only 35 in the tamoxifen arm.[79] These were the main propitious findings; unfortunately, the trial also revealed a large Achilles' heel in tamoxifen prophylaxis. The drug only reduced the incidence of ER-positive breast cancers—there was no significant difference between the two arms in the rate of ER-negative malignancies. While most breast cancers, especially postmenopausal ones, tend to be at least somewhat hormonally responsive, ER-negative tumors which are totally nonresponsive behave more aggressively and contribute mightily to mortality. Since tamoxifen does not prevent these tumors, any assumption that a five-year prophylaxis with this drug could reduce our overall mortality rate by 50% is probably unwarranted. We should rejoice in the P-1 finding that tamoxifen reduced the annual rate of ER-positive breast cancers "by 69%"; but until we have a way of predicting whether a future tumor is going to be ER-positive or ER-negative, we should caution young women with family histories of devastating early-onset malignancies that tamoxifen prophylaxis cannot offer the same degree of protection as prophylactic mastectomy.

One subset of women in the tamoxifen arm fared especially well—those with the high-risk cellular proliferations dubbed atypical hyperplasia and lobular carcinoma *in situ* (LCIS). Dr. Fisher and his colleagues point out that these lesions are usually ER-positive, a fact which explains why "tamoxifen administration dramatically reduced the risk of invasive cancer." According to the NSABP calculations, the drug reduced that risk by 56% in the women with LCIS. For the trial's 1,193 participants with atypical hyperplasia, the risk reduction was stunning. The annual rate of invasive cancer was 10.11 per 1,000 women in the placebo arm, but only 1.43 per 1,000 in the tamoxifen arm.[80]

The most unexpected disappointment from Protocol P-1 was the trial's failure to confirm that major protective effect against coronary artery disease which had been suggested by the Scottish trial's 1991 report. The best thing the NSABP team could say is that "at least during the P-1 study, the drug did not have a detrimental effect on the heart." In fact, the two arms ran neck-and-neck in the cardiovascular competition, with the placebo takers (28 heart attacks) appearing to beat the tamoxifen takers (31 heart attacks) by a nose. "Overall," calculated Fisher et al, "the average annual rate of ischemic heart disease was 2.37 per 1,000 women in the placebo group and 2.73 per 1,000 in the tamoxifen group." With regard to the prevention of osteoporotic bone fractures, the drug did a slightly better job in achieving the anticipated benefits—137 women in the placebo group suffered fractures affecting the hip, lower spine, or radius, while 111 women in the tamoxifen group had comparable fractures. Dr. Fisher and his colleagues pointed out that "this represents a 19% reduction in the incidence of fractures, a reduction that almost reached statistical significance."[81]

While the results from Protocol P-1 failed to support the most enthusiastic projections of tamoxifen proponents, neither did they vindicate the dire suspicions of the naysayers. There was not a single case of liver cancer recorded in either arm of the trial. The annual rate of cataract formation was only slightly elevated in the tamoxifen arm, at 24.82 per 1,000 women compared to 21.72 per 1,000 women in the placebo arm. More than twice as many endometrial carcinomas occurred in the tamoxifen arm (36 compared to only 15 in the placebo arm), but all were detected while still localized and curable. Thus the fear that tamoxifen might promote unusually aggressive endometrial

malignancies proved to be unfounded. The incidence of other types of cancer (colon, lung, ovarian, etc.) was equivalent in the trial's two arms, providing further evidence that tamoxifen, while mitogenic in the endometrium, is not at all carcinogenic.

From the standpoint of scientific knowledge, it is regrettable that this double-blinded trial was halted in April 1998 so that participants from the placebo arm could have an opportunity to start taking tamoxifen. Does a five-year course of this drug really "imprint the breast" (as Dr. Jordan says) and therefore continue to prevent malignant transformation twenty years later? Protocol P-1 with its mean follow-up of four years cannot answer this question—Dr. Fisher and his NSABP colleagues had to cite data from Protocol B-14 to demonstrate that "the benefit remains through ten years of follow-up."[82] In the fall of 1998 the Food and Drug Administration approved the prophylactic use of tamoxifen, but the drug is hardly the ideal chemopreventive agent we would like to see. It seems probable that tamoxifen could prevent a substantial percentage of postmenopausal breast cancers—however, the fact that Protocol P-1 has as yet failed to demonstrate decisive protective effects against cardiovascular disease and osteoporosis should make us hesitate before recommending its routine use in a postmenopausal population which is typically at much greater risk of disability or death from heart attacks and bone fractures than from breast tumors. The prophylactic application which the P-1 results appear to support most convincingly might be for premenopausal women diagnosed with premalignant conditions like atypical hyperplasia or lobular carcinoma *in situ*, or with ductal carcinoma *in situ*. In these instances the risk of invasive breast cancer is noticeably elevated, yet bilateral mastectomy to achieve "the cure" usually strikes both physicians and patients as an excessively drastic measure. Insofar as the abnormal mammary cells are ER-positive, they receive a powerful hormonal stimulus with each menstrual cycle; tamoxifen can block that stimulus.

When Tamoxifen Fails—
Some Second-line Strategies

Tamoxifen can be called a "miracle drug" only by comparison to earlier hormonal manipulations like additive estrogens and androgens. While many patients with ER-positive breast cancer who would otherwise promptly relapse are going to enjoy extended disease-free survival because of tamoxifen, any exact "cure rates" are hard to pin down. American oncologists seem to cite more optimistic statistics than their British and Canadian counterparts; however, as yet neither tamoxifen nor cytotoxic chemotherapy has produced a really dramatic decline in breast cancer mortality. The overall effect of systemic therapies has been modest. And tamoxifen in particular is best viewed as a "management drug," proven to be helpful in controlling subclinical micrometastases for long periods of time. That tamoxifen by itself ever totally eradicates these micrometastases is open to question. We know for a fact that the drug cannot eliminate established metastatic disease, though it can often induce temporary remissions.

A significant number of breast cancer patients given adjuvant tamoxifen will eventually experience **failure** or **resistance**. Oncologists employ these two terms interchangeably to say much the same thing— viz., the drug is not working. We must draw that unhappy conclusion when a patient prescribed tamoxifen after surgery develops either a local recurrence or a distant metastasis, or when a patient taking tamoxifen to combat existing metastases reveals disease progression. There are three main explanations for tamoxifen failure. The first of these is **patient noncompliance**. A therapeutic level of the drug has not been present in the bloodstream because the patient, feeling well enough, has not been taking the pills on a regular basis or has discontinued them altogether. Under the heading of noncompliant behavior, we should perhaps quote V. Craig Jordan's observation that "weight increases" can contribute to treatment failure, "because tamoxifen is extremely lipophilic and may depot in the body fat, thereby reducing bioavailability to the tumor."[83] The second possible explanation for failure is **the emergence of an ER-negative phenotype**. Unlike the cancer cells in the primary breast tumor, those found in the recurrence are predominantly ER-negative and therefore not responsive to the drug. We might surmise that the original tumor shed a few ER-negative cells prior to diagnosis, and that these cells continued to multiply in the presence of tamoxifen, eventually becoming numerous enough to cause symptoms. A third possible explanation is **tamoxifen stimulation of ER-positive tumor cells**. For some reason this drug (which acts like estrogen on bone cells and endometrial cells) has started to exert comparably estrogenic effects on the breast cancer cells, thereby causing their proliferation instead of stymieing it. This phenomenon is occasionally encountered in the laboratory when cell lines or tumor-bearing mice are given tamoxifen. C. Kent Osborne has long suspected that it lies behind most cases of treatment failure. Writing in the *New England Journal of Medicine*, he points out that "tamoxifen-stimulated growth explains the 'withdrawal response' that occurs in some patients when the drug is stopped because of tumor progression. At least two thirds of the tumors that become resistant to tamoxifen continue to express estrogen receptors, and many of these regress when second-line hormonal therapy is initiated."[84]

Whenever a patient taking tamoxifen suffers a recurrence, her physician needs to discover which of the three aforementioned mechanisms is at fault. This knowledge is not just academic; it should dictate the choice of a second-line therapy. A treatment failure due to noncompliance does not necessarily indicate drug resistance—tamoxifen may still prove effective if the patient will take the medicine as directed. On the other hand, a tumor recurrence which is assayed as ER-negative and PgR-negative not only points toward tamoxifen resistance, but strongly suggests that all hormonal strategies will prove futile—the patient should now be offered cytotoxic chemotherapy. A positive receptor reading on the tumor recurrence (either ER or PgR present, preferably both) opens the door for second-line hormonal therapies; there are several options.

In the 1980s **additive progestins** (synthetic versions of progesterone) became the hormonal therapy of choice after ta-moxifen failure in postmenopausal patients. Both medroxyprogesterone acetate and megestrol acetate were convenient oral drugs which often induced remissions in metastatic breast cancer. The response rates correlated with the degree of PgR positivity, higher assay readings being indicative of better odds. In the United States postmenopausal patients with recurrent disease typically received a prescription for **Megace** (Mead Johnson's popular brand of megestrol ace-tate) calling for "40 mg q.i.d." (four tablets daily). The most common side effects were an improved appetite and a tendency to gain weight. Higher doses of Megace were also well-tolerated; unfortunately, they upped the weight gain as well as the response rates. One study of patients given 800 milligrams daily (five times the standard 160 mg dose)

found that 43% gained over 20 pounds![85]

Ablative strategies can also play a role after tamoxifen failure—drugs which act to diminish the body's estrogen production have largely replaced the surgical excision of endocrine glands. As recently as the 1970s the standard maneuver for postmenopausal patients was **adrenalectomy**, removal of the adrenal glands (these produce androgens which are converted to estrogen in fatty tissues containing the enzyme aromatase). Adrenalectomy prevented estrogen synthesis in older women; but by the early 1980s we had learned that a drug called **aminoglu-tethimide** was just as effective, shutting down adrenal function and thus accomplish-ing a "medical adrenalectomy."[86] Aminoglu-tethimide was the crude forerunner of an increasingly important class of drugs known as **aromatase inhibitors**. It never became as popular as Megace because it could produce troublesome side effects (fatigue, skin rash, dizziness) and required the concurrent ad-ministration of a corticosteroid.

Aromatase inhibitors have not been given to premenopausal women because they cannot stop the ovaries from producing estrogen. Either **surgical oophorectomy** or **ovarian irradiation** could be used to achieve this end, and either maneuver would stand a good chance of inducing tumor regression in ER-positive breast cancer which no longer responds to tamoxifen. Oophorectomies and many other abdominal surgeries are now done laparoscopically—that is, by means of flexible tubes and tiny instruments inserted through small incisions in the abdominal wall. This technical advance has greatly reduced hospital costs and recovery times; and it should make oophorectomy a more palatable alternative for patients who are already suffering from painful metastatic disease. Oncologists naturally tend to think in terms of pharmaceutical solutions rather than surgical ones. An efficient "medical oophorectomy" can be accomplished by a monthly injection of a **gonadotropin-releasing hormone agonist** (GnRH agonist), which would shut down ovarian function and bring the estrogen content of the blood down to postmenopausal levels within a few days. This pharmaceutical maneuver is reversible, and thus it may be less distressing to some patients than oophorectomy. The Southwest Oncology Group and allied organizations conducted a pertinent clinical trial, assigning 136 premenopausal patients with "receptor-positive" metastatic breast cancer to undergo surgical oophorectomy or to receive monthly injections of the GnRH agonist **goserelin**. The trial results revealed no significant differences between the two arms either in disease-free survival or in overall survival: "Hot flashes and tumor flare were more common with goserelin."[87]

Looking for a Better *SERM*

The aforementioned second-line strategies were typically used for "salvage"—that is, to buy a few months of symptomatic relief in advanced metastatic disease. Drugs like Megace or aminoglutethimide were not suitable for adjuvant therapy, much less for prophylaxis. Pharmacologically-minded researchers have therefore dreamed of discovering a truly revolutionary **Selective Estrogen Receptor Modulator** (SERM) suitable for prevention as well as for therapy. The ideal SERM would combat diseases associated both with excessive estrogenic stimulation (e.g., mammary carcinomas) and with diminished estrogen levels (e.g., atherosclerosis and osteoporosis). Tamoxifen, our prototypical SERM, was proposed as that ideal agent; but as we've seen, it did not quite measure up to its advance billing. Would a newer SERM—or perhaps a combination of several SERMs—do a better job?

Our drug companies continue to experiment with synthetic compounds which seem likely to exert beneficial effects by modulating cellular ER protein.[88] We have just space to discuss two compounds which excited a great deal of enthusiasm and which are now available as prescription drugs.

Toremifene, synthesized in Finland in 1981, is almost identical to tamoxifen in its chemical structure. But this drug does not bind to the ER protein quite as avidly as tamoxifen; consequently, the recommended daily dose (60 mg) is three times that of tamoxifen (20 mg). The amount of clinical data we have for toremifene looks like a molehill compared to the Himalayas of data available for tamoxifen. In an American trial involving 648 postmenopausal patients with metastatic breast cancer, toremifene proved to be as effective as tamoxifen in prolonging survival. A small Finnish trial found that toremifene raised postmenopausal levels of high-density lipoprotein (the good cholesterol) slightly more efficiently than tamoxifen.[89] The Food and Drug Administration has approved toremifene for use in metastatic breast cancer, and since 1997 the drug has been readily available from the Schering Corporation under the brand name **Fareston**.[90] Is toremifene better than tamoxifen? The laboratory results on the newer drug look promising; but currently we do not know whether it will be as good as tamoxifen in preserving bone mineralization, or whether it will be equally well-adapted for long-term adjuvant therapy. And the very fact that toremifene is so similar to tamoxifen poses an obstacle to its widespread use as a second-line therapy. Aman U. Buzdar and Gabriel N. Hortobagyi of Houston's M. D. Anderson Cancer Center suspect that toremifene could be relatively ineffective in patients previously treated with tamoxifen "due to the likelihood of cross resistance."[91] In other words, any breast cancer cells which are resistant to tamoxifen will probably be resistant to toremifene as well.

The new SERM which seemed most promising for breast cancer prophylaxis has been **raloxifene**. Preliminary laboratory tests demonstrated that this drug could preserve bone mineral density in rats whose ovaries had been removed, without exerting estrogenic effects on the mammary gland and the uterus. Eli Lilly and Company consequently developed raloxifene as an osteoporosis prophylaxis for postmenopausal women who might be reluctant to take estrogen replacement therapy. Since gaining FDA approval for this application in 1997, Lilly has been energetically marketing raloxifene under the brand name **Evista**.[92] Although the early clinical trials naturally focused on raloxifene's ability to maintain bone density, they also revealed two noteworthy incidental findings—first, that the drug reduced the number of breast cancers diagnosed among trial participants, and second, that it seemed to improve the participants' lipid profiles, lowering the bad LDL cholesterol while elevating the good HDL variety.[93] Is raloxifene that long-sought-after drug which simultaneously—and amazingly!—combines estrogenic and antiestrogenic effects in such a way as to prevent osteoporotic fractures, heart attacks, and breast malignancies? We would certainly like to think so; the problem is that we have only small molehills of suggestive data when we need unshakeable mountains of proof.

Raloxifene has not been approved for any therapeutic indication involving breast malignancies, but we should soon know whether this drug can be used to prevent them. In 1998 the NSABP finalized its plans for **Protocol P-2**, also known as the **STAR Trial** or **"Study of Tamoxifen and Raloxifene."** This mammoth prevention trial was expected to enroll 22,000 healthy women who were either postmenopausal or otherwise deemed at higher risk for breast carcinogenesis. Participants were to be randomly assigned to receive either tamoxifen or raloxifene, with the principal end point being a reduction in the incidence of breast cancers.[94] V. Craig Jordan believes that on the basis of laboratory experiments, "one could predict that raloxifene and tamoxifen will not be completely cross-resistant. Raloxifene treatment to prevent osteoporosis could be considered after the appropriate course of adjuvant tamoxifen treatment for node-negative breast cancer."[95] While we are waiting for clinical trials to establish the validity of these hypotheses, we should be grateful for that very mature drug tamoxifen, whose properties we know so well. Cost-conscious consumers now have a choice between the famous brand product (Nolvadex) or a less expensive generic one.

AROMATASE INHIBITORS
Some Postmenopausal Strategies

However impractical aminoglutethimide had been as a second-line hormonal drug, its success in suppressing postmenopausal estrogen production spurred pharmaceutical companies to develop improved **"third-generation" aromatase inhibitors**. Taken orally, these new agents are largely free of short-term side effects. Aromatase inhibitors (AIs) have no role in the treatment of premenopausal patients or of ER-negative tumors. They are indicated only for **postmenopausal ER-positive patients**. By the year 2000 it seemed probable that they would prove superior to tamoxifen in certain subgroups of patients; in any event, they were already being aggressively promoted by their respective manufacturers. AIs act by a different mechanism from that found in anticancer SERMs like tamoxifen and toremifene.

SERMs act on the individual tumor cells by binding to the ER protein and blocking its stimulus to cellular division; they do not lower the level of estrogen in the blood. In contrast, AIs shut down postmenopausal estrogen production by disabling the enzyme **aromatase**, which is needed to convert adrenal androgens into estrone and estradiol. The new drugs are very effective. Paul E. Goss and Kathrin Strasser of Toronto's Princess Margaret Hospital point out that "peripheral aromatization in postmenopausal women is almost completely inhibited by third-generation inhibitors."[96] The fact that AIs prevent estrogenic stimulation of tumor cells explains why they quickly became the therapy of choice after tamoxifen failure. As we have seen, that failure most frequently occurs because tamoxifen has begun to provide an estrogenic stimulus to ER-positive breast cancer cells. The new AIs painlessly terminate the body's supply of estrogen; and since they do not share cross-resistance with tamoxifen, they may well achieve tumor regressions in tamoxifen-resistant disease if the cancer cells still remain estrogen dependent.

The earliest clinical trials involving the new aromatase inhibitors were conducted in metastatic breast cancer; they typically pitted a third-generation AI against Megace (megestrol acetate), the prevalent second-line drug of the 1980s and 1990s. In 1996 Aman U. Buzdar of Houston's M. D. Anderson Cancer Center and his international colleagues reported that **anastrozole**, "a potent and selective aromatase inhibitor," was as effective as Megace in postmenopausal breast cancer patients who had "progressed following tamoxifen treatment." Anastrozole caused more gastrointestinal disturbances than Megace, but seemed preferable because it "avoided the weight gain associated with megestrol acetate treatment."[97] In 1998 a double-blinded clinical trial reported that

letrozole was not only better tolerated than megestrol acetate, but achieved a "higher objective response rate" (24%) compared with the progestin (16%) in postmenopausal breast cancer patients "previously treated with antiestrogens."[98] **Exemestane**, a steroidal AI, has slightly different attributes from anastrozole and letrozole. A well-designed European trial randomized 769 postmenopausal patients with tamoxifen-resistant metastatic breast cancer to receive either exemestane (25 mg daily) or Megace (40 mg four times daily). The results published in 2000 indicated a definite but modest advantage for exemestane therapy. The "objective" (measurable) response rate was slightly higher in the exemestane group (15.0% versus 12.4% for Megace), as was the median "time to tumor progression" (20.3 weeks versus 16.6 weeks for Megace).[99]

Third-generation aromatase inhibitors have been a welcome addition to the breast cancer armamentarium. Oncologists soon learned to refer to these FDA-approved agents by their commercial names— **Arimidex** (AstraZeneca's brand of anastrozole tablets), **Femara** (Novartis Pharmaceuticals' brand of letrozole tablets), and **Aromasin** (Pfizer's brand of exemestane tablets). Of course, those early trials had also shown us that the new AIs were no more likely to achieve the long-term suppression of metastatic breast cancer than any other of our available pharmaceuticals. Consequently, we have been most concerned to learn about their utility in adjuvant therapy—that is, when they would be incorporated into hormonal regimens given after the initial surgery with a view to preventing local recurrences in a preserved breast, *de novo* tumors in the contralateral (opposite) breast, and distant metastases. The new AIs looked promising for these adjuvant applications because they were as convenient and as well-tolerated as tamoxifen but acted through an entirely different mechanism. Would not there be additional antitumor activity beyond that achievable by tamoxifen alone? These hopes were tempered by a concern that AIs, by sending estrogen levels plummeting, might eventually lead to an unacceptably high incidence of osteoporotic bone fractures. An emerging strategy addressed this concern by **sequential scheduling**. That is, begin the adjuvant hormonal therapy with two to three years of tamoxifen since this drug tends to preserve bone density—then switch to a potent estrogen-ablative AI before tamoxifen has any chance to evolve into an estrogenic agent for breast cancer cells. This type of sequential regimen seemed to offer an advantageous combination of possible osteoporosis prophylaxis and presumably enhanced antitumor activity.

Paul E. Goss of Princess Margaret Hospital headed a large clinical trial which randomized 5,187 postmenopausal breast cancer patients who had just completed "approximately five years of adjuvant tamoxifen therapy" to receive five years of subsequent adjuvant letrozole (Femara), or to take look-alike placebo tablets. An "interim analysis" after "a median follow-up of 2.4 years" appeared in the *New England Journal of Medicine* on November 6, 2003. "The estimated four-year disease-free survival rate," reported Dr. Goss and his colleagues, "was 93 percent in the letrozole group and 87 percent in the placebo group." Altogether there had been "207 local or metastatic recurrences of breast cancer or new primary cancers in the contralateral breast—75 in the letrozole group and 132 in the placebo group."[100] Of course, that 87% disease-free rate estimated for the placebo group still speaks well for the standard tamoxifen regiment. Did the long-term benefits of five more years on letrozole outweigh any possible long-term risks? Aman U. Buzdar wrote

the *Journal* to express his concern: "Goss et al present their results in a manner that could influence treatment decisions more strongly than is merited by the data provided." Dr. Buzdar observed that "two years of safety data" were not sufficient to define the risks of adjuvant letrozole "regarding fractures, osteoporosis, and cardiovascular events."[101]

The London oncologist R. Charles Coombes headed an international trial in which 4,742 postmenopausal breast cancer patients were randomly assigned to the standard five years of adjuvant tamoxifen, or to just "two to three years of tamoxifen therapy" before being switched to exemestane (Aromasin) "for the remainder of the five years of treatment." A preliminary report published in the *New England Journal of Medicine* on March 11, 2004, revealed an advantage in disease-free survival for the exemestane arm. There had been 33 local recurrences in the tamoxifen arm, but only 21 in the group switched over to exemestane. *De novo* tumorigenesis in the contralateral breast had occurred in 20 patients who were taking the standard tamoxifen regimen, but only in 9 patients who were taking sequential exemestane. Distant metastases had been detected in 174 tamoxifen patients and in 114 exemestane patients.[102] Some researchers believe that exemestane as a steroidal agent should do a better job of preserving postmenopausal bone mass than the other AIs; however, Dr. Coombes and his co-workers acknowledged that more fractures occurred in the exemestane arm (72 recorded) than in the tamoxifen arm (53 recorded).[103]

The ATAC Trial

In terms of its sheer size, the most impressive investigation of aromatase inhibition has been the London-based **ATAC trial**. The initials stand for **Arimidex, Tamoxifen,**

Alone or in Combination. This trial drew upon the resources of "381 centers in 21 countries"; it recruited 9,366 postmenopausal breast cancer patients who "had completed primary surgery" and "were candidates to receive hormonal adjuvant therapy." These patients were randomly assigned between three treatment arms—(1) the standard five years of adjuvant tamoxifen (20 mg daily), or (2) five years of adjuvant Arimidex (anastrozole, 1 mg daily), or (3) five years of both drugs taken concurrently. Begun in 1996, the ATAC trial has already given us some plausible answers regarding the use of AIs in the adjuvant setting. The trial's initial report, published in the *Lancet* in 2002, revealed that the combination of concurrent anastrozole and tamoxifen was not any more effective than tamoxifen alone in preventing tumor recurrences. Thus we now have good reason to believe that AIs should not be given at the same time as tamoxifen; but if we have to choose between one of the newer AIs and the venerable SERM, which drug should we give? That initial ATAC report at a median follow-up of 33.3 months revealed that anastrozole alone had slightly outperformed tamoxifen in disease-free survival—89.4% DFS in patients taking the potent AI as compared to 87.4% DFS in patients taking tamoxifen. While that's not much of a difference percentage-wise, there were more striking contrasts in performance between the two drugs. Anastrozole did a noticeably better job of suppressing *de novo* tumorigenesis in the contralateral breast—only 14 new tumors were detected in the anastrozole arm as compared to 33 tumors detected in the tamoxifen arm. But the venerable SERM did a better job of heading off bone fractures. Only 115 fractures occurred in the tamoxifen arm, while 183 were recorded in the anastrozole arm.[104] A second analysis of the ATAC results, done after a median follow-up of 47 months, appeared in 2003. Anastrozole still remained ahead in disease-free survival, 86.9% DFS as compared to 84.5% DFS in the tamoxifen arm. And once again this AI demonstrated its superior ability to suppress contralateral tumorigenesis—only 25 cancers detected as compared to 40 in the tamoxifen arm. But the drug's association with an increased rate of bone fractures also became more apparent. While only 137 fractures had been counted in the tamoxifen arm, 219 were recorded for the anastrozole arm.[105]

By December 2004 the ATAC collaborators were sufficiently satisfied with their results that they held a press conference at the San Antonio Breast Cancer Symposium and announced the superiority of anastrozole over tamoxifen as a first-line adjuvant treatment. This opinion was immediately and uncritically trumpeted in the newspapers and TV newscasts. The official ATAC report "after a median follow-up of 68 months" appeared in the *Lancet* on January 1, 2005. It repeated that enthusiastic endorsement of anastrozole as "the preferred initial treatment" of ER-positive postmenopausal breast cancer, but not all the data presented would seem to support a rush to this judgment. "Overall survival," the ATAC trialists conceded, "was similar for anastrozole and tamoxifen."[106] The fact that more distant metastases were detected in the tamoxifen arm (375 recorded) than in the anastrozole arm (324 recorded) suggested that a modest survival advantage favoring anastrozole would be eventually demonstrated—but the balance of benefits-to-risks in long-term anastrozole therapy needed to be defined by more comprehensive and more mature data.

We should remember that tamoxifen won universal acceptance as an adjuvant not because it was predictably curative, but because with hormonally-responsive invasive breast tumors, the balance of potential benefits clearly outweighed the known risks.

Of course, tamoxifen proponents managed to make the drug sound like the Fountain of Youth, and some trials produced data suggesting that it could reduce the incidence of cardiovascular disease. The <u>mature</u> <u>data</u> generated by NSABP Protocol P-1 showed us that tamoxifen does not protect against heart attacks. Unfortunately, we have no comparably mature data on the likely side effects of prolonged anastrozole therapy. The short-term findings from the ATAC trial published in the January 1, 2005, *Lancet* point toward superior antitumor activity, but otherwise present us with the enigma of disease substitution. Are the 24 fewer contralateral breast tumors and the 51 fewer distant metastases seen in the anastrozole arm worth the 103 additional fractures which were also recorded?

Whither Hormonal Therapy?

Recently there has been a momentary sighting of a fabulous creature more elusive than any unicorn. *Yes!*—there would seem to be **<u>a</u> <u>broad</u> <u>consensus</u>** that a third-generation aromatase inhibitor should be tried as salvage therapy after tamoxifen failure in postmenopausal ER-positive breast cancer. But perhaps that is the extent of the consensus—the mythic beast of our desiring has already vanished into the mist. We really do not know which of the three current AIs will eventually prove to be the most effective agent. Conceivably, there could be subtle differences in efficacy or tolerability between these drugs, and these differences might well dictate the choice of one drug rather than another. The principal investigators in the ATAC trial portray anastrozole as the preferred agent; but as all of them received financial support from the manufacturer of Arimidex tablets, perhaps their phraseology tends to be slightly rosier on that account

than warranted by the bare-bones data. We should be curious to see the results of future trials featuring letrozole (Femara) and exemestane (Aromasin) in the adjuvant setting.

As yet we do not know as much about the long-term consequences of aromatase inhibition as we know about the long-term consequences of tamoxifen therapy. Insofar as AIs are going to be prescribed as adjuvants for breast cancer patients who may be actually at greater risk of dying from cardiovascular disease or hip fracture, hard data on these consequences would be appropriate. One of tamoxifen's selling points has been that it confers a modest survival advantage which persists even years after therapy is ended. Will this also be true of the new AIs? Is there a survival advantage, how big is it, and how long does it persist?

For the time being, the wise oncologist should continue to look closely at the individual patient's overall state of health and personal circumstances as well as at her pathology report. A node-negative patient with a small "good-risk" tumor may well be better served by the traditional tamoxifen regimen, which—as far as we know—does not elevate the risk of fractures or heart attacks. Now that this drug is available in a generic version, it stands to be the most economical therapy. A family history of osteoporosis or disabling fractures should give us pause when considering aromatase inhibition. Some researchers have suggested that AIs could be taken concurrently with bisphosphonates, drugs known to preserve bone mass; but the efficacy of this strategy has not yet been demonstrated. Currently, the most logical candidates for adjuvant AI therapy would seem to be patients who are node-positive or otherwise deemed at some risk of developing systemic disease. Metastatic breast cancer has not been curable, and of course the dissemination of cancer cells to the bone marrow may rapidly lead to devastating fractures of the hip, femur, vertebrae, or other weight-bearing structures. With high-risk patients we would naturally be more concerned with quickly obtaining the maximum antitumor activity than with protecting against a gradual loss of bone density. Whether high-risk patients should be given anastrozole or some other AI as a single agent—or whether they should first be placed on tamoxifen and then later switched to an AI—are intriguing questions whose resolution will surely keep our clinical trial organizations busy for some years to come.

Chapter Twenty-three

Breast Cancer Chemotherapy

ytotoxic chemotherapy was first envisioned in the 1890s by the Berlin physician Paul Ehrlich. In an era when many people died of bacterial infections, Ehrlich dreamed of "magic bullets"—that is, of potent chemicals which could be injected into the body to destroy the culprit microorganisms. He himself pioneered the use of Salvarsan, an unpleasant arsenical compound which became the first effective treatment for syphilis. Subsequent pharmacologists developed antimicrobial agents which far exceeded Ehrlich's expectations, notably the sulfa drugs of the 1930s and the mold-derived antibiotics of the 1940s (penicillin, streptomycin, aureomycin, and terramycin). These products truly merited the nickname **wonder drugs**. Since they were much more toxic to the infectious organisms than to the human host, they led to seemingly miraculous cures. Patients dying from overwhelming septicemia would be rescued by a single injection; a day or two later they could walk out of the hospital.

Unfortunately, anyone who expects that cancer chemotherapy can duplicate the aforementioned miracles will be terribly disappointed. The treatment tends to be complex and prolonged. The drugs used are toxic—the best we can hope for is that they will prove more toxic to the genetically unstable cancer cells than to normal cells, but this is not always the case. Some commonplace tumors—notably those arising in the brain, kidneys, liver, pancreas, and prostate—have proven so resistant to cytotoxic chemotherapy that it is not often attempted. While our current regimens may induce remissions in disseminated lung or ovarian malignancies, they are not curative and do not prevent an eventual recurrence. Breast cancer patients are usually in a better position than if they had been diagnosed with one of the other solid tumors; most of them do not need cytotoxic chemotherapy, and those who do need it generally stand to benefit from it. But breast cancer chemotherapy is a perpetually evolving field fraught with uncertainties and unanswered questions. Of the several standard regimens and the numerous variations on them, we cannot truthfully describe any one as "the best" or as "predictably curative." And while we have learned what tumor characteristics point toward an elevated risk for metastatic dissemination, we have no convenient assays for predicting the effect of chemotherapy on individual patients. These deficiencies must be chalked up to biological complexity rather than to a lack of initiative; there has been no shortage of effort. The present chapter briefly details the progress we have made.

Leukemia Leads the Way

Penicillin and the sulfa drugs silenced those skeptics who doubted that medicines to cure systemic bacterial infections could ever be developed. But skepticism about the prospects for cancer chemotherapy remained pervasive. Why, you might as well try to design a medication which would dissolve one ear while leaving the other untouched! Prior to the Second World War, surgeons were the only cancer doctors around, though they might be aided on occasion by radiologists. Nobody contemplated treating solid tumors with drugs—the surgeons had to cut them out, and that was about all you could do. Cancer chemotherapy thus evolved from attempts to forestall the relentless and often terribly rapid progress of the **hematologic malignancies**—that is, the **leukemias and lymphomas**. There was virtually no role for surgery in these cancers, and not much of a role for radiotherapy, because the malignant white blood cells were almost always disseminated throughout the body at presentation. Since it was impossible to excise these multitudinous cells and not practical to irradiate them, a few researchers started to wonder whether drugs might not be designed which would stymie their reproduction. Indeed, during the First World War a synthetic chemical had been introduced which did a splendid job of destroying white blood cells: it was **mustard gas**. Autopsies performed on soldiers killed by German gas attacks revealed that they had few remaining white cells. Mustard gas was an **alkylating agent**—the chemical bound avidly to the bases of DNA, interfering with chromosomal replication. During the 1930s researchers discovered that **nitrogen mustard**, another alkylating compound derived from the mustard plant, could shrink tumors in mice. In 1942 a team at Yale University gave this experimental drug to a 48-year-old man with a lymphoma so advanced that his trachea (windpipe) was virtually closed shut by tumor masses. Within a week the tumors receded, and the patient could breathe again. Unfortunately, the malignant masses grew back whenever the nitrogen mustard injections were discontinued; eventually they ceased to respond to the drug, and the patient died.[1] This famous Yale experiment illustrated a pattern which remains distressingly familiar in cancer chemotherapy—the dramatic remission followed by the development of irremediable drug resistance.

In the late 1940s Sidney Farber and his colleagues at the Boston Children's Hospital turned their attention to the most poignant of the hematologic malignancies, those acute leukemias which killed children and adolescents with devastating rapidity.[2] There had never been a treatment for these disorders; they were always fatal. **Acute lymphoblastic leukemia** (ALL), the most prevalent variety, originates from a single immature lymphocyte (or "blast") which has suffered a genetic mutation causing it to multiply uncontrollably. Soon the malignant "clones" (the leukemic cells) overrun the bone marrow and saturate the peripheral blood. At this point the body's production of normal blood cells begins to shut down, and the patient's parents become alarmed at the symptoms they see. An affected child will suddenly appear listless and lethargic: this is due to profound anemia—there are not enough red blood cells carrying oxygen to the tissues. And the child's body gets covered with purplish bruises: this is due to thrombocytopenia—there are not enough platelets to seal up and repair the subcutaneous blood vessels which start leaking after bumps and falls. Before Sidney Farber came along, children with ALL and other acute hematologic malignancies usually did not live more than a few weeks after their diagnosis. They would typically die from hemorrhaging in the brain (since they had no platelets), or from massive infections (since those nonfunctional leukemic cells had also supplanted the normal white cells which could fight off invading bacteria and viruses). Dr. Farber and his co-workers extended the life expectancies of these children with a new drug called **aminopterin**; it is remembered as the first **antimetabolite** to be used in cancer medicine. More specifically, aminopterin was a **folic acid antagonist**—its molecular structure closely resembled that of folic acid, an essential metabolite which cells need to synthesize DNA. A leukemic cell engaged in DNA synthesis during the S-phase of the cell cycle would thus absorb aminopterin in lieu of folic acid; but this particular "building block" turned out to be a pharmacological monkey wrench which stopped cellular reproduction altogether. By 1950 the Farber team and other cancer specialists were using an improved folic acid antagonist to induce remission in acute leukemia. That drug, initially called amethopterin, later became known as **methotrexate**; it still remains an important component of many cytotoxic regimens.

Additional drugs soon proved valuable. In 1951 researchers at a pharmaceutical company (Burroughs Wellcome) synthesized an antimetabolite specifically designed to interfere with leukemic cells: it was **6-mercaptopurine**, called **6-MP** for short. Like aminopterin and methotrexate, this drug was a monkey wrench disguised as a DNA building block; but since it interfered with a cell's use of the purines (guanine and adenine) rather than with its use of folic acid, it was not cross-resistant to the first two drugs. In other words, a cancer cell which proved resistant to aminopterin and methotrexate might well respond to 6-MP because this drug relied on a different mechanism for its cytotoxicity. The steroid **prednisone** seemed

to prolong those remissions induced by the several antimetabolites; since the early 1950s this convenient oral drug has been routinely given to leukemia patients. In the late 1950s **vincristine**, a vinca alkaloid derived from the periwinkle plant, became available. This drug interferes with mitosis (the act of cellular division), damaging the fibrous spindle which separates the two sets of chromosomes into two identical daughter cells.

The induction of complete remissions in childhood leukemia soon became fairly common. Physicians were gratified to find that the leukemic cells seemed to have vanished from blood samples and bone marrow biopsies. The problem was that these apparent cures were not permanent. After a few months or years the disease recurred, and this time the drugs did not work.

Combination Chemotherapy:
How They Cured Leukemia

By 1960 the pharmaceutical ingredients to cure acute lymphoblastic leukemia were on hand, but as yet nobody had a recipe for success. Obviously, it was not enough to kill 99.999% of the leukemic cells. If just one malignant clone remained, the disease would recur. Therefore all the cells had to be killed, and as quickly as possible, before drug resistance developed. Since several drugs had pronounced activity against ALL but no single agent could eradicate the disease, why not combine several agents to create a more potent cytotoxic cocktail? That drug combination ought to be delivered rapidly and at full strength, in much the same way as a prize fighter might combine a quick succession of powerful punches to kayo his opponent when no single blow would suffice.

Credit for the first curative leukemia regimens must be liberally assigned to the researchers at the National Cancer Institute. The campus of the National Institutes of Health at Bethesda, Maryland, offered unparalleled facilities for medical research; the most visible landmark was a large modern hospital known as the Clinical Center (or simply "Building 10"), which opened in 1953. But the people who came to Bethesda (physicians, patients, scientists) were more important than the imposing structures. In 1954 the NCI acquired the services of C. Gordon Zubrod as the Clinical Director who supervised its treatment programs. A gifted administrator as well as a compassionate physician, Zubrod entertained the novel notion that leukemia might someday be cured; to this end he established a separate Leukemia Service at the Clinical Center. Two young doctors whom Zubrod enlisted for the NCI's Leukemia Service were Emil ("Tom") Frei and Emil J. ("Jay") Freireich. The chemotherapeutic principles which this NCI trio (Zubrod, Frei, and Freireich) formulated to cure leukemia merit our attention because they would soon be applied to breast cancer and other solid tumors. The first principle is **the combination of non-cross-resistant agents**, amply illustrated by the **VAMP regimen** introduced in 1962. The acronym stands for <u>v</u>incristine, <u>a</u>methopterin (methotrexate), <u>m</u>ercaptopurine (6-MP), and <u>p</u>rednisone. These four drugs have different mechanisms for killing cancer cells and different dose-limiting side effects. Thus, if a leukemic cell should prove resistant to one drug, the odds are still good that it will be susceptible to another VAMP agent which uses a different means of attack. Because the side effects of each drug are different, there are no overlapping toxicities which would require a reduction in dose levels—all the drugs can therefore be given at a therapeutic dosage. Dr. Freireich later explained that the NCI team decided to give VAMP "in combination" because when these leukemia drugs

were given sequentially, "those patients who failed to respond to the first drug often died before they had the opportunity to get the second." VAMP produced some impressive results. "We got all the patients into remission," Freireich remembered: "40 or 50 percent were in remission with just a single course of chemotherapy, and when we gave them a second course, almost all of them were."[3]

In the long search for a curative leukemia regimen, VAMP did not mark the end of the journey, but it was a light at the end of the tunnel. VAMP is also noteworthy as an illustration of our second fundamental principle of cancer chemotherapy—**cyclical treatments**. The drugs in VAMP worked well on rapidly dividing leukemic cells, with methotrexate and 6-MP targeting those in S-phase, and vincristine disrupting those in the act of mitosis. Thus a single treatment with this drug combination often achieved a clinical remission—that is, the apparent disappearance of the leukemic clones from the bloodstream. But one treatment could not obtain a cure, because not all the malignant cells happened to be dividing at the time the drugs were administered. A few cells always survived that first attack, which faded away as soon as the drugs were cleared from the body. The NCI team sought to solve this problem by giving repeated cycles of VAMP; they reasoned that sooner or later the drugs would catch the surviving cells in S-phase or undergoing mitosis. With each cycle there would be fewer and fewer leukemic cells in the body, until finally there were none; then the patient would be cured. For our purposes **a cycle** may be defined as a unit of time (so many calendar days) encompassing both the administration of the cytotoxic drugs and an ensuing rest period without treatment. That rest period is scheduled to allow the patient's bone marrow (the organ responsible for producing blood cells) and any other affected organs to recover from the drug toxicities. A cycle of VAMP was about three weeks long, with the drugs being given for ten days "separated by ten-day or longer intervals of recovery." The original regimen called for one or two cycles to achieve remission, followed by five or more additional cycles administered for "consolidation"—that is, to be sure of destroying any remaining leukemic cells.[4]

No medical historian can tell us the exact year in which acute lymphoblastic leukemia became curable. The cure did not come with a single dramatic breakthrough, but rather with a continual series of small improvements. Supportive care got much better, allowing acutely ill children to live long enough to receive the chemotherapy. Dr. Freireich and his NCI co-workers discovered that they could control the constant hemorrhaging of advanced ALL by giving their patients transfusions of platelets. Antibiotics helped to banish the specter of bacterial infections. The chances of long-term survival increased exponentially when we finally realized that most treatment failures were caused by residual leukemic cells lingering in the central nervous system, an anatomic location which the drugs did not adequately penetrate. Methotrexate was injected directly into the cerebrospinal fluid to solve this problem—patients deemed at high risk of relapse might also be given cranial irradiation. Our chemotherapy regimens became much more effective through the addition of several new drugs, notably cytosine arabinoside (Ara-C) and the potent anthracycline antibiotics doxorubicin (Adriamycin) and daunorubicin.

During the late 1960s the remissions being induced in ALL patients started to last much longer; and at some point—nobody knows exactly when—they became cures! Children who had been treated as toddlers became teenagers, became adults, then got married and had children of their own! Readers who wish more information on this complex miracle may enjoy John Laszlo's book *The Cure of Childhood Leukemia*. As of 1995, Dr. Laszlo informs us, 75% to 80% of the children diagnosed with ALL were being cured: "Treatment now included seven or eight agents, VAMP plus asparaginase, daunorubicin, cytosine arabinoside or others."[5] Children diagnosed with **acute myelogenous leukemia** (a less common variety) usually obtained remissions, but the cure rate was not nearly so impressive, with the majority of patients eventually suffering disease progression. Chemotherapy often extended survival in the leukemias and lymphomas (usually chronic) which afflicted adults; but only **allogeneic bone marrow transplantation**—that is, the replacement of the patient's diseased blood cells with someone else's— offered the promise of cure. Notwithstanding these shortfalls, the decisive victory over the prevalent juvenile leukemia gave a tremendous boost to the proponents of cancer chemotherapy. "The cure of childhood leukemia indicated that it can be done," Emil Frei recalled in 1999. "If in childhood leukemia, why not lung cancer?"[6]

Curing *Exceptional* Tumors

The first attempt to treat a disseminated solid tumor with chemotherapy achieved a wonderful success which can only be described as "exceptional." The rare cancer involved, **choriocarcinoma**, is not at all typical of adult tumors; it arises from the placenta during pregnancy. Of course, the malignant choriocarcinoma cells retain certain characteristics of normal placental cells, including an extremely rapid rate of multiplication and the ability to induce angiogenesis (blood vessel formation) in the surrounding tissues.

In the days before chemotherapy, these characteristics translated into terribly aggressive metastases and early death. By the mid-1950s, however, they suggested a probable sensitivity to methotrexate, that antimetabolite which works so well on cancer cells in the S-phase. In late 1955 and early 1956 Min Chiu Li, an endocrinologist at the National Cancer Institute, demonstrated that methotrexate given directly into the bloodstream could rescue even those choriocarcinoma patients who were dying from extensive pulmonary (lung) metastases. The drug went right to the well-vascularized tumor masses and started to shrink them. Were these impressive remissions really cures? Dr. Li knew that choriocarcinoma cells (like the placenta) secrete abundant quantities of the pregnancy-sustaining hormone called **human chorionic gonadotropin** (hCG); and he soon surmised that the presence or absence of hCG in a patient's urine indicated whether or not choriocarcinoma cells remained active in her body. If the hCG assay was positive, he simply gave intermittent doses of intravenous methotrexate until the reading turned negative; this usually meant that the patient was cured. In most cases she was!

Dr. Li died in 1980; no doubt we would remember him as "the man who cured cancer" if choriocarcinoma had not been such an exception to the rule. The more common cancers, both solid and hematologic, do not display such an exquisite sensitivity to a single agent, or offer such broad vascular avenues into metastatic deposits, or feature a convenient and reliable marker like hCG. The NCI researcher who gathered the most laurels for "curing cancer" was Vincent T. DeVita, Jr., who headed the team which developed the famous **MOPP regimen for advanced Hodgkin's disease**. This strange malignancy had been baffling physicians ever since that versatile Englishman Thomas Hodgkin described its clinical symptoms in 1832. Hodgkin's disease is classified as a lymphoma because its large distinctive cells—called **Reed-Sternberg cells** after two pathologists who studied them—are derived from a transformed lymphocyte of B-cell lineage.[8] But Hodgkin's behaves more like a solid tumor than the other hematologic malignancies. The disease usually begins locally in a single lymph node, often one in the chest (above the diaphragm); the malignant cells then spread contiguously to adjacent lymph nodes. Later the visceral organs (e.g., the liver) and the bone marrow are affected. Early-stage Hodgkin's, limited to a few lymph nodes in the same area, has long been curable by a short course of radiation therapy. But advanced Hodgkin's, with disease disseminated to several nodal chains, to the liver, or to the bone marrow, was previously regarded as untreatable. Most patients have advanced disease at the time of their diagnosis. Prior to the 1970s almost all patients with disseminated Hodgkin's died; since this disease tends to afflict young adults between the ages of 20 and 30, many lives were cut short.

The MOPP regimen that Dr. DeVita and his NCI colleagues introduced in August 1964 was modeled after VAMP—it featured a combination of four non-cross-resistant agents to be delivered at full doses in repetitive cycles. The acronym stands for the alkylating agent mechlorethamine (technical name for nitrogen mustard), Oncovin (a brand name for vincristine), and the oral drugs procarbazine and prednisone. Like many later regimens, MOPP called for 28-day cycles. Most patients in the NCI's initial trial achieved remission after the first or second cycle; but treatment was continued for another five or six cycles, with a view to eradicating every malignant cell. "The cyclic use of combination chemotherapy for six months," DeVita and his associates recalled, "exceeded the duration of any prior treatment of adult tumors." In 1970 the NCI team reported that 81% of the advanced Hodgkin's patients treated with MOPP had achieved complete remission (no sign of disease). Most of these remissions eventually proved to be cures; relapses more than four years after the completion of treatment were uncommon. In 1993 DeVita et al gave the results of a twenty-year follow-up on the NCI trial: "Of those patients obtaining complete remissions, 64% remain continuously disease-free."[9]

During the 1980s MOPP was often supplemented or replaced with the newer regimen **ABVD** (Adriamycin, bleomycin, vinblastine, dacarbazine). Some oncologists preferred to alternate the two regimens, giving MOPP one cycle and ABVD the next; others chose to integrate the drugs into a single hybrid regimen designated with the acronym **MOPP/ABV**. The death rate from Hodgkin's plummeted; now patients who relapsed after one regimen might still be rescued by salvage chemotherapy with a second regimen. In 1991 the radiation oncologist Samuel Hellman summed up this therapeutic revolution: "A disease that was curable perhaps 10% or 15% of the time thirty years ago is now being cured 75% or 80% of the time."[10]

The next demonstration of the curative potential of cytotoxic chemotherapy was made possible by a single drug, a salt of the metal platinum called **cisdiamminedichloroplatinum**. That ponderous chemical moniker soon got shortened to **cisplatin**—the prevalent brand name **Platinol** (Bristol-Myers) may also be used. Approved by the Food and Drug Administration in 1978, cisplatin works much like the traditional alkylating agents, by binding to the DNA of actively dividing cells. Oncologists quickly learned to appreciate this drug's antitumor activity and to fear its toxicity. The nausea and vomiting associated with cisplatin therapy are proverbial. The kidneys, principally responsible for clearing the drug from the body, start to suffer subtle but irreparable damage with repeated exposures to it. Fortunately, just a little bit of cisplatin will suffice to cure **germ-cell tumors**—that is, those ovarian and testicular cancers which arise in the cellular forerunners of the ova or sperm. Ovarian germ-cell tumors are relatively rare, occurring mainly in young premenopausal women; they need to be distinguished from the more common epithelial ovarian tumors, which tend to afflict postmenopausal women and which cannot be easily eradicated once they have spread throughout the abdomen. But a very large majority of testicular tumors (about 95%) are of germ-cell origin; over 7,000 American men are diagnosed with these germ-cell malignancies each year.[11]

Before cisplatin-based chemotherapy became available, testicular tumors were the principal cause of cancer deaths in young men between the ages of 15 and 35. These fast-growing malignancies usually have metastasized by the time they are diagnosed; patients often present with grossly enlarged abdominal lymph nodes and multiple tumor nodules in the lungs. In the early 1970s disseminated testicular cancer was always fatal, but by the mid-1980s it became apparent that three or four cycles of **BEP** (bleomycin, etoposide, Platinol) could cure even advanced cases. The same regimen worked equally well against germ-cell ovarian tumors.[12] Those testicular patients who experienced disease progression after BEP might still be rescued with the slightly more toxic **VIP** (vinblastine, ifosfamide, Platinol). In testicular cancer as in Hodgkin's disease, salvage chemotherapy offered a second chance at survival. By the 1990s over 98% of testicular patients with early-stage disease were being cured; amazingly, so were over 80% of the patients with distant metastases.[13]

Optimistic oncologists like to cite testicular cancer as evidence that chemotherapy ought to be able to eradicate other solid tumors, even after widespread systemic dissemination. More cautious oncologists resist this conclusion: they will argue that the cells of the indisputably curable cancers—the transformed placental cells of choriocarcinoma, the strange Reed-Sternberg cells of Hodgkin's, and the malignant germ-cell precursors—are not comparable to the differentiated somatic cells which give rise to breast, prostate, or colon cancers. One obvious difference between the routinely curable malignancies and the other less susceptible tumors has to do with **doubling time**—that is, the length of time it takes for a cancer cell to reproduce itself. We are indebted to the English oncologist C. J. Williams for some representative statistics. Choriocarcinoma, Dr. Williams informs us, has a doubling time of 1.5 days—Hodgkin's disease, 3 to 4 days—and testicular cancer, 5 to 6 days. These rates stand in sharp contrast to the doubling time of a colon cancer cell, which is 80 days.[14] We cannot generalize about breast cancer cells in this matter: some of them might have as short a doubling time as testicular cancer cells, while others could be as slow as colon cancer cells. Needless to say, we need to know whether the individual breast tumor is a tortoise or a hare before prescribing any systemic therapy. The tortoise variety of breast tumor will probably prove unresponsive to S-phase-specific agents like methotrexate and, indeed, to most other cytotoxic drugs.

The Early NSABP Trials

By the mid-1950s researchers at the National Cancer Institute were beginning to wonder whether nitrogen mustard or methotrexate could alter the natural history of breast cancers. Those obligatory preclinical studies involving cancer cells grown in Petri dishes or injected into immunodeficient mice had already suggested that breast tumors might be vulnerable to cytotoxic agents. The fledgling **National Surgical Adjuvant Breast and Bowel Project**, begun in 1957, was given the task of generating data on human subjects. Its first two trials sought to evaluate the potential of "perioperative" adjuvant therapy: the drugs were to be administered immediately after surgery, before the patients left the hospital. Between 1958 and 1961 the NSABP randomly assigned 826 breast cancer patients to radical mastectomy alone or to radical mastectomy followed by intravenous **thiotepa** (an alkylating agent related to nitrogen mustard) "on each of the first two postoperative days." The only patients who benefited from this little experiment were premenopausal women with substantial nodal involvement (four or more positive axillary nodes)—after five years of follow-up they had "a 33 percent greater survival rate" than comparable patients in the control group. A second trial begun in the early 1960s randomized 1,725 mastectomy patients to three consecutive days of intravenous thiotepa or to four consecutive days of intravenous **fluorouracil** (5-FU) or to a placebo. As in the first NSABP trial, those high-risk premenopausal patients (four or more positive nodes) benefited from thiotepa, having 21% fewer recurrences than comparable patients in the placebo group. But the patients assigned to 5-FU did not seem to benefit, and they suffered undesirable side effects. The NSABP's chairman Bernard Fisher was forced to characterize this trial's results as "disappointing."[15]

The NSABP took a different tack in its third trial, Protocol B-05, which looked at the potential of prolonged therapy with a convenient oral drug, **L-phenylalanine mustard**. This was an alkylating agent popularly known as **L-PAM**. Between 1972 and 1974 the NSABP assigned 269 node-positive mastectomy patients to two years of L-PAM or to a placebo. Adjuvant therapy was commenced "no sooner than two weeks and not later than four weeks after operation." Patients took an L-PAM pill or a placebo tablet at bedtime, "for five consecutive days every six weeks." The *New England Journal of Medicine* published the NSABP's report on this trial on January 16, 1975. Premenopausal patients given the drug appeared to benefit, regardless of whether they had limited nodal involvement (one to three positive nodes) or extensive nodal involvement (four or more positive nodes). Only 3% of the premenopausal patients taking L-PAM pills experienced a recurrence during the brief follow-up period, but 30% of the premenopausal patients taking placebo tablets did so. At the very least, L-PAM was helping to prolong disease-free survival in these younger women.[16]

While the early NSABP trials now look naive, we must remember that they were designed at a time when nobody had any experience with adjuvant chemotherapy for breast cancer. Dr. Fisher and his colleagues proceeded cautiously because they really did not know if their patients would benefit. Accordingly, they chose mild single-agent regimens—just a little chemo given in the most convenient fashion, either during that initial hospitalization for the mastectomy or as an intermittent bedtime pill. Yet the three trials clearly demonstrated that even these mere dabs of chemo could benefit premenopausal patients whose nodal status bespoke occult micrometastases. Since the postmenopausal patients in these trials did not appear to benefit significantly, the NSABP team took pains to dismiss any suspicions that the premenopausal benefit was mediated solely by ovarian suppression—i.e., that the alkylating agents had shut down the ovaries, and that this hormonal effect explained the observed benefits. In Protocol B-05, Fisher et al pointed out, the premenopausal patients under age 40 getting L-PAM typically maintained ovarian function—yet this subgroup benefited even more than the premenopausal patients between 40 and 49 getting the drug, who usually lost ovarian function.[17] Obviously, the L-PAM had been killing the disseminated cancer cells outright, apart from any indirect endocrine effects it might have had on them.

Adjuvant CMF
The Milan Trial

Audacity gathers more laurels than caution. Erring on the side of caution, those early NSABP trials were not to foreshadow subsequent trends in breast cancer medicine. The laurels went to Gianni Bonadonna and his colleagues at Milan's *Instituto Nazionale Tumori*, who convincingly demonstrated that rigorous combination chemotherapy can alter the natural history of breast malignancies. The Milan team elaborated on prior American accomplishments, taking hints from the NCI researchers who had developed the VAMP regimen for childhood leukemia and the MOPP regimen for Hodgkin's disease. The combination of drugs the Italians adopted—cyclophosphamide, methotrexate, and fluorouracil—had originally been advocated in the late 1960s by Richard Cooper, an American oncologist who also favored the addition of vincristine and prednisone. In the early 1970s George P. Canellos, Vincent T. DeVita, Jr., and other NCI oncologists had used a cyclical CMF regimen to treat metastatic breast cancer. Dr. Bonadonna and his colleagues were to prove the worth of this regimen in the adjuvant setting.

Between 1973 and 1975 the Milan team randomly assigned 391 node-positive breast cancer patients, all of whom had previously undergone mastectomy, to receive no further treatment or to receive twelve cycles of the regimen now known as **classical CMF**. The cornerstone drug in this regimen was the synthetic alkylating agent **cyclophosphamide**, which can kill metabolically active cancer cells even if they are not in S-phase or undergoing mitosis. Introduced in the late 1950s, cyclophosphamide quickly became one of the most widely used cytotoxic agents because its gastrointestinal side effects were relatively mild and because it caused only modest bone marrow (blood cell) suppression. This drug can be given intravenously (to achieve high exposure to it during a short period), or taken orally in convenient tablet form (to achieve sustained exposure over several weeks). The Bristol-Myers brand name **Cytoxan** is also used for cyclophosphamide, which acts through a different mechanism from—and is non-cross-resistant to—the S-phase-specific antimetabolites **methotrexate** and **fluorouracil**. In the classical (or standard) CMF regimen which Dr. Bonadonna and his colleagues began to use in 1973, patients took daily cyclophosphamide tablets during the first two weeks (days 1 through 14) of a 28-day cycle; and they received intravenous methotrexate and fluorouracil on days 1 and 8. No treatment was given during the last two weeks (days 15 through 28), thus allowing for bone marrow recovery.

The publication of the initial results from the Milan trial was a landmark event which marked the beginning of widespread adjuvant chemotherapy for early-stage breast cancer. In the *New England Journal of Medicine* for February 19, 1976, Bonadonna et al reported that after a 27-month follow-up the patients in their untreated control group

had a recurrence rate more than four times that of the patients who received CMF. There was no subgroup in the CMF arm which failed to benefit; and in contrast to those early NSABP trials, the postmenopausal patients seemed to benefit as much as the premenopausal ones. The relapse rates for premenopausal patients were 24.3% in the control group and 5.2% in the CMF arm. For postmenopausal patients the rates were almost identical—23.7% for the controls and 5.3% for the CMF arm. What Bonadonna et al had to say about the regimen's toxicity was also encouraging. True, most CMF patients experienced "various degrees of nausea and vomiting within a few hours of the intravenous drug administration." And the CMF patients tended to suffer "abdominal disturbance" and "loss of appetite" caused by the cyclophosphamide tablets, so much so that about a third of them wanted to discontinue the drug and had to be "encouraged to take it regularly." But by and large the gastrointestinal side effects were not disabling: "Most working women continued to work during the entire period of chemotherapy." Alopecia (hair loss) was moderate: "The loss of hair usually started after the first cycle and in most cases stopped after the fifth to the sixth cycle. In some patients we noticed a regrowth of hair before the end of therapy."[18]

The impact of the Milan report on the *Journal*'s readers and on the news media was greatly enhanced by an accompanying editorial written by James F. Holland, the long-time chairman of Acute Leukemia Group B, a task force of physicians who were struggling to improve the survival rates in childhood leukemia. Dr. Holland already knew that a proper combination of cytotoxic drugs could cure juvenile leukemia, and he was understandably predisposed to welcome evidence that chemotherapy could cure other forms of malignancy. Praising the Milan report as "a work of monumental importance," he pointed out that most node-positive breast cancers are disseminated at presentation and thus not curable by surgery. If chemotherapy is to be administered, it should be given while the tumor burden is still small and the patient "better able to withstand the drug effects," rather than waiting on the appearance of metastatic disease. "The CMF treatment," Dr. Holland observed, "has produced results nothing short of spectacular." These results are "consistent with cellular cure in at least a portion of the cases."[19] Did somebody actually use that word cure?

Ironing Out the Wrinkles

Gianni Bonadonna and his colleagues maintained a conscientious follow-up on their patients. After five years they noticed that the postmenopausal CMF patients, who had initially enjoyed a distinct advantage in disease-free survival (DFS), were starting to experience more recurrences. Bonadonna et al reviewed their records from the trial, looking for a plausible explanation. In 1981 they published a second report in the *New England Journal of Medicine*, explaining that "CMF was useful only when given in a full or nearly full dose." Overall, those CMF patients who received at least 85% of the planned dose "had a five-year relapse-free survival of 77 percent, as compared with 45 percent for patients treated only with radical mastectomy." But those CMF patients who received less than 65% of the planned dose had a five-year DFS of 48%, only 3% better than the control group. And most of the CMF patients receiving reduced doses were postmenopausal—the Milan investigators had intentionally given the trial's older women lower doses of methotrexate and fluorouracil. The level of exposure to

cyclophosphamide was deemed especially important, because the response of cancer cells to this agent "decreases exponentially as the dose decreases." Cyclophosphamide being administered by mouth, "peak drug levels were never very high. Another factor that could have reduced exposure is the lack of compliance that was observed repeatedly, particularly in elderly women."[20]

The Milan team's 1981 reanalysis of their data provided us with one of the few self-evident truths in breast cancer chemotherapy. Viz., if <u>chemo is to be given at all, it should be given at optimal dose levels</u>. "Menopausal status itself," Dr. Bonadonna and his colleagues concluded, "should probably no longer be regarded as an important prognostic factor."[21] Another result from the reanalysis was a modification to the CMF regimen—henceforth the Milan team would give cyclophosphamide intravenously so as to be sure of obtaining adequate dose levels. Some American oncologists adopted this revision, while others stayed with classic CMF. Our clinical trials have not established whether the intravenous administration of cyclophosphamide is more efficacious than the convenient tablets, though many oncologists have definite opinions on this matter.

One modification to classic CMF did meet with almost unanimous acceptance—**the number of cycles was reduced from twelve to six**. In September 1975 the Milan trial began randomizing its newly accrued node-positive patients to receive six CMF cycles or to receive twelve. The five-year results published in 1983 revealed apparent advantages for those patients whose treatment stopped upon completion of the sixth cycle. Their disease-free and overall survival rates were 65.6% and 76.9% respectively, as compared with 59% (DFS) and 72.7% (OS) for those patients who received twelve CMF cycles.[22] With breast cancer chemotherapy, more is not necessarily better—any benefits are likely to be achieved with the first few cycles.

Would three CMF cycles do as well as six? A large European trial attempted to answer this question, randomly assigning 1,554 node-positive breast cancer patients to three cycles of classic CMF or to six. The five-year results published in 1996 were mixed. Patients under age 40 fared better if given six cycles—DFS was 49% on six cycles, only 37% on three—but the patients over age 40 ran neck and neck, DFS being 60% for those getting six cycles and 61% for those getting three. The European investigators concluded that "three courses of adjuvant CMF are not sufficient in younger women and in patients with ER-negative primary tumors."[23]

Some Skeptical Reactions
(And the Reasons for Them)

For all practical purposes, the Milan CMF trial of the 1970s was the last trial involving node-positive breast cancer patients which pitted adjuvant chemotherapy against no further postsurgical treatment. By the early 1980s the proposition that node-positive patients benefit from systemic therapy had become an entrenched dogma, but even some professional oncologists wondered whether there should not have been more clinical trials featuring untreated control groups. Patient activists and physicians in other specialties (e.g., surgery) were often publicly skeptical about this rush to embrace chemotherapy. No one could have been more articulate or more outspoken in protest than the writer Rose Kushner, who feared that cytotoxic cocktails would amount to **"a new Halsted"**—viz., an excessively rigorous treatment which might benefit the few, but

which would be indiscriminately prescribed for the many. Writing in 1984, Kushner argued that "the media blitz" following the publication of the Milan results had discouraged impartial evaluations of these emerging strategies: "It took almost a century to abandon the Halsted radical, but fewer than five years to embrace adjuvant chemotherapy. Doctors feared malpractice suits if they did not refer all stage II breast cancer patients for such state-of-the-art treatment."[24] In 1986 the public health physicians John C. Bailar III and Elaine M. Smith hurled a weighty gauntlet into the oncologists' camp, publishing a skeptical review entitled **"Progress Against Cancer?"** in the *New England Journal of Medicine*. Doctors Bailar and Smith saw very little in the way of meaningful progress. Current treatments have not reduced the mortality rates for most malignancies, they argued; consequently more attention should be paid to instituting good preventive measures instead of devising marginally effective therapies. Breast cancer was their case in point: "There has been no apparent change in mortality since 1950."[25] These opinions elicited heated replies from Vincent T. DeVita, Jr., and other oncologists, who intimated that Bailar and Smith were using outdated statistics. Not so, retorted the public health duo: "Major improvements in survival should be clearly visible in the data now available; they are not there."[26]

In truth, any significant effect that adjuvant chemotherapy might have on breast cancer survival rates cannot be plausibly assessed with short-term follow-up. We need a decade or two for this assessment. The reasons for this will become clearer if we briefly contrast acute lymphoblastic leukemia (ALL) with those tumors arising from the mammary gland. With the former malignancy we know that sophisticated multidrug regimens usually prove curative;

but with the various and sundry breast malignancies, systemic therapy amounts to a shot in the dark. ALL cells are clonal, and they presumably share the same degree of sensitivity to chemo. The cells from any individual breast tumor are more likely to be heterogeneous—thus the fact that some cells may be susceptible to chemo is no guarantee that others will be so. ALL cells will be found swimming in the bloodstream or in the cerebrospinal fluid; therefore any drugs given intravenously or intrathecally (put in the cerebrospinal fluid) stand an excellent chance of coming into contact with them. With early-stage breast tumors, we typically cannot determine the extent of dissemination beyond the regional lymph nodes—there may be cancer cells elsewhere in the body, but we really do not know where they could be hiding. Intravenous drugs would readily contact any breast cancer cells found swimming in the bloodstream or lurking in the bone marrow, but any tumor cells which had sequestered themselves in soft tissues like the liver or lungs could be relatively inaccessible. Tumor metastases, even if only a few millimeters in diameter, may have an avascular core containing poorly oxygenated cancer cells which are living in a state of suspended animation and which are highly resistant to cytotoxic agents. We cannot be sure that our drugs will reach these isolated cells, much less kill them. With ALL a tiny blood specimen from a finger prick can give us solid evidence of a drug's cytotoxic action on the leukemic cells, and a negative bone marrow sample demonstrates a complete response. We have no comparable assays for use in the adjuvant therapy of breast cancers. We usually do not know what effect the drugs are having.

Theoretically, any disseminated cancer, hematologic or solid, could be cured if we could kill all the malignant cells. Oncology textbooks are full of optimistic graphs purporting to show how "total cell kill" can be accomplished. Yet with the notable exceptions of the childhood leukemias, the germ-cell tumors, and Hodgkin's disease, this total eradication of malignant cells does not seem to be done very often, at least not in a way we can verify. If 99% of the disseminated cancer cells are destroyed, the patient may benefit greatly, possibly even enjoy a normal life span; but should that surviving 1% acquire drug resistance and start to multiply again, the reprieve will be short-lived. We can assume that a child or young adult with ALL who stays in remission for several years has been cured—the reason being that if a single leukemic cell had remained active, by this time it would surely have multiplied itself a millionfold, exponentially, and filled the bloodstream with daughter cells. But no comparable assumption can be made for early-stage breast cancers—the course of disease is unpredictable, with or without chemotherapy, and it may be prolonged. A ten-year period with no sign of recurrence is encouraging, but it does not prove that the treatment has produced a cure. Our best indicator of therapeutic effect remains the long-term follow-up on patients enrolled in clinical trials. That follow-up may tell us that a group of patients randomized to Treatment A fared—as a group—better or worse than a comparable group of patients randomized to Treatment B. The twenty-year follow-up on the Milan CMF trial which Gianni Bonadonna and his colleagues published in 1995 is particularly instructive. Since many postmenopausal patients who were assigned to CMF did not receive the optimal dose, we will consider only those patients who were premenopausal or perimenopausal at the time of randomization. The survival rate at twenty years was 24% for patients in this subgroup who received no further treatment after surgery and 47% for those who received CMF.[27] These statistics indicate that adjuvant chemotherapy in node-positive patients tends to translate into more prolonged survival; but they also remind us that even among younger node-positive patients, a significant minority (24% in this case) may become long-term survivors without any systemic therapy. For reasons we do not fully understand, some breast cancer cells are able to migrate to the regional lymph nodes, but still do not possess those elusive additional characteristics needed to establish metastatic colonies. Patients with these particular node-positive tumors are in effect "cured" by local therapy. They do not need systemic chemotherapy; but since they usually get it, their favorable outcomes are wrongly attributed to this or that regimen. "Pre-cured" patients are a large worm (one of several) in the survival statistics which are so glibly quoted.

ADRIAMYCIN
The Big <u>Red</u> One

Notwithstanding the inherent uncertainties of breast cancer chemotherapy, the demonstration that CMF could help many patients gave a tremendous boost to the oncologic profession. Prior to the 1960s oncology did not exist as a separate, well-defined medical specialty. The American Society of Clinical Oncology, the most important professional organization, was not founded until 1964; in the mid-1970s it had a mere 800 members. By the early 1990s the Society's membership had jumped to 8,000—a tenfold expansion.[28] All these new professionals could not hope to support themselves by curing the handful of patients with ALL or Hodgkin's disease; it was the treatment of breast malignancies which provided the first major economic incentive. Each year tens of thousands of

American women would be diagnosed with these unpredictable tumors, and oncologists could now promise to better the odds of long-term survival. By the early 1980s they could also offer their breast cancer patients potent new regimens based on the anthracycline antibiotic **doxorubicin**. This drug, isolated from bacteria in the late 1960s, was approved by the Food and Drug Administration in 1974. It is often referred to as **Adriamycin**, a brand name of Adria Laboratories; and it figures as that prominent "A" in current regimens for Hodgkin's disease (ABVD), lung cancer (CAP, CAV), bladder cancer (M-VAC), stomach cancer (FAM), and breast cancer (AC, CAF, FAC).

Adriamycin (doxorubicin) can only be given intravenously—great care must be taken to avoid extravasation (seepage of the drug into tissues surrounding the infusion site). This drug binds to the chromosomes in a cell's nucleus, interfering with the synthesis of DNA and RNA, and stopping mitotic activity. Like most cytotoxic agents, it works best on cells in S-phase or undergoing mitosis; but it is not "phase specific," meaning that it can kill metabolically active cells even if they are not preparing to divide. Adriamycin quickly became popular among oncologists because it is so powerful and so versatile, doing efficient duty against many different malignancies. The drug's downside is toxicity. Adriamycin places a close second to cisplatin in its potential to induce nausea and vomiting that patients never forget. Some years ago the interior decorators at Boston's Dana-Farber Cancer Institute learned about this drug the hard way; they had put a cheerful-looking red rug in the hospital's entrance foyer, hoping to brighten the patients' spirits. This is not what happened. No sooner did patients enter the hospital than they began to throw up, illustrating a phenomenon which oncologists call **anticipatory vomiting**. The association which triggered this Pavlovian response had to do with the rug's color. Adriamycin is supplied as *a cheerful-looking red liquid.*[29]

Another prominent side effect of doxorubicin therapy which disturbs patients is hair loss. Unlike CMF, regimens containing Adriamycin can result in total or near-total alopecia—hair tends to fall out in clumps, so rapidly that patients may become completely bald in just a few days. There is no satisfactory regrowth of hair until several months after the end of therapy. But patients are blissfully unaware of the most dangerous side effect, which is inconspicuous and rarely becomes apparent during treatment. Adriamycin is absorbed by—and is quite toxic to—the myocardium (heart muscle). This effect is cumulative, meaning that after a certain level of drug exposure the heart cannot be exposed again without risking permanent damage. Oncologists have generally regarded the safe lifetime exposure to Adriamycin as 550 milligrams per square meter of body surface area.[30]   However, susceptible individuals should not receive this drug at all, a lesson we learned tragically from the occasional doxorubicin-treated child who survived leukemia or osteosarcoma only to die of congestive heart failure as a teenager. Adult patients with a history of heart attacks, angina, liver disease, or high blood pressure are not good candidates for Adriamycin.[31]

During the 1990s we made some headway in muting these prevalent toxicities. Improved antiemetic drugs, given to patients before and after doxorubicin chemotherapy, considerably reduced the severity and duration of vomiting. And the newer anthracycline antibiotics, notably **daunorubicin** and **epirubicin**, seemed to be slightly less cardiotoxic than doxorubicin. In the United States daunorubicin replaced Adriamycin in many leukemia regimens; in Europe and Canada epirubicin has often been used in lieu of Adriamycin in breast cancer regimens. Higher doses of doxorubicin can be safely given if accompanied by an infusion of the cardioprotective drug **dexrazoxane**, marketed under the brand name **Zinecard** by Pharmacia & Upjohn. Nobody is altogether sure how dexrazoxane works, but oncologist Sandra M. Swain and her colleagues conducted two clinical trials which demonstrated its effectiveness in doxorubicin-based chemotherapy for breast cancer.[32]

Adjuvant FAC
The M. D. Anderson Regimen

Adriamycin (doxorubicin) first appeared in breast cancer chemotherapy as a salvage agent—it was given to patients with metastatic disease. These early studies established Adriamycin's reputation as the most powerful drug in the armamentarium, because it consistently produced more responses in advanced breast cancer than any other single agent. For discovering Adriamycin's value in the adjuvant setting, we are indebted to Aman U. Buzdar and his colleagues at Houston's M. D. Anderson Cancer Center. The regimen they popularized was **FAC**, which reminds us of the Texas hospital in much the same way that CMF reminds us of Milan. Like classic CMF, FAC ran on a 28-day cycle, but it was administered altogether intravenously—fluorouracil on days 1 and 8, Adriamycin (doxorubicin) on day 1, and cyclophosphamide on day 1. Needless to say, that first day with all three drugs represented an unforgettable triple whammy. The regimen was repeated every 28 days for about seven months, stopping when the cumulative dose of doxorubicin reached 300 milligrams per square meter of body surface area. Between 1974 and 1977 Dr. Buzdar and his M. D. Anderson co-workers gave FAC to 222 patients with Stage Two (node-positive) or Stage Three (locally advanced) breast cancer. These researchers sang the praises of FAC at the Consensus Development Conference on breast cancer chemotherapy held in September 1985.[33] In 1989 Buzdar et al published some impressive statistics on their FAC patients based upon a median follow-up of 133 months: "Estimated ten-year disease-free survival was 58% and 36% for stage II and III disease, respectively. Estimated ten-year survival was 62% for patients with stage II disease and 40% for those with stage III disease." Dr. Buzdar and his colleagues concluded that FAC "was effective in improving disease-free and overall survival regardless of age, stage of disease, or extent of nodal involvement."[34]

How much better were these FAC results than those seen in the untreated control group? Unfortunately, there was no control group, because the M. D. Anderson studies of this regimen were not randomized trials—all the patients got chemotherapy. For comparison Dr. Buzdar and his colleagues relied on "historical controls"; they looked at the outcomes recorded for comparably staged M. D. Anderson patients from the years 1971 through 1973 who were given the same surgical therapy (mastectomy), but who did not receive FAC or any other systemic therapy. Normally we should be suspicious of historical controls, since they may have had more advanced disease than the recent study participants—that is, yesterday's "Stage Two" patient might be diagnosed as Stage Three or Four if seen today and given a more thorough examination. In this case, however, such "stage migration" would seem to have been minimal, and the statistics Buzdar et al give us are plausible. Overall survival at ten years for Stage Two patients under age 50 was 30% for the historical controls and 66% for the FAC recipients. For Stage Two patients over age 50, the ten-year survival rates were 42% for the controls and 57% for the FAC recipients.[35]

Are the "A" Regimens Better?

During the 1980s those American oncologists who believed that cytotoxic therapy could really cure breast malignancies flocked to Adriamycin like flies to honey. Many oncology groups now favored a second doxorubicin-based regimen dubbed **CAF**—oral cyclophosphamide (tablets) on days 1 through 14, intravenous Adriamycin and fluorouracil on days 1 and 8, repeat the cycle every 28 days.[36] Much tinkering was done with both FAC and CAF, blurring the original recipes. The dose levels and mode of administration might be altered; the cycles might be shortened to 21 days or lengthened to 35 days, and the number of cycles might be increased or decreased. Additional drugs like methotrexate, prednisone, tamoxifen, or vincristine might be given concurrently or tacked on afterwards as maintenance therapy. The comparison of results obtained at different institutions using different recipes soon became a mind-boggling exercise.

<u>Did</u> <u>the</u> <u>more</u> <u>toxic</u> <u>Adriamycin</u> <u>regimens</u> <u>generally</u> <u>achieve</u> <u>better</u> <u>results</u> <u>than</u> <u>the</u> <u>familiar</u> <u>CMF</u>? This fundamental question does not seem to have arisen at M. D. Anderson, where almost all breast cancer patients at risk of recurrence were steered toward FAC. Elsewhere it provoked considerable controversy. One of the more outspoken Adriamycin proponents was the veteran oncologist Ezra M. Greenspan of New York's Mount Sinai Medical Center. In a 1986 letter to the *New England Journal of Medicine*, Dr. Greenspan complained: "Most oncologists use only the mild convenience regimen consisting of cyclophosphamide,

methotrexate, and fluorouracil (CMF) for premenopausal women. I estimate that 10,000 lives could be saved by the early aggressive use of polychemotherapy in breast cancer, as compared with the negligible number of lives, perhaps several thousand, now being saved. Corresponding with the *Journal of the National Cancer Institute*, Greenspan observed that "doxorubicin-containing regimens" can achieve "virtual and apparent clinical cure" in "25% to 35% of stage III breast cancers, even inflammatory cancers."[37] I. Craig Henderson of Boston's Dana-Farber Cancer Institute was far more reserved about the curative potential of cytotoxic chemotherapy and of doxorubicin in particular. Speaking to the San Antonio Breast Cancer Symposium in 1988, Dr. Henderson admitted that "some patients may be cured" by chemotherapy, but argued that "there is at present no evidence that this ever happens, let alone that it happens frequently." He recommended that all node-positive premenopausal patients receive "some form of chemotherapy," but he found the clinical data suggesting a survival advantage for Adriamycin-based regimens to be inconsistent and premature: "No program has been reproducibly shown to be superior to CMF administered for six months."[38]

Although the clinical trials reported during the 1990s did not end "The Battle of the Regimens," several of them merit our attention. Adriamycin proponents received a boost from **NSABP Protocol B-15**, a big trial which compared a short doxorubicin-based regimen with classic CMF. The breast cancer patients in Protocol B-15 had undergone mastectomy or lumpectomy between two and five weeks prior to beginning their chemotherapy. They were all node-positive and regarded as "tamoxifen-nonresponsive"; about 80% were under age 50. Between 1984 and 1988 the NSABP assigned 781

trial participants to receive four cycles of **AC** (high-dose doxorubicin and cyclophosphamide given intravenously on day 1 every 21 days), and 776 trial participants to receive six cycles of **CMF** (oral cyclophosphamide on days 1 through 14, intravenous methotrexate and fluorouracil on days 1 and 8, repeat every 28 days). The three-year results which the NSABP published in September 1990 revealed "no significant difference" between AC and CMF, either in disease-free survival or in overall survival. Notwithstanding this statistical dead heat, Bernard Fisher and his colleagues concluded that AC "seems preferable" because the treatment is "completed on day 63 versus day 154 for conventional CMF." The AC patient makes four visits to her oncologist's office; the CMF patient must make twelve. While conceding that alopecia (hair loss) and vomiting were more severe with AC, the NSABP team pointed out that "nausea without vomiting, diarrhea, and weight gain" were more frequently encountered with CMF.[39]

During the 1990s AC became the NSABP's regimen of choice for node-positive breast cancer. The Southwest Oncology Group (SWOG) went its own way, in the opposite direction from the NSABP. The SWOG oncologists evaluated long-term therapy (52 weeks) with a souped-up version of CMF—low-dose oral cyclophosphamide every day for one year, intravenous methotrexate and fluorouracil once a week, with added oral prednisone every day for the first 70 days, and added intravenous vincristine once a week for the first 10 weeks. This potent **CMFVP** was pitted against four longish cycles of **FAC-M**—fluorouracil, doxorubicin, and cyclophosphamide given intravenously on day 1, fluorouracil again on day 8, and intravenous methotrexate on day 22, the cycle being repeated every 35 days. Between 1984 and 1990, the SWOG team randomly assigned 531 patients "with hormone receptor-negative, node-positive breast cancer" to receive either CMFVP or FAC-M. In the five-year results published in 1995, the CMFVP group fared slightly better than the FAC-M group, both in freedom from recurrence (55% as compared to 50% for FAC-M) and in overall survival (64% versus 61% for FAC-M). "Because the disease-free survival produced by CMFVP is marginally superior," the SWOG team concluded, "we do not recommend FAC-M. Our trial is consistent with the general experience that doxorubicin-containing combinations are not superior to effective non-doxorubicin regimens."[40] Of course, the CMF variant tested, with its 52 office visits for intravenous therapy and 365 days of ongoing treatment, is not one of those "mild convenience regimens" that Dr. Greenspan complained about.

The prolonged controversy over the role of Adriamycin in breast cancer chemotherapy did not escape the notice of Gianni Bonadonna and his colleagues at the *Instituto Nazionale Tumori*. The Milan group had a different idea—why not give *both Adriamycin and CMF* to those patients at the highest risk of metastatic disease? Between 1982 and 1990 they recruited 402 breast cancer patients who had four or more positive nodes for a trial of this combined therapy. All the drugs were given intravenously on day 1 of a 21-day cycle; there were four cycles of high-dose doxorubicin and eight of the modified CMF. The trial sought to determine whether it was better to give the combination sequentially (four cycles of doxorubicin followed by eight cycles of the modified CMF), or in alternation (two cycles of CMF and then one of doxorubicin, repeat four times). The ten-year results which Dr. Bonadonna and his colleagues published in the *Journal of the American Medical Association* revealed significant advantages for the sequential arm. Overall survival at ten years for the patients who received Adriamycin followed by CMF

was 58%. Their disease-free survival rate was 42%. If we reflect that historically most patients with substantial nodal involvement, especially younger ones, have died within ten years of their original diagnosis, we will appreciate the benefit apparent in the Milan statistics. The median age of patients in this trial was 47; several were still in their twenties.

In 1998 the Early Breast Cancer Trialists' Collaborative Group, headquartered in England, published a meta-analysis of 58 chemotherapy trials involving some 24,000 patients. The international collaborators concluded that "adjuvant polychemotherapy" either with CMF or with a regimen based on an anthracycline antibiotic (doxorubicin or epirubicin) has been shown to produce "an absolute improvement of about 7% to 11% in ten-year survival for women aged under 50 and of about 2% to 3% for those aged 50 to 69." Looking at eleven trials specifically pitting CMF variations against regimens based on doxorubicin (Adriamycin) or epirubicin, the Trialists' Group detected a slight advantage for anthracycline combinations. According to their meta-analysis, the estimated disease-free survival at five years has been 57.3% for anthracycline-based regimens as compared to 54.1% for CMF variations. The estimated overall survival at five years was 71.5% for the anthracyclines as compared to 68.8% for CMF.[42]

The preceding statistics taken from the British medical journal *Lancet* are conservative; almost all American oncologists would give higher estimates of the likely benefits to be had from breast cancer chemotherapy. Needless to say, the recommendation a patient receives will depend largely upon whose door she happens to open. American oncologists in private practice have traditionally leaned toward CMF because this regimen's side effects are predictable and relatively mild. The vomiting and loss of body hair associated with Adriamycin therapy are emotionally disturbing to many patients; and every so often a patient receiving this drug will unexpectedly display symptoms of cardiac distress, a medical emergency that few private practitioners relish dealing with. The large cancer hospitals have tended to emphasize Adriamycin: with their round-the-clock staffing they are better equipped to deal with this drug's physical and psychological side effects. The most appropriate candidates for doxorubicin-based chemotherapy are younger node-positive patients who have been diagnosed with aggressive breast tumors but who have no chronic conditions affecting the function of the heart, the liver, or the kidneys.

Multidrug Resistance

There are three reasons why chemotherapy cannot routinely and predictably eradicate disseminated cells from solid tumors. We have already touched briefly on two of them—**pharmaceutical sanctuaries** (this means that some cancer cells may be sequestered in the center of metastatic colonies or in the central nervous system so that they are protected from drug exposure), and **kinetic factors** (this means that some cancer cells are not in a vulnerable phase of the cell cycle when the drugs are administered). If our problems were limited to these two situations, we might not be able to cure metastatic malignancies, but we could presumably control them because our drugs would still kill any metabolically active tumor cells they came in contact with. A third problem, entirely distinct from the first two, is the principal reason why chemotherapy patients often relapse and die—**multidrug resistance** (MDR). This phenomenon tends to make our cytotoxic agents useless—they can no longer kill the cancer cells, at least not in concentrations which would not also prove lethal to patients. MDR is frequently observed in laboratory Petri dishes—cultivated cancer cells which had previously been vulnerable to a particular cytotoxic agent will suddenly become resistant not only to that drug, but to other drugs to which they had not previously been exposed. Practicing oncologists have to deal with the human consequences of this phenomenon. Patients with metastatic breast cancer sometimes respond dramatically to chemotherapy, but then after a year or two they may not respond either to the initial salvage regimen or to any new drugs which are administered.

What changes are occurring inside the individual tumor cells to bring about multidrug resistance? The first clue came back in the 1970s. Researchers discovered that cancer cells exhibiting MDR typically expressed a protein on their outer membranes called **P-glycoprotein** (P-gp) which was lacking in chemosensitive cells. That "P" in P-gp stands for "permeability." It is believed that P-gp functions as a kind of efflux pump—that is, the protein presumably binds to any incoming toxic molecules, enabling the cell in question to pump them out. In the mid-1980s the gene responsible for encoding P-gp was tracked to the long arm of chromosome seven, isolated, and finally cloned. Laboratory experiments have shown us that when this gene known as *MDR1* is inserted into chemosensitive cancer cells, they will become multidrug resistant. Additional investigations revealed that the *MDR1* gene and its protein are widely conserved in living organisms, present in the lowly bacterium as well as in *Homo sapiens*. They constitute a commonplace biological mechanism which has evolved to protect cells from toxins.[43]

By the 1990s immunostaining assays using monoclonal antibodies reactive with

P-glycoprotein gave us a simple tool to determine which cells were producing the drug-resisting protein. We soon learned that healthy cells in the liver and kidneys normally produce high levels of P-gp, because these organs have the chore of neutralizing and removing any toxins present in the bloodstream. Colon cells also produce large quantities of this protein as a way of protecting themselves against toxic substances in the feces. Needless to say, when liver, kidney, or colon cells turn malignant, they will continue to express high levels of P-gp—this fact does much to explain why malignancies arising in these organs have been so notoriously resistant to cytotoxic chemotherapy. Hematologic malignancies affecting adults, notably chronic lymphocytic leukemia, chronic myelogenous leukemia, and multiple myeloma, are far more likely to express this protein than the acute juvenile leukemias; consequently they are not likely to be cured by chemotherapy.[44] P-glycoprotein came to the attention of breast cancer specialists as a mechanism which could disarm even the mighty Adriamycin.[45] Bruce J. Trock and other researchers at Georgetown University's Lombardi Cancer Center have published a meta-analysis of 31 studies on this protein's role in breast malignancies. Dr. Trock and his colleagues concluded that even before systemic therapy, a few breast tumors are already producing detectable levels of the protein: "Patients with tumors expressing *MDR1* and P-glycoprotein were three times more likely to fail to respond to chemotherapy than patients whose tumors were negative. Treatment with chemotherapeutic drugs or hormonal agents was associated with an increase in the proportion of tumors expressing *MDR1* and P-glycoprotein."[46] The cells of the mammary gland typically do not produce P-gp because unlike hepatic, renal, or gastrointestinal cells, they usually do not have to deal with toxic substances. But breast cancer cells retain functional *MDR1* genes; and if these cells are not killed by the first few cycles of chemotherapy. additional exposure to cytotoxic drugs may well lead to *MDR1* activation and P-gp expression. This biological mechanism does much to explain the most surprising finding from the Milan CMF trial—viz., that breast cancer patients receiving twelve cycles of CMF actually had slightly poorer outcomes than those patients who received only six cycles.

Can we ever reverse multidrug resistance? In the mid-1980s oncologists entertained hopes for a drug called **verapamil**, which has been commonly used to treat hypertension. Given intravenously, verapamil can also reduce drug resistance caused by P-gp expression, apparently by binding to the protein and interfering with its efflux activity. But the results from the first clinical trials were hardly encouraging. Verapamil must be administered in heavy doses to mute P-gp activity; and at these dose levels it causes unacceptable cardiovascular side effects, including "heart block, hypotension, sinus bradycardia, and junctional rhythms."[47] The immunosuppressive drug **cyclosporine** has also been studied. It effectively inhibits P-gp function in drug-resistant cell lines; but when given to patients along with chemotherapy, it leads to excessive bone marrow suppression (i.e., an unacceptable reduction in blood cell production).[48] **Valspodar**, an analog of cyclosporine, has seemed more promising because it inhibits P-gp without causing so much marrow suppression. To date, our problems with P-gp suppressors have been that excessively large doses are required, and that when these agents succeed in suppressing the antitoxin protein in cancer cells, they will also suppress it in healthy liver, kidney, and gastrointestinal cells. Thus their dose-limiting side effect is an unacceptable increase in drug toxicity affecting these vital organs. But even if we had a service-able P-gp inhibitor, we would not be out of the woods. Cell lines revealing multidrug resistance without any evidence of the membranous P-glycoprotein demonstrate that this protein, while important, is not the only mechanism involved in this phenomenon. By the late 1990s researchers on MDR postulated that human cells had the potential to produce several dozen "transporter proteins" which might interfere with cytotoxic agents.[50] Thus the mechanism responsible for resistance to one drug could be different from the mechanism causing resistance to another. Conceivably, a multidrug-resistant cancer cell could be employing several of these efflux pumps at the same time. The expectation of an easy solution to MDR faded away after these new revelations of biological complexity. Jeffrey Moscow, a pediatric oncologist at the University of Kentucky in Lexington, reflected the growing skepticism in a 1998 interview: "What we've learned both about the multitude of drug transporters and about their physiologic roles raises a question whether multidrug resistance reversal is ever going to be a useful paradigm in the clinic."[51] At least it would seem prudent to assay tumor specimens for P-glycoprotein expression before prescribing Adriamycin and certain other drugs. Cancer cells expressing P-gp stand a good chance of being resistant to the anthracycline antibiotics (doxorubicin and epirubicin), the vinca alkaloids, and the taxoid drug paclitaxel.

Dose and Dose Intensity

Having no useful chemosensitizer to fight drug resistance, oncologists pondered strategies which might prevent this problem from developing in the first place. The strategies most frequently advocated have been **dose escalation** and **dose intensity**—in other words, give the drugs in the highest doses possible, and as rapidly as possible, so as to kill the disseminated cancer cells before they become drug resistant. We'll have more to say about dose escalation for high-risk breast cancer patients in Chapter Twenty-five; at the moment we can profitably consider dose intensity, since this strategy tends to modify the outpatient regimens offered to the more numerous moderate-risk patients. "Dose" refers to the total quantity (cumulative dosage) of a drug administered, while "dose intensity" refers to the interval of time in which that dose is given. When we give the same dose over a shorter time period, we are practicing dose intensity. The increased therapeutic benefits that we might achieve with this strategy have to be carefully weighed against the increased side effects that inevitably accompany it.

American oncologists who believe in dose intensity now favor adjuvant regimens for breast cancer which are considerably shorter than the six-month courses of therapy prevalent in the 1980s. The 63-day **AC** regimen used in NSABP Protocol B-15 is a good example of dose intensity; but for a big trial testing the validity of the strategy itself, we are principally indebted to the **Cancer and Leukemia Group B** (CALGB). These researchers did not experiment with new drug combinations—they simply adopted the intravenous **FAC** regimen popularized by the M. D. Anderson Cancer Center. Their trial sought to determine how differences in the dose and the dose intensity of FAC affected patient outcomes. Between 1985 and 1991 CALGB randomly assigned 1,550 patients with Stage Two (node-positive) breast cancer to one of three treatment arms. The first was standard FAC, with the cumulative dose being administered in six cycles of 28 days each. The second was dose-intense FAC, with the same dose being administered in four cycles instead of six, so that on any treatment day patients received 50% more of the drugs than those patients assigned to the standard regimen. The third arm was <u>low-dose FAC</u>, with the cumulative dose being only half of that used in the standard and dose-intense arms. This reduced dose was given in four cycles.

The first report from the CALGB dose-intensity trial appeared in the *New England Journal of Medicine* on May 5, 1994. After a median follow-up of 3.4 years, the patients who received dose-intense FAC were faring slightly better than those assigned to standard FAC, while the low-dose patients experienced noticeably more recurrences. Disease-free survival (freedom from all recurrences) was 74.3% in the dose-intense arm, 71.6% in the standard arm, and 62.7% in the low-dose arm. William C. Wood of Emory University and his CALGB colleagues concluded that "a reduction in chemotherapy doses reduces the benefit of adjuvant therapy." This finding held true for both premenopausal and post-menopausal patients. The downside of dose-intense FAC proved to be toxicity. Only 16% of the patients getting the standard regimen experienced leukopenia (dangerously low levels of the infection-fighting white blood cells); but 65% of those patients receiving dose-intense FAC did so, and 4% of them required hospitalization. Stomatitis (painful irritation of the oral cavity with difficulty eating and swallowing) affected 10% of the dose-intense patients, who also reported more nausea (39% affected) than the patients on standard FAC (35% affected).[52]

The CALGB trial unequivocally indicated the superiority of full dosage. When you reduce the dose to lessen toxicity, you are reducing the patient's chances of survival. This trial also demonstrated the feasibility of dose intensity on an outpatient basis: you can up the dose by 50% without having to put too many people in the hospital. A survival advantage for four-cycle dose-intense FAC over the standard six-cycle regimen was not immediately apparent, but the slight trend favoring dose intensity persisted through nine years of follow-up. The updated report published by the CALGB team in 1998 had the dose-intense patients edging ahead in overall survival with 66.5% still alive, compared to 65.5% in the standard FAC group and 58.1% in the low-dose group. The disease-free statistics also hinted at advantages to be had from dose-intensity: 57.6% of these patients showed no sign of recurrent cancer, as compared to 53.6% in the standard FAC group and 46.9% in the low-dose group.[53]

Talking with an Oncologist

It is better not to develop cancer. And if a malignancy does occur, it is better to have a tumor which gives no sign of systemic dissemination or of metastatic potential. In this case there would be no need to consult an oncologist. But all patients who have infiltrating (invasive) carcinomas known to have spread to one or more regional lymph nodes should do so. Not one of medicine's joyous specialties, oncology ranks among its most intellectually challenging. Practitioners are spared the steady stream of hypochondriacs with minor aches and pains—any patients who come for an oncology consultation have good reason to be worried. Unfortunately, with many adult malignancies there is little evidence that cytotoxic chemotherapy can significantly alter the course of disease, and these patients must be given the bad news at the outset. With breast malignancies the potential benefit can be very great; however, since oncologists cannot surely predict who will benefit, every consultation becomes a difficult balancing act. On the one hand, the possible benefit must be enthusiastically depicted; on the other, the treatment's toxicities must be realistically described, and the uncertainty of outcome honestly admitted. Dr. I. Craig Henderson has given his fellow oncologists a prescription for breast cancer consultations. He recommends that patients be informed that the effect of chemotherapy can vary from individual to individual: "The change in survival may be only a few months (or even a shortening of life) or may be measured in decades." Dr. Henderson reasons that "a large reduction in tumor burden will result in a prolongation of life even if the eventual growth of resistant cells finally causes death."[54]

Understandably, breast cancer patients want to know what their personal odds of survival are and how chemotherapy might change these odds. Merle O'Rourke Thompson, a patient with a Ph.D. in a nonmedical field, observes that this information is not always forthcoming: "I remember being so frustrated that no doctor would give me even a good guess on my future. Eventually the oncologist, direct as those doctors usually are, told me that my stage II cancer gave me a 35% chance of survival, but he could make that 65% with his chemotherapy. Tough as that was to hear, I was grateful for the truth."[55] In breast cancer matters, nobody's statistics are sacrosanct, but those quoted to Dr. Thompson qualify as plausible estimates of the ten-year survival rates we might expect for most node-positive patients. As we've seen, the updated report from the big CALGB trial pegged the long-term survival rate for patients given standard or dose-intense FAC at around 65%; and M. D. Anderson's ten-year survival estimates for Stage Two patients under age 50 were 30% without chemotherapy and 66% with FAC. The statistics for Stage Three patients are less propitious. Larger primary tumors or greater numbers of positive nodes point toward a substantial tumor burden—viz., many more

cancer cells in systemic dissemination, with a stronger probability that some of them will not respond to chemotherapy because they are sequestered in hypoxic metastases or have become drug resistant.

Oncologists entertain honest differences of opinion as to which regimen might be generally superior, or as to which regimen might be preferable for this or that patient, given the individual's state of health, her age, and her personal circumstances. But not all divergences in oncologic practice can be described as "honest." Our clinical trial organizations—Milan, NSABP, SWOG, CALGB—have consistently demonstrated that adjuvant chemotherapy for breast malignancies is most effective when administered at full dose levels over a limited period of time, usually no longer than six months. David Young, a California physician, complains that certain oncologists with "very lucrative private practice" willfully disregard these fundamental principles: "Patients are routinely continued on ineffective chemotherapy despite obvious progression of disease. Others are given adjuvant chemotherapy for long periods, even extending to five years. Patients are sometimes treated with doses as little as one fourth of those in recommended regimens in order to facilitate sustained compliance."[56] We sincerely hope that Dr. Young's whistle-blowing will not be necessary in the future—readers of this book should know enough to be suspicious of any adjuvant cytotoxic regimen which seems unduly prolonged or not especially toxic. Until that future day when we have wonder drugs which selectively target only the disseminated cancer cells, any regimen powerful enough to change the course of disease stands to cause unpleasant side effects. Patients who are in doubt as to whether chemotherapy is advisable, or as to which regimen might be most appropriate, should obtain a second opinion. Michael Van Scoy-Mosher, an oncologist practicing in Beverly Hills, California, reports that his rich and famous clientele need little encouragement in this regard: "My patients usually seek out two to three opinions, and I had one get eight. They also consult multiple cancer centers."[57]

The controversies in breast cancer chemotherapy are profound and enduring. On the one hand, all this debate is bewildering to patients and physicians alike; on the other, it bears witness to a continuing effort to find better treatments. As the list of drugs with activity against breast malignancies has gradually lengthened, the number of potential drug combinations has increased exponentially. The dose levels of these drugs, their mode of administration, and their sequencing offer a boundless field for experimentation. Of course, the conclusive demonstration that one combination is superior to another typically requires a large well-designed clinical trial and ten years of follow-up—thus it is not surprising that such demonstrations have been infrequent. During the 1990s the newer taxoid drugs **paclitaxel** and **docetaxel** were found to have significant antitumor activity when used as salvage agents against metastatic breast cancer; they are now being incorporated into adjuvant regimens for early-stage disease. We might hope that the taxoid-containing combinations will deliver a higher survival rate than the 65% estimate hitherto bandied about for node-positive patients receiving cytotoxic chemotherapy.

Chapter Twenty-four

Undergoing Chemotherapy

reast cancer chemotherapy has traditionally been given postoperatively, in a timely fashion. Patients normally begin receiving chemotherapy somewhere between two and four weeks after lumpectomy or mastectomy—the convenient interval between treatments allows time for pathological analysis of the tumor specimen and for extended consultations. Chemotherapy given before surgery (preoperatively) is sometimes referred to as neoadjuvant. Back in the 1980s Bernard Fisher and his co-workers in the National Surgical Adjuvant Breast and Bowel Project wanted to know whether neoadjuvant chemotherapy would be more effective in reducing the likelihood of distant metastases; the experiments they had conducted with tumor-bearing mice suggested that it might.[1] **NSABP Protocol B-18** randomly assigned 1,523 breast cancer patients to receive four cycles of AC (Adriamycin and cyclophosphamide) either before or after their surgery. All the tumors had previously been diagnosed as malignant by fine-needle aspiration or by core-needle biopsy. About 72% of them were larger than two centimeters in diameter and thus would have been classified as Stage Two disease on the basis of size alone. The five-year results which Dr. Fisher and his colleagues published in 1998 failed to reveal any significant differences between the trial's two arms

either in disease-free survival or in overall survival.[2] Protocol B-18 did not provide a rationale for changing our basic practice— viz., surgery and pathology analysis first, with the chemotherapy soon afterwards—but the trial did demonstrate that preoperative chemo can increase the proportion of patients who will be eligible for breast-conserving surgery. According to the NSABP team, "12% more lumpectomies were performed in the preoperative group; in women with tumors 5.1 cm or larger there was a 175% increase."[3]

Gianni Bonadonna and other oncologists at Milan's *Instituto Nazionale Tumori* have also promoted neoadjuvant chemotherapy as a way to avoid mastectomy. Between 1988 and 1995 they treated 536 breast cancer patients with tumors 2.5 cm or larger in diameter: "Following primary (preoperative) chemotherapy, 85% of patients could be subjected to breast-sparing surgery; in 14 patients (3% of the group), surgical specimens failed to show any residual cancer cells."[4] Neoadjuvant chemotherapy is particularly indicated for inflammatory breast cancers—i.e., those poorly differentiated tumors which mimic acute infections in their presentation and which have typically spread throughout the body by the time they are diagnosed. In these unfortunate cases, doing the surgery first tends to make matters worse;

but rigorous preoperative chemo usually produces an impressive response, which is sometimes so complete that no cancer cells can be detected on subsequent biopsies of the tumor area. Mastectomy performed after such neoadjuvant therapy stands a much better chance of achieving local control.

Whether given before or after surgery, breast cancer chemotherapy has become considerably more tolerable than it was in the 1970s and 1980s. Patients can continue to work and to maintain their normal routines. But the months of treatment necessarily remain stressful. This is not a propitious time to make major changes in one's life—to get married or start a business, to move to a new house or learn a new job. It is instead a time to learn about cytotoxic drugs and their side effects, and to pay close attention to any written or oral instructions that may be given. The nurses who work in the oncologist's office are often a patient's most accessible sources of information; they can usually answer all those questions that inevitably arise.

DOSE CALCULATION
And Drug Administration

Oncology offices are designed for comfort. Patients lie back in cozy recliners while they listen to soft music, read books and magazines, or just doze off. The metal "drip stand" adjacent to each recliner is the only sign of the serious business at hand; it suspends a vial of liquid medication overhead, allowing the fluid to drip down an intravenous line. There is no room for error either in the calculation of the drug dosage or in the placement of that intravenous line—false steps can lead to dire consequences. With cytotoxic agents the amount of medication a patient receives must be precisely measured

according to his or her body size; thus a larger patient will be given more medication than a smaller one. Back in the 1950s drug doses were meted out simply on the basis of body weight. Current practice relies on a more complicated method which takes into account both weight and height. A standardized computation yields the patient's **Body Surface Area** (BSA), which is expressed in **square meters** (m^2). Chemotherapy regimens typically call for so many <u>milligrams of the drug to be given per square meter of BSA</u>: this is abbreviated as "mg/m^2" in the prescribing information.[5] The prescription for the FAC regimen which we discussed in the last chapter would be written in this fashion—"fluorouracil 400 mg/m^2 i.v. on days 1 and 8, doxorubicin 40 mg/m^2 i.v. on day 1, and cyclophosphamide 400 mg/m^2 i.v. on day 1, repeat every 28 days."

The abbreviation "i.v." means "intravenously." Only a few cytotoxic drugs are given "p.o." (abbreviation for *per os*, Latin for "by mouth"). Access to the circulatory system is of paramount importance—we want the infused drugs to be promptly carried away by the bloodstream, not to pool up in tissues surrounding the injection site. In outpatient chemotherapy, venous access is typically obtained by using a vein in the hand or forearm. The injection area is first cleansed with an antiseptic; and a needle is inserted into the vein selected, being secured in place with a nonirritating tape. The flexible tubing of the intravenous line (the catheter) is then attached to the needle—the lower portion of the catheter is also taped into position, so as to further reduce the chances that the needle might be dislodged. The relatively small quantities of cytotoxic drugs may be diluted with a harmless carrier fluid (e.g., saline) as they flow down the catheter into the vein.

From the patient's point of view, intravenous drug administration might be best described as *slow-drip*, because it often requires one to stay put in a recliner for hours on end. But oncologists describe concentrated infusions of relatively short duration as *bolus* (the Greek word for "lump"). **Continuous infusions** which may last a day or more are usually given through a **central venous catheter**. In this instance a catheter is inserted into a large vein deep beneath the skin, typically the subclavian vein under the collarbone. Venous access may then be easily obtained through a port located at or near the skin surface. The catheter and its port are left in place throughout the treatment period. Such indwelling catheterization offers decided advantages when frequent or constant access to the circulatory system is required. Cytotoxic drugs, powerful antibiotics and painkillers, or parenteral (intravenous) nutrition may be infused round-the-clock if need be. Ambulatory patients can go home wearing little battery-operated reservoirs under their clothing: these devices automatically pump a measured amount of medication into the catheter.[6]

Although some experimental regimens may call for continuous infusion of this or that drug, adjuvant chemotherapy in early-stage breast cancer relies principally on bolus infusions which require only temporary venous access. The risk of infection at the access site is far lower than with indwelling catheters, but there are other problems. Some patients have small or elusive veins in their hands and forearms, so that finding a suitable one becomes a Grail quest. To avoid phlebitis (vein inflammation), a new access site should be selected on each day that chemotherapy is given. Often the oncology nurse can use the same vein as in the preceding session, only moving the access site a little bit higher up toward the elbow. If the patient has not had an extensive axillary dissection on the contralateral (opposite)

side, it may be advantageous to use a new vein in the contralateral hand or forearm. The principal danger with temporary venous access is **extravasation**—i.e., seepage of the toxic drugs into the surrounding tissues. This can easily occur if the needle should slip out of position. Adriamycin and certain other drugs are vesicants with the potential to do great damage if they should be locally concentrated. Known or suspected needle displacement must therefore be handled as a medical emergency. The infusion has to be stopped immediately, the needle aspirated and removed, and the patient's arm elevated to promote the drainage and dissemination of any extravasated drugs. Depending on the particular drug involved, a warm compass or an ice pack would be applied to the access site. If an antidote to the drug exists, it would be injected into the affected area. Steroid creams may help to mute the local inflammatory reactions caused by extravasation, but prevention is always better. Patients should be instructed to report any discomfort at the access site either during chemotherapy administration or afterwards. Symptoms of unnoticed extravasation may not appear until several days later; they could include pain, redness, or swelling at or near the access site, as well as difficulty in moving the affected hand or arm.[7]

While adverse reactions during intravenous drug administration are uncommon, oncologists and oncology nurses have to be prepared for every contingency. Some patients may have mild allergic reactions manifested by localized urticaria (hives) near the access site. Every now and then a patient will have a severe hypersensitivity reaction with dizziness and generalized urticaria, or even go into anaphylactic shock with difficulty in breathing and loss of consciousness. Unfortunately, we cannot always identify patients prone to hypersensitivity reactions before therapy; oncology offices therefore contain anaphylaxis kits with oxygen canisters, epinephrine (Adrenalin) injections, and potent antihistamines.[8]

Nausea and Vomiting

Emesis, the act of vomiting, is a chemotherapy side effect which everybody knows about and which most people wrongfully regard as unavoidable. True enough, back in the 1970s and 1980s many breast cancer patients did experience terrible bouts of vomiting, especially those treated with doxorubicin (Adriamycin) and intravenous cyclophosphamide (Cytoxan). Usually the actual administration of chemotherapy proceeded without a hitch, and the patient went home feeling well enough. But sometime between six and twelve hours after therapy, the cytotoxic drugs would begin to affect the rapidly multiplying cells lining the gastrointestinal tract; and the patient would be overwhelmed by sudden nausea, then racked by vomiting and retching (dry heaves) lasting for hours on end. In her book *Winning the Chemo Battle*, Joyce Slayton Mitchell graphically recounted her experiences after her first day of FAC chemotherapy in late 1984. She was treated in the afternoon, and in the evening she went out (most unwisely) to a Chinese restaurant for a big meal of wontons and mixed vegetables. Around 11:00 PM she awoke from an uneasy sleep: "My feet hit the floor, I bounded into the bathroom. I threw up, retched, vomited, heaved, and retched some more and just couldn't stop. My body felt bloated in every direction, my skin stretched and punctured as if I'd thrown up through each pore in my body. Every grain of rice, every sip of water, that horrendous wonton taste made me shudder to my soul, and I got sicker and sicker."[9]

The 24-hour bouts of nausea and vomiting which Mitchell described were not always the rule, but a decade or two ago most patients receiving rigorous chemotherapy experienced comparably nauseous awakenings the night after they were first exposed to cytotoxic drugs. These days oncologists take pains to minimize such occurrences, prescribing antiemetic drugs to be taken before, during, and after chemotherapy administration. There are compelling reasons why we wish to prevent that initial episode of nausea and vomiting, or at least to lessen its severity and duration. Vomiting quickly leads to dehydration and electrolyte depletion, with subsequent impairment of renal (kidney) function. This situation is unacceptable—adequate hydration and smoothly functioning kidneys could not be more important. Patients are routinely instructed to drink plenty of fluids after receiving cisplatin, cyclophosphamide, or methotrexate, because these drugs can cause damage if they linger in the kidneys or elsewhere in the urinary tract.[10] Cyclophosphamide has been implicated in hemorrhagic cystitis—a painful inflammation of the bladder with blood in the urine. We naturally want cyclophosphamide and other cytotoxic agents to be flushed out of the body in a timely fashion. Patients who become dehydrated due to intractable vomiting may have to be given fluids intravenously. Moreover, patients who suffer mightily during their first exposure to chemotherapy may be reluctant to complete the planned course of treatment. And some of them will also suffer from that strange phenomenon known as **anticipatory nausea and vomiting**, whereby something or somebody they have mentally associated with that first unpleasant experience has the potential to trigger a spontaneous emetic response. Patients so "conditioned" have been known to throw up upon encountering their oncologist in the supermarket—a reaction which is hardly conducive to cordial doctor-patient relationships![11]

Our recent progress in controlling emesis has been largely due to an improved understanding of the biochemical processes responsible for it. Mother Nature designed the reflexes which cause nausea and vomiting as an involuntary protective mechanism, an automatic way of preventing *Homo sapiens* and other mammals from absorbing too much of any irritating or poisonous substances they might chance to eat. Back in the 1950s researchers applied electrodes to the brains of cats and dogs in an effort to locate the region which controls these reflexes. More recent research implicates two distinct regions in the **medulla oblongata** (the lower brain stem), that area where the brain merges into the spinal cord. The medulla oblongata plays an important role in regulating breathing, swallowing, the heart rate, and other vital functions that our bodies perform without our conscious volition. The two regions involved in chemotherapy-related emesis have been named the **vomiting center** and the **chemoreceptor trigger zone**. The vomiting center promptly initiates the emesis reflex after it receives afferent impulses (i.e., ascending nerve-borne distress signals) from the cells lining the gastrointestinal tract. In the case of anticipatory (or "conditioned") vomiting, the nerve-borne signals acting on the vomiting center emanate from the highest region of the brain, the cerebral cortex which holds out memories and our thoughts. The chemoreceptor trigger zone (CTZ) does not directly initiate emesis, but this region of the brain stem can detect the presence of toxic substances in the bloodstream. When aroused by toxins, the CTZ forwards subtle biochemical messages to the nearby vomiting center, which then transmits the appropriate efferent impulses (descending nerve signals) to bring about an emptying of the stomach.[12]

We could avoid nausea and vomiting altogether by putting the patient under general anesthesia, thereby suppressing the activities of the brain stem. As this alternative is not practical, we needed to find other ways of disrupting the biochemical chain of events. The first step was the discovery that the neurotransmitter **dopamine** plays a ubiquitous role in the transmission of stimulatory impulses to the vomiting center. Steven M. Grunberg of the University of Southern California Cancer Center reminds us that "dopamine receptors are found in both the chemoreceptor trigger zone (humoral pathway) and the gastrointestinal tract (peripheral pathway)."[13] Since the 1960s **dopamine antagonists** have been a mainstay of antiemetic therapy; these drugs bind to dopamine receptors and block their activity. The most widely prescribed dopamine antagonist has long been **prochlorperazine** (one of the phenothiazines); it is often referred to as **Compazine** (a SmithKline Beecham brand name). At low doses Compazine's side effects are mild; this inexpensive drug may be given intravenously, injected into a muscle, inserted as a rectal suppository, or taken orally as a tablet, as a capsule, or as syrup. Other phenothiazines are marketed under the brand names **Tigan** and **Torecan**. Even more potent dopamine antagonists may be prescribed for highly emetic chemotherapy: **haloperidol** and **metoclopramide** are available under the brand names **Haldol** and **Reglan**, respectively.

Corticosteroids and **sedatives** have proven effective when used in conjunction with dopamine antagonists. The steroid **dexamethasone**, available under the brand name **Decadron**, may be given intravenously or taken orally; it is frequently administered together with Compazine (prochlorperazine). The sedative most widely prescribed by oncologists has been **lorazepam**, a benzodiazepine marketed under the brand name **Ativan**. Lorazepam can induce a mild amnesia which allows patients to forget about the unpleasant aspects of chemotherapy administration and about any subsequent episodes of nausea and vomiting. The mechanisms through which corticosteroids act to reduce nausea and vomiting have not been clearly defined. Sedatives like lorazepam or **diazepam** (a drug best known under the brand name **Valium**) act by depressing the central nervous system.

Back in the 1980s oncologists and government officials sat on the horns of a dilemma after chemotherapy patients learned that **marijuana**, an illegal agricultural product, possessed antiemetic properties. No one could deny that smoking marijuana lessened patients' anxieties about chemotherapy; in some cases it prevented anticipatory nausea and vomiting when nothing else seemed to help. Libertarians in the oncology community pushed for the plant's legalization, and at one point the Public Health Service (PHS) was distributing government-grown marijuana to patients whose "compassionate-need" applications had been reviewed (most carefully!) and approved (reluctantly) by the Food and Drug Administration. The PHS quickly ceased marijuana distribution when the psychoactive ingredient in this plant, **tetrahydrocannabinol** (THC), was synthesized and marketed under the brand name **Marinol** by Roxane Laboratories. The firm's product information cautions that this legal but closely controlled drug is "highly abusable" and that "prescriptions should be limited to the amount necessary for a single cycle of chemotherapy."[14] The Marinol pills work as well as smoking marijuana, without adding the lung-threatening carcinogens found in the smoke. But because Marinol is expensive and may have adverse effects on mental status (e.g., drowsiness, muddled thinking, and easy laughter), it has been viewed mainly as a second-line therapy for patients who do poorly on the prevalent

phenothiazines (Compazine, Tigan, and Torecan).

The 1990s saw the introduction of an important class of antiemetics, the **serotonin antagonists**. Like dopamine, serotonin is a neurotransmitter intimately involved in the transmission of emetic stimuli to the vomiting center. Michael B. Tyers, a pharmacologist with Glaxo Group Research, points out that serotonin receptors are "densely located in areas important in the emetic reflex, including the chemoreceptor trigger zone."[15] The serotonin antagonists **ondansetron** and **granisetron**, marketed under the brand names **Zofran** and **Kytril**, bind to these receptors and stymie the emetic reflex. The advantages of these new drugs are their relative freedom from side effects and their proven efficacy with extremely emetic agents like cisplatin. Writing in 1993, Steven M. Grunberg and his colleague Paul J. Hesbeth observed that "fifteen years ago patients receiving cisplatin for the first time had a median of 12 vomiting episodes within the first 24 hours, whereas now more than 50 percent have no vomiting at all."[16] Serotonin antagonists have been a godsend for cisplatin patients; but several studies suggest that for moderately emetic regimens like those typically prescribed for early-stage breast cancer, the combination of a potent dopamine antagonist like metoclopramide (Reglan) and a corticosteroid like dexamethasone (Decadron) may be equally effective and considerably less expensive.[17] Like the dopamine antagonists, serotonin antagonists can be administered intravenously or taken orally, and they can be given concurrently with corticosteroids and sedatives.

The specter of nausea and vomiting has not been completely banished from cancer chemotherapy, but it is not nearly as fearsome as it used to be. Oncologists have realized that just as there are diverse mechanisms for activating these reflexes, combination of diverse antiemetics stand a better chance of deactivating them. These days the prescription for an antiemetic regimen may be longer than that for the chemotherapy. A few minutes before patients receive their cytotoxic drugs, they are usually given a dopamine or serotonin antagonist, a corticosteroid, and a sedative. This antiemetic regimen may be administered intravenously. Afterwards patients are sent home with a supply of pills to take every four to six hours, "p.r.n." (abbreviation for *pro re nata*, Latin for "as needed").[18] The most likely side effect of these antiemetic combinations is a drowsiness which fortuitously puts patients to sleep and dulls their memories of any emetic episodes. Carol Ann H. Peters, an oncology nurse at the University of Pennsylvania Hospital, explains that "the goal is for the patient to sleep through the nausea and emetogenic peaks of the chemotherapy. The patient will awaken to vomit, thus protecting the airway, and then fall back to sleep. The following day the patient is able to recall the number of emeses but not the feeling of nausea, so conditioning is avoided."[19]

There is no reason why today's chemotherapy patients need to suffer terribly from emesis; our antiemetic drugs do not interfere with the anticancer activity of our cytotoxic drugs. Therefore the matter of emesis prevention should be discussed at every consultation, and patients should not hesitate to ask questions if they do not fully understand their oncologist's instructions. Besides preemptive antiemetic medication, a modicum of restraint also helps to forestall nausea and vomiting. The day on which chemotherapy is administered and the day following it are not an auspicious time for heavy meals, for greasy or spicy foods, or for alcoholic beverages. Patients should opt instead for light meals featuring bland cool foods (cottage cheese, toast, crackers) and innocuous beverages (chicken soup, soft drinks).

Certain practical matters must not be overlooked. Any patient receiving an antiemetic regimen concurrently with chemotherapy should have someone else—a friend, a relative, or a volunteer from a support group—drive her to and from the oncologist's office. Antiemetic drugs, especially potent sedatives like lorazepam, impair one's ability to drive a car and to perform other tasks requiring mental alertness. Usually chemotherapy is most advantageously scheduled for afternoon administration, so that the patient will be enjoying sedative-assisted sleep during the time (six to twelve hours later) when we anticipate the strongest emetic impulses. Oncology practices tend to be especially busy on Friday afternoons—people who work on weekdays naturally want to use the weekend to recover from their chemotherapy session. Fortunately, almost all of them will be feeling fine by Monday morning.

Hair Today—Gone Tomorrow?

Alopecia (hair loss) is the other chemotherapy side effect that everybody knows about. To professional oncologists, alopecia is only of incidental concern since it is reversible and does not affect a patient's overall health or require an alteration to the chemotherapy regimen. To many patients, however, hair loss is a devastating event which damages their self-esteem and poses all sorts of annoying dilemmas. Jane Poulson, an experienced physician on the University of Toronto Faculty of Medicine, learned to appreciate the patients' point of view when she herself was diagnosed with breast cancer in 1996. "Losing my hair," she recalls, "was more upsetting than any of the other physical consequences of cancer therapy. There I was, engaged in a battle for my life, and weeping on day 21 of the first cycle of chemotherapy because my hair—which would grow back—was slithering away down the drain." Dr. Paulson soon discovered that the conventional hair prostheses had their limitations: "Yes, there were some very cute cotton hats or scarves. Yes, my wig was a dead ringer for my natural hair. But both hats and wigs felt suffocating. Regular people do not wear hats indoors. Out of doors, the first puff of wind struck terror to my heart. I had to choose between walking along with my hand on my head or chasing after a truant wig."[20]

Chemotherapy does not affect hair which has already grown out—this hair has no blood supply, and it is in any case fully keratinized and quite dead. Drugs like Adriamycin and high-dose cyclophosphamide attack the rapidly multiplying cells in the multitudinous hair follicles embedded in the skin. The scalp is affected first, since the hair-making cells are more active here than in the other hairy regions of the body (e.g., eyebrows, axillae, groin). Once these cells are damaged, the shafts of any newly-formed hairs will be abnormally fragile and thin. Thus a week or two after a patient is exposed to certain drug combinations, scalp hairs will begin to break off at the skin's surface and fall out.

Cytotoxic drugs vary widely in their potential to cause alopecia. Some agents have little effect on the hair follicles; but Adriamycin-based regimens like AC or FAC have the potential to produce total alopecia, with the eyebrows, eyelashes, and pubic hair being affected as well as the scalp hair. In contrast, breast cancer patients assigned to classic CMF usually do not lose their scalp hair, although after a cycle or two they might notice that it has become thinner and seems to have lost its luster. Neither fluorouracil nor methotrexate has been implicated in severe alopecia, and low-dose oral cyclophosphamide is relatively gentle on the hair follicles. Alopecia is not permanent because a few "stem cells" in each individual hair follicle tend to lie dormant—they will not be actively dividing during chemotherapy administration, and thus they will survive to produce a new crop of hair. But patients who have suffered substantial alopecia should not expect an adequate regrowth of hair until several months after the end of therapy, and then they should be prepared for the possibility that their new hair will be somewhat different in color and in texture than their original hair.

Our efforts to find a reliable way of preventing hair loss during chemotherapy have been disappointing. Back in the 1970s researchers at the University of Arizona Cancer Center reported that local hypothermia (i.e., chilling the scalp) seemed to help, and soon several manufacturers were producing "chemocaps" (scalp ice packs) for patients to wear before and during drug infusions.[22] The idea here was that chilling the scalp ought to reduce the blood flow to the hair follicles and therefore restrict their exposure to the cytotoxic agents. But the effectiveness of this technique has not been demonstrated in randomized clinical trials, and most oncologists are skeptical of it.[23] Wigs remain popular. The prudent patient will determine beforehand how much alopecia is likely to result from her chemotherapy regimen, then anticipate the problem by purchasing a wig or two in advance. In her book *The Race Is Run One Step at a Time*, chemotherapy veteran Nancy Brinker points out that wigs made from "virgin hair" (natural hair that has never been colored) are the most natural-looking, but that "synthetic wigs are usually less expensive and much easier to take care of." Wig prices can range from under \$100 to \$3,000 or more; the cost is often covered by health insurance if the oncologist has previously written a prescription for a "hair prosthesis." Mrs. Brinker suggests that chemotherapy patients have their hair cut short before alopecia begins: "Many women find it easier to make the adjustment from short hair to no hair rather than from long hair to no hair."[24] Closely cropped hair is also an asset when shopping for hats, scarves, and wigs—one gets a much better idea of how these items will subsequently look, feel, and fit.

Patients concerned with their appearance may wish to consult Nancy Brinker's book; it abounds in hints on how to look stylish while undergoing chemotherapy. For referrals to local beauticians and wig retailers, they should contact their city's chapter of the American Cancer Society. The ACS has long been promoting a sophisticated program called **"Look Good—Feel Better"**: it is intended to respond to the sudden cosmetic dilemmas created by chemotherapy.

Bone Marrow Suppression:
Controlling the Risk of Infection

Prospective patients and other laypersons are usually unaware of the really dangerous side effect of chemotherapy—the cytotoxic drugs destroy the newly-formed blood cells being created in the bone marrow. Since chemotherapy has little effect on the mature blood cells already in circulation (they are not actively dividing and therefore not especially vulnerable), **bone marrow suppression** does not become apparent until a week or two after drug administration. The cellular deficiencies may manifest themselves in several ways. Patients undergoing chemotherapy typically complain of increasing fatigue, not without reason. After a few cycles of chemo they begin to suffer from **anemia**, a shortage

of the red blood cells which carry energizing oxygen to the body's tissues. **Thrombocytopenia**, a shortage of the platelets necessary for blood to clot, could lead to hemorrhaging. For all practical purposes, however, neither anemia nor thrombocytopenia poses much of a problem in breast cancer chemotherapy—the former condition tends to be mild, the latter does not often become severe enough to cause symptoms. **Neutropenia** is a more immediate concern. The term indicates a deficiency of **neutrophils** or (as they are sometimes called) **polymorphonuclear granulocytes**. Neutrophils are the expendable foot soldiers of the immune system: far more numerous than other white cells, they readily engage invading bacteria in mortal combat. They have been dubbed "neutrophils" because their cytoplasmic granules (or vesicles) appear to stain a neutral color when viewed under the microscope.

The extent to which oncological office procedures are dictated by fears of neutropenia is not generally appreciated. First of all, there are those incessant finger pricks to obtain teeny-tiny blood specimens, performed as soon as the patient walks through the door. The idea behind this practice is to verify that there are sufficient numbers of circulating neutrophils before administering additional chemotherapy. As neutrophils have a lifespan of only a few hours, a deficiency in their numbers quickly becomes apparent. Our cytotoxic regimens have tended to run on 21-day or 28-day cycles because the lowest neutrophil count—this is called **"the nadir"** in oncological parlance—normally occurs sometime between 10 and 14 days after drug administration, with adequate recovery of neutrophil numbers sometime between day 21 and day 28. Different drugs and different dose levels produce different degrees and durations of bone marrow suppression—recovery from that dangerous nadir takes longer with some regimens than with others.[25]

Neutropenia is conventionally diagnosed when the neutrophil count drops below 1,000 per microliter of blood. An older definition of neutropenia—fewer than 1,000 neutrophils per cubic millimeter of blood—still appears in many textbooks. These two measurement units (microliters and cubic millimeters) are essentially identical. Any reading below 1,000 means that chemotherapy cannot be administered because the patient is now extremely vulnerable to bacterial and fungal infections. A reading under 500 has long been interpreted as a minor medical emergency—patients with neutrophil counts this low have often been confined to restricted-access hospital rooms specially designed to keep out pathogens. When neutropenic patients start to run a fever, physicians must assume the presence of infection and a potential for deadly septicemia. Traditionally patients with fever were hospitalized and given intravenous broad-spectrum antibiotics before anything else was done, so urgent did the situation seem to be. Those laboratory analyses of blood and urine samples and of throat swabbings, which might tell us which particular microorganism was running amuck, just had to wait.

In the 1990s oncologists began to consider the different degrees of neutropenia, with a view to distinguishing between those neutropenic patients who required emergency hospitalization and those who might be simply "observed" (followed closely without treatment) or treated on an outpatient basis. Neutropenia without fever and lasting only a few days is now perceived as "low-risk." A study done at Houston's M. D. Anderson Cancer Center involving the newer drug paclitaxel (Taxol) found that 100% of the participating breast cancer patients experienced neutrophil counts lower than 500; but of these patients only 36% developed fevers, and only 8% had documented infections.

The bone marrow suppression, while considerable, usually proved transient.[26] The recent availability of powerful oral antibiotics like ciprofloxacin should lead to inexpensive outpatient management of this condition. Alison Freifeld of the National Cancer Institute and her colleagues randomly assigned 232 chemotherapy patients with fever and severe neutropenia (neutrophil counts less than 100) to receive "either oral ciprofloxacin plus amoxicillin-clavulanate or intravenous ceftazidime." In this trial the patients receiving the convenient oral antibiotics fared as well as those given the traditional intravenous therapy. "None of the patients died," Freifeld et al report, "and fever disappeared within five days in over 90 percent of all episodes."[27]

Several neutropenia and consequent infections requiring hospitalization are relatively uncommon in breast cancer chemotherapy, but all patients need to be aware of this danger. Jeffrey H. Silber of the University of Pennsylvania Cancer Center and his colleagues point out that an excessively low nadir (i.e., an unusually depressed neutrophil count) after the first cycle of chemotherapy is "an excellent predictor" of subsequent neutropenia : "the bone marrow becomes less resilient the longer the duration of chemotherapy."[28] Patients should therefore observe commonsense precautions throughout the time they are receiving cytotoxic drugs and for several weeks afterwards. They need to avoid physical overexertion (which may depress the immune response) and to get plenty of rest. Insofar as possible, they should also avoid exposure to large crowds and to persons with upper respiratory infections (colds and influenzas). Diligent hand-washing with a mild soap may reduce the risk of microbial infection, but then it should not be done so much that the skin starts to dry out and become cracked. Small cuts and fissures in the skin offer pathogens an entry portal. Excessive sun exposure during chemotherapy would be unwise. Fresh fruits and vegetables, unequivocally recommended for healthy persons, must now be consumed with caution—raw produce can carry bacteria or fungi. Undercooked eggs, meat, chicken, or seafood also pose a hazard of possible bacterial contamination. Chemotherapy patients should opt for soft bland foods which have been thoroughly cooked. Peeled or processed fruits (apples, bananas, oranges, pears, prunes) and cooked vegetables are much less likely to harbor microorganisms.

The Gastrointestinal Gamut

Cytotoxic drugs have their greatest effect on rapidly dividing cells. Besides the ever-active cells in the hair follicles and the ever-evolving blood cells being born in the bone marrow, another cellular species sure to be affected is represented by the epithelial cells which line the oral cavity and the gastrointestinal tract. These cells are also extremely active. Because they are subject to constant wear and tear, they have to be replaced every few days. Chemotherapy's effect on them is not as dramatic as sudden alopecia or as precisely measurable as neutropenia, but it is inevitable. After a cycle or two of cytotoxic drug administration, the entire food processing apparatus becomes mildly inflamed—mouth, tongue, esophagus, stomach, small intestine, colon, and rectum. The taste buds are an early casualty: patients notice that foods begin to taste differently. Adriamycin is a major culprit in this transformation; this drug leaves a metallic flavor in the mouth. Some patients also find that their sense of smell is affected in strange ways; odors they never noticed before may suddenly become offensive.[29]

Stomatitis, inflammation of the oral cavity, can occasionally be so troubling as to necessitate a postponement of chemotherapy, but most cases are mild. The buccal mucosa (moist membranes of the interior cheek) may become reddish, and the patient might experience a slight burning sensation when eating. In severe cases the oral cavity turns as red as a fire-engine and becomes covered with ulcers; patients so afflicted could have difficulty swallowing water. Fluorouracil has been strongly implicated in stomatitis. Researchers at the Mayo Clinic and other Midwestern hospitals discovered that patients who swished ice chips in their mouths while receiving intravenous fluorouracil subsequently had a lower incidence of oral cavity irritations. The apparent side effects caused by this prophylactic measure included "temporary mouth numbness or a headache," both of which "resolved after cessation of cryotherapy."[30] This inexpensive remedy would seem harmless enough.

Treatments for symptomatic stomatitis rely heavily on systemic or topical analgesics, prescribed to lessen the pain so that patients can eat and drink normally. Appropriate antibiotics may be given to combat the bacterial, fungal, or viral (herpes) infections which tend to erupt in the mouths of immunosuppressed persons with ulcerated oral mucosa. But prevention is the best strategy: we want to reduce the likelihood of oral complications developing in the first place. Needless to say, pre-existing dental problems (cavities, missing fillings, poorly fitting dentures) should be attended to before chemotherapy begins. Oral hygiene is of paramount importance during treatment; patients should remember to brush their teeth gently, using a soft brush and a mild toothpaste. Flossing, if done at all, has to be accomplished carefully; toothpicks or other pointed instruments should not be used to clean the spaces between the teeth. Gargling with a lukewarm saline solution (a teaspoon salt in a glass of water) helps to keep the mouth clean and to ameliorate minor discomforts; this can be done before and after meals, and at bedtime. Variations on this home remedy may be recommended for specific purposes. Adding a little hydrogen peroxide to the saline solution (or to plain water) gives us a mouth rinse with germicidal properties. Adding sodium bicarbonate (baking soda) gives us a rinse which reduces mouth acidity. Commercial mouthwashes which contain a great deal of alcohol should be avoided because they have a drying effect. Patients should inspect their mouths once a day and report any problems to their oncologist. Persistent bleeding from the gums is suggestive of thrombocytopenia, while soft whitish patches on the tongue and buccal mucosa are usually indicative of an overgrowth of the commonplace fungus *Candida albicans*.[31]

Daily visual inspections of the stomach are not practical. We should therefore assume that the gastric lining has been irritated by the cytotoxic drugs, and we should try not to irritate it further. The identification of foods to avoid during treatment is best given in general terms. Roughage should be minimized: this is not the time to nibble on raw broccoli at the salad bars—or to fill up on popcorn at the movies! In addition to "the raw and the rough," warnings need to be sounded against *the fried, the greasy, the highly seasoned, and the exotically spiced*. Don't visit that neighborhood Pakistani restaurant for a hot and spicy specialty which flows through your bowels like a river of fire—the meal would be even more memorable than usual! The preferred diet for chemotherapy patients can be summed up in a very few words—*the bland and the thoroughly digestible*. This recipe is dull, but the cost of deviating from it may be registered in discomfort. Many manuals on cancer nursing also propose to prohibit alcohol and coffee.

We are not sure that a total prohibition is necessary, but anyone can imagine that potent martinis or strong black coffee hitting an empty pre-irritated stomach may produce the wrong kind of jolt. Aspirin and products containing aspirin (e.g., many cold remedies) should not be taken during chemotherapy. Not only does aspirin have the potential to irritate the gastric mucosa, but it tends to reduce the blood's ability to clot, an undesirable attribute in patients whose platelet counts are low.

Diarrhea, the passage of multiple soft or liquid stools each day, is the most frequent intestinal complaint reported during chemotherapy. Occasionally, diarrhea may be due to a bacterial infection in the intestines; but the vast majority of episodes among breast cancer patients are caused by the antimetabolites fluorouracil and methotrexate, or by Adriamycin. These drugs are known to irritate the intestinal mucosa. Within a week or two after the first chemotherapy session, the inflamed gastrointestinal membranes will not be doing an efficient job of absorbing the water and nutrients passing by, and they will be secreting abnormally large quantities of mucus.[32] Both these factors strongly predispose to diarrhea, and any ensuing loss of fluids and nutrients can quickly lead to dehydration and malnutrition. A patient with severe diarrhea may have to be placed on an all-liquid diet and given a prescription for a powerful antidiarrheal drug—yet most cases can be handled with more conservative measures. Popular over-the-counter products like Kaopectate (a brand name for kaolin and pectin) or Imodium A-D (a brand name for loperamide hydrochloride) usually suffice to end the acute misery. Thereafter patients should be counseled to maintain adequate fluid intake and to stay on a low-residue diet. In this instance high-fiber foods are best avoided—refined cereal products (e.g., white bread, corn flakes, noodles) can be served in lieu of bran muffins and granola bars. Broiled fish or baked chicken accompanied by mashed potatoes might qualify as an appropriate main dish. Only well-cooked and totally digestible vegetables should be consumed—e.g., tender green peas rather than the more fibrous cabbage. Bananas, rich in potassium, can help to remedy electrolyte deficiencies.

Constipation can also occur during chemotherapy, possibly due to reduced peristalsis (i.e., fewer wavelike motions in the intestines). As with diarrhea, adequate fluid intake should be maintained, but the dietary advice is just the opposite. In this case a high-residue diet ought to be followed. We still don't want irritating roughage like popcorn or raw broccoli, but fibrous content would otherwise be desirable. A breakfast cereal rich in bran or wheat fiber might be a good beginning to the day. Peeled apples, canned pears, and stewed prunes figure prominently on the list of acceptable fruits; and well-cooked string beans or Brussels sprouts are representative of efficacious vegetables. Stool softeners like Colace (brand name for docusate) and gentle bulk-forming laxatives like Metamucil (brand name for psyllium) may be helpful in reestablishing regularity. Fast-acting stimulant laxatives like Ex-Lax (brand name for phenolphthalein) are probably best avoided.

What we've said about sore mouths and diarrhea may lead the casual reader to assume that patients typically emerge from chemotherapy as thin as rails, having lost considerable weight. But insofar as breast cancer chemotherapy is concerned, the converse tends to be true. Six months of CMF has typically translated into **weight gain**, sometimes as much as twenty pounds or more.[33] Several factors could be cited to explain this well-documented phenomenon. First of all, those episodes of diarrhea and

stomatitis, if they occur at all, are likely to be mild and transient. Secondly, patients typically increase their food intake while undergoing chemotherapy, either because they want to maintain their strength or because they want "compensation" for feelings of depression. They may preferentially select high-calorie foods like ice cream or custard, which are easy on the oral cavity and gastrointestinal tract but hard on the waistline. Thirdly, patients may reduce their level of physical activity during chemotherapy, either because they feel fatigued or because they too readily fall into the role of invalids. None of these behavioral modifications is desirable—excess weight gain poses almost as many hazards as severe malnutrition. Chemotherapy patients should thus avoid overeating and check their weight several times a week. While strenuous exertion is not prudent, neither is lying on the couch. For their psychological well-being and overall health, patients should engage in moderate exercise on a daily basis.

Fertility and Sexuality

Breast cancer chemotherapy frequently has adverse effects on the ability of premenopausal women to engage in sexual intercourse and to bear children. Yet for all their frankness in discussing chemo's other side effects, oncologists and oncology nurses tend to shy away from meaningful discussions of these extremely personal matters. As a result many patients in their thirties and forties are "surprised" when, after a cycle or two of chemotherapy, they stop menstruating or experience dyspareunia (painful intercourse) due to insufficient vaginal lubrication. But these effects have been thoroughly documented in medical literature. While the statistics on newer adjuvant regimens like the NSABP's dose-intense AC or combinations emphasizing the taxoid drugs (paclitaxel and docetaxel) are still being compiled, we have long known what the traditional six-month courses of CMF and FAC can do—they accomplish chemical oophorectomy, sending most premenopausal patients into the menopause a decade ahead of time. Gianni Bonadonna and his colleague Pinuccia Valagussa published some sobering statistics on 549 premenopausal women given CMF at Milan's *Instituto Nazionale Tumori*. Amenorrhea (cessation of the menses) occurred in 54% of the patients aged 40 or younger; it proved to be reversible in 23% of the affected patients. In the CMF patients over age 40, amenorrhea was virtually universal (96% affected) and usually permanent—only 4% of the affected patients resumed menstruating after the completion of chemotherapy.[34] At the Consensus Development Conference on breast cancer chemotherapy held in 1985, Gabriel N. Hortobagyi and his co-workers presented comparable data on the premenopausal patients treated with FAC at Houston's M. D. Anderson Cancer Center. While patients under age 30 continued to menstruate normally, "33% of those between 30 and 39 years of age, 96% of those 40 to 49, and all patients older than 50 became amenorrheic during therapy." After chemotherapy about half of the women under age 40 started menstruating again, but "few patients over 40 resumed menses."[35]

The prospect of permanent ovarian suppression may not be upsetting to breast cancer patients in their forties who have already had all the children they wish to bear. It is naturally disturbing to patients in their twenties and thirties who aspire to motherhood. As a rule of thumb we would anticipate that women under age 35 will recover fertility and again be able to have children; unfortunately, there have been no adequate follow-up studies on such women or on any subsequent pregnancies they might have.

Will those chemotherapy patients who resume menstruating eventually enter the menopause a few years earlier than their contemporaries who were not exposed to cytotoxic agents? Will the infants conceived by former chemotherapy patients be at greater risk of genetic defects? At present we do not have hard data on these important questions; however, we do know which drug is principally responsible for the ovarian suppression. Bonnie S. Reichman and Karen B. Green of the New York Hospital and Cornell University Medical Center remind us that cyclophosphamide, that versatile mainstay of breast cancer regimens, is the main culprit: "Alkylating agents cause cytotoxicity independent of the cell cycle and affect the resting oocyte. Ovarian biopsies in patients undergoing cyclophosphamide-based treatment reveal complete absence of ova or small numbers of inactive ova with fibrosis and no evidence of follicular maturation."[36] Cyclophosphamide also has depressive effects on sperm production in male chemotherapy patients. Women over age 40 fare so badly because they have only a limited number of follicles remaining; and when these are destroyed, the ovaries will cease to produce ova as well as the hormones estrogen and progesterone.

Avant-garde researchers have proposed several novel techniques to preserve fertility in young women facing chemotherapy for breast cancer or other malignancies. Roger Gosden of the University of Leeds in England suggests that one ovary might be surgically removed prior to drug administration and "cryopreserved" (frozen), thus protecting the undeveloped follicles from damage. After chemotherapy the ovary left in the body would be sterile; but because the blood vessels supplying it would be intact, it would offer an excellent location for an ovarian graft. That sterile ovary could now be taken out, and the cryopreserved ovary grafted in its place and reactivated. This technique has worked well in sheep—the experimental animals subsequently had successful pregnancies.[37]

At the moment, however, the only solution tested in large-scale clinical trials has been the most obvious one—viz., *drop the culprit cyclophosphamide from CMF!* Around 1980 the National Cancer Institute and the National Surgical Adjuvant Breast and Bowel Project joined forces to explore this possibility. As former NCI director Vincent T. DeVita, Jr., recalls, "one program (methotrexate and fluorouracil) was actually designed to test a treatment option that did not include alkylating agents in order to avoid their effects on the ovary."[38] Like classic CMF (parent regimen), **MF** ran on a 28-day cycle, with intravenous methotrexate and fluorouracil being given on days 1 and 8. The differences were an increased dose of methotrexate (100 mg/m^2 on each treatment day instead of 40 mg/m^2) and the omission of the cyclophosphamide tablets. Beginning in 1981 **NSABP Protocol B-13** randomly assigned 679 breast cancer patients diagnosed with "node-negative, estrogen receptor-negative tumors" to receive twelve cycles of MF or to receive no adjuvant therapy. The patients enrolled in this trial were at moderate risk for metastatic progression—although node-negative, they were all ER-negative, and they tended to be young (about 59% under age 50) and to have had large primary tumors (about 55% over two centimeters in diameter). The four-year results which the NSABP published in 1989 revealed a significant advantage for the MF arm: 80% of these patients remained free of recurrences, but only 71% of those who received no adjuvant therapy were still disease-free. As breast cancer regimens go, MF was well-tolerated. There was no hair loss to speak of, but patients reported various degrees of nausea

(37% affected), vomiting (47% affected), diarrhea (45% affected), and stomatitis (31% affected).[39]

NSABP Protocol B-19 asked the really important question—is MF as good as classic CMF in fighting disseminated breast cancer, or would patients who opted for the less toxic regimen be inviting metastases? Between October 1988 and July 1990 the NSABP randomly assigned 1,095 node-negative, ER-negative patients to receive six cycles of MF or six cycles of CMF. The majority of patients enrolled in this trial (slightly over 60%) were under age 50. In 1996 Bernard Fisher and his NSABP colleagues published their five-year results: the CMF arm had fared significantly better than the MF arm in disease-free survival (DFS), with 82% of the CMF patients being free of recurrences compared to 73% of the MF patients. When the analysis was restricted to patients under age 50, the CMF advantage became even more apparent—84% DFS on CMF, but only 72% DFS on MF.[40] We would expect that the DFS advantage seen at five years would eventually translate into an advantage in long-term survival. "In the early stages of breast cancer," Dr. DeVita reminds us, "long-term trends are reproducibly predicted by what happens to relapse-free survival between eighteen months and three years."[41]

There is as yet no easy answer to the problem of reduced fertility after chemotherapy. Persons who undergo such extensive therapeutic interventions to save their lives are no doubt expecting too much if they want their "reborn lives" to be exactly normal. Survival comes at a price—this is as true for chemotherapy patients as it is for persons dying of heart disease or kidney failure whose lives are rescued by organ transplants. While the MF regimen does avoid the worst ovarian toxicity, NSABP Protocol B-19 indicates that cyclophosphamide cannot be omitted from breast cancer regimens without sacrificing considerable antitumor activity. Moreover, functional ovaries secreting estrogen may be deemed undesirable in high-risk patients with ER-positive tumors, since the hormone has the potential to stimulate the growth of any disseminated cancer cells. We have some reason to worry that continued fertility and subsequent pregnancies might increase the risk of metastatic progression in this patient subset. As yet we do not know whether antiestrogenic drugs like tamoxifen can altogether counteract the presumably stimulatory effect of functional ovaries. These troubling uncertainties were not a concern in NSABP Protocols B-13 and B-19, because enrollment in both trials was scrupulously limited to ER-negative patients.

Cytotoxic chemotherapy affects sexual activity in various ways. The loss of hair makes patients feel undesirable; fatigue drains away their desire and physical energy, and feelings of depression inevitably accompany treatment. Sexual intercourse may become difficult due to vaginitis (inflammation of the vaginal lining). The drugs will damage any replicating cells in the vaginal mucosa just as they damage replicating cells in the oral cavity and gastrointestinal tract. Ovarian suppression, even if only temporary, nonetheless stops that production of estrogen which accomplishes vaginal lubrication in premenopausal women.

The most accessible remedy for vaginal dryness is Johnson and Johnson's familiar lubricant **K-Y jelly**, available without prescription at drugstores and supermarkets. Stacey Young-McCaughan, an officer in the U. S. Army Nurse Corps, points out that newer products like **Replens**, **Gyne-moistrin**, and **Lubrin** (brand names) "are designed to be used regularly to maintain vaginal moisture." **Astroglide** (brand name), "a water-based, glycerin lubricant," has been "designed to be used with intercourse." Unfortunately, problems with sexual expression tend to linger long after the completion of chemotherapy, and they are usually too complex to be adequately remedied by over-the-counter products. "Human sexuality," Young-McCaughan perceptively writes, "is influenced by various physiologic, psychologic, and interpersonal events, and women treated for breast cancer can suffer multiple insults to their sexual self in each of these areas."[42]

An important step toward recovery would seem to be better communication between patients and healthcare professionals. Oncologists who quickly become alarmed at falling neutrophil counts and slight fevers need to recognize the more subtle warnings that personal lives are in disarray. And patients should not fear to discuss sexual dysfunctions with their physicians and nurses. Some form of hormonal replacement might be considered for former chemotherapy patients whose lives are made miserable by hot flashes and vaginitis. It is unlikely that low-dose estrogen therapy would increase the risk of metastatic progression in ER-negative patients, and the application of estrogenic vaginal creams might not affect the prognosis of ER-positive patients who are taking tamoxifen or some other systemic antiestrogen. Testosterone, the principal androgen, could be given systemically to improve the libido or topically to combat vaginitis; neither form of therapy seems likely to have an adverse effect on prognosis.[43]

Chapter Twenty-five

High-Dose Therapy and the Taxoid Drugs

During the 1990s two innovations in breast cancer medicine held the attention of oncologists and the public alike; both seemed to foreshadow chemotherapy regimens which could cure a much larger percentage of patients, even some with widespread metastatic disease. Laypersons often referred to the first innovation as a **"bone marrow transplant"**: this was an erroneous and misleading description. The proper terminology is **high-dose chemotherapy with autologous bone marrow support** or (after the mid-1990s) **with peripheral blood stem cell support**. This particular innovation bespeaks enormous advances in biological knowledge and medical technology, but its application to the treatment of breast malignancies has been extremely controversial. In contrast, the recently available taxoid drugs **paclitaxel** and **docetaxel** represent a long overdue innovation in pharmacology whose addition to breast cancer chemotherapy is universally applauded. Hitherto our adjuvant regimens have principally relied on drugs introduced way back in the 1950s (e.g., cyclophosphamide, fluorouracil, methotrexate) or in the 1970s (e.g., Adriamycin and tamoxifen). But however welcome the taxoid drugs may be, we have much to learn before we can be sure that we are using them in the most efficient way.

The Bone Marrow Strategies

All higher life forms owe their existence to **cellular differentiation**. In humans this amazing process is most strikingly displayed during embryonic development, when a single pluripotential cell (the fertilized ovum) gives rise to the hundreds of specialized cell types which make up the body's diverse tissues. Once differentiated, our somatic cells do not undergo further evolution; and some of them—for example, the neurons of the brain and spinal cord—cannot even reproduce themselves, so that any appreciable cellular destruction causes irreparable injury to the tissue involved. While the process of cellular differentiation is not a prominent feature of the adult body, the jelly-like bone marrow constitutes an exception. Here this process is perpetual, constantly ongoing from embryonic development until death. In the bone marrow, **pluripotential stem cells** have the awesome task of fulfilling the body's unrelenting demands for new blood cells. When a stem cell divides in two, one of the daughter cells will remain an undifferentiated stem cell identical to its parent. But the other daughter cell must proceed down a pathway leading to differentiation—it may evolve into an erythrocyte (red blood cell), or a megakaryocyte (platelet forerunner), or any of the various white cells (neutrophils, basophils, eosinophils, monocytes and macrophages, and lymphocytes). The speed of **hematopoiesis** (blood cell production) and the precise lineage of the cells being produced are determined by the body's needs at the moment. Anemic conditions tend to stimulate the production of red blood cells, and bacterial infections will result in a larger output of neutrophils. Elevated basophil counts are usually indicative of allergic reactions, and eosinophilia (too many eosinophils) is sometimes a physician's only clue to subtle parasitic infestations with intestinal worms or blood flukes.

As we have seen in the preceding chapter, the rapidly multiplying and evolving cells in the bone marrow are especially vulnerable to cytotoxic chemotherapy. Oncologists have long regarded the marrow as the main obstacle to therapeutic success, because the dose-limiting side effect of many cancer drugs is **myelosuppression** (marrow toxicity). In other words—just when the blood level of a drug begins to be high enough to kill any circulating cancer cells, the dose must often be sharply reduced lest the stem cells in the bone marrow be so decimated that they cannot reconstitute hematopoiesis. Without an adequate hematopoietic recovery, the chemotherapy patient would soon die from infections or from internal hemorrhaging. Understandably, many oncologists have believed that they could cure many more malignancies if only the cytotoxic dose levels .could be escalated beyond the narrow limits dictated by bone marrow tolerance. But prior to the 1970s we had no way to accomplish this dose escalation without destroying the vital stem cells. In that decade, however, physicians at Seattle's Fred Hutchinson Cancer Research Center and other institutions perfected techniques for marrow cryopreservation (i.e., freezing). Henceforth a small portion of the patient's bone marrow could be extracted before the high-dose

chemotherapy, cryopreserved, and then reinfused afterwards. The thawed-out stem cells remained fully viable. Frederick R. Appelbaum of Fred Hutchinson reminds us of "the remarkable regenerative capacity" of these cells: "In mice the transfer of a single stem cell can result in hematopoietic reconstitution of a lethally irradiated recipient. While human bone marrow has never been put to this test, transplantation of considerably less than ten percent of total body marrow regularly results in complete replacement of a patient's hematopoietic system. After intravenous infusion, marrow cells have the capacity to home to the marrow space."[1] Of course, the word transplant is inappropriately used when the marrow cells being infused are autologous (the patient's own). What the newspaper and TV reporters might call "a bone marrow transplant" is in this instance no more than a dodge to permit the administration of cytotoxic doses which would otherwise prove lethal. By the end of the 1970s, **high-dose chemotherapy with autologous marrow support** was curing cases of Hodgkin's disease and the non-Hodgkin's lymphomas which had proven resistant to standard-dose regimens. This technique was really very simple—extract a little bone marrow and freeze it, then give the massive dose of chemo destroying tumor cells and stem cells alike, then reinfuse the cryopreserved marrow so that hematopoiesis can be reestablished just in the nick of time.

Allogeneic bone marrow transplantation should not be confused with the aforementioned autologous strategy. In this instance the term transplant is entirely appropriate, as the patient is receiving someone else's bone marrow (*allogeneic* derives from the Greek word *allos*, meaning "other"). Allogeneic marrow transplantation has the potential to cure any and all genetic diseases arising in the pluripotential stem cells. When successful, it is curative for chronic myelogenous leukemia (the prevalent leukemia among adults) as well as for nonmalignant disorders like sickle-cell anemia and aplastic anemia. Allogeneic transplantation has occasionally been used to rescue patients with acute leukemias or with non-Hodgkin's lymphomas who did not respond to chemotherapy. Yet this strategy is so fraught with toxicity and uncertainty that only a desperately ill patient would chance it. First of all, the patient's own diseased marrow (i.e., the defective stem cells) must be destroyed—such "conditioning" has traditionally been accomplished by a combination of high-dose cyclophosphamide and total-body irradiation. After conditioning is completed, the patient will be extremely vulnerable to infections and hemorrhaging until the infused allogeneic marrow achieves engraftment (i.e., starts to produce blood cells). Long-term recovery is likely to be uncomplicated only with **syngeneic transplants**—that is, those in which the donor marrow derived from the patient's genetically identical twin brother or sister. Transplant patients who receive marrow from other relatives or from unrelated donors are prone to suffer from **graft-versus-host disease** (GVHD). In this syndrome the donor lymphocytes of the T-cell variety perceive the recipient's tissues as foreign and begin to attack them—the liver, the gastrointestinal tract, and the skin are typically affected. GVHD is no longer as threatening as it once was, because we now take pains to match the patient's tissue-identity markers—these are cell-surface proteins called **human leukocyte antigens** (HLA)—with those of any prospective marrow donor. Nonetheless, many recipients of allogeneic transplants must be maintained on immunosuppressive drugs like cyclosporine or prednisolone to head off this condition. E. Donnall Thomas, who won a Nobel prize for his work on allogeneic transplantation, concedes that as

a group transplant recipients tend to have shortened life expectancies; but he points out that "the slightly increased risk of death may not be so bad when one considers the alternative."[2]

Autologous Marrow Support:
The Early Experiments

Breast cancer patients are not candidates for allogeneic marrow transplantation. Although breast malignancies regularly metastasize to the bone marrow, they do not arise from the hematopoietic stem cells and therefore would not be curable by this strategy. But because breast malignancies tend to be more chemosensitive than other solid tumors, researchers quickly became interested in autologous strategies. Around 1980 Patricia S. Stewart and her colleagues at Fred Hutchinson gave high-dose cyclophosphamide and total-body irradiation to five young patients with metastatic breast cancer, rescuing them afterwards with infusions of their cryopreserved bone marrow. Two patients obtained a **complete response**, by which is meant that all evidence of malignancy seemed to vanish. No traces of disease could be detected after therapy either by clinical (physical) examination or by diagnostic imaging (e.g., by X-rays and CAT scans). Unfortunately, this early experiment did not herald a cure. One patient died of septicemia (systemic infection) before her reinfused marrow could achieve engraftment. Within a year the other four patients also died, either from progressive cancer or from opportunistic infections.[3]

During the early 1980s William P. Peters, Karen Antman, and their colleagues at Boston's Dana-Farber Cancer Institute worked hard to develop a high-dose regimen which could be routinely used for refractory solid tumors. The drug the Dana-Farber team pinned their hopes to was **cyclophos-phamide**, that versatile chemotherapeutic workhorse also known by the brand name **Cytoxan**. There were two good reasons for this choice. Alkylating agents like cyclo-phosphamide are principally dose-limited by myelosuppression. If this initial limitation is removed, much higher doses—say, anywhere from three to fifteen times higher—can be given before we encounter another life-threatening toxicity which requires us to reduce the dose or to discontinue treatment altogether. Cyclophosphamide also exhibits a pronounced **dose-response curve**—that is to say, the more medication you give, the more anticancer activity you get. In labora-tory experiments involving mice and cell cultures, higher doses of cyclophosphamide are consistently able to kill cancer cells which can survive at lower doses. Would cyclophosphamide dose escalation cure breast cancer as efficiently in patients as in test tubes? The first study the Dana-Farber team conducted did not directly address this question; as a so-called "Phase One" trial, it sought to record any toxic side effects and to determine a tolerable dose level. Bone mar-row was aspirated under general anesthesia from the iliac crests (the top of the hip bones) of 29 patients with various metastatic can-cers. These patients were subsequently hospitalized in sterile private rooms, given central (indwelling) venous catheters, and then administered a four-day intravenous regimen consisting of cyclophosphamide, the potent platinum drug cisplatin, and car-mustine (a second alkylating agent). The total cyclophosphamide dose was 5,625 milligrams per square meter of body surface area; we can begin to understand its magni-tude by comparing it to the cyclophos-phamide dose in the familiar outpatient regimen **FAC**. As explained in the preceding chapter, FAC calls for 2,400 mg/m^2 of the drug; yet this dose is spread out over some

six months, with only 400 mg/m^2 being infused every 28 days. The experimental Dana-Farber regimen called for one-hour infusions of 1,400 mg/m^2 cyclophosphamide on each of four successive days. Cisplatin was administered by continuous infusion, the dose being limited to 165 mg/m^2 because of this drug's potential to cause kidney damage. Carmustine was reserved for the final day, with 5 mg/m^2 being infused every minute to achieve the total dose of 600 mg/m^2 within two hours. Three days after this massive cytotoxic assault, the patients were reinfused with their cryopreserved bone marrow.[4]

The side effects from the Dana-Farber regimen were of a magnitude far surpassing anything observed in outpatient chemother-apy. All 29 patients suffered severe nausea and vomiting. By the conclusion of the four-day regimen, their hematopoietic stem cells had been decimated; and even the vigilant support services of the Dana-Farber staff could not prevent serious complications. All the patients became feverish. Culture-proven infections were documented in 18 patients, ranging from "bacteremias" (11 cases) to outbreaks of viral herpes (6 cases). One patient died of *Candida* (fungal) septicemia; and before their reinfused marrow cells could restore hematopoiesis, two additional pa-tients died of "thrombocytopenia-associated hemorrhage." These short-term complica-tions arising from myelosuppression were not the only danger. In some patients high-dose regimens may induce chronic fibrosis in the liver and lungs. Characteristic symptoms like hepatomegaly (liver enlargement) and progressive loss of liver function point to a diagnosis which the high-dose oncologists came to call **hepatic veno-occlusive disease**. Two patients in the Dana-Farber Phase One trial eventually died from this syndrome. Shortness of breath, fever, and hypoxemia (inadequate oxygenation of the blood) may be indicative of pulmonary (lung) fibrosis.

The high-dose oncologists use the term **interstitial pneumonitis** to describe this late sequela—two patients in the Dana-Farber trial eventually developed its troublesome symptoms.[5]

The aforementioned toxicity and horrendous treatment-related mortality (five of the 29 patients died from complications) would be altogether unacceptable in a chemotherapy regimen given—as are most regimens for metastatic carcinomas—simply for palliation. We can ease a terminal patient's symptoms with a far milder outpatient regimen, albeit with no expectation of changing the outcome. The rationale behind a chemotherapy so toxic that it required protracted hospitalization was, as William P. Peters explained, "to treat to the limits of tolerance with the intent to cure." With the cure of metastatic cancer as their endpoint, the Dana-Farber team felt that they had to discount partial responses. "Anything short of a complete response," Dr. Peters observed, "would be unlikely to contribute to long-term remissions."[6] Unfortunately, only a minority of the 29 patients in this first Dana-Farber trial obtained even a temporary disappearance of metastatic lesions. The two patients with colon cancer showed no response at all. Of the thirteen melanoma patients, eight experienced partial responses, and one had a complete response. The nine breast cancer patients fared better than most. Although one patient died from infection early on, all the others had measurable responses to this treatment—five partial and three complete. Most encouragingly, one of these complete responders still revealed no trace of cancer two years later in 1986, when Dr. Peters and his colleagues published the results of their Phase One trial.[7] Whether cured or not, that single case looked like a beacon of hope in the darkness.

The Duke University Program

In 1985 William P. Peters left Dana-Farber to become director of the Bone Marrow Transplant Program at the Duke University Medical Center in Durham, North Carolina. Under his guidance the Duke program soon gained a national reputation for its willingness to attempt the cure of seemingly hopeless breast cancer cases. The first Duke study recruited 22 premenopausal women with documented metastases from estrogen receptor-negative breast tumors; they were given the regimen developed at Dana-Farber (cyclophosphamide, cisplatin, carmustine), with their cryopreserved marrow extracts being subsequently reinfused to restore hematopoiesis. Mortality from this treatment remained high; several patients died of complications. But more than half of these young women (54%) obtained complete responses—no results even approaching this response rate had hitherto been reported . Although most of the complete responders soon relapsed, three of them were still alive and free of recurrences in 1995, more than eight years after they received the high-dose regimen.[8] No further treatment had been given—had these three patients actually been *cured* of metastatic breast cancer?

Before beginning their second study, Dr. Peters and his Duke colleagues tried to learn from those previous patients (the majority) who either did not achieve a complete response or who quickly relapsed after having done so. One factor strongly associated with treatment failure was bulky metastatic disease. Patients who relapsed usually had their recurrences at previously involved sites, suggesting that the brief exposure to high-dose chemotherapy was insufficient to eliminate hypoxic (poorly oxygenated) cancer cells in the center of large metastases. Patients who had previously been given multiple cytotoxic regimens also did not fare well, suggesting that the prior development of drug resistance constituted yet another barrier to success. The Duke team's plan to circumvent these obstacles was twofold. First of all, they wanted to treat patients earlier in the course of disease, before metastatic tumors had a chance to grow so large. Secondly, they would henceforth give patients several cycles of outpatient chemotherapy just before the inpatient high-dose regimen. They hoped to shrink any existing metastatic deposits to microscopic size, thereby improving the odds that a brief exposure to a massive cyclophosphamide dose would eradicate all the malignant cells.

Between 1987 and 1991 Dr. Peters and his co-workers applied their new strategy to 85 young breast cancer patients (median age 38) who had ten or more positive axillary nodes. We should emphasize that this time the high-dose regimen was being used as adjuvant therapy instead of salvage therapy. These patients had not yet developed distant metastases, although we would have expected them to do so owing to their youthful age and the extent of axillary involvement. For their outpatient "induction therapy," all patients received four cycles of dose-intense FAC (50% more of the drugs administered at each treatment session than in the standard six-cycle FAC). Bone marrow was harvested from each patient's iliac crests after the third cycle of FAC. When the patients recovered from the fourth cycle, they were hospitalized to receive their high-dose regimen of cyclophosphamide, cisplatin, and carmustine, with subsequent hematopoietic rescue by autologous marrow. The initial results of this study were published in the *Journal of Clinical Oncology* in 1993. With a median follow-up of 2.5 years, the rate of disease-free survival (DFS) for these Duke patients was 72%. By way of comparison, Dr. Peters and his colleagues cited the big randomized trial of

dose-intense FAC then being conducted by the Cancer and Leukemia Group B. Those patients in the CALGB trial with ten or more positive nodes who received the same four-cycle FAC regimen—but not the inpatient high-dose regimen—achieved only a 52% rate of DFS after 2.5 years of follow-up. Thus it seemed that the addition of a high-dose inpatient regimen offered a significant DFS advantage over even the most rigorous conventional chemotherapy, but was that advantage being purchased at too high a price? Dr. Peters and his colleagues frankly admitted their treatment's drawbacks. While suffering from the profound myelosuppression it induced, the Duke patients had to remain in rooms equipped with elaborate air filtration systems designed to keep out pathogens. Both visitors and staff members took precautions to preserve the sterile environment: "Access to rooms required masks, gloves, gowns, and shoe covers." Yet all these measures were not enough to prevent ten of the 85 patients (12%) from dying because of treatment-related complications.[9]

The Controversy Begins

Notwithstanding the toxicity of high-dose therapy with marrow support, hospitals across the United States quickly hopped on the bandwagon. Oncologists are naturally attracted to the idea of dose escalation, and they felt they had nothing better to offer the most desperate breast cancer cases. This procedure seemed to hold out the promise of cure. In 1989 only 261 American breast cancer patients received it; the tally for 1992 stood at 893 patients.[10] Houston's M. D. Anderson Cancer Center reported a 53% complete response rate in metastatic breast cancer, while conceding that about 9% of patients died from the therapy itself.[11] No patients died in the small study conducted at the Johns Hopkins Oncology Center in the late 1980s. The Center reported a 33% complete response rate in metastatic breast cancer, but this involved terribly protracted hospitalizations: "Patients were hospitalized a median of 41.5 days."[12] William P. Peters reminds us that in the late 1980s high-dose chemotherapy routinely led to "refractory thrombocytopenia" (severe platelet deficiencies), causing runs on hospital blood banks: "The average patient required more than 30 platelet transfusions and over 25 units of red blood cells."[13]

Any therapy for breast malignancies is likely to produce at least a simmering controversy. When Dr. Peters and other American oncologists started to talk about "curing" metastatic disease with a treatment involving unparalleled morbidity, they were sure to ignite a firestorm! The Harvard breast surgeon Blake Cady opined that "bone marrow and stem cell transplantation" represented "a dangerous and illusory idea."[14] No doubt many surgeons shared Dr. Cady's suspicions; the oncologists themselves were sharply divided on the potential of—and the indications for—this new strategy. Writing in 1991, I. Craig Henderson of the Dana-Farber Cancer Institute observed that "despite the impressive complete response rates, the duration of response and survival has been disappointingly short." Dr. Henderson complained that the high-dose oncologists "have raised the public's expectations far beyond what is supported by the published data."[15] The weightiest objections came from the veteran oncologist George P. Canellos. As the editor of the *Journal of Clinical Oncology*, Dr. Canellos commanded the attention of his fellow professionals. He observed that the explosive increase in the number of these procedures being performed provided "a good example of technology and its dissemination having outpaced clinical scientific investigation."[16] There had been no large-scale clinical trials which might conclusively demonstrate the superiority of the high-dose strategies—the "trials" being reported in the late 1980s and early 1990s might be more accurately described as "feasibility studies." As these studies enrolled only a few patients and were conducted by physicians deeply involved with the treatment being tested, suspicions of possible bias could not be easily dismissed. Did the high-dose regimens show better response and survival rates because these studies tended to exclude patients who were in poor overall health or had metastases to the brain? Gabriel N. Hortobagyi of the M. D. Anderson Cancer Center made no bones about saying that he thought so.[17]

Who Pays the Bill?

Besides toxicity, the question of expense also figured largely in the ongoing debate about high-dose chemotherapy and autologous marrow support. That month spent in a private hospital room and the extensive support services required (nursing, antibiotics, transfusions) did not come cheap. In the late 1980s and early 1990s, the bill ranged somewhere between $100,000 and $200,000 for each "transplant." Bruce E. Hillner and his colleagues at the Medical College of Virginia analyzed the pertinent literature in 1992; they concluded that high-dose therapy typically gave patients with metastatic breast cancer "a survival benefit of 6.0 months at an incremental cost of $115,800 per year of life saved, a cost that may be untenable."[18] The private insurance companies, health maintenance organizations (HMOs), and other third party payers were dismayed by the prospect of having to pay for thousands, maybe even tens of thousands, of these new procedures every year just to treat breast malignancies.

Taking note of the divisions among professional oncologists regarding the strategy's value, many insurance companies refused to pay for it; they cited the escape clauses in their contracts disclaiming any coverage of experimental or unproven treatments. This posture on the part of third-party payers infuriated the high-dose oncologists and their patients. Writing in the *New England Journal of Medicine*, Karen Antman and her Dana-Farber colleagues warned that the future of clinical cancer research was "in jeopardy." Antman et al admitted that the strategy's status remained investigational, but argued that it nonetheless represented "the best available care." How could cancer medicine hope to progress if insurance companies would not pay for patient care in trials of promising therapies? "The available curative treatments for childhood and adult cancers were all initially considered investigational."[19]

The anguish of breast cancer patients whose claims for insurance coverage were denied knew no bounds. In the early 1990s newspapers in every sizable American city began to publish heart-wrenching stories about their plight. All these reports seemed to have been based on the same script, with only minor variations in detail. The patients were typically young women in their thirties. For most of them, the diagnosis of breast cancer had been unduly delayed because their personal physicians (well-meaning gynecologists mainly) did not adequately appreciate that women so young could be afflicted with this disease. Lumps and other symptoms which would have prompted mammograms and biopsies in women over fifty were thus ignored, overlooked, or pooh-poohed as "nothing serious." The belated diagnosis and the disfiguring breast surgery had come as a terrible shock; then these young patients had endured the standard outpatient chemotherapy, which did not

work. Now the cancer had metastasized, and they were (as the newspaper reports always said) "fighting for their lives." The doctors had recommended "a bone marrow transplant" as the best chance for survival, but the insurance would not pay for it. At this point the newspaper reports diverged in one of two directions. By way of concluding the story, they might describe (1) an effort to raise $150,000 through charitable contributions, or (2) a lawsuit being brought against an insurance company.

The vast majority of these poignant articles had to be followed up a few months later with an obituary notice. The breast cancers depicted were metastatic tigers, as uncharacteristically aggressive as the patients were uncharacteristically young. Some of these patients died before they could undergo the high-dose chemotherapy. The development of intracranial metastases (a frequent event) meant automatic disqualification from transplant programs, as the thrombocytopenia the high-dose regimens inevitably produced would have predisposed these individuals to brain hemorrhages. Many other patients died after receiving their "transplant," which was (as we have seen) hardly the sure-fire cure that the newspapers and TV stations seemed to be describing. Only in the courtroom did high-dose chemotherapy win unequivocal victories. Those lawsuits which went to trial featured dueling doctors. The insurance company's physicians would testify that the procedure in question was unproven and could kill the patient, while the physicians testifying for the plaintiff would assert that it was the best available treatment and potentially curative. Not knowing what to make of these arcane controversies, juries usually gave patients the benefit of a doubt. So did state legislatures. By 1995 Massachusetts and several other states had passed laws requiring insurers to pay for this costly treatment.[20] But while the lawyers and politicians squabbled, the issues of expense and morbidity suddenly became less compelling. Thanks to advances in basic science, high-dose therapy and hematopoietic reconstitution was rapidly becoming a largely outpatient procedure, with far lower costs and considerably less danger.

Peripheral Blood Stem Cells

During the 1990s bone marrow transplantation was gradually relegated to that dustbin reserved for effective but overly cumbersome therapies. Although marrow aspirated from the hip bones could reconstitute hematopoiesis, this technique was never very efficient. What we needed for the task was not marrow *per se*, but pluripotential stem cells. These "progenitor cells" (as they are sometimes called) are capable of perpetual self-renewal and unrestricted differentiation; theoretically at least, any one of them has the potential to re-create all the necessary blood cells in a patient whose marrow has been destroyed by irradiation or by cytotoxic drugs. While the marrow is the body's richest source of hematopoietic stem cells, only 1% or 2% of the cells normally found there are true progenitors. The remaining 98% or 99% of the marrow's cells have lost that power of pluripotential differentiation—they are more mature and more restricted, "committed" (as the oncologists say) "to a particular lineage." In other words, they have begun the process of evolving into granulocytes (white cells), erythrocytes (red cells), or megakaryocytes (platelet forerunners). Marrow cells already committed to granulocytic lineage cannot differentiate into erythrocytes or megakaryocytes, and vice versa. Hematopoietic reconstitution using bone marrow required numerous transfusions and a month in the hospital because the reinfused marrow contained comparatively few stem cells. Engraftment

took a long time.

Whether performed for autologous support (rescue after chemotherapy) or for allogeneic transplantation, hematopoietic reconstitution promised to be safer, faster, and cheaper if our researchers could devise a way to deliver larger quantities of stem cells. Unfortunately, back in the early 1980s we did not know how to identify these progenitor cells, much less how to isolate and concentrate them. Kenneth F. Mangan of Philadelphia's Temple University Cancer Center reminds us that under a traditional microscope these cells appeared as "nondescript small to medium-sized round lymphoid mononuclear cells."[21] They could not be distinguished from marrow cells already committed to a particular lineage. In 1984, however, Curt I. Civin of Johns Hopkins and his colleagues demonstrated that those marrow cells capable of unrestricted differentiation carried a distinct protein on their surface membranes called **CD34**. We still do not know what function this protein serves; but since it is not expressed by other blood cells, it has given us a splendid way of identifying stem cells. Reagents using monoclonal antibodies directed against the CD34 protein will bind to the true progenitor cells but not to more differentiated blood cells. After reagents are added to a specimen of blood or bone marrow, that specimen can be run through an automated flow cytometer—those CD34-positive stem cells will shine brightly under the light source, and a nearby computer will deliver a printout telling us what percentage of the specimen they represent. Those hematopoietic cells which are only weakly CD34-positive shine dimly under the light source. While they are descended from pluripotential stem cells, these cells have already begun to commit themselves to particular lineages and are therefore ceasing to express the telltale protein.[22]

Prior to the mid-1980s nobody thought

that stem cells would be found in the peripheral blood—that is, in the blood coursing throughout the body. But flow cytometric analysis of peripheral blood samples using CD34 reagents revealed that, yes, stem cells do circulate in the bloodstream, though not in sufficient numbers to be useful in hematopoietic reconstitution. Normally stem cells comprise considerably less than one-half of one percent of the cells found in peripheral blood. Oncology researchers soon discovered an exception to the rule. When cancer patients are given a hefty dose of cyclophosphamide or some other myelosuppressive drug, about three weeks later their peripheral blood will be temporarily swarming with stem cells. Diane S. Krause of Johns Hopkins and her colleagues point out that "the percentage of CD34-positive cells may increase to 1% to 5%."[23] What happens in this situation is easy to understand. Since the cytotoxic drug has destroyed the majority of the developing blood cells, the marrow's stem cells must multiply furiously to replace them. Inevitably, some cells from this rapidly expanding stem-cell population will spill over into the general circulation. For a short time the peripheral blood thus becomes a repository of hematopoietic progenitors—we can now "harvest" (as the oncologists say) our **peripheral blood stem cells** (PBSCs).

The term **mobilization** has come to be used to describe that necessary prelude to PBSC harvesting, whereby we create a spill-over of stem cells into the bloodstream. During the 1990s mobilization was increasingly accomplished by **colony-stimulating factors** (CSFs), which could be administered with or without a preliminary dose of cyclophosphamide. CSFs, also known as "hematopoietic growth factors," are elusive proteins produced by the marrow's blood cells. These proteins spur the stem cells into proliferation and then channel the newly-born daughter cells into this or that lineage which the body urgently requires. During the 1980s the genes responsible for the production of several important CSFs were located, cloned, and inserted into compliant bacteria. Thanks to recombinant DNA technology, we now have abundant supplies of **granulocyte colony-stimulating factor** (G-CSF) as well as **granulocyte-macrophage colony-stimulating factor** (GM-CSF).[24] Both these CSFs were approved by the Food and Drug Administration in 1991. Along with **erythropoietin** (a red-cell CSF approved in 1989), they may be prescribed for chemotherapy patients who are suffering from severe neutropenia or anemia. G-CSF, also known as **filgrastim**, has proven especially efficient at stem cell mobilization prior to PBSC harvest. GM-CSF, also known as **sargramostim**, has likewise proven effective for this purpose, although G-CSF tends to be preferred since it has fewer side effects.[25]

The mobilization and harvest of PBSCs can be accomplished in about ten days, on an outpatient basis. The risk of complications is slight. For the first five days or so, a patient will be given injections of G-CSF (filgrastim). Twice-a-day injections using higher doses have been shown to mobilize more CD34-positive cells than the hitherto conventional once-daily injections. The percentage of CD34-positive cells in the blood is monitored by flow cytometry. When it is high enough, harvesting of PBSCs begins with a procedure called **apheresis** or (more precisely) **leukapheresis**. Here the patient's blood is circulated out of his or her body so as to be able to remove the small white cells (which would include the PBSCs). The red cells, platelets, and plasma are then returned to the bloodstream.

Venous access must be obtained before apheresis—an indwelling central catheter is typically inserted into the subclavian vein beneath the collarbone. The patient's blood flow can then be diverted through a **cell separator**, an automated device which yields a PBSC product with a relatively high proportion of CD34-positive cells. During apheresis the patient must remain hooked up to the hospital's cell separator for several hours. As each apheresis procedure may cost $2,000 or more, PBSC harvesting is not exactly cheap. Fortunately, we can usually get all the PBSCs we need from two to five aphereses, performed on as many successive days. The extracted PBSCs are cryopreserved; after completion of the high-dose chemotherapy, they are thawed and then reinfused into the patient to reconstitute hematopoiesis.[26]

The PBSC Advantages!

There are three reasons why the high-dose oncologists treating advanced breast malignancies so quickly embraced the new PBSC technology. The first is the relative ease of harvest. Unlike bone marrow extraction, the collection of PBSCs did not entail general anesthesia or overnight hospitalization. Secondly, the PBSC product posed considerably less risk of malignant contamination. Since breast tumors tend to metastasize to the bone marrow, oncologists worried that cryopreserved marrow might contain occult cancer cells along with the hematopoietic stem cells. What would be the purpose of curing metastatic disease if the reinfused marrow reinfected the patient with the deadly cancer? In the early 1990s the transplant centers experimented with various methods intended to "purge" (remove) any malignant cells which might be contaminating the aspirated marrow. A team at Duke reported that treating the marrow with 4-HC (a cyclophosphamide derivative) before cryopreservation "can efficiently remove breast cancer cells"; the cytotoxic drug had no apparent

effect on the subsequent engraftment.[27] But PBSCs looked like an even better idea. The peripheral blood was much less likely to harbor colonies of metastatic cancer cells; and the CD34 surface protein gave us a way to separate the stem cells from any intermingling cancer cells by *positive selection*, without recourse to cytotoxic purging. In this instance, the PBSC harvest undergoes further refinement. After being removed from the cell separator, it is incubated with CD34-specific monoclonal antibodies and then passed over "immunoaffinity" or "immunomagnetic" columns. The upshot is that the pluripotential stem cells (which have bound the CD34 antibodies) will adhere to the columns, while any intermingling cancer cells (which would not have bound the antibodies) can be washed away. Any of the several variations on this method will give us a PBSC product composed almost entirely of CD34-positive cells, with minimal risk of malignant contamination.[28]

The third PBSC advantage was by far the most persuasive—**rapid engraftment**. In 1995 a nationwide survey of 692 patients receiving PBSCs after high-dose chemotherapy yielded a gratifying statistic: the median time to hematopoietic recovery was only nine days. After a week or ten days, patients usually had sufficient neutrophils and platelets circulating in their blood that they no longer required antibiotics to prevent infections or transfusions to prevent hemorrhages.[29] Of course, such patients no longer needed to be quarantined in sterile hospital rooms; the era of protracted hospitalizations was over. As early as 1992 William P. Peters and his colleagues in Duke's transplant program had begun to treat their breast cancer patients in a modified outpatient setting. The patients were still hospitalized while receiving the four days of high-dose chemotherapy, Peters et al explained, because the regimen (cyclophosphamide, cisplatin, and carmustine) required "aggressive hydration with an average of 14 liters of fluid daily, continuous use of multi-agent antiemetics, and intensive physiologic monitoring." But a day or two after completing chemotherapy, patients could usually be discharged to a nearby residence facility (e.g., a suitably equipped hotel). Subsequently they had to return each day to the hospital's outpatient clinic, where they could be "supported with electrolytes, antiemetics, and red blood cell and platelet transfusions as necessary." Those patients who started to run a fever or to experience other complications were rushed back into the hospital until their condition stabilized; most patients required only outpatient services. Within three weeks of the PBSC reinfusion, "90% of patients were discharged to home."[30]

The cost savings accomplished by the rapid-engrafting PBSCs and outpatient management were substantial. In 1990 the breast cancer patients treated at Duke required a median of 37 days of hospitalization; by 1993 the hospitalization period had been shortened to a median of seven days. In 1990 a Duke patient receiving high-dose chemotherapy and autologous marrow support typically incurred hospital charges between $100,000 and $150,000—by 1993 that bill had been reduced to $60,000. As Dr. Peters and his colleagues pointed out, these savings could be obtained without endangering patients only at cancer centers which were large enough to maintain a round-the-clock outpatient clinic.[11] The Scripps Clinic in La Jolla, California, took the Duke innovation a step further, giving the entire treatment (high-dose chemo, PBSCs, and supportive care) in an intensely monitored outpatient setting. The Scripps patients were allowed "to reside at their private homes if less than 45 minutes from the clinic by car."[32]

It would be misleading to convey the impression that high-dose myelosuppressive chemotherapy had become altogether risk-free. Patients still died from treatment-related complications. Even with PBSCs engraftment might take longer with some patients than with others, and in a few cases infections or hemorrhaging might intervene before the patients achieved hematopoietic independence. Yet the mortality rate during or shortly after treatment, which hovered at about 20% in the late 1980s, had dropped to about 5% by the mid-1990s.[33] Some institutions reported even lower rates. Of 125 breast cancer patients treated in Emory University's autologous transplant program between 1992 and 1994, only one died from complications, representing a mortality rate of less than 1%.[34] Previously used mainly for metastatic breast cancer, high-dose chemotherapy with marrow or PBSC support was now being used just as often as adjuvant therapy for patients with ten or more positive axillary nodes. Once largely restricted to youngish patients in their thirties and forties, the therapy was now being offered to patients in their fifties and sixties, a more typical breast cancer population. The Johns Hopkins transplant program set age 65 as its uppermost age limit.[35]

The most radical change to high-dose strategies envisioned in the late 1990s was a drug administration scheduling which would be—as cancer chemotherapy has traditionally been—cyclical. As performed in the late 1980s and early 1990s. dose escalation with marrow support deviated from the fundamental principle of repetitive cycles—it was seen as a dramatic one-shot, all-or-nothing intervention which would either cure the patient or kill her. Oncologists soon realized that PBSCs offered an opportunity to experiment with cyclical high-dose regimens. After the marrow's stem cells had been adequately mobilized by a growth factor like G-CSF, the harvest obtained from two to five daily aphereses provided an abundance of PBSCs. In fact, hematopoiesis could be reconstituted three or four times over—therefore why not do the high-dose chemo three or four times over? If some of the disseminated tumor cells were not in cycle during drug administration (i.e., neither dividing nor preparing to divide), they might be relatively resistant to the cytotoxic onslaught. Perhaps they would be in cycle—and therefore more vulnerable—during a second or third drug administration.

In 1997 Charles L. Shapiro and his colleagues reported an experimental cyclical modification they had made to Dana-Farber's newest high-dose regimen for metastatic breast cancer. When given in a single administration, that regimen consisted of cyclophosphamide (6,000 mg/m^2) together with the platinum drug carboplatin (800 mg/m^2) and the second alkylating agent thiotepa (500 mg/m^2). Shapiro et al gave 18 breast cancer patients four cycles of this regimen at one-quarter dose: "Each cycle consisted of cyclophosphamide (1,500 mg/m^2), thiotepa (125 mg/m^2), and carboplatin (200 mg/m^2). PBSCs were reinfused 48 hours after the completion of each. Cycles were repeated every 21 to 42 days." By way of comparison we should point out that each "one-quarter-dose" cycle still provided almost four times the cyclophosphamide dose given in a FAC cycle—that is, 1,500 mg/m^2 as compared to FAC's 400 mg/m^2. This multi-cycle high-dose regimen achieved a complete response rate of 22%. Three patients did not receive all four cycles due to "cumulative hematologic toxicity," which "appeared to be greater than with a single high-dose cycle." Dr. Shapiro and his team modestly concluded that their study demonstrated only the feasibility of cyclical high-dose chemotherapy: "Randomized trials are required to determine whether a multiple-cycle intensification regimen might offer a therapeutic advantage over a single cycle."[36]

Waiting on the Clinical Trials

A standing ovation is due to the scientists and medical equipment manufacturers who gave us that wondrous PBSC technology! Thanks to their efforts, we now have unprecedented freedom to escalate the doses of those cytotoxic drugs whose dose-limiting side effect is myelosuppression. There is little doubt that high-dose chemotherapy with PBSC support sometimes betters the odds of long-term survival in refractory hematological malignancies (i.e., certain leukemias and lymphomas). That this technique conveys any benefit in those sluggish solid tumors emanating from the colon, pancreas, and prostate seems very unlikely; but it has looked promising in the treatment of certain lethal but somewhat chemosensitive carcinomas, most notably ovarian tumors and small-cell lung cancer.[37] Of course, by the mid-1990s the therapy was being performed far more often for breast cancers than for any other type of malignancy.[38] The "rub" here was that the practice of cyclophosphamide dose escalation had been widely adopted before we had conclusive proof that it really worked better than the commonplace breast cancer regimens (CMF, FAC, AC) which were much less toxic and far less expensive. Skeptical oncologists like I. Craig Henderson and Gabriel Hortobagyi took pains to point out that the estimates of improved survival coming from the transplant centers were not based on randomized (Phase Three) clinical trials, but on feasibility studies (Phase One trials) which tended to enroll patients with favorable prognostic features. These patients had subsequently been compared with heterogeneous groups of "historical controls." Thus we did not have a proven cure on our hands so much as one humdinger of a controversy. An analogous situation prevailed back in the late 1960s, when the Halstedian breast surgeons could cite oodles of nonrandomized studies which purported to demonstrate that radical mastectomy improved survival compared to less mutilative operations. This viewpoint was eventually refuted by NSABP Protocol B-04, a trial which randomly assigned 1,665 patients to radical mastectomy or to the less disfiguring simple (total) mastectomy. Where was the NSABP now that we needed it? Actually, Bernard Fisher and his far-flung collaborators had been preoccupied with the merits (or demerits) of cyclophosphamide dose escalation throughout the 1990s—they conducted two big clinical trials which tested various dose levels of this drug in their favored AC regimen. **NSABP Protocol B-22**, begun in 1989, enrolled and randomized 2,305 node-positive breast cancer patients. **NSABP Protocol B-25**, begun in 1992, enrolled and randomized another 2,548 patients. The dose and the dose intensity of Adriamycin (doxorubicin) were held constant in both trials—60 mg/m^2 every 21 days, four times, to achieve 240 mg/m^2 (total dose). But in Protocol B-22 the standard AC dose of cyclophosphamide (600 mg/m^2 every 21 days, four times, to total 2,400 mg/m^2) was <u>intensified</u> (1,200 mg/m^2 twice, in the first two cycles), and then <u>intensified</u> <u>and</u> <u>increased</u> (1,200 mg/m^2 four times to total 4,800 mg/m^2). Protocol B-25 featured further intensification and escalation—one arm received 2,400 mg/m^2 every 21 days for two cycles to total 4,800 mg/m^2 (an intensification over Protocol B-22), while another arm got 2,400 mg/m^2 every 21 days for four cycles to total 9,600 mg/m^2 (the largest escalation). The five-year follow-ups on both trials appeared in the *Journal of Clinical Oncology*, the B-22 findings in May 1997 and the B-25 findings in November 1999. Try as they might, Bernard Fisher and his

NSABP co-workers were unable to find any statistically significant differences between the various dose levels. In their second report they observed that the disease-free survival (DFS) and the overall survival (OS) of the B-25 patients getting that big cyclophosphamide escalation (2,400 mg/m^2 four times) were not much better than the results recorded for the B-22 patients who received the standard AC dose (600 mg/m^2 four times). At five years DFS stood at 66% for that highest-dose arm and at 62% for the standard-dose arm—OS was 79% and 78% respectively. About the only thing Dr. Fisher and his colleagues were sure that cyclophosphamide dose escalation accomplished for breast cancer patients was toxicity: almost 50% of the B-25 patients getting that highest dose eventually required blood transfusions, and four of them died from treatment-related complications.[39]

The findings from NSABP Protocols B-22 and B-25 ought to convince us that cyclophosphamide escalation *per se* is no more likely to be a miracle cure for progressive breast carcinomas than anything else; yet these trials did not directly evaluate the high-dose regimens with PBSC support being offered by Duke, Dana-Farber, and other transplant centers. The biggest cyclophosphamide administration in B-25 (2,400 mg/m^2) was still noticeably below the single dosing with 6,000 mg/m^2 that transplant regimens might call for. Moreover, in the NSABP trials the drug was given concurrently (at the same time) with Adriamycin and, for patients over 50, with tamoxifen. The transplant centers did not use this combination. In 1991 two American trials got under way with a view to pitting high-dose chemotherapy with marrow or PBSC support as administered by the transplant centers against the standard CMF and FAC regimens. The **Philadelphia Intergroup trial**, headed by Edward A. Stadtmauer of the University of Pennsylvania, sought to enroll and randomize patients with metastatic breast cancer. The **Cancer and Leukemia Group B trial**, headed by Duke's William P. Peters, limited its enrollment to high-risk primary breast cancer—patients were to have ten or more positive axillary nodes, but no evidence as yet of distant metastases. Alas, the Intergroup and CALGB trials soon got bogged down in the recruitment process; enrollment was tortuously slow. Although there was no shortage of prospective patients, most of them had been influenced by newspaper or TV reports which conveyed the impression that "bone marrow transplants" could cure breast cancer. The upshot was that few patients would accept a randomization which gave them a fifty-fifty chance of getting CMF or FAC instead of the desired high-dose regimen. Many patients simply shopped around until they found an ongoing Phase One trial which gave a high-dose regimen to all participants. In 1995 William Vaughn of the University of Alabama at Birmingham aptly described the recruiter's dilemma: "It takes three times as long to explain to a patient referred for a transplant that a transplant may not be in her best interest as to say, 'Sure, transplants R us.'"[40]

While the American trials moved ponderously forward, Werner R. Bezwoda and his colleagues rushed to announce their encouraging results from a little clinical trial conducted at the University of Witwatersrand in Johannesburg, South Africa. Bezwoda et al had assigned 90 young women with metastatic breast cancer (average age about 38) to receive two cycles of a high-dose regimen with marrow or PBSC support, or to receive six to eight cycles of a conventional-dose regimen. The high-dose chemotherapy consisted of <u>cyclophosphamide</u> (2,400 mg/m^2), a drug that stymies DNA synthesis called <u>mitoxantrone</u> (35 to 45 mg/m^2), and

the mitotic inhibitor <u>etoposide</u> (2,500 mg/m^2). The conventional-dose regimen consisted of <u>cyclophosphamide</u> (600 mg/m^2), <u>mitoxantrone</u> (12 mg/m^2), and the mitotic inhibitor <u>vincristine</u> (1.4 mg/m^2). In 1995 Bezwoda et al reported that after three years of follow-up the high-dose arm had revealed several statistically significant advantages, most notably a complete response (CR) rate of 51% (23 of 45 patients). The CR rate they reported for the conventional-dose arm was only 4.4% (two of 45 patients). "In the high-dose arm," said Bezwoda et al, "CRs were seen at all disease sites, including viscera, and also in four of 18 patients (22%) with bone metastases. Among patients who received conventional-dose treatment, CRs were seen only at soft tissue sites of disease and in one instance of pulmonary metastatic disease."[41] In 1998 Bezwoda announced that nine complete responders from the high-dose arm still remained in remission, with no evidence of recurrent disease, more than five years after their treatment.[42]

During the late 1990s American proponents of high-dose chemotherapy often cited the aforementioned South African trial as evidence of the strategy's potential. But at the May 1999 meeting of the American Society of Clinical Oncology, it was the skeptics' turn to gloat—the early results from the Philadelphia Intergroup and CALGB trials had given no indication that high-dose chemotherapy with stem cell support improved survival over the conventional regimens. In the Intergroup trial involving metastatic breast cancer, the two-year survival rate was actually lower in the 101 patients assigned to the high-dose regimen (46% surviving) than in the 79 patients assigned to CMF (52% surviving). The CALGB trial had eventually randomized 783 patients with ten or more positive nodes to receive Duke's high-dose regimen (cyclophosphamide 5,625 mg/m^2, cisplatin 165 mg/m^2, carmustine 600 mg/m^2), or to receive an intermediate-dose version of it (these doses were 900 mg/m^2, 90 mg/m^2, and 90 mg/m^2 respectively). Unfortunately, after a median follow-up of 37 months, William P. Peters and his CALGB colleagues had to report that the trial data generated were "currently inconclusive for policy decisions." The high-dose arm had done better in disease-free survival (68% DFS compared to 64% for the intermediate-dose arm)—but it had experienced 29 treatment-related deaths, whereas the intermediate-dose arm had not experienced any treatment-related deaths. Thus the overall survival rate was actually better in the intermediate-dose arm, with 80% surviving compared to 78% surviving in the high-dose arm.[43]

That the May 1999 ASCO meeting did not resemble a complete Waterloo for the high-dose oncologists was due to the continuing efforts of Werner R. Bezwoda and his South African colleagues. The Johannesburg group released very encouraging data from a new clinical trial involving high-risk primary breast cancer. Its enrollment had been limited to patients with ten or more positive axillary nodes or with other dire prognostic features. Of the 154 patients recruited, 79 were assigned to receive six cycles of a standard adjuvant regimen (intensified FAC); and 75 were assigned to receive two cycles of a high-dose regimen (cyclophosphamide 4,400 mg/m^2, mitoxantrone 45 mg/m^2, and etoposide 1,500 mg/m^2), each cycle being followed by PBSC rescue. Bezwoda et al reported that, after a median follow-up of 278 weeks (5.3 years), the trial's high-dose arm was enjoying statistically significant advantages both in freedom from recurrences and in overall survival. In the standard-regimen arm, 52 of the 79 patients (66%) were said to have experienced recurrences, and 28 (35%) to have died. In the high-dose arm, only 19 of the 75 patients (25%) were said to have experienced recurrences, and only eight (9.4%) to have died.[44]

The Johannesburg trial headed by Dr. Bezwoda was inevitably compared with the larger CALGB trial headed by Dr. Peters. Both trials recruited comparable patients (all with high-risk primary breast cancer), yet the results announced in May 1999 were strikingly discordant. An obvious difference between the two trials was that the CALGB trial, like the Philadelphia Intergroup trial, had used induction chemotherapy before randomization. All the CALGB patients received four cycles of intensified FAC *before* they were randomized to the Duke high-dose regimen or to the intermediate-dose version of it. Did that extra induction regimen have the unwanted effect of promoting drug resistance? Would it be more efficacious to give high-risk patients that massive dose of alkylating chemotherapy as the *initial* systemic treatment? By late 1999 the National Cancer Institute had begun thinking about a big clinical trial which might answer these questions. Before proceeding with this trial, however, the NCI took the prudent step of dispatching an auditing team to Johannesburg to examine the South African data. ***HORRORS!!*** What these auditors discovered was—as the NCI later reported— "evidence of serious improprieties and breaches of acceptable research practices." The upshot was that the University of Witwatersrand publicly rescinded the study involving high-risk primary breast cancer. On January 30, 2000, Werner R. Bezwoda wrote his University colleagues to acknowledge "a serious breach of scientific honesty and integrity."[45] The semblance of Waterloo which Dr. Bezwoda's "results" narrowly averted in May 1999 was fully accomplished by his admissions the following January. The high-dose proponent Jeffrey Abrams, coordinator of the NCI's breast cancer trials, tried to minimize the damage. "The falsification of the South African study," said Dr. Abrams, "is devastating. However, an even greater tragedy could result if this news causes patients and doctors to avoid clinical trials of transplants altogether. The basic research this treatment is based on remains solid."[46] Aetna, the nation's largest health insurer, quickly announced that it would no longer pay for high-dose chemotherapy with stem cell support in the treatment of breast cancer, unless the patient receiving therapy was enrolled in a clinical trial "sponsored or authorized by the National Cancer Institute or the Food and Drug Administration."[47] Coming after the South African debacle, Aetna's change of policy seemed rational rather than discriminatory.

What Have We Learned?

What has long been true of breast cancer surgery has recently become *notoriously true* of cytotoxic chemotherapy for those patients who have—or are expected to develop—metastatic disease. Viz., the therapy recommended varies according to which doctor's door a patient happens to open. Granted, oncologists generally concede the importance of adequate dosing and dose intensity; but there is no consensus regarding the use of doses so high that hematopoietic reconstitution is required. And there is no standard high-dose regimen—the drugs, the doses, and the scheduling have varied from one transplant center to the next. In November 1999 the high-dose proponent Karen Antman collaborated with the skeptic Gabriel N. Hortobagyi to review nine randomized trials of high-dose regimens for the *Journal of the American Medical Association.* Drs. Antman and Hortobagyi both agreed that because these breast cancer trials had "different designs and follow-up," it was premature to reach any conclusion: "The hints of benefit from some of the trials suggest that more, and perhaps better, information is needed."[48]

No doubt more breast cancer cases hitherto deemed hopeless could be rescued if we could develop an optimal high-dose regimen. For the time being, concerned patients would do well to remember these Golden Rules: **"Get a second opinion! Hit it early!"** An appropriate regimen, if given early enough, may well alter the course of disease. But the odds of long-term survival seem to be principally determined by that first exposure to cytotoxic agents. Patients who have relapsed after prior chemotherapy are difficult to save. Richard J. O'Reilly, a pediatric oncologist, aptly summarizes the rationale for an aggressive initial strategy: "If you're going to cure cancer, the time to hit it is early and you hit it intensively. In some ways cancer is not so different from a bacterial infection. If you treat a bacterial infection with low doses of antibiotics, you should expect to see drug-resistant bacteria. The same holds true for cancer cells."[49] Prior exposure to lower-dose regimens may be one reason why the Philadelphia Intergroup trial involving metastatic breast cancer failed to show any benefit from high-dose therapy: over half of the patients assigned to the high-dose arm had already received—and failed—adjuvant chemotherapy before their enrollment.[50] David A. Rizzieri and his colleagues in Duke's transplant program looked for prognostic indicators in the files of 425 patients with metastatic breast cancer whom they had previously treated: "Our review shows that any prior chemotherapy exposure is associated with worse outcome. The administration of high-dose chemotherapy early in the course of treatment may be important."[51]

*   *   *   *   *   *   *   *

TAXOL:
A New Drug from the Old Yew

The high-dose regimens of the 1980s and 1990s revealed new ways of using old drugs (e.g., cyclophosphamide); but the most promising developments during these decades involved two new drugs, **paclitaxel** and **docetaxel**. The adjective "taxoid" and the noun "taxane" are frequently applied to these powerful cytotoxic agents, giving us a clue to their botanical origins. The genus *Taxus* includes various evergreen trees commonly called yews. Back in 1963 a screening program sponsored by the National Cancer Institute discovered that extracts from the bark of the Pacific yew, *Taxus brevifolia*, could induce remissions in tumor-bearing mice. Given the fact that all sorts of natural products seem to have anticancer properties in mice experiments, it is hardly surprising that the NCI felt no great sense of urgency about yew bark. The compound responsible for the bark's activity was not isolated until 1969; its complex molecular structure was deciphered two years later. The pharmaceutical development of **Taxol** (as the compound came to be called) did not shift into high gear until the early 1980s. Interest in this agent suddenly increased after researchers demonstrated in 1979 that it had a novel mechanism for killing cancer cells.[52] Most of our cytotoxic agents accomplish this either by damaging DNA outright (e.g., alkylating agents) or by interfering with its synthesis (e.g., antimetabolites). In contrast, Taxol acts to disrupt the mitotic spindle which enables the actual division of a multiplying cell. That spindle consists of filamentous microtubules, thin strands of a protein called tubulin; they draw the condensed chromosomes apart into two daughter cells. Microtubules also serve various other functions—for our purposes it is important to remember that they are not

intended to be stable and permanent, but rather to be flexible and collapsible. These structures must be quickly assembled or disassembled, depending on a cell's needs at the moment. When added to active cell cultures, Taxol results in the production of abnormally rigid microtubules: this stops cells from completing mitosis. Eric K. Rowinsky and Ross C. Donehower of the Johns Hopkins Oncology Center observe that Taxol "promotes the polymerization of tubulin" and thereby "inhibits the disassembly of microtubules." Any microtubules formed in the drug's presence will be "extraordinarily stable and dysfunctional, causing the death of the cell by disrupting the normal dynamics required for division and vital interphase processes."[53]

This novel cytotoxic mechanism led the NCI to single out Taxol from hundreds of other natural compounds. The transformation of a crude bark extract into a convenient therapeutic drug stood to involve the expenditure of prodigious amounts of time and money. Would the final product justify that enormous cost? The NCI hoped that since Taxol worked differently from other cytotoxic agents, it would not be "cross-resistant" with them—i.e., that it would work in cancer cells resistant to those other drugs. Perhaps it could even produce responses in patients whose metastatic tumors had developed an apparently insurmountable multidrug resistance.

The Early Experiments

The initial obstacle to testing Taxol in human patients was drug scarcity. The complex molecule of this natural compound proved difficult to synthesize, leaving the bark of *Taxus brevifolia* as the only practical source. Yet extraction posed a logistical nightmare because the yield was so low. Susan G.

Arbuck and her NCI colleagues observe that about 20,000 pounds of bark had to be processed to obtain one kilogram of clinically usable Taxol: "Each tree yielded enough drug to provide only two to three doses."[54] With time the extraction process would become more efficient, but in the 1980s no one knew how to obtain a bountiful supply. *Taxus brevifolia* took many years to grow to maturity; and the existing trees were not especially numerous, being found mainly in the ancient forests of the Pacific Northwest. The yew's bark contained almost four times as much Taxol as its needles, but stripping the bark away effectively killed the donor tree.

Notwithstanding these difficulties, the National Cancer Institute persisted. By the mid-1980s researchers at the NCI and other institutions had enough Taxol on hand to begin **Phase One trials**. The new drug was given to a few patients with metastatic disease and short life expectancies, simply with a view to discovering its side effects and gaining some notion of its therapeutic potential. The most troubling finding from these early trials was a high incidence of **hypersensitivity reactions**. Within minutes after receiving intravenous Taxol, patients might break out in hives, experience shortness of breath and precipitous drops in blood pressure, or even go into irreversible anaphylactic shock. Symptoms like these are not caused by a drug's cytotoxic action but rather by the body's immune system overreacting to a substance perceived as terribly foreign. Taxol is prone to elicit hypersensitivity reactions because it has a bulky chemical structure and, being insoluble in water, must be administered with Cremophor, a potentially irritating combination of alcohol and castor oil which serves as a carrier vehicle. The solution to hypersensitivity reactions proposed in the 1980s is still used today— give a hefty dose of immunosuppressive

drugs before infusing the Taxol. A standard premedication regimen calls for patients to begin with the corticosteroid <u>dexamethasone</u> (taken orally) twelve hours in advance; then right before the Taxol infusion they are started on the antihistamines <u>cimetidine</u> and <u>diphenhydramine</u>, both given intravenously. Bruce A. Chabner of the NCI's Division of Cancer Treatment observes that "although fewer than 10% of patients premedicated with corticosteroids and antihistamines will have a hypersensitivity reaction, this risk is sufficiently high to mandate the initial administration of the drug in the setting of inpatient monitoring."[55]

Having learned to cope with hypersensitivity, the oncologists conducting the Phase One trials soon began to appreciate Taxol's therapeutic potential. The drug had produced noteworthy responses in patients with melanoma and non-small-cell lung cancer, two tumors which are notoriously resistant to cytotoxic chemotherapy. The results in epithelial ovarian cancer were even more promising. The platinum drug cisplatin usually extended the life expectancies of women with disseminated ovarian tumors; but once resistance to cisplatin developed, there had been little hope of slowing disease progression. In 1989, however, a team at Johns Hopkins reported that Taxol was not cross-resistant with cisplatin. When given to forty patients whose metastatic ovarian tumors had progressed during or after cisplatin therapy, Taxol produced nineteen verifiable responses—one complete, eleven partial, and seven "minor."[56] Breast cancer specialists paid particular attention to a trial conducted at Houston's M. D. Anderson Cancer Center in 1990. Frankie Ann Holmes and her colleagues gave high-dose Taxol (250 mg/m^2 by 24-hour infusion every 21 days) to 25 patients with metastatic cancer who had failed previous chemotherapy. Three patients were to experience complete responses, meaning that all traces of disease seemed to disappear; and eleven patients had partial responses, defined as a shrinkage of existing metastases by 50% or more.[57] At a September 1992 workshop on Taxol hosted by the National Cancer Institute, Dr. Holmes and her colleagues told us what they had learned about this drug's customary side effects. The major dose-limiting effect is bone marrow suppression—at high doses Taxol drops that crucial tally of neutrophils (infection-fighting white cells) down to frighteningly low levels (500 or fewer per microliter of blood). The marrow usually recovers rapidly, before patients develop serious infections. But to be on the safe side, the M. D. Anderson team began giving their Taxol-treated patients two weeks of granulo-cyte colony-stimulating factor (G-CSF) to boost neutrophil production. Nausea and vomiting, a considerable problem with DNA-damaging drugs like Adriamycin and cis-platin, tend to be mild with Taxol; but alope-cia (hair loss) is often total. Taxol may also result in "peripheral neuropathies," a side effect not usually encountered in breast cancer chemotherapy. Within a day or two after treatment, patients may experience numbness, tingling, or burning sensations in a "stocking-and-glove distribution"—that is, the feet and hands are principally affected. Although not often disabling, this side effect is cumulative. Patients given several cycles of Taxol may begin to have difficulties with activities which require agile and sensitive fingers (e.g., buttoning blouses, tying shoe laces, or playing the piano). Myalgias and arthralgias (muscle and joint aches) are a common occurrence after Taxol infusions, being more pronounced at higher doses. Dr. Holmes and her colleagues found that these aches typically "began three to six days after treatment and lasted three to six days." Over-the-counter pain relievers like Tylenol (acetaminophen) "proved useful" in most

cases.[58] All these side effects tend to resolve after Taxol therapy is discontinued.

Save the Yew!

Prior to 1990 few Americans other than professional oncologists had ever heard of Taxol. By late 1991 cancer patients at least were becoming increasingly aware of the new drug. The mass media had pounced on this pharmaceutical development with a vengeance. Newspapers and TV stations were running optimistic stories about patients at death's door who seemed to have been rescued by Taxol—just in the nick of time! Of course, relatively few patients in those early trials had experienced complete remis-sions, and almost all responses had been of limited duration—but you would not get that impression from hearing or reading these reports. *Life* magazine ran a long feature article entitled "Tree of Hope," which paid homage to the yew and repeatedly alluded to Taxol as a "miracle drug."[59]

At the time there was not enough Taxol to go around, a fact which made splendid grist for the journalistic mills. Soon the telephones at the American Cancer Society and the National Cancer Institute were ring-ing off their hooks. Anxious patients wanted to know how they might obtain the drug. Property owners in Oregon and Washington State announced their willingness to donate (or to sell) any yew trees which might be found on their land. But the snafus were occurring mainly in the extraction and purifi-cation process—the NCI was already back-logged with the bark of *Taxus brevifolia*, thanks to the efforts of the United States Forest Service. Up through the year 1990 the Forest Service had sent the NCI a mere 200,000 pounds of yew bark from the public lands under its management. In 1991 it furnished a whopping 750,000 pounds, fulfilling this quota again in 1992. Environmentalists now saw red—were the NCI and the Forest Service fixing to harvest *Taxus brevifolia* to extinction? Didn't these agencies know they were destroying the habit of the Northern spotted owl? Congress quickly enacted the **Pacific Yew Act**, legislation which was designed to prevent anyone from cutting down a yew tree *by accident*.[60]

In the meantime the NCI had implemented a "compassionate-need program," whereby Taxol would be provided free of charge to appropriate patients who had failed previous chemotherapy. For practical purposes Taxol was pretty much reserved for metastatic ovarian tumors which no longer responded to cisplatin and for metastatic breast cancers which could not be treated with Adriamycin (doxorubicin) because of drug resistance or cumulative cardiotoxicity. In 1990 there had been only enough Taxol to treat 500 women; by late 1992 more than 4,600 women had been treated at NCI-designated cancer centers.[61]

Paclitaxel and Docetaxel:
The Taxoid Drugs Go Online

The worries about running out of Taxol or yew trees were soon to fade away. In January 1991 the NCI had signed an agreement allowing Bristol-Myers Squibb to develop and market the promising new drug—the name "Taxol" was to be retained as the company's registered trademark. Henceforth articles about the drug appearing in medical and scientific journals would use the generic name **paclitaxel**. Although Bristol-Myers Squibb had access to enough stockpiled yew bark for several years of paclitaxel production, the company promptly sought to find a more reliable source of raw materials. Could renewable parts of the yew—say, its needles

or its leaves—be used instead of its bark? Researchers in France had discovered that a taxoid precursor compound could be isolated from the leaves of the plentiful European yew *Taxus baccata*. The French scientists subsequently demonstrated that this precursor compound could be converted not only into paclitaxel, but also into a powerful analog drug which they dubbed "Taxotere." Following up on these important discoveries, Bristol-Myers Squibb decided to use the European yew for raw material, but opted to process the tree's needles instead of its leaves. Careful processing proved essential to preserve that precursor compound; the needles had to be left attached to their stems and then dried at temperatures ranging between 40 and 50 degrees centigrade.[62] In mid-1995 Bristol-Myers Squibb brought out its new semisynthetic paclitaxel made from *Taxus baccata* needles; the bark of the Pacific yew would not be used again.[63]

In late 1992 the Food and Drug Administration had already approved paclitaxel (Taxol) for use in relapsed ovarian cancer. The FDA sanction meant that henceforth any oncologist could prescribe the drug for this indication. On April 12, 1994, the FDA similarly approved paclitaxel for the treatment of breast carcinomas "after failure of combination chemotherapy for metastatic disease or relapse within six months of adjuvant therapy." Jeffrey Abrams and his colleagues point out that paclitaxel is one of "only a few single agents with proven activity for doxorubicin-resistant breast cancer." Of course, the drug had not been shown to be a sure-fire cure for these cases. An NCI-sponsored trial headed by Dr. Abrams recorded a modest 23% response rate when paclitaxel was given to 172 "heavily pretreated" patients with "chemotherapy-refractory metastatic breast cancer."[64]

By the mid-1990s American oncologists were curious to know whether that analog drug developed in France would be any better than paclitaxel. The French pharmaceutical firm Rhône-Poulenc Rorer was now marketing this second semisynthetic taxane in Europe under the brand name **Taxotere**; the medical journals usually referred to it by its generic name **docetaxel**. Like paclitaxel, docetaxel promoted the formation of abnormally stable, nonfunctional microtubules in metabolically active cells; but this second drug seemed more potent, was more water-soluble, and had a much longer half-life in the body (11.8 hours as compared to paclitaxel's 4.3 hours).[65] Docetaxel produced the same short-term side effects (profound but temporary neutropenia, alopecia, peripheral neuropathies); but after three to five cycles—when the cumulative dose reached 300 to 500 mg/m^2—it also tended to induce a troubling **fluid retention syndrome** not seen with paclitaxel therapy. Patients would gain weight and suffer from swollen hands and feet; occasionally, their breathing might be impaired because of pleural effusions (fluid retention in the chest cavity). This syndrome caused many patients to discontinue docetaxel therapy; in December 1994 it led an FDA panel to postpone approval of the drug, citing a need for more convincing data on safety issues. Further clinical experience demonstrated that the incidence both of fluid retention and of hypersensitivity reactions sharply diminished after patients were premedicated with the corticosteroid dexamethasone. The standard prophylaxis is simple—take a dexamethasone pill (8 mg) twice a day for five days, beginning the day before the docetaxel infusion.[66] In May 1995 the FDA approved docetaxel for the treatment of metastatic breast cancer. The new drug was the focus of attention at the San Antonio Breast Cancer Symposium in December 1997. Researchers from several countries enthusiastically reported that it seemed to be as potent as

Adriamycin (doxorubicin), without causing so much nausea, vomiting, and cardiotoxicity.[67] Rhône-Poulenc Rorer now filled the American oncology journals with colorful full-page advertisements for Taxotere—they depicted a vibrant young woman whose uplifted face was bathed in golden light. Lest unwary readers suspect that suntan lotion or a beach resort was being advertised, the ad's small print provided a sobering warning: "The incidence of treatment-related mortality is increased in patients receiving higher doses and in patients with abnormal liver function."[68] Docetaxel is mighty serious cancer medicine, a cytotoxic hammer on the order of Adriamycin or cisplatin.

Dose and Scheduling

Now that oncologists had paclitaxel and docetaxel firmly in their armamentarium, they needed to discover the best ways of using these weapons. Clinical trials were promptly initiated to generate more precise information on **dose**—(how much of the drug should be given?)—and on **scheduling**—(are longer infusions more effective than short ones?). These matters remain under investigation. Both paclitaxel and docetaxel have generally been given in **21-day cycles**—that is, only one infusion every three weeks, thus allowing time for bone marrow recovery. The Phase One trials involving docetaxel suggested that the maximum tolerable dose for this drug fell somewhere between 80 and 115 mg/m^2 per cycle. Oncologists pretty much agreed on the basic prescription—100 mg/m^2 docetaxel by one-hour infusion every 21 days.[69] But there have been considerable variations in the dosage and scheduling of paclitaxel. Oncologists wanted to tinker with Taxol because animal experiments suggested that both the dose used and the duration of drug exposure had a great deal to do with the amount of antitumor activity. Nobody knew whether dose and scheduling would prove equally important in human patients. Three different dose levels of paclitaxel have been frequently used. The lowest dose (135 mg/m^2) may sometimes be selected for those patients who have previously received extensive irradiation or multiple chemotherapy regimens—it produces milder side effects, though sufficing to cause alopecia. Bristol-Myers Squibb as well as most American oncologists have recommended an intermediate dose (175 mg/m^2) for metastatic breast cancer. Even more paclitaxel can be tolerated if neutrophil recovery is accelerated by injections of granulocyte colony-stimulating factor (G-CSF); but at the highest dose currently used (250 mg/m^2), side effects start to present an obstacle. Andrew D. Seidman and his colleagues at New York's Memorial Sloan-Kettering Cancer Center treated 76 patients with doxorubicin-resistant metastatic breast cancer with doses ranging from 200 to 250 mg/m^2. Although these patients also received eight days of G-CSF, 40 of them (52.6%) eventually required dose reductions, usually because of "neutropenia and fever."[70]

During the early 1990s paclitaxel was most often given by 24-hour infusions. Oncologists felt that a gradual administration of this drug would minimize the risk of hypersensitivity reactions. Wyndham H. Wilson and his colleagues at the National Cancer Institute experimented with a 96-hour infusion, giving a moderate dose (120 to 140 mg/m^2) to 33 patients whose metastatic breast tumors had progressed in spite of previous therapy with Adriamycin (doxorubicin) or mitoxantrone. Almost half of these patients (16 of the 33) achieved a partial response—this is a better rate than typically encountered in second-line salvage regimens. Wilson et al concluded that "the activity of paclitaxel may be schedule-dependent" and that "very short infusion schedules, such as

three hours, may be less effective."[71] Notwithstanding these concerns, oncologists have recently leaned toward shorter infusions, because longer ones (24 hours or more) mandate that patients either be hospitalized or fitted out with central venous catheters and ambulatory infusion pumps. In a word, shorter infusions are much more convenient.

Dr. Seidman and his Sloan-Kettering colleagues have tried a different tack to increase the cumulative paclitaxel dosage and to prolong tumor exposure to the drug. They used one-hour infusions but gave them every week instead of every three weeks; they achieved a 53% response rate in a small study (only 30 patients) of metastatic breast cancer. Although that weekly dose was held at 100 mg/m^2 or less, Seidman et al discovered that "peak plasma paclitaxel concentrations were similar to those observed with a dose of 135 to 175 mg/m^2 delivered over three hours."[72] Bristol-Myers Squibb paid little heed to the alternative schedules developed by the NCI and Sloan-Kettering teams. The company's advertisements emphasized the three-hour infusion with 175 mg/m^2 every 21 days, a "dose and schedule" which "allows for convenient administration in an outpatient setting."[73] The three-hour infusion also tended to produce less neutropenia than longer infusions, another factor which accounted for its acceptance by community-based oncologists. But Dr. Seidman wonders whether "a young woman who desires an aggressive treatment approach" might not be better served by longer scheduling: "It is compelling that responses can be found merely by prolonging the infusion from 3 to 96 hours."[74]

Did longer infusions of paclitaxel improve the outcome and thereby warrant the inconvenience? The NSABP pursued hard data on this question with **Protocol B-26**.

This little trial recruited 563 women with locally advanced or frankly metastatic breast carcinomas. They all received high-dose paclitaxel (250 mg/m^2) every three weeks, but were randomized to three-hour infusions or to 24-hour infusions. The initial report from this trial tended to support longer scheduling—the 24-hour arm achieved a response rate of 50%, while the group given the three-hour infusions registered only a 40% response rate. The response advantage was particularly pronounced in patients who were under age 50, who had distant metastases, or who had received prior adjuvant chemotherapy.[75]

Taxane-Based Regimens

In the 1990s paclitaxel and docetaxel were typically given as single agents to patients whose metastatic tumors had ceased to respond to other types of chemotherapy. These small trials revealed that the taxoid drugs were not intrinsically cross-resistant with the agents hitherto used in breast cancer regimens. Sometimes they could shrink drug-resistant metastases to the point of apparent disappearance. The next step was to learn how to combine the new taxoid drugs with the older agents. At the Fox Chase Cancer Center workshops held in 1996 and 1997, oncologists from many different countries described their experimental combinations: paclitaxel with cyclophosphamide—with fluorouracil—with cisplatin or carboplatin—with epirubicin—or with mitoxantrone.[76] But one combination elicited more interest than any other—paclitaxel with the mighty Adriamycin (doxorubicin), long the biggest cannon in breast cancer chemotherapy and the drug of choice as a first-line therapy for metastatic disease. Paclitaxel had produced response rates comparable to those produced by Adriamycin—wouldn't the two drugs together do even better? Combining these

highly toxic drugs safely was no simple matter, as demonstrated by a small Phase One trial conducted at the M. D. Anderson Cancer Center. Frankie Ann Holmes and her colleagues gave ten patients with metastatic breast tumors a 24-hour infusion of paclitaxel followed by a 48-hour infusion of doxorubicin. The result was more neutropenia than either drug would cause if given alone as a single agent. Severe mucositis (inflammation of the mucous membranes) affected the mouth and gastrointestinal tract. These unacceptable side effects came about because of **schedule-dependent toxicity**. In this instance, paclitaxel (which was given first) had interfered with the liver's ability to eliminate doxorubicin.[77] Thanks to Dr. Holmes and her co-workers, we now know to give Adriamycin first and to await its clearance from the body before giving paclitaxel.

Oncologists soon became aware of a second danger related to Adriamycin's long-recognized potential to induce congestive heart failure—that is, to weaken the heart muscle's ability to pump blood. Normally symptoms of impaired cardiac function do not appear until after patients have received a cumulative doxorubicin dose of 550 mg/m^2; but when paclitaxel is given simultaneously with doxorubicin, a hefty percentage of patients (20% in one trial) will have trouble at much lower doses. Interference with hepatic metabolism again looked like the culprit. A clever pharmacologist reckoned that a doxorubicin dose of 480 mg/m^2 given together with paclitaxel exerted the equivalent cardiotoxicity of precisely 624 mg/m^2 doxorubicin given as a single agent. This threatening drug interaction did not seem to occur if you waited at least 24 hours after the Adriamycin infusion before giving the paclitaxel; nonetheless, some oncologists decided to limit the cumulative doxorubicin dose to 360 mg/m^2 as a safety measure.[78]

Breast cancer specialists took note

when Luca Gianni and his colleagues at Milan's *Instituto Nazionale Tumori* reported encouraging findings. The Italian team had given Adriamycin and paclitaxel to 32 patients with metastatic breast cancer "who never received chemotherapy of any type." The combination shrank metastases at all sites except those in the central nervous system (a sanctuary not readily penetrated by the bulky paclitaxel molecules). Measurable responses were recorded for 30 of the 32 patients, and 13 patients (41%) achieved a complete response. "Patients with symptomatic bone metastases," observed Gianni et al, "had an often dramatic and rapid control of pain."[79] The American oncologists attending the Fox Chase workshops were quite impressed by the Italian pilot study, but wanted corroboration before endorsing this new drug combination. Fortunately, an Intergroup trial headed by George W. Sledge, Jr., soon provided more mature data. This trial sought to evaluate first-line therapies for metastatic breast cancer, randomizing 739 patients to receive Adriamycin or to receive paclitaxel or to receive both drugs. The preliminary results suggested that these two agents were comparable in effectiveness, with a 34% response rate being achieved by Adriamycin and a 33% response rate being achieved by paclitaxel; yet the combination did much better than either drug alone, achieving a 46% response rate.[80]

By the late 1990s many oncologists were beginning to suspect that docetaxel might be the most appropriate taxane to combine with Adriamycin. There were several reasons for this supposition. On a milligram-by-milligram basis, docetaxel was a stronger drug than paclitaxel. Moreover, whenever docetaxel had been pitted against Adriamycin in clinical trials, this newest taxane usually appeared to outperform Adriamycin, an upset no one had anticipated.

Stephen Chan of the Nottingham City Hospital (England) and other European oncologists conducted an important clinical trial to verify this finding. They enrolled 326 patients with metastatic breast cancer who had previously been treated with alkylating agents (e.g., the cyclophosphamide in CMF), but who had not yet been exposed either to an anthracycline (e.g., doxorubicin or epirubicin) or to a taxane. These patients were randomly assigned to receive high-dose Adriamycin (75 mg/m^2 every three weeks) or to receive high-dose docetaxel (100 mg/m^2 every three weeks), "for a maximum of seven cycles." The dose levels chosen, Dr. Chan and his colleagues observe, were "the highest feasible" without recourse to neutrophil growth factors like G-CSF. The trial results published in 1999 gave the nod to docetaxel, which had produced a 47.8% rate of objective response as compared to the 33.3% rate achieved by Adriamycin (doxorubicin). In certain subgroups, the docetaxel advantage was even more pronounced. Patients who had displayed drug resistance during their previous chemotherapy recorded a 47.4% response rate if assigned to docetaxel, but only a 24.7% rate if assigned to doxorubicin. Those troublesome liver metastases proved almost twice as likely to shrink in the presence of docetaxel (54.3% response rate) as in the presence of doxorubicin (25.8% response rate).[81]

Perhaps it would be premature to depose Adriamycin as the most active agent in breast cancer chemotherapy, though we must now recognize docetaxel as a plausible contender for that throne. Oncologists have wanted to combine these two drugs for reasons of convenience as well as of therapeutic efficacy. The Phase One trials suggested that docetaxel could be given immediately after doxorubicin without significantly increasing the anthracycline's cardiotoxicity. This finding meant that the two drugs could be administered together during one office visit. For example, Adriamycin might be given by a very quick infusion that oncologists call a <u>bolus</u> (Greek for "lump"), to be followed shortly thereafter by the customary one-hour infusion of docetaxel. Jean-Marc Nabholtz and his co-workers at Edmonton's Cross Cancer Institute (Canada) tried out a convenient outpatient regimen they dubbed **TAC** (the "T" stands for the brand name Taxotere). Given every three weeks, TAC called for "doxorubicin 50 mg/m^2 as a three-to-five minute intravenous bolus followed by cyclophosphamide 500 mg/m^2 as an intravenous bolus and (within an hour) by docetaxel 75 mg/m^2 as a one-hour infusion." An impressive 79% response rate was achieved when Dr. Nabholtz's team gave TAC to 42 breast cancer patients with measurable metastases who had received "no prior chemotherapy for metastatic disease and no prior exposure to anthracyclines." Two patients experienced complete responses. TAC proved particularly effective against "visceral metastases" in the liver (11 of 15 patients responding, a 73% rate) and in the lungs (17 of 20 patients responding, an 85% rate).[82]

Testing Adjuvant Regimens:
The NSABP Trials

By the mid-1990s paclitaxel and docetaxel had already been established as the drugs to use after Adriamycin resistance developed in metastatic breast tumors. Speaking at a Fox Chase workshop in 1996, George W. Sledge, Jr., observed that paclitaxel was "a standard off-protocol salvage agent for all our patients now, basically having tossed out mitomycin and vinblastine, or at least put them into third-line therapy."[83] If the results from the clinical trial conducted by Dr. Chan and his colleagues are confirmed, docetaxel might

well replace Adriamycin as the drug of choice for the initial treatment of metastatic breast cancer. But the main task facing oncologists in the year 2000 was to learn how to use paclitaxel and docetaxel in adjuvant regimens. Treatment for metastatic carcinomas tends to become a palliative exercise—salvage chemotherapy usually improves the quality of a patient's life, but it does not often alter the course of disease. Adjuvant therapy given before metastatic disease takes hold stands a much better chance of extending life expectancy. We already have solid evidence that the standard adjuvant regimens of the 1980s and 1990s (CMF, FAC, AC) did exactly that for a noteworthy percentage of patients with early-stage breast cancer who would have otherwise relapsed and died. Considering the impressive responses that paclitaxel and docetaxel achieved when used as salvage agents, we have assumed that their addition to adjuvant regimens ought to improve the survival rates of newly-diagnosed patients who are node-positive or otherwise deemed at risk for systemic disease. Of course, in the year 2000 we did not actually know for a fact that adjuvant taxanes could improve long-term survival, nor did we have an optimal regimen which had been proven superior to others we might devise.

The inevitable consequence of the aforementioned uncertainties is sure to be experimentation. We may anticipate that our cancer centers and clinical trial organizations will want to test different drug combinations, different dose levels, and variant scheduling. It might be foolhardy to hazard a guess as to which adjuvant regimen (or regimens) will eventually emerge from this experimentation, to be offered as standard therapy for the next generation of breast cancer patients. As far as the NSABP is concerned, however, any new drug regimens ought to feature a taxane in combination with those old workhorses

Adriamycin and cyclophosphamide. In the year 2000 our preeminent data-generating organization had four adjuvant trials under way which were designed to test paclitaxel or docetaxel in this or that scheduling together with the familiar AC regimen (doxorubicin 60 mg/m^2 i.v., cyclophosphamide 600 mg/m^2 i.v., repeat every 21 days for four cycles).

NSABP Protocol B-28 was projected to enroll 3,050 patients with node-positive breast cancer. After undergoing definitive surgery (lumpectomy or mastectomy), they were to be randomized to four cycles of AC or to four cycles of AC followed by four cycles of paclitaxel (225 mg/m^2 i.v. over three hours, repeat every 21 days). **NSABP Protocol B-31**, a smaller trial, stood to enroll 1,000 or more node-positive patients whose tumors overexpressed the stimulatory onco-gene HER-2/*neu*. All trial participants were to receive AC and paclitaxel sequentially (as in the second arm of Protocol B-28), but half of them were also to be given weekly infu-sions (52 weeks) of the therapeutic mono-clonal antibody **Herceptin** (brand name for **trastuzumab**). This new drug has produced significant responses in some breast cancer patients with HER-2/*neu* overexpression.

When designing **Protocol B-27**, the NSABP returned to a question previously explored in Protocol B-18—viz., does neoad-juvant (preoperative) chemotherapy lead to better survival rates than the customary adjuvant (postoperative) chemotherapy? The 1,500 or so women expected to enroll in this trial were to have been diagnosed with inva-sive breast cancer by core-needle biopsy—a high risk for systemic tumor dissemination being assumed by the presence of "clinically positive" (palpable) axillary lymph nodes or

by a primary tumor larger than one centime-ter in diameter. These high-risk patients were then to be randomized to one of three treatment arms: (1) four cycles of preopera-tive AC and subsequent surgery, <u>or</u> (2) four cycles of preoperative AC combined with docetaxel (all three drugs being given on the same day) and subsequent surgery, <u>or</u> (3) four cycles of preoperative AC, subsequent surgery, and four cycles of postoperative docetaxel.

NSABP Protocol B-30, the largest of these taxane-oriented trials, will no doubt make—or break—the case for adjuvant docetaxel. The projected enrollment called for 4,000 women with node-positive breast cancer. After undergoing surgery these patients were to be randomized to one of three treatment arms: (1) four cycles of AC followed by four cycles of docetaxel, <u>or</u> (2) four cycles of doxorubicin and docetaxel given together (do we really need the cyclo-phosphamide if we are pounding away with those cytotoxic sledgehammers Adriamycin and Taxotere?), <u>or</u> (3) four cycles of AC and docetaxel given together, followed by daily injections of granulocyte colony-stimulating factor (is G-CSF really all that good at pre-venting neutropenic fevers?).[84]

Professional oncologists will probably quibble over the details of these four trials, but no one is likely to ignore the findings which will emerge from them. Unlike small pilot studies conducted at this or that hospi-tal, the nationwide NSABP trials bespeak our greatest desiderata—freedom from bias and statistical power. Sooner or later they should tell us whether the taxoid drugs can really help to alter the natural history of breast malignancies.

Chapter Twenty-six

STAGE FOUR
The Management of Metastatic Disease

The majority of breast malignancies currently being diagnosed in the United States and other industrial nations have an excellent prognosis. Thanks to mammographic screening and increased public awareness, we are seeing large numbers of tiny *in situ* (noninvasive) lesions and of small low-grade invasive tumors; most of these cancers can be cured by appropriate local therapy. And a certain percentage of those high-grade tumors which have shed malignant cells into systemic circulation are now being cured by adjuvant chemohormonal therapies. Unfortunately, we cannot often use the word "cure" with respect to metastatic disease; the encouraging cure rates reported by some institutions may be due to the characterization of soft-tissue recurrences in the regional lymph nodes or in the skin near the tumor site as "metastases." Recurrences like these do not always foreshadow a poor prognosis; and they can usually be managed by surgical excision, with or without local irradiation. Properly speaking, the term "metastatic disease" should be reserved for **distant metastases**—that is, for recurrences occurring in organs or tissues which have no immediate anatomical connection to the mammary gland. A single metastatic lesion discovered in the skeletal framework

or in the liver or in the lungs warrants an emphatic classification as Stage Four, not without reason. Even the smallest distant metastasis looms as a large problem. We may be justly proud of our recent progress in diagnostic imaging—CAT and MRI scans can often detect metastatic tumors as small as half a centimeter in diameter. From a clinical perspective this would be a modest-sized lesion; but from a molecular viewpoint it is enormous, involving millions of cancer cells. Ant the fact that these cells have demonstrably been able to establish themselves in tissues so unlike the mammary gland—as it were, to take root and flourish in foreign soil—is ominous.

With most breast cancer cases, the appearance of one or more distant metastases marks the onset of a complex, progressive, and relentless process which we do not fully understand and which we have hitherto been unable to reverse. The appropriate word to describe the intent behind our interventions is **management**—that is, they are undertaken to prevent complications which would interfere with the patient's ability to function. We always hope that our interventions will also extend life expectancy; sometimes they do. But when metastatic disease spreads throughout the body and ceases to respond to chemotherapy, the intent behind our interventions changes to **palliation**—that is, they are done simply to alleviate pain and to provide as dignified a death as possible.

Most breast cancer patients who develop distant metastases will eventually succumb to the host of complications that result from uncontrollable systemic disease. The long-term outlook for these patients continues to be bleak. The Sloan-Kettering oncologists Gabriella M. D'Andrea and Andrew D. Seidman observe that "despite a wide array of chemotherapeutic regimens with documented activity against advanced breast cancer, less than one in five patients are alive five years after diagnosis of metastatic disease."[1] Yet there are wide variations in the course of disease and in survival times. Gabriel N. Hortobagyi of the M. D. Anderson Cancer Center reminds us that "metastatic breast cancer is a heterogeneous disease with protean manifestations. Some patients develop rapidly progressing and metastasizing disease that results in death less than six months after diagnosis, while others live in apparent symbiosis with their disease for many years, sometimes decades, almost irrespective of the therapy administered."[2] Breast cancer specialists like Dr. Hortobagyi have long used simple rules of thumb to distinguish between those Stage Four patients who are likely to have a very bad time and those who may well be able to coexist with their cancer. These rules are based on the **disease-free interval** and on the **number and location of the distant metastases**. As a rule, the more time that has elapsed between the surgical treatment of the primary tumor and the appearance of a detectable metastasis, the better the patient's outlook. And as a rule, a single isolated metastasis bodes for longer survival than multiple metastases which seem to have appeared almost simultaneously. On the one hand, a Stage Four patient who went five or more years without recurrence and then presented with a small osseous (skeletal) lesion may be no more than inconvenienced by this metastatic event. A few sessions of radiotherapy might well take care of her problem. On the other hand, a Stage Four patient who developed multiple metastatic nodules in the liver and lungs within a year or two of her surgery would be viewed as gravely ill—and we could not predict whether any current therapy would necessarily extend her survival. Osseous metastases, especially if limited in extent, are associated with longer survival than the so-called "visceral" metastases (those occurring in the abdominal and chest cavities). Metastases affecting the brain usually foreshadow an early demise.

Current Systemic Therapies

Hormonal agents continue to play a significant role in the management of metastatic breast cancer, for the simple reason that cytotoxic chemotherapy is unpleasant and that as yet no cytotoxic regimen has been shown to be curative. **Tamoxifen**, that tried-and-true antiestrogen, might still be the drug of choice if the patient has not previously been exposed to it. Of course, if she developed metastases during or after tamoxifen therapy, some other agent should probably be used. Older patients with sluggish, hormonally responsive disease have often fared well on **Megace** (brand name for megestrol acetate), a synthetic progestin which has mild side effects. As we have seen in Chapter Twenty-two, our newer hormonal drugs for breast cancer include **aromatase inhibitors** for postmenopausal patients and **gonadotropin-releasing hormone agonists** for premenopausal patients.

Before contemplating any hormonal therapy, it is prudent to determine the estrogen and progesterone receptor status of the metastatic lesions. The fact that the primary tumor was receptor-positive is no guarantee of continued hormonal responsiveness—the metastatic cells could have undergone mutations which rendered them receptor-negative and therefore resistant to hormonal manipulations. Fine-needle aspiration can often provide an adequate cellular specimen of distant metastases, while a simple immunostaining assay will suffice to determine receptor content. Traditionally, oncologists have assumed that a long disease-free interval and a modest metastatic presentation limited to the skeleton would be associated not only with hormone receptor positivity, but also with a low S-phase (i.e., slow rate of cellular multiplication). Breast malignancies with these characteristics, whether primary or metastatic, are obvious candidates for hormonal therapy. A short disease-free interval and multiple visceral metastases have traditionally been interpreted as an indication of hormone receptor negativity and a high S-phase, two characteristics which define the need for cytotoxic chemotherapy. When a patient presents with life-threatening respiratory difficulties or with imminent hepatic failure, chemotherapy is the appropriate option even if the lung or liver metastases should assay receptor-positive. In this case we need an immediate response to prevent complications. Hormonal drugs may take two or three months to shrink tumors; consequently they are not indicated for rapidly progressive disease, regardless of its hormone receptor status.

Sooner or later, virtually all Stage Four patients will become candidates for chemotherapy, either upon the diagnosis of metastatic disease or after disease progression (treatment failure) during hormonal therapy. While our cytotoxic regimens cannot routinely cure metastatic disease, they have nonetheless proven extremely useful, often

heading off complications and occasionally producing a lengthy remission. Adriamycin (doxorubicin) has historically been the agent of choice. Paul A. C. Greenberg and his colleagues went through the well-maintained database at Houston's M. D. Anderson Cancer Center and retrieved the case histories of 1,581 Anderson patients who received rigorous chemotherapy for metastatic breast cancer between 1973 and 1982. The Adriamycin-based FAC regimen had been given first, followed by CMF as maintenance therapy. Patients received up to two years of chemo. You might ask, "Was anyone cured?" The exceptionally long follow-up provided by Greenberg et al gives us some sobering insights. Of the 1,581 patients, 263 (16%) achieved complete remissions (no evidence of disease detectable) from the potent FAC and CMF combination. But only 49 of these patients (3.1% of the 1,581) still remained in remission five years after completing chemotherapy. In 1996, with a median follow-up of 191 months (15.9 years), 26 of the complete responders still revealed no trace of recurrent cancer. If we assume that these 26 patients will remain disease-free, we might claim an apparent cure rate of 1.64% for this large series. Patients in the series who achieved such durable responses had several distinguishing characteristics—"younger age, lower tumor burden, and better performance status." Dr. Greenberg and his M. D. Anderson colleagues suggest that patients with these characteristics "should be approached with potential cures in mind," yet they concede an unhappy truth: "Response rates to salvage regimens, once hormonal and first-line chemotherapy have been exhausted, are extremely poor and short-lived."[3]

It would seem that every cytotoxic agent in existence has been tried out as second-line therapy for metastatic breast tumors which no longer responded to the standard adjuvant regimens. **Mitoxantrone**, a powerful drug that acts much like doxorubicin but with less cardiotoxicity, has been prominently featured in salvage regimens. The antitumor antibiotic **mitomycin** has also been frequently employed, as have the vinca alkaloids **vinblastine** and **vinorelbine**. During the 1990s **paclitaxel** and **docetaxel** established their worth as salvage agents; some oncologists began to suspect that these taxoid drugs might prove more effective than Adriamycin, though as yet nobody had an impressive verification of long-term results comparable to that available for the M. D. Anderson series on FAC with CMF maintenance.

All the aforementioned drugs have produced responses in metastatic breast cancer, but no drug or combination of drugs always does so, and the durable remission remains an exception to the rule. Stage Four patients who experience disease progression after responding to a first-line salvage regimen are considerably less likely to obtain a significant response when a second-line regimen is given. The odds of response to a third or fourth salvage regimen become smaller and smaller. Yet the willingness of American oncologists to employ third or fourth regimens has long been proverbial. Not everybody applauds this practice. In his fatalistic bestseller *How We Die*, the Yale surgeon Sherwin B. Nuland wryly observes that oncologists will "try almost any last-ditch effort to stave off inevitability—they can be seen on the barricades when other defenders have furled their flags."[4] Lee N. Newcomer, an oncologist turned cost-conscious director of a managed care plan, has a more pointed criticism: "In oncology, you were always raised to say, 'Well, what the heck, I'm out of standard therapy, let's just try something else.' And that's bad medicine. We wouldn't allow that in any other specialty."[5] Of course, the expectations of patients and their family members have a great deal to do with this freewheeling therapeutic empiricism. Very few laypersons realize how remote the chances of a meaningful response to a third salvage regimen really are. Breast tumors which have spawned distant metastases in spite of adjuvant chemotherapy and then continued to progress through salvage attempts with Adriamycin and a taxoid drug have already demonstrated intractable drug resistance. Until we learn how to reverse that resistance, we must at some point conclude that the side effects of additional cytotoxic therapy will probably outweigh any conceivable benefit.

Waiting on New Modalities:
Angiogenesis Inhibitors

Stage Four patients and their oncologists desperately need new systemic drugs which rely on some other mode of action than indiscriminate cytotoxicity and which do not elicit multidrug resistance. **Angiogenesis inhibitors** represent a novel class of agents which seem likely to avoid both the toxic side effects and the drug resistance associated with traditional chemotherapy. As we have seen in Chapter One, malignant tumors cannot grow beyond minuscule size without significant **angiogenesis**—that is, without the formation of additional blood vessels in the surrounding tissues. Physicians as far back as Hippocrates noticed those prominent blood vessels feeding the growth of tumors—the process was often visible to the naked eye, especially in the case of advanced breast malignancies. Only in the 1990s, however, did biomedical scientists and pharmaceutical companies finally devote massive amounts of time and money to studying the molecular mechanisms behind this neovascularization, with a view to discovering or designing chemical compounds which could prevent it. The angiogenesis researcher Judah Folkman of the Harvard Medical School points out that the progression of a solid tumor, whether primary or metastatic, depends on two different types of cells—firstly, the transformed tumor cells, and secondly, the normal endothelial cells lining the nearby blood vessels. For a tumor to grow, the cancer cells must stimulate the endothelial cells, and vice versa.[6] When a formerly *in situ* malignancy becomes invasive, lytic enzymes called **matrix metalloproteinases** begin to degrade the surrounding basement membrane, the extracellular matrix, and the underlying connective tissue (*stroma*).[7] At the same time the tumor cells secrete angiogenic growth factors which prod the adjacent endothelial cells to proliferate and create new blood vessels. This process of matrix dissolution and neovascularization is complex, and our scientists are still counting all the lytic enzymes and growth factors involved. Writing in the *New England Journal of Medicine*, Dr. Folkman observed that twelve angiogenic factors had been identified.[8] Two of these elusive proteins—**basic fibroblast growth factor** (bFGF) and **vascular endothelial growth factor** (VEGF)—play an important role in the progression of many different tumors; consequently, they have prompted the most intensive investigations. Assays recently developed to detect bFGF in the blood and urine may give us an early warning of disease recurrence. The urine samples provided by cancer patients often have bFGF levels 100 to 200 times higher than normal.[9] VEGF, which acts specifically on endothelial cells, seems to have particular significance for breast malignancies. Giampietro Gasparini and his colleagues in Italy and Japan found that node-negative breast cancer patients whose tumors had high VEGF levels were far more likely to experience disease recurrence than comparable

patients whose tumors had lower levels. Similar findings have been reported by teams in Sweden, Switzerland, and other European countries.[10]

Many pharmaceutical researchers think that angiogenesis inhibition will eventually prove to be a better strategy than simply trying to kill cancer cells outright, that long prevalent approach which has resulted in cytotoxic cannons like Adriamycin, cisplatin, and docetaxel. For one thing, angiogenesis is physiologically negligible in adults, who have no great need for new blood vessels unless they happen to be pregnant or are recovering from serious wounds or burns. Therefore drugs which interfere only with neovascularization should not have those toxic life-threatening consequences—indeed, they should have minimal side effects. And drug resistance ought to be a minor problem, because the endothelial cells being targeted would be far less prone to mutate into drug-resistant phenotypes. Metastatic cancer cells are moving targets—genetically unstable to begin with, they tend to divide frequently and to acquire new mutations as they do so. Thus the cytotoxic drug which worked yesterday may be ineffective today, because resistant cells have evolved in the meantime. Normal endothelial cells do not divide unless prompted to do so; it is much less likely that they would acquire mutations leading to drug resistance.

The growing interest in antiangiogenic strategies led to Judah Folkman's selection as a keynote speaker at the May 1996 meeting of the American Society of Clinical Oncology. Dr. Folkman told the crowded assembly that 26 pharmaceutical firms were vying to develop clinically useful angiogenesis inhibitors.[11] The public at large learned about these developments two years later. On May 3, 1998, the *New York Times* ran a front-page story focusing on **angiostatin** and

endostatin, two naturally occurring angiogenesis inhibitors which had been isolated in Folkman's lab. Both molecules had produced remissions in immunodeficient mice which had been inoculated with human tumor cells.[12] The enthusiastic *Times* piece left anxious patients and other laypersons with the impression that wonder drugs for cancer were just around the corner, likely to be ready in a year or two at most. The reality was different—angiostatin and endostatin had not been produced in quantity, nor had they been tested on human subjects. But **combretastatin**, an angiogenesis inhibitor made from the bark of a South African willow tree, had already entered human trials; and at least one patient with metastatic thyroid cancer had experienced a complete remission after receiving this drug.[13]

Several of the new agents being studied targeted matrix metalloproteinases, those enzymes responsible for creating an environment in which tumor-related angiogenesis can take place. The synthetic agents **batimastat** and **marimastat** achieved impressive results in mice. While batimastat was the first to enter human trials, it was soon supplanted by the more soluble marimastat, which offered the advantage of convenient oral administration. Both these drugs are well-tolerated, but neither has induced remissions in metastatic human cancers. Amy R. Nelson and her colleagues at the Vanderbilt University Medical Center believe that matrix metalloproteinase inhibitors might be more effective if given earlier in the course of disease, when the tumor burden is still small.[14]

One of the angiogenesis inhibitors being evaluated in the 1990s was neither new nor unknown. In the late 1950s physicians in England, Germany, and other European nations had liberally dispensed prescriptions for a synthetic sedative called **thalidomide**. This drug was deemed so safe that it was unhesitatingly prescribed for pregnant women. This practice led to the most notorious pharmacological disaster of the twentieth century—thousands of infants were born with shocking deformities, flippers taking the place of hands and arms, stumps being found where the legs should have been. Nobody knew it at the time, but thalidomide could act as an angiogenesis inhibitor as well as a sedative. In this instance the drug had suppressed angiogenesis in first-trimester embryos right at the time when the extremities (the arms and legs) were supposed to be formed. While the precise mechanism of thalidomide's antiangiogenic action remains unknown, cancer researchers have recently been lining up to test the drug because it has virtually no side effects in nonpregnant patients. Clinical trials of thalidomide in metastatic breast cancer, in Kaposi's sarcoma (a rare skin cancer associated with AIDS), and in gliomas (malignant brain tumors) attracted much attention. Howard Fine of Boston's Dana-Farber Cancer Institute headed a preliminary trial of thalidomide for recurrent gliomas. "If thalidomide works," observed Dr. Fine in 1997, "it will become one of the first antiangiogenics in the clinic. It is a great drug. We are used to using incredibly toxic drugs that cause all kinds of organ dysfunction and discomfort."[15]

From the 1950s to the present, cancer chemotherapy has relied on brief intermittent exposures to cytotoxic agents, with the aim being to eradicate all the malignant cells. Angiogenesis inhibition would not work like that—it would aim at long-term suppression of tumor growth rather than total eradication. Consequently, any antiangiogenic drugs must be safe enough for constant and prolonged therapy. Ideally, they would be taken as a daily pill or nasal spray, without recourse to bothersome intravenous administration. The measure of an antiangiogenic's effectiveness would not necessarily be the destruction of existing metastases (they might persist), but rather the prevention of new ones. James M. Pluda of the National Cancer Institute's antiangiogenic program explains that the real goal is "to convert cancer into a chronic disease whereby patients can live for thirty years in a symbiotic-type relationship with their tumor, where the tumor doesn't bother them and drugs keep the tumor in check."[16]

Unfortunately, we have miles to go before we can sleep on angiogenesis inhibition. Dozens of potential agents are being investigated, but it seems unreasonable to expect that any one of them will do for diverse malignancies what penicillin once did for diverse bacterial infections. The biggest stumbling block lies in the fact that tumors have numerous pathways through which they can accomplish matrix dissolution and angiogenesis. A metastasis principally secreting vascular endothelial growth factor might be deprived of its neovascularization by an anti-VEGF drug, but a second metastasis principally secreting another growth factor would be unaffected. Those famous mice experiments done in Dr. Folkman's lab often revealed a troubling pattern of tumor shrinkage followed by subsequent regrowth. The phenomenon suggests that when an antiangiogenic drug shuts down one pathway to neovascularization, the tumor cells may start to rely on another. This is not the same thing as the intractable multidrug resistance which we encounter with cytotoxic chemotherapy; however, it does suggest that multiple antiangiogenic agents may be required to maintain tumor suppression. Isaiah Fidler of the M. D. Anderson Cancer Center suspects that the innate diversity among blood vessel cells will pose an obstacle to the development of a broad-spectrum antiangiogenic: "You have to remember that the endothelial cells of different organs are phenotypically different. Some of these agents therefore

may be active in some organs, but not others. We may have to learn how to tailor our antiangiogenic therapy to that reality."[17]

For the time being, patients with metastatic breast cancer will continue to receive cytotoxic chemotherapy or hormonal drugs as their main treatment. Yet we can anticipate that in the future these patients will be given an antiangiogenic agent or two along with the traditional regimens. When we have better evidence that antiangiogenic therapy really works in human malignancies, perhaps we could begin to "tailor" the drugs and the dose levels to the particular tumors.

Immunotherapeutic agents represent another class of essentially noncytotoxic drugs whose cancer-fighting potential seems substantial. Some of these **biological response modifiers** (as they are also called) have already entered the clinic. Patients with metastatic breast tumors which overexpress the HER-2/*neu* oncogene are now receiving Genentech's drug **Herceptin** (brand name for **trastuzumab**). Approved by the FDA in 1998, this agent is a humanized monoclonal antibody which binds to the HER-2 protein found on the outer membranes of the tumor cells. In a very few cases, it has rescued patients at death's door; most responses have been less dramatic. Genentech has also developed a monoclonal antibody which targets VEGF; in a preliminary trial involving patients with metastatic cancer, this drug rapidly decreased the amount of VEGF in the blood, without appreciably shrinking the metastases.[18]

The subject of prospective immunotherapies is so important that it deserves a chapter of its own. Therefore we must postpone the extended discussion of this topic until Chapter Twenty-seven, though it necessarily merits at least a passing mention in any paragraphs touching on new modalities. In general, we can only applaud the ongoing research on angiogenesis inhibitors and biological response modifiers, yet the unwary reader must be cautioned against the assumption that these agents will soon vanquish metastatic disease. Nude mice inoculated with human cancers are sitting ducks—any drug which doesn't cure them is not selected for further development. In contrast, the metastatic tumors seen in patients are more apt to be leaping tigers—and the biological mechanisms behind this behavior have hitherto defied our attempts at explication. While we may hope that our pharmaceutical ingenuity will someday transform metastatic disease into an easily controllable illness, we cannot predict just when this will happen. Therefore we must in prudence return to this chapter's main subject matter—viz., **the prevention of complications and the relief of pain in end-stage disease**.

SKELETAL METASTASES
The Prevention of Fractures

Breast malignancies can metastasize to all sorts of unexpected sites: the ovaries, the gastrointestinal tract, the spleen, or the uvea (vascular layer of the eye).[19] In the interest of brevity, however, we must limit our discussion of symptoms and their management to those sites which are most frequently involved—the skeleton, the lungs, the liver, and the central nervous system. Skeletal metastases are by far the most common; they are typically **osteolytic**—that is, they tend to destroy bone and to precipitate fractures. The bones likely to be involved are the spinal vertebrae, the marrow-rich ilia (hip bones), the femur (thigh bone), the humerus (upper arm bone), and the ribs. The presenting symptom is usually pain—a chronic aching which persists and intensifies, often interfering with sleep or with daily activities. The

pain associated with osseous metastases needs to be distinguished from that of muscular backaches or of swollen or arthritic joints. The cancer pain tends to be localized to the spot of involvement—for example, to the middle of the back if the spinal vertebrae are involved. And that spot may be tender to the touch. A sharp or sudden pain in a weight-bearing bone like the femur or hip, brought on by standing up or by other physical activity, has often been the harbinger of an impending fracture.

Needless to say, any persistent skeletal discomfort ought to be thoroughly investigated. A **bone scan** has traditionally been the first examination ordered, because it gives us an image of the entire skeleton. Plain radiographs (ordinary X-rays) may then be taken of any areas of unusual activity seen on the scan as well as of any spots which the patient has identified as painful. What these X-ray close-ups show us is the extent of erosion in the **cortical bone**—i.e., in the hard outer layer of bone which gives the skeleton its strength. If too much cortical bone has been lost, an orthopedic surgeon would be called upon to insert an internal pin in the bone involved, so as to head off a fracture. Kristine A. Nelson and her colleagues at the Cleveland Clinic recommend that "weight-bearing bones should be stabilized surgically before radiotherapy when the metastatic lesion is greater than three centimeters in length."[20] Smaller lesions usually do not require surgical fixation; they are given external-beam radiotherapy as the initial treatment.

Irradiation remains our principal tool in the management of osseous metastases, for the simple reason that bone is relatively radioresistant. It can safely absorb doses which would destroy other tissues. The size of the dose to be aimed at any involved area, and the number of fractions (treatment sessions) over which the dose is administered, are left to the judgment of the attending radiation oncologist. Irradiation is highly effective in relieving bone pain; and for terminal patients, when palliation is the only goal, a single fraction of 800 rads (8 grays) may be sufficient.[21] Pain relief, while not instantaneous, normally occurs within a week or two. In patients with a better prognosis, we would use larger cumulative doses and more protracted scheduling (more fractions), with a view to sterilizing the tumor cells and hopefully allowing healing (reossification) to occur. Salvatore Veltri of the Medical College of Ohio (Toledo) observes that "most patients receive optimal results from courses of 30 grays (3,000 rads) in 10 fractions, or 40 grays (4,000 rads) in 15 fractions."[22]

Back in the 1980s half-body irradiation was often used to relieve pain in patients who had numerous metastatic lesions at different skeletal locations. The drawback was that these "broad fields" (i.e., the irradiation of large areas of the body) tended to produce unwanted side effects, including bone marrow suppression, pneumonitis (inflammation of the lungs), and nausea and vomiting. The 1990s saw the introduction of the useful radioisotope **strontium 89**, which has been marketed under the brand name **Metastron**. Given intravenously, the radioactive strontium is preferentially absorbed at sites of osseous activity. While the drug may take several weeks to act, a single brief infusion can ultimately provide up to three months of relief from the pain of widespread skeletal metastases. And subsequent infusions are usually just as effective as the first one.[23] We should stress that strontium 89 is used exclusively for palliation. External-beam irradiation which delivers a high dose to individual skeletal lesions not only relieves pain, but also causes tumor regression. Consequently it remains our first-line therapy.

Molecular Mechanisms: The Advent of Bisphosphonates

Our pharmacologists have been trying to decipher the biochemical processes behind cancer-related bone destruction, in hopes of someday designing drugs which can prevent it. The mechanical events are easy to understand. A primary tumor in the breast or elsewhere sheds malignant cells into systemic circulation, which eventually come to rest amid the latticelike structures of the porous interior bone (cancellous bone). While the blood flow here is sluggish and eddying, the jellylike marrow constitutes a site of intense mitotic activity, with untold millions of new blood cells being born every day. Consequently the marrow is awash with cellular growth factors, a fact which helps to explain why it serves as fertile soil for many diverse tumors. But what particular circumstances explain why breast cancer cells seem to thrive at this location?

Gregory Mundy, an endocrinologist at the University of Texas in San Antonio, observes that "bone is like fertilizer to tumor cells, particularly breast cancer cells. Breast cancer cells love bone."[24] Dr. Mundy points out that the actual resorption (breakdown) of bone is not done by the newly arrived malignant cells, but by native marrow cells called **osteoclasts**, which play a leading role in the remodeling of bone that goes on all the time, even in elderly adults. What the metastatic cells provide is an inappropriate stimulus to the osteoclasts, shifting them (so to speak) into perpetual high gear. This stimulus has long been thought to be "humoral" in nature; that is, to be a substance (or substances) found in bodily fluids. In the late 1990s American researchers cited **parathyroid hormone-related protein** (PHrP) as the most likely culprit. This protein is structurally similar to the hormone secreted by the parathyroid glands, which do much to regulate the body's metabolism of calcium and phosphorus. A major difference between these two humoral factors is that parathyroid hormone circulates throughout the body, while PHrP is basically a local messenger within tissues, serving to transmit a stimulus from one set of cells to an adjacent group of cells.[25]

The osteolytic scenario that Dr. Mundy and his colleague Toshiyuki Yoneda proposed in the *New England Journal of Medicine* begins with the metastatic cancer cells secreting increasing quantities of PHrP. The surfeit of PHrP prods the nearby osteoclasts into misguided action. "When bone is resorbed," Mundy and Yoneda point out, "transforming growth factor beta and other peptides are released, causing further bone destruction and stimulating the proliferation of tumor cells."[26] A vicious cycle is thus established, with the colonizing cancer cells stimulating the native osteoclasts, and vice versa. In osteolytic malignancies like metastatic breast cancer, the upshot is not only bone pain and eventual fractures, but a pernicious condition called **hypercalcemia** (too much calcium in the blood), which quickly leads to serious complications.

Our emerging knowledge of the molecular mechanisms causing cancer-related bone dissolution has not as yet led to new designer drugs which specifically target and suppress the misguided osteoclasts. Breast cancer specialists have been looking instead to chemical compounds called **bisphosphonates**, which were discovered over a century ago and which have hitherto been used principally as water softeners. Only in the 1990s did important medical applications begin to be perceived. When given to patients, bisphosphonates adhere to the calcium crystals in bone, inhibiting their breakdown by osteoclasts. Bone resorption, whether due to

osseous metastases or to osteoporosis, does not occur so readily. Gentle bisphosphonates like **alendronate**, **etidronate**, and **risedronate** have attracted attention as promising therapies to prevent osteoporosis or to slow its progression; any of these drugs can be taken as a convenient daily pill, with few side effects beyond the occasional upset stomach. Merck & Co. has been promoting its alendronate sodium tablets under the brand name **Fosamax**, touting them as "the first non-hormonal treatment for postmenopausal osteoporosis."[27]

Considerably stronger bisphosphonates are needed to combat the rapid osteolysis sometimes associated with metastatic breast carcinomas. In the United States the preferred drug has been **pamidronate**; it is typically given as a two-hour infusion (90 milligrams) every three or four weeks. As most patients receiving pamidronate are also receiving chemotherapy, intravenous administration has not posed a great inconvenience. And we have firm evidence that pamidronate really delays the progression of osteolytic skeletal metastases, at least to a certain extent. Gabriel N. Hortobagyi and other American oncologists conducted a clinical trial in which 380 breast cancer patients with osseous metastases were randomly assigned to receive a monthly infusion of pamidronate or of a placebo. The results revealed that pamidronate significantly reduced the number of fractures. The median time to "the first skeletal complication" was 13.1 months in the pamidronate arm, as compared to 7.0 months in the placebo arm. The patients getting pamidronate reported less bone pain. After three monthly infusions they had fewer episodes of hypercalcemia; after six, they made fewer trips to the hospital for palliative irradiation. Pamidronate proved to be well-tolerated; however, it did not appreciably increase the median survival times, which were 14.8 months in the pamidronate arm and 14.2 months in the placebo arm.[28]

Some oncologists in Europe and Canada have been enthusiastic about **clodronate**, a bisphosphonate which can be taken by mouth. Ingo J. Diel and other German physicians conducted an early trial of clodronate as adjuvant therapy. They enrolled 302 women treated for breast cancer at the Heidelberg University Hospital between 1990 and 1995; none of these patients had metastatic disease at diagnosis, but all had isolated tumor cells in bone marrow (as detected by marrow sampling and immunostaining) and were therefore presumed to be at high risk for osseous metastases. All these patients received chemotherapy and tamoxifen; but 157 of them were also assigned to two years of clodronate therapy, which involved no more than taking four pills (400 milligrams each) every morning before breakfast. In 1998 Dr. Diel and his colleagues published their encouraging findings in the *New England Journal of Medicine*. After a median follow-up of 36 months, the clodronate arm had fewer patients diagnosed with distant metastases (only 21) than the control arm (42 patients diagnosed). There were also tantalizing hints of a survival benefit—only six patients died in the clodronate arm, while 22 died in the control arm.[29]

Can a nontoxic bisphosphonate pill both reduce the odds of developing osseous metastases as well as extend survival in those patients who do develop these metastases? Obviously, we'd like to believe so; but we should remember that "the jury is still out" with regard to adjuvant clodronate. And palliative pamidronate has not been altogether uncontroversial. The FDA approved this intravenous bisphosphonate in 1996, for the treatment of osteolytic lesions due to metastatic breast cancer. American oncologists have tended to endorse pamidronate because it is a more potent drug than clodronate, has a more lasting effect, and seems

better at reducing hypercalcemia.[30] Sales of pamidronate, marketed under the brand name **Aredia**, jumped 80% in 1997 and then increased another 61% in 1998. The drug was not cheap, and breast cancer patients with osseous metastases required ongoing monthly infusions. Since there is insufficient evidence that pamidronate extends survival times, the therapy has been criticized for its lack of cost-effectiveness. Writing in 1997, Gary Kao of the University of Pennsylvania Hospital offered some dollar figures: "The acquisition cost of a single 90-mg dose of pamidronate at our pharmacy is approximately $700; a one-year course thus costs at least $8,400."[31] The ultimate economic impact of pamidronate therapy remains open to question, because patients taking this drug may require fewer painkillers, less irradiation, and fewer surgical fixations.

There should be more day to dawn on the bisphosphonates. While these agents have no direct effect on metastatic cancer cells, they do seem to stymie the osteoclasts, at least in laboratory simulations. Pharmaceutical researchers have recently been looking at **ibandronate** and **zoledronate**, two second-generation bisphosphonates which are far more powerful than clodronate or pamidronate.[32] An optimistic long-range goal is that a bisphosphonate or two, if given early enough, will prevent osteolytic metastases from developing in the first place.

Spinal Cord Compression

The word **crisis** was very much current in early nineteenth-century American medicine. "Thank heaven! the crisis is past" began a famous poem by Edgar Allan Poe. The verse was written for a reading public accustomed to hearing doctors prattle about pernicious fevers and the crucial "crisis," an event which supposedly spelled the difference between life and death.[33] Today's physicians no longer employ the term, unless they happen to be oncologists treating patients with metastatic tumors. In this instance the term remains valid coinage, being used to designate an emergency in which a patient needs an immediate intervention to forestall catastrophic complications. The most urgent crisis that might be faced by breast cancer patients with osteolytic metastases is **spinal cord compression**. If this condition is not immediately diagnosed and treated, an affected patient may lose not only the ability to walk, but also control over bladder and bowel functions. A lamentable outcome!

The spinal cord is the central conduit of nerves which runs downward from the brain, passing through an open canal in each of the spinal vertebrae. The cord contains both motor nerves, which stimulate the muscles into action, and sensory nerves, which transmit sensations back to the brain. While protected by the surrounding vertebrae, the cord is nonetheless extremely vulnerable. An injury which severs it or otherwise destroys any portion of it cannot be remedied. Prolonged compression of the cord will also result in permanent loss of function. Once cancer patients lose control over their legs due to spinal cord compression, they do not often become ambulatory again, regardless of what therapeutic measures might be taken. The spinal nerves, while intact, have been excessively traumatized.

Spinal cord compression typically comes about in one of two ways. The first is **vertebral fracture**, also termed **vertebral collapse**. In this instance osteolytic metastases to the spine have caused so much resorption in a vertebra that it begins to disintegrate, with resulting impingement of the cord. **Epidural tumors** represent a second mechanism—in this instance malignant cells growing right outside the cord's outer membrane (the *dura*) are beginning to put

pressure on the enclosed nerves. These epidural lesions may originate either in tumor outgrowths from affected vertebrae, or in adjuvant lymph nodes which are swollen with metastatic cancer cells. An inflammatory reaction, with localized swelling and fluid accumulation, tends to aggravate any episode of cord compression, whether due to vertebral collapse or to epidural tumor or to both. It is crucial that we control that inflammatory reaction and prevent further compression of the cord if paraplegia (lower body paralysis) is to be avoided. Every Stage Four patient should know this syndrome's warning signs, because a few hours' delay in getting help may make an unfortunate difference in outcome.

Any lingering pain in the middle of the back should be regarded with suspicion, and painful tenderness elicited by a physician's examining hand always indicates an urgent need for diagnostic tests. Certain neurological symptoms should be regarded as alarm bells warning of probable cord compression: they include unexplained weakness affecting the legs, difficulty in controlling the anal and urinary sphincter muscles, and paresthesias (numbness or tingling) anywhere in the lower body. The English oncologist C. J. Williams and his colleagues point out that these symptoms may be "insidious in onset" and can vary "depending on the level of compression."[34] Nowadays the diagnosis of cord involvement can be made with remarkable accuracy. Plain X-rays will reveal any loss of mineralization in the individual vertebrae; any vertebral body which has recently diminished in height can be presumed to have suffered a fracture. The specific site or sites at which cord compression is occurring can be located with a **myelogram** (from the Greek *myelos*, "marrow"). In this exam a contrast agent (radio-opaque dye) is first injected into the spinal fluid; the spinal column is then X-rayed to pinpoint the areas of impingement on the cord. **Magnetic resonance imagery** (MRI) has supplanted CAT as the diagnostic tool of choice for identifying epidural tumors. These soft-tissue masses are not well visualized on X-rays or CAT scans because of radiographic glare coming from the nearby bony structures. Douglas J. Quint of the University of Michigan Medical Center (Ann Arbor) reminds us that MRI is safer than a myelogram, which carries "the additional risks of contrast material and spinal needle placement."[35]

The treatment of spinal cord compression usually begins with the synthetic corticosteroid **dexamethasone**. A high initial dose—the so-called "loading dose"—is given intravenously, with a view to reducing the inflammatory swelling and fluid accumulation as fast as possible. Most patients are subsequently maintained on low-dose dexamethasone tablets (e.g., four to six milligrams every six hours). **Irradiation** is the main treatment—often several different areas of the spinal column need to be irradiated because the X-rays or MRI have revealed multiple epidural tumors or structurally weakened vertebrae. As with steroid therapy, a high initial dose—say, 400 rads daily—may be used for the first few days. Salvatore Veltri observes that "radiation therapy is most frequently given to a total dose of 40 to 45 grays (4,000 to 4,500 rads), with daily dose fractions of 200 to 250 centigrays (200 to 250 rads)."[36]

Surgery plays a secondary role in treating spinal cord compression. The collapsing portions of the vertebrae and the epidural tumors are almost always located on the anterior (front) of the spinal column, where they are difficult to access. Nonetheless, if a patient is on the verge of paralysis and unable to wait for radiotherapy to take effect, a skilled neurosurgeon may be called upon to remove a crumbling vertebral body and the adjacent intervertebral disks. Once decompression of the spinal cord is achieved, the spinal column can be stabilized with an implanted vertical rod and methyl methacrylate cement. Neurosurgeons have also been asked to debulk large epidural tumors prior to radiotherapy. All these procedures are risky, with considerable loss of blood and the possibility of postoperative morbidity.[37] In the 1990s avant-garde specialists experimented with a less invasive technique called **percutaneous vertebroplasty**, whereby liquid methyl methacrylate is injected directly into vertebrae weakened by osteolytic metastases. Open surgery is thus avoided. Anne Cotton and her colleagues in France have enthusiastically reported that the hardening cement tends to stabilize the vertebral body, with marked or complete pain relief: "Most patients stand upright the next day; hospitalization time is short."[38] One of the first American hospitals to offer this procedure was the Milton S. Hershey Medical Center in Hershey, Pennsylvania. Writing in 1998, Michelle S. Barr and John D. Barr of the Hershey Center complained that American insurance companies often would not pay for the procedure because they did not know about it: "Education of insurance companies remains vital to the success of a percutaneous vertebroplasty program."[39]

Visceral Complications:
The Problematic Lungs and Liver

Oncologists sometimes refer to **visceral metastases**, by way of distinction from purely osseous ones and those in the central nervous system. The term is comprehensive enough, *viscera* being Latin for "inner organs" and therefore embracing the entire contents of the abdominal and thoracic (chest) cavities. The viscera most likely to be affected by metastatic breast cancer are the lungs and the liver. These two organs have different functions—the lungs oxygenate blood while the liver plays so many vital roles in the body's digestive and metabolic processes that even the largest textbook seems inadequate to describe them all. Yet it is the similarities between these disparate organs which do much to explain why metastatic tumors take root in them and why the resulting lesions are so difficult to manage. These tissues of both organs are fragile, easily injured, and highly vascularized. Any cancer cells circulating in the blood will necessarily pass through the lungs and the liver; in either organ they can easily come to rest in the elaborate networks of minute capillaries and venules. Once metastatic colonization has taken place, our treatment options are often limited. In most cases of pulmonary or hepatic involvement, cytotoxic chemotherapy will be the treatment of choice. As we have seen in the preceding chapter, the new taxoid drugs have proven remarkably effective in shrinking these metastases. But irradiation, our principal tool for managing osseous involvement, has only a few applications in the lungs and liver, for the simple reason that both these organs are too radiosensitive. A radiation dose high enough to eliminate metastatic disease would also bring about their destruction. By way of comparison, we might point out that the whole-organ tolerance of the lungs has been estimated at about 1,500 rads; that of the liver, at about 2,500 rads; and that of bone, at over 6,000 rads.[40] Surgery also tends to have few practical applications. A complete resection (surgical removal) of the lungs or liver is out of the question, since both organs are absolutely essential to life. Of course, the removal of isolated tumor nodules—or even of large organ segments—is quite possible; and it would not usually impair a patient's ability to function. Such partial resections

have occasionally been reported to extend survival times for patients with limited metastatic disease in the lungs or liver. The problem is that metastases in these organs rarely occur at just one or two spots; they are much more likely to be multifocal. The few lesions that we might see on an X-ray or CAT scan are typically the unhappy harbinger of other widespread lesions which are still too small to be detected. Therefore candidates for surgery must be thoughtfully selected; as a rule of thumb, they should not have rapidly progressive disease or substantial metastases in other organ systems (e.g., the skeleton). Ideally, the tumor nodules in the lungs or liver would be well-defined, not too numerous, and seemingly stable.

The **symptoms of lung involvement** usually appear gradually. **Dyspnea** (difficulty in breathing), especially during physical exertion, is often the first clue. Some patients may experience a dry nonproductive cough or a growing feeling of heaviness on the chest. On rare occasions **hemoptysis** (coughing up blood) can occur if metastatic tumor has invaded one of the larger bronchial tubes. Chest X-rays, so cheap and so fast, are the initial diagnostic exam; they should reveal any sizable tumor nodules, as well as any areas of exceptional density or of fluid accumulation. Then a CAT scan would be indicated to provide more detailed information on the number and location of the nodules, as well as on the status of the thoracic lymph nodes. Fine-needle aspiration of one of the nodules normally suffices to confirm the diagnosis.

Occasionally a cancer patient will present with rapidly worsening dyspnea, but neither the X-rays nor the CAT scan reveal anything suggestive of metastatic disease. In this circumstance we must suspect an acute condition known as **lymphangitic carcinomatosis**, in which the lymphatic vessels throughout the lungs are being obstructed by proliferating cancer cells. This diagnosis can often be confirmed by extending a flexible fiberoptic tube—**a bronchoscope**—down a large airway (a bronchus) and taking a small tissue sample. Aggressive chemotherapy is the only treatment for lymphangitic carcinomatosis, which carries an extremely poor prognosis.[41] In contrast, the prognosis with the nodular lesions commonly encountered in metastatic breast cancer can vary considerably. Edgar D. Staren and other thoracic surgeons have reported a five-year survival rate of 36% for a small group of patients whose pulmonary tumor nodules were resected with wide margins (one to two centimeters) of normal tissue. Even multiple nodules can be advantageously removed, Dr. Staren and his colleagues advise, so long as the patient has "a satisfactory workup indicative of no extrapulmonary disease."[42]

Radiotherapy comes into play for the crisis (severe dyspnea) which ensues when metastatic tumor begins to obstruct a large bronchial branch. This obstruction can be brought about either by direct tumor invasion of the airway or by compression of the airway due to adjacent tumor masses. Fortunately, <u>small</u> areas of the lung can be subjected to high doses of radiation (about 4,000 rads or so) without immediate complications. We call the preferred method of irradiating these small areas **brachytherapy** (from the Greek word *brachys*, meaning "short"). In this instance, a slender tube containing radioactive pellets would be carefully positioned in the airway so that only the obstructed portion receives the high-dose radiation.

Another crisis which can occur when breast cancer metastasizes to the lungs is called **a pleural effusion**. For readers unversed in thoracic anatomy, we must explain that the *pleurae* are flexible lubricated membranes which cover the lungs and then double back on the inside of the rib cage. The surfaces of these membranes are always wet with a thin layer of fluid, which acts as a cushion to reduce friction between the ever-expanding lungs and the rigid rib cage. The pleurae secrete several liters of fluid daily; under normal circumstances it does not accumulate, being drained off by the thoracic lymphatics. What happens in a pleural effusion is that metastatic cancer cells have infiltrated between the two pleural surfaces, thereby stimulating the production of more fluid at the same time they are clogging up the lymphatic drainage vessels. All of a sudden an affected patient will begin to have difficulty breathing, because her lungs are struggling to expand against several liters of fluid trapped between the pleural membranes. This condition can be easily diagnosed by X-rays or by ultrasound; and prompt relief can be obtained by **thoracentesis**, whereby a needle is inserted into the chest cavity to remove the offending fluid. Thoracentesis is a safe procedure; the only drawback is that by itself this remedy can never be permanent. After aspiration the fluid immediately begins to accumulate again, so that several weeks later the patient will again be suffering from severe dyspnea. Thus for patients who are not obviously near death, oncologists often seek to obtain a more permanent solution by injecting a sclerosing agent between the two pleural surfaces. The idea is to promote adhesions between these surfaces and thereby to obliterate the space which is constantly filling with fluid. We call this technique **pleurodesis** (from the Greek word *desis*, meaning "a binding together"). The antibiotic tetracycline has traditionally been used as the sclerosing agent, with reported success rates ranging up to 75%. Some oncologists have advocated the infusion of cisplatin or some other cytotoxic drug instead of tetracycline, arguing that this would not only induce the necessary adhesions but should have an antitumor effect as well.[43]

Pericardial effusions are occasionally seen with breast carcinomas and other malignancies which metastasize to the chest cavity. In this case that troublesome fluid gets trapped underneath the **pericardium**, the membrane covering the heart muscle. Presenting symptoms include dyspnea, chest pain, and tamponade (cardiac insufficiency due to compression of the muscle). An ultrasound technique called echocardiography usually suffices to establish the diagnosis, and **pericardiocentesis** (fine-needle aspiration of the fluid) serves to forestall the crisis. Therapeutic options if the effusion recurs include sclerotherapy with tetracycline as well as partial resection of the membrane itself (we call this "pericardiectomy").[44]

Cancer patients suffering from **vena cava syndrome** are not so acutely ill as those who present with pleural or pericardial effusions. This visceral complication occurs when tumor masses either infiltrate or compress the *superior vena cava*, the large vein which carries blood back from the head and arms to the heart. The earliest symptoms may be nonspecific (e.g., headaches); but they are soon succeeded by the telltale clinical signs—facial swelling and distended veins in the neck. Vena cava syndrome is more common with primary lung cancers than with metastatic breast cancer, but every oncologist and oncology nurse knows to watch out for it in both types of malignancy. Once the location of a vena cava obstruction has been determined by X-rays or by a CAT scan, the preferred treatment is external-beam radiotherapy.[45]

Malignant tumors which arise in the colon or rectum and spread beyond their site of origin almost invariably metastasize to the liver, since both the blood and lymph coming from the pelvis flow directly toward that vulnerable organ. **Hepatic metastases** also represent a major management challenge in disseminated breast cancers. The liver is a large organ, second only to the brain in weight and size. Metastatic colonization in the liver typically begins without noticeably affecting its function or otherwise causing symptoms that would attract our attention. When symptoms finally appear, they are apt to be nonspecific—a nauseous queasy feeling, vague gastrointestinal complaints, and an elevated level of alkaline phosphatase in the blood (a laboratory finding that could result from problems unrelated to cancer). Only when large segments of the organ have been replaced by tumor does the diagnosis become unmistakable. The liver no longer produces enough bile to allow the intestinal digestion of fats; an affected patient will start to lose weight. Serum (blood) levels of **bilirubin**, a yellowish component of bile, soon soar to pathological heights. Eventually the patient's skin and eyes will take on a yellowish tint, that excess bilirubin having been deposited in the body's superficial tissues. This condition called **jaundice** (from the French *jaune*, "yellow") is a visible sign of liver failure. By now the organ may be enlarged and unusually firm, owing to the inflammation and fibrosis brought about by the invading tumor cells. Under these circumstances an examining physician can readily palpate the liver's lower edge in the upper right quadrant of the abdomen, just below the rib cage.

Diagnostic imaging can often tell us whether hepatic symptoms are caused by metastatic cancer or by one of the many nonmalignant diseases which can affect the liver (e.g., cirrhosis, hepatitis, cysts). The same ultrasound equipment which gives us those familiar images of developing fetuses can be brought to bear on the troubled liver. Ultrasound is by far the fastest and cheapest exam; but while it readily distinguishes cysts from solid lesions, it cannot reveal tumors smaller than one centimeter in diameter. In the year 2000 a team of Scottish researchers reported that Doppler ultrasonography, a sophisticated technique for imaging blood flow, could detect small occult metastases by measuring "changes in liver blood flow."[46] As yet, however, this application has not been validated in American clinical practice. Since the 1980s the most trusted exam for liver imaging has been contrast-enhanced CAT. After administration of an intravenous contrast agent, CAT can routinely detect lesions as small as half a centimeter in diameter. Contrast-enhanced MRI has been regarded as more expensive and not necessarily more accurate, thought it may be preferred for some indications. PET (positron emission tomography), our most sensitive tool for detecting liver metastases, is not available at many American hospitals. Since PET is very expensive, it probably should be reserved for those cases in which a CAT scan has detected a suspicious lesion too small for convenient needle biopsy, but whose nature (benign or malignant) needs to be determined.[47] Two imaging techniques widely used in the 1970s find only a few applications today. A liver scan involves the injection of a mildly radioactive isotope, followed by radiographic imaging of the organ. Like a bone scan, a liver scan is relatively cheap and will reveal areas of abnormal activity, without positively distinguishing between benign disorders and malignancy. Angiography involves the injection of a contrast agent so that an X-ray picture of the liver's blood vessels can be taken. Sometimes angiography will point to the location of metastatic deposits; it may be helpful before a planned resection, since it provides the surgeon with detailed information on the individual patient's vascular anatomy.

Cytotoxic chemotherapy is the most plausible treatment for breast cancer which has metastasized to the liver. The regimen of choice would probably include Adriamycin (doxorubicin) and a taxoid drug. An outpatient regimen emphasizing Adriamycin and docetaxel achieved a 73% response rate in one study involving breast cancer patients with hepatic metastases.[48] Some recent experiments have used **regional perfusion techniques** for drug administration—the cytotoxic agents are infused directly into the hepatic artery or into the portal vein by means of an implantable pump or a subcutaneous catheter. The idea here is to achieve high drug concentrations in the liver while minimizing drug exposure to the rest of the body. Some oncologists argue that since both the hepatic artery and the portal vein supply the liver with blood, both should be accessed during chemotherapy so as to ensure that the drugs are uniformly diffused throughout the organ.[49]

Liver surgery has long been a risky business because the organ is so fragile and so vascular. Hemostasis (control of bleeding) can be difficult. The advent of contrast-enhanced CAT in the 1980s improved things a little, but not much. What often happened is that metastatic lesions which appeared to be resectable on the CAT scan proved to be inoperable at **laparotomy**—that is, during the operation in which the surgeon opened the abdomen and exposed the liver. Palpation and close visual inspection of the organ might reveal minute tumor nodules dispersed throughout, or tumor masses infiltrating or wrapped around the major blood vessels or bile ducts. Findings like these tend to extinguish our hopes for a successful resection. In the 1990s the selection of appropriate candidates for surgery improved greatly, thanks to the refinement of **laparoscopic techniques**. We could now visually inspect over two-thirds of the liver's surface area before laparotomy, simply by inserting a flexible fiber-optic tube through a small puncture made in the abdominal wall.[50]

These days all sorts of abdominal operations which formerly required open surgery are being done laparoscopically—gall bladder removals, hernia repairs, ovariectomies, splenectomies, you name it! Laparoscopic resections of benign hepatic lesions (e.g., cysts) are often possible, and laparoscopic biopsies of apparent hepatic malignancies are routine. But laparotomy is still preferred for the attempted resection of metastatic disease. In this circumstance surgeons want to palpate the liver, and they want to reduce its blood flow during resection by compressing the hepatic artery and the portal vein. Most importantly, they want an opportunity to roll an ultrasound transducer over the liver's exposed surface. Intraoperative ultrasonography can detect occult metastases within the liver, even those as small as three or four millimeters in diameter. And we now have increasingly effective tools to deal with multiple lesions in this size range. The surgeon Steven A. Curley of Houston's M. D. Anderson Cancer Center favors **radiofrequency ablation** (RFA) to destroy small hepatic metastases which are not accessible to the scalpel. This technique grew out of those electrocautery needles that surgeons apply to control intraoperative bleeding. The RFA needle used by Dr. Curley and his colleagues differs in that it has ten retractable tines in its tip. First the needle's tip is guided into a malignant lesion by ultrasound. Then the tines are expanded and the current turned on, heating as much as several cubic centimeters of tumor tissue to a lethal temperature (over 50 degrees centigrade). RFA is remarkably versatile in that it simultaneously accomplishes lesion ablation and hemostasis, and that it can be applied at multiple sites without unduly compromising liver function. Percutaneous RFA with ultrasound guidance—i.e., just inserting the needle through the skin—may be considered

for an accessible lesion on the liver's surface; however, Dr. Curley and his colleagues caution that laparotomy is indicated for multiple tumors, large tumors, or "tumors near major intrahepatic blood vessels."[51]

Other cancer surgeons have used **cryoablation** to destroy hepatic metastases. In this technique a slender probe placed into a malignant lesion releases liquid nitrogen to freeze it and a small area of surrounding tissue. Like RFA, cryoablation can sterilize numerous lesions during one operation. Both techniques are associated with a low rate of postoperative complications.[52] We should be hopeful that RFA or cryoablation, especially if combined with chemotherapy, will improve the survival times for patients with diffuse metastatic disease in the liver. Hitherto these times have been quite short.

The Central Nervous System

Metastatic dissemination to the brain or elsewhere in the central nervous system (CNS) is a late and exceedingly ominous event in the natural history of solid tumors. Carcinomas of the lung frequently metastasize to the brain, as do aggressive breast cancers and some melanomas. But even when a brain lesion derives from a sluggish colon cancer, the patient's life expectancy is apt to be short. We may surmise that any cancer cells which can penetrate and colonize the CNS are an undifferentiated and highly proliferative lot, because the brain, its covering membranes (the meninges), and the cerebrospinal fluid constitute the body's sanctuary site. The CNS does not receive lymphatic drainage from other organ systems; therefore metastatic dissemination can only occur hematogenously (through the blood). Yet the process by which a cancer cell leaves a blood vessel to implant in a target tissue—we call this **extravasation**—is surely more difficult in the brain than in the lungs or liver. Mother Nature did not want bacterial cells or large toxic molecules to obtain ready access to the brain; accordingly, she established the **blood-brain barrier**, whereby the junctions between the endothelial cells lining blood vessels and the surrounding connective tissues are much tighter—and therefore less permeable—than elsewhere in the body.

The earliest symptom of metastatic disease in the CNS is often a headache which—unlike the ordinary tension and migraine headaches—persists and intensifies over many successive days. Kristine A. Nelson and her colleagues at the Cleveland Clinic point out that "early morning headache upon awakening with resolution 20 to 30 minutes after arising suggests increased intracranial pressure."[53] Unrelieved intracranial pressure eventually leads to overt and distressing symptoms—dizziness, nausea, and vomiting. The neurological functions which will be lost are determined by the particular cranial or spinal nerves being compressed by metastatic tumor. Patients may have impaired speaking ability (aphasia) or experience various visual abnormalities (e.g., reduced field of vision, double vision, photophobia). If the cerebellum is affected, they may have difficulty walking or keeping their balance. The initial intellectual deficits may be subtle (e.g., memory loss or personality change); but without treatment they are apt to be succeeded by more dramatic phenomena (e.g., seizures).

Prompt diagnosis is essential if we hope to control the aforementioned symptoms. The tests we relied upon in the 1970s—radioisotope brain scans and cranial angiograms—tended to be uninformative. By the 1980s they had been largely supplanted by contrast-enhanced CAT scans, which could reveal the location of sizable metastases and of edematous (fluid-swollen)

areas as well as any displacement of the intracranial structures. The neurologist Carlos S. Kase reminds us that with CAT it became easy to distinguish hematogenous metastases to the brain from those tumors which originate there (e.g., benign meningiomas and malignant gliomas). Dr. Kase observes that metastases are commonly located in "the superficial, corticosubcortical portions of the hemispheres rather than the deep white-matter predominance of gliomas." Low-density areas on a CAT scan are "consistent with the prominent vasogenic edema that frequently surrounds metastatic tumors."[54] Unlike primary brain tumors, metastatic disease often presents as multiple lesions of various sizes scattered across the cerebral cortex. By the 1990s contrast-enhanced MRI had replaced CAT as the imaging modality of choice—it did a much better job of detecting small metastases. CAT was still used for those patients who had implanted pacemakers or other metallic prostheses (and thus could not be exposed to a magnetic field), as well as for those who could not remain motionless during the long MRI exam.[55]

Occasionally a Stage Four patient will suffer from rapidly progressive neurological symptoms, yet the CAT or MRI scan of the brain reveals nothing abnormal. Under these circumstances we should suspect a dire condition known as **meningeal carcinomatosis**, in which metastatic cancer cells are proliferating between the thin CNS membranes and spilling over into the cerebrospinal fluid. This finding has recently become more frequent in breast cancer patients who have undergone adjuvant chemotherapy. While the cytotoxic drugs may have killed malignant cells elsewhere in the body, they would seem to have had little or no effect on those cells sequestered in the meninges, a sanctuary site behind the blood-brain barrier. The diagnosis of meningeal carcinomatosis can often be confirmed by withdrawing a sample of cerebrospinal fluid and subjecting it to microscopic analysis—any malignant epithelial cells present would be easily recognized because they bear little resemblance to the white cells which are normally found in the fluid.[56] Intrathecal chemotherapy is the principal treatment for this complication: methotrexate and possibly other drugs would be delivered directly into the fluid. Radiotherapy plays a secondary role. The radiation oncologist Jay R. Harris and his colleagues point out that irradiation of the entire spinal column "is generally not recommended because it would involve more than 40% of the bone marrow."[57]

When dealing with the more common intracranial metastases, the aforementioned situation is reversed—irradiation is our main tool, especially in the case of radiosensitive tumors like breast cancer. The results from intravenous chemotherapy have usually been disappointing. Those bulky-molecule taxoid drugs paclitaxel and docetaxel, so effective against metastatic disease in the lungs and liver, are hardly able to transverse the blood-brain barrier. Irradiation works well in the brain because the cerebral neurons are more radioresistant than the invading cancer cells; they can tolerate doses of 5,000 rads or more without loss of function.[58] But the first task in managing symptomatic brain metastases is to control the elevated intracranial pressure by administering high-dose corticosteroids. Jane B. Alavi of the University of Pennsylvania observes that a large loading dose of intravenous dexamethasone (10 mg), followed by smaller maintenance doses by mouth (e.g., 4 mg every six hours), "reduces or eliminates the lethargy, headaches, visual blurring, and nausea caused by cerebral edema."[59] Dexamethasone therapy is continued while the patient undergoes irradiation, then tapered off afterwards. The dose and scheduling for **whole-brain radiotherapy**

have varied considerably. A frequent prescription calls for 3,000 rads in ten fractions (i.e., delivered over ten daily sessions). The treatments themselves are not painful, but all patients should be informed that alopecia (hair loss) and fatigue are predictable short-term side effects. Neurological deficits also may occur as a result of whole-brain radiotherapy, but usually not until a year or two afterwards. Nonetheless, some radiotherapists advise irradiating patients with longer life expectancies (over six months) on a more protracted schedule (with more fractions), a strategy which may possibly produce more durable responses and reduce the risk of subsequent deficits.[60]

Surgery is not employed as frequently for metastases to the brain as it is for primary brain tumors. Occasionally a **craniotomy** (incision in the skull) will be done to permit the resection of a single large metastasis which is causing troublesome symptoms. To destroy multiple metastases, we have been increasingly relying on a noninvasive technique called **stereotactic radiosurgery**. The patient's head is first immobilized in a stereotactic frame; then a contrast-enhanced CAT or MRI scan is performed so as to plot the precise location of the intracranial metastases, with an accuracy down to a millimeter or two. Narrow beams of radiation are now aimed at the metastases from several different angles. The upshot is that the tumor sites, where these beams intersect, will receive a high dose of radiation, while the surrounding normal tissues receive relatively little exposure. The painless treatment can sometimes be completed within an hour; the patient is observed briefly, then discharged. Boston's Joint Center for Radiation Therapy began to emphasize this technique in the late 1980s. Jay S. Loeffler and his Joint Center colleagues explain that "brain metastases are physically and biologically ideal to treat with radiosurgery," being "conveniently spherical, relatively small, and minimally invasive." Consequently "the entire extent of disease can be encompassed in the treatment field."[61]

Stereotactic radiosurgery for brain metastases has not been available at all American hospitals. This is unfortunate because it unquestionably helps to control symptoms and it may increase the survival times for some patients. In 1998 radiation oncologists at Heidelberg University (Germany) reported a median survival time of 15.4 months for cancer patients with brain metastases who received radiosurgery to destroy the detectable lesions, together the conventional whole-brain irradiation given to control subclinical disease.[62]

Paraneoplastic Syndromes

Metastatic progression in any one of the four vital organs we have discussed—skeleton, lungs, liver, brain—will eventually produce death. But cancer patients may actually be less likely to die from tumor growth in this or that organ than from those subtler systemic manifestations of malignancy which we call **paraneoplastic syndromes**. These syndromes bespeak metabolic processes gone haywire. Since they affect the entire body, they can be said to be above and beyond (Greek *para*, "beyond") the local destruction caused by tumors (neoplasms) in specific organs. We cannot "see" a paraneoplastic syndrome on a CAT or MRI scan in the same way that we might see a metastatic deposit. What we see are troublesome symptoms in patients, which are partially explained by laboratory blood workups revealing pathological elevations of certain hormones or other biologically active proteins. On a molecular level, various and sundry genes are being inappropriately expressed, much to the patient's detriment. Sometimes the culprit genes will be found in the increasingly

undifferentiated cancer cells; but they might also be traced to normal cells which have been spurred into misguided gene expression by encroaching malignancy.

Dozens of paraneoplastic syndromes have been described in the vast oncologic literature. Readers who wish to learn about all of them must be referred to a weighty textbook like the *Principles & Practice of Oncology*.[63] We have only space to discuss three common syndromes which are routinely associated with metastatic carcinomas. The first is **hypercalcemia**, a morbid excess of calcium in the blood. A generation ago oncologists believed that this pathological complication came about through tumor-related bone resorption and a concomitant release of calcium. These days we look at hypercalcemia not simply as a localized osteolytic event, but rather as a systemic syndrome caused by the ectopic (abnormal) production of parathyroid hormone-related protein and possibly of other substances (e.g., prostaglandins). We now know that this condition can occur even with malignancies which do not metastasize to the skeleton. But in tumors like breast cancer which tend toward osseous involvement, hypercalcemia is terribly frequent. Since it can give rise to life-threatening complications, its prompt diagnosis and treatment are highly advisable.

The earliest symptoms of hypercalcemia are nonspecific and may easily be mistaken for the side effects of chemotherapy or irradiation. Affected patients will typically experience fatigue, muscular weakness, and constipation as rising calcium levels begin to inhibit the function of neurons which activate both the voluntary skeletal muscles and the involuntary smooth muscles of the gastrointestinal tract. Soon the kidneys will be working overtime, vainly trying to remove the excess calcium from the blood and producing symptoms reminiscent of diabetes—e.g., polyuria (frequent urination) and polydipsia (excessive thirst). Nausea and vomiting follow, making matters a lot worse. Since patients now have difficulty consuming liquids, they quickly become dehydrated; and serum calcium levels soar to toxic concentrations. At this point patients will show signs of mental confusion; they will subsequently lapse into coma. Death is inevitable in untreated hypercalcemia; it typically occurs because of renal failure (the kidneys shut down) or cardiac arrhythmias (the heart muscle malfunctions due to decreased nerve-impulse conduction).[64]

Oncologists can make the diagnosis of hypercalcemia when serum (blood) calcium exceeds 11 mg/dl—that is, over eleven milligrams calcium per tenth of a liter. Readings over 14 mg/dl are regarded as severely elevated. Breast cancer patients who have mild elevations and no nausea may just be advised to drink plenty of fluids, to avoid calcium-rich foods or supplements, and to stay physically active (bed rest promotes bone resorption and constipation). At the other extreme, a patient suffering from mental confusion, vomiting, and oliguria (diminished urine output) represents an oncologic crisis—she would have to be hospitalized and given intravenous hydration. Except for patients who should not be exposed to sodium (e.g., those with congestive heart failure), saline is the preferred fluid for hydration. The sodium helps the kidneys to excrete calcium. Raymond P. Warrell, Jr., of the Cornell University Medical College cautions that "few hospitalized patients actually achieve normocalcemia with hydration alone. For acute emergencies, the combination of short-course high-dose calcitonin plus a potent antiresorptive drug (gallium nitrate, pamidronate, or alendronate) is recommended."[65] These strategies usually prove effective in the short-term management of severe hypercalcemia; of course, so long as an affected patient's tumor burden remains high, this condition can easily recur.

Anorexia is an inevitable paraneoplastic syndrome in advanced metastatic cancer. The term designates a loss of appetite (from the Greek *an*, "without," and *orexis*, "appetite"). Affected patients do not want to eat; and when they do, they are apt to suffer from early satiety—that is, they feel satisfied after several mouthfuls, a situation which alarms family members. The profound anorexia of cancer can have diverse causes. A few patients will be found to have tumor-associated obstructions in the gastrointestinal tract; others will be suffering from aftereffects of treatment, which can be psychological (e.g., mental depression) as well as physiological. But in any patient with a large tumor burden, we must also suspect that the metastatic cancer cells are stimulating the release of unspecified humoral factors which act to inhibit the appetite.

While not an acute crisis, anorexia is ultimately life-threatening. Malnutrition and loss of weight substantially contribute to cancer mortality. Fortunately, we have several drugs which can be used to combat anorexia. Corticosteroids, especially dexamethasone, have frequently been given to anorectic patients, who then experienced a sense of well-being, improved appetite, and some weight gain. The drawbacks are that ever-larger doses of steroids will be required to maintain appetite stimulation and that their long-term use will result in troublesome side effects, including fluid retention, hyperglycemia (too much sugar in the blood), and an unacceptable suppression of the immune system. During the 1990s American oncologists increasingly prescribed **Megace** (brand name for **megestrol acetate**) for appetite stimulation and weight gain in advanced cancer. This synthetic progestin had few side effects beyond occasional nausea and a slightly enhanced risk of thromboembolic complications (blood vessel clots). A dose of

800 milligrams daily was thought to provide the maximum benefit; the drug could be taken either in the familiar tablets (40 mg each) or in a new liquid formulation. Charles L. Loprinzi and his colleagues at the Mayo Clinic (Rochester, Minnesota) conducted a clinical trial in which 317 anorectic cancer patients were randomly assigned to receive dexamethasone or megestrol acetate. The trial's results, published in 1999, indicated that the two drugs had "similar appetite stimulating efficacy," though megestrol acetate seemed to have "a slight edge in nonfluid weight gain." Dexamethasone was a better choice from a financial standpoint, the dose used in this trial costing about $0.60 per day compared to $10.25 per day for megestrol acetate in the liquid formulation. Dr. Loprinzi and his colleagues concluded that while dexamethasone might be appropriate for short-term treatment ("days to a couple of weeks"), megestrol acetate should be preferred for longer therapy because of "better patient acceptance" and "fewer corticosteroid-type toxicities."[66]

Cachexia is the Great Sphinx of paraneoplastic syndromes. The term denotes a "bad condition" (from the Greek *kachexia*); in cancer medicine it is applied to the puzzling wasting which afflicts terminal patients. Anorexia and cachexia are discussed together in textbooks and may be hard to distinguish clinically, yet the latter condition is far more complicated than a failure of appetite or an inadequate caloric intake. Cachexia represents a profound derangement of the body's metabolism. When a caloric restriction is imposed on normal individuals, they principally lose weight from adipose (fatty) tissue. Cachectic weight loss occurs most prominently from muscular tissue. Moreover, this loss continues even when affected patients are given supplemental nutrition; it is irreversible. Giovanni Mantovani and other oncologists at the University of Cagliari in Italy list a host of metabolic abnormalities associated with cancer cachexia, including "catabolism of skeletal muscle, decreased protein synthesis, insulin resistance, and enhanced lipid mobilization." This complex syndrome is always a late development, indicative of established metastatic disease and a large tumor burden. Dr. Mantovani and his colleagues suggest that the humoral factors inducing cachexia might be "a set of cytokines that work in concert."[67] Cytokines are those extremely potent molecules—for example, the interferons and interleukins—which our immune cells release in response to bacterial or viral infections or to other major challenges to the body's integrity. In laboratory experiments with cachectic mice, the administration of monoclonal antibodies which interfere with specific cytokines has sometimes slowed the loss of body weight. As yet we have no comparable therapies for human cachexia.

Who Dares to Say "Terminal"?

Cancer physicians, surgeons and oncologists alike, have long used the adjective *terminal* to designate patients with advanced systemic disease who could be expected to die within six months. Terminal patients are not candidates for further therapeutic interventions, either pharmaceutical or surgical. Indeed, these patients are deemed "terminal" only because we do not have any practical therapy for them—at least no therapy which would be likely to extend their life expectancies. The dire prognostic features which warrant the use of this term vary from one type of malignancy to the next, and even from patient to patient. With breast malignancies, the word has come to be synonymous with drug resistance. Although multiple cytotoxic regimens have been given, we have radiological portraits of progressive, ever-growing metastases which are affecting one or more (usually several) vital organs. The patient's overall physical condition also figures in terminal equations—intractable anorexia and cachectic weight loss are outward symptoms which run parallel to the distressing radiological findings. All manner of irremediable complications can now ensue. Day by day the terminal patient will grow weaker and more dependent on others to fulfill his or her basic needs; the will to live is gradually replaced by a sense of resignation. It is not always possible to predict exactly when a terminal patient will die, and predicting the cause and manner of death is much more problematic. We do know that a sufficiently large tumor burden will lethally derange the body's metabolism, even when vital organs are spared from overt destruction. One postmortem of patients who died from metastatic breast cancer found that a surprising 24% actually died from infections, a fact which points to a concomitant suppression of the immune system. Other causes discovered in this study included respiratory insufficiency (26%), hepatic failure (14%), central nervous system dysfunction (9%), hypercalcemia (3%), and cardiovascular disease or hemorrhaging (24%).[68]

Telling a patient that the available therapeutic options have been exhausted and that he or she has only a few weeks or months left to live is never easy. Of late, those ubiquitous articles in oncology journals purporting to set guidelines for this consultation have counseled semantic delicacy—*whatever you say, don't use that T-word!* The reason, usually unstated in print, is that this particular word can provoke strong, even explosive emotional reactions—sometimes from the patient, but just as frequently from distraught family members. Most laypersons do not comprehend the woeful inadequacy of our present therapeutic tools when applied

to metastatic solid tumors. For their part, oncologists are reluctant either to concede the failure of all those unpleasant regimens or to say something which would destroy a patient's remaining hope. Gentle evasions have thus become *de rigueur*. Dexamethasone is prescribed, without comment, for cerebral edema or involuntary weight loss. The family members applaud because the patient no longer has those terrible headaches, feels much better, and is eating more. Corticosteroid pills usually mark the boundary between therapeutic interventions and purely palliative measures, but laypersons cannot be expected to know this.

Experienced physicians in any specialty are careful in what they say to their patients. The information imparted must be tailored to fit what the individual patient is emotionally ready to accept and what he or she is capable of understanding. Notwithstanding this truism, evasiveness should be avoided in cancer medicine. Most children over the age of ten can comprehend the concept of mortality; and once past the age of thirty, most adults can name a growing list of relatives, friends, and acquaintances who have died from cancer. If that traditional time frame is extended slightly beyond six months, there would be no one alive who would not be "terminal." The dissolution of the body is God's law and Nature's necessity. And all medicine must ultimately be viewed as palliative. Oncology differs from the more joyous specialties in that its most obvious role is palliation, the relief of suffering in patients who cannot be cured.

For the year 2000 the American Cancer Society forecast that 552,200 Americans would die from cancer, "more than 1,500 people a day."[69] Even greater numbers die from heart attacks and strokes, or from Alzheimer's disease and other forms of senile dementia. Unlike heart attack and stroke victims, most terminal cancer patients will know several months in advance that they are going to die; and unlike Alzheimer's sufferers, they will fully understand their situation. The advance warning gives them time to put their affairs in order and to make their peace with God and their neighbor. Unfortunately, it also gives them plenty of time to worry about some important questions which have not been addressed in their previous consultations with physicians. Will the terminal stages of disease be painful and, if so, how will that pain be controlled? Will dying be difficult? How can I maintain my dignity during a debilitating illness which will eventually render me helpless and dependent?

The Control of Pain

George Crile, Jr., that doughty fighter against the cancerphobia of the 1950s, argued that our fears of painful cancer deaths were grossly exaggerated. "Most patients with terminal cancer do not complain of excessive pain," he wrote in 1973. "Terminal cancer, like old age, gives its own analgesia."[70] It is tempting to dismiss these sentiments as preposterous baloney that only a famous Harvard-educated M.D. (such as Crile was) could make without being laughed out of court. But we must concede an element of truth in Crile's observations. Paraneoplastic syndromes sometimes kill patients in a painless fashion. Once the nausea and vomiting are past, hypercalcemia allows patients to slip into a peaceful coma. The lethal wasting of anorexia and cachexia, so distressing to family members, is not at all painful to patients. Unfortunately, there seem to be many more ways in which metastatic tumors can cause pain than in which they produce anesthesia. Breast cancer patients with osseous metastases typically suffer moderate to severe bone pain, which may intensify

with disease progression. Whenever tumor masses start to compress individual nerves or to infiltrate nerve plexuses, pain is sure to ensue. Whenever disseminated cancer cells obstruct a blood vessel, a lymphatic channel, a bronchial branch, or a segment of intestine, pain is a probable byproduct. The labored breathing brought about by lung involvement is terrifying, giving rise to psychological distress as well as considerable physical discomfort. The inflammation and edema which may accompany any malignant infiltration of soft tissues can contribute both to localized pain and to systemic malaise.

The relevant truism about pain from metastatic carcinomas is the same as the truism about the behavior of these entities generally—**every case is different**. Some patients may have little or no pain, while others may suffer from such severe pain that only the most sophisticated interventions can bring relief. Since we cannot predict how much pain individual patients will suffer during the terminal phase of their illness, we should be prepared for every contingency. During the 1980s and 1990s this preparedness took center stage as the large cancer hospitals established pain management services, and more and more doctors and nurses began to school themselves in palliative techniques. The neurologist Kathleen Foley has long been involved with pain management at New York's Memorial Sloan-Kettering Cancer Center. Dr. Foley has estimated that "two thirds of patients with advanced disease have significant pain."[71] Her assessment is more realistic than Dr. Crile's. We should therefore anticipate that most terminal patients will eventually need **analgesics**—that is, drugs whose purpose is simply to suppress pain (from the Greek *an*, "without," and *algos*, "pain"). Analgesics can be divided into two main categories, the milder **nonopioid drugs** (like aspirin) and the stronger **opioid drugs** (like morphine).

Our medicine chest also contains assorted **adjuvant agents**. When pain management specialists use that word "adjuvant," they mean a drug which is not primarily an analgesic but which nonetheless lessens the patient's perception of pain. Adjuvants are extremely useful because they enable us to use lower doses of analgesics. At higher doses any analgesic, whether aspirin or morphine, can produce serious side effects. Modern palliative regimens consequently tend to combine an analgesic with one or more adjuvants. **Pamidronate**, the intravenous bisphosphonate, qualifies as an adjuvant because it may reduce the pain of osseous metastases. Corticosteroids like **dexamethasone**, **prednisolone**, and **prednisone** are often employed as adjuvants because they reduce edema and inflammation. Sedatives like **Valium** (brand name for **diazepam**) or **lorazepam** also figure largely in palliative cocktails, since they raise a patient's pain threshold. Under certain circumstances the attending oncologist may have recourse to the psychiatrist's armamentarium. Antidepressant drugs like **amitriptyline** can help to alleviate such neurological phenomena as burning sensations or skin hypersensitivity. Antipsychotic drugs like **haloperidol** can help to combat agitation, nausea, and the hiccups.[72]

The WHO Analgesic Ladder

In 1986 the World Health Organization (WHO) issued educational guidelines for the pharmaceutical management of cancer pain. WHO took the position that almost all patients could have adequate pain relief if healthcare professionals throughout the world would "learn how to use a few effective and relatively inexpensive drugs," which could be given "by mouth, on a regular basis."[73] These guidelines were embodied in a three-step plan known as the **WHO Analgesic Ladder**. This "ladder" has been widely cited; while it is short on specific instructions, it does give us a good framework to discuss the basics of cancer pain control.

The first rung on the ladder deals with **mild pain**, for which nonopioid analgesics should be given together with any adjuvants deemed appropriate. These analgesics tend to be familiar over-the-counter products like aspirin, acetaminophen (Tylenol), ibuprofen, or naproxen. They may also be referred to as **nonsteroidal anti-inflammatory drugs** or **NSAIDs**; they have virtually no side effects at low dose levels. Of course, when they are "prescribed" for cancer pain, the oncologist may recommend doses considerably above those indicated on the bottle labels. Laypersons may not fully appreciate that there are subtle differences between the biological effects of different NSAIDs, and that different individuals may fare better on one drug than on another. Naproxen works well against the pain caused by osseous inflammation. So does aspirin, but large doses of this NSAID can cause gastric irritation and the inhibition of blood clotting. The versatile acetaminophen (which is not technically a NSAID) avoids these particular problems, but then it has little anti-inflammatory action and may prove toxic to persons with liver disease. A common limitation of nonopioid drugs is that they have a "low ceiling"—that is to say, after a certain dose level is reached, giving a still larger dose will not provide additional pain relief.[74]

Moderate pain unrelieved by NSAIDs constitutes the second rung on the WHO ladder. At this stage we would add a low-dose opioid drug to the analgesic cocktail. These agents are also referred to as **opioid agonists**. They act directly on the central nervous system, producing analgesia by binding to and stimulating opioid receptors expressed by neurons in the brain and spinal cord. It is important to continue the NSAID prescribed on the ladder's first rung if the patient has skeletal metastases. Because the pain from osseous disease typically has an inflammatory component, it usually requires a NSAID or a corticosteroid as well as the opioid agonist for adequate relief.[75] Codeine, a weak opioid commonly prescribed after tooth extractions and minor surgeries, may not be the best choice for cancer patients; with long-term use it has a high incidence of constipation. Most American oncologists prefer **oxycodone** for moderate cancer pain. This drug binds to cellular opioid receptors just as avidly as morphine—and it is therefore as potent as morphine—yet its name carries no negative "narcotic associations" which might alarm laypersons. Those convenient tablets combining oxycodone and acetaminophen are available generically as well as under the brand name **Percocet**.

In the United States the drug of choice for **severe pain**, the third rung of the WHO ladder, continues to be **morphine**. This analgesic is potent and fast-acting, and it has no ceiling. Raising the dose always provides additional pain relief. Other opioid agonists frequently used in American palliative medicine (e.g., fentanyl, hydromorphone, and oxycodone) share these characteristics; the perceived advantage of morphine has more to do with convenience and familiarity. <u>Distributed under many brand names, this drug comes in a formulation to suit every purpose</u>. There are immediate-release morphine tablets and capsules (15 or 30 mg); twelve-hour sustained-released tablets (15, 30, 60, 100, 200 mg) and capsules (20, 50, 100 mg); liquid solutions for patients who have difficulty swallowing pills; injectable solutions for intravenous or intramuscular administration; and rectal suppositories.[76] Morphine's analgesic action and its side effects are fairly predictable, so that oncologists have little trouble adjusting the dose upwards (a frequent necessity when the drug is given for terminal cancer). Dose increases tend to intensify the side effects, but these usually remain manageable. When morphine is given initially, or whenever the dosage is increased, patients may experience mild nausea and considerable drowsiness; these effects typically vanish within a day or two. Unfortunately, tolerance does not develop to those gastrointestinal effects mediated by the drug's action on the autonomic nervous system. Patients taking morphine inevitably experience decreased gastric secretions and reduced peristalsis (less intestinal motility). They are thus powerfully disposed to constipation, to dry stools, and eventually to fecal impaction. A daily laxative regimen should therefore be commenced along with the drug. A stool-softener like Colace (brand name for docusate sodium) and an osmotic laxative like Phillips' Milk of Magnesia (brand name for magnesium hydroxide) may forestall the need for stronger measures.[77] The risk of overdose is relatively small with morphine because the drug tends to induce the desired analgesia long before it produces sedation (unconsciousness) or respiratory depression (slow, irregular breathing). Should either of these potentially life-threatening conditions be observed, the patient can be rescued by **naloxone**, an antagonist drug which binds to opioid receptors but does not stimulate them.

Around-the-Clock Dosing

Terminal cancer patients experiencing pain unrelieved by Percocet-type combinations (rung two on the WHO ladder) are often reluctant to request stronger doses of opioids (rung three on the ladder). Many patients believe that they should "save the powerful drugs for when they really need them"—viz., for the intense pain that may occasionally develop during the last few days of life. In reality, pain control is much easier if it is established early during the illness and maintained throughout. Patients need to remember that while tolerance to opioid drugs does occur, it can be overcome by adjusting the dose upward. Declan Walsh, a pain management specialist at the Cleveland Clinic, points out that the old practice of giving analgesics "reactively"—i.e., only after the patient has experienced severe pain—is now discredited: "The preferred approach is small doses of analgesic administered on a fixed around-the-clock schedule to prevent pain." Dr. Walsh cautions that misconceptions about opioid analgesics abound among pharmacists as well as among laypersons. He recommends that a family member, "preferably a caretaker," be present at the initial consultation on pain control, "so that questions can be answered and anxieties reduced." Any prescription given by the oncologist "must be supplemented by specific detailed written instructions about analgesic dose, timing, and side effects."[78]

In American practice the initial prescription for severe cancer pain usually calls for immediate-release morphine tablets. Particularly in the generic product ("morphine sulfate"), they can be inexpensive, providing most patients with relief for a dollar or two each day. Patients may be surprised when their pharmacist hands them two different bottles—for example, one containing 30 mg tablets and another with 15 mg tablets. This is not an error, but it does require an explanation. Pain control is best maintained when the amount of the drug in the bloodstream reaches a certain appropriate level and stays at that level. Pharmacologists refer to this desired level as the "steady state." With a view to maintaining steady-state effectiveness, modern palliative practice calls for analgesics to be given in **around-the-clock dosing** (ATC dosing). That's what

the 30 mg tablets are for—a patient would typically take one tablet every four hours, punctually, regardless of whether he or she perceived significant pain. The daily ATC dose would thus be six tablets (180 mg). The constant level of morphine thereby obtained in the bloodstream ought to keep the patient pain-free most of the time, especially during sleep.

But that regular ATC dose may need to be supplemented. While immediate-release morphine tablets can produce analgesia within thirty minutes, the drug's half-life is limited. Its pain-killing action starts to wane somewhere between two and four hours after oral administration. When a cancer patient experiences renewed pain an hour or two before the next scheduled ATC dose, we speak of **end-of-dose failure**. If a patient on ATC dosing should experience sudden pain brought on by physical activity (e.g., doing housework), we would employ the term **breakthrough pain**. Unfortunately, both end-of-dose failure and breakthrough pain are common occurrences. To alleviate them, patients taking opioid analgesics are given a second prescription for a **rescue dose**—that is, for a smaller dose of the drug which could be taken supplementally whenever the ATC dose fails to maintain pain control. Declan Walsh advises that the rescue dose may be "calculated as 25% to 50% of the four-hourly ATC dose."[79] Of course, that aforementioned bottle of 15 mg morphine tablets was intended as the rescue dose, which might also have been called the **PRN dose** (from the Latin *pro re nata*, "as needed"). The important thing to remember about rescue (PRN) doses is that they are not to be taken on a fixed ATC schedule, but only when needed because of recurrent pain, and then usually no more than one rescue dose in each ATC dosing interval. For example, a patient taking a 30 mg morphine tablet at 2:00 PM might be directed to take a 15 mg tablet sometime between 4:00 PM and 6:00 PM (during the last two hours of the ATC dosing interval), if he or she experienced end-of-dose failure.

Once pain control has been established using immediate-release formulations, those patients who find the four-hour dosing intervals bothersome have the option of switching to sustained-release capsules or tablets. Michael H. Levy of Philadelphia's Fox Chase Cancer Center observes that with sustained-release formulations of morphine or oxycodone, "relief should begin in one hour, peak in two to three hours, and last for twelve hours." While the ATC dosing interval has been extended from four to twelve hours, rescue dosing still runs on the traditional four-hour interval. The PRN prescription would typically call for a fast-acting liquid or tablet formulation at about one-third the strength of the twelve-hour ATC dose. By way of illustration, Dr. Levy suggests that a patient taking 90 mg of sustained-release morphine as the ATC dose "should be given 30 mg of immediate-release morphine every four hours for unrelieved breakthrough pain."[80] Patients should be aware that brand-name sustained-release capsules and tablets tend to be considerably more expensive than generic immediate-release tablets. And it is essential that they know that the long-acting pills must be swallowed whole—the tablets should not be chewed or crushed, nor should the capsules be broken open and the contents mixed with food. Such practices may cause excessively rapid drug absorption and result in an overdose.[81]

Regardless of the formulation used or the dosing schedule selected, analgesia with morphine or other opioid agonists usually requires periodic dose increases because of drug tolerance or disease progression. We refer to the process by which the new dose level is determined as **titration** (from the French *titre*, "a standard"). Declan Walsh advises that the ATC dose and the rescue dose should be considered "simultaneously but separately."[82] If the patient reports numerous episodes of end-of-dose failure, the ATC dose needs to be titrated upwards. If he or she reports breakthrough pain unrelieved by the rescue prescription, then that PRN dose should be increased. In most titrations, however, both the ATC dose and the PRN dose will be increased. Since we have no laboratory tests to measure a cancer patient's perception of pain or an analgesic's effectiveness in a particular individual, the golden rules for the prescribing physician could not be clearer: **pain is what the patient says it is—a drug's effectiveness is what the patient says it is**. The doses necessary for satisfactory analgesia can vary tremendously. Michael H. Levy reminds us that "although pain can be controlled in most patients with 240 mg of oral morphine per day or less, patients with severe cancer pain may require 1,200 to 1,800 mg per day."[83]

Switching Drugs and Routes

Ideally, terminal cancer patients would be maintained on the same oral formulation of the same opioid analgesic throughout the course of their illness. But when faced with persistent side effects, oncologists will try another drug. **Oxycodone** is the most obvious alternative to morphine. Dr. Walsh and his Cleveland Clinic colleagues suspect that oxycodone "may cause less gastrointestinal disturbance than morphine" and thus be more suitable for "frail elderly patients."[84] But when American oncologists want a strong concentrated opioid, they usually think of **hydromorphone**, now available generically as well as under the brand name **Dilaudid**. Dr. Levy observes that hydromorphone is "six times as soluble in aqueous solutions as morphine and four times as potent, allowing for smaller injection or infusion volumes."[85] This drug is often given intravenously to patients in severe pain who need immediate relief.

Naturally we want to maintain the oral administration of drugs for as long as possible, because it is so much simpler and cheaper than injections and infusions. A few patients who could not swallow morphine tablets have still been managed via the oral route, by virtue of sublingual wafers. Placed in the mouth, the drug-impregnated wafers dissolve, and enough of the released morphine gets swallowed to produce analgesia.[86] But morphine and most other opioids are not really suited for sublingual (under the tongue) or buccal (in the cheek) administration, because they are not sufficiently lipophilic for good absorption by the oral mucosa. In the year 2000 pain management specialists looked optimistically to a new product called **Actiq** (brand name), which delivered **fentanyl**—a potent and highly lipophilic opioid—via buccal absorption. Actiq resembles a little lollipop on a plastic stick; the patient places the pleasant-tasting wafer (lollipop end) between the gum and cheek, and then sucks gently to release the fentanyl.[87] A transdermal fentanyl system has been marketed under the brand name **Duragesic**. In this case the patient simply affixes a drug-impregnated adhesive patch to a relatively hairless area of skin. The fentanyl is first absorbed by the subcutaneous fat, then gradually released into the bloodstream. Although a fentanyl patch may initially take twelve hours to produce analgesia, it will continue working for up to three days. After this time it must be removed and a new patch applied. The dose of fentanyl delivered can be controlled by the number and the size of the patches used—larger ones contain more of the drug.[88] The Duragesic system can serve as around-the-clock dosing for patients who cannot remember to take their morphine tablets on time. Actiq is intended as a rescue dose; it can be used either in conjunction with the fentanyl patches, or simply to provide convenient PRN analgesia for a bedridden patient who has difficulty swallowing pills. The Duragesic patches and Actiq "lollipops" are much more expensive than morphine or oxycodone tablets, but then they are less costly and less time-consuming than arranging an infusion every time a forgetful or incapacitated patient needs pain control.

Intelligent, highly motivated patients who are alert and ambulatory, but who have constant pain from sluggish visceral metastases, are the most appropriate candidates for **portable infusion pumps**. A variety of these devices were brought on the market in the 1980s and 1990s. Most are small and light enough to be worn under loosely-fitting clothing. In essence, an infusion device consists of a drug reservoir (usually filled with space-saving hydromorphone) and a battery-operated pump which delivers the analgesic into the bloodstream through an indwelling catheter. The newer models can be electronically programmed so that the pump automatically delivers a fixed ATC dose at preset intervals, while the patient can push a button for smaller rescue doses PRN. Normally that rescue button will have a physician-ordered "lockout time," meaning that it can be operated only once in a given interval (e.g., once every thirty minutes). This feature is intended as a safeguard against accidental overdoses. But since patients actually order their own rescue infusions, the medical literature discussing these pumps comes under the heading of **patient-controlled analgesia** (PCA). The main advantage of PCA pumps is that they instantaneously deliver a potent painkiller through a faster and more efficient route than oral administration—patients can get relief within a minute or two. The disadvantages include a considerable expense and inconvenience as well as the necessity of educating patients about their proper use. When PCA is used in an outpatient setting, the ever-present risks of infection or obstruction involving the indwelling catheter, or of a malfunction involving the pump itself, mandate that patients not wander too far away from qualified medical assistance.[89]

Stopping Intractable Pain

The vast majority of terminal cancer patients with increasing pain can obtain adequate relief from the upward titration of a single opioid drug and the judicious use of several familiar adjuvants (e.g., naproxen, dexamethasone, Valium). Only an occasional patient will have pain which is refractory to the convenient pharmaceutical regimens. That exceptional case warrants consultation with a skilled neurosurgeon. The surgical remedies for intractable pain can be effective, but they are tricky and risky, requiring the most precise knowledge of the nervous system. What the surgeon must do is to sever or otherwise disable the sensory nerve fibers relaying painful sensations to the brain. At the same time the nearby motor fibers which activate muscles must be preserved, lest the patient suffer unwanted paralysis. A relatively safe procedure which might be used in advanced breast cancer is called **dorsal rhizotomy**. In this instance the surgeon severs the sensory branch of a spinal nerve at its root (Greek *rhiza*, "root"), just as it emerges from the spinal cord. Kathleen Foley observes that "in patients with chest wall pain from tumor invasion, improved analgesia in 50% to 80% has been reported with dorsal rhizotomy."[90] **Nerve blocks** are less invasive; they can be accomplished by injecting a neurolytic agent like alcohol or phenol into the relevant plexus—that is, into

the cluster of nerves principally involved with the transmission of pain. Blockade of the celiac plexus in the upper abdomen has been a boon to patients suffering from end-stage pancreatic cancer, with success rates approaching 90%.[91] Nathan I. Cherny, a cancer pain specialist in Jerusalem, advises that celiac plexus blockade may also be useful against pain arising from "neoplastic infiltration of the liver, gall bladder, and proximal small bowel."[92]

Spinal opioids represent a last-ditch pharmaceutical alternative to rhizotomies and nerve blocks. While the risk of motor nerve damage is reduced, the spinal administration of analgesics involves more hazards than any other route; consultation with a neurosurgeon remains advisable. The spinal route is characterized by the placement of the catheter which delivers the drugs. **Epidural analgesia** means that the catheter is positioned outside of the tough protective membrane (the *dura*) covering the spinal cord. The epidural administration of opioids may be considered either for short-term or for long-term analgesia; it can mute cancer pain originating from multiple sites. Dr. Foley points out that epidural analgesia has fewer systemic side effects, since it "minimizes distribution of drugs to the brain stem and cerebral hemispheres" while "suppressing noxious stimuli at the spinal cord level."[93] When a patient suffering from intractable pain is already receiving substantial oral or intravenous opioids, epidural catheterization may be used to deliver a potent local anesthetic like **bupivacaine** rather than additional opioids. In this instance the goal is to anesthetize the sensory branches of the relevant spinal nerves.[94] **Intrathecal analgesia** involves putting the catheter underneath the dura; it carries the greatest risk of complications, but it is marvelously efficient. Because the infused opioid goes directly into the cerebrospinal fluid, a very low dose will suffice to produce analgesia. Only a very few patients are candidates for long-term spinal opioids; and most of them can now be managed on an outpatient basis, thanks to the recent development of implantable infusion pumps like the Infusaid and SynchroMed systems (brand names). These devices are considerably smaller than the PCA pumps which are worn underneath clothing. Typically, a surgeon inserts the miniaturized pump beneath the skin of the abdomen, while extending a subcutaneous catheter around the patient's flank to reach an epidural or intrathecal access site. Patients can take baths and perform other light activities while fitted with these implantable devices, but cost is a major drawback. Since the surgeon's bill is added to the little pump's hefty price tag, outpatient spinal analgesia involves an initial expense of $10,000 or more. Appropriate candidates for it must be ambulatory and psychologically stable, have severe pain poorly managed by the oral or intravenous routes, and at the same time have an estimated life expectancy of several months.[95]

SOCIETAL CONSTRAINTS
Why Pain Control Is So Hard

The pharmaceutical management of cancer pain is easier in some cases than in others. Some patients do not need opioids, and a few who do may remain pain-free on the same regimen throughout the course of their illness. More often, however, cancer pain will prove to be a moving target. The type of pain, the level of pain, and the response to analgesics can change from day to day, requiring considerable tinkering with drug combinations, doses, and the schedules and routes of administration. It is mandatory that the prescribing oncologists be thoroughly schooled in a wide variety of palliative agents and in the possible interactions between these agents. It is equally important that they be constantly available for consultation with patients, yet this requirement has yet to be legislated in any country. Pain control can be time-consuming and labor-intensive; unfortunately, the physician who has the authority to alter the previously prescribed drugs and dose levels may not be present at the precise moment when a patient urgently needs help.

The aforementioned circumstances are inherent and universal—they contribute to the suffering of terminal cancer patients in every nation of the world. In the United States these difficulties are compounded by popular prejudices about opioid agonist drugs and by governmental restrictions on their distribution and use. The word *narcotic* evokes terrible connotations for laypersons. Many cancer patients worry about becoming "addicted," without realizing that the type of drug dependence which develops among persons who consume opiates illegally does not occur among the terminally ill who need them for pain control. **Addiction** is as much a psychological phenomenon as a physiological one. It is born of an economic or intellectual impoverishment which leads naive young persons to consume drugs to achieve a chemical euphoria ("a high") when they are denied emotional and spiritual satisfactions. Addicts will engage in criminal activity or in other self-destructive behavior to support their habit. Cancer patients are usually much older and much wiser; when they take opiates for severe pain, they do not experience euphoria, simply analgesia. The two characteristics which principally define addiction in our society—psychological dependence and asocial behavior—do not develop.

There are neither words nor statistics to convey the extent of illegal drug consumption in the United States, or to depict the havoc that this consumption wreaks on the fabric of American life. In 1999 *Time* magazine reported that one of every ten adults in Baltimore was "a drug addict."[96] Perhaps this estimate is exaggerated, yet its accuracy is a moot point. True or not, the report speaks volumes about prevalent societal trends which make opioid analgesia unnecessarily difficult. Hospital pharmacies do stock the pertinent agents; but these days many of them operate behind locked doors, while closed-circuit TV cameras keep the premises under constant surveillance. Commercial pharmacies in some urban neighborhoods do not carry any opioid analgesics stronger than Percocet-type combinations, out of fear of robbery attempts. In New York, California, Texas, and several other states, physicians have been required to write narcotic prescriptions on special multiple-copy forms, with one copy being forwarded to the state drug-enforcement agency. Minor errors on these forms or even a seemingly excessive number of prescriptions have been known to prompt embarrassing investigations.[97]

American oncologists look with envy toward England, a country where opioid analgesia for cancer pain is accepted as a matter of course and largely unfettered by governmental regulations. Many English oncologists regard **diamorphine** as the opiate of choice because it is more soluble than morphine and seems to cause less nausea.[98] This highly effective agent is not available in American pharmacies, though it has been openly hawked on street corners throughout the land. The common name for it is **heroin**. Oncologists in Canada and continental Europe sometimes sing the praises of **methadone**, a wondrously cheap and long-acting analgesic. While this opiate is available in the United States, it has never recovered from the stigma attached to it from its use in heroin detoxification programs. Mark A. O'Rourke and other oncologists

practicing in Greenville, South Carolina, have complained that in their state "the prescribing physician must write a letter to the Department of Health and Environmental Control for each patient starting and stopping methadone." Access to methadone should be increased, Dr. O'Rourke and his colleagues urge, for the sake of "patients with anguish over the cost of pain relief." They point out that daily analgesia with methadone costs about fifty cents, while equivalent treatment with sustained-release morphine formulations can cost three dollars or more.[99]

The average American is blissfully ignorant of the subtle ways in which state and federal regulations affecting the distribution of opiates can interfere with pain control for cancer patients. Most people find out about this problem the hard way, when they must watch a friend or family member suffer needlessly. The syndicated columnist Mona Charen has written forcefully about her mother, who "ran into trouble" during several hospitalizations for cancer-related complications. "The nurses, even on the cancer ward, were shockingly, almost sadistically stingy with pain injections," recalls Ms. Charen. "I used to have to raise my voice to get them to respond to my mother's calls. And when they did respond, it was only after dilatory tactics like reviewing the chart, calling the doctor, and checking on a few other things. While we waited, my blood would boil, because pain is like a locomotive. It is relatively easy to arrest when it first gets going, but once it builds momentum, it becomes extremely hard to stop."[100]

One solution to the tragic and all-too-common situation described by Ms. Charen would be to train more nurses in the varied techniques of pain management and to give certain nurses, those with special and undeniable credentials, considerably more authority in dispensing opioid analgesics. A fledgling organization of service providers called the

American Society of Pain Management Nurses would seem to represent a large step in the right direction.

Doctors at the Deathbed:
Is There "A Right to Die"?

Lewis Thomas, the physician and essayist, has given us a memorable anecdote. In the early 1950s Dr. Thomas attended an awards banquet somewhere in Mississippi, at which the guest of honor, a general practitioner, rushed out in the middle of the ceremony because one of his longtime patients had just died. That small-town doctor felt an overwhelming obligation to be with his patient's family at that particular moment, even if it meant walking out on a medical society convened in his honor.[101] This anecdote takes us back to simpler times, before the era of CAT scans and molecular biology, when American doctors made house calls equipped with little more than a black bag and a stethoscope. The science behind our contemporary medicine is more sophisticated, but in bedside manners those old-time docs had a decided edge. They knew their patients; they knew their patients' families; and they established doctor-patient relationships which were deep and abiding. Under these circumstances, the family doctor's attendance at the deathbed became almost an obligatory duty. The doctor was expected "to be there" when his patient died, not necessarily for therapeutic purposes, but rather to lend a sense of order to Nature's proceedings and to assure the family that "everything possible had been done."

The idea that physicians should play an important role in the terminal event faded away in the 1970s and 1980s. American society had become much more mobile; doctors and their patients did not always stay in the same community for a lifetime. The representative American physician was no longer a general practitioner who made house calls, but a specialist who practiced with a group of other specialists and who never visited patients' homes. A patient with a serious illness (like cancer) was apt to be briefly seen by a succession of specialists, none of whom would form a personal relationship strong enough to prompt a subsequent deathbed vigil. Paradoxically, the 1990s saw an amazing resurgence of the idea that physicians should be intimately involved in their patients' final hours, and this time the proposed involvement went far beyond simply being present to offer consolation. Indeed, it revolved around a single explosive question—**under what conditions, if any, can a physician take steps to hasten the death of a terminally ill patient who wishes to die?**

Our new medical technologies seem more of a curse than a blessing when they serve to keep alive persons with incurable disease whose quality of life rapidly deteriorates from poor to horrible. Terminal cancer patients have always tended to comprise the majority of this unfortunate population; yet in the 1980s its ranks were significantly increased by AIDS sufferers kept alive with sophisticated antibiotic regimens, and by victims of **multiple sclerosis** (MS) and **amyotrophic lateral sclerosis** (ALS, "Lou Gehrig's disease"), two devastating neurological disorders which paralyze the body while leaving the mind in tact. Most patients with the aforementioned illnesses (terminal cancer, AIDS, MS, and ALS) will remain fully cognizant in spite of their physical degeneration. While it is conceivable that some of them would welcome a doctor's help to end their suffering, the topic of **physician-assisted suicide** (PAS) had long been avoided by mainstream American medical journals. For one thing, PAS ran counter to the Hippocratic oath and to the physician's instinct to preserve life; for another, it was illegal in the United States. And before **Timothy E. Quill**, few doctors wanted to admit helping a patient to shorten his or her life, at least not in print.

Dr. Quill, a physician in Rochester, New York, broke the conspiracy of silence in 1991, when he published an account of his dealings with "Diane" in the *New England Journal of Medicine*. Diane was a middle-aged woman who had battled alcoholism and depression before being diagnosed with acute myelomonocytic leukemia. Although this disease in adults can sometimes be cured with allogeneic bone marrow transplantation, the odds of long-term survival are not good. Dr. Quill frankly told Diane about the protracted chemotherapy and its life-threatening toxicities, estimating her chances of a durable remission at no more than 25%. She declined treatment. In a subsequent interview with Dr. Quill, she stated that when she could no longer "maintain control of herself and her own dignity," she preferred "to take her life in the least painful way possible." At this point Quill referred her to the **Hemlock Society**, an activist organization which holds that terminally ill persons should have a legal right to take their own lives if they choose. What ensued in Diane's case was yet another consultation with Dr. Quill, this time about insomnia, and a resulting prescription for barbiturates, ostensibly given to solve that problem. "I made sure," Quill recalled, "that she knew how to use the barbiturates for sleep, and also that she knew the amount needed to commit suicide."[102]

Dr. Quill's advice seems to have gone up to the very border of criminal activity as defined in New York State, without exactly crossing over it. He was not charged for his admitted (albeit limited) role in Diane's death. Since 1991 he has continued to argue the case for legalized PAS in a steady stream

of books and articles. He is a restrained spokesman, conceding that many terminally ill patients who approach their physicians with suicide requests might be better served by adequate pain control and thoughtful counseling.[103] Restraint is not an attribute of *Final Exit* (1991), a best seller written by Hemlock Society founder Derek Humphry. The book abounds with recipes for self-destruction. When Quill reviewed it for the *New England Journal of Medicine*, he complained that "current law creates a paradox by prohibiting a physician's participation under any circumstances while allowing explicit information about methods of suicide to flow through the impersonal, uncontrolled, and potentially dangerous format of a book."[104]

Since Dr. Quill has principally sought to persuade medical professionals to accept PAS, few laypersons have heard of him. But almost every American came to know about **Jack Kevorkian**, who became not only the nation's most visible PAS advocate but also its best-known physician. A retired pathologist, Dr. Kevorkian chose the path of civil disobedience—he defied the prosecutors in his home state of Michigan by assisting in several dozen suicides. *Time* magazine put a picture of Kevorkian on its cover, alongside the caption "Doctor Death." The accompanying story described his famous suicide machine (the patient pulled a string to inhale a lethal dose of carbon monoxide).[105] Outraged Michigan authorities made a habit of putting him on trial, once in 1994 and twice in 1996; but all three juries declined to convict him, accepting his argument that he intended only to relieve human suffering. In November 1998, however, Dr. Kevorkian overstepped the bounds of good taste by permitting the popular TV program "60 Minutes" to televise an assisted suicide he conducted. This time the Michigan authorities had ample evidence—a film showing him personally injecting lethal drugs into a paralyzed ALS sufferer who had trouble breathing and frequently choked on his own saliva. In the ensuing trial for first-degree murder, Kevorkian threw caution to the winds by acting as his own attorney. The jury eventually convicted him of second-degree murder on March 26, 1999; he was subsequently sentenced to 10-to-25 years imprisonment.[106]

However much we may applaud Dr. Kevorkian's courage in challenging overly restrictive state laws, he has not given us a useful model of strategies by which physicians might safely intervene to shorten terminal suffering. Most Americans have strong opinions on this topic—yet these are not based so much on "reason" or "common sense" (as we might all like to think of our own opinions) as on upbringing, mindset, temperament, and personal experiences. Members of the principal religious denominations often object to PAS *in toto*; they argue that assisted suicide at the patient's request would quickly evolve into indiscriminate euthanasia, whereby elderly or handicapped persons would be put to death without being asked for consent. On the other hand, freethinkers and skeptics take the denominations to task for presuming to dictate the civil laws of a largely secular and quite pluralistic society. They will argue that rational persons should be able to choose their manner of dying with the same freedom that they have to choose their associates or their place of residence. Intelligent persons on both sides of the debate are aware of the abuses which might result from unrestricted PAS. Physicians who did not adequately investigate their patients' medical or psychiatric backgrounds might wind up assisting the suicides of persons who were mentally unbalanced or simply depressed rather than terminally ill. Self-serving family members might attempt to expedite the death of an elderly relative who had become a burden or who stood to leave an inheritance behind.

While the techniques of PAS are not complicated, designing right-to-die legislation with plausible safeguards is very much so. Referendums which would have established legal PAS for the terminally ill were narrowly defeated by voters in Washington State (1991) and California (1992). In 1994, however, an initiative sponsored by the Hemlock Society entitled the **Oregon Death with Dignity Act** won approval from the voters in that state, by a margin of 52% to 48%.[107] Implementation was immediately stalled by injunctions and court appeals; in 1995 a federal district judge declared the new Oregon law unconstitutional. The controversial issue made its way up the judicial ladder. On June 26, 1997, the United States Supreme Court unanimously ruled that there is no constitutional right to assisted suicide, while emphasizing the authority of the separate states to outlaw it or to decriminalize it. The high court's decision left in tact 35 state laws specifically prohibiting PAS as well as the unique Oregon statue legalizing it. On October 14, 1997, the Court reaffirmed this stance when it declined to hear an appeal protesting the Death with Dignity Act. Oregon thus became the first state in the nation where PAS could be openly performed without fear of prosecution.[108]

The Oregon experiment seems to have avoided those potential abuses cited by PAS opponents. The Death with Dignity Act does not permit euthanasia—a physician cannot administer a lethal medication to a demented or unconscious person. It does permit a physician to issue a prescription for a lethal medication as well as appropriate advice on taking it, but only under certain conditions. The patient who receives this prescription must be an adult, an Oregon resident, and mentally competent. Moreover, two M.D.'s (the patient's primary physician and a consulting physician) must certify that the patient's illness is indeed terminal—that is, that it would normally be expected to cause death within the next six months. The patient must make three separate requests for the prescription, one in writing and two oral requests separated by at least fifteen days. Arthur E. Chin and his colleagues in the Oregon Health Division, the agency supervising these matters, point out that the primary physician is also obligated to inform any patient requesting a lethal prescription "of all feasible alternatives, such as comfort care, hospice care, and pain-control options." And if a lethal prescription is actually handed to a patient, the physician must report it to the Oregon Health Division. Only when all these conditions are fulfilled is the prescribing physician protected from prosecution.[109]

The reporting proviso of the Death with Dignity Act has enabled Dr. Chin and his colleagues to give us some noteworthy statistics for 1998, the first full year of legalized PAS in Oregon. Only 23 Oregonians received lethal prescriptions during the entire year. Of these, 21 had died before the end of the year. Chin et al record that "15 died after taking their lethal medications" and "6 died from their underlying illnesses." Most of the dying patients (18 of the 21) had terminal cancer. "With one exception," Chin et al observe, "all prescriptions were for 9 grams of a fast-acting barbiturate and an antiemetic agent." Secobarbital was the preferred barbiturate (19 of 21 prescriptions). Patients taking the lethal medications were typically "unconscious within 20 minutes"; but the time to death was "not always rapid or predictable," ranging from less than one hour to 11.5 hours.[110]

The preceding modest statistics (only 15 actual suicides in one year) suggest that Oregonians are no more anxious to quaff the hemlock than anybody else. As the Death with Dignity Act encourages considerable forethought on the patient's part and mandates pre-event counseling, it may have the effect of preventing impulsive suicide attempts, particularly those messy ones involving firearms or crude drug overdoses which are not uncommon in American society. The vast majority of terminal cancer patients would not be at all interested in PAS if they knew that their last days would be dignified and pain-free; unfortunately, an assurance to this effect cannot always be given. Most Americans are rightly appalled by the prospect of elaborate interventions which serve only to add a few days of marginal existence at an astronomical cost in human suffering and in hospital bills. The excesses of physicians bent on preserving life can become every bit as distasteful as Dr. Kevorkian's suicide machine.

Readers of this book must be cautioned not to draw broad inferences from Oregon's Death with Dignity Act. American statutes touching on right-to-die issues are heterogeneous. They vary from state to state, and how they might be interpreted by different physicians or applied at different hospitals is anybody's guess. But certain basic principles are well-established throughout the nation and have been upheld by the courts. Every patient has a legal right to refuse treatment, either the entire proposed treatment or any aspect of it. Healthy persons as well as those diagnosed with terminal illnesses often consult their attorneys to complete **a living will** in advance of need. One of these documents simply declares that the person signing it does not want to be kept alive "by extraordinary means" if he or she should become incapacitated. What might constitute extraordinary means has never been precisely defined—therefore a living will is most likely to be effective if an attorney or family member has been legally empowered beforehand to represent the patient's interests. This empowerment is easily accomplished by completing another advance directive known as **a durable power of attorney for health care**.

At some time in their careers, most oncologists will have occasion to do something which shortens a terminal patient's life. Such actions or omissions are not always entered on patient charts; and when they are recorded, they are never identified as life-shortening. **Withholding aggressive treatment** is not to be equated with assisted suicide or euthanasia; but every oncologist knows that if severe hypercalcemia is not aggressively combated, the patient will lapse into coma and die peacefully.[111] Other crises commonly associated with terminal cancer—infections, cerebral hemorrhages, renal failure—will likewise hasten death. For a dying patient who is in no discomfort, the best intervention may be none at all. **Aggressive pain management** often has the effect of shortening a terminal patient's life. While this strategy does require an active intervention by the attending physician, the Supreme Court rulings of June 1997 specifically permitted aggressive palliation of pain, even to the point of "terminal sedation"—that is, rendering the patient unconscious during any unacceptably painful final days. David Orentlicher, a physician who is also a lawyer, points out that sedation followed by the withholding of nutrition and hydration—"a second step that is typically part of terminal sedation"—amounts to "slow euthanasia."[112] True enough, but since terminal sedation is described on the chart only as necessary analgesia, it does not ruffle the sensibilities of the patient's family members or of the local prosecutors.

HOSPICE

These days terminal cancer patients may feel somewhat abandoned by their busy physicians, who often seem to lose interest once it becomes clear that no additional therapeutic measures are indicated. Giving comfort and support to the dying, however essential this service may be, is not the stuff of which Nobel prizes are made, nor is it headlined in the medical journals. For patients with short life expectancies, the hospice movement has thus come to represent an alternative to traditional care, which all too frequently involves a string of rather pointless hospitalizations. The modern hospice was conceived as a different kind of institution from the modern hospital, that familiar multistory temple of healing epitomized by million-dollar diagnostic machines and by proficient, often spectacular surgical interventions. A hospice is a much smaller and far more intimate facility devoted to palliation. The diagnosis has already been determined as has the outcome—all hospice patients have chronic progressive diseases which can be expected to cause their death. The hospice's goal is not to extend life expectancy, but rather to enhance the quality of the remaining life and to provide a dignified setting for the process of dying.

While the first hospice opened its doors in London in 1967, this new concept in patient care found its fullest expression on American soil. Florence S. Wald, dean of the Yale School of Nursing, helped to establish the prototypical institution in 1974, the Connecticut Hospice at Branford. When Mrs. Wald was interviewed in 1999, she recalled that "at the time the patient had no choice in terms of the care given. Physicians would sometimes forbid nurses to answer questions from a patient about his condition." The hospice movement changed all that—it called for disclosure of the prognosis, freedom to accept or reject treatment, and attentiveness to the dignity and humanity of terminal patients. We may gather some inkling of the vast need that hospices fulfilled from their astonishing proliferation: by the year 1998 there were upwards of 3,000 operational hospice programs in the United States.[113]

While individual hospices are as diverse as the local communities which support them, they share a common egalitarianism: any terminal patient, rich or poor, is eligible for their services. Hospices are far less expensive than hospitals, because they have much lower overhead expenses to begin with, and because they attract volunteer workers as well as monetary contributions. Hospice charges tend to be based on a sliding scale, adjusted to the patient's financial resources. Private insurance companies have generally found it cost-effective to pay for hospice care. Medicare and Medicaid also pay benefits, but federal regulations stipulate that both the attending physician and the hospice's medical director must certify that the patient being referred has less than six months to live. Ira Byock, a palliative care physician at the University of Montana, fears that this rule may discourage hospice programs from accepting patients with "Alzheimer's dementia, congestive heart failure, or chronic pulmonary disease," illnesses whose progression to death may be prolonged beyond six months. The federal timetable poses no barrier to most cancer patients being referred; but Dr. Byock points out that when cancer patients require "expensive palliative interventions" like whole-brain radiotherapy or neurolytic blocks, "the capitated, per diem payment structure of the Medicare Hospice Benefit imposes severe financial strains on hospice programs."[114]

The majority of patients who utilize hospice services, 60% or more, have terminal cancer. A common complaint among hospice professionals is that cancer patients are referred much too late, usually only during the last few weeks of life—in other words, that they get abruptly "dumped at hospice" when their oncologists are finally forced to concede defeat. Earlier referrals would be easier on all parties concerned. Ideally, hospice services will be divided into two distinct phases: **outpatient care** for patients who can still live at home, and **inpatient care** for severely incapacitated patients who are near death. If a terminal patient has a family member or other able-bodied caregiver at home, the local hospice program can arrange for frequent house calls by a nurse or by a trained volunteer. The hospice-affiliated visitor typically provides essential instruction to the home caregiver—how to give sponge baths to a bedridden patient, how to manage personal hygiene and other small dilemmas, how and when to administer pain medications, when to call for outside assistance. The preparation of meals requires a great deal of foresight. Terminal cancer patients are prone to suffer from dysphagia (difficulty in swallowing) as well as from the inevitable anorexia (loss of appetite). Frequent small meals—say, five or six daily—can help to compensate for the patient's early satiety (feeling "full" after several mouthfuls). Soft or pureed foods may help to overcome dysphagia; the best strategy is to let the patient eat what he or she likes.

Bedridden cancer patients receiving opioid analgesia are going to suffer from severe constipation, due to insufficient intestinal secretions and lessened motility. Rectal impaction of fecal matter should be anticipated; in many cases the judicious use of enemas will suffice to soften the stool and permit defecation. Occasionally a patient will have to be sedated while the hospice physician performs manual disimpaction. Dyspnea (difficulty in breathing) is almost universal among cancer patients with metastatic tumor in the lungs or elsewhere in the chest cavity. Analgesic drugs can often provide relief, the opioids by reducing air hunger and the tranquilizers by reducing anxiety. A room humidifier may help some patients; others will require supplemental oxygen administered through a nasal cannula.

Inpatient care at the hospice's residence facility should be considered whenever a patient's condition becomes unstable or whenever a home caregiver's emotional and physical resources start to be overtaxed. Patients and their family members are often surprised when they first pass through the hospice doors—the experience is usually more like entering a well-appointed resort hotel than walking down the sterile corridors of a hospital. The architects who designed our new hospices took pains to create quiet residential atmospheres. The design typically calls for cheerful patient rooms, with a small cafeteria providing visitors with food and drink. A nearby chapel offers opportunities for spiritual reflection. With respect to layout and accommodations, hospices are pleasant places to visit, intentionally so. The hospice director has the essential task of explaining more significant matters to new arrivals and their family members. Patients must be assured that their needs will be foremost, and that they will not be allowed to linger in pain or to die alone. Family members should be told that the hospice staff is always ready to answer their questions and to provide advice and counsel, both before and after their loved one's death.

Whenever a patient is transferred to the residence facility, the hospice physician or another qualified staff member should review the previously prescribed medications with a critical eye. Joni Berry, a pharmacologist affiliated with the Hospice of Wake County in North Carolina, explains that she looks "for duplications or any unnecessary drugs" as well as "for drugs the patient needs but is not receiving."[115] Pain control by means of opioid analgesics and appropriate adjuvant agents remains paramount. Oral administration is used as long as possible; but in the last weeks of life, some hospice patients may become so enfeebled that they cannot swallow pills or even sip liquids. They may also be so emaciated that finding a suitable vein for an intravenous catheter becomes next to impossible. Rectal suppositories or intramuscular injections can be used to deliver painkilling medications under these difficult circumstances.

Those inspirational deathbed scenes which we have all seen in the movies or read about in romantic novels are best regarded as a convention of fiction. In a matter-of-fact article entitled "The Dying Cancer Patient," Kristine A. Nelson and her knowledgeable colleagues at the Cleveland Clinic remind us that the last 48 hours of life are often characterized by distressing cognitive changes, which can include "somnolence, delirium, and agitation." They recommend that caregivers "anticipate the common end-stage symptoms and have medications on hand to provide prompt relief." Antipsychotic drugs like **chlorpromazine** or **haloperidol** are effective against agitation and hallucinations. Delirium in terminal cancer, if it does occur, usually gives way to a somnolence which should not be interrupted. Dr. Nelson and her colleagues point out that although an unconscious patient will feel no pain, it is unwise "to abruptly stop opioid analgesics as withdrawal may occur." They advise that "one quarter of the prior daily dose" will suffice to prevent withdrawal under these circumstances.[116]

The indications that a terminal cancer patient will die within the next few hours are hard to mistake. The senses of sight and hearing start to fail, followed by a complete loss of consciousness. The production of urine ceases while the extremities become cool to the touch; at this point the skin will appear mottled. Family members standing vigil are sure to be disappointed if they hope to hear a final statement or a last goodbye. What they hear is what deathbed watchers have always heard—**"the death rattle."** This is the sound of slow labored breathing, of air being drawn over uncleared respiratory secretions in the throat and bronchial tubes. The auditory phenomenon requires no treatment; the patient is beyond pain. But for those who must live, that relentless rasping sound can be a more powerful invitation to prayer than all the Sunday sermons ever written.

The Emerging Immunotherapies

Back in the 1950s the eminent Australian immunologist Macfarlane Burnet proposed the concept of **immune surveillance**. Burnet's hypothesis holds that malignant cells frequently appear in humans, but that our immune cells are constantly searching out and destroying them before they can develop into dangerous tumors. Of course, this would explain why we are not all plagued with continuous malignant transformations. And any tumor which does develop may thus be attributed to an inefficient or weakened immune response.

How much do we want to believe in this attractive theory! And how often have writers on cancer felt impelled to cite it, usually with nods of approval! The truth is that if this hypothesis had been put forth by anybody except an illustrious Nobel prize winner, it would have been regarded as exuberant speculation rather than as a possibly plausible explanation. Perhaps the immune surveillance envisioned by Burnet plays a role in preventing certain types of human malignancy, but we really don't know under what circumstances this subtle intervention might occur—or even if it ever does.[1] The immunological principle most obviously demonstrated in oncology is not surveillance but **self tolerance**. Our immune cells do not seem to be overly concerned about malignant transformation; as far as we can tell, neither early nor late do they mount an effective defense against the misguided cancer cells. Unfortunately, the **leukocytes** (white cells) which constitute our immune system are not designed to do so; they have evolved over millions of years to fulfill a different and very specific purpose—viz., to protect us against a world of potentially harmful microorganisms. And usually our assorted leukocytes do a fine job of fending off the multitudinous bacteria, viruses, fungi, protozoa, and worms which would otherwise spell our doom. In this instance, immune surveillance is no fanciful hypothesis but an ongoing phenomenon whose most minute aspects can now be observed and recorded. But the same immune cells which routinely recognize and attack invading microorganisms must also recognize—*and refrain from attacking*—the body's own tissues. When this or that subset of leukocytes goes astray and starts to react to this or that molecular component found in the body's own tissues, the end result will be one of those chronic debilitating disorders we now classify as **autoimmune diseases**. Rheumatoid arthritis, lupus, multiple sclerosis, and myasthenia gravis are well-known examples of autoimmune pathology. The properly functioning immune system does not react with self (i.e., the body's own tissues). It normally remains a bystander even if the self-tissues manifest abnormal growth patterns. As a rule of thumb, **neoplasms** (Latin for "new forms") do not elicit a noteworthy immune response; this is as true for the deadly carcinomas and sarcomas as it is for the innocent moles, warts, and freckles. The outward signs of leukocyte activity which we have all experienced from time to time—e.g., the <u>fever</u> which accompanies colds and the flu (common viral infections), or the <u>inflammation</u> which develops around boils and pimples (superficial bacterial infections)—are conspicuously absent during the presentation and progression of malignant tumors.

Immunologists will explain that the overwhelming majority of tumors fail to elicit an immune response because they are not sufficiently "antigenic." That Greek term **antigen** is miscellaneously applied to any substance which causes the production of antibodies or which stimulates any other immune function. Common antigens include the plant pollens, mold spores, house dust, and animal dander associated with sneeze-and-cough allergies, as well as certain proteins found in seafood and peanuts which can provoke hypersensitivity reactions in susceptible individuals. However, when we speak of antigens in tumor immunology, we are referring to **<u>molecules</u> <u>expressed</u> <u>on</u> <u>the</u> <u>outer</u> <u>surface</u> <u>of</u> <u>cancer</u> <u>cells</u>**. Our immune cells are perpetually checking the surface markers (the "credentials," as it were) of all cells in the body. If they encounter a marker perceived as foreign—i.e., not self—they will attempt to eliminate the cells carrying it. This surveillance works like a charm with invading bacteria because the molecules on their outer membranes are so antigenic, so obviously not self, that every leukocyte quickly perceives the threat. Tumor cells are a different matter. They often do express surface molecules which differ from those on

normal cells, and considerable efforts have been made to identify and catalogue these **tumor-associated antigens** (TAAs). The problem is that TAAs are less antigenic in the patient's body than in test-tube simulations. Writing in 1999, the immunologist Lawrence G. Lum conceded an unhappy truth: "Unfortunately, most tumor-associated antigens are overexpressed self-antigens."[2]

We have learned that some varieties of cancer are potentially more antigenic than others. **Melanomas**, those dangerous skin cancers, derive from peculiar and highly specialized cells called melanocytes, whose function is to impart pigmentation to the skin. This means that melanomas carry TAAs not widely expressed on other cells. The identification of reasonably unique melanoma antigens has prompted ongoing efforts to create an effective vaccine against this type of cancer. But long before we knew about TAAs, melanomas were recognized as the most immunogenic human malignancy because of well-documented **spontaneous remissions**. In these rare cases, all traces of disease vanish without treatment, even in patients who have widespread metastases. Such phenomena suggest that the immune system by itself can vanquish cancer, at least under the proper extraordinary conditions. And although melanoma regressions are infrequent, they do occur with a certain regularity. A report in the *Journal of the National Cancer Institute* estimated that "one out of every 2,000 cases of metastatic melanoma will undergo complete spontaneous remission." Donald L. Morton, a melanoma specialist at the John Wayne Cancer Center (Santa Monica, California), believes that an immune response must be involved because "the spontaneous regression events were all triggered by some sort of natural assault to the immune system." Melanoma patients have experienced these dramatic recoveries after fighting off bacterial infections, after becoming pregnant, and after receiving blood transfusions.[3]

Renal cell carcinomas which arise in the kidney also tend to display distinct TAAs, and like melanomas they have been associated with occasional spontaneous remissions. While cancer specialists never doubted that these wondrous self-cures could sometimes come to pass, they had no formula for inducing them. Only in the 1990s did we have an immunostimulatory drug which could induce with some regularity the regressions seen in nature. As we will see later in this chapter, **interleukin-2** has achieved durable remissions (apparent cures) in about 5% to 10% of patients treated for metastatic melanomas and renal cell carcinomas. While that cure rate may sound *under*-whelming, we must keep in mind that no other therapy has been shown to achieve any cures whatsoever. These two malignancies rarely respond to cytotoxic chemotherapy, and they generally cause death within a year or two after the onset of metastatic disease.

Spontaneous remissions are not a recognizable feature in the natural history of other solid tumors. Most reports of inexplicable regression may be better described as "anecdotal" rather than "documented"—they are more likely to be due to an initial misdiagnosis than to an aroused immune system. We should stress that the diverse malignancies which arise in the mammary gland are not known to be immunogenic. There is no reliable evidence that any type of breast cancer routinely, or even occasionally, elicits an immune response which might alter the course of disease. In the 1970s Maurice M. Black and other pathologists speculated that increased numbers of leukocytes in the vicinity of a primary breast tumor might be a favorable prognostic marker.[4] But the data gathered from the NSABP trials of that era failed to confirm this supposition. In 1980

the pathologist Edwin R. Fisher and his NSABP co-workers reported that they had "consistently observed that a brisk cell reaction within a breast cancer does not indicate a favorable prognosis. Indeed, such reactions are more significantly observed in poorly differentiated tumors and are attended with a greater incidence of treatment failure."[5] The surreptitious way in which aggressive breast tumors infiltrate the axillary lymph nodes is another indication of antigenic invisibility. Regional lymph nodes are the very places where immune responses develop! Any bacterial antigens reaching a lymph node will spur the resident leukocytes into frantic activity. Within hours the affected node will become swollen and tender, easily discernible by an examining physician. Nothing like this ever happens with breast malignancies— they can spread to dozens of lymph nodes over a period of several years, without producing a single outward sign of their presence. Node-positive breast cancer patients often hesitate to take chemotherapy or an antiestrogenic drug like tamoxifen because they want "to keep their immune system strong to fight cancer." This attitude has no scientific basis and may prove to be unwise. While chemotherapy does temporarily suppress the immune system, it favorably alters the course of disease in many cases. Antiestrogenic drugs are not noticeably immunosuppressive.

The casual belief that the immune system fights cancer, so passionately espoused by laypersons and by vitamin salesmen, is untenable. It simply does not happen 99.99% of the time. On the other hand, the possibility that we might duplicate those extraordinary spontaneous remissions either by making cancer cells more antigenic, or by making immune cells more tumor-antigenresponsive, offers a valid field for scientific inquiry. It is the most exciting prospect in cancer research. While our therapeutic successes to date have been modest, our hopes are justifiably high because of the vast expansion of immunological knowledge in recent decades. There was relatively little a cancer surgeon in the year 2000 could do that a surgeon in 1950 could not do. In contrast, the leading immunologists of the 1950s now strike us as denizens of the Dark Ages, who were fundamentally ignorant of basic principles that every medical student has long since memorized. Immunology has increasingly looked like the most promising and relevant biomedical discipline. Some of our researchers seek to learn how to damper the immune response, so as to halt the progression of autoimmune diseases or to prevent the rejection of transplanted organs. For malignancies as well as the immunodeficiency syndromes, the goal is to learn how to stimulate a purposeful immune response. Immunodeficiency has proven a fortuitous teacher. That terrible AIDS virus which preferentially attacks and decimates immune cells forced us to learn more about the functions of these cells than we had hitherto dreamed possible. By the year 2000 the techniques of molecular biology enabled us to understand the genetic mechanisms behind those distressing immunodeficiencies occasionally encountered in young children. We could now demonstrate that a tiny point mutation in this or that gene resulted in the production of an abnormal protein, which in turn adversely affected the performance of this or that subset of leukocytes, with catastrophic results. Afflicted children will fall prey to recurrent infections; the type of pathogen which gains the upper hand is determined by which element of the immune system has been disabled.[6]

For convenience, writers discussing the immune response divide that broad topic into two distinct but overlapping fields. Our first line of defense against invading microbes is called **innate immunity**. This consists primarily of protective barriers such as the skin and various mucosal surfaces awash with antimicrobial fluids, and of neutrophils and macrophages, those ravenous phagocytes programmed to recognize and devour bacteria. The role of protective barriers and phagocytes was adequately understood by the Russian pathologist Elie Metchnikoff, who observed phagocytic activity in primitive invertebrates (sponges and starfish) during the 1870s. Modern researchers on tumor immunology are principally concerned with the second and far more sophisticated line of antimicrobial defense, which we call **adaptive (or specific) immunity**. This type of immunity is well-developed in higher life forms, notably *Homo sapiens* and other mammals. Adaptive immunity explains why if you contract chicken pox or mumps or measles during childhood, you will never again experience these particular illnesses, no matter how old you might live to be. From time to time, you will inevitably be reexposed to the causative viruses; but since you carry a small number of long-lived immune cells which are specifically programmed to react with them, any viruses gaining entry to the body will be squelched before they can cause disease.

This marvelous lifelong immunity is brought about by a subset of leukocytes known as **lymphocytes**. These relatively small and nondescript white cells are plentiful in the lymph nodes and lymph fluid (hence their name), but scarce in the bloodstream and in other bodily tissues. As seen under a microscope, their activities are less spectacular than those of the phagocytes and not readily comprehensible. The immunologists of the 1950s did not know much about lymphocytes. By the 1970s we knew enough to recognize three main subsets of lymphocyte, which have different functions. **B cells** secrete antibodies, tiny bits of protein which bind to specific pathogens, hamper their reproduction and movement, and mark them for destruction by phagocytes. **Cytotoxic T cells** are lymphocytes which can lyse (kill) bodily cells infected by viruses. A "killer T cell" will press against a cell expressing viral or other extraneous not-self particles on its outer membrane, binding to it just long enough to release lytic molecules called **perforin** and **granzymes**. The perforin produces small holes (pores) in the target cell's membrane. While this alone would eventually cause the target cell's death, the process of apoptosis (cellular disintegration) is greatly hastened by the granzymes which float through the perforin-induced pores.[7] At least in test-tube simulations, cytotoxic T cells can also be made to recognize and lyse cancer cells. Popular-science writers tend to dwell on these laboratory demonstrations, without mentioning that they occur under controlled and highly artificial conditions.

A third subset of lymphocytes is less heralded but terribly important. **Helper T cells** function as the maestros of the immune response, releasing molecules which direct all the phagocytes, B cells, and killer T cells into coordinated activity. Later, after the pathogens are vanquished, the helper T cells will release a different set of molecules which has the effect of turning off that frenzied immune response.

Our hope is in the lymphocytes! They have been the starting point for our recent efforts to develop cancer immunotherapies. We have tried to churn out antibodies which would bind firmly to malignant cells (the proposed B cell contribution), and to excite killer T cells into a tumor-specific fury. While neither strategy has as yet lived up to our expectations, the story of these ongoing experiments merits our attention.

Dr. Coley and his Toxins

The idea that the immune system might somehow be stimulated to destroy malignant tumors is not new. Impressive cures brought about by immunologic manipulation were achieved over a century ago by **William B. Coley**, a well-known surgeon practicing in New York City.[8] Born in 1862, Coley had barely completed his medical training in the fall of 1890, when he attempted to cure a pretty seventeen-year-old girl named Bessie Dashiell, who had a painful bump on her right hand. The "bump" proved to be an aggressive sarcoma. In November 1890 Coley amputated Bessie's arm below the elbow, but this did not slow the progression of disease. By early December Bessie had metastatic nodules in both breasts; then her liver and lungs became involved. She died a horrible death on January 23, 1891, emaciated, vomiting blood, and covered from head to foot with tiny cutaneous nodules. Yet Bessie did not die in vain. Her tragic case gave Dr. Coley an indelible lesson in the limitations of surgery against rapidly metastasizing tumors. Indirectly, Bessie also gave Coley—as well as many subsequent cancer researchers—a generous financial patron. Her teenage boyfriend John D. Rockefeller, Jr., had been shaken by her illness and death, so much so that he had to forego his first term at Yale College. Young Rockefeller, the heir to the Standard Oil fortune, eventually recovered his equilibrium, but he never forgot Bessie. He later became an enthusiastic backer of her surgeon's efforts to develop a workable cancer immunotherapy.

The spring of 1891 found Dr. Coley in a medical library, poring over published reports of sarcomas and other malignancies. These tended to foreshadow his own experience—viz., surgery did little to slow disease progression, and the patient soon died. Paradoxically, the few rays of hope in these stories had been provided by the then deplorable sanitary conditions in hospitals, which left patients vulnerable to infection with *Streptococcus pyogenes*. This bacterium can cause an acute febrile illness called **erysipelas**, whose course is characterized by very high fever, chills, and a widespread skin rash. What excited Coley's curiosity was a mere handful of reports about hospitalized cancer patients who seemed to be dying, but who had experienced wondrous recoveries after contracting erysipelas. In October 1891, a year after he first saw Bessie Dashiell, Coley encountered another sarcoma patient. An Italian immigrant named Mr. Zola had a tumor in his neck so large that it blocked his throat and prevented him from eating. Coley tried a desperate gambit—he injected the tumor mass with an especially virulent strain of *Streptococcus pyogenes*. Mr. Zola now came down with a furious case of erysipelas. He shook uncontrollably with chills, his temperature shot up to 105 degrees, and a red rash spread over his neck and face. Zola almost died from this infection; but as his fever subsided, so did his tumor. Within two weeks it had vanished completely. That tremendous immune response aroused by the streptococci had somehow carried off the sarcoma in its wake. The patient recovered and went back to Italy. His physician was possibly less fortunate, because he fell into the trap of believing too strongly in the curative potential of an unorthodox treatment. Stephen S. Hall, an astute historian of cancer immunotherapies, observes that "Coley had the good and bad fortune of achieving a remarkable success in his very first case."[9]

The other patients Coley injected with *Streptococcus pyogenes* in 1891 and 1892 had less felicitous outcomes. His four carcinoma patients did not respond; and while his eight sarcoma patients all responded to some extent, only two were to experience complete remissions. Unfortunately, two of the twelve patients died from erysipelas. By 1893 Coley had decided to abandon the use of live bacteria. For one thing, erysipelas proved surprisingly difficult to induce; and when successfully induced, the disease could easily get out of hand. For another, Coley suspected that the tumor regressions were not caused by the bacteria *per se*, but rather by elusive humoral factors that they produced. He referred to these unknown substances as **toxins**. In the future he would treat his cancer patients with an extract obtained by growing bacteria in a culture medium and then passing the resulting liquid through a fine-pore filter. "Coley's toxins" thus consisted of bacterial byproducts (antigens) which would elicit a strong immune response, without the bacteria which might actually cause disease (the filter had excluded them). *Streptococcus pyogenes* was an obvious choice for culture; Coley also included the gram-negative bacterium *Bacillus prodigiosus*, which he believed would increase the virulence of the streptococci.

On January 24, 1893, Coley began to inject his bacterial broth into a teenage boy with a large abdominal tumor. At first nothing happened; but Coley persisted for several months, giving one injection after another, directly into the tumor as well as in the nearby muscles. With this case as with later ones, he gradually upped the dose of toxins until his patient developed a raging fever. The higher the fever Coley had discovered, the better the odds of tumor regression. And a series of feverish reactions generally yielded better results than a solitary episode. On May 13, 1893, Coley discontinued the injections—the boy's abdominal tumor no longer protruded, and it was continuing to shrink. This patient would eventually die 26 years later, from a heart attack.

By the end of 1893 Coley had published an account of his early cases, predicting that "further investigation along these lines will be followed by even more brilliant results than those already obtained." But other surgeons who fumblingly tried to reproduce his methods obtained only failures. The upshot was that on December 15, 1894, the *Journal of the American Medical Association* carried an editorial which damned the toxins as worthless and did not spare Coley's feelings. "The seeker after notoriety," opined the *Journal*, "may enjoy a temporary celebrity by a very easy process. He has only to announce the sure cure of some hitherto incurable disease by some foreign chemic product, or microbic mystery and the thing is done."[10] This editorial condemnation did much to stigmatize Coley's approach as controversial and to discourage investigation of its merits. But the toxins continued to be used for several decades, because they represented the only therapy for inoperable or metastatic cancer that had any claim to efficacy. Coley was no obscure quack but a highly respected surgeon, the confidant of John D. Rockefeller, Jr., and a close associate of the influential pathologist James Ewing.

What biological mechanisms could explain the remarkable remissions that the toxins occasionally produced? Why did they work in some cases but not in most others? Coley had no answer to these questions, but he did leave behind detailed case records. An analysis published in 1953 concluded that out of 1,200 cancer patients he eventually treated with the toxins, 270 achieved complete remissions. This success rate of 22.5% compares favorably with those reported for interleukin-2 therapy in the 1980s and 1990s. Coley obtained his best results with sarcomas, those aggressive tumors arising in bone or other connective tissues. A few carcinomas and melanomas also seem to have been cured.[11] Modern attempts to explain these therapeutic successes have focused on *Bacillus prodigiosus*, which (like other gram-negative bacteria) secretes an extremely antigenic substance called <u>endotoxin</u> (a bacterial lipopolysaccharide). This antigen prompts leukocytes to churn out **tumor necrosis factor** (TNF), a molecule which exerts pronounced inflammatory effects. TNF has been implicated in septic shock and rheumatoid arthritis. Its anticancer activity may be related to its ability to cause intravascular thrombosis (clotting inside the nearby blood vessels); this would shut off the blood supply that sarcomas and other rapidly growing tumors depend upon.[12] But local necrosis at and around the tumor site seems insufficient to explain the most striking aspect of Dr. Coley's work—viz., that some of his terminally ill patients were still alive twenty or thirty years later. We may suspect that in these few cases the toxin-induced immune response had somehow generated memory cells, long-lived B and T cells which could identify any residual cancer cells and act to destroy them.

Coley died in 1936. While he may have demonstrated the potential of immunological interventions, he did not create a practical cancer treatment. There was neither a prescribed dose for the toxins nor a schedule for administering them. Dr. Coley had improvised upon these matters in each case. Other physicians were not schooled in his methods; and even if they had been interested in toxin-based immunotherapy, they did not have reliable pharmaceutical agents to use. Several drug companies marketed their own versions of the toxins, but these commercial products were of uneven quality, and they all lacked the antigenic potency of the extracts whose preparation Coley had personally supervised. Cancer immunotherapy did not catch on during Coley's lifetime because there were no organized groups of health professionals dedicated to it. The trends in cancer therapeutics were determined by surgeons who sought to improve cure rates by devising increasingly radical operations.

THE FABLED INTERFERON
Learning about Cytokines

The 1950s, those immunological Dark Ages, did produce at least one stunning breakthrough. That was the discovery of **interferon** in 1957 by Alick Isaacs and Jean Lindenmann, two young biologists working in London.[13] In the late 1930s scientists had already described the phenomenon of "viral interference"—i.e., after a live cell in a test tube is infected with one virus, it cannot be subsequently infected with another kind of virus. At the time everybody suspected that the first virus entering the cell somehow prevented other viruses from gaining entry. What Isaacs and Lindenmann demonstrated in an elegant experiment using chicken embryo cells is that the infecting virus has nothing to do with creating viral interference. The infected cell is solely responsible. It responds to an initial viral infection by secreting an elusive protein which will protect itself and any nearby cells from attacking viruses. Isaacs and Lindenmann named this protein interferon. Their discovery raised hopes of obtaining a "viral penicillin" (a drug which could combat viral infections), but there was not enough interferon on hand to conduct additional experiments. The protein proved almost impossible to extract from cell cultures.

By the early 1960s, however, we had learned that leukocytes exposed to viruses will secrete much more interferon than other cells. The task of isolating and purifying this protein assumed an unprecedented urgency in 1969, when a sometime Harvard researcher named Ion Gresser made a remarkable discovery. *Interferon could cure cancer in mice!* The newspapers and science fiction writers pounced on this revelation—in the next decade interferon took on the luminous aura of a wonder drug waiting just over the horizon. In the popular imagination as well as in the comic strips, it promised to cure metastatic cancer, multiple sclerosis, rheumatoid arthritis, and all other dread diseases for which medical science had no solution. If only it were available in quantity!

A researcher in Finland named Kari Cantell found out that the Sendai virus (which normally infects birds) is quite efficient in prodding human leukocytes to churn out interferon. Soon he was supplying the elusive protein to researchers throughout the world. But Cantell's methods were cumbersome—swimming pools full of blood had to be expended to obtain a gram or two of interferon, and that blood had to be human. Since interferon is species-restricted, white blood cells taken from lower animals could not serve as a source of the protein. So much blood was required because even when fighting off viral infections, leukocytes produce only trace amounts of interferon. By the late 1970s, however, Cantell's lab in Helsinki was extracting enough interferon for a team of physicians in Sweden to test it on a few cancer patients. The results, while not definitive, seemed to point toward substantial benefits. In 1979 the National Cancer Institute announced plans to buy nine million dollars worth of Finnish interferon, so as to be able to conduct larger trials in the United States. Yet within two years the advent of recombinant DNA technology would consign the Helsinki enterprise to the history books. An important interferon gene was tracked to the ninth human chromosome, cloned, and then inserted into *Escherichia coli* bacteria, which multiplied happily while churning out ever-greater quantities of the desired protein.[14]

The problem of supply being solved, the next task was to establish that interferon was more than a laboratory phenomenon—that it really offered therapeutic benefits in human disease. But physicians testing this agent at Houston's M. D. Anderson Cancer Center in the early 1980s came up empty-handed. Evidently interferon was no universal passkey which unlocked the immune response, just one piece of a much larger puzzle. What Isaacs and Lindenmann had stumbled across was not a broad-spectrum wonder drug, but one of many short-range effector molecules which direct cells into this or that activity. Immunologists now refer to these molecules as **cytokines**. Unlike endocrine hormones such as estrogen or insulin, cytokines do not have systemic effects on diverse tissues throughout the body; and they are not normally detectable in the general circulation. Yet they may be found in high concentrations at sites of inflammation (i.e., where an active immune response is taking place). Secreted by individual cells rather than by endocrine glands, cytokines act either in a *paracrine* fashion (on the adjacent cells) or in an *autocrine* fashion (on the cells which are themselves secreting the cytokines). Often cytokines will mediate several paracrine and autocrine effects at the same time—of course, these effects would occur only after the cytokine molecules bind to and activate specific receptors expressed on the outer membranes of the responding cells. While other cells besides leukocytes secrete cytokines, these effector molecules represent the main means of communication between the different white cells. In the 1980s they were sometimes referred to as **lymphokines**, a term that was later felt to be too narrow in its implications.

Other pertinent nomenclature has also been modified because of expanding immunological knowledge. The term "interferon," originally used as the designation for a single protein, is now understood to refer to a family of related molecules encoded by different genes. The cytokine authority Frances R. Balkwill observes that there are "at least 23 different genetic loci" for **interferon alpha**,

"of which 15 correspond to functional genes."[15] Interferon alpha, secreted by leukocytes, has been the subject of most investigations; but two other types of interferon are also recognized. Fibroblasts (connective tissue cells) can secrete **interferon beta**, and activated immune cells in the spleen and bloodstream produce **interferon gamma**. Different types of interferon mediate different biological effects. By and large, interferons are <u>cytostatic</u> rather than cytotoxic; they simply tend to inhibit the reproduction of cancer cells. Various mechanisms have been proposed to explain the anticancer effects produced by interferons in laboratory experiments—they include disruption of tumor angiogenesis, enhancement of differentiation, and stimulation of lymphocytes and phagocytes.[16]

Translating the tantalizing laboratory observations into treatments for human cancer took some time. Eventually the frustrated researchers at M. D. Anderson tried their interferon alpha on a patient with **hairy cell leukemia**, a rare B cell malignancy that afflicts middle-aged or elderly men. The result was a durable remission—this came as a complete surprise because no previous therapy had ever produced any regression in this sluggish but relentless form of leukemia. Subsequent clinical studies reported response rates of 90% or more in patients with hairy cell leukemia who were given interferon alpha. While the treatment did not cure this disease—(leukemic cells persisted in the bone marrow)—it improved the quality of patients' lives and extended their life expectancies.[17] Hairy cell leukemia thus became the first indication for interferon approved by the FDA. In 1986 drug company Hoffmann-LaRoche ran sumptuous advertisements in the *New England Journal of Medicine* to promote **Roferon-A**, its brand of interferon alpha-2a, which was touted as the "first recombinant interferon into the clinic" and as "a new modality in cancer therapy." To induce remission in hairy cell leukemia, Hoffmann-LaRoche recommended a daily injection of three million units continued for 16 to 24 weeks. The subsequent "maintenance" regimen given to maintain remission called for three injections per week.[18]

The antiviral activity of interferon alpha led to FDA approval for its use in condylomata acuminata (genital warts caused by human papilloma viruses) and in Kaposi's sarcoma, a skin malignancy frequently encountered in AIDS patients who have been infected with HHV-8 (human herpes virus 8) as well as with HIV. The 1990s saw the increasing use of interferon alpha to treat hepatitis B and other chronic viral infections of the liver.[19] Clinical trials established that interferon alpha, while not curative, could produce improved disease-free and overall survival in diverse hematological malignancies. The best-known indication was in the treatment of **chronic myelogenous leukemia**, where interferon alpha-2a extended patients' survival by "slowing the progression from the chronic phase to an accelerated or a blastic phase."[20] Interferon therapy found wide acceptance as the best alternative for patients who were not good candidates for allogeneic bone marrow transplantation. **Melanoma** proved to be a more controversial indication. The Eastern Cooperative Oncology Group (ECOG) conducted a clinical trial whose results, published in 1996, revealed improved survival rates for node-positive melanoma patients receiving a year of high-dose interferon alpha-2b. FDA approval followed, and the Schering Corporation advertised its **Intron-A** (brand name for interferon alpha-2b) as "a matter of life and death" for melanoma patients at risk of relapse.[21] Preliminary findings from a follow-up trial failed to demonstrate a survival benefit; but in October 2000 John M. Kirkwood of the University of Pittsburgh made

public the results of an ECOG-Intergroup trial, which "confirmed the overall survival benefit in a decisive and unequivocal manner."[22]

Interferon gamma, structurally different from the other interferons, has distinct stimulatory effects on phagocytes. In 1990 the FDA approved it for **chronic granulomatous disease**. This catchall term refers to the recurrent childhood infections which develop when a patient's phagocytes (due to this or that genetic defect) are unable to kill the bacteria they ingest. Interferon gamma promotes the production of antimicrobial oxygen metabolites within macrophages and other phagocytes, thus greatly reducing the incidence of serious infections in afflicted children.[23] Interferon beta was the last type of interferon to find a clinical application. During the late 1990s it was increasingly used to treat multiple sclerosis. Although neurologists agreed that for many patients this cytokine could reduce the frequency of relapses and delay the onset of disability, nobody knew exactly what biological mechanism might lie behind these therapeutic benefits.[24]

By the year 2000 it had become clear that while the several interferons did not represent curative therapy for any disorder, they could be useful in the management of certain malignancies and some chronic infections. These indications had been discovered empirically, simply by giving the drug to patients and observing the outcome. The chief side effect of high-dose interferon was likely to be flu-like symptoms (chills, fever, headache, nausea, fatigue, and sore muscles), which resolved as soon as the drug was discontinued. Yet cost and inconvenience argued against the casual use of interferons. In 1994 a correspondent writing to the *New England Journal of Medicine* complained that the cost of interferon therapy for chronic myelogenous leukemia was "two hundred times higher" than chemotherapy.[25] Because the interferons had a short half-life (eight hours or less) and could not be taken orally, therapy typically required daily intramuscular or subcutaneous injections. While patients could be taught to administer the drug themselves, the fact that these injections had to be given every day, for months on end, was one of the least attractive aspects of interferon therapy. A modified interferon alpha called **peginterferon** may simplify treatment, as this formulation has a much longer half-life. Researchers in Germany, Canada, and other nations have reported that once-weekly injections of peginterferon are effective in treating hepatitis C, a leading cause of liver disease in the industrialized world.[26]

Steven A. Rosenberg:
Adoptive Immunotherapy

The most obvious successor to William B. Coley has been Steven A. Rosenberg of the National Cancer Institute.[27] Born in 1940 to an Orthodox Jewish family, Rosenberg studied science at Johns Hopkins and medicine at Harvard. In 1968, while serving as a surgical resident at a veterans' hospital near Boston, he treated a patient who had experienced a spontaneous remission of inoperable stomach cancer after developing an abdominal infection. Like Coley before him, Rosenberg realized that an aroused immune system can sometimes cure even disseminated and highly lethal malignancies. Also like Coley, Rosenberg did not hesitate to try out potentially dangerous therapies if he thought they might help patients who would otherwise die from cancer. He became the NCI's chief of surgery in 1974, at the age of thirty-four. This post brought with it ample funding, a large supportive staff (nurses, scientists, and technicians), an unending stream of terminal cancer patients, and media coverage that can only be described as excessive.

Rosenberg's forte has been **adoptive immunotherapy**. In this case that term means that the immune cells intended to battle the tumor have been prepared outside of the patient's body. These cells could be either the patient's own white cells which have been removed and modified in some way, or cells taken from a donor. The first experiment tried by Dr. Rosenberg and his colleagues now strikes us as naive and crude—the donor cells used were not merely *allogeneic* (taken from some other person), but downright *zoogenous* (of animal origin). In October 1977 the NCI team excised tumor nodules from the lungs of a young woman dying from an aggressive sarcoma; this malignant tissue was then sown into the mesentery (abdominal lining) of a pig. The animal's lymphocytes would naturally recognize and reject the implanted tissue, not because it was malignant, but because it came from a different species. Would pig lymphocytes sensitized in this way specifically recognize and attack the tumor if they were to be infused into the patient? No small hospital or private practitioner would have the audacity to test this novel idea; but being relatively immune from malpractice suits, Rosenberg and his NCI co-workers went ahead. In November 1977 they removed the pig's abdominal lymph nodes, so as to "harvest" (obtain) tumor-sensitized lymphocytes. These cells were then infused into the patient. Unfortunately, no therapeutic benefit was observed either with this patient or with five other patients who subsequently received the procedure.[28]

The discovery that gave the greatest impetus to adoptive immunotherapy was not made in Dr. Rosenberg's lab, but in that of another famous NCI researcher, the virologist Robert Gallo. In 1975 a cell biologist working in Gallo's lab discovered a new cytokine which was a potent growth factor. **Interleukin-2** or **IL-2** (as this factor came to be known) especially stimulates the reproduction and differentiation of cytotoxic T cells, those lymphocytes which could conceivably kill any cancer cells they learned to recognize as "not self." While Gallo and his close associates did not fully appreciate the potential applications of IL-2, Rosenberg immediately grasped this molecule's importance. He knew that if only a few lymphocytes reactive to a malignant tumor could be isolated, IL-2 would enable physicians to culture them in quantity. Animal experiments had already convinced him that vast numbers of tumor-reactive killer cells would be necessary to mediate significant anticancer effects. At first purified IL-2 was hard to come by; but by the mid-1980s the pharmaceutical company Cetus had solved the supply problem, bringing out a recombinant cytokine generated by E. coli bacteria. The preclinical tests with this drug gave Dr. Rosenberg and his co-workers cause for optimism. They discovered that mononuclear white cells separated from blood samples and then briefly incubated with IL-2 acquired extraordinary properties. At least in test-tube experiments, these cells would consistently lyse (kill) tumor cells while leaving adjacent normal cells unharmed. The Rosenberg team called these IL-2-primed leukocytes **LAK cells**. The moniker was an abbreviation standing for **lymphokine-activated killer cells**. Subsequent analyses revealed that LAK cells originating in the peripheral (circulating) blood are, to begin with, mainly immature lymphocytes. They will lack the characteristic surface markers found on mature B and T cells because they have not yet undergone antigen exposure and differentiation in the regional lymph nodes.[29]

Those obligatory tests performed with nude (immunodeficient) mice indicated that LAK cells stood to be most effective if given together with a large dose of IL-2. Writing in 1985, Rosenberg recounted the results of a representative experiment involving mice which had been injected with human tumor cells and were brimming over with metastatic nodules. The control mice (those receiving no treatment) averaged 227 metastases each; those mice receiving LAK cells alone averaged 210 metastases each, while the mice receiving LAK cells together with high-dose IL-2 averaged only six (6) metastases each.[30] Rosenberg and his co-workers now tested LAK cells and high-dose IL-2 on 25 NCI patients with various metastatic tumors. All these patients underwent leukaphereses (procedures to remove blood and separate the white cells). The lymphocyte precursors thus obtained were cultured in IL-2 for three or four days, then reinfused in the patients together with high-dose IL-2. Since IL-2 has an extremely short half-life, Rosenberg et al gave the drug as a fifteen-minute infusion every eight hours. These infusions were continued for several days after each LAK cell administration. Depending on their individual tolerance, patients received from four to fourteen cycles of LAK cells and high-dose IL-2.

On December 5, 1985, the *New England Journal of Medicine* published the preliminary results of this first human trial. Rosenberg et al reported that "objective regression of cancer (more than 50 per cent of volume) was observed in 11 of the 25 patients." Melanomas and renal cell carcinomas, the immunogenic tumors, responded best—seven of ten patients experienced objective regression. But two colorectal tumors also responded, as did a lung carcinoma. One of the melanoma patients had a complete remission (the disappearance of all traces of disease), and it was "sustained." The Rosenberg team conceded that the side effects caused by high-dose IL-2 amounted to "severe toxicity," but pointed out that they "disappeared promptly after administration ended." Besides chills, fever, and malaise (effects generally associated with cytokine therapy), IL-2 caused a troublesome capillary permeability. Fluid tended to escape from the small blood vessels into the surrounding tissues, and the inevitable weight gain was more than a nuisance. As the cumulative dose of IL-2 increased, fluid retention began to adversely affect the function of the heart and lungs, so much so that intensive support measures were sometimes necessary. In this initial NCI trial, twenty patients developed dyspnea (difficulty in breathing) due to "pulmonary interstitial edema"; and two of them required intubation for "severe respiratory distress."[31]

While the Rosenberg team's article in the *Journal* was judicious and restrained, the public media's coverage of the new treatment smacked of hoopla and hyperbole. Was Dr. Rosenberg himself partly to blame for these excesses? He had already enjoyed considerable celebrity as the surgeon who, in July 1985, operated on President Ronald Reagan for colon cancer. Now he almost seemed to court representatives of the media, giving interviews both to print journalists and to TV news anchors. A melanoma patient who was responding to therapy appeared on the nightly newscasts, bubbling over with confidence and enthusiasm. Some ten days before the *Journal* article was published, the business magazine *Fortune* had broken the story with a lead article headlined "Cancer Breakthrough." The photograph on the magazine's cover portrayed a small vial of liquid beside the caption "Cetus Corp.'s tumor-zapping interleukin-2." Newspapers throughout the world now put the story on their front pages, and *Newsweek* put a picture of Dr. Rosenberg on its cover. NCI director Vincent DeVita appeared with him to answer reporters' questions on the popular CBS program "Face the Nation."[32]

Because these inflated news reports seemed to bear an official NCI imprimatur, the public reaction to them was pronounced. During the month of December 1985, the NCI's toll-free information number averaged more than a thousand calls a day. And every American oncologist had to answer his share of urgent phone calls and anxious inquiries. Most practitioners were privately annoyed that so much publicity had been given to an experimental treatment whose effectiveness had not been properly evaluated in randomized clinical trials. Charles G. Moertel, the Mayo Clinic's estimable oncologist, dashed off a letter to the *New England Journal of Medicine*, condemning "the public media" for raising "unrealistic expectations among patients with advanced cancer." Moertel found the response rates reported by the Rosenberg team to be "relatively commonplace." As yet no evidence had been presented that LAK cells and IL-2 could cure metastatic cancers, or even increase the life expectancies of patients.[33] Dr. Moertel expanded his objections in a December 12, 1986, editorial in the *Journal of the American Medical Association*. High-dose IL-2 therapy as given by the NCI team, he argued, was "an awesome experience" requiring "weeks of hospitalization." The "unacceptably severe toxicity and astronomical costs" were "not balanced by any persuasive evidence of true net therapeutic gain."[34]

In 1987 Rosenberg and his NCI colleagues published a follow-up report in the *New England Journal of Medicine*, describing the administration of LAK cells and IL-2 to 106 patients with various metastatic cancers. This time there had been eight complete responses (7.5%) and fifteen partial responses (14.2%). Renal cell carcinomas responded best (12 of 36 patients responding, a 33% rate), followed by melanomas (6 of 26 patients responding, a 23% rate). The second article by Rosenberg et al did not provoke a media extravaganza, possibly because the authors described the toxic side effects at length and conceded that most responses did not last more than a few months.[35]

Almost all the toxicity in these early NCI trials had been due to the large doses of interleukin-2; the LAK cells by themselves were well-tolerated. Rosenberg and his team hoped to make adoptive immunotherapy less toxic by using lower doses of IL-2, and more effective by using immune cells which were more reactive to the tumor than LAK cells derived from peripheral blood. They now focused on the mature T cells which often infiltrate solid tumors in great numbers, albeit without displaying the desired cytotoxicity. Would not lymphocytes found in the immediate vicinity of a malignant tumor be somewhat sensitized to it? And could not that sensitivity be enhanced with IL-2, so as to result in tumor-specific cytotoxicity? The preclinical experiments with mice led to a relatively simple technique for obtaining **tumor-infiltrating lymphocytes**—or **TILs** for short. Writing in *Science* in 1986, Rosenberg and his colleagues described how you excised a tumor specimen and minced it into tiny pieces, which were then digested with several enzymes. The resulting cell suspension was passed through a fine sterile filter to remove debris, then cultured in Petri dishes awash with IL-2. "After several days," Rosenberg et al recalled, "small colonies of lymphoid cells could be seen among the tumor cells. The number of lymphoid cells increased and that of tumor cells decreased until about day eight, when nearly all of the remaining cells were lymphocytes." By day fifteen of culture, the number of living TILs had been increased "approximately hundred-fold," and there were no viable cancer cells. When the NCI team tested these TILs against tumor-bearing mice, they discovered that "TILs are 50 to 100 times more effective than LAK cells." These new cells could "mediate the regression of large metastatic tumors" even "in the absence of administered IL-2, although low doses of IL-2 can enhance their therapeutic efficacy."[36]

Metastatic melanoma was the first choice for human TIL trials, because this malignancy produces cutaneous nodules which are easy to excise and which tend to be heavily infiltrated by lymphocytes. In 1988 Rosenberg and his NCI co-workers published a preliminary report in the *New England Journal of Medicine*, describing the administration of TILs and IL-2 to twenty melanoma patients. The TILs obtained from the excised tumor nodules had been "expanded in culture for four to eight weeks"; they were then given to patients in "one to seven infusions," over the course of "one to two days." After the first TIL infusion, patients began receiving intravenous IL-2 every eight hours—this was continued "until dose-limiting toxicity occurred." Rosenberg et al were pleased to report that eleven of the twenty patients responded, a noticeably higher rate (55%) from this single course of treatment than previously obtained in the NCI melanoma patients given multiple courses of LAK cells. TILs were deemed more effective because they were "predominately T lymphocytes and often capable of lysing autologous melanoma in a highly specific fashion." Yet only one of the responding patients had a complete remission which persisted for over a year; the others had partial responses which usually faded away sometime between two and nine months after therapy. The Rosenberg team cautioned that the task of culturing adequate numbers of TILs is "complex and laborious," and that treatment with them "should be considered highly experimental."[37]

IL-2 as Standard Therapy

Those fascinating NCI experiments with LAK cells and TILs, so highly publicized in the 1980s, were not to evolve into a standard therapy of the 1990s. Ensuing events did much to reaffirm the validity of the great caveat in clinical cancer research—**"Don't use laboratory simulations with nude mice to leap to sweeping conclusions about human disease!"** The response rates seen in the pilot studies were not sustained in the larger follow-up trials which the NCI sanctioned. A trial of LAK cells and IL-2 for renal cell carcinoma, conducted at six leading cancer centers, reported a modest 16% response rate, significantly down from the 44% rate Rosenberg et al cited in their initial publication. Subsequent trials of TILs also yielded disappointing results.[38] By the early 1990s everybody knew that interleukin-2 infusions could produce anticancer effects in certain patients, but there was no consensus regarding the *ex vivo* (out-of-body) expansion of lymphocyte populations. Did you really have to remove immune cells and culture them? The multiple leukaphereses required for LAK cell generation were costly, time-consuming, and distressing to patients. Those rarer TILs could not be readily isolated from many types of tumor; and even when they were isolated, they could not always be grown in culture. Would it not be simpler and cheaper just to give patients intravenous IL-2, and let the cytotoxic T cells multiply *in vivo*?

In 1992 the Food and Drug Administration agreed to this proposition, approving the recombinant cytokine as a treatment for metastatic renal cell carcinoma. IL-2 was now readily available under the Cetus brand name **Proleukin**, the generic name for it being **aldesleukin**. The FDA soon added metastatic melanoma as a second approved indication.[39] IL-2 therapy became noticeably

safer after Dr. Rosenberg and his colleagues learned to combat the fluid retention syndrome by giving prophylactic vasopressors (drugs which constrict the blood vessels, such as dopamine and phenylephrine). In 1994 Rosenberg et al described their administration of high-dose IL-2 to 283 patients with metastatic melanoma or renal cell carcinoma. The objective response rates were 17% for melanoma (23 of 134 patients responding) and 20% for renal cell carcinoma (30 of 149 patients responding).[40] A follow-up report detailing the IL-2 therapy given to 409 consecutive patients appeared in 1998. This time Rosenberg and his colleagues provided noteworthy data on the durability of the complete responses. Some 6.6% of the melanoma patients (12 of 182) and some 9.3% of the renal cell patients (21 of 227) enjoyed a gratifying disappearance of all traces of disease. And these regressions were seemingly proving to be permanent. Twelve patients had been in remission, without any detectable disease recurrence, for more than four years—and "fifteen for more than seven years"! Those patients who obtained only partial responses eventually suffered tumor regrowth; but Rosenberg et al observed that that the majority of the complete responders (27 of 33, or 82%) had experienced "perhaps curative tumor regression."[41]

Can IL-2 therapy consistently <u>cure</u> a small but not insignificant percentage of patients with these two immunogenic malignancies? The maturing NCI data strongly suggested that it could do exactly that. And we must assume that all these tumor regressions, whether complete or partial, had been mediated by immune stimulation. IL-2 does not kill cancer cells—it prods lymphocytes into action, which can sometimes be verified. Dr. Rosenberg explains that his team takes sequential biopsy samples of any shrinking metastatic nodules: "We see increasing infiltration of lymphocytes into the lesions as they regress."[42] In those patients who have enjoyed sustained remissions, it would seem that not only did the T lymphocytes acquire tumor-specific cytotoxicity, but that some of them evolved into long-lived memory cells which would go on killing any recurrent cancer cells for years afterward. If this is indeed the fact, we will finally have a believable demonstration of that immune surveillance postulated by Macfarlane Burnet in the 1950s.

Of course, the aforementioned modest successes ought not to make us forget that well over 75% of the NCI patients failed to obtain a significant response to IL-2 therapy. The response rates for the more common tumors (breast, colon, prostate) have been much lower than those recorded for melanoma and renal cell carcinoma. And even when we are dealing with these two immunogenic malignancies, we have no way of predicting which patients will respond to therapy. The best counsel the Rosenberg team has to offer is that most responders can be identified after a single course of IL-2, and that patients who have not responded after two courses are not going to do so and should not be given further treatment.[43] IL-2 fails most of the time because it is—like Coley's toxins and interferon alpha—a crude tool with which to fine-tune an immune response against cancer. By the year 2000, upwards of twenty different interleukins had been isolated and characterized. As the name of this cytokine family implies, these signaling molecules help to coordinate activity "between the leukocytes." But no single interleukin or interferon does the job. An effective immune response comes about through the subtle interplay of dozens of cytokines, some of which intensify leukocyte activity while others serve to modulate it. Immunologists employ the term **cytokine cascade** to characterize these close-knit molecular reactions, but <u>orchestration</u> might be a more descriptive word. "Monotherapy" with this or that cytokine is much like trying to create a symphony by blowing mightily on a single horn. The resulting blast certainly stirs things up, but it usually does not possess the therapeutic properties of great music.

Cancer Vaccines

A vaccine can be just about anything which educates lymphocytes to recognize and combat an agent of disease. The first vaccine that really improved the human lot was itself a pathogen, the **vaccinia virus** which causes mild skin eruptions (cowpox) in diary cows and in persons who milk them. In 1798 the English physician Edward Jenner demonstrated that children inoculated with this pathogen became immune to the disfiguring and often lethal disease smallpox. The relatively benign cowpox virus was structurally similar to the deadly smallpox virus, so much so that an immune system conditioned to reject the former pathogen would also reject the latter. In the 1880s Louis Pasteur proved that even the terrible rabies virus could serve as a preventive vaccine if its virulence was muted by attenuation. Vaccines made from attenuated (weakened) or killed viruses cannot cause disease, but the immunity they produce may be incomplete or short-lived. Those familiar flu vaccines have to be taken every year, because they are based on killed viruses and thus elicit only a brief **humoral immunity**. That is, the body's B cells temporarily produce antibodies to the viral strains involved, giving at best a few months of protection. While most of our vaccines work by stimulating antibody production, an ideal vaccine would elicit **cell-mediated immunity** as well. That is, it would also give rise to a population of cytotoxic T cells which would seek out and destroy any cells infected with the virus or other pathogen causing the disease in question. Lasting protection against any infectious disease depends on a vaccine's ability to generate **memory cells**, a tiny subset of long-lived B or T lymphocytes (or both) which are specifically reactive to the pathological agent and which can rapidly expand their numbers if they should encounter it again.

Our efforts to develop vaccines against viral diseases have been gratifyingly successful. Epidemic scourges like yellow fever, polio, and measles have faded into dim recollection; and juvenile nuisances like chickenpox and mumps are no longer an inevitable part of growing up. The reason for these triumphs has to do with the nature of viruses. They are biologically simple constructs, displaying only a few antigens (surface molecules) which might arouse the immune system. And with the aforementioned viral diseases, the relevant antigens are invariably expressed—(they do not change over time)—and strongly immunogenic. In contrast, influenza viruses are prone to "antigenic drift" (slight alterations in immunogenicity), making the development of a broad-spectrum vaccine extremely difficult. The task of cancer vaccination would seem even more problematic. Any cancer cell is incomparably more complex than the largest virus. The number of surface molecules a cancer cell might display is almost limitless; but none of them is likely to be strongly immunogenic, since they are of self origin and (in most cases) not unique to the tumor. Variability is the rule rather than the exception. Cancer antigens vary from one tumor type to the next, and from one patient to the next—and, yea, even from one malignant cell to the next. Under these circumstances, our hopes for a vaccine depend largely on identifying an antigen or antigens expressed solely or predominantly on the cancer cells, and then of finding some way to intensify that

antigenic element so that the immune system can recognize it.

During the 1980s and 1990s research on cancer vaccines ceased to be regarded as a fool's errand, because we had become much more adept at sorting out the protein molecules expressed on the surface of cells. We had also learned much about how lymphocytes respond to such antigens. Melanoma inspired more vaccine studies than any other type of malignancy. The incidence of this dangerous skin cancer was increasing, as was the mortality from it. Chemotherapy had little effect on metastatic melanoma, which could be rapidly fatal. But now the techniques of DNA analysis and immunostaining led to the identification of some twenty antigens overexpressed by melanoma cells. Donald L. Morton and his colleagues at the John Wayne Cancer Institute (Santa Monica, California), assayed the existing cell lines— that is, the permanent cultures of melanoma cells taken from different patients. Eventually Morton et al selected three cell lines, which together expressed at least fifteen tumor-associated antigens, to produce a **whole-cell vaccine**.[44] The rationale for basing a vaccine on complete cancer cells is to provide the maximum number of antigenic proteins, thereby bettering the odds that one or more of them will evoke the desired immune response. Scientists already knew that the membranous proteins found on one patient's cancer cells are sometimes identical to those on cancer cells from other patients— this is especially apt to be true with melanomas.

In 1984 Dr. Morton and his co-workers began giving **CancerVax**, as they called their live-cell vaccine, to patients with metastatic melanoma. The vaccine was irradiated before use, with a view to making it more antigenic and to removing any chance that the cancer cells might proliferate. During the first two treatments, CancerVax was injected together with *bacille Calmette-Guérin* (BCG), an attenuated (nonvirulent) strain of the tuberculosis bacillus. Although BCG could not specifically elicit an immune response against melanoma, the John Wayne team hoped that it would function as **an adjuvant**—viz., that it would attract lymphocytes and other immune cells to the injection site and enhance their activity. Writing in 1996, Dr. Morton and his colleague Andreas Barth explained that since melanoma antigens are only weakly immunogenic, patients were "immunized repeatedly for prolonged periods." The side effects from CancerVax were far milder than those associated with chemotherapy, typically consisting of localized reactions at the injection sites. Since the vaccine did not kill cancer cells directly, it never produced rapid shrinkage of metastatic lesions. Morton and Barth pointed out that the documented tumor regressions depended on "humoral and cell-mediated immune responses, which evolved over a period of twelve to fourteen weeks." Any slowing of tumor growth could not be detected in the first three or four months of therapy; but once a response occurred, it was "usually durable, lasting from months to years."[45]

Conscientious scientists that they are, Morton and his John Wayne colleagues have been careful not to overstate the effectiveness of CancerVax. In a 1998 survey of their results, they cited a response rate of only 15% to 20%, while claiming that the responding patients did enjoy "significantly longer survival than historical control patients." Morton et al also reported that they had developed assays which accurately distinguished between responders and nonresponders. Circulating antibodies to the prevalent melanoma antigen TA90 ("a 90-kilodalton tumor-associated glycoprotein") were deemed good evidence of a humoral

response to the vaccine. And a positive result on a skin test for delayed-type hypersensitivity (DTH) provided adequate evidence of a T cell-mediated response. Those John Wayne patients who did not develop antibodies to TA90 or any DTH reactions proved to have noticeably shortened life expectancies. The five-year survival rate for this group was only 8%; in contrast, the rate for those patients who assayed positive on both tests was 75%.[46]

CancerVax has not been a sure-fire cure for melanoma, nor has its true level of effectiveness been properly evaluated in large-scale randomized trials. But the data coming from the John Wayne Cancer Institute have spurred efforts to develop vaccines for other tumor types. Elizabeth M. Jaffee and her colleagues at Johns Hopkins also focused on whole-cell vaccines. They think that **autologous tumor cells**—those taken from the patient—"would be the best source of immunizing proteins, since they would likely display all of the relevant tumor antigens for inducing antitumor immunity in the patient." Unfortunately, adequate numbers of autologous tumor cells are "rarely available because of the reactive processes that are found infiltrating many common cancers." In designing an experimental vaccine for pancreatic cancer, Dr. Jaffee and her team relied on two allogeneic cell lines, both of which had been "stably transfected" with the gene for granulocyte-macrophage colony-stimulating factor (GM-CSF). The rationale for this particular gene transfer lies in the fact that GM-CSF attracts and powerfully stimulates many immune cells, especially the dendritic cells which play an important role in T cell activation. As with other cytokines, GM-CSF given intravenously will cause side effects and will be rapidly cleared from the bloodstream; moreover, it would not approximate the physiological secretion of this cytokine by the individual cells during a spontaneous immune response. By putting the GM-CSF gene in the pancreatic cancer cells being used as a vaccine, Jaffee et al hoped to obtain physiological cytokine secretion at and around the injection site—viz., at the very spot where immune cells would come into contact with the tumor antigens.[47]

Dr. Jaffee and her colleagues gave their experimental vaccine to fourteen patients who had undergone surgery for pancreatic cancer at Johns Hopkins. Different doses, consisting of larger or smaller numbers of the allogeneic tumor cells, were given to different patients. All injections were administered "intradermally into three different limbs," with a view to involving several different groups of lymph nodes (axillary and inguinal) in an antitumor response. Afterwards Jaffee and her colleagues sought to determine whether the vaccine really had generated a population of tumor-reactive T cells. To this end they injected patients with their own tumor cells, which had been frozen immediately after surgery. Three patients who received large doses of the vaccine displayed pronounced delayed-type hypersensitivity (DTH) to this challenge, manifested by skin reactions greater than one centimeter in diameter. This finding was deemed indicative of numerous tumor-reactive T cells. When reporting the results of their vaccine trial in 2001, Jaffee et al observed that although the other eleven patients had already suffered disease recurrence, the three patients with the vigorous DTH reactions still remained disease-free.[48]

The aforementioned findings from the John Wayne Cancer Institute and Johns Hopkins should encourage us to anticipate that allogeneic whole-cell vaccines, perhaps enhanced by immunogenic adjuvants or by inserted cytokine genes, will soon play a role in treating chemotherapy-resistant solid tumors. Researchers at Johns Hopkins have

also experimented with autologous whole-cell vaccines for prostate cancer and renal cell carcinoma. This technique is considerably more time-consuming. Some of the patient's own tumor cells must first be grown (expanded) in culture, then transfected with an immunostimulatory cytokine gene and subsequently irradiated, before being injected intradermally (within the skin).[49] Other methodologies being investigated by cancer researchers include **lysate vaccines**, made from tumor cells which have been mechanically disrupted (broken up), and **peptide vaccines** using those tiny bits of protein which are what T cells actually recognize as foreign and react against. Peptide vaccines are also known as "pure antigen vaccines."[50]

Vigorous experimentation aimed at developing **breast cancer vaccines** did not get underway until the 1990s, but by the year 2000 several research groups were conducting Phase One trials of innovative therapies. Such trials typically recruit a handful of patients suffering from advanced disease, with a view more to learning about a proposed treatment's side effects than to establishing its effectiveness. John W. Smith II and his co-workers at the Providence Portland Medical Center in Portland, Oregon, were testing a whole-cell vaccine. They took an allogeneic breast cancer cell line and transfected it with the gene for CD80 (also known as B7-1). When other leukocytes need to activate helper or cytotoxic T cells, they switch on the CD80 gene—it produces a potent costimulatory molecule which helps T cells to respond to antigens.[51] Donald W. Kufe of the Dana-Farber Cancer Center and allied Boston researchers decided a base an experimental vaccine on vaccinia, that highly immunogenic but relatively benign cowpox pathogen. This time the well-known virus had been genetically modified so as to express DF3 and MUC-1, antigenic proteins associated with many breast carcinomas. Mary L. Disis of the University of Washington in Seattle led a team which put peptides from the HER-2/*neu* protein into tiny microspheres also containing GM-CSF. Eligibility for this trial was limited to those patients whose breast tumors overexpressed the HER-2/*neu* gene.[52]

In the year 2000 the only breast cancer vaccine that seemed on the verge of commercial distribution was **Theratope** (brand name), a drug that had been in the works at the Canadian pharmaceutical company Biomira for almost a decade. Theratope grew out of research on **mucins**, glycoproteins that are found in the outer membranes of normal ductal cells in the breast as well as on the surfaces of normal cells in other organs. When mammary cells turn malignant, however, they tend to express an abnormal mucin with an exposed protein core. This has been named **mucin-1** or simply **MUC-1**. Since the early 1990s researchers have known that MUC-1 was sufficiently antigenic that it could, under the appropriate circumstances, activate helper and cytotoxic T cells. Theratope combines a synthetic version of MUC-1 with an adjuvant rife with bacterial antigens. The results from preliminary trials suggested that this vaccine might induce disease remission in some patients. Biomira subsequently recruited 950 women with metastatic breast cancer for a randomized Phase Three trial, to be conducted at numerous hospitals in the United States, Canada, Australia, and several European nations.[53]

If Theratope and other breast cancer vaccines prove to have at least minimal therapeutic activity, we may anticipate that they will win FDA approval and then be enthusiastically marketed by their manufacturers. Yet it seems unrealistic to expect that any current vaccine strategy will lead to predictable cures for breast malignancies.

Vaccines, like chemotherapy, may well help certain patients while doing nothing of value for others. The strongest selling points for immunogenic agents will probably be that they are nontoxic and that they can easily be combined with chemotherapy regimens or with hormonal drugs.

Dendritic Cells:
The Key to T Cell Activation?

The reason why most vaccines evoke only humoral (antibody-mediated) immunity is that B cells are relatively easy to activate. If equipped with appropriate receptors, B cells can respond to circulating antigens on their own initiative, without interacting with other leukocytes. T cell activation, deemed so important in cancer immunotherapy, is much more difficult. Those NCI experiments with LAK cells and tumor-infiltrating lymphocytes showed us that it is not enough simply to multiply vast numbers of T cells—nothing will happen unless those T cells are specifically "educated" to recognize the tumor cells as foreign. And before T cells can respond to a malignancy or to a microbial pathogen, they must first be activated by **antigen-presenting cells** (APCs). In theory, virtually any cell in the body could function as an APC; in practice, leukocytes do most of the work. Macrophages exemplify the APC's routine task, which is phagocytose (swallow up) a bacterium, disassemble it in the cytoplasm, and then present protein fragments from it (peptides) on the outer membrane for T cell recognition. Contemporary immunologists postulate that a T cell must receive three unmistakable signals from an APC before becoming sensitized to a particular antigen. The first is a copious display of MHC molecules on the APC's surface—i.e., those specialized proteins of the **major**

histocompatibility complex (MHC) which mark a body cell as self rather than as an outside invader. The second signal is provided by an antigenic peptide complexed (bound) to the APC's MHC molecules. Given the presence of these two signals, what a T cell would perceive is a friendly cell reporting a serious problem—that antigenic peptide sticks out like a sore thumb in the cluster of MHC molecules.[54] But before the T cell can move to eliminate the antigen, the APC must provide yet another signal (the third) in the form of **costimulatory molecules**. These are membrane proteins which promote temporary adhesion between the APC and the T cell, and which typically stimulate both cells into a purposeful immune response. Tim F. Greten and Elizabeth M. Jaffee of Johns Hopkins remind us that "the context in which the antigen is presented to the immune system seems to determine whether or not a T cell becomes activated. In the absence of appropriate costimulatory signals, engagement of the T cell receptor itself can lead to ignorance, anergy, or even apoptotic death of the T cell, scenarios that are the complete opposite of what one might wish."[55]

We may gain some inkling of the vast explosion in our immunological knowledge by pondering **dendritic cells** (DCs). In the year 1970 even our Nobel-prize-winning immunologists could not tell us what function these highly specialized leukocytes performed. By the late 1990s researchers throughout the world had begun to regard DCs as the most plausible key to T cell activation and the successful immunotherapy of cancer. A 1998 review in the British journal *Nature* went so far as to state that the functions of both B and T cells are "under the control of dendritic cells."[56] While this may be a slight exaggeration, no one questions that DCs do a splendid job of presenting

antigens to T cells. Indeed, that is their principal function—*they are the body's professional APCs!*

Though long neglected, dendritic cells were recognized as early as 1868, when the pathologist Paul Langerhans described the large leukocytes he saw scattered throughout the epidermis (outer layer of the skin). These cells were loosely associated with, but not attached to, the neighboring keratinocytes (skin cells). Their distinctive feature was the dendritic processes (branchlike projections) which they sent into the adjacent intercellular spaces. **Langerhans cells** (as these epidermal DCs came to be called) did not seem to be doing anything. We now know that DCs will remain immature and quiescent until they come into contact with microbes, which they would phagocytose, or with antigenic particles, which they would absorb. Once a DC has been exposed to an antigen, however, it becomes exceptionally active. The cell's expression of MHC and costimulatory molecules increases at the same time it is sending peptide fragments of processed antigen to its outer membrane. Meanwhile, the cell leaves its tentative mooring in the peripheral tissues and starts to migrate toward the nearby lymph nodes, which contain naive B and T lymphocytes awaiting instructions. Upon its arrival in a lymph node, the DC is fully mature and easily recognizable by its distinctive morphology. It is now a large, roughly star-shaped cell with thin veil-like projections extending out in all directions. The immunologists Jacques Banchereau and Ralph M. Steinman observe that "the shape and motility of DCs fit their functions, which are to capture antigens and select antigen-specific T cells."[57]

The idea of using dendritic cells in cancer therapy seems to have occurred to everybody all at once. Could not DCs be multiplied *ex vivo* and then loaded down with tumor-derived peptides? That might educate

A Mature Dendritic Cell

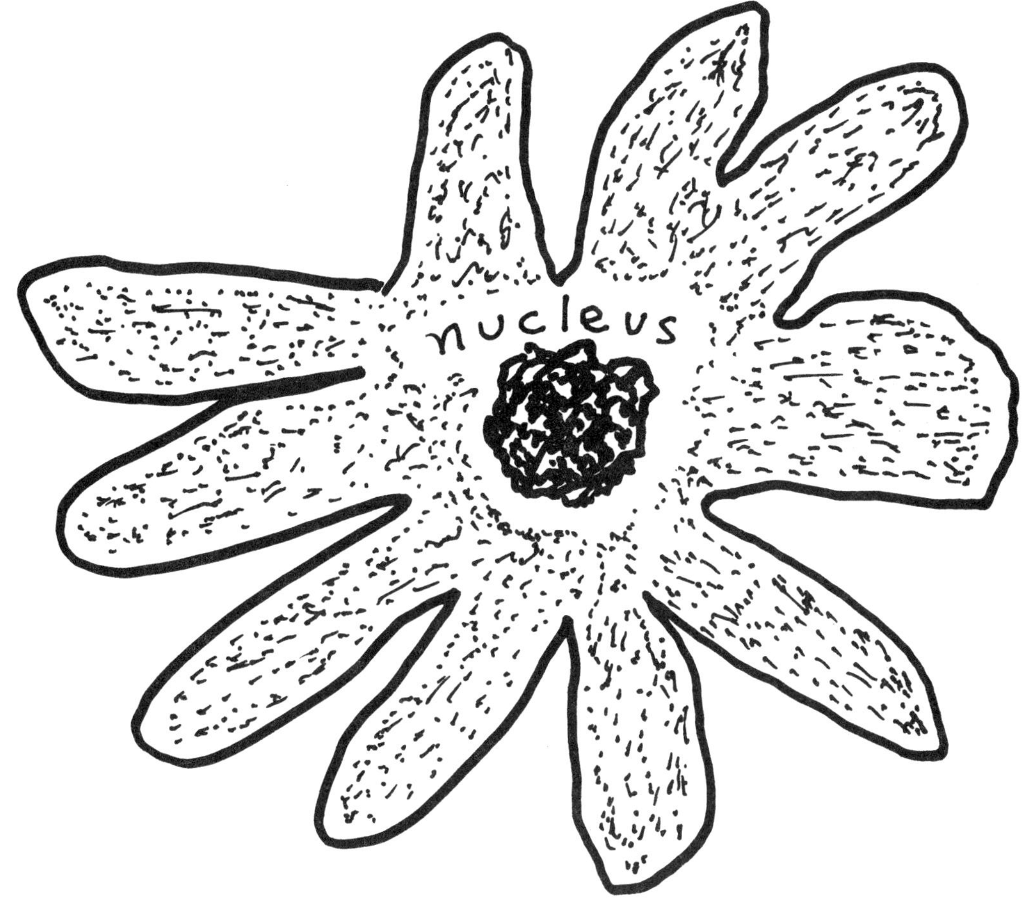

Dendritic cells are characterized by large irregular nuclei and by numerous dendritic (branching) projections. They play a crucial role in generating immune responses to microbial pathogens, first capturing antigens (foreign particles) and then presenting them to lymphocytes (white cells) in the regional lymph nodes. Cultivated dendritic cells which are "pulsed with" (exposed to) tumor-associated antigens may possibly prove useful in stimulating an immune response to cancer.

those T cells to recognize the tumor! And what about transfecting DCs with oncogenes like *ras*, *p53*, or HER-2/*neu*? That might put the tumor-initiating proteins on the surface of DCs, in a context where they would become immunogenic. But before such strategies could be tried in patients, methods of harvesting and culturing human DCs had to be developed. Immature dendritic cells can be detected in tissues throughout the body, notably in the epidermis, the respiratory tract, and the spleen; yet these sites do not lend themselves to cellular harvests. Like other leukocytes, DCs evolve from the hematopoietic stem cells of the bone marrow. By the mid-1990s we knew that an appropriate mix of cytokines and growth factors would cause stem cells growing in culture to differentiate into DCs, but the method required a troublesome extraction of marrow. Researchers soon developed a simpler technique—it relied upon **peripheral blood mononuclear cells** (PBMCs), partially differentiated leukocytes in the general circulation which retain the capacity to evolve either into DCs or into macrophages. All you had to do was to draw blood, separate the PBMCs by mechanical means such as centrifugation or sedimentation, and then incubate them with GM-CSF and interleukin-4. After a week or so the cultured PBMCs will assume the characteristic stellate morphology of DCs; more importantly, they will express the CD83 surface molecule, which is unique to cells of dendritic lineage. Anita Reddy and her colleagues at Rockefeller University caution that DCs cultured in GM-CSF and IL-4 alone are unstable: they tend to "revert to a more adherent form" and "take on macrophage characteristics."[58] Other cytokines must be added to culture to approximate the natural differentiation of PBMCs into DCs which occurs in the body. Michael A. Morse and his team at Duke University emphasize that tumor necrosis factor alpha (TNF-alpha) is essential to produce mature DCs, yet they advise that its addition to culture should be delayed. "Immature DCs may be more effective at antigen processing," Morse et al opine, "whereas mature DCs may be better at T cell stimulation. Consequently, one approach to using DCs in a vaccination protocol would be to generate immature DCs with GM-CSF and IL-4, pulse the DCs with antigen, and then briefly treat the DCs with TNF alpha before inoculation."[59]

Dendritic cells represent an exciting development in cancer immunotherapy. The treatment strategies in the offing propose to blend the methodologies of adoptive immunotherapy and its *ex vivo* cell expansion with those of antigen-based vaccination. While we do not know how effective these strategies will be in routine clinical practice, we are optimistic about their prospects. Writing in the year 2000, Jan Baggers and other physicians at the Memorial Sloan-Kettering Cancer Center confidently observed that "tumors have antigens, and dendritic cells have everything else needed to stimulate T cell immunity. The challenge then is how best to combine the two, now that sufficient numbers of dendritic cells are obtainable."[60]

Clinical trials presently being conducted with melanoma patients may be the first to tell us whether we really know as much about tumor antigens, T cells, and DCs as we think we do. Several Phase One trials have been designed to test DC-based strategies in breast malignancies. Samir N. Khleif and other investigators at the National Cancer Institute selected a peptide encoded by a mutant *p53* gene as their antigen. In one arm of their breast cancer trial, patients were to receive DCs cultured in GM-CSF and IL-4 which had been exposed to "pulses" (intermittent doses) of the *p53* peptide. In the other arm, patients were to receive the

the peptide vaccine simultaneously with GM-CSF, but no DCs.[61] Perhaps this trial will help to determine whether the *ex vivo* generation and peptide pulsing of DCs is necessary, or whether just giving patients the tumor antigen together with GM-CSF would produce equivalent results. Dr. Baggers and the Sloan-Kettering team remind us that GM-CSF "has consistently proven to be the most pivotal cytokine for dendritic cell growth, differentiation, and survival."[62]

In the year 2000 cancer immunologists, including Michael A. Morse of Duke, were investigating the potential of a newly discovered cytokine known as **Flt3 ligand** (Flt3L). Dr. Morse and his colleagues demonstrated that daily Flt3L injections could increase the number of DC precursors in the blood of cancer patients, without causing troublesome side effects.[63] Perhaps cytokine "cocktails" of GM-CSF and Flt3L given directly to patients will become the first standard DC therapy. We would naturally expect the simplest and least expensive approach to triumph, unless *ex vivo* techniques prove to have decided therapeutic advantages. At the moment few immunologists believe that any manipulation of dendritic cells will emerge as a primary treatment for cancer. However, there is considerable expectation that one or more approaches will soon be used as adjuvant therapy, given to better the odds of survival after the traditional modalities (surgery, irradiation, and chemotherapy) have reduced the tumor burden.

Monoclonal Antibodies:
The B Cell Contribution

Our hopes for effective immunotherapies have naturally tended to focus on T cells, whose potential ability to kill cancer cells provides vivid copy for science writers. But we should not forget those B cells which represent the other half of the adaptive immune response—viz., **antibody-mediated immunity**. An immature B lymphocyte which has been activated by a particular antigen will quickly differentiate into a **plasma cell**. The task of a plasma cell (i.e., the mature and fully functional B cell) is to secrete antibodies which specifically bind to the particular activating antigen. Each plasma cell (cellular clone) will produce multitudinous copies of the same identical antibody—that is, **monoclonal antibodies** or **MAbs**. Antibodies are minuscule bits of protein floating in the bloodstream. They do not kill pathogens outright; but by sticking to the surface of bacteria or viruses, they hamper the movement and reproduction of these microorganisms, and help to mark them for destruction by effector leukocytes (neutrophils, macrophages, and killer T cells). Blood tests for the presence of specific antibodies have long been used to determine whether individuals have been infected with *Treponemia pallidum*, the spirochete which causes syphilis, or with HIV, the human immunodeficiency virus which causes AIDS.

No comparable assays exist to detect subclinical malignancy, for the simple reason that cancer cells do not normally activate B cells any more than they normally activate T cells. Notwithstanding this fact, we knew that tumor-specific antibodies would have numerous applications in cancer medicine if only we could learn how to produce them. By the early 1970s experiments with laboratory mice had taught us that, yes, tumor cells sometimes express immunogenic molecules on their outer membranes, and that, yes, B cells will sometimes secrete antibodies which bind to these antigens. But there was a large obstacle to any practical application of this knowledge. We would need enormous quantities of tumor-specific MAbs for diagnostic assays or therapeutic drugs—and this meant that we would have to grow the antibody-producing B cells in permanent artificial cultures. Unfortunately, B cells do not normally multiply in culture; they die.

In 1975 Georges Köhler and Cesar Milstein, two biologists at Cambridge University, announced a novel solution to the problem of antibody production. First they had injected mice with a strong antigen (in this case, red blood cells taken from sheep). Then they had extracted B cells from the spleens of the immunized mice—these cells were producing MAbs specific for the antigen, but of course they could not be maintained in culture. What Köhler and Milstein did next was to culture these B cells with a line of mice myeloma cells, in the presence of the Sendai virus. Myeloma cells are B cells which have undergone malignant transformation; like other cancer cells they are "immortalized" and can be grown in culture. The Sendai virus is an agent which can occasionally induce cell infusion. In this famous experiment, some of the antibody-producing B cells successfully fused with the immortalized myeloma cells. **Hybridomas**, as these new hybrid cells were dubbed, proved to have the very attributes everybody was looking for. Like mature B cells, they secreted antibodies specific for a particular antigen; like malignant myeloma cells, they could be artificially maintained. When announcing this discovery in the journal *Nature*, Köhler and Milstein modestly pointed out that hybridomas "can be grown *in vitro* in massive cultures to provide specific antibody. Such cultures could be valuable for medical and industrial use."[64]

Köhler and Milstein received a Nobel prize for their work in 1984. Hybridoma cultures now strike us as a crude way to manufacture MAbs, this approach having been largely superseded by the more sophisticated techniques of genetic engineering. Yet we should never forget what a sweeping

revolution in diagnostics came about because of hybridomas. Suddenly we had MAb reagents which could identify the tiniest traces of a sought-after protein. The home pregnancy test was perhaps the most familiar example—a reagent placed in a urine sample would change color if its constituent MAb bound to the pregnancy-associated hormone hCG (human chorionic gonadotropin). Pathology reports on tumors soon became more informative, because the new MAb-based "immunostains" gave us visual evidence as to whether the cancer cells expressed estrogen receptors or as to whether they harbored defects in the *p53* and HER-2/*neu* genes. If not precisely quantitative, at least these assays promised to be rapid and inexpensive.

The prospect of therapeutic applications excited pharmaceutical companies. Here was a new and seemingly nontoxic modality for cancer! What if disseminated tumor cells could be bombarded with those sticky MAbs? That might slow the chain of events we call metastasis. And protein antibodies which bound to the malignant cells would actually become cytotoxic if they could be "labeled with"—that is, *made to carry*—radioactive isotopes or molecules of cytotoxic drugs. Assuming the MAbs bound exclusively to the cancer cells, this strategy promised to vastly reduce the toxicity associated with irradiation and chemotherapy. Labeled MAbs would become (as it were) guided missiles which delivered their deadly warheads only to precisely-targeted tumor cells.

The malignancies offering the most fertile field to test these hypotheses seemed to be low-grade B cell lymphomas. Chemotherapy is of limited value against these sluggish tumors. But the surfaces of B cells, normal or malignant, are studded with antigen receptors and distinctive molecular markers, providing an easy target for MAb interventions. In 1982 the *New England*

Journal of Medicine reported the case history of a terminal lymphoma patient who achieved a durable remission after treatment with MAbs specially prepared for his tumor cells.[65] In the 1990s efforts to develop practical lymphoma drugs were intensified. The new MAbs targeted the CD20 surface molecule, which is heavily expressed on B cells but not on other cells. Some investigators labeled their anti-CD20 MAbs with the radioisotope iodine-131. Radiation-emitting MAbs promised to be more effective—they would not necessarily need to bind to every lymphoma cell, since they could kill malignant cells simply by being nearby. This attribute could prove important in cases where a percentage of lymphoma cells strongly express the CD20 molecule while others have variable or minimal expression. In 1993 the *New England Journal of Medicine* reported an experiment done at the University of Michigan in Ann Arbor. An iodine-131-labeled MAb had been given to nine patients with "CD20-positive B cell lymphomas" who had failed chemotherapy. Four patients achieved complete remissions, and the side effects from therapy proved to be mild.[66]

The encouraging results with a handful of lymphoma patients provided the inspiration for Grant Fjermedal's *Magic Bullets* (1984), Marshall Goldberg's *Cell Wars* (1988), and other ebullient books which tended to leave naive readers with the impression that MAb-based therapies would soon be able to cure most cancers. This was hardly the fact. In the late 1980s and early 1990s, research on therapeutic applications almost seemed to get bogged down as we became more familiar with the inherent biological obstacles. Variability of antigen expression was a fundamental problem. For the vast majority of malignancies, we did not have a convenient membranous target like the CD20 molecule. Labeling MAbs with

isotopes, drugs, or toxins worked better in the test tube than in patients, where these conjugations typically proved to be unstable and unwieldy. An experiment done at the Duke University Medical Center illustrated the necessity of doing one's homework. In 1987 a MAb conjugated with ricin, a potent plant toxin, was given to five patients with metastatic breast cancer. The trial had to be stopped prematurely when these patients developed "debilitating plexopathies and neuropathies."[67] The Duke team belatedly discovered that the immunoconjugate not only bound to breast cancer cells, but to nerve cells as well!

Pharmacokinetics posed a question mark, regardless of whether the infused MAbs were labeled or unlabeled. Antibodies are teeny-weeny objects compared to cells, but they are monstrously large molecules compared to most drugs used in cancer medicine. Because of their bulk, they cannot penetrate into the interior of poorly vascularized tumors; and they are prone to be arrested and degraded in the liver. James L. Mulshine of the National Cancer Institute observes that MAbs are "passive jellyfish floating through the bloodstream. The chance of one meeting up with the appropriate tumor antigen is small. At least 99.99% are degraded or cleared without ever finding their desired target."[68] An obvious response to this inefficiency would be to give larger doses and repeated administrations of MAbs, so that the 0.01% of the drug which is not degraded would eventually achieve therapeutic levels. In the early 1990s, however, this strategy was not feasible. Human cells did not lend themselves to hybridoma creation; the upshot was that the MAbs then being used were of murine origin—that is, made in mice cells. After the first MAb infusion, the patient's immune system would start to manufacture antibodies directed against the murine proteins. This immune reaction would cause unpleasant symptoms and block the antitumor activity of the murine MAbs; it became more pronounced with each additional dose, eventually necessitating the discontinuance of therapy.

By the mid-1990s pharmaceutical companies were racing to design MAbs which would be less likely to elicit disabling immune reactions. These new agents were designated as **chimeric MAbs** (part murine, part human) or as **fully humanized MAbs** (no significant murine elements). Various strategies were used to produce them. Human immunoglobulin genes could be inserted into specially-bred mice which lacked their own antibody-producing genes. Another option was to put the cloned human genes into that bacterial workhorse *Escherichia coli*.[69] Between November 1997 and September 2000, no fewer than eight of these less immunogenic MAbs were approved by the Food and Drug Administration.[70] The pharmaceutical company Genentech, based in South San Francisco, scored a coup with its **rituximab**, the first MAb to become a standard cancer therapy. Marketed under the brand name **Rituxan**, this agent is a chimeric MAb indicated for "relapsed or refractory low-grade, CD20-positive, B cell non-Hodgkin's lymphoma." In 2001 Genentech estimated that some 38,000 Americans had already received Rituxan. The firm's advertisements cited a clinical trial which had reported an overall response rate of 48%, with 11.6 months being the "median duration of response."[71]

Several labeled MAbs also seem likely to play a growing role in the treatment of hematologic malignancies. **Mylotarg** (a Wyeth-Ayerst brand name) combines a MAb against the CD33 surface molecule found on myeloid leukocytes with a potent antibiotic; the FDA has approved this agent for the treatment of relapsed acute myelogenous leukemia. Coulter Pharmaceuticals' **Bexxar**

(brand name) combines an anti-CD20 MAb with iodine-131—a Phase Three trial using this agent has reported a 70% response rate in relapsed low-grade B cell lymphomas.[72] Since it would be misleading to convey the impression that oncology is the only medical specialty standing to benefit from the new therapeutic MAbs, we can profitably mention several important applications which have nothing to do with malignancy. Recipients of transplanted hearts, kidneys, and other organs now have a better chance of achieving a normal life span because of **daclizumab**. This humanized MAb binds to the interleukin-2 receptor, thereby muting the activity of T cells which would otherwise attack the transplanted tissues. Patients with rheumatoid arthritis and Crohn's disease, two debilitating autoimmune disorders, can be grateful for **infliximab**. This chimeric MAb binds to and neutralizes tumor necrosis factor alpha, an inflammatory cytokine which has been implicated in both maladies.[73]

HERCEPTIN
Targeting a Breast Cancer Gene

The first antibody drug to become standard therapy for a solid tumor was **trastuzumab**. This is an unconjugated humanized MAb. It acquired considerable celebrity in late 1998 after the FDA approved it for metastatic breast cancer, and Genentech began to market it under the brand name **Herceptin**. Just as the first vials of trastuzumab had started to arrive in oncologists' offices, their patients were rushing to acquire a new book entitled *Her-2: The Making of Herceptin, a Revolutionary Treatment for Breast Cancer* (Random House, 1998). Written by the NBC science correspondent Robert Bazell, this book provided a behind-the-scenes look at the American pharmaceutical industry in the

1990s. But its most compelling stories are those of a few terminal patients whose lives were saved by Herceptin.

Attentive readers of *The Breast Cancer Epidemic* will recognize that the title *Her-2* refers to the HER-2/*neu* gene located on chromosome 17, which we discussed in Chapter Three. This gene encodes a growth factor receptor for the cell's outer membrane. The HER-2 protein is closely related to several other growth factor receptors situated on that plasma membrane, whose collective function when activated is to send signals to the nucleus calling for cell division. These related proteins include the **epidermal growth factor receptor** (also called HER-1) and two receptors dubbed HER-3 and HER-4 respectively. Mark X. Sliwkowski and his co-workers at Genentech point out that these HER family receptors are "rarely, if ever, expressed alone within a given tissue, but are found in various combinations." HER-2/*neu* and its protein got singled out for intensive research at Genentech because in some 25% to 30% of breast carcinomas, this particular gene is amplified. In other words, during the numerous divisions leading to full-fledged malignancy, an affected cancer cell will have somehow accumulated multiple copies of the HER-2/*neu* gene. And the upshot is that the tumor cell's outer membrane will eventually become saturated with growth-stimulating protein. "Gene amplification," Sliwkowski et al observe, "results in HER-2 protein levels that are tenfold to a hundredfold greater than those found in the adjacent normal breast epithelium."[74] We have never identified the growth factor which binds to the HER-2 receptor—the ligand (binding molecule) may actually be interacting more with the EGF receptor (HER-1) or with HER-3 or HER-4. But this is a moot point. Since the pioneering studies of Dennis J. Slamon and his UCLA colleagues in the late 1980s, we have known that amplification of

the HER-2/*neu* gene and an excess of its protein product will necessarily translate into aggressive breast malignancies and shorter survival times. The same situation seems to prevail in ovarian, gastric, lung, and prostatic carcinomas with HER-2/*neu* overexpression. That pathological excess of receptor protein means that signals to divide are constantly being sent to a tumor cell's nucleus.[75]

By 1990 researchers at Genentech had demonstrated that an unconjugated murine MAb known as 4D5 could interrupt the aforementioned signals. Simply by binding to the HER-2 protein, the antibodies nullified its growth stimulatory effects. In laboratory experiments, 4D5 consistently reduced the number of cancer cells in S-phase when added to HER-2-positive cultures. Paul Carter and his Genentech colleagues reported the successful "humanization" of 4D5 in 1992. Not only was the humanized MAb less immunogenic, but it "bound its antigen threefold more tightly than the parent antibody."[76]

Genentech called its drug Herceptin for marketing purposes. Several Phase One trials quickly established that Herceptin was reasonably safe for humans, and a larger Phase Two trial headed by José Baselga of the Memorial Sloan-Kettering Cancer Center showed us how remarkably well-tolerated this agent could be. Baselga et al gave weekly infusions to 43 breast cancer patients with HER-2 overexpression and "extensive metastatic disease." Five of these patients did develop "fever and chills" after the first dose of Herceptin, but "the fever lasted less than eight hours and did not recur on subsequent administrations." Those dreaded chemo-type side effects (nausea, vomiting, hair loss) simply did not occur. Reporting the trial's results in 1996, Baselga et al sounded a note of optimism about the drug's therapeutic potential. One of their patients achieved a complete response and had remained in remission (no evidence of disease) for over two years. Four other patients had partial responses (tumor shrinkage by 50% or more), which lasted from one to 7.7 months. While the demonstrable response rate was a modest 11.6% (only five of the 43 patients responding), Baselga et al pointed to 16 additional patients who had experienced minor responses or stable disease. They felt that almost half the treated patients did in fact benefit from Herceptin, suggesting that "stable disease may be an authentic reflection of the biologic action of the drug, which differs markedly from conventional anti-cancer agents."[77]

The Chicago oncologist Melody A. Cobleigh headed an important international trial which began in April 1995 and which eventually treated 213 breast cancer patients with the weekly infusions of Herceptin. Responses were evaluated by an independent committee whose members had been "blinded to treatment" when reviewing X-rays and CAT scans. Even with these stringent criteria, the committee identified eight complete responders (3.8%) and 26 partial responders (12.2%), for an overall response rate of 16%. Dr. Cobleigh and her colleagues found this response rate encouraging in view of the patients' advanced metastatic disease: "The study population had a very poor prognosis. Most patients had visceral disease because of the requirement for bidimensionally measurable disease. Patients were heavily pretreated. The great majority had received multiple chemotherapy regimens, and approximately one-fourth had undergone bone marrow or stem cell transplantation."[78]

The trials headed by Drs. Baselga and Cobleigh should convince us that while Herceptin as a single agent can sometimes induce complete remissions of HER-2-positive tumors, it is unlikely to be curative in cases of widespread metastatic disease.

In the year 2000 several correspondents to the *Journal of Clinical Oncology* emphasized its pharmacokinetic limitations. A bulky molecule like other MAbs, Herceptin does not readily transverse the blood-brain barrier. Peripheral infusions of it would therefore be ineffective against brain metastases.[79] But few oncologists wanted to use Herceptin as a single agent. Dennis J. Slamon headed the Phase Three trial which demonstrated that Herceptin combined with chemotherapy was more effective than chemotherapy alone as a first-line treatment for metastatic breast cancer. Between June 1995 and March 1997, Dr. Slamon and his international co-workers enrolled 469 patients whose pathology work-ups had revealed at least moderate staining of tumor cell membranes for the HER-2 protein. These patients were then randomly assigned to receive the popular AC regimen (doxorubicin and cyclophosphamide) or the taxoid drug paclitaxel (if they had previously been treated with doxorubicin), or to receive the identical chemotherapy together with concurrent weekly infusions of Herceptin. The preliminary results from this trial were made public at the May 1998 meeting of the American Society of Clinical Oncology—only 36.2% of the patients getting chemo alone had responded to treatment, but fully 62% of those getting chemo plus Herceptin had done so.[80] By the time the trial's final report appeared in the *New England Journal of Medicine* on March 15, 2001, it was clear that the new MAb drug had produced a modest but statistically significant improvement in survival times. The median duration of response was 6.1 months in the patients given chemotherapy alone, but 9.1 months in those patients who also received Herceptin. At one year after the completion of treatment, 33% of the patients in the chemo arm had died, compared to only 22% of those in the Herceptin arm. "Few studies of metastatic breast cancer," wrote Dr. Slamon and his colleagues, "have demonstrated a survival advantage of this magnitude in association with the addition of a single agent."[81]

Unfortunately, that big Phase Three trial also exposed a hidden worm in the Herceptin apple—a dangerous side effect which had not been suggested by the pre-clinical tests or by the earlier trials. When given together with an anthracycline like Adriamycin (doxorubicin), this well-tolerated antibody drug can contribute mightily to cardiac dysfunction, which typically manifests itself by a reduced ability of the heart's left ventricle to pump blood. We have already discussed Adriamycin's potential to surreptitiously damage the heart muscle. The 8% incidence of cardiac dysfunction in the Phase Three patients receiving the AC regimen had not been unexpected—what was surprising was the 27% incidence recorded in those patients who received AC concurrently with Herceptin. The most plausible explanation for this finding would be that Adriamycin exposure causes an initial injury to the myocytes (heart cells), which is then compounded by Herceptin's binding to their surface membranes. The distressed heart cells apparently express just enough of the HER-2 protein to cause this unwanted drug interaction.[82] Oncologists now know that Herceptin should be given cautiously to patients who are elderly, who have cardiovascular disorders, or who have had prior anthracycline exposure.

We may be justly proud of the vast acumen illustrated by the development of Herceptin. First our scientists arrived at a sufficient understanding of a genetic defect which promotes the progression of malignancy. And then they came up with a drug which specifically targets this defect. *That's the sort of cancer medicine we want to see!!* Drugs which combat the malignant cells— and by and large don't bother normal cells!

Unhappily, Herceptin does have one thing in common with the indiscriminately cytotoxic chemotherapy—viz., it only works for a minority of patients, and we are not sure how to identify that minority. Those durable remissions written up in Robert Bazell's book *Her-2* have been exceptions to the rule. To begin with, this drug stands to be useless in the 70% to 75% of breast cancer cases which do not have HER-2/*neu* overexpression. And the objective response rates seen in the single-agent trials done by Baselga et al and by Cobleigh et al (11.6% and 16% respectively) show us that even when we are treating supposedly HER-2-positive patients, therapeutic effectiveness is not a foregone conclusion. We do know that increasing levels of the HER-2 protein correlate with an increasing likelihood of response, but there is no consensus as to what assay reading indicates adequate positivity or even as to what type of assay should be used. The assay cited most frequently has been the Dako Corporation's convenient **HercepTest** (brand name). In this exam an immunostaining reagent is applied to pathology slides to highlight any HER-2 protein present in tumor cell membranes; the reading's accuracy depends on the expertise of the pathologist who looks at the slides. Dennis J. Slamon and his UCLA colleagues favor another assay called **fluorescence *in situ* hybridization** (FISH), which reveals the number of copies of the HER-2/*neu* gene in tumor specimens.[83] FISH is more expensive and requires special equipment. With either the HercepTest or FISH, the assay result tends to be more believable if the tumor specimen used is fresh or frozen rather than previously "fixed" (treated for preservation) and embedded in paraffin. Mark X. Sliwkowski of Genentech suggests that both assays should be performed for maximum accuracy, FISH for a quantitative estimate of gene amplification, and immunostaining to identify those occasional cases where the protein is overexpressed without multiple gene copies. In the latter instance, the usually reliable FISH would give false-negative readings.[84]

It behooves women newly diagnosed with invasive breast cancer to query their oncologists and pathologists about their HER-2 status, and to insist upon assay standardization. Assuming that history is prone to repetition, we might naturally worry that an intervention which benefits the few would be rather casually prescribed for the many, in much the same way that radical mastectomy was once mindlessly prescribed for all. Herceptin is neither mutilative nor toxic; but since the weekly treatments involve considerable expense and bother, this drug should be reserved for patients who are strongly HER-2-positive. If only we could be certain about this matter! Gabriel Hortobagyi has lamented that a patient's HER-2 status may depend upon which cancer center she happens to visit. "There are centers that call any staining positive," Dr. Hortobagyi observes. "The HercepTest kit calls 10% or more of the cells with membrane staining positive. There are others who call 50% or more stained cells positive. This is in addition to all of the other technical variations."[85]

The next step for Herceptin is its integration into adjuvant regimens. We would naturally assume that this gentle antibody drug will be most effective if it is given early in the course of disease—i.e., to newly diagnosed patients who have only a few disseminated cancer cells floating about in the bloodstream and the bone marrow, rather than to Stage Four patients with visceral metastases large enough to be seen on CAT scans. American oncologists are excited by the prospect of combining Herceptin with chemotherapy. Laboratory tests have suggested that the concurrent administration of Herceptin would actually increase the effectiveness of several cytotoxic drugs, notably cisplatin, cyclophosphamide, and docetaxel. But Herceptin probably should not be given at the same time as the most familiar breast cancer regimens—with AC or FAC it would increase the risk of doxorubicin-related cardiotoxicity, and with CMF it would be antagonistic to fluorouracil.[86]

Such drug interactions were carefully pondered by the planners at the National Cancer Institute who approved **NSABP Protocol B-31**. This clinical trial should tell us how much of a contribution adjuvant Herceptin will make toward improving the long-term survival rates in node-positive, HER-2-positive breast cancer—a patient population at high risk for the development of distant metastases. Those Protocol B-31 patients randomized to the trial's Herceptin arm were to start with the NSABP's 63-day AC regimen. Some three weeks after finishing it, they were to begin receiving concurrent Herceptin and paclitaxel—the antibody against HER-2 being infused once a week for a year, while the taxane drug was given once every three weeks for four courses (four infusions in 63 days).[87] The rationale behind this scheduling was to decimate the ranks of the circulating cancer cells with that fast-acting AC howitzer, then to use maintenance drugs with different cytotoxic mechanisms to mop up any malignant stragglers.

One important question that Protocol B-31 does not address is the duration of Herceptin therapy. How long should you continue the weekly infusions to achieve optimal results? A year? Two years? Three or more? The "full prescribing information" made available on Genentech's Internet website did not touch on this point so potentially pregnant with profits. It did warn physicians to monitor patients receiving this drug for fever, chills, and possible hypersensitivity reactions. Caution is indicated during the initial Herceptin infusion—this is a larger "loading dose" (four milligrams per kilogram of body weight), to be administered over ninety minutes. If there are no adverse side effects from this first exposure to the drug, the smaller maintenance doses (2 mg/kg) would be given as thirty-minute infusions.[88]

Chapter Twenty-eight

Screening Mammography

The preceding six chapters have dealt with our ongoing attempts to develop systemic therapies for metastatic or potentially metastatic breast tumors. These efforts have been constantly expanded since the late 1960s. Today we can say with confidence that a drug regimen properly tailored to the characteristics of the individual tumor stands to better the odds of long-term survival for any patient at risk of metastatic disease. Unfortunately, neither our hormonal drugs nor our chemo sledgehammers, nor our newer modalities (angiogenesis inhibitors, monoclonal antibodies, vaccines), have as yet delivered that certainty of cure we so desperately want. With breast cancers as with other solid tumors, it remains far, far better to discover and treat the disease before the malignant cells have had a chance to develop metastatic potential and spread beyond their original location. Early detection offers the best hope of cure—this principle is self-evident. In theory at least, any and all cancers would be completely curable if we could detect them as soon as the first few cells started to undergo malignant transformation. In practice, looking for cancers at their very earliest stages is fraught with pitfalls, owing to the considerable imperfections in our screening assays.

From the 1970s onward, the American Cancer Society, the American College of Radiology, the National Cancer Institute, and other advisory organizations have advocated periodic mammograms to catch breast malignancies while still localized and easily curable. As explained in Chapter Ten, **"diagnostic" mammography** is a wonderful tool for evaluating breast symptoms; it can usually distinguish between palpable masses ("lumps") which are clearly benign, like cysts and fibroadenomas, and those which are probably malignant. **"Screening" mammography** is a different matter—in this instance we are not using that imaging technology to evaluate symptoms which have come to our attention, but to evaluate vast numbers of women who have no symptoms that can be seen or felt. Occasionally a screening mammogram will discover a small localized lesion which is in the process of evolving into an aggressive metastatic tumor. More often these exams turn up occult abnormalities which might possibly be caused by malignancy—*and which therefore require follow-up*—but which subsequently prove to be harmless. The aging mammary gland can give rise to all manner of radiological false alarms. If we also remember that periodic mammography for the early detection of breast malignancies is one of the most expensive and cumbersome public health measures ever proposed, we will not be surprised that it continues to generate multiple controversies. Whom do we screen, and how often? At what age do we start the regular mammograms, and at what age should they be discontinued? How effective is mammographic screening in reducing the overall mortality from breast cancers? This chapter presents findings from randomized clinical trials which have sought to answer these urgent questions.

The Basics of Screening

Before we can even think about screening asymptomatic individuals for cancer, we need two things—(1) **a population at risk** and (2) **a curative intervention**. Nobody has ever proposed screening teenagers for colon cancer, because this population is not at risk for the disease. Similarly, it would not make sense to screen elderly nuns who have practiced lifelong celibacy for cervical cancer; we now know that this disease is likely to arise only in women who have been infected with certain sexually-transmitted papillomaviruses. But screening for these two malignancies has become a growth industry in American medicine, because we do have large populations at some degree of risk (all persons over age 50 for colon cancer, young women with multiple sexual partners for cervical carcinomas), and because we anticipate that surgery can cure early-stage disease in both cases.

Assuming a population at risk and a curative intervention, it would still make no sense to subject seemingly healthy persons to periodic examinations unless we have an effective screening assay for the malignancy in question. The effectiveness of any assay intended for cancer detection can be measured by its **sensitivity** and its **specificity**. By "sensitivity," we mean that the test will routinely give a positive reading when occult early-stage disease is present. "Specificity"

means that the test will not give a positive reading unless the disease is present. If a screening assay is not sensitive enough, it will be prone to give **false-negative readings**. In other words, the test would often show us green lights (no disease) when red lights would have been appropriate. And the upshot would be that occult tumors would be allowed to progress until they produced obvious symptoms, by which time they could be incurable. If a screening assay is sensitive enough but not sufficiently specific, it will tend to give **false-positive readings**. In other words, the test would frequently show us red lights (disease possibly present) when green lights would have been appropriate. And the upshot would be that healthy persons would be subjected to fruitless follow-up tests (always) and to needless biopsies (sometimes), with the accompanying burdens of psychological distress and financial expense.

Cancer screening has not been one of the great triumphs of modern medicine. We may dream of that ideal screening assay which would be perfect in sensitivity and specificity, as well as being inexpensive, painless, and fast, and involving no risk of any kind. Unfortunately, what we have actually had at our disposal is a hodgepodge of diverse assays for different malignancies. Each of these tests has its selling points, but none of them begins to approach the aforementioned ideal. The **digital rectal examination** (DRE), long proposed for the early detection of prostate cancer, is cheap and fast enough; but what sensitivity it might have depends largely on the examiner's expertise. We may hypothesize that an experienced urologist would be able to discern, via palpation, subtle changes in the texture of a prostate gland which had started to undergo malignant transformation—but any survival advantage to be had from periodic DRE remains to be demonstrated. The newer blood tests which measure the levels of **prostate-specific antigen** (PSA) are considerably more sensitive to prostatic disorders; but they are hardly specific for carcinomas, because elevated readings also occur with benign prostatic hypertrophy.

For persons over age 50, the American Cancer Society has recommended annual screening for **fecal occult blood** as an aid in detecting colorectal malignancies early. This assay is painless and cheap—you only need a stool specimen and a reagent which changes color in the presence of blood—but its sensitivity and specificity leave a great deal to be desired. Early-stage colorectal tumors do not always bleed on cue, raising the specter of false-negative results. And false-positive readings are frequent, because the test reacts to blood in the gastrointestinal tract regardless of its source. A bleeding stomach ulcer or a half-digested piece of rare beefsteak will also set off alarm bells. Two examinations which allow visual inspection of the interior colorectal mucosa are far more sensitive and specific. **Sigmoidoscopy** involves the use of a flexible fiberoptic tube to inspect the lower third of the colon—it's uncomfortable for the patient, but it gives us a close-up view of the lumen (hollow interior) of the sigmoid colon. **Colonoscopy** allows visualization of the entire colon. Patients must be sedated during this more extensive endoscopic procedure. While colonoscopy carries a slight risk of complications (e.g., perforation of the colon), it is vastly superior to the old-fashioned **barium enema**. Putting a radio-opaque substance like barium in the colon enables us to take an X-ray which would reveal any obstructions or any large tumors jutting out into the lumen, but not much else. Endoscopic exams let us see tiny lesions, and they give us an opportunity to take biopsy samples at the same time. Researchers at Johns Hopkins and other institutions have studied a stool-based assay for colorectal cancer which promises to be more specific than fecal-blood screening. They isolate DNA from stool samples and then amplify it by polymerase chain reaction (PCR), so as to look for telltale mutations in *ras* and other genes implicated in colorectal tumorigenesis.[1]

Johns Hopkins physicians have also been studying PCR amplification of cellular DNA present in urine specimens, as a noninvasive assay for early-stage bladder and renal (kidney) tumors.[2] The surgeon Steven A. Ahrendt of the Medical College of Wisconsin (Milwaukee) collaborated with a Hopkins team to produce an experimental screening assay for lung cancer. Ahrendt et al used a flexible bronchoscope to inject lavage fluid (warm saline) into suspect areas of patients' lungs. Some of the fluid was then suctioned out and centrifuged, yielding "a pellet" of bronchial cells. After being amplified by PCR and subjected to molecular analysis, the cellular DNA sometimes revealed tumor-associated mutations in the *ras* and *p53* genes.[3] While the suitability of such DNA examinations for mass screening has not been established, no one would question the need for a more effective assay to intercept lung malignancies, which have been so common and so lethal. Back in the 1970s the American Cancer Society (ACS) urged habitual smokers (the population at highest risk) to have annual chest X-rays and annual microscopic examinations of their sputum (coughed-up bronchial secretions). But the clinical trials conducted in that decade failed to show any significant reduction in lung cancer mortality from this screening strategy, and in 1980 the ACS withdrew its recommendation. By the year 2000, however, some proponents of screening argued that sputum examinations could be beneficially combined with low-dose helical CAT scans. They reasoned that sputum analysis has the potential to detect cancer cells shed from tumors located in the larger central airways, while CAT scans can often detect tiny nodules located in the smaller bronchi or in peripheral areas of the lungs.[4] But whatever level of effectiveness this expensive strategy might prove to have, it could never save as many lives as the successful implementation of the most obvious public health measure— viz., *persuading smokers to quit!*

At the moment, our most practical screening assay continues to be the **Pap smear**. Mortality from cervical cancer in the United States plummeted 70% between 1947 and 1984—that striking decline presumably had much to do with the widespread adoption of the Pap smear for screening, which took place during this period.[5] The Pap smear is so effective because it amounts to a minimal biopsy, giving us a sample of the cells we're concerned about. Assuming an adequate swabbing of the uterine cervix and a proficient microscopic examination, this assay's sensitivity for overt cancer approaches 100%. Unfortunately, it is relatively nonspecific. Screening turns up tremendous numbers of atypical cells and of low-grade epithelial lesions. Although the vast majority of these cells and lesions never progress to become invasive carcinomas, we have had no good way to predict their future behavior. And the upshot has been a need for repeated smears and for incisional biopsies. While these particular follow-up exams are not terribly expensive, they have occasioned considerable anguish to women who often are told only that "something is wrong."

Skin self-examination tops the list of screening assays which are cheap and fast. Since it is performed by laypersons, it can make no especial claims to sensitivity or specificity. Nonetheless, Marianne Berwick and other cancer epidemiologists have estimated that regular self-examinations of the skin ought to reduce melanoma mortality by 63%. Berwick et al cite evidence that melanomas "progress in a stepwise fashion," from superficial cutaneous lesions which are readily curable, to "a vertical growth stage," which can give rise to distant metastases. "Patients with thin lesions have a better prognosis, suggesting that early detection protects against the development of lethal melanoma." Alas, the study Berwick and her colleagues did with Connecticut residents found that no more than 15% of them performed thorough skin self-examinations.[6]

In terms of the publicity it has been given, the **mammogram** is far and away America's foremost screening assay. Unfortunately, publicity is the only superlative we can think of. Breast radiographs do not approach the sensitivity of Pap smears or even of visual skin examinations. Unlike the Pap smear, a mammogram cannot show us that handful of malignant cells which marks the start of tumorigenesis. What we see is at best a small tumor, which may be quite large in molecular terms. The veteran oncologist David Plotkin has estimated that the average tumor discovered by mammography is "a bit more than a quarter of an inch across" and contains "about 600 million cells."[7] While most tumors in this size range (under one centimeter) have not yet acquired metastatic potential, a few will have already sown the seeds of systemic disease. Not even the most ardent proponents of screening mammography would claim that it can prevent every death from breast cancer.

The sensitivity and specificity of mammography vary from individual to individual. We assume that this assay will be both more sensitive and more specific in postmenopausal breasts with their increasing fat content than in densely glandular premenopausal breasts, which are less radiolucent. Mammography is doubly operator-dependent. Its value depends as much on the technician who positions breasts for X-ray as on the radiologist who must interpret the resulting images.   Those spicular or stellate masses we see illustrated in textbooks are not the measure of a breast radiologist's discrimination—these familiar "red flags" bespeak infiltrating ductal carcinomas, many of which will have already metastasized by the time they give us this obvious radiological presentation.   Mammographers win their laurels in those gray areas where the signs of malignancy are indirect or indistinct.   Subtle changes in breast architecture, ill-defined densities, and tiny flecks of calcification represent the acid tests of specificity, because such findings are often due to biological mechanisms other than malignancy.

Does cancer screening really reduce death rates?   Laypersons typically assume that any survival advantage to be had from a screening assay would be easy to demonstrate.   This is hardly the case.   A convincing demonstration requires a massive clinical trial in which many thousands of asymptomatic volunteers are recruited without bias and randomized without bias, half to pursue the particular screening strategy and half to serve as unscreened controls.   Moreover, all those thousands of trial participants would need to be scrupulously followed for twenty years or so, to verify that the screened group had actually experienced fewer deaths from the malignancy in question.   In any trial of a cancer screening strategy, short-term follow-ups of five or ten years usually produce misleading results.   There are two reasons for this phenomenon—**lead time** and **overdiagnosis**.   The term "lead time" refers to the amount of time gained by detecting an occult cancer with a screening assay rather than waiting for it to present symptomatically.   By way of illustration, we may envision an aggressive breast cancer which will kill the patient exactly ten years after the first few

cells turn malignant.   Let's assume that the tumor will produce clinical symptoms (e.g., a hard lump) leading to its diagnosis at year six, but that with screening mammography we can detect and diagnose it at year three.   That would give us an impressive lead time of three years.   If our hypothetical tumor does not begin to shed metastatic cells until year four, then its detection and eradication at year three will translate into a cure—that's a real survival benefit!   On the other hand, if the tumor begins to shed metastatic cells at year two, then its detection at year three will not necessarily alter the course of disease or change the outcome.   And thus we might have no real benefit from screening but simply an artifact—viz., "improved" five-year survival due to lead-time bias.   True, our screened patient would be alive five years after her diagnosis, while a comparable control patient would be dead five years after diagnosis—but the apparent survival benefit obtained by screening is illusory, since both patients would ultimately die in the tenth year after the onset of tumorigenesis.

Most people who are skeptical about cancer screening worry more about overdiagnosis than about lead-time bias.   By the term "overdiagnosis," we mean that the screening assay tends to discover low-grade lesions which may look bad under the microscope, but which do not have metastatic potential and which will not necessarily acquire it during an average lifespan.   Overdiagnosed cancers are those which—save for the screening assay—we might not have become aware of, because they progress so slowly that most patients will die from non-malignant causes before developing clinically obvious tumors.   And the more slow-growing a breast tumor is, the more likely it is to be picked up by periodic mammograms.   If you don't catch the little lesion this year, you've got another chance at detection next year, and then still another the year after that!

Lead time and overdiagnosis distort the data coming from our cancer screening trials in slightly different ways. Lead-time bias may have played a role in the Mayo Lung Project, which recruited 9,211 male smokers between 1971 and 1983. The early results pointed to increased survival for lung cancers diagnosed by the screening intervention, which consisted on chest X-rays and sputum microscopy every four months. But the twenty-year follow-up published in 2000 revealed that the intervention arm actually went on to have a higher death rate than the controls.[8] When overdiagnosis is the culprit distorting our screening data, the newspapers and TV networks will report frightening increases in the number of cancer cases as well as gratifying increases in the percentage of patients being cured. Unwary laypersons are thus led to believe that the tumor in question is on an epidemic rampage, but that our healthcare industries are making tremendous progress in combating it. Alas, both the epidemic and the progress would seem to be largely artifacts, and they pose a riddle worthy of the Sphinx: "When cure is possible, is it really necessary?"

Overdiagnosis probably played a considerable role in the surge of prostate cancers being reported in the late 1980s and early 1990s, at the time when testing for PSA levels first became widespread. Data collected by the National Cancer Institute suggested that the incidence of prostatic tumors among American men aged 65 and older leaped 82% from 1986 to 1991, with an amazing 20% increase occurring in the year 1990 alone.[9] Overdiagnosis overtly impacted the incidence statistics for breast cancer in the early 1980s—but with these tumors an artifactual epidemic would seem to have gotten underway several decades before. In 1940 the American Cancer Society estimated that one American woman out of twenty would develop breast cancer during her lifetime. In 1991 the Society announced, with much media fanfare, that the lifetime risk of disease was one in nine.[10] Of course, the absolute death rate stayed fairly constant between 1940 and 1991. In 1992 the Centers for Disease Control in Atlanta reported that "from 1980 through 1987, the incidence of breast cancer increased from 94.6 to 124.3 per 100,000 women." The fact that disease mortality did not increase—(it stood at a modest 31.1 per 100,000 in 1988)—suggests either than more lethal cases are being cured, or that more cases are being diagnosed which are not likely to become lethal.[11]

Being cured of a malignancy which is not going to cause symptoms during one's lifetime is a regrettable event. Unfortunately, that has been the worst side effect of mass screening for breast and prostate cancers, though nobody has plausible statistics on the extent of this overtreatment. Few physicians will welcome even a gentle insinuation that some patients may have been subjected to unnecessary therapy. Of course, the problem lies not with the morals of our doctors, but with screening assays and pathology workups which cannot predict the future behavior of early-stage neoplasms. For breast malignancies, nobody questions the urgent need to treat all palpable lesions (those which produce a lump) as well as any nonpalpable lesions which show evidence of infiltration (invasion of the surrounding tissues). Our treatment dilemmas are generated almost entirely by **ductal carcinoma *in situ*** (DCIS), where the transformed cells are confined to the ducts of origin and give no hint of infiltration. As we have seen in Chapter Twelve, DCIS lesions do not often produce palpable masses which could lead to self-discovery; but since they tend to secrete tiny calcifications, they are frequently detected by screening mammograms. Thus a type of breast cancer which was rarely mentioned before the mammography era has come to represent our biggest challenge in differential diagnosis. According to the National Cancer Institute, the reported incidence of DCIS rose from 2.4 cases per 100,000 American women in 1973 to 15.8 cases per 100,000 in 1992, almost a sevenfold increase.[12] This diagnosis always needs additional clarification. DCIS lesions range from relatively uniform cells which are hard to distinguish from atypical hyperplasia (a benign finding), to poorly-differentiated cells with adjacent necrosis, the so-called *comedo* variety which tends to evolve into infiltrating carcinomas.

Treating some cases of DCIS is therefore a presumably lifesaving measure, while treating others probably accomplishes little except to label perfectly functional individuals as "cancer patients" and to inflict upon them all manner of psychological anguish and monetary expense. Yet all DCIS lesions discovered by screening mammography are going to be referred to surgeons, for reasons that possibly have less to do with cancer biology than with fears of malpractice litigation. No radiologist or surgeon wants to stand before a jury accused of having ignored the little lesion which—a year or two later—blossomed into a deadly carcinoma. So if there seems to be even the slightest chance that the tiny cluster of calcifications could represent a seedbed of malignancy, the process of diagnosis and treatment will be set in motion. One breast surgeon quoted in the *New England Journal of Medicine* lamented that he was himself a victim of these new circumstances: "I am biopsying abnormalities that I wouldn't touch in my spouse. The difference is that she won't sue me."[13]

The HIP Clinical Trial

Screening mammography did not get established as an early-detection assay overnight. In the United States it had its origins in the work of Robert L. Egan. As a young radiologist at Houston's M. D. Anderson Cancer Center in the late 1950s, Dr. Egan began to take mammograms of the contralateral breasts of breast cancer patients who had previously undergone mastectomies. These women knew that they were at risk for the development of malignancy in the remaining breast, and they readily consented to the new radiological exams. Dr. Egan's results, first published in 1960, indicated that mammography could often detect breast tumors before they became palpable. Other radiologists now hastened to study his techniques, but it remained to be demonstrated that periodic screening of asymptomatic women could save lives. The first American trial which tested this proposition was called the **Health Insurance Plan Project**—or the **HIP trial** for short.[14] It still commands our attention because it used a representative cross section of the American population, randomized its subjects without bias, and monitored their outcomes with a prolonged and scrupulous follow-up. The HIP trial was conducted by a constellation of competent researchers, including the epidemiologist Sam Shapiro and the radiologist Philip Strax. Between 1963 and 1966, some 62,000 women aged 40 to 64 were recruited from subscribers to the Health Insurance Plan of New York, a prepaid health plan covering almost 700,000 government employees and their family members. Half of these women were randomly assigned to serve as controls; the other half became the study group. The screening intervention offered the study group consisted of a physical examination (breast palpation) by an experienced physician (usually a surgeon), as well as two-view mammography with a craniocaudal (top-to-bottom) exposure and a mediolateral (side) exposure. The HIP trial was brief—a woman being screened received an initial physical exam and set of mammograms, followed by three repeat screenings at annual intervals. All screening was completed by June 1970.

While the HIP trial represents a landmark event in the history of screening mammography, it did not establish the superiority of this particular assay. On the contrary, the physical exams did a better job of catching tumors. The final HIP tally stood at 304 diagnosed breast cancers in the study group, compared to 295 in the control group. For the study group as a whole, 44.7% of the malignancies detected by screening had been picked up by palpation alone, only 33.3% by mammography alone. The primitive mammography machines of the 1960s did not work well on the premenopausal breast. Of those malignancies detected by screening in women aged 40 through 49, only 19.4% had been found by mammography alone, while 61.3% owed their discovery exclusively to palpation.[15]

Long-term follow-up on the breast cancer cases diagnosed in HIP participants eventually revealed a modest survival benefit for the study (screened) group. In 1982 Sam Shapiro and his colleagues reported that "by the end of ten years after entry, the study group's mortality due to breast cancer was about 30% below the control group's." That estimate—an "about 30%" reduction in deaths accomplished by screening—has often been bandied around as the most pertinent statistic to come out of the HIP trial. In fact, the survival benefit observed varied dramatically according to the length of follow-up. The earliest results, computed at five years from trial entry, showed an impressive benefit for women aged 50 through 59 at entry. There had been 33 breast cancer deaths among the controls, but only 15 in the study group—a 55% reduction in mortality. But the fourteen-year computation revealed a greatly diminished benefit—68 deaths from breast cancer had occurred in the control group, but now there were 53 deaths in the study group, and therefore only a 22% mortality reduction attributable to screening.[16] In this instance we might attribute most of that apparent "five-year survival benefit" in the 50-to-59 age bracket to lead-time bias.

Dr. Shapiro and his HIP co-workers spent a long, long time looking for a survival advantage in the screened women who had entered the trial between the ages of 40 and 49. For over a decade the HIP team complained that there had been too few cancer deaths in these younger women to draw any firm conclusions. In 1988. however, Kenneth C. Chu and other statisticians at the National Cancer Institute announced that they had analyzed the HIP trial data "after at least eighteen years of follow-up using different statistical methods than those previously employed." Then Chu et al dropped a bombshell—not only was there a statistically significant reduction in breast cancer mortality for the screened women aged 40 to 49 at entry, but that reduction at 24% was actually greater than the 21% reduction now calculated for the study group women aged 50 to 64 at entry.[17] In September 1988 newspaper and TV reporters throughout America pounced on the NCI revelations, churning out enthusiastic stories about mammography saving the lives of forty-year-olds. This ebullient assumption was hardly warranted by the HIP data, which (as we have seen) indicated that the clinical breast examination (palpation) discovered far more tumors in the 40-to-49 age group than mammography did.

What valuable lessons can we gather today from the old HIP trial? We certainly can conclude that periodic screening stands to detect a certain percentage of breast malignancies which might otherwise prove deadly while they are still in a localized and therefore curable stage. And the HIP experience ought to instill a healthy respect for old-fashioned palpation of the breast, a cheap and fast assay which can be quite useful in skilled hands. Unfortunately, the survival benefits from screening seem to shrink with the passage of time. The final computation by Sam Shapiro and his HIP collaborators, performed at eighteen years from entry, put the mortality reduction for the entire study group at no more than "23 to 24 percent."[18] Why did it take so long for a mortality reduction to become evident for the women screened in their forties. We normally assume that premenopausal breast cancers tend to be more aggressive than postmenopausal breast cancers; by this reasoning, any reduction in mortality ought to become evident *earlier* in premenopausal women than in postmenopausal women. Yet this did not happen in the HIP trial, nor has it ever happened in any subsequent trial of breast cancer screening. An alternate explanation tailored to the HIP results would be that the benefits of screening younger women are largely due to the early detection of a subset of sluggish breast cancers which would take many years to produce death. Dr. Chu and his NCI colleagues embraced this hypothesis, pointing out that the survival benefit they detected for the 40-to-49 age bracket derived from Stage One (node-negative) tumors and that it did not become statistically significant until the ninth year of follow-up.[19]

BCDDP:

Testing Mammography's Potential

While the **Breast Cancer Detection Demonstration Project** (BCDDP) was not a clinical trial, it generated mountains of data which we cannot afford to ignore.[20] The National Cancer Institute and the American Cancer Society joined forces to organize and fund this enormous project, whose goals were to explore the potential of the rapidly improving mammographic technology and to popularize screening mammograms among physicians and the public alike. From 1973 to 1975 the BCDDP enlisted 283,222 American women between the ages of 35 and 74, all of whom were offered five years of annual examinations. Screening was conducted at 29 medical centers distributed throughout the United States; the assays used were the standard two-view mammography (craniocaudal and mediolateral exposures) and the clinical breast exam. While palpation was retained in the BCDDP, it played second fiddle to radiology. The palpatory and visual exams were not performed by veteran physicians but by "paraprofessionals" (often nurses) who had received instruction for this purpose yet were presumably less experienced. The population screened in the BCDDP, while vast, may have been a less representative cross section than that screened in the HIP trial. Relying on volunteers attracted by newspaper and television publicity, the BCDDP probably tended to enroll more women who had a family history of breast cancer or who otherwise perceived themselves to be at higher risk. The BCDDP's greatest demographic strength was its balanced distribution of participants by age. When screening began, roughly half the women were under age 50, and half were age 50 or older. This balance naturally shifted toward "over 50" as the project progressed; but even at the fifth (last) annual examination, 45.6% of the participants were still under age 50.[21]

All screening was completed by early 1981. The following year the BCDDP published detailed statistics comparing the efficiency of its two principal assays. In contrast to the HIP trial of the 1960s, mammography had far outperformed breast palpation in the detection of early breast cancers. This was true for all age brackets, but more so in postmenopausal women. Yet mammography now clearly demonstrated its value as a tool to evaluate the premenopausal breast. Of the cancers detected in women aged 40 to 49, only 13.1% had been discovered by palpation alone, while 35.4% had been apparent solely on the mammograms. Using the two assays together achieved the greatest sensitivity— 50% of the cancers found by screening in this age group set off alarm bells both on the mammographic exam and on the physical exam.[22]

While the BCDDP illustrated mammography's growing sensitivity for the premenopausal breast, it did not bear witness to specificity. The number of false positives leading to needless biopsies was appalling. For women who entered the BCDDP at ages 35 through 39 and who later had biopsies, the ratio of benign to malignant findings was 16.4 to one. For women aged 45 through 49 at entry, that ratio still stood at 6.5 to one. Even the women aged 55 through 59 at entry, all presumably postmenopausal, proved 3.8 times more likely to have a benign finding at biopsy than a diagnosis of malignancy. The ratio fell below three-to-one only for women who were age 70 or older at entry.[23]

Larry H. Baker, chairman of the BCDDP, attributed the elevated "surgical recommendation rates" for premenopausal women to "fibrocystic disease."[24] Dr. Baker's explanation recalls an unfortunate diagnostic term current in the 1970s which stuck a disease label on a normal aging process. The mammary glands of women in their thirties begin to reveal increasing fibrosis. When pronounced, this benign process often results in areas of nodular density or in pockets of entrapped fluid (cysts). Both the lumpy densities and the cysts are easy to confuse with those dominant masses which

suggest malignancy. Fortunately, the number of surgical biopsies has fallen dramatically in recent years. Fine-needle aspiration frequently enables us to rule out malignancy without resorting to the operating room. But the basic lesson from the BCDDP remains as valid as ever. Women in their thirties and forties who begin breast cancer screening are much more likely to have benign abnormalities which will mimic malignancy and which will therefore require additional examinations to establish the diagnosis. And as for cancer, these younger women are much less likely to have it than women in their fifties and sixties. The BCDDP gave us some compelling statistics which illustrate how the incidence of breast malignancies gradually creeps upward with advancing years. For women who entered the project at ages 35 through 39, the true-positive rate (cancer actually detected) was 0.9 per 1,000 annual screenings. That rate stood at 2.0 per 1,000 screenings for women aged 40 through 44 at entry, and at 3.2 per 1,000 screenings for women aged 45 through 49 at entry. There was never a dramatic surge in the true-positive rate—just a little step upward with each five-year age bracket. For the 50-to-54 age group, the rate was 3.7; for the 55-to-59 group, 4.5; for the 60-to-64 group, 5.1; and for the 65-to-69 group, 5.4. Women who entered the BCDDP at ages 70 through 74 had a very high rate of true positives on their initial screening (12.9 per 1,000 screenings), but their overall rate for the project stood at a relatively modest 6.6 per 1,000 screenings.[25]

With the benefit of hindsight, we can see some troublesome deficiencies in the BCDDP's otherwise admirable collection and presentation of data. This project represents the first time that mammography was able to identify large numbers of tiny breast malignancies which would never have been detected by palpation alone. Unfortunately, the BCDDP lumped all these lesions together under the heading **"minimal cancer"**—another vague diagnostic term from the 1970s. That thoroughly mixed up the sheep and the wolves, putting noninvasive neoplasms like lobular carcinoma *in situ* (always sheep) and ductal carcinoma *in situ* (mostly sheep) in the same corral with infiltrating carcinomas less than one centimeter in diameter (always presumed to be potentially wolves). Only one statistic from the BCDDP's data on "minimal" cancers seems worth quoting here. Of the 195 invasive tumors detected by mammography alone, just 15 (or 7.7%) proved to be node-positive (Stage Two disease).[26] We cannot currently form plausible estimates of the mortality reductions to be had from detecting and eradicating noninvasive neoplasms; however, with the aforementioned 195 nonpalpable invasive tumors, we might anticipate a cure rate of about 90% for lesions which would probably tend to shorten life expectancies.

The BCDDP did not give us solid data on any mortality reductions obtained by its screening strategy, because it had no unscreened control group for comparison, and because there was no comprehensive long-term follow-up. Only about one-fifth of the 283,222 participants were followed after the screening ended, and these only for nine years from the date of entry. In 1988 the epidemiologist Alan S. Morrison and his colleagues compared the outcomes in a subset of 55,053 BCDDP participants who received follow-up surveillance with the probable outcomes suggested by the National Cancer Institute's mortality database. Morrison et al found that "breast cancer mortality among BCDDP participants was about 20% less than the level expected from national data." But the ratio of observed-to-expected mortality varied according to the age of the participants. For women who began screening at ages 60 through 74, Morrison et al

calculated a 26% reduction in mortality. The estimated reduction slipped slightly to 24% for women who entered at ages 50 through 59, and plunged down to 11% for those who entered at ages 35 through 49.[27]

The ACS Guidelines:
Building on Shifting Sands

While the American Cancer Society (ACS) does much to support basic research on cancer, its most visible function is public education. More than any other organization, the ACS has spread the gospel that the early detection of malignancies will lead to their cure. From the 1920s through the 1960s, its pamphlets and flyers instructed Americans about clinically evident symptoms which everyone could understand—lumps in the breast or elsewhere, alterations in bowel habits, sores that did not heal, unexplained bleeding, etc., etc. Of course, the problem with this educational strategy was that such overt presentations do not necessarily indicate malignancy, and that when they do, they often indicate late-stage disease past the point of any curative intervention. The ACS has therefore been extremely interested in screening assays which promise to detect malignancies months or years before they would cause symptoms. From the 1970s onward the Society has increasingly sought to convince the public of the necessity for periodic cancer screening. An important tool for this purpose has been the **ACS Guidelines on Screening**. They contain definite recommendations on which early-detection assays are appropriate for this or that type of malignancy, and on which subgroups of the population at large should undergo testing. Gerald D. Dodd, a former President of the Society, points out that its first specific guidelines for breast cancer screening were not issued until 1977, a year marked by such undue worries about radiation carcinogenesis that even the BCDDP suspended mammography for women under age 50. Influenced by the radiation scare as well as by the early findings from the HIP trial, the ACS limited its recommendation for annual mammograms to women aged 50 and older. Women aged 40 to 49 were advised to have mammography only if they had a strong family history of breast cancer (a mother or sister diagnosed). Women aged 35 to 39 were advised to have it only if they had "a personal history of breast cancer." The 1977 guidelines saw much value in palpation, recommending monthly breast self-examination and periodic exams by a physician for all women aged 20 and older.[28] The revised guidelines the ACS issued in 1980 retained this emphasis on palpation, urging women over 40 to have a doctor's exam every year. But the question of regular mammography before age 50 was sidestepped—these younger women were counseled "to consult their physicians about the need in their individual situation." The 1980 edition of the guidelines saw the first endorsement of the **baseline mammogram**, a screening stratagem much beloved by the ACS. Women in their thirties were urged to have a single set of mammograms taken sometime between the ages of 35 and 39, so as to provide a "baseline" (frame of reference) for comparison in the event that mammograms taken in later years seemed to reveal abnormalities.[29]

By the mid-1980s almost all cancer specialists agreed that periodic screening mammography could lower the risk of death from breast cancer in women over age 50. The HIP trial had pointed to a substantial mortality reduction for this age bracket, as did the early results from several trials done in Sweden. The big "Two County" trial had recruited and randomized 134,867 Swedish

women between the ages of 40 and 74. The only screening assay used was single-view mammography (mediolateral oblique exposure), offered every two to three years. The first report from this trial, published in 1985, indicated that the women over age 50 randomized to screening were experiencing 40% lower mortality from breast cancer than their compeers in the control group. For the screened women who entered the trial between the ages of 40 and 49, no reduction in mortality had as yet been observed.[30]

The voluminous BCDDP data provided ammunition both to those who advocated screening women in their forties and to those who did not. For the proponents, all those false positives and that low rate of disease incidence tended to be counterbalanced by the fact that mammography by itself had detected a significant number of small tumors in the 35-to-49 age group. In 1983, as the fear of radiation carcinogenesis subsided, the ACS cast its lot with the proponents. The Society's well-known guidelines were now modified to include a recommendation that women between 40 and 49 undergo mammography "at intervals of one to two years."[31]

Notwithstanding the ACS recommendation, the idea of universal screening mammography for women in their forties evoked skepticism in some quarters. David M. Eddy of Duke University and his colleagues prepared a carefully researched estimate of the potential benefits, risks, and costs which this policy might entail. As their estimate was endorsed by the Council of Scientific Affairs of the American Medical Association, it attracted much attention when it was published in March 1988. Eddy et al observed that about 16% of the breast malignancies then being diagnosed occurred in women between the ages of 40 and 49. For that age group, adding annual mammography to the annual physical exams ought to reduce the risk of dying from breast cancer from about 82 in 10,000 to about 60 in 10,000—"a reduction of about 26%." The risk of having a biopsy "for a lesion that is not cancer" was estimated to be one in ten. Dr. Eddy and his colleagues were models of fairness. They agreed that screening mammography should be made available to younger women "who understand the limits of its benefits," but they felt that the question of whether the benefits outweighed the risks had not been conclusively answered. "It might be inappropriate," Eddy et al argued, "to make a blanket recommendation that all women in this age group be screened with mammography." Persons who would offer such a recommendation "should recognize that they are projecting their own values on others."[32]

The ACS did not take the hint. In September 1988 the recalculation of the HIP trial data, which now revealed a mortality reduction for women screened in their forties, cleared the way for those bent on making blanket recommendations. This time the ACS acted in conjunction with eleven other organizations, including the National Cancer Institute, the American Medical Association, and the American College of Radiology. The **"Glorious Consensus of 1989"** (as we might dub this display of unprecedented unanimity) resulted in a screening recommendation which bore almost everybody's imprimatur, save for the mavericks in the American College of Surgeons. The consensus guidelines were unveiled with much publicity on June 27, 1989; they urged American women to begin breast cancer screening by age 40, getting "annual clinical examinations with screening mammography performed at one-year to two-year intervals."[33]

The ACS paid a high price to create this unified front. The new guidelines said not a word about baseline mammograms at age 35, because several cosignatory organizations had objected that the stratagem's

value had never been established. Yet the ACS was undaunted, and it kept this concept alive by means of an advertising campaign. A public service message repeated over and over in the 1990s specifically targeted the 35-year-old woman: "If you haven't had a mammogram, you need more than your breasts examined."[34]

Interval-Surfacing Tumors

Consensus in breast cancer matters is much like the snow in north Florida—it never gets very deep, and it melts away as soon as the temperature rises up a degree or two. In the case of screening mammography, discordant opinions voiced by well-known physicians and scientists go far beyond the issue of whether forty-year-olds should be assayed. The veteran surgeon John S. Spratt, co-editor of a standard textbook on breast cancer, has long been critical of the optimistic messages put out by the ACS and some professional mammographers. In a 1986 letter to the *New England Journal of Medicine*, Dr. Spratt worried that "the effectiveness of screening may be exaggerated fraudulently, particularly when any universal benefit is implied." He proposed that any guidelines for periodic mammography should "contain disclaimers that recognize the extreme variations in the lethality of breast cancers, the extreme variations in growth rates, and the imperfections of screening techniques."[35] To illustrate his point, Dr. Spratt cited the phenomenon of **interval-surfacing tumors**. That term refers to the biggest worm in the mammographic apple. If a woman undergoing annual screening has a perfectly normal examination one year, and then before her next scheduled examination discovers a breast malignancy on her own, we would have an example of an interval-surfacing tumor. These lesions mock all our efforts at early detection; they are not picked up by our supposedly sensitive screening assays, but emerge without warning to produce symptoms which send women running to their doctors. We first became aware of this problem during the HIP trial— 25% of the breast cancers recorded in the screened group were not detected at the annual examinations, but became symptomatic in the intervals between examinations.[36] The BCDDP of the 1970s made an especial effort to gather information on this phenomenon. The project's chairman Larry H. Baker later reported that 744 tumors were "detected within one year after an annual screening at which no surgical recommendation was made." About 20% of all breast cancers discovered during the BCDDP presented symptomatically between the annual examinations—this rate is a tad lower than that seen in the HIP trial, possibly because no records were kept of any interval-surfacing tumors which presented after the fifth and final screening.[37]

Breast cancer specialists have traditionally assumed that interval-surfacing tumors are not detected by periodic screening mammography because they grow so fast. Speaking at a surgical meeting, Dr. Spratt argued that "the biological behavior" of these lesions set them apart: "Some breast cancers are so acute that they can go from inception to the death of the host in as brief a period as 120 days. Other breast cancers are so chronic that the patient might live 23 years with no treatment at all. These chronic cancers would be picked up by the annual mammography, while the acute cancers would be interval cancers."[38] Yet this grim scenario is not always in evidence. Several studies have suggested that a substantial minority of interval-surfacing tumors are overlooked at the annual screenings simply because they are relatively "invisible." In 1999 Peggy L. Porter and her colleagues at Seattle's Fred Hutchinson Cancer Research Center pointed out that breast tumors with "lobular or mucinous histology" are prone to be missed because they often do not evoke a "stromal response," that fibrosis in the surrounding tissues which sets off alarm bells both on mammography and on palpation.[39] Mucinous tumors have a good prognosis, as do many lobular carcinomas. We have long known that younger women undergoing periodic mammography are more likely to have interval-surfacing tumors than older women. In some cases, however, the problem lies not so much with tumor growth rates as with dense glandular breasts, which can mask even the distinctive radiological silhouette of an infiltrating ductal carcinoma. A study done in Washington State in the 1990s found that screened women with "extremely dense breasts" had about six times the number of cancers detected between examinations as screened women with "predominantly fatty breasts."[40]

In those cases where we do not find lobular or mucinous histology, or a masking effect caused by breast density, Dr. Spratt's assumption is probably correct. Malignancies which pop up unexpectedly between screening examinations do tend to be more aggressive. The New Mexico Mammography Project of the early 1990s recorded a 20% rate of interval-surfacing tumors. Frank D. Gilliland of the University of Southern California and his colleagues used immunostaining to contrast the molecular aberrations in 64 interval-surfacing tumors from this project with 63 cancers detected at its annual examinations. Those breast tumors which presented between examinations proved to be more than twice as likely to have overexpression of a mutated *p53* gene, indicative of "dysregulation of the cell cycle and potential genetic instability." They were also twice as likely to have one-fifth or more of their cells in cycle—that is, either dividing or preparing to divide.[41] These findings give some support to Dr. Spratt's hypothesis that interval-surfacing tumors typically experience a period of rapid growth just before they come to our attention with a symptomatic presentation. This sudden growth spurt does much to explain why any strategy calling for periodic screening will be relatively ineffectual at catching them preclinically.

The Heretical CNBSS:
A Cold Wind from Canada

By the early 1990s screening mammography had become big business in the United States, providing gainful employment to thousands of radiologists and their assistants. The idea that radiological imaging of asymptomatic breasts could prevent death from mammary carcinomas was now an orthodox dogma, constantly being hammered into American consciousness by the litany of ACS public service announcements. But a terrible heresy was afoot just across the Canadian border, in Toronto. A massive clinical trial, the largest ever of screening mammography in North America, constituted the instrument of iconoclasm—the **Canadian National Breast Screening Study**, or the **CNBSS** for short. Conducted under the auspices of Canada's National Cancer Institute and other Canadian health-oriented organizations, the CNBSS was headed by Anthony B. Miller, an epidemiologist at the University of Toronto who had worked on the old HIP trial and who had considerable respect for breast palpation as a screening assay. Essentially, the CNBSS protocols asked a single question appropriate in an atmosphere of socialized medicine and cost containment, but which understandably offended American radiologists whose economic livelihood and professional integrity depended on the assumed survival benefit conferred by screening mammography. Viz., **do you really need all those expensive mammograms if you do the palpation properly?**

Between 1980 and 1985 the CNBSS recruited 50,430 women aged 40 to 49 as well as 39,405 women aged 50 to 59. All 89,835 participants were instructed in the techniques of breast self-examination (BSE) and advised to examine their breasts monthly. The women in their forties at entry were randomly assigned to receive five years of annual mammograms (two exposures) as well as annual breast examinations (palpation) by a physician or a nurse (this was the intervention group)—or simply to receive an initial breast examination and no further screening assays except monthly BSE (this was the control group). The women in their fifties at entry were randomly assigned to five years of annual mammograms and breast examinations (this was the intervention group)—or simply to five years of annual breast examinations (this was the control group).[42]

Those American radiologists who served as consultants to the CNBSS could never suppress their suspicions that its mammography was substandard. Were not many of the machines being used antiquated? And how many of the people taking and interpreting the breast images actually had credentials as full-time mammographers? In 1985 the Canadians replaced the mediolateral exposure with the mediolateral oblique at the Americans' urging—the latter view usually did a better job of imaging the axillary tail of the mammary gland, where tumors may spring up surreptitiously. Yet the American radiologists still wanted to see more evidence of quality control; two of them eventually resigned from the CNBSS, a gesture of protest which quickly became more public than private.[43]

In May 1992 Anthony B. Miller and his colleagues leaked the seven-year CNBSS results to the news media, months before the official publication in a medical journal. The American radiologists' worst fears were confirmed as the magnitude of the heresy became clear. The CNBSS reported no survival advantage gained by annual mammography, either in the 40-to-49 age group or in the 50-to-59 age group. Even worse, the younger women who got mammograms had experienced more deaths from breast cancer (38) than the younger women who merely practiced BSE (28). Pressed by journalists for an explanation, Dr. Miller and his CNBSS co-workers speculated that the breast compression required for mammography might have forced cancer cells into the bloodstream and thereby hastened the process of metastasis. This wild hypothesis was repeated by the London *Times* and many other newspapers in England and Canada. On May 18 *Time* magazine broke the story for American readers under the quizzical headline "Are Mammograms Bad for Your Health?"[44]

Open warfare quickly ensued—the American radiologists lobbed anathema after anathema across the Canadian border. The Cincinnati mammographer Myron Moskowitz felt that the Canadians had committed every radiographic sin in the book: "I seem to recall that many of the films suffered from poor compression to no compression, low contrast, fuzzy detail, motion, and other artifacts." Daniel B. Kopans of Boston's Massachusetts General Hospital was the most vocal of the inquisitors attempting to squelch the heresy. In a series of thoughtfully composed letters and editorials, he sought to explain why the CNBSS results should not be taken seriously: "The trial was designed from an epidemiological perspective to test the benefit of a screening technology (mammography), but the importance of the technology as well as the quality of the mammography itself was discounted. At best the results may tell us whether there is any benefit from poor-quality mammography." Dr. Kopans calculated that over 50% of the mammograms taken in the trial's first four years were "unsatisfactory." The Canadians did not tolerate this arithmetic for an instant. Dr. Miller countered that only 2% of all the mammograms taken in the trial were unsatisfactory.[45] His colleague Cornelia J. Baines argued that the trial's mammography compared favorably to that in other large trials: "In both age groups, mammography was associated with higher cancer detection rates." Dr. Baines opined that the CNBSS findings were simply "unwelcome" in an atmosphere where both the lay public and many health professionals automatically equated earlier detection with a cure.[46]

Besides antiquated equipment and faulty technique, American radiologists also took the CNBSS for that striking peculiarity which no one could fully explain—the excess of breast cancer deaths in the 40-to-49-year-old women who were randomized to receive annual mammography. How did it happen that during the trial's first year 19 advanced tumors, with four or more positive axillary nodes, were diagnosed in the mammography arm, while only five comparably advanced tumors were detected in the control group? Stephen A. Feig of Philadelphia's Thomas Jefferson University Hospital, suspected that this circumstance came about because of **allocation bias**—in other words, that women with existing breast lumps or other symptoms at entry had been "preferentially assigned to the study group."[47] Nonsense, retorted Dr. Miller and his CNBSS colleagues; the trial's randomization was above board. They hinted that the imbalance might have occurred through **diagnostic bias**—in other words, that some of the Canadian medical centers may not have performed thorough axillary dissections, thereby allowing extensive nodal involvement to go undetected in a few breast cancers diagnosed in the control group. When the CNBSS team presented revised results based on an average follow-up of 10.5 years, they pointed out that the mortality rate for the control group in the 40-to-49 age bracket was rapidly catching up with the rate seen in the mammography arm. Now there were 72 breast cancer deaths recorded for the controls, as compared to 82 recorded for the women who received annual mammograms. Thus the apparent reduction in mortality favoring the controls had declined from the 26% reported at seven years to a modest 12%. Dr. Miller and his colleagues opined that the CNBSS controls diagnosed with breast cancer had fared so much better than comparable controls in earlier mammography trials because they tended to have smaller tumors and, if node-positive, they were almost always given adjuvant chemotherapy.[48] No doubt that reduction in tumor size owed something to the CNBSS emphasis on breast self-examination. Did the controls do their monthly BSE more conscientiously than the women in the intervention arm who might have been lulled into a false sense of security by less-than-optimal mammograms?

The "Under 50" Battles

The personal integrity of the CNBSS collaborators remained unchallenged; but the same cannot be said for the very sweeping conclusion they continued to promulgate— viz., that periodic mammography would add little, if anything at all, to the reduction in breast cancer mortality achievable by proficient clinical examinations. In the United States battle lines were forming around the issue of whether mammograms should be recommended for women in their forties.

Daniel B. Kopans and allied radiologists searched the record room of the Massachusetts General Hospital for case histories of breast carcinomas diagnosed in women under age 50. The survival statistics were then fired off like cannonballs aimed at the CNBSS. For 846 women who had palpable invasive tumors, the five-year survival rate was 72%. For 70 women who had nonpalpable invasive tumors detected by mammography alone, the five-year survival rate was 91%. Who says that you get the same odds of survival if you wait for tumors to become palpable? Who says that women under 50 don't benefit from screening mammography? In truth, the survival statistics in the Massachusetts General series were unremarkable, just about what you would expect; but they seemed to come as a revelation to General Electric, a major manufacturer of mammographic equipment. That company began running a TV commercial touting "a remarkable 91% cure rate" for breast cancer, made possible by early detection with mammograms.[49] The implication of vital and almost universal benefit was even less subtle than the ACS messages!

The National Cancer Institute now sought an antidote to the plague of exaggeration. In February 1993 the NCI hosted an "International Workshop" on breast cancer screening at its Bethesda, Maryland, campus. A blue-ribbon panel heard much testimony from epidemiologists and radiologists, but its main task was to evaluate the results from the eight clinical trials to date—the old HIP trial, the two protocols of the CNBSS, four trials done in Sweden, and one done in Scotland. The upshot from this workshop was the "Fletcher report," so dubbed after the panel's chairperson Suzanne W. Fletcher, editor of *Annals of Internal Medicine*. Dr. Fletcher and her fellow panelists agreed that the evidence from these trials supported "the scientific observation that screening leads to reduced breast cancer mortality in women aged 50 to 69." The panel offered a ballpark estimate of "about a third" (30% to 35%) for the probable mortality reduction; but they had no clue whether screening mammography in this age group should be performed yearly, as recommended in the United States, or every two years, as practiced in several European countries. "The Swedish studies," Fletcher et al observed, "suggest that a mammogram as infrequently as every 33 months reduces mortality." With regard to women over age 70, the panel felt that the previous trials had included "too few women for adequate analysis." A mortality reduction obtainable by screening women aged 40 to 49 also remained to be demonstrated. "For this age group," Dr. Fletcher and her colleagues concluded, "there is no reduction in mortality in the first five-to-seven years after study entry. There is an uncertain and, if present, marginal reduction in mortality at about ten-to-twelve years."[50]

The portions of the Fletcher report touching on the effectiveness of screening mammography before age 50 were not well received in all quarters. Dr. Kopans and the San Francisco radiologist Edward A. Sickles leaped on the barricades, blasting the report for "discounting the importance of nonrandomized controlled data." Drs. Kopans and Sickles plausibly asserted that, insofar as women aged 40 to 49 were concerned, all the randomized trials had "flaws in experimental design and technical deficiencies in implementation" which "severely limit both statistical validity and clinical applicability." With the exception of the CNBSS, none of these trials was specifically designed to detect a benefit for women in their forties; and all of them suffered from poor-quality mammography. "As a result, mammographic images from the eight randomized trials are not at all comparable with today's real-world mammography." Kopans and

Sickles concluded that "it is scientifically unjustified to claim that screening women aged 40 to 49 is ineffective. The only reason not to screen is economic."[51]

Dr. Fletcher and her fellow panelists launched a proper counterattack. They explained that they could form conclusions only on results from clinical trials, not on "the unpublished findings" cited by Kopans and Sickles. And there were other reasons besides economics to advise against routine mammography for women in their forties. To name a few, Fletcher et al cited "the lack of evidence supporting screening and the potential for negative side effects, including false-positive test results and overdiagnosis."[52] The battle intensified during October 1993, as proponents and opponents of screening mammography before age 50 argued their respective cases before an NCI advisory committee. Peter Greenwald, director of the NCI's Division of Cancer Prevention and Control, calculated that an enormous clinical trial would be necessary to demonstrate an unequivocal survival advantage in women aged 40 to 49. "If we need a million women and ten years to detect a benefit," quipped a committee member, "the benefit must be extremely small."[53]

On December 3, 1993, the NCI finally issued an official statement clarifying its position: "Experts do not agree on the role of routine screening mammography for women ages 40 to 49. To date, randomized clinical trials have not shown a statistically significant reduction in mortality for women under the age of 50."[54] While not cast as a screening recommendation, the NCI's "statement of evidence" had the effect of rescinding its previous guidelines which had endorsed mammography for women both over and under age 50. That terse statement not only handed the laurels of victory to Dr. Fletcher's panel, but—*oh horrid schism!*—placed the NCI in direct opposition to the American

Cancer Society. Whatever happened to the Glorious Consensus of 1989?

For its part, the ACS did not yield an inch of ground. The Society reaffirmed its previous guidelines, calling upon American women aged 40 to 49 to undergo screening mammography "every one to two years." Curtis Mettlin and Charles R. Smart, members of the ACS Detection and Treatment Committee, acknowledged that women over age 50 were at greater risk for breast malignancies, and that "in this age group mortality reductions from annual screening have been of greater magnitude and more uniformly observed across different studies." Yet Mettlin and Smart pointed out that "23% of all breast cancer deaths occur in women diagnosed when they were younger than 50 years." There are no early-detection strategies for these younger women "with as much supporting evidence as there is for mammography and clinical breast examination."[55]

Still on the ramparts, Daniel B. Kopans objected that the whole idea of using age 50 as an arbitrary dividing line was silly. "The breast tissues do not turn to fat at age 50 or at menopause," he explained. That was just a myth with no biological basis. In fact, the replacement of glandular tissues by fat is a gradual process which occurs over several decades. Insofar as mammographic accuracy is concerned, Dr. Kopans asserted, the differences between women in their forties and women in their fifties are relatively insignificant.[56]

The Consensus Conference:
Agreeing to Disagree

The release of the CNBSS findings and the NCI's retraction of its guidelines probably left many women uncertain about the value of screening mammography. Worse than that, however, was the fact that these highly publicized and imprimatur-stamped events emboldened the really aggressive iconoclasts, those complete nonbelievers who wanted to dispense with the assay altogether. In 1995 the English medical journal *Lancet* published a blistering commentary written by two Canadians, who concluded that screening mammography has been associated with "marginal benefit, substantial harm, and enormous costs." The skeptical duo argued that public funds should not be used for "mass unselected screening" in any age group—the money would be better spent if "channeled into more realistic public education along with casefinding in targeted high-risk groups."[57] We may perhaps wonder whether any medical journal in the United States would dare to publish such a violent dismembering of a sacred cow. The *Atlantic Monthly*, a prestigious literary journal, had no qualms; in 1996 it published a thoroughly irreverent piece by David Plotkin, a Los Angeles oncologist who had worked on several NSABP trials. "Mammography," wrote Dr. Plotkin, "is only leading physicians to diagnose an ever-larger number of harmless tumors. Patients who otherwise would never have known they have cancer may needlessly suffer. For all we know, the chief effect has been to disguise our inability to cure the old cancer, by burying it in cases of new cancer."[58]

As the published opinions of leading experts became more and more contradictory, the authorities at the National Cancer Institute dreamed of that fantastical celestial paradise called *Consensus*, so alluring yet so terribly elusive! The goal of the **Consensus Development Conference** (CDC) held in Bethesda, Maryland, on January 21, 22, and 23, 1997, seemed modest enough—to come up with a new NCI guideline on screening mammography for women aged 40 to 49. The twelve-member panel charged with this task and an audience numbering over a thousand listened to the presentations made by 32 speakers. The CDC soon came to focus on that pathological enigma called ductal carcinoma *in situ*. While DCIS is always curable, the necessity of always curing it remains open to question. Karla Kerlikowske and John Barclay, epidemiologists at the University of California in San Francisco, told the panel and audience that DCIS is more likely to be detected in women in their forties than in older women. By way of proof, they presented data generated by their University's Mobile Mammography Screening Program. Of the participating women aged 40 through 49 who had positive biopsy reports after an initial screening exam, 44% had DCIS. The DCIS portion of the diagnosed breast cancers dropped to 30% for women aged 50 to 59, and still further to 18% for women aged 60 to 69. "The natural history of DCIS is unknown," Kerlikowske and Barclay observed. "The current clinical dilemma lies in not being able to distinguish which lesions will progress to invasive cancer. Numerous studies have shown that only 15% to 25% of DCIS lesions progress to invasive cancer over five to ten years, and maybe as few as 7%."[59]

Given the fact that DCIS is more prevalent in premenopausal women than in postmenopausal ones, we might even suspect that some of these lesions may regress of their own accord when the hormones acting on the mammary gland become less plentiful. In the United States, of course, no physician is going to adopt a wait-and-see policy for DCIS—all lesions discovered by mammography will be referred for definitive local therapy (i.e., mastectomy or lumpectomy). Maryann Napoli of the Center for Medical Consumers (New York City) emphasized to the CDC panel and audience that the public should be warned about the dangers inherent in discovering "cancers" so early that their future behavior cannot be predicted: "I have met many a woman who has had a mastectomy for DCIS, who regards herself as a cancer survivor, who worries about recurrence like every other cancer patient, who believes her daughters are at high risk, and who has no idea of the uncertainties that surround her diagnosis." American women, observed Ms. Napoli, "have received such one-sided and distorted information about early detection that most probably don't know what they should be asking about mammography screening in their forties."[60]

The frequently expressed concerns about overdiagnosis seem to have weighed heavily on the CDC panel. When the presentations were finished, ten of its twelve members issued a majority statement concluding "that the data currently available do not warrant a universal recommendation for mammography for all women in their forties. Each woman should decide for herself whether to undergo mammography." In a striking departure from tradition, the panel majority suggested that DCIS and other slow-growing cancers "could be detected by mammograms after age 50 and treated at that time. Earlier detection may cause additional months or years of cancer-related anxiety, affecting personal and workplace relationships, as well as insurance coverage." *What on earth!!* Did somebody actually say that cancer detection should be delayed? Two members of the CDC panel refused to go along with this blatant heresy; they released a separate minority report which endorsed routine screening mammography for "all healthy women" aged 40 through 49. "Biologically," the minority panelists wrote, "all invasive ductal and lobular cancers must begin as *in situ* lesions; it is potentially dangerous to suggest that DCIS could safely be left undetected until women are in their fifties."[61]

Notwithstanding the open schism on the CDC panel, the thoughtfully worded majority opinion represented a great victory for those skeptics who believed that universal mammography for asymptomatic women in their forties would create far more problems than it solved. The breast surgeon Susan Love hailed the CDC verdict as "right on target" in a *Newsweek* article: "The real challenge isn't deciding whether to screen women between 40 and 50; it's to go beyond imaging and come up with really early detection."[62] The syndicated columnist Mona Charen also applauded: "We have all been over-terrified about breast cancer and over-sold on mammograms. Of course, any individual woman who believes that she is at higher than average risk should go ahead and be X-rayed. Why is it so difficult to be told to make our own decisions? Women make these decisions all the time, weighing benefit against risk."[63]

The United States Senate, a male-dominated organization, placed considerably less confidence in the individual woman's judgment. In early February 1997 the Senate passed a nonbinding resolution with a lop-sided vote (98 to 0), calling on the National Cancer Institute to "reinstate the pre-1993 screening guidelines." The timely detection of breast malignancies would seem to have become as much a political litmus test in the 1990s as the containment of communism used to be in the 1950s—simply whisper the word and you've got a Senator's vote! Alas, the laurels of victory crowning the skeptics' brows quickly withered away in the intense heat surreptitiously emanating from Capitol Hill and the White House. On February 25, 1997, the National Cancer Advisory Board (NCAB), whose members are Presidential appointees, convened in a two-hour session to consider screening mammography.[65] And just one month later, on March 27, the NCI director Richard D. Klausner held a press conference to announce that the National Cancer Institute had accepted new guidelines as recommended by the NCAB. Henceforth the NCI would advise women at "average risk" aged 40 through 49 to undergo screening mammography "every one to two years." Dr. Klausner, who had previously expressed some sympathy for the CDC's majority position, now sounded apologetic. "The data are complex," he conceded, "and the evidence is not transparent." President Bill Clinton entertained no such doubts. Speaking from the Oval Office, he hailed the new NCI guidelines: "The federal government is doing its part to make sure women have both coverage and access to this potentially life-saving test."[66]

For their part, the skeptics felt that scientific deliberation had been summarily sacrificed on the altar of political expediency. Suzanne W. Fletcher wrote an article for the *New England Journal of Medicine*, pleading that recommendations for "clinical policies that affect large segments of the population" should be the responsibility of qualified scientists: "Congress should stay out of this process. When the discussion of medical science moves from an NIH auditorium to a hearing room in the Senate Office Building, the ground rules change. Whereas anecdotes constitute weak evidence in medical science, personal stories are powerful persuaders in a Senate hearing."[67] Two correspondents to the *Journal of the National Cancer Institute* offered a monetary analysis based on a Bureau of the Census estimate that there were 20,050,000 American women between the ages of 40 and 49. Assuming a price tag of $125 for each set of mammograms, the cost of screening all these women for just one year would amount to 2.5 billion dollars. And that would be about eight times the sum (300 million dollars) that the NCI had allotted for breast cancer research in its annual budget.[68]

Hard Opinions, Soft Data

By the year 2000 the splendid illusion of unanimity created by the twelve-imprimatur guidelines of 1989 had melted into thin air and left not a rack behind. Polarization reigned supreme. On one side were professional mammographers who felt that their technology's potential to reduce breast cancer mortality had hardly been explored. On the other side stood an alliance of assorted non-radiologists who felt that screening mammography had been shamelessly overpromoted and that it principally led to unnecessary interventions. The solid data which could produce accord simply did not exist. In the year 2000 no one could cite any clinical trial which had reported that periodic screening reduced breast cancer mortality by 50% or more. As we have seen, the HIP trial of the 1960s and the BCDDP of the 1970s gave us plausible evidence that the combination of physical examinations and mammograms could eventually reduce mortality by about 25%. We might have logically expected that subsequent refinements in breast imaging technology would have improved that percentage somewhat, but as yet there has been no sweeping reduction in the death rate comparable to the 70% plunge in cervical cancer mortality after the introduction of the Pap smear. Writing in 1996, the NCI statistician Kenneth C. Chu and his colleagues pointed out that breast cancer mortality in the United States actually increased a little in the mid-1980s, prior to a 6.8% drop from 1989 through 1993. During this period "a significant decrease of approximately 2% per year was observed in every decade of age, from 40 to 79 years of age." Chu et al concluded that the reduction in mortality was "too rapid to be explained only by the increased use of mammography; likewise, there has been no equivalent dramatic increase in survival rates that would implicate therapy alone."[69]

Earlier detection and systemic therapy do seem to be making small inroads in that long-constant mortality rate for breast carcinomas, but how much credit should be proportioned to mammography? We really need the NSABP to do a big authoritative trial of screening mammography—say, a million participants, with ten years of annual mammograms and twenty years of follow-up. If well-designed, a trial like this ought to tell us for sure how effective mammography is in preventing premature death. For the time being, we are left with lesser trials and with that embarrassing question asked by the CNBSS protocols—viz., do annual mammograms really lower long-term mortality all that much better than diligent palpation? In the year 2000 American radiologists were lauding recent results from the Gothenburg trial, which had randomized 25,941 Swedish women aged 39 through 49 to receive two-view mammography every eighteen months (intervention group), or to an unscreened control group. After some eleven years of follow-up, the mammography arm was enjoying a 45% reduction in breast cancer mortality compared to the control group.[70] Stephen A. Feig cited the "relatively short screening interval" and "improved image contrast" as the reasons why the Gothenburg trial found a much greater mortality reduction than any previous trial involving women in their forties. Mammographic screening at annual intervals, Dr. Feig opined, should do even better.[71]

Unfortunately, those devilish Canadians were not yet done with making mischief. In the *Journal of the National Cancer Institute* for September 20, 2000, Anthony B. Miller and his CNBSS colleagues published the survival statistics from their trial protocol for women aged 50 through 59 at entry, the very age group where annual mammography is supposed to be so effective in saving lives. Miller et al conceded that mammography had indeed detected more cancers than palpation, and had detected cancers at smaller sizes; but they reported that the lead time gained did not translate into a reduction in mortality. After a follow-up of thirteen years, the two arms were experiencing almost identical mortality—107 deaths from breast cancer among those women who received both annual mammograms and annual physical exams, as compared to 105 deaths among the women who received only annual physical exams. The CNBSS team confidently concluded that "the addition of annual mammography to physical examination has no impact on breast cancer mortality."[72]

There would seem to be two possible explanations for the extraordinary CNBSS findings. The first is that they are an artifact created by poor mammography and the otherwise bungled execution of an ill-conceived trial (American radiologists have tended to espouse this hypothesis). A second possibility is that they are a logical consequence of differences in tumor biology. This hypothesis assumes that the most lethal breast carcinomas do not necessarily produce radiological clues years in advance of metastatic dissemination, but rather would tend to present without warning, sometimes in the intervals between screening examinations. For these tumors, neither mammography nor palpation would predictably alert us in time for a curative surgical intervention. Any other potentially-lethal tumors must be assumed to be so slow-growing that it would make little difference whether they are detected earlier by mammography or somewhat later by palpation—there would still be time for effective interventions. As we have seen, Dr. Spratt hinted at this heretical idea many years ago. The CNBSS findings give it

renewed currency; if it should ever become orthodoxy, all those high-volume breast imaging centers which opened in American cities during the 1980s would no doubt go the way of the tuberculosis sanitariums of the 1920s and the iron-lung polio wards of the 1950s. Cornelia J. Baines of the CNBSS cared not a fig about the employment prospects of American radiologists. "If you can't afford mammography or don't like it," she advised women in an Associated Press interview, "go get a good clinical physical exam and you will be protecting yourself against breast cancer death." Her remarks appeared in many American newspapers, together with a strong caveat from Robert A. Smith of the American Cancer Society. "The problems with the Canadian study," observed Dr. Smith, "are well known."[73]

Author Trying to Play Solomon

We should be grateful to the CNBSS for reminding us that simple old-fashioned palpation confers a degree of protection, but at present it would seem unwise to regard this trial's controversial results as the final word on breast cancer screening. Mammography remains the gold standard of early detection, with a sensitivity which is usually far superior to palpation. That ability to detect tiny infiltrating carcinomas and poorly differentiated DCIS lesions several years before they would become palpable must be assumed, in at least some cases, to translate into reduced mortality. The problem is that we have no really convincing statistics about the extent of this reduction. We do know from long experience that when solid tumors become palpable or otherwise clinically apparent, they often have already metastasized. This knowledge gives us a perpetual incentive to develop methods of preclinical detection. While mammography is nowhere near as sensitive as the Pap smear, its most troublesome shortcoming has been its lack of specificity for nonpalpable abnormalities. Back in the BCDDP days, this flaw was manifested by benign-to-malignant biopsy finding ratios ranging as high as 16.4 to one. More recently, we have been troubled by the fact that mammography has become sensitive enough to detect ever-growing numbers of DCIS lesions, but not specific enough to tell us which lesions are going to pose an imminent threat.

In most countries, public health strategists cannot even dream of widespread screening mammography. The disease in question principally afflicts women past childbearing age; it does not cause immediate disability, nor does it appreciably shorten the lifespans of most victims. The entire world has been sold on the Sabin polio vaccine, because a single vaccination costing a few pennies provides lasting protection. In contrast, screening mammography is perceived as a necessity only in very rich and very healthy nations like Sweden and the United States. This public health measure must be repeated at regular intervals. A recommendation to screen all women between the ages of 40 and 79 translates into forty years of annual mammograms—the expense and inconvenience involved would be more palatable if the disease were slightly more prevalent or slightly more lethal, or if we had slightly better evidence of the strategy's effectiveness in reducing morbidity and mortality. Financial considerations prompt efforts to restrict mass screening of asymptomatic individuals to those age groups where it seems most likely to be productive. The American Cancer Society has not recommended an upper age limit for periodic mammography, but most other organizations have hinted that at some point the rationale for this assay must cease to exist. Eighty-year-old women, for example, continue to be

at risk of developing breast cancer, yet their risk of actually dying from it is getting smaller and smaller. Breast malignancies in octogenarians usually behave sluggishly; patients diagnosed in this decade are more likely to die *with* cancer than *from* cancer—the cause of death typically being an unrelated and nonmalignant malady. There can be little justification for taking routine mammograms of elderly women with morbid conditions like Alzheimer's disease or congestive heart failure; in most cases they would not live long enough to complete the screening process.

In 1995 a task force of experts convened by the Public Health Service (PHS) looked at the pros and cons of cancer screening, eventually producing a very conservative set of guidelines. The PHS panel concluded that there was "insufficient evidence" that the current screening assays for lung, prostatic, and ovarian cancers were achieving mortality reductions. For breast cancer the panel recommended mammography "every one to two years for women aged 50 to 69." The American Cancer Society and the American College of Radiology protested that the PHS mammography guideline "discriminated" against both younger (under 50) and older (over 70) women.[74] Of course, the idea was not to discriminate, but rather to designate the age group where the mass screening of asymptomatic women with no exceptional risk factors seems most warranted. Only a few nonbelievers would oppose mammography for women aged 50 to 69. Whether screening at two-year intervals will achieve mortality reductions comparable to those produced by annual screening remains to be demonstrated; obviously it would cut the radiology bill in half.

Women aged 35 to 49 were included in the BCDDP. This age group stands to lose the most years of life in the event of malignant transformation, yet it is at considerably less risk of disease than the 50-to-69-year-olds. Most American women in their thirties and forties vastly overestimate their risk, thanks to all those public service messages and magazine articles which target this age group instead of more grandmotherly types. A survey published in the *Journal of the National Cancer Institute* found that women under age 50 overestimated their probability of dying from breast cancer by more than twentyfold.[75] So much for "educating" the public about cancer! There is, however, a small subset of premenopausal women who are at very high risk of disease occurrence and premature death—namely, those with a family history of aggressive early-onset breast carcinomas. These women stand to benefit from the earliest possible detection and therapeutic intervention; the problem is that as yet we have scant evidence that periodic mammography will substantially reduce their risk level. Writing in 2001, the Australian oncologist Kelly-Anne Phillips observed that breast malignancies associated with hereditary mutations in the *BRCA1* gene "have a relatively homogeneous phenotype that generally includes high grade, *p53* positivity, and estrogen receptor negativity." In other words, they might tend to be interval-surfacing tumors—Dr. Phillips expresses concern "that mammography may be of less value than hoped for in this situation."[76]

Not all mutations in the *BRCA1* gene are equally dangerous. Nonetheless, the clinical trials of screening mammography have consistently reported that any reductions in breast cancer mortality take several years longer to become apparent in women under age 50 than in older women. And this fact demonstrates that mammography has historically done a poor job of providing sufficient early warning of fast-moving premenopausal breast cancers. Stephen A. Feig, Daniel B. Kopans, and other radiologists argue that women in their forties must

be screened at more frequent intervals if such tumors are to be detected in time for curative interventions. Accepting this logic, the American Cancer Society changed its screening guidelines in March 1997, recommending annual mammograms for women aged 40 to 49 instead of mammography "every one to two years."[77] The rationale for shorter screening intervals is clear enough. But the best we can say for any cancer screening strategy is that it betters the odds of survival in the event of malignant transformation. With our improvements in genetic analysis, those young women who have watched a mother or a sister die from early-onset breast cancer will often have to live with the knowledge that they too carry the culprit mutation in the *BRCA1* or *p53* gene. Unfortunately, even the most frequent screening with mammograms and clinical examinations cannot begin to offer these women the same degree of protection as that afforded by prophylactic bilateral mastectomy.

Some Practical Advice

Screening mammography is unlikely to vanish from the American scene—indeed, it may even become more popular if technical advances make it more accurate and less cumbersome. Our radiologists are anxiously awaiting the perfection of **full-field digital mammography**, that long-awaited wedding of traditional imaging to the new computer technology. Those familiar black-and-white films of the 1980s and 1990s may soon be replaced by color images displayed on computer monitors. How much this electronic revolution will contribute to diagnostic accuracy remains to be seen. Stephen A. Feig believes that "digital mammography, especially when used in conjunction with computer-aided detection and digital tomosynthesis, could be particularly useful for dense fibroglandular breasts that now pose a major problem."[78] Ease of manipulation would head the list of digital mammography's advantages—images could be immediately enlarged, made brighter, or given more contrast. Preservation and transmission would also be a snap—numerous mammograms could be stored on a single computer disk, and selected images could be instantaneously transmitted to distant consultants via the Internet. In the long run, digital mammography would probably prove cheaper than the old film-screen methodology. There would be no costs for film processing, and the task of visual evaluation would be expedited by computer programs which automatically scanned the breast images and highlighted any seeming abnormalities. One of these programs had already won FDA approval in 1998.[79] Yet additional technical refinements and some price reductions will be needed before the promise of digital mammography can be fully realized. In the year 2000 the initial cost of a digital breast-imaging system was about five times that of a film-screen system.

While the era of digital mammography may soon be at hand, no computer program will entirely eliminate the possibility that healthy women may be harmed by screening, either by false positives leading to unnecessary biopsies, or by the detection and treatment of low-grade neoplasms whose clinical course would have been benign. A few hints on avoiding pitfalls are in order. Dr. Kopans reminds us that the risk of radiation carcinogenesis due to mammography has often been exaggerated by the popular media: "Risk to the breast is related to the age at exposure, with likely no risk among women in their forties."[80] An exception to this rule is provided by **ataxia-telangiectasia**, a recessive hereditary disorder. Women who carry the culprit genetic defect may be put at risk of

mammary and other tumors by any exposure to radiation. While the actual disease is quite rare, about one percent of the American population are suspected to be carriers.[81]

Premenopausal women, particularly those just beginning annual screening, are at the greatest risk of unnecessary biopsies. Their mammographic and physical examinations will be most accurate and least painful if performed within a week after menstruation—that is, in the early follicular phase, when breast engorgement is minimal. The CNBSS reported an increased percentage of false-negative results for those mammograms taken during the luteal phase (last half of the menstrual cycle).[82] Edward A. Sickles offers practical advice to all women undergoing screening mammography on how to avoid needlessly repeated imaging. "The false-positive rate," Dr. Sickles assures us, "is reduced by more than half when current mammograms are compared with previous screening mammograms." He cites "cysts, calcified fibroadenomas, and intramammary lymph nodes" as examples of benign lesions which can arouse suspicion of malignancy. Since these lesions usually "do not change in appearance over time," comparison with previous mammograms will often enable the radiologist to recognize their true nature. Sickles urges "women scheduling appointments for screening to bring their previous mammograms with them to the examination, if these films were taken at another practice." This circumstance occurs frequently because "insurance carriers now change radiology providers on a regular basis."[83]

Not only should women undergoing periodic mammography be mindful of the location of previous images, but they need to know more about the art and science of breast radiology. In 1999 the Food and Drug Administration took a step toward promoting meaningful public awareness, by requiring mammography clinics to send a written report on each exam directly to the patient. The radiologist's evaluation of the mammograms must be written in terms a layperson can understand and forwarded no later than thirty days after the exam. If the exam suggests the presence of malignancy, the FDA recommends that the results be forwarded to the referring physician within three days and then to the patient within five. The doctor's two-day advance notification is intended to give him or her the time to prepare responses to the patient's anxious inquiries.[84]

Consultations about infiltrating breast tumors tend to be comparatively straightforward, but the question of what to tell patients about ductal carcinoma *in situ* is problematic. The term "breast cancer" has the effect of an electric prod, and it is typically an overstatement when used to describe small DCIS lesions discovered by mammography. Even evasive gobbledygook about "neoplasms of uncertain behavior" might be preferable— certainly patients should be made aware that the risk of DCIS lesions evolving into invasive tumors is highly variable and hard to express in exact percentages. The pathological findings from the NSABP's clinical trial on DCIS singled out "comedo necrosis" as an indicator associated with local recurrences after lumpectomy.[85] Patterns of linear or branching calcifications seen on mammograms often foreshadow this comedo variety of DCIS. The radiologist Paul C. Stomper

and his colleagues at the Roswell Park Cancer Institute (Buffalo, New York) remind us that any suspected DCIS lesion should be imaged a second time with **magnification mammography**, so as to gain a better idea of its extent and nature. They caution that the presence or absence of invasive foci "cannot be predicted with a high degree of accuracy on the basis of mammographic appearance."[86]

Treatment for DCIS is intended solely to obtain local control. Mastectomy remains a reasonable option for an extensive comedo or otherwise poorly differentiated lesion which affects several breast quadrants. Focal excision (lumpectomy) followed by surveillance would seem adequate for smaller and less ominous lesions. When the breast is preserved, radiation therapy can better the odds against local recurrence—it tends to be especially valuable when a poorly differentiated lesion is excised with narrow or possibly involved margins. Chemotherapy is not indicated for DCIS, but tamoxifen or some other hormonal agent could be logically prescribed after the diagnosis of an estrogen receptor-positive lesion. In this instance the hormonal agent would not be intended to stymie metastatic disease, but simply to prevent recurrent or new DCIS lesions from arising either in the affected breast or in the contralateral breast.[87]

Chapter Twenty-nine

Breast Self-Examination

In past decades **breast self-examination** (BSE) on a monthly basis was a screening tool prominently recommended in the brochures on breast cancer distributed by the American Cancer Society and the National Cancer Institute.   This traditional advice would seem harmless enough. Who could quibble with the ideas that women should be knowledgeable about those clinical symptoms which might possibly be caused by malignancy, and that they should be aware of changes occurring in their breasts, with a view to detecting any suspicious symptom in a timely fashion and bringing it to medical attention? Unfortunately, like other matters pertaining to breast cancer, BSE has lately managed to become controversial. The NCI no longer prints a BSE guide, and the ACS has noticeably downplayed BSE in its educational materials. The spokespersons for these two organizations will take pains to explain that there is no solid evidence that BSE reduces breast cancer mortality, and that an undue emphasis on this technique might deter some women from getting those annual mammograms whose potential to save lives seems much greater.[1] Professional radiologists have been especially hard on BSE. Writing in the *Journal of the American Medical Association* in the year 2000, Daniel B. Kopans conceded "that clinical breast examination can detect a number of small cancers undetected by mammography," yet he argued that this practice "can lead to significant harms, including false alarms, anxiety, and unnecessary biopsies."[2]   Dr. Kopans' objection would seem overwrought and misplaced. Those concerns about "false alarms" and "unnecessary biopsies" are more properly related to screening mammograms which discover clusters of suspect but innocent calcifications. Any persistent abnormal presentation involving the breast that we can actually see and feel always demands a diagnosis. Now we may not need to treat the underlying condition—it usually proves to be benign—but we always need to know its nature. While overt symptoms discovered by BSE may lead to anxiety, BSE *per se* cannot be said to produce anxiety. Surgical biopsies have historically been more common—and more difficult—with those nonpalpable lesions discovered by mammography than with the palpable ones found by visual and manual examinations. Clinical presentations are usually easy to diagnose. As discussed in Chapter Ten, diagnostic mammography can often tell us whether a palpable breast mass is simply a harmless cyst or fibroadenoma (the most frequent diagnoses), or whether it has a radiographic silhouette suggestive of malignancy. If in doubt, we could do a fine-needle aspiration or a core-needle biopsy to establish the diagnosis before deciding on a surgical intervention.

While BSE cannot approach the sensitivity of mammography, it can be a useful supplement to radiology. More than that, however, monthly BSE is one screening procedure which could be recommended to women of all ages, from nineteen to ninety-nine. BSE's potential to detect palpable but as yet unobtrusive breast masses depends upon how diligently it is performed by the individual woman. If done knowledgeably and conscientiously, it should better the odds of survival in the event of malignant transformation. The smallest masses that might be predictably discovered by thorough palpatory examinations probably would range upwards of one centimeter in diameter—say, somewhere between one-quarter and one-half inch in diameter. Tumors in this size range are not exactly minuscule, but then they tend to have a good prognosis. The clinical trials conducted by the NSABP and other organizations have consistently reported that the majority of invasive tumors under one centimeter in diameter will prove to be node-negative—and therefore presumably curable by adequate local therapy. Whether node-negative or not, these small-diameter tumors more readily lend themselves to breast preservation. If they should have already shed malignant cells outside the breast, these cells might be more likely to respond to cytotoxic or hormonal drugs because the overall tumor burden in the body would still be rather modest. The benefits which we might anticipate from the timely detection of small breast masses and other clinical presentations are self-evident. Occasionally monthly BSE will detect palpable tumors which are missed by periodic mammography, either because they are radiographically invisible, or because they present in the intervals between screening examinations. Under these circumstances BSE obviously outperforms mammography. When we consider that BSE costs nothing, requires only a few minutes each month, and can be performed at home, we may not wish to shelve the practice, but rather to find ways in which it can be made more effective.

Some Ways to Approach BSE

Not many American breast specialists are prepared to entertain the heretical conclusion reached by Cornelia J. Baines and her colleagues of the Canadian National Breast Screening Study—namely, that visual and palpatory examinations of the breast can save just as many lives as annual mammograms. And nobody, not even Dr. Baines, believes that casually performed BSE is likely to be an effective screening tool. "In the same way that some people have urged that screening mammography must be of the highest technical standard," Dr. Baines and her CNBSS observe, "so too must it be urged that, when physical examination is done, it should be done well."[3] While an optimal technique for doing BSE has never been defined, learning to do a reasonably thorough exam requires more detailed instruction than that provided by those simplistic ACS illustrations of shower-stall palpation. Ideally, a woman motivated to follow a regimen of monthly BSE would receive personal coaching from a physician or registered nurse who had considerable experience with—and a strong belief in the value of—the clinical breast examination. Unfortunately, knowledgeable and enthusiastic BSE instructors are not likely to be identified in any city's Yellow Pages, though perhaps a local cancer support group or ACS chapter can provide the name of a qualified coach in the vicinity.

The few words of advice in this book are not intended to substitute for personalized BSE instruction, but simply to outline some basic principles. In general, the particular technique adopted for BSE would seem less important than a certain seriousness of intent. For a few minutes at least, you have to concentrate on the breast being examined and on the visual and tactile messages your eyes and fingers are sending to your brain. The exam normally begins with an attentive **visual inspection** of both breasts, which takes place before a mirror. Dr. Baines and her CNBSS colleagues advise that you could be either "seated or standing" (whichever is more comfortable), as you observe the changes in the breasts' appearance produced by three arm positionings. The arms are initially "relaxed and hanging," then raised above the head, and finally placed akimbo with "hands pressing into waist."[4] Attentive readers of Chapter Nine ("The Office Visit") will recall that raising the arms overhead tends to accentuate any changes of contour in the lower breast quadrants. Pressing down forcefully on the hips flexes the pectoralis major muscle, which should accentuate any area of retraction due to an underlying mass. Small differences in size and shape between the two breasts are normal. The idea behind monthly visual inspections is to look for **a newly apparent difference**—that is, to detect any change in size or shape, or in nipple or skin coloration, which affects only one breast and which was not noticeable the month before.

The most important element of the **palpatory examination** is thoroughness. The entire breast should be carefully palpated, as well as the axilla (armpit), with a view to detecting any dominant masses or areas of increased density. The left hand is used to palpate the right breast and axilla—the right hand for the left breast and axilla. Several **search patterns** have been used to ensure full coverage of the mammary gland and the axillary lymph nodes. The easiest to learn is the "concentric circle" pattern. In this instance the palpation begins at the nipple and moves out in gradually widening circles, eventually reaching the axilla. A second pattern is called the "vertical strip"— here the palpation begins in the axilla, then moves up and down over the breast in narrow vertical paths, eventually reaching the sternum (breastbone). The CNBSS used the "radial spoke" pattern. With this technique the nipple is envisioned as a central hub; and the palpation proceeds from the periphery toward it in straight lines, just like the spokes on a wheel.

We do not have plausible evidence that one search pattern is inherently better than another. But BSE proponents do agree on the **digital technique** for breast palpation. The end pads (not the tips) of the middle three fingers—i.e., the forefinger and the two adjacent long fingers—should be used as the palpatory instruments. Applying a mild lubricant on the breast surface and the finger pads makes palpation easier and probably improves sensitivity. Baby oil can be used for this purpose, or just the soap suds available during a shower or bath. Dr. Baines and her CNBSS colleagues inform us that the axilla should be palpated in the upright position—i.e., either sitting or standing—while the ipsilateral arm is held above the head. The breast can also be palpated in the upright position; but the supine position (lying on the back) is better for large-breasted women, because it tends to flatten unwieldy fatty tissues against the rib cage. Putting a pillow under the back on the side being examined is also helpful. Sticklers for arm positioning, Dr. Baines and her colleagues recommend that the ipsilateral arm be held above the head when examining the breast in the upright position. During BSE in the supine position, they recommend that the arm be held "above the head for the medial breast exam" (palpation of the central quadrants) and "at right angles to the body axis for the lateral breast exam" (palpation of the outer quadrants).[5]

Mary B. Barton of the Harvard Medical School and her colleagues offer a palpatory prescription which requires considerable attention to detail and some expenditure of time. They recommend "varying palpation pressure" during BSE—going from light pressure to medium pressure and finally to heavy (deep) pressure—"to ensure palpation of all levels of tissue." According to Barton et al, the breast should be "palpated by making small circles as if following the edge of a dime. At each spot, three circles using three different pressures are made." A careful palpation of an average-sized breast, Barton and her colleagues assure us, "takes at least three minutes (six minutes for both breasts). This is much longer than the average 1.8 minutes physicians spent in one study examining both breasts and giving instructions for breast self-examination."[6]

The Proper Mindset

Breast self-examination should never be thought of as a quest for occult malignancy. BSE has neither the sensitivity nor the specificity for this task. But it is quite worthwhile as **an exercise in breast awareness**. The woman who practices monthly BSE will come to know her breasts much better, and she will recognize what is normal for her. Therefore if something abnormal should appear, she stands to recognize it much sooner. Of course, the odds that any clinical presentation in the breast will prove to be the result of malignancy are comparatively low. Readers of Chapter Eight ("A Lump in the Breast") may perhaps recall the one-in-ten statistic cited there. About 90% of overt breast symptoms are due to conditions which have nothing to do with cancer and which are readily treatable. Moreover, the "symptoms" perceived by the beginning BSE practitioner usually turn out to be idiopathic rather than pathologic. "The normal breast," Dr. Barton and her colleagues caution us, "does not have a homogeneous texture but usually is somewhat lumpy on palpation."[7]

While BSE should not be performed in a casual or haphazard fashion, it may be unwise to invest too much mental energy on this exercise. But then BSE does need to be done on a regular basis. The traditional "once-a-month" prescription has been dictated by convenience rather than by any scientific evidence, yet it is not unreasonable. Premenopausal women should perform their BSE about a week after the onset of menstruation, when hormonally-related breast engorgement is minimal. Postmenopausal women may wish to do BSE on a monthly calendar date which is easy to remember—for example, the first of the month or the second Saturday.

Patient Resources

All cancer patients need to acquire information about their particular type of malignancy, so as to participate in treatment decisions and to cope with the side effects of treatment. Many of them will come to need other services besides those related to basic education. Fortunately, the available sources of information and assistance are numerous and easy to access. The refinement of the Internet in the 1990s has meant that anyone with a personal computer can instantaneously obtain sophisticated information about cancer medicine and enlist the services of support organizations. The following appendix is not intended to be comprehensive, but simply to identify those major resources which seem likely to prove consistently useful.

American Cancer Society

The ACS remains our most important support organization, reaching out into every community and providing a wide variety of services free of charge. The national headquarters is located in Atlanta (1599 Clifton Road NE, zip code 30329), but a glance in any telephone directory usually suffices to procure the address and phone number of a local chapter in your vicinity. Each state in the Union has its own ACS division. The easiest and fastest way to obtain information is to call the **toll-free number 1-800-ACS-2345**, or (for the hearing impaired) **1-866-228-4327**. A trained operator at the other end of the line will describe the ACS services available in your home community. Free brochures can also be ordered over the toll-free line; current titles include a "Breast Cancer Dictionary" (also available in Spanish) and "Breast Cancer Treatment Guidelines." The Society's printed materials for laypersons sometimes tend to be simplistic. To gain a better idea of what the ACS has to offer, you should visit its Internet home page at **http://www.cancer.org** (actually **cancer.org** will suffice as an address line on most browsers). The ACS home page works like a charm, providing breaking news on developments in breast cancer medicine as well as high-speed links to the Society's support programs. **Reach to Recovery**, a program established in the 1950s, remains a keystone service for breast cancer patients; it seeks to provide effective counseling for anyone facing breast surgery, chemotherapy, or radiation treatments. In larger communities this program relies on volunteers (all former patients) who make personal visits to newly-diagnosed women; in less populated areas the counseling may be given over the phone. **Look Good—Feel Better** provides detailed advice on wigs, make-up, and other cosmetic dilemmas to women undergoing cytotoxic chemotherapy. This popular program has taken on a life of its own, so much so that it has a separate toll-free number **1-800-395-LOOK** and a separate website (**lookgoodfeelbetter.org**). Like Reach to Recovery, the program emphasizes personalized instruction in larger communities—the volunteers in this instance have cosmetology credentials. Patients living in small towns or in rural areas can obtain a free instructional video by calling the program's toll-free number. Another ACS-affiliated service is the **tlc catalog**, a magazine which combines articles on cosmesis with advertisements for wigs, hats, breast prostheses, and related products. The abbreviation "tlc" stands for "tender loving care"; copies of the catalog can be ordered online at **www.tlccatalog.org** or by calling **1-800-850-9445**.

An exceptionally valuable service offered through the Society's Internet home page is **the identification of appropriate hospitals**. The ACS database lists some 1,400 hospitals which have met the criteria established by the American College of Surgeons, as well as the limited number of large **Comprehensive Cancer Centers** formally recognized by the National Cancer Institute. Patients or their family members wishing to participate in this ACS service must go through a confidential registration process. Afterwards they can use the "Treatment Center" link on the Society's home page to search for suitable facilities by geographical location or by the services offered. Registration is also required to participate in the ACS website's **Message Boards**. This feature amounts to a virtual "chat room" (discussion group) which allows cancer patients and their family members throughout the country to share information and exchange ideas in a perfectly secure and anonymous fashion. The breast cancer "Message Board" is especially active, with hundreds of ongoing discussions dealing with cancer drugs and their side effects, with breast reconstruction, with cosmesis during chemotherapy, with disease recurrence, and with numerous other topics.

National Cancer Institute

While the NCI is not a multifaceted support organization like the ACS, it is probably the best single source of information on tumors and their treatment. One way of accessing this information is to call the **NCI's toll-free number 1-800-4-CANCER**. A trained operator will be pleased to take your order for detailed "Fact Sheets" listing the principal support organizations and the potential sources of financial aid. But a visit to the NCI's home page at **http://www.cancer.gov** is highly recommended for anyone wishing to monitor ongoing developments in cancer medicine. While this website is rich in news items pertaining to breast cancer, its most valuable feature is easy access to an **extensive database on current clinical trials**. Simply click on the "Clinical Trials" link— or type **cancer.gov/clinicaltrials** in your address line—and you'll be carried away to an authoritative search engine which can identify and describe every randomized trial being conducted in the United States and Canada. Anyone with a computer can search through this database; there is no registration requirement. The basic search format lets you search for active trials by type and stage of cancer—e.g., breast cancer, Stage Two— and produces a longish list of relevant trials. The advanced search format lets you specify additional criteria—for example, you could search for breast cancer trials featuring a particular drug or being conducted at a particular hospital or in a particular city. An inquiry simply specifying the "NSABP" as the "lead organization" would result in a list of the randomized trials currently being conducted by the **National Surgical Adjuvant Breast and Bowel Project**. If you wanted further information on a particular trial like **Protocol B-35**, an additional mouse click would reveal that this NSABP trial seeks to determine whether **tamoxifen** or the aromatase inhibitor **anastrozole** is the most appropriate drug for preventing recurrences in postmenopausal women diagnosed with ductal carcinoma *in situ*. A little scrolling in the accompanying description would give you a fuller statement of the trial's objectives and its entry criteria, as well as the name and phone number of a contact person at each of the participating hospitals. Breast cancer patients at risk of recurrence often stand to benefit from participation in a clinical trial. The perceived disadvantage of being involuntarily randomized to this or that drug regimen is usually outweighed by the assurance of obtaining attentive care and of getting expensive pharmaceuticals free of charge.

Breast Cancer Organizations

There are more support groups and organizations devoted to breast cancer than to any other type of malignancy. Impromptu associations of patients have arisen in many communities, often being loosely affiliated with local hospitals which provide meeting rooms and other amenities. These informal groups provide companionship, psychological support, and a forum for the exchange of information and ideas. The nearest ACS chapter should be able to tell you if a grassroots association of patients exists in your area. But no one should overlook the substantial services provided by well-established national organizations whose goal is to assure that no patient in the country must face this diagnosis alone. The **Y-ME National Breast Cancer Organization**, established in 1978, has its headquarters in Chicago (212 West Van Buren, Suite 1000, zip code 60607-3908), with local affiliates in California and other states. It's on the Internet at **http://y-me.org**, but the communication tool it emphasizes is a **24-hour hotline** available

both in English, **1-800-221-2141**, and in Spanish, **1-800-986-9505**. The trained counselors answering the incoming calls are themselves breast cancer survivors. The **Susan G. Komen Breast Cancer Foundation** has its headquarters in Dallas (5005 LBJ Freeway, Suite 250, zip code 75244); there are over one hundred affiliate groups located elsewhere. This potent advocacy organization is best known for hosting the "Race for the Cure," an annual marathon held in various cities to promote public awareness of breast cancer issues. Like Y-ME, the Komen Foundation maintains a toll-free helpline in English and Spanish, **1-800-I'M AWARE**, as well as a sophisticated Internet website (**komen.org**). The **National Breast Cancer Coalition** in Washington, D.C., is another advocacy organization; it publishes a quarterly newsletter entitled *Call to Action* as well as various "Fact Sheets" which take positions on controversial issues. The Coalition is on the web (**natlbcc.org**), and its phone number is 202-296-7477.

For over sixty years **CancerCare** has provided free support services to "anyone affected by cancer." It conducts telephone and online support groups for patients who live in rural areas, who have limited mobility, or who are otherwise "unable to attend a more traditional group." CancerCare also promises to help with the financial burdens occasioned by treatment; its services range "from providing information to limited financial grants." This venerable nonprofit organization has its main office in New York City (275 Seventh Avenue, zip code 10001); it's on the web at **cancercare.org**, and its toll-free number is **1-800-813-HOPE**.

Going to the Library

Most municipal libraries in the United States do not have the space or funds to maintain a worthwhile collection of current books and journals on cancer medicine. Anyone who wants to "read up" on some aspect of this extremely broad topic would do better to visit a **hospital library** or a **medical school library**. Hospital libraries tend to be small; but then their holdings are focused on medicine, and their librarians usually knowledgeable and helpful. Patients who wish to locate a qualified specialist—or to find out about their doctor's credentials—can consult the *Directory of Physicians in the US*, based on the records of the American Medical Association, or the *Directory of Board Certified Medical Specialists*, published by Marquis Who's Who. Even the smallest medical libraries would normally hold one or more physician directories, but of course their other holdings may be quite modest. Fortunately, anyone with Internet access can now make a virtual visit to the unsurpassed collections of the **National Library of Medicine** (NLM) in Bethesda, Maryland. The Library's main address line is easy to remember (**nlm.nih.gov**), but then the serious researcher will want to enter its databases through its new **Gateway** page located at **http://gateway.nlm.nih.gov/gw/Cmd**. From the Gateway page you can proceed to browse through the NLM catalog of books and journals, or to consult the layperson-oriented **MedlinePlus** retrieval system for health topics and drug information. If you really want to know what the experts are saying today, **PubMed** is essential. This Gateway-accessible system lets you search through hundreds of medical and scientific journals from your home computer—just type in your topic of interest, and within seconds PubMed will deliver abstracts of the recently published articles touching on that subject. PubMed is user-friendly, up-to-date, and wondrously comprehensive.

The big Internet search engines **AltaVista** (**www.altavista.com**) and **Google** (**www.google.com**) offer advanced search criteria which let you browse the entire web for the most precise or obscure topics. If your arcane subject is mentioned in any accessible electronic document, AltaVista and Google will surely find it! Yet this level of inclusiveness merits a caveat as well as applause. Cancer patients browsing the web at large are likely to be confronted with quackish remedies, commercial hucksterism, and unproven hypotheses. The information appearing on websites hosted by universities or by the large cancer centers is not necessarily free from error, but then it may have a better claim to our attention.

Hereditary Breast Cancer

The evaluation of hereditary (familial) cancer syndromes is one area in which medical technology has made great strides. Yet an accurate estimate of an individual family member's level of risk still may depend as much on face-to-face consultations with a trained geneticist as on the results of DNA analysis. Henry T. Lynch's **Hereditary Cancer Institute** at Creighton University, founded in 1984, has been particularly interested in breast-ovarian syndromes. The Institute's "Prevention Clinic" advises that a determination of risk requires an initial analysis of "the pattern of cancer occurrences within the family," to be followed by "DNA testing to determine who actually has the genetic mutation." The Institute is located in Omaha, Nebraska (Creighton University, 2500 California Plaza, zip code 68178); it's on the Internet at **http://medicine.creighton. edu/hci/**, and its breast cancer resource has its own toll-free number **1-800-648-8133, extension 2634**.

Cancer-oriented hospitals in other parts of the country are also offering genetic counseling and screening for DNA mutations.

The **Thomas Jefferson University Hospital** in Philadelphia (111 South 11th Street, zip code 19107) has an active testing program for hereditary breast cancer. Its website is located at **www.jeffersonhospital.org**, and its toll-free number is **1-800-JEFF-NOW**. Many commercial laboratories offer screening for those mutations in the *BRCA1* and *BRCA2* genes known to predispose to mammary carcinogenesis. A search for these two genes or for "breast cancer testing" using the AltaVista or Google search engines is likely to turn up advertisements for labs which promise speedy DNA analysis and subsequent counseling by phone or e-mail. The toll-free number of DNA Direct, a lab based in San Francisco, is 1-877-646-0222.

End-of-Life Concerns

No issue is more important to patients and their family members than adequate pain control in terminal cancer. Yet this subject tends to get blurred by all manner of misconceptions, and patients and their family members often feel themselves to be at the mercy of doctors and nurses who are perceived as being "nonresponsive." The **American Pain Foundation** is an important educational resource. The Foundation's home page at **www.painfoundation.org** offers an online library for pain control topics and provides links to relevant cancer-oriented websites. The Foundation has its headquarters in Baltimore (201 North Charles Street, Suite 710, zip code 21201-4111); its toll-free number is **1-888-615-PAIN**.

When a patient with terminal cancer can no longer be maintained in the home environment, referral to a **hospice residence facility** is usually preferable to hospitalization. The proliferation of American hospice programs in recent decades is a success story of palliative medicine which speaks volumes about the limitations of our therapeutic strategies for cancer and other chronic diseases. The **Hospice Education Institute**, founded in 1985, seeks to educate physicians and the public "about the many facets of caring for the dying." Its home page is found at **http://hospiceworld.org**, and its toll-free number for referrals is **1-800-331-1620**. The **National Hospice and Palliative Care Organization** lets visitors to its website (**nhpco.org**) search for a nearby hospice by state or by zip code. Its headquarters is located in Alexandria, Virginia (1700 Diagonal Road, Suite 625, zip code 22314); and its toll-free number for referrals is **1-800-658-8898**.

Notes

Abbreviations Used for Books and Journals

Books mentioned in several chapters are cited by the surnames of the authors. The abbreviations used for medical and scientific journals conform to standard usage. In the interest of brevity, long rosters of co-authors affixed to journal articles have been shortened to "et al." The titles of journal articles, if lengthy, have often been shortened; but the relevant volume numbers, publication dates, and pages are given in their entirety.

Advances   abbreviation for *Important Advances in Oncology*, an annual edited by Vincent T. DeVita, Jr., et al, and published yearly by J. B. Lippincott Co.

Am J Clin Nutr   abbreviation for *American Journal of Clinical Nutrition*

Am J Clin Pathol   abbreviation for *American Journal of Clinical Pathology*

Am J Epidemiol   abbreviation for *American Journal of Epidemiology*

Am J Pathol   abbreviation for *American Journal of Pathology*

Am J Surg Pathol   abbreviation for *American Journal of Surgical Pathology*

Angier   Natalie Angier, *Natural Obsessions: The Search for the Oncogene*. Boston: Houghton Mifflin, 1988.

Ann Intern Med   abbreviation for *Annals of Internal Medicine*

Ann Surg   abbreviation for *Annals of Surgery*

Arch Intern Med   abbreviation for *Archives of Internal Medicine*

Arch Surg   abbreviation for *Archives of Surgery*

Ariel and Cleary   Irving M. Ariel and Joseph B. Cleary, *Breast Cancer: Diagnosis & Treatment*. New York: McGraw-Hill, 1987.

Bland and Copeland   Kirby I. Bland and Edward M. Copeland III, eds., *The Breast: Comprehensive Management of Benign and Malignant Diseases*. Philadelphia: W. B. Saunders Co., 1991.

Breast Cancer Res Treat   abbreviation for *Breast Cancer Research and Treatment*

Brinker   Nancy Brinker, *The Race Is Run One Step at a Time*. New York: Simon and Schuster, 1990.

Br Med J   abbreviation for *British Medical Journal*

CA   abbreviation for *CA: A Cancer Journal for Clinicians*

Chemotherapy Consensus   abbreviation for *Consensus Development Conference on Adjuvant Chemotherapy and Endocrine Therapy for Breast Cancer*, ed. Marc E. Lippman. Bethesda, Maryland: National Cancer Institute monograph, 1986.

Cibas and Ducatman   Edmund S. Cibas and Barbara S. Ducatman, *Cytology: Diagnostic Principles and Clinical Correlates*. Philadelphia: W. B. Saunders Co., 1996.

Cooper   Geoffrey M. Cooper, *Elements of Human Cancer*. Boston: Jones and Bartlett, 1992.

Crile   George Crile, Jr., *What Women Should*

Know About the Breast Cancer Controversy. New York: Macmillan, 1973.

Digest abbreviation for *The Breast Cancer Digest.* 2nd ed. Bethesda, Maryland: National Cancer Institute, 1984.

Donegan and Spratt William L. Donegan and John S. Spratt, eds., *Cancer of the Breast.* Philadelphia: W. B. Saunders Co. Third edition, 1988. Fourth edition, 1995.

Egan Robert L. Egan, *Breast Imaging: Diagnosis and Morphology of Breast Diseases.* Philadelphia: W. B. Saunders Co., 1988.

Epidemiol Rev abbreviation for *Epidemiologic Reviews*

Feldman Gayle Feldman, *You Don't Have to Be Your Mother.* New York: W. W. Norton & Co., 1994.

Freireich and Lemak Emil J. Freireich and Noreen A. Lemak, *Milestones in Leukemia Research and Therapy.* Baltimore: Johns Hopkins University Press, 1991.

Gribbin John Gribbin, *In Search of the Double Helix.* New York: McGraw-Hill, 1985.

Harris et al Jay R. Harris et al, eds., *Breast Diseases.* 2nd ed. Philadelphia: J. B. Lippincott Co., 1991.

Holtzman Neil A. Holtzman, *Proceed with Caution: Predicting Genetic Risks in the Recombinant DNA Era.* Baltimore: Johns Hopkins University Press, 1989.

Hughes et al L. E. Hughes et al, *Benign Disorders and Diseases of the Breast.* London: Baillière Tindall, 1989.

JAMA abbreviation for *Journal of the American Medical Association*

J Clin Oncol abbreviation for *Journal of Clinical Oncology*

J Clin Pathol abbreviation for *Journal of Clinical Pathology*

J Natl Cancer Inst abbreviation for *Journal of the National Cancer Institute*

Jordan (1986) V. Craig Jordan, ed., *Estrogen/ Antiestrogen Action and Breast Cancer Therapy.* Madison, Wisconsin: University of Wisconsin Press, 1986.

Jordan (1994) V. Craig Jordan, ed., *Long-term Tamoxifen Treatment for Breast Cancer.* Madison, Wisconsin: University of Wisconsin Press, 1994.

Kushner Rose Kushner, *Alternatives: New Developments in the War on Breast Cancer.* New York: Warner Books, 1985.

Laszlo John Laszlo, *Understanding Cancer.* New York: Harper & Row, 1987.

Lippman and Dickson Marc E. Lippman and Robert B. Dickson, *Breast Cancer: Cellular and Molecular Biology.* Boston: Kluwer Academic Publishers, 1988.

Lippman et al Marc E. Lippman et al, *Diagnosis and Management of Breast Cancer.* Philadelphia: W. B. Saunders Co., 1988.

Love Susan M. Love with Karen Lindsey, *Dr. Susan Love's Breast Book.* Reading, Massachusetts: Addison-Wesley, 1990.

N Engl J Med abbreviation for *New England Journal of Medicine*

Nichols and Sweeney David H. Nichols and Patrick J. Sweeney, *Ambulatory Gynecology.* 2nd ed. Philadelphia: J. B. Lippincott Co., 1995.

Noone R. Barrett Noone, ed., *Plastic and Reconstructive Surgery of the Breast.* Philadelphia: B. C. Decker, 1991.

Obstet Gynecol abbreviation for *Obstetrics and Gynecology*

Patterson James T. Patterson, *The Dread Disease: Cancer and Modern American Culture.* Cambridge, Massachusetts: Harvard University Press, 1987.

PPO abbreviation for *Cancer: Principles & Practice of Oncology*, ed. by Vincent T. DeVita, Jr., et al. 4th ed., 2 vols. Philadelphia: J. B. Lippincott Co., 1993.

Proc Natl Acad Sci USA abbreviation for *Proceedings of the National Academy of Sciences*

Rinzler Carol Ann Rinzler, *Estrogen and Breast Cancer: A Warning to Women.* New York: Macmillan, 1993.

Rosenthal et al Susan Rosenthal et al, *Medical Care of the Cancer Patient.* 2nd ed. Philadelphia: W. B. Saunders Co., 1993.

Semin Oncol abbreviation for *Seminars in Oncology*

Shapiro Robert Shapiro, *The Human Blueprint.* New York: St. Martin's Press, 1991.

Shorter Edward Shorter, *The Health Century.* New York: Doubleday, 1987.

Skeel　Roland T. Skeel, ed., *Handbook of Cancer Chemotherapy.* 5th ed. Philadelphia: Lippincott Williams & Wilkins, 1999.

Stoll　Basil A. Stoll, ed., *Approaches to Breast Cancer Prevention.* Dordrecht, Netherlands: Kluwer Academic Publishers, 1991.

Strömbeck and Rosato　Jan Olof Strömbeck and Francis E. Rosato, *Surgery of the Breast: Diagnosis and Treatment of Breast Diseases.* Stuttgart, Germany: Georg Thieme Verlag, 1986.

Surg Clin North Am　abbreviation for *The Surgical Clinics of North America*

Surg Gynecol Obstet　abbreviation for *Surgery, Gynecology and Obstetrics*

Taylor and Cote　Clive Roy Taylor and Richard J. Cote, *Immunomicroscopy: A Diagnostic Tool for the Surgical Pathologist.* Philadelphia: W. B. Saunders Co., 1994.

Therman　Eeva Therman, *Human Chromosomes.* 2nd ed. New York: Springer Verlag, 1986.

Trojani　Monique Trojani, *A Color Atlas of Breast Histopathology.* Philadelphia: J. B. Lippincott Co., 1991.

Taxol Workshop　abbreviation for *Proceedings of the Second National Cancer Institute Workshop on Taxol and Taxus.* Bethesda, Maryland: National Cancer Institute monograph, 1993.

Wadler　Joyce Wadler, *My Breast: One Woman's Cancer Story.* Reading, Massachusetts: Addison-Wesley, 1992.

Weatherall　D. J. Weatherall, *The New Genetics and Clinical Practice.* 3rd ed. Oxford and New York: Oxford University Press, 1991.

Williams　C. J. Williams, ed., *Cancer Biology and Management: An Introduction.* Chichester, England: John Wiley & Sons, 1990.

Younger Women　abbreviation for *Breast Cancer in Younger Women.* Bethesda, Maryland: National Cancer Institute monograph, 1994.

Chapter One

1. Shorter, p. 183. See also S. Jay Olshansky et al, "Human Longevity," *Science*, 250 (Nov. 2, 1990), pp. 634-640.

2. National Cancer Institute statistics cited in Rosenthal et al, p. 8.

3. Irving M. Ariel, "Preface," in Ariel and Cleary, p. xi.

4. Mature erythrocytes (red blood cells) are an exception. In the final stage of their development, they lose their nuclei. The reduction gives these cells more space to carry oxygen-binding hemoglobin; and it makes them smaller and more pliable, so that they can squeeze through the tiniest capillaries.

5. "Benign, High-Risk, and Premalignant Lesions of the Mamma," in Bland and Copeland, pp. 113-134.

6. William D. Dupont and David L. Page, "Risk Factors for Breast Cancer in Women with Proliferative Breast Disease," *N Engl J Med*, 312 (Jan. 17, 1985), pp. 146-151.

7. "Metastasis Suppressor Genes," *J Natl Cancer Inst*, 82 (Feb. 21, 1990), pp. 267-276.

8. Choriocarcinoma was the first malignancy to be routinely cured with chemotherapy, as recorded by Shorter, pp. 190-192. For the curability of germ-cell tumors, both ovarian and testicular, see Stephen D. Williams et al, "Treatment of Disseminated Germ-Cell Tumors," *N Engl J Med*, 316 (June 4, 1987), pp. 1435-1440, and Cornelius O. Granai, "Ovarian Cancer," *N Engl J Med*, 327 (July 16, 1992), pp. 197-200.

Chapter Two

1. McClintock received a Nobel Prize for her work in 1983, fifty years after the fact. Her contribution has been assessed by Gribbin, pp. 78-82, 299-303. For Morgan's work with *Drosophila*, see Shapiro, pp. 33-42.

2. Watson and Crick's landmark articles from *Nature*, April 25 and May 30, 1953, were reprinted on their fortieth anniversary in *JAMA*,

269 (Apr. 21, 1993), pp. 1966-1969.

3.   The genetic code is explained at length in the readable books by Gribbin and Shapiro.

4.   "Methods in Human Cytogenetics," Therman, pp. 32-44; Freireich and Lemak, pp. 140-145.

5.   Michael Gold gives an informative account of karyotyping procedures in *A Conspiracy of Cells* (State University of New York Press, 1986), pp. 56-60. Therman, pp. 36-41, explains banding techniques and chromosome nomenclature. Human chromosomes are numbered by decreasing size, chromosome 1 being the largest.

6. This adult leukemia is also referred to as "chronic myelocytic" and "chronic granulocytic." Nowell and Hungerford simply mentioned a shortened chromosome in their original report, which appeared in *Science*, 132 (Nov. 18, 1960), p. 1497. In 1973 Janet D. Rowley of the University of Chicago reported that the translocation consisted of a loss on chromosome 22 and a gain on chromosome 9; her article appeared in *Nature*, 243 (June 1, 1973), pp. 290-293.

7.   Gunnar Juliusson et al, "Prognostic Subgroups in B-Cell Chronic Lymphocytic Leukemia," *N Engl J Med*, 323 (Sept. 13, 1990), pp. 720-724.

8. Freireich and Lemak, pp. 151-152.

9.   George J. Bosl et al, "Chromosome 12 Marker for Male Germ-Cell Tumors," *J Natl Cancer Inst*, 81 (Dec. 20, 1989), pp. 1874-1878.

10. Jeffrey M. Trent et al, "Cytogenetic Abnormalities and Clinical Outcome in Metastatic Melanoma," *N Engl J Med*, 322 (May 24, 1990), pp. 1508-1511.

11. Early study cited by Freireich and Lemak, p. 153; Robert C. Bast, Jr., et al, "Ovarian Epithelium," *J Natl Cancer Inst*, 84 (Apr. 15, 1992), pp. 556-558.

12. I. U. Ali et al, "Chromosome 11 in Human Breast Neoplasia," *Science*, 238 (Oct. 9, 1987), pp. 185-188.

13. Razelle Kurzrock et al, "Molecular Genetics of Philadelphia Chromosome-Positive Leukemias," *N Engl J Med*, 319 (Oct. 13, 1988), pp. 990-998.

14. Arthur Kornberg, "Synthesis of DNA," *Scientific American*, 219 (Oct. 1968), pp. 64-70, 75-78.

15.   The Southern blot is explained by Holtzman, pp. 63-64, and by Williams, pp. 34-35.

16.   The defective allele causing cystic fibrosis was not isolated until 1989; its discovery was announced with much fanfare in *Science*, 245 (Sept. 8, 1989), pp. 1029, 1059-1080.

17.   Shapiro, pp. 243-251; Lee Tune, "Polymerase Chain Reaction," *J Natl Cancer Inst*, 82 (July 4, 1990), pp. 1093-1094; and J. Madeleine Nash, "Ultimate Gene Machine," *Time*, Aug. 12, 1991, pp. 54-56.

Chapter Three

1. "Molecular Basis of Cancer," *Scientific American*, 249 (Nov. 1983), pp. 126-142.

2. Cooper, pp. 126-127.

3.   The competition to clone the first human oncogene has been recounted by Angier, pp. 96-116.

4. Dennis J. Slamon observed that by the 1980s homologues to the important viral oncogenes had been discovered "in normal vertebrate DNA, including that of humans." See his article "Proto-Oncogenes and Human Cancers," *N Engl J Med*, 317 (Oct. 8, 1987), pp. 955-957.

5. Angier, pp. 117-139; Cooper, pp. 135-137.

6.   *Scientific American* (as in note 1), pp. 139, 142.

7.   Weatherall, pp. 242-243. See also articles on "Colorectal Tumor Development" by Bert Vogelstein et al, by Lisa A. Cannon-Albright et al, and by Peter C. Nowell, *N Engl J Med*, 319 (Sept. 1, 1988), pp. 525-537, 575-577.

8.   News report on "Novel Anticancer Agents" by John Travis, and research articles by Nancy E. Kohl et al, and by Guy L. James et al, *Science*, 260 (June 25, 1993), pp. 1877-1878, 1934-1942.

9.   Feig's editorial on "Strategies for Suppressing Oncogenic *ras* Protein," *J Natl Cancer Inst*, 85 (Aug. 18, 1993), pp. 1266-1268; report of mice immunization by Robert G. Fenton et al, pp. 1294-1302.

10. Cooper, pp. 146-147; Henry Harris et al, "Suppression of Malignancy by Cell Fusion," *Nature*, 223 (July 26, 1969), pp. 363-368.

11. "Statistical Study of Retinoblastoma," *Proc Natl Acad Sci USA*, 68 (Apr. 1971), pp. 820-823.

12. "Genetics of Cancer" in Williams, pp. 18-19.

13. Charis Eng et al, "Mortality from Second Tumors Among Long-Term Survivors of Retinoblastoma," *J Natl Cancer Inst*, 85 (July 21, 1993), pp. 1121-1128.

14. Articles on "Retinoblastoma Gene in Human Breast Cancers" by Eva Y.-H. P. Lee et al, *Science*, 241 (July 8, 1988), pp. 218-221, and by Anne T'Ang et al, *Science*, 242 (Oct. 14, 1988), pp. 263-266.

15. Stephen H. Friend et al on *Rb* cloning, *Nature*, 323 (Oct. 16, 1986), pp. 643-646, and Huei-Jen Su Huang et al on gene transfer experiment, *Science*, 242 (Dec. 16, 1988), pp. 1563-1566.

16. Abramson quoted by Angier, pp. 360-361.

17. "Tumor Suppressor Genes," *Science*, 254 (Nov. 22, 1991), pp. 1138-1146.

18. Monica Hollstein et al, "*p53* Mutations in Human Cancers," *Science*, 253 (July 5, 1991), pp. 49-53. See also Arnold J. Levine et al, "*p53* Tumor Suppressor Gene," *Nature*, 351 (June 6, 1991), pp. 453-456.

19. The genetic analysis of Li-Fraumeni families was reported by David Malkin et al, "Germline *p53* Mutations in a Familial Syndrome of Breast Cancer, Sarcomas, and Other Neoplasms," *Science*, 250 (Nov. 30, 1990), pp. 1233-1238.

20. Editorial on "*p53* Tumor Suppressor Gene," *N Engl J Med*, 326 (May 14, 1992), pp. 1350-1352. See also the accompanying articles on "Germline Mutations of the *p53* Gene" by Junya Toguchida et al, and by David Malkin et al, pp. 1301-1315.

21. Cooper, pp. 164-167, who cites earlier research by E. R. Fearon and Bert Vogelstein.

22. Suzanne J. Baker et al, "Suppression of Human Colorectal Carcinoma Cell Growth by Wild-Type *p53*," *Science*, 249 (Aug. 24, 1990), pp. 912-915.

23. Patricia S. Steeg et al, "Evidence for a Novel Gene," *J Natl Cancer Inst*, 80 (1988), pp. 200-204. See also Lance A. Liotta et al, "Metastasis Suppressor Genes," *Advances* (1991), pp. 85-100.

24. Liotta et al (as in preceding note), pp. 86-87.

25. Colm Hennessy et al, "Expression of the Anti-metastatic Gene *nm23* in Human Breast Cancer," *J Natl Cancer Inst*, 83 (Feb. 20, 1991), pp. 281-285.

26. Janice A. Royds et al, "*nm23* Protein Expression in Breast Carcinoma," *J Natl Cancer Inst*, 85 (May 5, 1993), pp. 727-731.

27. Quoted by Jean Marx, "Route to Metastasis," *Science*, 259 (Jan. 29, 1993), pp. 626-629.

28. Chiaho Shih et al, "Transforming Genes of Neuroblastomas," *Nature*, 290 (Mar. 19, 1981), pp. 261-264; mice experiment cited by Jean Marx, and by Dennis J. Slamon et al, *Science*, 244 (May 12, 1989), pp. 655, 712-713.

29. Alan L. Schechter et al, "The *neu* Oncogene: An *erb*B-related Gene," *Nature*, 312 (Dec. 6, 1984), pp. 513-516; and Adrian L. Harris and Stewart Nicholson, "Epidermal Growth Factor Receptors in Human Breast Cancer," in Lippman and Dickson, pp. 93-118.

30. Alan L. Schechter et al, "The *neu* Gene: An *erb*B-Homologous Gene Distinct from and Unlinked to the Gene Encoding the EGF Receptor," *Science*, 229 (Sept. 6, 1985), pp. 976-978; and Lisa Coussens et al, "Receptor with Extensive Homology to EGF Receptor," *Science*, 230 (Dec. 6, 1985), pp. 1132-1139.

31. Pier Paolo Di Fiore et al, "*erb*B-2 Potent Oncogene When Overexpressed," *Science*, 237 (July 10, 1987), pp. 178-182. See also Robert M. Hudziak et al, "Increased Expression [of HER-2] Causes Tumorigenesis," *Proc Natl Acad Sci USA*, 84 (Oct. 1987), pp. 7159-7163.

32. Therman, pp. 256-261, 268-269; N. R. Dennis on "Gene Amplification" in Williams, p. 17.

33. Dennis J. Slamon et al, "Human Breast Cancer: Correlation of Relapse and Survival with Amplification of the HER-2/*neu* Oncogene," *Science*, 235 (Jan. 9, 1987), pp. 177-182.

34. Iqbal Unnisa Ali et al, "Amplification of *erb*B-2," *Science*, 240 (June 24, 1988), pp. 1795-1796.

35. Dennis J. Slamon and Gary M. Clark, "Response," *Science*, 240 (June 24, 1988), pp. 1796-1798.

36. Dennis J. Slamon et al, "HER-2/*neu* Proto-oncogene in Human Breast and Ovarian Cancer," *Science*, 244 (May 12, 1989), pp. 707-712.

37. Soonmyoung Paik et al, "Prognostic Significance of *erb*B-2 Protein Overexpression in Primary Breast Cancer," *J Clin Oncol*, 8 (Jan. 1990), pp. 103-112.

38. D. Craig Allred et al, "Association of *p53* Protein Expression with Tumor Cell Proliferation Rate and Clinical Outcome in Node-Negative Breast Cancer," *J Natl Cancer Inst*, 85 (Feb. 3, 1993), pp. 200-206.

39. Immunostaining for *nm23* expression has been demonstrated by Robert Barnes et al, "Low *nm23* Protein in Breast Carcinomas Correlates with Reduced Survival," *Am J Pathol*, 139 (Aug. 1991), pp. 245-250.

40. *Science* (as in note 36), p. 712.

Chapter Four

1. Darcy V. Spicer et al, "Changes in Mammographic Densities," *J Natl Cancer Inst*, 86 (Mar. 16, 1994), pp. 431-436.

2. S. W. Hutson et al, "Age Related Changes in Normal Human Breast," *J Clin Pathol*, 38 (Mar. 1985), pp. 281-287.

3. The pathologist Carlos M. Perez-Mesa observes: "It has become increasingly accepted that ductal carcinoma originates from the terminal duct lobular units rather than from larger ducts" (Donegan and Spratt, 1988 ed., p. 206).

4. Donegan and Spratt (1988), p. 443.

5. Cited by John S. Spratt and Gordon R. Tobin, in Donegan and Spratt (1988), pp. 29-30.

6. Cited by Katherine Y. Y. Li and Z. Z. Shen, in Ariel and Cleary, p. 267.

7. Hiram S. Cody, III, et al, "Rotter's Node Metastases," *Ann Surg*, 199 (Mar. 1984), pp. 266-270.

8. Weatherall, p. 53.

9. Marc E. Lippman et al, "Estrogen Receptors and Response Rate to Cytotoxic Chemotherapy in Metastatic Breast Cancer," *N Engl J Med*, 298 (June 1, 1978), pp. 1223-1228.

10. Gary M. Clark et al, "Progesterone Receptors as a Prognostic Factor in Stage II Breast Cancer," *N Engl J Med*, 309 (Dec. 1, 1983), pp. 1343-1347; and Gary M. Clark and William L. McGuire, "Progesterone Receptors and Human Breast Cancer," *Breast Cancer Res Treat*, 3 (1983), pp. 157-163.

11. The principal events of the menstrual cycle were first described in 1923 by George W. Corner, an American researcher at Johns Hopkins University. As he explained in his autobiography *The Seven Ages of a Medical Scientist* (University of Pennsylvania Press, 1981), pp. 163-166, he used rhesus monkeys for his experiments.

12. What we know about the mitotic activity of the mammary gland during the menstrual cycle has been summarized by Malcolm C. Pike et al, "Estrogens, Progestogens, Normal Breast Cell Proliferation, and Breast Cancer Risk," *Epidemiol Rev*, 15 (1993), pp. 17-35.

13. Hannah Peters and Kenneth P. McNatty, *The Ovary* (University of California Press, 1981), p. 75.

14. Progesterone was isolated in 1929 by George W. Corner and the young biochemist Willard Allen. For a fuller account of the hormone and its medical applications, see Corner's autobiography (as in note 11), pp. 231-254.

15. Pike et al (as in note 12), pp. 22-23.

16. Estrogen levels also fall just prior to menstruation, but it is progesterone deprivation which principally initiates this event. Menstruation can be artificially induced by the drug mifepristone, popularly known as "RU 486," which counteracts the effects of progesterone. This antiprogestin synthesized in 1980 became famous as an abortion pill; by blocking progesterone, it can quickly terminate a beginning pregnancy.

17. Meyer's important study of "Cell Proliferation in Normal Human Breast Ducts" appeared in *Human Pathology*, 8 (Jan. 1977), pp. 67-81.

18. John S. Meyer, "Cell Kinetics," in Donegan and Spratt (1988), pp. 250-269.

19. Irma H. Russo et al, "Hormones and Proliferative Activity in Breast Tissue," in Stoll, pp. 35-51.

20. Irma H. Russo et al, "Human Chorionic Gonadotropin and Rat Mammary Cancer Prevention," *J Natl Cancer Inst*, 82 (Aug. 1, 1990), pp. 1286-1289. Rats have provided an instructive model for the protective effects of pregnancy; see the detailed study by Jose Russo et al, "Differentiation of the Mammary Gland and Susceptibility to Carcinogenesis," *Breast Cancer Res Treat*, 2 (1982), pp. 5-73.

21. "Cell Proliferation in Postmenopausal Breast Ducts," *Cancer*, 50 (Aug. 15, 1982), pp. 746-751.

22. "Life Without Estrogen," *N Engl J Med*, 331 (Oct. 20, 1994), pp. 1088-1089.

23. Eric P. Smith et al, "Estrogen Resistance in a Man," *N Engl J Med*, 331 (Oct. 20, 1994), pp. 1056-1061.

24. Arthur C. Guyton, *Textbook of Medical Physiology*, 6th ed. (W. B. Saunders Co., 1981), p. 1011.

25. American men with breast cancer have a median age of 65 years at diagnosis, compared to a median age of 63 years for newly diagnosed women. See the *Cancer Statistics Review, 1973-1987* (National Cancer Institute monograph, 1990), Table I-16.

26. Karin A. Rosenblatt et al, "Breast Cancer in Men: Aspects of Familial Aggregation," *J Natl Cancer Inst*, 83 (June 19, 1991), pp. 849-854.

27. David B. Thomas, "Breast Cancer in Men," *Epidemiol Rev*, 15 (1993), pp. 220-231.

28. W. H. Messerschmidt and Francis E. Rosato, "Male Breast Carcinoma," in Strömbeck and Rosato, pp. 325-331.

29. Early studies summarized by John S. Spratt et al, in Donegan and Spratt (1988), p. 56.

30. "Endogenous Hormones and Breast Cancer Risk," *Epidemiol Rev*, 15 (1993), pp. 48-65.

31. Dana P. Loomis et al, "Breast Cancer Mortality Among Female Electrical Workers," *J Natl Cancer Inst*, 86 (June 15, 1994), pp. 921-925.

32. John E. Vena et al, "Use of Electric Blankets and Risk of Postmenopausal Breast Cancer," *Am J Epidemiol*, 134 (July 15, 1991), pp. 180-185.

33. Mary S. Wolff et al, "Blood Levels of Organochlorine Residues and Risk of Breast Cancer," *J Natl Cancer Inst*, 85 (Apr. 21, 1993), pp. 648-652.

34. Nancy Krieger et al, "Breast Cancer and Serum Organochlorines," *J Natl Cancer Inst*, 86 (Apr. 20, 1994), pp. 589-599.

35. Henry I. Kohn and R. J. Michael Fry, "Radiation Carcinogenesis," *N Engl J Med*, 310 (Feb. 23, 1984), pp. 504-511; and studies of "Breast Cancer after Irradiation" by Nancy G. Hildreth et al, and by Anthony B. Miller et al, *N Engl J Med*, 321 (Nov. 9, 1989), pp. 1281-1289.

36. Daniel A. Hoffman et al, "Breast Cancer in Women with Scoliosis," *J Natl Cancer Inst*, 81 (Sept. 6, 1989), pp. 1307-1312.

37. Steven L. Hancock et al, "Breast Cancer after Treatment of Hodgkin's Disease," *J Natl Cancer Inst*, 85 (Jan. 6, 1993), pp. 25-31.

Chapter Five

1. Several epidemiological studies did in fact report increased rates of cervical cancer in oral contraceptive users. As a group, OC users have tended to have more sexual partners than nonusers and to undergo more frequent Pap smears—either of these confounding variables, or both, could explain the positive association.

2. "Meta-analysis/Shmeta-analysis," *Am J Epidemiol*, 140 (Nov. 1, 1994), pp. 771-778.

3. Eva Negri et al, "Risk Factors for Breast Cancer: Pooled Results from Three Italian Case-Control Studies," *Am J Epidemiol*, 128 (Dec. 1988), pp. 1207-1215.

4. American Cancer Society statistics cited by Donald R. Shopland et al, "Smoking-Attributable Cancer Mortality," *J Natl Cancer Inst*, 83 (Aug. 21, 1991), pp. 1142-1148. Smoking was implicated in 86.1% of lung cancer deaths.

5. Quoted by Patterson, p. 13.

6. Joseph F. Fraumeni et al, "Cancer Mortality among Nuns," *J Natl Cancer Inst*, 42 (Mar. 1969), pp. 455-468.

7. MacMahon's estimates cited by Jennifer L. Kelsey and Marilie D. Gammon, "Epidemiology of Breast Cancer," *CA*, 41 (May/June 1991), pp. 146-165.

8. Bernard Rosner, Graham A. Colditz, and Walter C. Willett, "Reproductive Risk Factors," *Am J Epidemiol*, 139 (Apr. 15, 1994), pp. 819-835.

9. Mats Lambe et al, "Transient Increase in the Risk of Breast Cancer after Giving Birth," *N Engl J Med*, 331 (July 7, 1994), pp. 5-9.

10. Summary of findings by Leslie Bernstein and Ronald K. Ross, *Epidemiol Rev*, 15 (1993), p. 52. The study of "Estrogen Levels in Nulliparous and Parous Women" appeared in *J Natl Cancer Inst*, 74 (1985), pp. 741-745.

11. Victoria C. Musey et al, "Long-term Effect of a First Pregnancy on the Secretion of Prolactin," *N Engl J Med*, 316 (Jan. 29, 1987), pp. 229-234.

12. Nicholas L. Petrakis, "Nipple Aspirate Fluid," *Epidemiol Rev*, 15 (1993), pp. 188-195.

13. CASH data reprinted by Jennifer L. Kelsey et al, "Reproductive Factors," *Epidemiol Rev*, 15 (1993), pp. 36-47 (see Table 4 on p. 39). Parity was defined as any pregnancy of more than six months' duration ending in "a single live birth, multiple births, or a stillbirth."

14. Correspondence on "Multiple Births" from Chung-Cheng Hsieh et al, and from Herbert I. Jacobson et al, *Am J Epidemiol*, 139 (Feb. 15, 1994), pp. 445-447.

15. Jose Russo and Irma H. Russo, "Pregnancy Interruption as a Risk Factor," *Am J Pathol*, 100 (Aug. 1980), pp. 497-512.

16. News report by Troy Perkins, "Does Abortion Increase Breast Cancer Risk?" *J Natl Cancer Inst*, 85 (Dec. 15, 1993), pp. 1987-1988.

17. Britt-Marie Lindefors Harris et al, "Risk of Cancer of the Breast after Legal Abortion during First Trimester: A Swedish Register Study," *Br Med J*, 299 (Dec. 9, 1989), pp. 1430-1432.

18. Janet R. Daling et al, "Risk of Breast Cancer among Young Women: Relationship to Induced Abortion," *J Natl Cancer Inst*, 86 (Nov. 2, 1994), pp. 1584-1592.

19. Daling quoted by Tara Weingarten, *Time*, Nov. 7, 1994, p. 61.

20. Stephanie J. London et al, "Lactation and Risk of Breast Cancer in a Cohort of U.S. Women," *Am J Epidemiol*, 132 (July 1990), pp. 17-26.

21. Jian-Min Yuan et al, "Risk Factors for Breast Cancer in Chinese Women in Shanghai," *Cancer Research*, 48 (Apr. 1, 1988), pp. 1949-1953.

22. Keun-Young Yoo et al, "Protective Effect of Lactation . . . Japan," *Am J Epidemiol*, 135 (Apr. 1, 1992), pp. 726-733.

23. "Breast-Feeding and Risk of Breast Cancer in Young Women," *Br Med J*, 307 (July 3, 1993), pp. 17-20.

24. C. Paul Yang et al, "Lactation and Breast Cancer Risk," *Am J Epidemiol*, 138 (Dec. 15, 1993), pp. 1050-1056.

25. Polly A. Newcomb et al, "Lactation and a Reduced Risk of Premenopausal Breast Cancer," *N Engl J Med*, 330 (Jan. 13, 1994), pp. 81-87.

26. The lactational suppression of ovulation by African women has been explained by Robert A. Hatcher et al, *Contraceptive Technology*, 14th ed. (Irvington Publishers, 1988), pp. 115-124. Hatcher et al, p. 116, suggest that the elevated prolactin level "decreases the level of luteinizing hormone necessary for maintaining the menstrual cycle."

27. Correspondence in *N Engl J Med*, 330 (June 9, 1994), pp. 1682-1684.

28. Leslie Bernstein et al, "Prospects for the Primary Prevention of Breast Cancer," *Am J Epidemiol*, 135 (Jan. 15, 1992), pp. 142-152.

29. Age at menarche cited by Eliot Marshall in *Science*, 259 (Jan. 29, 1993), pp. 618-621.

30. *Digest*, p. 24.

31. Rose E. Frisch et al, "Delayed Menarche in Ballet Dancers," *N Engl J Med*, 303 (July 3, 1980), pp. 17-19.

32. Research summarized by Bernstein and Ross (as in note 10), p. 52.

33. The "estrogen window" hypothesis was proposed by Stanley G. Korenman, "Endocrinology of Breast Cancer," *Cancer*, 46 (Aug.

1980), Supplement, pp. 874-878.

34. Brian E. Henderson et al, "Do Regular Ovulatory Cycles Increase Breast Cancer Risk?" *Cancer*, 56 (Sept. 1, 1985), pp. 1206-1208.

35. Subsequent studies cited by Bernstein and Ross (as in note 10), p. 51.

36. Pike's explanation described by Rinzler, p. 168.

37. Henderson quoted by Jan Ziegler, "Can Breast Cancer Be Avoided?" *J Natl Cancer Inst*, 86 (Sept. 21, 1994), pp. 1374-1375.

38. Cited by John S. Spratt et al, Donegan and Spratt (1988), p. 59.

39. Ronald K. Ross and Brian E. Henderson, "Prostate Cancer Risk," *J Natl Cancer Inst*, 86 (Feb. 16, 1994), pp. 252-254.

40. World Health Organization data reproduced in *J Natl Cancer Inst*, 84 (July 15, 1992), p. 1070.

41. Cori Vanchieri, "Western Europe Cancer Maps," *J Natl Cancer Inst*, 85 (Apr. 21, 1993), pp. 603-604.

42. "Cancer around the World," *CA*, 43 (Jan/Feb. 1993), pp. 22-23.

43. Data from the California Department of Health Services, cited by Jennifer L. Kelsey and Pamela L. Horn-Ross, "Breast Cancer," *Epidemiol Rev*, 15 (1993), pp. 7-16.

44. Robert H. Yonemoto, "Breast Cancer in Japan and the United States," *Arch Surg*, 115 (Sept. 1980), pp. 1056-1062.

45. Ernst L. Wynder et al, "Comparative Epidemiology of Cancer between the United States and Japan," *Cancer*, 67 (Feb. 1, 1991), pp. 746-763.

46. Diet and mortality statistics for the 1960s derive from the Seven Countries Study and the World Health Organization, as reproduced by Walter C. Willett, "Diet and Health," *Science*, 264 (Apr. 22, 1994), pp. 532-537.

47. David P. Rose et al, "International Comparisons of Mortality Rates for Cancer of the Breast, Ovary, Prostate, and Colon, and Per Capita Food Consumption," *Cancer*, 58 (Dec. 1, 1986), pp. 2363-2371.

48. Cited in *Digest*, p. 24.

49. Hugh McIntosh, "Far East's Cancer Mortality Patterns Shift," *J Natl Cancer Inst*, 84 (July 15, 1992), pp. 1069-1071.

50. "Cerumen Genetics and Human Breast Cancer," *Science*, 173 (July 23, 1971), pp. 347-349.

51. Barry R. Goldin et al, "Estrogen Levels and Diets of Caucasian American and Oriental Immigrant Women," *Am J Clin Nutr*, 44 (Dec. 1986), pp. 945-953.

52. Judith Glassman described Holland's wartime diet in *The Cancer Survivors* (Dial Press, 1983), pp. 157-158. For the British wartime diet and subsequent reduction in breast cancer mortality, see the discussion by Sharleen Johnson Birkimer, "Nutrition and Breast Disease," in Donegan and Spratt (1995), pp. 56-57.

53. Analysis by K. K. Carroll in *Cancer Research* (1975), discussed by John S. Spratt et al, Donegan and Spratt (1988), pp. 62-63.

54. Ross L. Prentice et al, "Dietary Fat Reduction and Plasma Estradiol Concentration," *J Natl Cancer Inst*, 82 (Jan. 17, 1990), pp. 129-134.

55. Jacques Brisson et al, "Diet, Mammographic Features of Breast Tissue," *Am J Epidemiol*, 130 (July 1989), pp. 14-24.

56. *Diet, Nutrition, and Cancer* (National Academy Press, 1982), pp. 14-16.

57. *Cancer Control Objectives*, pp. 21, 89.

58. The history and merits of the Women's Health Trial have been debated by Alice S. Whittemore et al, "Dietary Fat and Breast Cancer," *J Natl Cancer Inst*, 85 (May 19, 1993), pp. 762-765.

59. Walter C. Willett et al, "Dietary Fat and the Risk of Breast Cancer," *N Engl J Med*, 316 (Jan. 1, 1987), pp. 22-28.

60. Peter Greenwald (editorial) and Ross L. Prentice et al (article) on the "Women's Health Trial," *J Natl Cancer Inst*, 80 (Aug. 3, 1988), pp. 788-790, 802-814.

61. Correspondence on "Dietary Fat and Breast Cancer" by Rose E. Frisch et al, *N Engl J Med*, 317 (July 16, 1987), pp. 165-167.

62. Arthur Schatzkin et al, *JAMA*, 261 (June 9, 1989), pp. 3284-3287.

63. Walter C. Willett et al, "Dietary Fat and Fiber in Relation to the Risk of Breast Cancer," *JAMA*, 268 (Oct. 21, 1992), pp. 2037-2044.

64. "Estrogen Excretion Patterns and Plasma Levels in Vegetarian and Omnivorous

Women," *N Engl J Med*, 307 (Dec. 16, 1982), pp. 1542-1547.

65. Rose et al (as in note 47).

66. L. A. Cohen et al, "Modulation of Mammary Tumor Promotion by Dietary Fiber and Fat," *J Natl Cancer Inst*, 83 (Apr. 3, 1991), pp. 496-501.

67. Willett et al (as in note 63), p. 2043. For another major study disputing the idea that a low-fat, high-fiber diet can diminish breast cancer incidence, see Saxon Graham et al, "Diet . . . Postmenopausal Breast Cancer . . . New York State Cohort," *Am J Epidemiol*, 136 (Dec. 1, 1992), pp. 1327-1337.

68. David J. Hunter and Walter C. Willett, "Diet, Body Size, and Breast Cancer," *Epidemiol Rev*, 15 (1993), pp. 110-132.

69. Willett (as in note 46), p. 533; Willett et al (as in note 63), p. 2043.

70. Willett profile by Michael Mason, "The Man Who Has a Beef with Your Diet," *Health*, 8 (May/June 1994), pp. 52-58.

71. Walter C. Willett et al, "Relation of Meat, Fat, and Fiber Intake to the Risk of Colon Cancer," *N Engl J Med*, 323 (Dec. 13, 1990), pp. 1664-1672.

72. Shorter, pp. 158-164, describes how the Framingham Study "changed heart disease from an issue in the doctor-patient relationship to an issue of lifestyle."

73. Keys interview by David Schardt et al, "Going Mediterranean," *Nutrition Action Health Letter*, 21 (Dec. 1994), pp. 1, 5-7.

74. Willett (as in note 46), p. 532.

75. Antonia Trichopoulou et al, "Consumption of Olive Oil . . . Breast Cancer Risk in Greece," *J Natl Cancer Inst*, 87 (Jan. 18, 1995), pp. 110-116.

76. Ruth Kirschstein, "Largest U.S. Clinical Trial," *JAMA*, 270 (Oct. 6, 1993), p. 1521.

77. The results from this study and others were reviewed by Richard J. Hershcopf and H. Leon Bradlow, "Obesity . . . Risk of Hormone-Sensitive Cancer," *Am J Clin Nutr*, 45 (Feb. 1987), pp. 283-289.

78. Stoll, pp. 11, 230-231.

79. Alfredo Morabia and Ernst L. Wynder, "Natural History of Breast Cancer," *Surg Clin North Am*, 70 (Aug. 1990), pp. 739-752.

80. Randall E. Harris et al, "Breast Cancer Risk . . . Body Mass," *J Natl Cancer Inst*, 84 (Oct. 21, 1992), pp. 1575-1582.

81. Aaron R. Folsom et al, "Increased Incidence of Carcinoma of the Breast Associated with Abdominal Adiposity," *Am J Epidemiol*, 131 (May 1990), pp. 794-803.

82. "Abdominal Obesity and Breast Cancer Risk," *Ann Intern Med*, 112 (Feb. 1, 1990), pp. 182-186; and "Upper-Body Fat Distribution and Endometrial Cancer Risk," *JAMA*, 266 (Oct. 2, 1991), pp. 1808-1811.

83. Stephanie J. London et al, "Prospective Study of Relative Weight, Height, and Risk of Breast Cancer," *JAMA*, 262 (Nov. 24, 1989), pp. 2853-2858.

84. Marilie D. Gammon and W. Douglas Thompson, "Polycystic Ovaries and the Risk of Breast Cancer," *Am J Epidemiol*, 134 (Oct. 15, 1991), pp. 818-824.

85. Rose E. Frisch et al, "Amenorrhea of College Athletes," *JAMA*, 246 (Oct. 2, 1981), pp. 1559-1563.

86. "Lower Prevalence of Breast Cancer among Former College Athletes," *British Journal of Cancer*, 52 (1985), pp. 885-891. See also Frisch interview by Harriet Brown, "The Other Reward of Exercise," *Health*, 8 (July/Aug. 1994), pp. 34, 36.

87. "Physical Exercise and Reduced Risk of Breast Cancer in Young Women," *J Natl Cancer Inst*, 86 (Sept. 21, 1994), pp. 1403-1408.

88. Samuel M. Lesko et al, "Cigarette Smoking and the Risk of Endometrial Cancer," *N Engl J Med*, 313 (Sept. 5, 1985), pp. 593-596.

89. Laszlo, p. 116. See also Jon J. Michnovicz et al, "Anti-Estrogenic Effect of Cigarette Smoking," *N Engl J Med*, 315 (Nov. 20, 1986), pp. 1305-1309.

90. Julie R. Palmer et al, "Breast Cancer and Cigarette Smoking," *Am J Epidemiol*, 134 (July 1, 1991), pp. 1-13.

91. Stephanie J. London et al, "Smoking and the Risk of Breast Cancer," *J Natl Cancer Inst*, 81 (Nov. 1, 1989), pp. 1625-1631.

92. Walter C. Willett et al, "Coronary Heart Disease among Women Who Smoke Cigarettes," *N Engl J Med*, 317 (Nov. 19, 1987), pp. 1303-1309; and Graham A. Colditz et al,

"Cigarette Smoking and Risk of Stroke in Middle-Aged Women," *N Engl J Med*, 318 (Apr. 14, 1988), pp. 937-941.

93. "Breast Cancer and Alcoholic Beverage Consumption," *Lancet*, January 30, 1982, pp. 267-271.

94. Walter C. Willett et al, "Moderate Alcohol Consumption and the Risk of Breast Cancer," *N Engl J Med*, 316 (May 7, 1987), pp. 1174-1180.

95. "Alcohol Consumption," *N Engl J Med*, 316 (May 7, 1987), pp. 1169-1173.

96. Elizabeth B. Harvey et al, "Alcohol Consumption and Breast Cancer," *J Natl Cancer Inst*, 78 (Apr. 1987), pp. 657-661.

97. *JAMA*, 259 (May 20, 1988), pp. 2867-2871.

98. Boyd Gibbons describes such autopsy findings in "Alcohol, the Legal Drug," *National Geographic*, 181 (Feb. 1992), pp. 2-35.

99. Eric B. Rimm et al, "Alcohol Consumption and Risk of Coronary Disease in Men," *Lancet*, 338 (Aug. 24, 1991), pp. 464-468.

100. "Chewing the Fat," *N Engl J Med*, 324 (Jan. 10, 1991), pp. 121-123.

101. "Moderate Alcohol Consumption . . . Tissue-type Plasminogen Activator," *JAMA*, 272 (Sept. 28, 1994), pp. 929-933.

102. Meir J. Stampfer et al, "Moderate Alcohol Consumption and the Risk of Coronary Disease and Stroke in Women," *N Engl J Med*, 319 (Aug. 4, 1988), pp. 267-273.

103. Charles S. Fuchs et al, "Alcohol Consumption and Mortality among Women," *N Engl J Med*, 332 (May 11, 1995), pp. 1245-1250.

104. "Effects of Alcohol Consumption on Plasma and Urinary Hormone Concentrations," *J Natl Cancer Inst*, 85 (May 5, 1993), pp. 722-727.

105. Susan M. Gapstur et al, "Breast Cancer," *Am J Epidemiol*, 136 (Nov. 15, 1992), pp. 1221-1231.

106. Philip C. Nasca et al, "Alcohol Consumption . . . Estrogen Receptor Status," *Am J Epidemiol*, 140 (Dec. 1, 1994), pp. 980-987.

107. Lynch quoted by Teri Randall, "Hereditary Cancers," *JAMA*, 268 (Nov. 4, 1992), pp. 2348-2349.

108. Lynch and his colleagues at Creighton contributed articles on "Hereditary Breast Cancer" to *Surg Clin North Am*, 70 (Aug. 1990), pp. 753-774, and on "Monitoring High Risk Women" to Stoll, pp. 191-205.

109. Graham A. Colditz et al, "Family History, Age, and Risk of Breast Cancer," *JAMA*, 270 (July 21, 1993), pp. 338-343.

110. Martha L. Slattery and Richard A. Kerber, "Family History and Breast Cancer Risk: The Utah Population Database," *JAMA*, 270 (Oct. 6, 1993), pp. 1563-1568.

111. David L. Roseman et al, "Positive Family History of Breast Cancer," *Arch Intern Med*, 150 (Jan. 1990), pp. 191-194.

112. Colditz et al (as in note 109).

113. Jeff M. Hall et al, "Linkage of Early-Onset Familial Breast Cancer to Chromosome 17q21," *Science*, 250 (Dec. 21, 1990), pp. 1684-1689. King's contribution has been assessed by Leslie Roberts, "Breast Cancer Susceptibility Gene," *Science*, 259 (Jan. 29, 1993), pp. 622-625.

114. Yoshio Miki et al, "A Strong Candidate for the Breast and Ovarian Cancer Susceptibility Gene *BRCA1*," *Science*, 266 (Oct. 7, 1994), pp. 66-71.

115. P. Andrew Futreal et al, "*BRCA1* Mutations," *Science*, 266 (Oct. 7, 1994), pp. 120-122.

116. Futreal quoted by Rachel Nowak, "Breast Cancer Gene Offers Surprises," *Science*, 265 (Sept. 23, 1994), pp. 1796-1799.

117. "Susceptibility Genes for Breast Cancer," *N Engl J Med*, 331 (Dec. 1, 1994), pp. 1523-1524.

118. Donna Shattuck-Eidens et al, "A Collaborative Survey of Mutations in the *BRCA1* Gene," *JAMA*, 273 (Feb. 15, 1995), pp. 535-541.

119. Richard Wooster et al, "Localization of a Breast Cancer Susceptibility Gene, *BRCA2*," *Science*, 265 (Sept. 30, 1994), pp. 2088-2090. See also the news report on *BRCA2* researchers, *Science*, 265 (Sept. 23, 1994), p. 1798.

120. Pedigree of Family 16 in Hall et al (as in note 113), p. 1686.

121. Lynch et al, *Surg Clin North Am* (as in note 108), p. 758.

122. "Genetic Linkage Analysis in Familial Breast and Ovarian Cancer," *American*

Journal of Human Genetics, 52 (Apr. 1993), pp. 678-701. Easton et al found that 67% of the breast tumors diagnosed before age 45 were linked to the *BRCA1* locus, but only 38% of those diagnosed after age 55.

123.　Shattuck-Eidens et al (as in note 118).

124.　Hrafn Tulinius et al, "Risk of Prostate, Ovarian, and Endometrial Cancer among Relatives of Women with Breast Cancer," *Br Med J*, 305 (Oct. 10, 1992), pp. 855-857.

125.　Thomas A. Sellers et al, "Familial Clustering of Breast and Prostate Cancers," *J Natl Cancer Inst*, 86 (Dec. 21, 1994), pp. 1860-1865.

126.　Adalgeir Arason et al, "Breast-Ovarian Cancer . . . Possible Relationship to Prostatic Cancer," *American Journal of Human Genetics*, 52 (Apr. 1993), pp. 711-717.

127.　Deborah Ford et al, "Risks of Cancer in *BRCA1*-Mutation Carriers," *Lancet*, 343 (Mar. 19, 1994), pp. 692-695.

128.　That average age is increasing as more women live longer. In 1990 it was estimated at 63 years (see note 25 for Chapter Four).

129.　"Age Distribution of Breast Cancer Cases," *J Natl Cancer Inst*, 86 (Oct. 5, 1994), p. 1441.

130.　National survival estimates cited by Jill Waalen, "Breast Cancer in Young Women," *J Natl Cancer Inst*, 84 (Aug. 5, 1992), pp. 1143-1145.

131.　The epidemiology and treatment of early-onset breast cancers are discussed in *Younger Women*. See especially the article by Kathy S. Albain et al, "Outcome and Predictors of Outcome . . . Age Differentials" (pp. 35-42).

Chapter Six

1.　The history of DES has been documented by Diana B. Dutton in *Worse than the Disease: Pitfalls of Medical Progress* (Cambridge University Press, 1988).

2.　Quoted by Dutton (preceding note), p. 31.

3.　Risk estimate and reproductive problems described by Dutton (preceding notes), pp. 86-87.

4.　E. R. Greenberg et al, "Breast Cancer in Mothers Given Diethylstilbestrol in Pregnancy," *N Engl J Med*, 311 (Nov. 29, 1984), pp. 1393-1398. See also Theodore Colton et al, "Diethylstilbestrol . . . Further Follow-Up," *JAMA*, 269 (Apr. 28, 1993), pp. 2096-2100.

5.　Allen J. Wilcox et al, "Fertility in Men Exposed Prenatally to Diethylstilbestrol," *N Engl J Med*, 332 (May 25, 1995), pp. 1411-1416.

6.　"Nothing else is Premarin" (advertisement), *JAMA*, 273 (Apr. 5, 1995), after p. 977.

7.　Wilson's role has been described by Rinzler, pp. 45-50.

8.　Articles on "Estrogen and Endometrial Cancer" by Donald C. Smith et al, and by Harry K. Ziel and William D. Finkle, *N Engl J Med*, 293 (Dec. 4, 1975), pp. 1164-1170.

9.　Deborah Grady et al, "Hormone Replacement Therapy and Endometrial Cancer Risk," *Obstet Gynecol*, 85 (Feb. 1995), pp. 304-313.

10.　Malcolm L. Padwick et al, "Optimal Dosage of Progestin in Postmenopausal Women Receiving Estrogens," *N Engl J Med*, 315 (Oct. 9, 1986), pp. 930-934.

11.　"Menopause," Nichols and Sweeney, pp. 274-303.

12.　Ingemar Persson et al, "Risk of Endometrial Cancer," *Br Med J*, 298 (Jan. 21, 1989), pp. 147-151.

13.　Robert Hoover et al, "Menopausal Estrogens and Breast Cancer," *N Engl J Med*, 295 (Aug. 19, 1976), pp. 401-405.

14.　Ronald K. Ross et al, "A Case-Control Study of Menopausal Estrogen Therapy and Breast Cancer," *JAMA*, 243 (Apr. 25, 1980), pp. 1635-1639.

15.　Louise A. Brinton et al, "Menopausal Estrogen Use and Risk of Breast Cancer," *Cancer*, 47 (May 15, 1981), pp. 2517-2522.

16.　Paul C. Stomper et al, "Mammographic Changes Associated with Postmenopausal Hormone Replacement," *Radiology*, 174 (Feb. 1990), pp. 487-490.

17.　R. Don Gambrell, Jr., et al, "Decreased Incidence of Breast Cancer in Estrogen-

Progestogen Users," *Obstet Gynecol*, 62 (Oct. 1983), pp. 435-443.

18. Virginia L. Ernster and Steven R. Cummings, "Progesterone and Breast Cancer," *Obstet Gynecol*, 68 (Nov. 1986), pp. 715-717. See also "Invited Commentary" by Deborah Grady and Virginia L. Ernster, *Am J Epidemiol*, 134 (Dec. 15, 1991), pp. 1396-1400.

19. Percentages cited by Colditz et al (as in note 21), p. 1590.

20. Leif Bergkvist et al, "The Risk of Breast Cancer after Estrogen and Estrogen-Progestin Replacement," *N Engl J Med*, 321 (Aug. 3, 1989), pp. 293-297.

21. Graham A. Colditz et al, "The Use of Estrogens and Progestins and the Risk of Breast Cancer in Postmenopausal Women," *N Engl J Med*, 332 (June 15, 1995), pp. 1589-1593.

22. "Estrogen and Coronary Heart Disease in Women," *JAMA*, 265 (Apr. 10, 1991), pp. 1861-1867.

23. "Menopause," Nichols and Sweeney, p. 292.

24. Meir J. Stampfer et al, "Postmenopausal Estrogen Therapy and Coronary Heart Disease," *N Engl J Med*, 313 (Oct. 24, 1985), pp. 1044-1049.

25. Peter W. F. Wilson et al, "Estrogen Use and Cardiovascular Morbidity in Women over 50," *N Engl J Med*, 313 (Oct. 24, 1985), pp. 1038-1043.

26. Karen A. Matthews et al, "Menopause and Risk Factors for Coronary Heart Disease," *N Engl J Med*, 321 (Sept. 7, 1989), pp. 641-646.

27. Jay M. Sullivan et al, "Postmenopausal Estrogen Use and Coronary Atherosclerosis," *Ann Intern Med*, 108 (Mar. 1988), pp. 358-363.

28. Jay M. Sullivan et al, "Estrogen Replacement and Coronary Artery Disease: Effect on Survival," *Arch Intern Med*, 150 (Dec. 1990), pp. 2557-2562.

29. Graham A. Colditz et al, "Menopause and the Risk of Coronary Heart Disease," *N Engl J Med*, 316 (Apr. 30, 1987), pp. 1105-1110.

30. Meir J. Stampfer et al, "Postmenopausal Estrogen Therapy and Cardiovascular Disease," *N Engl J Med*, 325 (Sept. 12, 1991), pp. 756-762.

31. "Uncertainty about Postmenopausal Estrogen," *N Engl J Med*, 325 (Sept. 12, 1991), pp. 800-802.

32. Quoted by Leon Jaroff, "The Biggest Killer of Women: Heart Attack," *Time*, Nov. 9, 1992, pp. 72-73.

33. Azmi A. Nabulsi et al, "Hormone Replacement and Cardiovascular Risk Factors," *N Engl J Med*, 328 (Apr. 15, 1993), pp. 1069-1075.

34. Margareta Falkeborn et al, "Hormone Replacement Therapy," *Arch Intern Med*, 153 (May 24, 1993), pp. 1201-1209.

35. "Effects of Estrogen or Estrogen-Progestin Regimens on Heart Disease Risk Factors in Postmenopausal Women," *JAMA*, 273 (Jan. 18, 1995), pp. 199-208.

36. "PEPI in Perspective" (editorial), *JAMA*, 273 (Jan. 18, 1995), pp. 240-241.

37. Percentages cited by Stavros C. Manolagas and Robert L. Jilka, "Bone Marrow, Cytokines, and Bone Remodeling," *N Engl J Med*, 332 (Feb. 2, 1995), pp. 305-311.

38. "Consensus Conference: Osteoporosis," *JAMA*, 252 (Aug. 10, 1984), pp. 799-802.

39. "Consensus Conference" (as in preceding note). In 1994 a NIH panel issued more elaborate guidelines for dietary calcium, recommending that all women over age 65 take 1,500 milligrams daily. See "Optimal Calcium Intake," *JAMA*, 272 (Dec. 28, 1994), pp. 1942-1948.

40. "Thinking Straight about Calcium," *N Engl J Med*, 328 (Feb. 18, 1993), pp. 503-505.

41. Douglas P. Kiel et al, "Hip Fracture and the Use of Estrogens in Postmenopausal Women," *N Engl J Med*, 317 (Nov. 5, 1987), pp. 1169-1174.

42. David T. Felson et al, "The Effect of Postmenopausal Estrogen Therapy on Bone Density in Elderly Women," *N Engl J Med*, 329 (Oct. 14, 1993), pp. 1141-1146.

43. Jane A. Cauley et al, "Estrogen Replacement Therapy and Fractures in Older Women," *Ann Intern Med*, 122 (Jan. 1, 1995), pp. 9-16.

44. "A Meta-analysis of the Effect of Estrogen Replacement Therapy on the Risk of Breast Cancer," *JAMA*, 265 (Apr. 17, 1991), pp. 1985-1990.

45. Colditz et al (as in note 21).

46. Elaine Eaker and Robert A. Hahn, "Women's Health Initiative," *N Engl J Med*, 330 (Jan. 6, 1994), pp. 70-71, and (June 2, 1994), pp. 1619-1620.

47. Rena Vassilopoulou-Sellin and Richard L. Theriault, "Randomized Prospective Trial of Estrogen Replacement Therapy in Women with a History of Breast Cancer," in *Younger Women*, pp. 153-159.

48. Melody A. Cobleigh et al, "Estrogen Replacement Therapy in Breast Cancer Survivors: A Time for Change," *JAMA*, 272 (Aug. 17, 1994), pp. 540-545.

49. CIBA advertisement for Estraderm, *Health*, 4 (Mar/Apr. 1990), after p. 91.

50. Wyeth-Ayerst advertisement for Prempro, *JAMA*, 273 (May 3, 1995), after p. 1319.

51. Quoted by Brian Vastag, "Hormone Replacement Therapy Falls Out of Favor," *JAMA*, 287 (Apr. 17, 2002), pp. 1923-1924.

52. Stephen Hulley et al, "Randomized Trial of Estrogen Plus Progestin for Secondary Prevention of Coronary Heart Disease," *JAMA*, 280 (Aug. 19, 1998), pp. 605-613.

53. Writing Group for the Women's Health Initiative, "Risks and Benefits of Estrogen Plus Progestin in Healthy Postmenopausal Women," *JAMA*, 288 (July 17, 2002), pp. 321-333.

54. "Risks of Postmenopausal Hormone Replacement" (correspondence), *JAMA*, 288 (Dec. 11, 2002), pp. 2819-2825.

55. Sally A. Shumaker et al, "Estrogen Plus Progestin and the Incidence of Dementia and Mild Cognitive Impairment in Postmenopausal Women," *JAMA*, 289 (May 28, 2003), pp. 2651-2662.

56. Joan Stephenson, "FDA Orders Estrogen Safety Warnings," *JAMA*, 289 (Feb. 5, 2003), pp. 537-538.

57. Adam L. Hersh et al, "National Use of Postmenopausal Hormone Therapy," *JAMA*, 291 (Jan. 7, 2004), pp. 47-53.

58. Women's Health Initiative Steering Committee, "Effects of Conjugated Equine Estrogen in Postmenopausal Women with Hysterectomy," *JAMA*, 291 (Apr. 14, 2004), pp. 1701-1712.

Chapter Seven

1. The thromboembolic complications associated with the earliest OCs have been described by Rinzler, pp. 37-41, 51-54. The Pill may occasionally induce abnormal blood clotting, but not arteriosclerosis (long-term hardening of the arteries). The Nurses' Health Study found that any negative effects of OC use seem to vanish once the The Pill is discontinued; see especially Meir J. Stampfer et al, "Past Use of Oral Contraceptive Agents and Risk of Cardiovascular Diseases," *N Engl J Med*, 319 (Nov. 17, 1988), pp. 1313-1317.

2. Daniel R. Mishell, Jr., "Contraception," *N Engl J Med*, 320 (Mar. 23, 1989), pp. 777-787.

3. Elfriede Fasal and Ralph S. Paffenbarger, Jr., "Oral Contraceptives as Related to Cancer and Benign Lesions of the Breast," *J Natl Cancer Inst*, 55 (Oct. 1975), pp. 767-773.

4. J. T. Casagrande et al, "Incessant Ovulation and Ovarian Cancer," *Lancet*, July 28, 1979, pp. 170-173.

5. Noel S. Weiss and Tom A. Sayvetz, "Endometrial Cancer . . . Oral Contraceptives," *N Engl J Med*, 302 (Mar. 6, 1980), pp. 551-554.

6. David W. Kaufman et al, "Decreased Risk of Endometrial Cancer among Oral Contraceptive Users," *N Engl J Med*, 303 (Oct. 30, 1980), pp. 1045-1047.

7. "Oral Contraceptive Use . . . The Centers for Disease Control Cancer and Steroid Hormone Study," *JAMA*, 249 (Mar. 25, 1983), pp. 1591-1604. Barbara S. Hulka provided the accompanying editorial (pp. 1624-1625).

8. Kushner, p. 143.

9. Malcolm C. Pike et al, "Oral Contraceptives and Early Abortion as Risk Factors for Breast Cancer in Young Women," *British Journal of Cancer*, 43 (1981), pp. 72-76.

10. Malcolm C. Pike et al, "Breast Cancer in Young Women and Use of Oral Contraceptives," *Lancet*, Oct. 22, 1983, pp. 926-930.

11. "Oral Contraceptive Use and the Risk

of Breast Cancer," *N Engl J Med*, 315 (Aug. 14, 1986), pp. 405-411; editorial on pp. 450-451.

12. "Endometrial Cancer," *JAMA*, 257 (Feb. 13, 1987), pp. 796-800; and "Ovarian Cancer," *N Engl J Med*, 316 (Mar. 12, 1987), pp. 650-655.

13. Thomas P. Gross and James J. Schlesselman, "Oral Contraceptive Use . . . Risk of Ovarian Cancer," *Obstet Gynecol*, 83 (Mar. 1994), pp. 419-424.

14. Anastasia Toufexis, "New Perils of The Pill?" *Time*, Jan. 16, 1989, p. 73.

15. Donald R. Miller et al, "Breast Cancer before Age 45 and Oral Contraceptive Use," *Am J Epidemiol*, 129 (Feb. 1989), pp. 269-280.

16. "Oral Contraceptive Use and Breast Cancer Risk in Young Women," *Lancet*, May 6, 1989, pp. 973-982.

17. Hakan Olsson et al, "Oral Contraceptive Use and Breast Cancer . . . a Study in Southern Sweden," *J Natl Cancer Inst*, 81 (July 5, 1989), pp. 1000-1004.

18. Isabelle Romieu et al, "Prospective Study of Oral Contraceptive Use and Risk of Breast Cancer," *J Natl Cancer Inst*, 81 (Sept. 6, 1989), pp. 1313-1321.

19. Quoted by Kara Smigel, "The Pill and Breast Cancer," *J Natl Cancer Inst*, 81 (Feb. 15, 1989), pp. 256-257.

20. Isabelle Romieu et al, "Oral Contraceptives and Breast Cancer: Review and Meta-Analysis," *Cancer*, 66 (Dec. 1, 1990), pp. 2253-2263.

21. Phyllis A. Wingo et al, "Age-Specific Differences in the Relationship between Oral Contraceptive Use and Breast Cancer," *Obstet Gynecol*, 78 (Aug. 1991), pp. 161-170.

22. Phyllis A. Wingo et al, "Oral Contraceptive Use and Breast Cancer," *Cancer*, 71 (Feb. 15, 1993), Supplement, pp. 1506-1517. See Table 5 ("Risk by Age at First Use"), p. 1513.

23. Emily White et al, "Breast Cancer among Young U.S. Women in Relation to Oral Contraceptive Use," *J Natl Cancer Inst*, 86 (Apr. 6, 1994), pp. 505-514.

24. Louise A. Brinton et al, "Oral Contraceptives and Breast Cancer Risk among Younger Women," *J Natl Cancer Inst*, 87 (June 7, 1995), pp. 827-835.

25. Janet L. Stanford and David B. Thomas, "Exogenous Progestins and Breast Cancer," *Epidemiol Rev*, 15 (1993), pp. 98-107. See Table One ("Risk Estimates in Relation to Progestin-Only Contraceptives"), p. 100.

26. "Norplant System," Wyeth-Ayerst brochure for physicians, 1991.

27. Richard Stone, "Controversial Contraceptive Wins Approval from FDA Panel," *Science*, 256 (June 26, 1992), p. 1754.

28. Charlotte Paul et al, "Depot Medroxyprogesterone (Depo-Provera) and Risk of Breast Cancer," *Br Med J*, 299 (Sept. 23, 1989), pp. 759-762.

29. "Breast Cancer and Depot Medroxyprogesterone," *Lancet*, 338 (Oct. 5, 1991), pp. 833-838.

30. David C. G. Skegg et al, "Depot Medroxyprogesterone and Breast Cancer," *JAMA*, 273 (Mar. 8, 1995), pp. 799-804.

31. Polly A. Marchbanks et al, "Oral Contraceptives and the Risk of Breast Cancer," *N Engl J Med*, 346 (June 27, 2002), pp. 2025-2032.

32. Correspondence, *N Engl J Med*, 347 (Oct. 31, 2002), pp. 1448-1449.

33. Thomas J. Anderson et al, "Oral Contraceptive Use Influences Resting Breast Proliferation," *Human Pathology*, 20 (Dec. 1989), pp. 1139-1144.

34. "Combination Estrogen-Progestin Oral Contraceptives," *N Engl J Med*, 349 (Oct. 9, 2003), pp. 1443-1450.

Chapter Eight

1. Patterson, pp. 174-175.

2. "Diagnosis," Donegan and Spratt (1988), pp. 125-126, 162.

3. "Diagnosis" (as in preceding note).

4. Robert W. Crichlow and Douglas B. Evans, "Cancer in the Male Breast," in Ariel and Cleary, p. 516.

5. "Foreword" in Hughes et al, p. v.

6. "Tumors: Wounds that Do Not Heal,"

N Engl J Med, 315 (Dec. 25, 1986), pp. 1650-1659.

7. "Breast Trauma, Hematoma, and Fat Necrosis," Harris et al, pp. 43-46.

8. Hughes et al, pp. 17, 59-73.

9. Trojani, pp. 78, 84-89.

10. Jeanne A. Petrek, "Cystosarcoma Phyllodes," Harris et al, pp. 791-797; discussions of phyllodes tumors by David L. Page and Jean F. Simpson, and by Wiley W. Souba, in Bland and Copeland, pp. 128-131, 725-726.

11. "Localized Sclerosing Lesions," Bland and Copeland, pp. 121-125.

12. Egan, pp. 215-216, 299.

13. Bland and Copeland, p. 123.

14. Roy A. Jensen et al, "Invasive Breast Cancer Risk in Women with Sclerosing Adenosis," *Cancer*, 64 (Nov. 15, 1989), pp. 1977-1983.

15. Love, p. 112.

16. "Galactocele," Hughes et al, pp. 99-100.

17. These recommendations for excluding cystic malignancy are echoed by most writers. William L. Donegan emphasizes that "only bloody fluid should be submitted for cytologic examination"; see his article "Evaluation of a Palpable Breast Mass," *N Engl J Med*, 327 (Sept. 24, 1992), pp. 937-942.

18. Hughes et al, p. 98.

19. Donegan (as in note 17), p. 938.

20. Haagensen quoted by Trojani, p. 65.

21. Autopsy studies cited by Wiley W. Souba in Bland and Copeland, p. 718.

22. "The Duct Ectasia/Periductal Mastitis Complex," Hughes et al, pp. 107-131.

23. Study of discharges cited by Barbara L. Smith, "Duct Ectasia, Periductal Mastitis, and Breast Infections," in Harris et al, pp. 38-42.

24. Egan, pp. 211-212; Bland and Copeland, p. 125.

25. Smith (as in note 23), p. 39.

26. Hughes et al, p. 151.

27. "Diagnosis" (as in note 2), p. 135.

28. "Nipple Discharge and Paget's Disease," Strömbeck and Rosato, pp. 148-150.

29. "Diagnosis" (as in note 2), p. 126.

30. Robert E. Rothenberg of the New York Medical College has observed that women who take oral contraceptives "are likely to have this type of discharge," which may manifest itself by "a stain on a brassiere or nightgown" (Ariel and Cleary, p. 445). See also Nicholas L. Petrakis, "Nipple Aspirate Fluid," *Epidemiol Rev*, 15 (1993), pp. 188-195.

31. Survey cited by Rothenberg (as in preceding note), p. 446.

32. "Papillary Carcinoma," Harris et al, pp. 261-263.

33. H. E. Stegner, "Differential Diagnosis of Papilloma and Papillary Carcinoma," in Strömbeck and Rosato, pp. 58-60.

34. Cibas and Ducatman, pp. 189-190.

35. Survey cited by John S. Spratt et al, "Screening," Donegan and Spratt (1988), p. 574.

36. Quotation from Ariel and Cleary, p. 168; Hughes et al on male nipple discharges (pp. 172-173) and on bleeding during pregnancy (p. 134).

37. Tumor-related size alterations discussed by H. E. Stegner in Strömbeck and Rosato, pp. 75-76.

38. "Infection of the Breast," Hughes et al, pp. 143-147.

39. Bland and Copeland, p. 488.

40. Hughes et al, p. 145, on role of needle aspiration; Donegan in Donegan and Spratt (1988), pp. 156, 392-395.

41. Irving M. Ariel et al, "Fibrocystic Breasts," in Ariel and Cleary, pp. 60-74.

42. "Confusion from the Lumpy Breast," Donegan and Spratt (1988), p. 574.

43. Caffeine restriction and other remedies cited in *Digest*, pp. 16-17, and by Kushner, p. 54. Love, pp. 81-87, questions whether caffeine plays any role in breast symptoms.

44. Dupont and Page, "Risk Factors for Breast Cancer in Women with Proliferative Breast Disease," *N Engl J Med*, 312 (Jan. 17, 1985), pp. 146-151.

45. Dupont and Page (as in preceding note), Table 3, p. 149: entry for proliferative disease without atypia or a family history of breast cancer.

46. Dupont and Page (as in preceding notes), Table 4, p. 149. See also Dupont and Page's updated report in Bland and Copeland, pp. 292-298.

47. Christine L. Carter et al, "Prospective

Study of the Development of Breast Cancer in 16,692 Women with Benign Breast Disease," *Am J Epidemiol*, 128 (1988), pp. 467-477.

48.   Stephanie J. London et al, "Benign Breast Disease and the Risk of Breast Cancer," *JAMA*, 267 (Feb. 19, 1992), pp. 941-944.

49.   Carol A. Bodian et al, "Pathologic Classifications of Benign Breast Disease," *Cancer*, 71 (June 15, 1993), pp. 3908-3913.

50.   NCI survey by Carter et al (as in note 47); CASH results published by Robert W. McDivitt et al, "Histologic Types of Benign Breast Disease and the Risk for Breast Cancer," *Cancer*, 69 (Mar. 15, 1992), pp. 1408-1414.

51.   William D. Dupont et al, "Long-Term Risk of Breast Cancer in Women with Fibroadenoma," *N Engl J Med*, 331 (July 7, 1994), pp. 10-15.

52.   Jensen et al (as in note 14).

53.   Bland and Copeland, p. 292.

54.   Carol A. Bodian, "Benign Breast Diseases, Carcinoma *in Situ*, and Breast Cancer Risk," *Epidemiol Rev*, 15 (1993), pp. 177-187. See also the study results as published by Bodian and her colleagues, "Prognostic Significance of Benign Proliferative Breast Disease," *Cancer*, 71 (June 15, 1993), pp. 3896-3907.

55.   Bland and Copeland, pp. 115-116.

56.   Dupont and Page, Table 14-1, in Bland and Copeland, p. 293.

57.   Bodian (as in note 54), pp. 182-183, 185; Bodian et al (as in note 54), p. 3902.

Chapter Nine

1. Kushner, pp. 151-152.

2.   "Techniques of Breast Examination," Harris et al, p. 82.

3.   "Palpation," Donegan and Spratt (1988), pp. 139-143.

4.   Kushner, pp. 3-4, 7, 11, 15, 170-172. Henry Eisenberg recalled his problems with thermography machines in *Night Calls: The Personal Journey of an OB/GYN* (Arbor House, 1986), pp. 213-214.

5.   The applications for ultrasound have

been reviewed by Luz A. Venta et al, "Sonographic Evaluation of the Breast," *RadioGraphics*, 14 (Jan. 1994), pp. 29-50.

6.   "Hand-held Ultrasonography of the Breast," Donegan and Spratt (1995), p. 183.

7.   "Aspiration Cytology for Breast Disease," *Surg Clin North Am*, 70 (Aug. 1990), pp. 801-813.

8.   "Breast" (Chapter Eight), Cibas and Ducatman, pp. 189-215.

9.   "Breast Disease: Office Procedures," Nichols and Sweeney, pp. 450-456.

10.   "Evaluation of a Palpable Breast Mass," *N Engl J Med*, 327 (Sept. 24, 1992), pp. 937-942.

11.   Correspondence, *N Engl J Med*, 328 (Mar. 18, 1993), pp. 810-812.

12.   "Dear Abby," *Savannah Morning News*, Jan. 27, 1995, p. 4B.

13.   *Journey to Justice: A Woman's True Story of Breast Cancer and Medical Malpractice* (Catalyst, 1987).

14.   "When no free fluid is found on aspiration of a palpable mass, a specimen for cytology is always obtained" (William L. Donegan in Donegan and Spratt, 1995 edition, p. 187).

Chapter Ten

1.   "Mammography as a Radiographic Examination," *RadioGraphics*, 9 (July 1989), pp. 723-764.

2.   Richard H. Gold et al, "Highlights from the History of Mammography," *RadioGraphics*, 10 (Nov. 1990), pp. 1111-1131.

3.   "Mass Screening of Asymptomatic Women," in Ariel and Cleary, pp. 145-151.

4.   John E. Martin, "A Demonstration Comparing Film Mammography with Xeromammography," *RadioGraphics*, 9 (Jan. 1989), pp. 153-168.

5.   Lawrence W. Bassett et al, "Mammography," *Surg Clin North Am*, 70 (Aug. 1990), pp. 775-800.

6. Egan, p. 71.

7. Egan, p. 178.

8. Myron Moskowitz, "Clinical Utility of Mammographic Signs," Donegan and Spratt (1995), pp. 213-215.

9. Illustrations of calcifying fibroadenomas in Egan, pp. 178-183.

10. Moskowitz (as in note 8), p. 215.

11. Discussion of radial scars by David L. Page and Jean F. Simpson, and by Wiley W. Souba, in Bland and Copeland, pp. 123-125, 720.

12. "The Mammographic Spectrum of Fat Necrosis," *RadioGraphics*, 15 (Nov. 1995), pp. 1347-1356.

13. Egan, p. 196.

14. "Analysis of Breast Masses," *RadioGraphics*, 15 (July 1995), pp. 925-927.

15. Moskowitz (as in note 8), p. 215.

16. Discussion of medullary and mucinous carcinomas by Egan, pp. 405-425, and by Luisa P. Marsteller and Ellen Shaw de Paredes, "Well-defined Masses in the Breast," *RadioGraphics*, 9 (Jan. 1989), pp. 13-37.

17. "Sign of Asymmetry," Donegan and Spratt (1995), p. 216.

18. "Vascularity," Egan, pp. 232-235

19. M. C. Wilhelm et al, "Nonpalpable Invasive Breast Cancer," *Ann Surg*, 213 (June 1991), pp. 600-605.

20. *Younger Women*, pp. 123-124.

21. Electron microscope studies cited by H. E. Stegner, "Calcifications," in Strömbeck and Rosato, p. 75; Egan, p. 454.

22. Chapter on "Breast Calcifications," Egan, pp. 454-490 (see especially pp. 455-457, 465, and 480).

23. Daniel B. Kopans, "Breast Lesions," *Diagnostic Imaging*, 13 (Sept. 1991), pp. 94-101.

24. Egan, p. 475.

25. Kopans (as in note 23), p. 97.

26. Previous studies cited by Joseph Ragaz et al in Ariel and Cleary, p. 322, and by John S. Spratt and John A. Spratt in Donegan and Spratt (1988), pp. 284, 291.

27. Emory series described in Egan, pp. 478-484; Virginia series reported by Ellen Shaw de Paredes et al, "Mammographic and Histologic Correlations of Microcalcifications," *RadioGraphics*, 10 (July 1990), pp. 577-589.

28. Egan, p. 468.

29. Moskowitz on "Microcalcifications" in Donegan and Spratt (1995), pp. 215-216.

30. "Management of Probably Benign Lesions," *RadioGraphics*, 16 (Mar. 1996), p. 463.

31. "Results of Breast Biopsies," Donegan and Spratt (1995), pp. 196-198.

32. "Magnification Mammography," Bland and Copeland, p. 432.

33. Discussion of CAT by Egan, pp. 94-96, and by Donegan in Donegan and Spratt (1988), pp. 150-151.

34. Florence Antoine, "Diagnostic Imaging Techniques," *J Natl Cancer Inst*, 81 (Sept. 20, 1989), pp. 1347-1349.

35. "Three-dimensional MR Imaging of the Breast," *RadioGraphics*, 13 (Mar. 1993), pp. 247-267.

36. Catherine W. Piccoli et al, "Breast MR Imaging for Cancer Detection and Implant Evaluation," *RadioGraphics*, 16 (Jan. 1996), pp. 63-75.

37. Linda F. Anderson, "Large-Scale Effort Tests Digital Mammography's Potential," *J Natl Cancer Inst*, 86 (Apr. 20, 1994), pp. 580-582.

38. Carl J. D'Orsi et al, "Digital Mammography," *RadioGraphics*, 16 (Mar. 1996), p. 466.

39. Stanley Edeiken, "Mammography and Palpable Cancer of the Breast," *Cancer*, 61 (Jan. 15, 1988), pp. 263-265.

40. Bragg's estimate in *J Natl Cancer Inst*, 84 (Mar. 18, 1992), p. 446; Brenner quoted by Hilary A. Frazer, "Experts Strive to Raise Quality of Mammography," *Diagnostic Imaging*, 12 (Oct. 1990), pp. 83-84.

41. "Detecting Breast Cancer Not Visible by Mammography," *J Natl Cancer Inst*, 84 (May 20, 1992), pp. 745-747.

42. Cullen Ruff and Robert McLelland, "The Mammography Quality Standards Act of 1992," *JAMA*, 269 (June 23/30, 1993), p. 3110.

Chapter Eleven

1.　Arthur I. Holleb, "Two Decades of Reach to Recovery," *CA*, 40 (Jan/Feb. 1990), pp. 5-7.

2. Kushner, pp. 16-19, 181-183.

3.　Susan G. Nayfield et al, "Statutory Requirements for Disclosure of Breast Cancer Treatment Alternatives," *J Natl Cancer Inst*, 86 (Aug. 17, 1994), pp. 1202-1208.

4.　Edwin R. Fisher et al, "Biologic Considerations Regarding the One and Two Step Procedures," *Surg Gynecol Obstet*, 161 (Sept. 1985), pp. 245-249.

5.　Lucio Bertario et al, "Outpatient Biopsy of the Breast: Influence on Survival," *Ann Surg*, 201 (Jan. 1985), pp. 64-67.

6.　Kushner, p. 194.

7.　Laszlo, p. 36.

8.　Among other sources, the author is indebted to the accounts of breast biopsies given by Brinker (pp. 44-45), Feldman (pp. 81-84), and Wadler (pp. 31-34).

9.　"Open Biopsy," Donegan and Spratt (1995), pp. 191-192.

10.　"Surgical Biopsy of the Breast," Bland and Copeland, pp. 534-536.

11.　L. Uddströmer, "Excisional Biopsy," in Strömbeck and Rosato, p. 44.

12.　The edema resulting from FNA can create misleading artifacts on mammography, as explained in Chapter Nine. "An interval of two weeks is generally advised between FNA and mammography" (Edward J. Wilkinson et al in Bland and Copeland, p. 476).

13.　Several different types of core needles are marketed. The popular "Tru-Cut" needle from the Travenol Laboratories is illustrated in Bland and Copeland, pp. 532-533.

14.　Dianne Georgian-Smith and William E. Shiels, "Freehand Interventional Sonography in the Breast," *RadioGraphics*, 16 (Jan. 1996), pp. 149-161.

15.　Stuart S. Kaplan et al, "Ultrasound-Guided Core Biopsy of the Breast," *Radiology*, 194 (Feb. 1995), pp. 573-575.

16.　Feldman, pp. 79-80. See also David W. Kinne et al, "Needle Localization," in Harris et al, pp. 113-117.

17.　The Swedish experience was reported by E. Azavedo et al, "Stereotactic Fine-Needle Biopsy in 2,594 Mammographically Detected Nonpalpable Lesions," *Lancet*, May 13, 1989, pp. 1033-1036.

18.　Steve H. Parker et al, "Stereotactic Breast Biopsy with a Biopsy Gun," *Radiology*, 176 (Sept. 1990), pp. 741-747.

19.　Robert A. Schmidt, "Stereotactic Breast Biopsy," *CA*, 44 (May/June 1994), pp. 172-191.

20.　Hassaun Jones-Bey, "Clash Continues Over Breast Core Biopsy," *Diagnostic Imaging*, 17 (Mar. 1995), Supplement, pp. 11-14, 19-20.

21.　Laura Liberman et al, "Radiology of Microcalcifications in Stereotaxic Mammary Core Biopsy Specimens," *Radiology*, 190 (Jan. 1994), pp. 223-225.

22.　Laura Liberman et al, "Stereotaxic 14-gauge Breast Biopsy: How Many Core Specimens Are Needed?" *Radiology*, 192 (Sept. 1994), pp. 793-795.

23.　Laura Liberman et al, "Stereotaxic Core Biopsy of Breast Carcinoma: Accuracy at Predicting Invasion," *Radiology*, 194 (Feb. 1995), pp. 379-381.

24.　Roger J. Jackman et al, "Stereotaxic Needle Biopsy," *Radiology*, 193 (Oct. 1994), pp. 91-95.

25.　Steve H. Parker et al, "Percutaneous Large-Core Breast Biopsy," *Radiology*, 193 (Nov. 1994), pp. 359-364.

26.　John H. Yim et al, "Mammographically Detected Breast Cancer: Benefits of Stereotactic Core *Versus* Wire Localization Biopsy," *Ann Surg*, 223 (June 1996), pp. 688-700.

27.　Schmidt (as in note 19), pp. 179, 188-189.

28.　Parker et al (as in note 18), p. 746.

Chapter Twelve

1.   Edwin R. Fisher et al, "Pathologic Findings from the National Surgical Adjuvant Breast Project (Protocol No. 4)," *Cancer*, 46 (Aug. 1980), Supplement, pp. 908-918.

2. This hypothesis was argued by Maurice M. Black et al, "Prognosis in Breast Cancer Utilizing Histologic Characteristics of the Primary Tumor," *Cancer*, 36 (Dec. 1975), pp. 2048-2055. See also the discussions by Carlos M. Perez-Mesa, "Inflammatory Infiltrate," in Donegan and Spratt (1988), pp. 239-240, 243, and by H. E. Stegner ("Cellular Infiltration") and Henry P. Leis, Jr. ("Host Reactivity") in Strömbeck and Rosato, pp. 75, 115.

3. Harris et al, pp. 248-249. The NSABP also concluded that lymphocytic infiltration is associated with a poorer prognosis (Fisher et al, as in note 1, pp. 914-916).

4. Laszlo, p. 65.

5. Jean F. Simpson and David L. Page, "Prognostic Value of Histopathology in the Breast," *Semin Oncol*, 19 (June 1992), pp. 254-262.

6. Simpson and Page (as in preceding note), p. 257. See also the discussion of "Histological Grading" in Trojani, p. 154.

7. Black et al (as in note 2). Maurice M. Black and Reinhard E. Zachrau contributed a chapter on nuclear grade and "immune mechanisms" (lymphocytic infiltration of tumors) to Ariel and Cleary, pp. 128-142.

8. Fisher et al (as in note 1), pp. 910-912.

9. Bland and Copeland, pp. 193-194.

10.   John S. Meyer, "Cell Kinetics of Breast and Breast Tumors" in Donegan and Spratt (1995), pp. 279-308 (see p. 294 for quotation).

11.   Fisher's presentations at the Conference, June 19 and 21, 1990 (author's notes); CDC statement as published, "NIH Consensus Conference: Treatment of Early-Stage Breast Cancer," *JAMA*, 265 (Jan. 16, 1991), pp. 391-395.

12.   Paul Peter Rosen, "Microscopic Pathology," Harris et al, pp. 249-251.

13. Discussion of staining by Rosen (as in preceding note), pp. 251-252.

14.   NSABP studies cited by Henry P. Leis, Jr., "Blood Vessel Invasion," Bland and Copeland, p. 342.

15. Noel Weidner et al, "Tumor Angiogenesis and Metastasis—Correlation in Invasive Breast Carcinoma," *N Engl J Med*, 324 (Jan. 3, 1991), pp. 1-8.

16. Noel Weidner et al, "Tumor Angiogenesis: A New Significant and Independent Prognostic Indicator in Early-Stage Breast Carcinoma," *J Natl Cancer Inst*, 84 (Dec. 16, 1992), pp. 1875-1887.

17. Giampietro Gasparini et al, "Tumor Microvessel Density . . . Node-Negative Breast Carcinoma," *J Clin Oncol*, 12 (Mar. 1994), pp. 454-466.

18. Karen Axelsson et al, "Tumor Angiogenesis as a Prognostic Assay for Invasive Ductal Breast Carcinoma," *J Natl Cancer Inst*, 87 (July 5, 1995), pp. 997-1008. See also the correspondence about this article published in the Dec. 6, 1995, issue (vol. 87, pp. 1797-1802).

19. Tom Reynolds, "Breast Cancer Prognostic Factors," *J Natl Cancer Inst*, 86 (Apr. 6, 1994), pp. 480-483.

20.   This point of origin is cited in the standard textbooks—see Bland and Copeland, p. 193, Donegan and Spratt (1995), p. 240, and Trojani, pp. 14-15, 146-148.

21.   "Common Adenocarcinoma," Bland and Copeland, p. 197.

22.   "Tubular Carcinoma," Bland and Copeland, p. 200.

23. "Unusual Lesions and their Management," *Surg Clin North Am*, 70 (Aug. 1990), pp. 963-975.

24. David J. Winchester et al, "Tubular Carcinoma of the Breast," *Ann Surg*, 223 (Mar. 1996), pp. 342-347.

25.   "Medullary Cancer of the Breast Revisited," *Breast Cancer Res Treat*, 16 (1990), pp. 215-229.

26. Wadler. See especially pp. 33-36, 40-42, 102-104, 128-129, and 149-158.

27. "Mucinous (Colloid) Carcinoma" in

Cibas and Ducatman, pp. 208-209.

28. Carlos M. Perez-Mesa, "Mucinous Carcinoma," in Donegan and Spratt (1995), pp. 243-247.

29. Perez-Mesa (as in preceding note), p. 245.

30. "Papillary Carcinoma," Harris et al, pp. 261-263.

31. Robert T. Osteen, "Paget Disease of the Nipple," in Harris et al, pp. 797-804.

32. Paget's cells have been described by Trojani, p. 202, and by Carlos M. Perez-Mesa in Donegan and Spratt (1995), p. 262.

33. Osteen (as in note 31), p. 800.

34. "Inflammatory Breast Carcinoma," Bland and Copeland, pp. 851-857.

35. Osteen (as in note 31), pp. 802-803.

36. Invasive lobular carcinomas illustrated in Trojani, pp. 174-177.

37. Paul Peter Rosen, "Infiltrating Lobular Carcinoma," in Harris et al, pp. 272-276.

38. Carlos M. Perez-Mesa, "Invasive Lobular Carcinoma," in Donegan and Spratt (1995), pp. 248-250.

39. Rosen (as in note 37), p. 273.

40. K. Kendall Pierson and Edward J. Wilkinson observe that "the reported frequency of bilaterality approaches 30 percent in some series" (Bland and Copeland, pp. 203-204).

41. Timothy J. Yeatman et al, "Tumor Biology of Infiltrating Lobular Carcinoma," *Ann Surg*, 222 (Oct. 1995), pp. 549-561.

42. Perez-Mesa (as in note 38), p. 248. For the lower mitotic rates of lobular carcinomas, see the discussions by Trojani, p. 174, and by Stuart J. Schnitt in Harris et al, p. 232.

43. Simpson and Page (as in note 5), p. 256.

44. Rosen (as in note 37), p. 275, and Perez-Mesa (as in note 38), p. 250.

45. John Reynolds et al, "Cystosarcoma Phyllodes," Bland and Copeland, pp. 217-219; and Jeanne A. Petrek, "Cystosarcoma Phyllodes," Harris et al, pp. 791-797.

46. Jeanne A. Petrek, "Angiosarcoma: A Special Case," in Harris et al, pp. 805-806.

47. Sloan-Kettering experience cited by John Reynolds et al, "Malignant Lymphoma of the Breast," in Bland and Copeland, p. 219. For

the M. D. Anderson cases, see Ibrahim M. H. El-Ghazawy and S. Eva Singletary, "Primary Lymphoma of the Breast," *Ann Surg*, 214 (Dec. 1991), pp. 724-726.

48. Michael D. Lagios, "Duct Carcinoma *In Situ*: Biological Implications for Clinical Practice," *Semin Oncol*, 23 (Feb. 1996), Supplement Two, pp. 6-11.

49. "Premalignant Conditions and Markers of Elevated Risk in the Breast," *Surg Clin North Am*, 70 (Aug. 1990), pp. 831-851.

50. Stuart J. Schnitt, "Pathologic Features of Ductal Carcinoma *In Situ*," in Harris et al, pp. 229-232.

51. Perez-Mesa in Donegan and Spratt (1995), p. 252, and Rosen in Harris et al, p. 245.

52. As in preceding note.

53. Schnitt (as in note 50), p. 229.

54. "A 47-Year-Old Woman with Ductal Carcinoma *In Situ*," *JAMA*, 275 (Jan. 3, 1996), pp. 61-66.

55. William L. Betsill, Jr., et al, "Intraductal Carcinoma: Long-term Follow-up after Treatment by Biopsy Alone," *JAMA*, 239 (May 5, 1978), pp. 1863-1867.

56. Michael D. Lagios et al, "Duct Carcinoma *In Situ*: Relationship of Extent to Occult Invasion," *Cancer*, 50 (Oct. 1, 1982), pp. 1309-1314.

57. "Mammographically Detected Duct Carcinoma *In Situ*: Frequency of Local Recurrence Following Tylectomy [Lumpectomy] and Prognostic Effect of Nuclear Grade," *Cancer*, 63 (Feb. 15, 1989), pp. 618-624.

58. "Ductal Carcinoma *In Situ*," *N Engl J Med*, 318 (Apr. 7, 1988), pp. 898-903.

59. Gordon F. Schwartz et al, "Subclinical Ductal Carcinoma *In Situ*: Treatment by Local Excision," *Cancer*, 70 (Nov. 15, 1992), pp. 2468-2474.

60. Lawrence J. Solin et al, "Ductal Carcinoma *In Situ* Treated with Breast-Conserving Surgery and Definitive Irradiation," *Cancer*, 71 (Apr. 15, 1993), pp. 2532-2542.

61. Bernard Fisher et al, "Lumpectomy Compared with Lumpectomy and Radiation Therapy for the Treatment of Intraductal Breast Cancer," *N Engl J Med*, 328 (June 3, 1993), pp. 1581-1586.

62.   Edwin R. Fisher et al, "Pathologic Findings from NSABP Protocol B-17," *Cancer*, 75 (Mar. 15, 1995), pp. 1310-1319.

63.   "Counterpoint" by Page and Lagios, *Cancer*, 75 (Mar. 15, 1995), pp. 1219-1222; "Reply" by Fisher et al, pp. 1223-1227.

64.   Lagios (as in note 48).   Statistics released by the National Cancer Institute show that from 1983 to 1992 the percentage of American DCIS cases treated by mastectomy dropped from 71% to 43.8%.   In the year 1992, 23.3% of DCIS cases were treated by lumpectomy and radiation, 30.2% by lumpectomy alone, and 2.6% with no surgery.   See Virginia L. Ernster et al, "Treatment for Ductal Carcinoma *In Situ*," *JAMA*, 275 (Mar. 27, 1996), pp. 913-918.

65.   "Lobular Carcinoma *In Situ*: A Rare Form of Mammary Cancer" (1941), reprinted in *CA*, 32 (July/Aug. 1982), pp. 234-237.

66.   "Pathologic Features of Lobular Carcinoma *In Situ*," in Harris et al, p. 232.

67.   Robert V. P. Hutter and Frank W. Foote, Jr., "Lobular Carcinoma *In Situ*: Long-term Follow-up," *Cancer*, 24 (Nov. 1969), pp. 1081-1085.

68.   Carlos M. Perez-Mesa, "Lobular Carcinoma *In Situ*," Donegan and Spratt (1995), pp. 252-257.

69.   According to Perez-Mesa, "about 80%" of LCIS cases are multicentric, and "some 15% to 40%" are bilateral (as in preceding note).   Trojani, p. 108, gives estimates of 30% for bilaterality and 50% to 70% for multicentricity.

70.   Haagensen's results cited by David W. Kinne, "Clinical Management of Lobular Carcinoma *In Situ*," in Harris et al, pp. 239-242.

71.   "Lobular Carcinoma *In Situ*: Pathology and Treatment," *Surg Clin North Am*, 70 (Aug. 1990), pp. 873-883.

72.   Kinne (as in note 70), p. 242.

73.   Simpson and Page (as in note 5), p. 258.

Chapter Thirteen

1.   "Through the Looking Glass," *JAMA*, 276 (Nov. 20, 1996), pp. 1535-1536.

2.   As reported by Feldman, p. 102.

3.   "NIH Consensus Conference," *JAMA*, 265 (Jan. 16, 1991), pp. 391-395.

4.   Robert T. Osteen et al, "Regional Differences in Surgical Management of Breast Cancer," *CA*, 42 (Jan/Feb. 1992), pp. 39-43.

5.   Cyrus A. Kotwall et al, "Breast Conservation Surgery: A Statewide Analysis in North Carolina," *Ann Surg*, 224 (Oct. 1996), pp. 419-429.

6.   Kotwall et al (as in preceding note), p. 427.

7.   Quoted in Kotwall et al (as in preceding notes), p. 427.

8.   "Maumee: My Walden Pond," *JAMA*, 276 (Dec. 25, 1996), p. 1931.

9.   *Kiss Me, But Not Goodbye* (Circle M Publications, 1988), pp. 125-126.

10.   "Cancer Statistics, 2004," *CA*, 54 (Jan/Feb. 2004), pp. 8-29.

11.   Reminiscence in *J Natl Cancer Inst*, 88 (Nov. 6, 1996), pp. 1591-1592.

12.   "Cancer Rehabilitation," *J Natl Cancer Inst*, 85 (May 19, 1993), pp. 781-784.

13.   Cori Vanchieri, "Oregon Health System," *J Natl Cancer Inst*, 84 (July 15, 1992), pp. 1064-1066.

14.   "Advocating for the Woman with Breast Cancer," *CA*, 45 (Mar/Apr. 1995), pp. 114-126.

15.   Quoted by Laurel L. Northouse, "The Impact of Breast Cancer on Patients and Husbands," *Cancer Nursing*, 12 (Oct. 1989), pp. 276-284.

16.   Judge O'Connor quoted by Peggy Eastman, "Survivors' Meeting," *J Natl Cancer Inst*, 86 (Dec. 21, 1994), pp. 1822-1824.

Chapter Fourteen

1. C. D. Haagensen with Carol Bodian, "A Personal Experience with Halsted's Radical Mastectomy," *Ann Surg*, 199 (Feb. 1984), pp. 143-150. Haagensen's system of grave signs, somewhat revised, later became known as the "Columbia Clinical Classification."

2. These examples are taken from the 1986 revision of the TNM classification as given in Lippman et al, pp. 54-56. The TNM system has been repeatedly tinkered with, and some breast specialists have made their own adaptations.

3. Fisher's remarks at the Consensus Development Conference on June 19, 1990 (author's notes).

4. "Tumor Size" in Donegan and Spratt (1988), pp. 354-355, and (1995), pp. 392-393.

5. Christine L. Carter et al, "Relation of Tumor Size, Lymph Node Status, and Survival in 24,740 Breast Cancer Cases," *Cancer*, 63 (Jan. 1, 1989), pp. 181-187.

6. Paul Peter Rosen et al, "Factors Influencing Prognosis in Node-Negative Breast Carcinoma: Analysis of 767 Patients with Long-term Follow-up," *J Clin Oncol*, 11 (Nov. 1993), pp. 2090-2100.

7. Rosen et al (as in preceding note), p. 2090.

8. Bernard Fisher, "Surgical Adjuvant Therapy for Breast Cancer," *Cancer*, 30 (Dec. 1972), pp. 1556-1564.

9. Edwin R. Fisher, "Prognostic and Therapeutic Significance of Pathological Features of Breast Cancer," *Chemotherapy Consensus*, pp. 29-34. See especially Table Two ("Nodal Status and Treatment Failure"), p. 30.

10. Editorial on "High-Risk Breast Cancer," *J Natl Cancer Inst*, 82 (Apr. 4, 1990), pp. 542-543.

11. Coral A. Quiet et al, "Natural History of Node-Positive Breast Cancer," *J Clin Oncol*, 14 (Dec. 1996), pp. 3105-3111. See especially Table Seven on p. 3110.

12. Bernard Fisher et al, "Nodal Staging and Limited Axillary Dissection in Carcinoma of the Breast," *Surg Gynecol Obstet*, 152 (June 1981), pp. 765-772.

13. Bernard Fisher et al, "Relation of Number of Positive Axillary Nodes to the Prognosis of Patients with Primary Breast Cancer," *Cancer*, 52 (Nov. 1, 1983), pp. 1551-1557.

14. Ludwig Breast Cancer Study Group, "Occult Axillary Lymph Node Micrometastases," *Lancet*, 335 (June 30, 1990), pp. 1565-1568. See especially the summary of comparable studies on p. 1567 (Table III).

15. Paul P. Lin et al, "Impact of Axillary Lymph Node Dissection on the Therapy of Breast Cancer Patients," *J Clin Oncol*, 11 (Aug. 1993), pp. 1536-1544.

16. Maurice S. Fox, "On the Diagnosis and Treatment of Breast Cancer," *JAMA*, 241 (Feb. 2, 1979), pp. 489-494.

17. Elwood V. Jensen et al, "Estrogen Receptors and Breast Cancer Response to Adrenalectomy," in *Prediction of Response in Cancer Therapy* (National Cancer Institute monograph, 1971), pp. 55-70.

18. Fisher (as in note 9), p. 29.

19. Carl G. Kardinal has ably summarized the extensive research on "Estrogen and Progesterone Receptors" in Donegan and Spratt (1995), pp. 540-546.

20. Nady Roodi et al, "Estrogen Receptor Gene Analysis in Breast Cancer," *J Natl Cancer Inst*, 87 (Mar. 15, 1995), pp. 446-451.

21. Milan results cited by William L. McGuire et al, "Steroid Hormone Receptors as Prognostic Factors in Breast Cancer," *Chemotherapy Consensus*, pp. 19-23.

22. "Quantitation of ER and Response to Endocrine Therapy" (Table 22-7), Donegan and Spratt (1995), p. 541.

23. Marc E. Lippman et al, "The Relation between Estrogen Receptors and Response Rate to Cytotoxic Chemotherapy in Metastatic Breast Cancer," *N Engl J Med*, 298 (June 1, 1978), pp. 1223-1228.

24. Results of study cited by C. Kent Osborne, "Receptors," in Harris et al, p. 313.

25. "Immunohistochemical Detection of Steroid Hormone Receptors," Taylor and Cote,

pp. 277-291.

26. Gary M. Clark et al, "Progesterone Receptors as a Prognostic Factor in Stage II Breast Cancer," *N Engl J Med*, 309 (Dec. 1, 1983), pp. 1343-1347.

27. Gary M. Clark and William L. McGuire, "Progesterone Receptors and Human Breast Cancer," *Breast Cancer Res Treat*, 3 (1983), pp. 157-163. See Table Two ("Response to Endocrine Therapy"), p. 159.

28. Peter M. Ravdin et al, "Prognostic Significance of Progesterone Receptor Levels in Estrogen Receptor-Positive Patients with Metastatic Breast Cancer," *J Clin Oncol*, 10 (Aug. 1992), pp. 1284-1291.

29. "Mitotic Counts," Donegan and Spratt (1995), pp. 279-280.

30. "Duration of Cell Cycle and its Segments," Donegan and Spratt (1995), p. 284.

31. Meyer summarized his findings in "Cell Kinetics in Selection of Patients for Adjuvant Therapy," *Chemotherapy Consensus*, pp. 25-28.

32. Rosella Silvestrini et al, "Cell Kinetics as a Prognostic Marker in Node-Negative Breast Cancer," *Cancer*, 56 (Oct. 15, 1985), pp. 1982-1987.

33. "Thymidine Labeling Index as a Prognostic Indicator in Node-Positive Breast Cancer," *J Clin Oncol*, 8 (Aug. 1990), pp. 1321-1326.

34. An initial report on the "Spectrophotometer: New Instrument for Ultrarapid Cell Analysis," published in 1965, was reprinted in *CA*, 42 (Jan/Feb. 1992), pp. 57-63. John S. Meyer described more sophisticated machines in "Flow Cytometry," Donegan and Spratt (1995), pp. 286-289.

35. Jorma J. Isola et al, "Evaluation of Cell Proliferation in Breast Carcinoma: Comparison of Ki-67 Immunohistochemical Study, DNA Flow Cytometric Analysis, and Mitotic Count," *Cancer*, 65 (Mar. 1, 1990), pp. 1180-1184. The immunoassays which measure tumor proliferation rates have been reviewed by Taylor and Cote, pp. 214-215.

36. Mattia Barbareschi et al, "Quantitative Growth Fraction Evaluation with MIB-1 and Ki-67 Antibodies in Breast Carcinomas," *Am J Clin Pathol*, 102 (Aug. 1994), pp. 171-175.

37. "Emerging Impact of Flow Cytometry in Predicting Recurrence and Survival in Breast Cancer Patients," *J Natl Cancer Inst*, 75 (Sept. 1985), pp. 405-410.

38. Gary M. Clark et al, "Prediction of Relapse or Survival in Patients with Node-Negative Breast Cancer by DNA Flow Cytometry," *N Engl J Med*, 320 (Mar. 9, 1989), pp. 627-633.

39. "Correspondence," *N Engl J Med*, 321 (Aug. 17, 1989), pp. 473-474.

40. H. Beerman et al, "Correspondence" (as in preceding note).

41. Frédérique Spyratos et al, "Cathepsin D: An Independent Prognostic Factor for Metastasis of Breast Cancer," *Lancet*, Nov. 11, 1989, pp. 1115-1118.

42. Atul K. Tandon et al, "Cathepsin D and Prognosis in Breast Cancer," *N Engl J Med*, 322 (Feb. 1, 1990), pp. 297-302.

43. Author's notes from Conference, June 19, 1990.

44. Peter M. Ravdin et al, "Cathepsin D by Western Blotting and Immunohistochemistry: Failure to Confirm Correlations with Prognosis in Node-Negative Breast Cancer," *J Clin Oncol*, 12 (Mar. 1994), pp. 467-474.

45. Tom Reynolds, "Breast Cancer Prognostic Factors," *J Natl Cancer Inst*, 86 (Apr. 6, 1994), pp. 480-483.

46. "Detection of Bone Marrow Micrometastasis," Taylor and Cote, pp. 227-231.

47. While some researchers have relied on a single reagent to detect tumor cells in the bone marrow, Taylor and Cote recommend using "cocktails" of several different antibodies for the best results (pp. 227-228).

48. W. Howard Redding et al, "Detection of Micrometastases in Patients with Primary Breast Cancer," *Lancet*, Dec. 3, 1983, pp. 1271-1274.

49. Richard J. Cote et al, "Monoclonal Antibodies Detect Occult Breast Carcinoma Metastases in the Bone Marrow," *Am J Surg Pathol*, 12 (May 1988), pp. 333-340.

50. R. C. Coombes et al, "Prognostic Significance of Micrometastases in Bone Marrow in Patients with Primary Breast Cancer,"

Chemotherapy Consensus, pp. 51-53.

51. Janine L. Mansi et al, "Micrometastases in Bone Marrow . . . Early Predictor of Bone Metastases," *Br Med J*, 295 (Oct. 31, 1987), pp. 1093-1096.

52. Janine L. Mansi et al, "The Fate of Bone Marrow Micrometastases in Patients with Primary Breast Cancer," *J Clin Oncol*, 7 (Apr. 1989), pp. 445-449. See Table Two ("Repeat Marrow Aspirates"), p. 447. Eleven of the 21 patients received adjuvant chemotherapy; but cytotoxic therapy alone cannot explain this finding, because nine of the ten patients who received no systemic drugs also tested negative on re-examination.

53. Mansi et al (as in preceding note), p. 448.

54. Richard J. Cote et al, "Prediction of Early Relapse in Operable Breast Cancer by Bone Marrow Micrometastases," *J Clin Oncol*, 9 (Oct. 1991), pp. 1749-1756.

55. Ingo J. Diel et al, "Micrometastatic Breast Cancer Cells in Bone Marrow at Primary Surgery: Prognostic Value in Comparison with Nodal Status," *J Natl Cancer Inst*, 88 (Nov. 20, 1996), pp. 1652-1664.

56. The Sloan-Kettering sampling procedures have been described by Alisa C. Thorne et al, "Harvesting Bone Marrow in an Outpatient Setting," *J Clin Oncol*, 11 (Feb. 1993), pp. 320-323. The Heidelberg team reported only one hemorrhage requiring ligature in the 727 patients they assayed (Diel et al as in preceding note).

57. Sharon Begley, "The Cancer Killer," *Newsweek*, Dec. 23, 1996, pp. 42-47.

58. As explained in Chapter Three (p. 48).

59. D. Craig Allred et al, "Association of *p53* Protein Expression with Tumor Cell Proliferation Rate and Clinical Outcome in Node-Negative Breast Cancer," *J Natl Cancer Inst*, 85 (Feb. 3, 1993), pp. 200-206.

60. Rosella Silvestrini et al, "*p53* as an Independent Prognostic Marker in Node-Negative Breast Cancer," *J Natl Cancer Inst*, 85 (June 16, 1993), pp. 965-970.

61. J. M. Cunningham et al, "*p53* Gene Expression in Node-Positive Breast Cancer: Relationship to DNA Ploidy and Prognosis," *J Natl Cancer Inst*, 86 (Dec. 21, 1994), pp. 1871-1873.

62. Rosella Silvestrini et al, "*p53* Expression in Node-Positive Breast Cancer," *J Clin Oncol*, 14 (May 1996), pp. 1604-1610.

63. Paul Peter Rosen et al, "*p53* in Node-Negative Breast Carcinoma," *J Clin Oncol*, 13 (Apr. 1995), pp. 821-830.

64. Timothy W. Jacobs et al, "Loss of Tumor Marker-Immunostaining Intensity on Stored Paraffin Slides of Breast Cancer," *J Natl Cancer Inst*, 88 (Aug. 7, 1996), pp. 1054-1059.

65. "Clinical Practice Guidelines for the Use of Tumor Markers in Breast and Colorectal Cancer," *J Clin Oncol*, 14 (Oct. 1996), pp. 2843-2877. See especially pp. 2865-2866.

66. H. Tsuda et al, "Histologic Grade of Malignancy and Copy Number of *erb*B-2 Gene in Breast Carcinoma," *Cancer*, 65 (Apr. 15, 1990), pp. 1794-1800.

67. S. Soomro et al, "*erb*B-2 Expression in Different Histological Types of Invasive Breast Carcinoma," *J Clin Pathol*, 44 (Mar. 1991), pp. 211-214.

68. Marc J. Van de Vijver et al, "*Neu*-Protein Overexpression in Breast Cancer," *N Engl J Med*, 319 (Nov. 10, 1988), pp. 1239-1245.

69. D. Craig Allred et al, "HER-2/*neu* in Node-Negative Breast Cancer," *J Clin Oncol*, 10 (Apr. 1992), pp. 599-605. See especially Figure Three on p. 602. A contrary opinion has been registered by Paul Peter Rosen and his Sloan-Kettering colleagues, who concluded that HER-2 overexpression is "not a reliable prognostic indicator" for most node-negative patients. See Rosen et al, "Immunohistochemical Detection of HER-2/*neu* in Node-Negative Breast Carcinoma," *Cancer*, 75 (Mar. 15, 1995), pp. 1320-1326.

70. Allred et al (as in preceding note), p. 604.

71. Bernard Têtu and Jacques Brisson, "Prognostic Significance of HER-2/*neu* Oncoprotein Expression in Node-Positive Breast Cancer," *Cancer*, 73 (May 1, 1994), pp. 2359-2365.

72. Hyman B. Muss et al, "*erb*B-2 Expression and Response to Adjuvant Therapy in Women with Node-Positive Early Breast Cancer," *N Engl J Med*, 330 (May 5, 1994),

pp. 1260-1266.

73. The contradictions in the published research on HER-2/*neu* have been summarized by Rosen et al (as in note 69), pp. 1324-1325.

74. "Breast Cancer Therapy," *N Engl J Med*, 326 (June 25, 1992), pp. 1774-1775. This issue contained a review article on "Prognostic Factors and Treatment Decisions in Axillary-Node-Negative Breast Cancer" by William L. McGuire and Gary M. Clark (pp. 1756-1761).

75. "NIH Consensus Conference: Treatment of Early-Stage Breast Cancer," *JAMA*, 265 (Jan. 16, 1991), pp. 391-394.

76. Compare the recommendation for aggressive chemotherapy given to Nancy Brinker, diagnosed with a small node-negative tumor at age 36 (Brinker, pp. 47-48).

Chapter Fifteen

1. "Edwin Smith Surgical Papyrus," quoted opposite the title page in Donegan and Spratt (1995).

2. Hippocrates and Galen quoted by William L. Donegan, "Introduction to the History of Breast Cancer," Donegan and Spratt (1995), pp. 1-2.

3. Mastectomy procedure of Scultetus described by Frederick W. Wagner in Bland and Copeland, p. 67, and by Irving M. Ariel in Ariel and Cleary, pp. 11-12.

4. Vienna mastectomy series and Alice James diagnosis discussed by Patterson, pp. 29, 34.

5. For the facts of Halsted's life, the author is indebted to John L. Cameron's sketch "William Stewart Halsted," *Ann Surg*, 225 (May 1997), pp. 445-458.

6. Halsted quoted by Kirby I. Bland and Edward M. Copeland, "Halsted Radical Mastectomy," Bland and Copeland, pp. 583-594 (see p. 583).

7. Bland and Copeland (as in preceding note), p. 584.

8. Donegan (as in note 2), p. 7.

9. Patterson, pp. 71-72, 77, 83.

10. Crile quoted by his son George Crile, Jr., in "Breast Cancer: A Personal Perspective," *Surg Clin North Am*, 64 (Dec. 1984), pp. 1145-1149.

11. M. Vera Peters, "Local Treatment of Early Breast Cancer," *Surg Clin North Am*, 64 (Dec. 1984), pp. 1151-1154. See also the obituary of Peters in *J Clin Oncol*, 12 (Feb. 1994), pp. 239-240.

12. Keynes reminisced about his career in "A Historical Perspective," collected by Jeffrey S. Tobias and Michael J. Peckham, eds., *Primary Management of Breast Cancer: Alternatives to Mastectomy* (London: Edward Arnold, 1985), pp. xiii-xvii.

13. Robert Calle, "Experience with Breast-Conserving Approaches at the Curie Institute," in Tobias and Peckham (as in preceding note), pp. 59-79.

14. Hiram S. Cody III and other Sloan-Kettering surgeons have analyzed Dr. Urban's choice of procedures for 1,288 patients he operated upon between 1965 and 1978. See Cody et al, "Have Changing Treatment Patterns Affected Outcome for Operable Breast Cancer?" *Ann Surg*, 213 (Apr. 1991), pp. 297-307.

15. Urban and the Swiss surgeon R. A. Egeli contributed a chapter on "Extended Radical Mastectomy" to Strömbeck and Rosato, pp. 138-147.

16. George Crile, Jr. (as in note 10), p. 1145.

17. Crile's article and the opposing viewpoints appeared in *Life*, 39 (Oct. 31, 1955), pp. 128-142.

18. Crile cited laboratory experiments supporting this hypothesis in his article "Possible Role of Uninvolved Regional Nodes in Preventing Metastasis from Breast Cancer," *Cancer*, 24 (Dec. 1969), pp. 1283-1285.

19. "Important Do's and Don't's," in Crile, p. 163.

20. As recounted in Chapter Eleven, p. 202.

21. Fisher recalled his involvement with the NSABP in "Thoughts from a Journey," *J Clin Oncol*, 11 (Dec. 1993), pp. 2298-2305.

22. Bernard Fisher and Edwin R. Fisher, "Transmigration of Lymph Nodes by Tumor

Cells," *Science*, 152 (June 3, 1966), pp. 1397-1398. See also Bernard Fisher, "Personal Contributions to Breast Cancer Research and Treatment," *Semin Oncol*, 23 (Aug. 1996), pp. 414-427.

23. As documented in Chapter Fourteen ("Bone Marrow Sampling"), pp. 278-280.

24. Bernard Fisher et al, "Location of Breast Carcinoma and Prognosis," *Surg Gynecol Obstet*, 129 (Oct. 1969), pp. 705-716.

25. As explained in Chapter Fourteen, p. 265, and at greater length by Bernard Fisher et al, "Axillary Dissection," *Surg Gynecol Obstet*, 152 (June 1981), pp. 765-772.

26. "Number of Nodes Examined by Protocol" (Figure 5), in Richard Margolese et al, "Lumpectomy and Axillary Dissection: A Syllabus from the National Surgical Adjuvant Breast Project," *Surgery*, 102 (Nov. 1987), pp. 828-834.

27. Bernard Fisher et al, "The Contribution of Recent NSABP Clinical Trials to an Understanding of Tumor Biology," *Cancer*, 46 (Aug. 1980), Supplement, pp. 1009-1025. See also Blake Cady's article "Lymph Node Metastases: Indicators, but Not Governors of Survival," *Arch Surg*, 119 (Sept. 1984), pp. 1067-1072.

28. Bernard Fisher, "Laboratory and Clinical Research in Breast Cancer—A Personal Adventure," *Cancer Research*, 40 (Nov. 1980), pp. 3863-3874.

29. Bernard Fisher et al, "Postoperative Radiotherapy in the Treatment of Breast Cancer: Results of the NSABP Clinical Trial," *Ann Surg*, 172 (Oct. 1970), pp. 711-732.

30. The indications for postmastectomy radiotherapy have been reviewed by the radiation oncologists J. Frank Wilson and James D. Cox in Donegan and Spratt (1988), pp. 465-469, and (1995), pp. 509-512.

31. Patient enrollment and treatment arms as described by Fisher et al (following note).

32. Bernard Fisher et al, "Comparison of Radical Mastectomy with Alternative Treatments for Primary Breast Cancer: A First Report of Results from a Prospective Randomized Clinical Trial," *Cancer*, 39 (June 1977), Supplement, pp. 2827-2839.

33. Bernard Fisher et al, "Ten-Year Results of a Randomized Clinical Trial Comparing Radical Mastectomy and Total Mastectomy with or without Radiation," *N Engl J Med*, 312 (Mar. 14, 1985), pp. 674-681.

34. Survey by the American College of Surgeons, cited in Ariel and Cleary, pp. 256-257.

35. John H. Moxley III et al, "Treatment of Primary Breast Cancer: Summary of the National Institutes of Health Consensus Development Conference," *JAMA*, 244 (Aug. 22/29, 1980), pp. 797-800.

36. Urban's "Minority Report" in *JAMA*, 244 (Aug. 22/29, 1980), pp. 800-803.

37. R. Robinson Baker, ed., *Current Trends in the Management of Breast Cancer* (Johns Hopkins University Press, 1977), p. 113.

38. "Urban's Double Check," *Time*, Dec. 9, 1974, pp. 90, 93.

39. Harold J. Wanebo et al, "Treatment of Minimal Breast Cancer," *Cancer*, 33 (Feb. 1974), pp. 349-357.

40. Edwin R. Fisher et al, "Pathologic Findings from the National Surgical Adjuvant Breast Project: Observations Concerning the Multicentricity of Mammary Cancer," *Cancer*, 35 (Jan. 1975), pp. 247-254.

41. Paul Peter Rosen et al, "Residual Mammary Carcinoma Following Simulated Partial Mastectomy," *Cancer*, 35 (Mar. 1975), pp. 739-747.

42. Frank E. Gump et al, "The Extent and Distribution of Cancer in Breasts with Palpable Primary Tumors," *Ann Surg*, 204 (Oct. 1986), pp. 384-390.

43. John Hayward and Maira Caleffi reviewed the Guy's Hospital trial in *Arch Surg*, 122 (Nov. 1987), pp. 1244-1247. It is also described in Ariel and Cleary, by Florence F. C. Chu (pp. 237-239) and Richard E. Wilson (p. 352).

44. The experiences at the Cleveland Clinic and M. D. Anderson were recalled by George Crile, Jr., et al, "Results of Partial Mastectomy in 173 Patients," *Surg Gynecol Obstet*, 150 (Apr. 1980), pp. 563-566, and by Eleanor D. Montague, "Conservation Surgery and Radiation Therapy in Operable Breast Cancer," *Cancer*, 53 (Feb. 1, 1984), Supplement, pp. 700-704.

45. The Joint Center regimen has been described by Scott A. Triedman et al, "Factors

Influencing Cosmetic Outcome of Conservative Surgery and Radiotherapy for Breast Cancer," *Surg Clin North Am*, 70 (Aug. 1990), pp. 901-916.

46.   Results cited by Jay R. Harris and Abram Recht in Harris et al, p. 393.

47.   Harris and Recht, Harris et al, p. 394.

48.   There have been several articles by Joint Center physicians discussing the adverse effect of an "extensive intraductal component." See Jay R. Harris et al in *Ann Surg*, 201 (Feb. 1985), pp. 164-169; Robert T. Osteen et al in *Arch Surg*, 122 (Nov. 1987), pp. 1248-1252; and Frank A. Vicini et al in *Ann Surg*, 214 (Sept. 1991), pp. 200-205.

49.   Harris et al, p. 399.

50.   Stuart J. Schnitt et al, "The Relationship between Microscopic Margins of Resection and the Risk of Local Recurrence in Patients with Breast Cancer Treated with Breast-Conserving Surgery and Radiation Therapy," *Cancer*, 74 (Sept. 15, 1994), pp. 1746-1751.

51.   Protocol description as given by Fisher et al (as in note 53).

52.   "Thoughts from a Journey" (as in note 21), p. 2305.

53.   Bernard Fisher et al, "Five-Year Results of a Randomized Clinical Trial Comparing Total Mastectomy and Segmental Mastectomy with or without Radiation in the Treatment of Breast Cancer," *N Engl J Med*, 312 (Mar. 14, 1985), pp. 665-673.

54.   "Surgery for Breast Cancer: Less May Be as Good as More," *N Engl J Med*, 312 (Mar. 14, 1985), pp. 712-714.

55.   "Treatment of Breast Cancer" (correspondence), *N Engl J Med*, 313 (July 11, 1985), pp. 116-118. For more information on Dr. Ferguson's views, see Paul Meier, Donald J. Ferguson, and Theodore Karrison, "A Controlled Trial of Extended Radical Versus Radical Mastectomy," *Cancer*, 63 (Jan. 1, 1989), pp. 188-195.

56.   Urban's remarks on "Nightline" quoted by Avrum Z. Bluming et al, "Treatment of Primary Breast Cancer," *Ann Surg*, 204 (Aug. 1986), pp. 136-147 (see p. 137).

57.   Bernard Fisher et al, "Eight-Year Results of a Randomized Clinical Trial Comparing Total Mastectomy and Lumpectomy with or without Irradiation in the Treatment of Breast Cancer," *N Engl J Med*, 320 (Mar. 30, 1989), pp. 822-828.

58.   Poisson's letter published in *N Engl J Med*, 330 (May 19, 1994), p. 1460. See also the editorial in this issue, "Setting the Record Straight in the Breast Cancer Trials" (pp. 1448-1450), as well as related correspondence (pp. 1458-1462).

59.   Bernard Fisher et al, "Reanalysis and Results after Twelve Years of Follow-Up in a Randomized Clinical Trial Comparing Total Mastectomy with Lumpectomy," *N Engl J Med*, 333 (Nov. 30, 1995), pp. 1456-1461.

60.   Michaele C. Christian et al, "National Cancer Institute Audit of NSABP Protocol B-06," *N Engl J Med*, 333 (Nov. 30, 1995), pp. 1469-1474.

61.   "Survival after Breast-Sparing Surgery Versus Mastectomy," *J Natl Cancer Inst*, 86 (Nov. 16, 1994), pp. 1672-1673. The "Ten-Year Results" from the NCI's own trial were reported by Joan A. Jacobson and her colleagues: "At ten years overall survival was 75 percent for the patients assigned to mastectomy, and 77 percent for those assigned to lumpectomy plus radiation." See Jacobson et al, *N Engl J Med*, 332 (Apr. 6, 1995), pp. 907-911.

62.   "NIH Consensus Conference: Treatment of Early-Stage Breast Cancer," *JAMA*, 265 (Jan. 16, 1991), pp. 391-395.

63.   See the discussion of lumpectomy rates in Chapter Thirteen, pp. 248-250.

64.   Letter in *N Engl J Med*, 313 (July 11, 1985), pp. 117-118.

Chapter Sixteen

1.   "Are Breasts Redundant Organs?" *Br Med J*, 304 (Apr. 18, 1992), p. 1060.

2.   "Introduction" to Philip Strax's *Make Sure You Do Not Have Breast Cancer* (St. Martin's Press, 1989), pp. xi-xii.

3.   As explained in Chapter Ten, p. 196.

4. John M. Kurtz et al, "Breast-Conserving Therapy for Macroscopically Multiple Cancers,"

Ann Surg, 212 (July 1990), pp. 38-44.

5. See the discussion of calcifications in Chapter Ten, pp. 189-195.

6. Deborah Schrag et al, "Effects of Prophylactic Mastectomy and Oophorectomy on Life Expectancy among Women with *BRCA1* or *BRCA2* Mutations," *N Engl J Med*, 336 (May 15, 1997), pp. 1465-1471; and Lynn C. Hartmann et al, "Bilateral Prophylactic Mastectomy in Women with a Family History of Breast Cancer," *N Engl J Med*, 340 (Jan. 14, 1999), pp. 77-84.

7. The converse is true of juvenile and adolescent breasts, which are prone to radiation carcinogenesis. See the discussion in Chapter Four, pp. 77-78.

8. Important studies have been published by Bernard Fisher et al, "Leukemia in Breast Cancer Patients Following Adjuvant Chemotherapy or Postoperative Radiation: The NSABP Experience," *J Clin Oncol*, 3 (Dec. 1985), pp. 1640-1658; and by Rochelle E. Curtis et al, "Risk of Leukemia after Chemotherapy and Radiation Treatment for Breast Cancer," *N Engl J Med*, 326 (June 25, 1992), pp. 1745-1751.

9. "NIH Consensus Conference: Treatment of Early-Stage Breast Cancer," *JAMA*, 265 (Jan. 16, 1991), pp. 391-395.

10. "It's Too Soon to Know" (editorial), *J Natl Cancer Inst*, 82 (Feb. 21, 1990), pp. 250-251.

11. Hermann quoted by Blake Cady et al, "New Therapeutic Possibilities in Primary Invasive Breast Cancer," *Ann Surg*, 218 (Sept. 1993), pp. 338-349.

12. Robert E. Hermann et al, "The Cleveland Experience," in Sharon Grundfest-Broniatowski and Caldwell B. Esselstyn, Jr., *Controversies in Breast Disease* (Marcel Dekker, 1988), pp. 287-306.

13. Hermann (as in note 11), p. 347.

14. Roy M. Clark et al, "Randomized Clinical Trial to Assess the Effectiveness of Breast Irradiation Following Lumpectomy and Axillary Dissection for Node-Negative Breast Cancer," *J Natl Cancer Inst*, 84 (May 6, 1992), pp. 683-689.

15. Roy M. Clark et al, "Update," *J Natl Cancer Inst*, 88 (Nov. 20, 1996), pp. 1659-1664.

16. Harris and Clark quoted by Kara Smigel, "Workshop Affirms Value of Breast Conserving Treatments," *J Natl Cancer Inst*, 86 (Dec. 21, 1994), pp. 1824-1825.

17. H. Stephen Gallager and John E. Martin applied this term to breast cancers "no greater than 0.5 cm in diameter," in which "invasion either has not occurred or is little more than microscopic in extent." See their article "An Orientation to the Concept of Minimal Breast Cancer," *Cancer*, 28 (Dec. 1971), pp. 1505-1507.

18. Abram Recht et al, "Follow-up after Conservative Surgery and Radiotherapy," *Surg Clin North Am*, 70 (Oct. 1990), pp. 1179-1186.

19. Margolese quoted by John H. Glick et al, "Meeting Highlights: Adjuvant Therapy for Primary Breast Cancer," *J Natl Cancer Inst*, 84 (Oct. 7, 1992), pp. 1479-1485.

20. "Breast-Preservation Therapy for Primary Invasive Breast Carcinoma," *Surg Clin North Am*, 70 (Oct. 1990), pp. 1047-1059. See also Cady et al (as in note 11).

Chapter Seventeen

1. At the Consensus Development Conference of 1990 (author's notes for June 18 session).

2. Richard G. Margolese et al, "Lumpectomy and Axillary Dissection: A Syllabus from the National Surgical Adjuvant Breast Project," *Surgery*, 102 (Nov. 1987), pp. 828-834.

3. Margolese et al (as in preceding note), p. 829.

4. Bernard Fisher's presentation at the Consensus Development Conference of 1990 (author's notes for June 18), and Margolese et al (as in preceding notes), p. 833.

5. Margolese et al (as in preceding notes), pp. 829, 831-832.

6. "Carcinoma of the Breast" (editorial), *Ann Surg*, 217 (Mar. 1993), pp. 205-206.

7. The Joint Center guidelines for breast preservation have been reviewed by Asa J. Nixon et al, "Local Management of Invasive Breast Cancer," *Semin Oncol*, 23 (Aug. 1996), pp. 453-463. Quadrantectomy has not been popular in

in the United States. Veronesi and his colleagues reported the Milan experience with this procedure in *Ann Surg*, 211 (Mar. 1990), pp. 250-259, and *N Engl J Med*, 328 (June 3, 1993), pp. 1587-1591.

8. The experiences at these two institutions are described in Chapter Sixteen, pp. 320-321.

9. "NIH Consensus Conference," *JAMA*, 265 (Jan. 16, 1991), pp. 391-395.

10. Joseph A. Brennan et al, "Molecular Assessment of Histopathological Staging in Squamous-Cell Carcinoma of the Head and Neck," *N Engl J Med*, 332 (Feb. 16, 1995), pp. 429-435. See also the article on "Molecular Margins" by Vincent T. DeVita, Jr., and Albert B. Deisseroth, *JAMA*, 275 (June 16, 1996), pp. 1833-1834.

11. Tracy Hampton, "Surgeons 'Vote with Their Feet' for Sentinel Node Biopsy for Breast Cancer Staging," *JAMA*, 290 (Dec. 17, 2003), pp. 3053-3054.

12. Margolese et al (as in note 2), pp. 831-832.

13. Paul Peter Rosen et al, "Discontinuous or 'Skip' Metastases in Breast Carcinoma: Analysis of 1,228 Axillary Dissections," *Ann Surg*, 197 (Mar. 1983), pp. 276-283.

14. Blake Cady and Michael D. Stone, "Breast-Preservation Therapy for Primary Invasive Breast Carcinoma," *Surg Clin North Am*, 70 (Oct. 1990), pp. 1047-1059.

15. The details of axillary surgery are explained and illustrated in Donegan and Spratt (1988), pp. 403-461, and (1995), pp. 443-504. Kirby I. Bland and other surgeons discussed "Neurovascular Structures of the Axilla" in Strömbeck and Rosato, p. 160.

16. Margolese et al (as in note 2), pp. 831, 834.

17. Cady and Stone (as in note 14), p. 1052; Haagensen's memoir in *Ann Surg*, 199 (Feb. 1984), pp. 143-150.

18. Armando E. Giuliano et al, "Lymphatic Mapping and Sentinel Lymphadenectomy for Breast Cancer," *Ann Surg*, 220 (Sept. 1994), pp. 391-401.

19. Armando E. Giuliano et al, "Improved Axillary Staging of Breast Cancer with Sentinel Lymphadenectomy," *Ann Surg*, 222 (Sept. 1995), pp. 394-401.

20. Giuliano et al (as in note 18).

21. John J. Albertini et al, "Lymphatic Mapping and Sentinel Node Biopsy in the Patient with Breast Cancer," *JAMA*, 276 (Dec. 11, 1996), pp. 1818-1822.

22. Giuliano et al (as in note 18), p. 397.

23. Umberto Veronesi et al, "Sentinel Node Biopsy to Avoid Axillary Dissection in Breast Cancer," *Lancet*, 349 (June 28, 1997), pp. 1864-1867.

24. Advertisement in *Ann Surg*, 223 (Feb. 1996).

25. Correspondence, *JAMA*, 277 (Mar. 12, 1997), pp. 791-792.

26. Remarks by Lawrence and Giuliano quoted in Giuliano et al (as in note 19), pp. 398-401.

27. "Discussion" in Carlson et al (as in note 33), pp. 575-578.

28. As explained by David W. Kinne, "Modified Radical Mastectomy," in Harris et al, pp. 350-354.

29. The mastectomy modifications of Patey, Auchincloss, and Madden are discussed by Eric R. Frykberg and Kirby I. Bland, "Emergence of Lesser Operative Procedures," Bland and Copeland, pp. 558-564.

30. The NSABP techniques for retracting (and thus preserving) the chest muscles during axillary dissection are explained by Margolese et al (as in note 2), pp. 833-834.

31. The technique of subcutaneous mastectomy is illustrated by R. Robinson Baker in *Current Trends in the Management of Breast Cancer* (Johns Hopkins University Press, 1977), pp. 97-101.

32. Wood (as in note 6).

33. Grant W. Carlson et al, "Skin-sparing Mastectomy: Oncologic and Reconstructive Considerations," *Ann Surg*, 225 (May 1997), pp. 570-578.

34. "Blood Transfusions," Donegan and Spratt (1995), pp. 443-444.

35. "General Principles of Mastectomy," Bland and Copeland, pp. 569-583 (see p. 577).

36. Eileen P. Lynch et al, "Thoracic Epidural Anesthesia Improves Outcome after

Breast Surgery," *Ann Surg*, 222 (Nov. 1995), pp. 663-669.

37. Christina R. Weltz et al, "Ambulatory Surgical Management of Breast Carcinoma Using Paravertebral Block," *Ann Surg*, 222 (July 1995), pp. 19-26.

38. Weltz et al (preceding note). See also the letter from these authors in *Ann Surg*, 225 (Mar. 1997), p. 341.

39. Drain placement illustrated in Donegan and Spratt (1995), p. 466.

40. Margolese et al (as in note 2), p. 834. See also Robert G. Somers et al, "Closed Suction Drainage after Lumpectomy and Axillary Node Dissection for Breast Cancer," *Ann Surg*, 215 (Feb. 1992), pp. 146-149.

41. Kirby I. Bland et al, "The Postmastectomy Patient," in Strömbeck and Rosato, pp. 158-160.

42. "Complications of Mastectomy," Donegan and Spratt (1995), pp. 485-493.

Chapter Eighteen

1. Ivalon implants and contracture have been discussed by George T. Grace and I. Kelman Cohen, "Silicones and Breast Surgery," in Noone, pp. 38-47.

2. Grace and Cohen (as in preceding note), p. 40.

3. Ross Rudolph, "Unfavorable Results of Augmentation Mammoplasty," Noone, pp. 167-186 (see p. 169).

4. "Breast Reconstruction after Mastectomy," *N Engl J Med*, 317 (Dec. 31, 1987), pp. 1711-1714.

5. The suspected role of subclinical infections in contracture has been discussed by Ross Rudolph (as in note 3), pp. 169-170, 180.

6. T. Roderick Hester, Jr., and his colleagues at Emory University favorably reported their "Five-Year Experience with Polyurethane-Covered Mammary Prostheses," *Clinics in Plastic Surgery*, 15 (Oct. 1988), pp. 569-585.

7. Andrew Purvis, "Time Bombs in the Breasts?" *Time*, Apr. 29, 1991, p. 70. The one-in-a-million estimate came from the Food and Drug Administration, as recorded by Louise A. Brinton and S. Lori Brown, "Breast Implants and Cancer," *J Natl Cancer Inst*, 89 (Sept. 17, 1997), pp. 1341-1349.

8. Estimate given by Marcia Angell in "The Breast Implant Story" (address to the American Medical Writers Association, Boston, Nov. 14, 1997).

9. Andrew Purvis, "A Strike Against Silicone," *Time*, Jan. 20, 1992, pp. 40-41; and Stuart L. Nightingale, "Moratorium on Silicone Gel Breast Implants," *JAMA*, 267 (Feb. 12, 1992), p. 787.

10. David A. Kessler, "The Basis of the FDA's Decision on Breast Implants," *N Engl J Med*, 326 (June 18, 1992), pp. 1713-1715.

11. "Woman Says She Removed Breast Implants Herself" (Associated Press report), Savannah *Evening Press*, Apr. 17, 1992, p. 1.

12. Michael Morykwas quoted by Teri Randall, "Silicon Is No Stranger to the Body," *JAMA*, 267 (May 13, 1992), pp. 2442, 2444.

13. Marcia Angell, "Breast Implants—Protection or Paternalism?" (editorial), *N Engl J Med*, 326 (June 18, 1992), pp. 1695-1696.

14. "Council Report: Silicone Gel Breast Implants," *JAMA*, 270 (Dec. 1, 1993), pp. 2602-2606.

15. David A. Kessler et al, "A Call for Higher Standards for Breast Implants," *JAMA*, 270 (Dec. 1, 1993), pp. 2607-2608.

16. Gary Solomon et al, "Breast Implants and Connective-tissue Diseases" (correspondence), *N Engl J Med*, 331 (Nov. 3, 1994), pp. 1231-1235. For the Texas findings, see Randall M. Goldblum et al, "Antibodies to Silicone Elastomers," *Lancet*, 340 (Aug. 29, 1992), pp. 510-513.

17. Nancy Bruning, *Breast Implants: Everything You Need to Know*, 2nd ed. (Hunter House, 1995), p. 78.

18. "Breast Suit Plaintiff Wins 7.34 Million" (Associated Press report), Savannah *Evening Press*, Dec. 16, 1991, p. 5.

19. *Vogue* advertisement quoted by Marsha F. Goldsmith, "Medical News," *JAMA*, 267 (May 13, 1992), pp. 2439-2442. The spelling errors appeared in the original advertisement.

20. Estimates given by Marcia Angell (as in note 8).

21. Jay Reeves, "Expanded Settlement in Implant Lawsuit" (Associated Press report), Savannah *Morning News*, Apr. 15, 1994, p. 11A.

22. Jay Reeves, "Questions Raised in Implant Settlement" (Associated Press report), Savannah *Morning News*, Oct. 4, 1995, p. 2C.

23. Angell (as in note 8). See also her "Shattuck Lecture—Evaluating the Health Risks of Breast Implants," *N Engl J Med*, 334 (June 6, 1996), pp. 1513-1518.

24. Sherine E. Gabriel et al of the Mayo Clinic, "Risk of Connective-tissue Diseases and Other Disorders after Breast Implantation," *N Engl J Med*, 330 (June 16, 1994), pp. 1697-1702. For the remarks on "free silicone gel" by John O. Naim et al and other correspondence critical of the Mayo Clinic study, see *N Engl J Med*, 331 (Nov. 3, 1994), pp. 1231-1235.

25. Jorge Sánchez-Guerrero et al, "Silicone Breast Implants and the Risk of Connective-tissue Diseases and Symptoms," *N Engl J Med*, 332 (June 22, 1995), pp. 1666-1670.

26. Kessler's testimony quoted by Lauran Neergaard, "Breast Implants" (Associated Press report), Savannah *Morning News*, Aug. 2, 1995, p. 3D.

27. Charles H. Hennekens et al, "Self-reported Breast Implants and Connective-tissue Diseases in Female Health Professionals," *JAMA*, 275 (Feb. 28, 1996), pp. 616-621.

28. The question of "Breast Implants and Cancer" has been examined by Brinton and Brown (as in note 7).

29. "Augmentation Mammoplasty: Normal and Abnormal Findings with Mammography and Ultrasound," *RadioGraphics*, 12 (Mar. 1992), pp. 281-295.

30. Neal Handel et al, "Mammographic Visualization of the Breast after Augmentation Mammoplasty," *JAMA*, 268 (Oct. 14, 1992), pp. 1913-1917.

31. Dr. Noone has discussed immediate reconstruction at length (Noone, pp. 344-371). See also Daniel J. T. Webster et al, "Immediate Reconstruction of the Breast after Mastectomy," *Cancer*, 53 (Mar. 15, 1984), pp. 1416-1419.

32. Noone, p. 347.

33. Louis C. Argenta, "Reconstruction by Tissue Expansion," in Noone, pp. 387-395.

34. These procedures are illustrated in Paul K. McKissock's *Color Atlas of Mammaplasty* (Thieme, 1991).

35. John B. McCraw et al, "Breast Reconstruction Following Mastectomy," in Bland and Copeland, pp. 656-693 (quotation from p. 659).

36. J. Brien Murphy, "Complications of Breast Reconstruction," in Noone, pp. 448-454.

37. McCraw et al (as in note 35), p. 675.

38. Dr. Hartrampf recorded his "Seven-Year Experience" with the TRAM flap in *Clinics in Plastic Surgery*, 15 (Oct. 1988), pp. 703-716.

39. "Immediate Reconstruction after Mastectomy," *Ann Surg*, 218 (July 1993), pp. 29-36.

40. "Breast Reconstruction with Rectus Abdominis Flaps," Noone, pp. 420-436.

41. Noone, p. 423.

42. Noone, p. 423.

43. Shaw quoted in "Medical News," *JAMA*, 268 (Nov. 18, 1992), p. 2627.

44. "Bilateral Breast Reconstruction with the TRAM Free Flap," *Ann Surg*, 226 (July 1997), pp. 25-34.

45. "Breast Reconstruction with Free Flaps," Noone, pp. 437-447.

46. "The Nipple-Areola Complex," Harris et al, pp. 494-495.

47. Various tissue grafts which have been used in nipple-areola reconstructions are illustrated in Strömbeck and Rosato, pp. 252-253.

48. "Nipple-Areola Reconstruction," Noone, pp. 467-480.

Chapter Nineteen

1. H. Rodney Withers, "Biological Basis of Radiation Therapy for Cancer," *Lancet*, 339 (Jan. 18, 1992), pp. 156-159.

2. See Chapter Fifteen, pp. 306-309, for information on *rads* and *grays*, and on the Joint Center regimen.

3. Carl M. Mansfield et al, "A Review of Radiation Therapy in the Treatment of Breast

Cancer," *Semin Oncol*, 18 (Dec. 1991), pp. 525-535.

4. Nancy Price Mendenhall, "Overview: Irradiation Following Breast-Conserving Surgical Procedures," in Bland and Copeland, pp. 781-798 (see p. 782).

5. Mansfield et al (as in note 3), p. 526.

6. "Radiotherapy Techniques," Harris et al, pp. 411-412.

7. Mendenhall (as in note 4), pp. 781-782; Mansfield et al (as in note 3), pp. 529-530.

8. Jay R. Harris and Abram Recht, "Treatment of the Axilla and Other Nodal Areas," in Harris et al, pp. 413-414.

9. The utility of CAT scans in planning treatment has been superbly illustrated by Mendenhall (as in note 4), pp. 787-788.

10. Carrie F. Dunne-Daly, "Adverse Reactions of External Radiation Therapy," *Cancer Nursing*, 17 (June 1994), pp. 236-256.

11. Dunne-Daly (as in preceding note), p. 240.

12. Dunne-Daly (as in preceding note), p. 241; Kathleen L. McGowan, "Radiation Therapy: Saving Your Patient's Skin," *RN*, June 1989, pp. 24-27.

13. Mary Ann Rose et al, "Conservative Surgery and Radiation Therapy for Early Breast Cancer: Long-term Cosmetic Results," *Arch Surg*, 124 (Feb. 1989), pp. 153-157.

14. Abram Recht et al, "Follow-up after Conservative Surgery and Radiotherapy," *Surg Clin North Am*, 70 (Oct. 1990), pp. 1179-1186.

15. Kathleen M. Harris et al, "The Mammographic Features of the Post-lumpectomy, Post-irradiation Breast," *RadioGraphics*, 9 (Mar. 1989), pp. 253-268.

16. Mendenhall (as in note 4), p. 796; Recht et al (as in note 14), p. 1184.

17. Kathleen M. Harris et al (as in note 15), pp. 253, 268.

18. See Chapter Fifteen, pp. 309-310, as well as the description of Protocol B-06 by Bernard Fisher et al, "Five-Year Results," *N Engl J Med*, 312 (Mar. 14, 1985), pp. 665-673.

19. Abram Recht et al, "The Sequencing of Chemotherapy and Radiation Therapy after Conservative Surgery for Early-Stage Breast Cancer," *N Engl J Med*, 334 (May 23, 1996),

pp. 1356-1361.

20. Mendenhall (as in note 4), p. 789.

21. "Combining Irradiation with Systemic Therapy," Bland and Copeland, pp. 868, 870.

22. Frederick C. Ames et al, "Conservation Surgery and Radiation: The M. D. Anderson Cancer Center Experience," in Bland and Copeland, pp. 798-800.

23. "Carcinoma of the Breast in Pregnancy and Lactation," in Bland and Copeland, pp. 1034-1040.

24. The therapeutic dilemmas have been reviewed by Jill Waalen, "Pregnancy Poses Tough Questions for Cancer Treatment," *J Natl Cancer Inst*, 83 (July 3, 1991), pp. 900-902, and by Jeanne A. Petrek, "Breast Cancer and Pregnancy," in *Younger Women*, pp. 113-121.

25. Allen S. Lichter and Marc E. Lippman, "Breast Cancer Occurring during Pregnancy," in Lippman et al, pp. 414-419.

26. Petrek (as in note 24), p. 115.

27. Lichter and Lippman (as in note 25), pp. 417-418.

28. Petrek (as in note 24), p. 116.

Chapter Twenty

1. Kushner, p. 179.

2. NCI recommendations cited by Kirby I. Bland et al, "The Physician's Role in Follow-up," in Strömbeck and Rosato, pp. 163-166.

3. C. D. Haagensen, "A Personal Experience with Halsted's Radical Mastectomy," *Ann Surg*, 199 (Feb. 1984), pp. 143-150.

4. This estimate is repeated by Arthur J. Donovan, "Bilateral Breast Cancer," *Surg Clin North Am*, 70 (Oct. 1990), pp. 1141-1149.

5. Edwin F. Fisher et al, "Pathologic Findings from NSABP Protocol No. 4: Bilateral Breast Cancer," *Cancer*, 54 (Dec. 15, 1984), pp. 3002-3011.

6. Paul Peter Rosen et al, "Contralateral Breast Carcinoma: An Assessment of Risk and Prognosis," *Surgery*, 106 (Nov. 1989), pp. 904-921.

7. Fisher et al (as in note 5). For more

information on lobular histology, see Chapter Twelve, pp. 229-231, 243-245.

8. For *p53* involvement in hereditary breast cancers, see Chapter Three, pp. 47-48. For the *BRCA1* and *BRCA2* genes, see Chapter Five, pp. 113-116.

9. "Metastases to the Opposite Breast," Strömbeck and Rosato, p. 166.

10. See Chapter Fifteen, pp. 309-312, for these NSABP findings.

11. Abram Recht et al, "Local Recurrence Following Breast Conservation," in Harris et al, pp. 541-546.

12. John M. Kurtz et al, "Local Recurrence after Breast-Conserving Surgery: Frequency, Time Course, and Prognosis," *Cancer*, 63 (May 15, 1989), pp. 1912-1917.

13. See Chapter Sixteen, p. 320.

14. Kurtz et al (as in note 12). See also an earlier study by John M. Kurtz et al, "Wide Excision for Mammary Recurrence after Breast-Conserving Therapy," *Cancer*, 61 (May 15, 1988), pp. 1969-1972.

15. "Radiation Therapy in the Treatment of Breast Cancer," *Semin Oncol*, 18 (Dec. 1991), pp. 525-535.

16. Recht et al (as in note 11), pp. 543-544.

17. Jay R. Harris and Rebecca Gelman of the Joint Center for Radiotherapy discussed the prognostic implications of these presentations in "What Have We Learned about Local Recurrence?" (editorial), *J Clin Oncol*, 12 (Apr. 1994), pp. 647-649.

18. "Management of Local and Regional Recurrence after Mastectomy or Breast-Conserving Treatment," *Surg Clin North Am*, 70 (Oct. 1990), pp. 1115-1124.

19. Nancy Price Mendenhall et al, "Management of Local/Regional Recurrence," in Bland and Copeland, pp. 863-875.

20. Mendenhall et al (as in preceding note), p. 868.

21. Robin Miller-Catchpole, "Hyperthermia as Adjuvant Treatment for Recurrent Breast Cancer," *JAMA*, 271 (Mar. 9, 1994), pp. 797-802.

22. Tom Reynolds, "Photodynamic Therapy," *J Natl Cancer Inst*, 89 (Jan. 15, 1997), pp. 112-114.

23. "Local and Regional Recurrence," Donegan and Spratt (1995), pp. 666-681 (see pp. 674-675 for axillary recurrences).

24. This technique is described by Irving M. Ariel, "Intravascular Irradiation of the Internal Mammary Lymph Nodes," in Ariel and Cleary, pp. 274-279.

25. "Local Recurrent Mammary Carcinoma," *Arch Surg*, 124 (Feb. 1989), PP. 158-161.

26. Ian S. Fentiman et al, "Supraclavicular Node Recurrence after Radical Mastectomy," *Cancer*, 57 (Mar. 1, 1986), pp. 908-910.

27. NSABP findings cited by David V. Schapira and Nicole Urban, "A Minimalist Policy for Breast Cancer Surveillance," *JAMA*, 265 (Jan. 16, 1991), pp. 380-382. See also the counterpoint in this issue by Michael D. Wertheimer, "Against Minimalist in Breast Cancer Follow-up," pp. 396-397.

28. "Hepatic Function and Liver Scanning," Donegan and Spratt (1995), pp. 383-384.

29. Robert R. Edelman and Steven Warach, "Magnetic Resonance Imaging," *N Engl J Med*, 328 (Mar. 11 and Mar. 18, 1993), pp. 708-716, 785-791.

30. Hugh McIntosh, "Serum Tumor Markers," *J Natl Cancer Inst*, 84 (Mar. 18, 1992), pp. 387-389.

31. "Guidelines for the Use of Tumor Markers in Breast and Colorectal Cancer," *J Clin Oncol*, 14 (Oct. 1996), pp. 2843-2877 (see pp. 2855-2859 for CEA and CA 15-3).

32. "Impact of Follow-up Testing on Survival in Breast Cancer" by the GIVIO Investigators, and "Intensive Diagnostic Follow-up after Primary Breast Cancer" by Marco Rosselli Del Turco et al, *JAMA*, 271 (May 25, 1994), pp. 1587-1597.

33. "Cost-effective Follow-up of Breast Cancer Patients" (letter), *J Clin Oncol*, 12 (Sept. 1996), p. 1996.

34. Wertheimer (as in note 27), p. 397.

Chapter Twenty-one

1. The conquest of scurvy and pellagra has been described by Shorter, pp. 10-13, 31-32.

2. Rima D. Apple, *Vitamania: Vitamins in American Culture* (Rutgers University Press, 1996), pp. 4, 9.

3. Miles and Kroger advertising quoted by Apple (as in preceding note), pp. 57, 96-97.

4. "Chemoprevention of Breast Cancer" in Stoll, pp. 169-180.

5. Meir J. Stampfer et al, "Vitamin E Consumption and the Risk of Coronary Disease in Women," *N Engl J Med*, 328 (May 20, 1993), pp. 1444-1449.

6. Eric B. Rimm et al, "Vitamin E Consumption and the Risk of Coronary Heart Disease in Men," *N Engl J Med*, 328 (May 20, 1993), pp. 1450-1456.

7. "Antioxidant Vitamins and Coronary Heart Disease," *N Engl J Med*, 328 (May 20, 1993), pp. 1487-1489.

8. Hoffmann-La Roche's two-page advertisement in *JAMA*, 272 (Sept. 14, 1994). A one-page advertisement appeared in *Time*, May 8, 1995.

9. Victor Herbert, "The Antioxidant Supplement Myth," *Am J Clin Nutr*, 60 (Aug. 1994), pp. 157-158.

10. "Antioxidants, Pro-oxidants, and their Effects" (correspondence), *JAMA*, 272 (Dec. 7, 1994), pp. 1659-1660.

11. Herbert (as in note 9), p. 158.

12. Pauling's career has been chronicled by Anthony Serafini, *Linus Pauling: A Man and his Science* (Simon & Schuster, 1989).

13. Cameron's work and the California mouse experiment described by Serafini (as in preceding note), pp. 245, 254-257. The RDA of vitamin C for adult men has been set at 60 milligrams per day, as documented in *Recommended Dietary Allowances*, 10th ed. (National Academy Press, 1989), p. 118.

14. Charles G. Moertel et al, "High-dose Vitamin C Versus Placebo in the Treatment of Advanced Cancer," *N Engl J Med*, 312 (Jan. 17, 1985), pp. 137-141.

15. The symposium presentations were reported by Donald Earl Henson et al, "Ascorbic Acid: Biologic Functions and Relation to Cancer," *J Natl Cancer Inst*, 83 (Apr. 17, 1991), pp. 547-550.

16. Serafini (as in note 12), pp. 254-265.

17. Allan H. Smith and Kim D. Waller cited many of these studies in "Serum Beta Carotene in Persons with Cancer," *Am J Epidemiol*, 133 (Apr. 1, 1991), pp. 661-671.

18. "Oncology," *JAMA*, 265 (June 19, 1991), pp. 3141-3143.

19. Frank L. Meyskens, Jr., et al, "Randomized Trial of Vitamin A Versus Observation in High-Risk Melanoma," *J Clin Oncol*, 12 (Oct. 1994), pp. 2060-2065; and the ATBC Prevention Study Group, "Effect of Vitamin E and Beta Carotene on the Incidence of Lung Cancer and Other Cancers in Male Smokers," *N Engl J Med*, 330 (Apr. 14, 1994), pp. 1029-1035.

20. Charles H. Hennekens et al, "Lack of Effect of Long-term Supplementation with Beta Carotene," *N Engl J Med*, 334 (May 2, 1996), pp. 1145-1149.

21. Gilbert S. Omenn et al, "Effects of a Combination of Beta Carotene and Vitamin A on Lung Cancer and Cardiovascular Disease," *N Engl J Med*, 334 (May 2, 1996), pp. 1150-1155.

22. "Council Report: Vitamin Preparations," *JAMA*, 257 (Apr. 10, 1987), pp. 1929-1936.

23. Herbert (as in note 9).

24. M. J. Xu et al, "Reduction in Plasma Vitamin E with Long-term Administration of Beta Carotene," *J Natl Cancer Inst*, 84 (Oct. 2, 1992), pp. 1559-1565.

25. Frank L. Meyskens, Jr., and his colleagues at the University of Arizona reported the "Regression of Cervical Neoplasia with All-*trans*-retinoic Acid," *J Natl Cancer Inst*, 86 (Apr. 6, 1994), pp. 539-543.

26. Martin S. Tallman et al, "All-*trans*-retinoic Acid in Acute Promyelocytic Leukemia," *N Engl J Med*, 337 (Oct. 9, 1997), pp. 1021-1028.

27. David P. Rose et al, "Effect of Dietary Fat on Human Breast Cancer Growth and Lung

Metastasis in Nude Mice," *J Natl Cancer Inst*, 83 (Oct. 16, 1991), pp. 1491-1495.

28. Meera Jain et al, "Premorbid Diet and the Prognosis of Women with Breast Cancer," *J Natl Cancer Inst*, 86 (Sept. 21, 1994), pp. 1390-1397.

29. L. E. Holm et al, "Treatment Failure and Dietary Habits in Women with Breast Cancer," *J Natl Cancer Inst*, 85 (Jan. 6, 1993), pp. 32-36.

30. L. A. Cohen et al, "Modulation of Mammary Tumor Promotion by Dietary Fiber and Fat," *J Natl Cancer Inst*, 83 (Apr. 3, 1991), pp. 496-501.

31. Wallace quoted by Tom Reynolds, "5-a-Day for Better Health," *J Natl Cancer Inst*, 83 (Nov. 6, 1991), pp. 1538-1539; estimated spending for program cited in "News," *J Natl Cancer Inst*, 84 (Aug. 5, 1992), pp. 1149-1150.

32. American Cancer Society Advisory Committee, "Guidelines on Diet, Nutrition, and Cancer Prevention," *CA*, 46 (Nov/Dec. 1996), pp. 325-341.

33. "Broccoli and the Breast," *Nutrition Action Health Letter*, 17 (Sept. 1990), p. 4.

34. Yanhong Zhou and Amy S. Lee, "Genistein, an Anticancer Phyloestrogen from Soy," *J Natl Cancer Inst*, 90 (Mar. 4, 1998), pp. 381-388.

35. Reported by Tom Reynolds, "Foods for Cancer Prevention," *J Natl Cancer Inst*, 83 (Aug. 7, 1991), pp. 1050-1052.

36. Meishiang Jang et al, "Cancer Chemopreventive Activity of Resveratrol, a Natural Product Derived from Grapes," *Science*, 275 (Jan. 10, 1997), pp. 218-220.

37. Hugh D. Crone, *Chemicals & Society: A Guide to the New Chemical Age* (Cambridge University Press, 1986), p. 220. The NCI program has been described by Reynolds (as in note 35).

38. Patterson, p. 162.

39. The Simontons' regimen was sympathetically depicted by Judith Glassman in *The Cancer Survivors* (Dial Press, 1983), pp. 278-289.

40. Laszlo, pp. 207-212; Holland quoted by Glassman (as in preceding note), p. 289.

41. Steven J. Schleifer et al, "Suppression of Lymphocyte Stimulation Following Bereavement," *JAMA*, 250 (July 15, 1983), pp. 374-377.

42. This self-evident truth was reaffirmed by Sheldon Cohen et al, "Psychological Stress and Susceptibility to the Common Cold," *N Engl J Med*, 325 (Aug. 29, 1991), pp. 606-612.

43. Atsushi Uchida et al, "Prediction of Postoperative Clinical Course by Autologous Tumor-Killing Activity in Lung Cancer Patients," *J Natl Cancer Inst*, 82 (Nov. 7, 1990), pp. 1697-1701.

44. "Influences on Prognosis," Donegan and Spratt (1988), p. 357.

45. Bernie S. Siegel, *Love, Medicine & Miracles* (Harper & Row, 1986), p. 41.

46. Laszlo, pp. 215-217; Moertel quoted by Francis X. Mahaney, Jr., "Psychoneuroimmunology: Can the Brain and Immune System Communicate?" *J Natl Cancer Inst*, 82 (May 2, 1990), pp. 738-739.

47. Siegel (as in note 45), p. 28.

48. Ruth Shereff, "Wish Me Well," *Ms.*, Oct. 1989, pp. 26-30.

49. Norman Cousins, *Head First: The Biology of Hope* (E. P. Dutton, 1989).

50. David Spiegel et al, "Effect of Psychosocial Treatment on Survival of Patients with Metastatic Breast Cancer," *Lancet*, Oct. 14, 1989, pp. 888-891.

51. Negative results were reported by Susan Tross et al, "Psychological Symptoms and Disease-free and Overall Survival in Women with Stage II Breast Cancer," *J Natl Cancer Inst*, 88 (May 15, 1996), pp. 661-667.

52. "The Laughter Connection" (Chapter Ten) in Cousins (as in note 49), pp. 125-153.

Chapter Twenty-two

1. Beatson's experiments have been described by Carl G. Kardinal in Donegan and Spratt (1988), pp. 503-504, and by Frederick B. Wagner, Jr., in Bland and Copeland, p. 14.

2. See Chapter Fourteen, p. 270, for representative measurements of ER.

3. Ovarian irradiation and other strategies

have been reviewed by N. O. Theve et al, "Different Ablative Procedures," in Strömbeck and Rosato, pp. 203-207.

4. For DES, see Chapter Six, pp. 120-121.

5. N. O. Theve et al, "Additive Hormonal Treatment," Strömbeck and Rosato, pp. 207-208; Carl G. Kardinal, "Estrogens," Donegan and Spratt (1988), pp. 525-526.

6. AMA Council on Drugs, "Androgens and Estrogens in the Treatment of Disseminated Mammary Carcinoma," *JAMA*, 172 (Mar. 19, 1960), pp. 1271-1283.

7. For more information on ER and PgR assays, see Chapter Fourteen, pp. 267-272.

8. The drug's history has been ably summarized by V. Craig Jordan, "The Development of Tamoxifen for Breast Cancer Therapy," in Jordan (1994), pp. 3-26.

9. Jordan (as in preceding note), p. 7.

10. Michael Fritsch and Douglas M. Wolf, "Symptomatic Side Effects of Tamoxifen Therapy," in Jordan (1994), pp. 235-255.

11. Richard R. Love, "Tamoxifen Therapy in Primary Breast Cancer: Biology, Efficacy, and Side Effects," *J Clin Oncol*, 7 (June 1989), pp. 803-815.

12. V. Craig Jordan et al, "Laboratory and Clinical Research on the Hormone Dependence of Breast Cancer," in Jordan (1986), pp. 501-522 (see especially p. 513).

13. Fritsch and Wolf (as in note 10), pp. 245-246.

14. David Plotkin et al, "Tamoxifen Flare in Advanced Breast Cancer," *JAMA*, 240 (Dec. 8, 1978), pp. 2644-2646.

15. Richard R. Love, "Toxicity of Tamoxifen in Postmenopausal Women," in Jordan (1994), pp. 51-81 (see especially pp. 70-71).

16. Bernard Fisher et al, "Treatment of Primary Breast Cancer with Chemotherapy and Tamoxifen," *N Engl J Med*, 305 (July 2, 1981), pp. 1-6.

17. Nolvadex Adjuvant Trial Organization, "Controlled Trial of Tamoxifen as Single Adjuvant Agent in Early Breast Cancer," *Lancet*, Apr. 13, 1985, pp. 836-840.

18. "Adjuvant Tamoxifen in the Management of Operable Breast Cancer: The Scottish Trial," *Lancet*, July 25, 1987, pp. 171-175.

19. Tommy Fornander et al, "Adjuvant Tamoxifen in Early Breast Cancer: Occurrence of New Primary Cancers," *Lancet*, Jan. 21, 1989, pp. 117-120.

20. Stuart L. Nightingale, "Tamoxifen Labeling Includes Stronger Warning," *JAMA*, 271 (May 18, 1994), p. 1472.

21. "Effects of Adjuvant Tamoxifen and of Cytotoxic Therapy on Mortality in Early Breast Cancer," *N Engl J Med*, 319 (Dec. 29, 1988), pp. 1681-1692.

22. "Systemic Treatment of Early Breast Cancer by Hormonal, Cytotoxic, or Immune Therapy," *Lancet*, 339 (Jan. 4 and Jan. 11, 1992), pp. 1-15, 71-85. See especially Figures 5 and 6 (pp. 10-11) as well as the article abstract (p. 1).

23. "Tamoxifen for Early Breast Cancer: An Overview of the Randomized Trials," *Lancet*, 351 (May 16, 1998), pp. 1451-1467.

24. "An Overview" (as in preceding note), pp. 1455-1456.

25. Consensus Development Panel, "Introduction and Conclusions," *Chemotherapy Consensus*, pp. 1-4.

26. Kara Smigel, "Doctors Change Breast Cancer Treatment Practices," *J Natl Cancer Inst*, 84 (June 17, 1992), pp. 924-925.

27. Marc E. Lippman and Bruce A. Chabner, "Editorial Overview," *Chemotherapy Consensus*, pp. 5-10.

28. Early Breast Cancer Trialists' Collaborative Group, "Ovarian Ablation," *Lancet*, 348 (Nov. 2, 1996), pp. 1189-1196.

29. Gerald Ribeiro and M. K. Palmer, "Adjuvant Tamoxifen for Operable Carcinoma of the Breast," *Br Med J*, 286 (Mar. 12, 1983), pp. 827-830.

30. James N. Ingle et al, "Bilateral Oophorectomy Versus Tamoxifen in Premenopausal Women," *J Clin Oncol*, 4 (Feb. 1986), pp. 178-185.

31. "Treatment of Breast Cancer," *N Engl J Med*, 339 (Oct. 1, 1998), pp. 974-984.

32. V. Craig Jordan et al, "Endocrine Parameters in Premenopausal Women during Long-term Tamoxifen," *J Natl Cancer Inst*, 83 (Oct. 16, 1991), pp. 1488-1491.

33. Bernard Fisher et al, "Influence of Tumor Estrogen and Progesterone Receptor

Levels on the Response to Tamoxifen and Chemotherapy in Primary Breast Cancer," *J Clin Oncol*, 1 (Apr. 1983), pp. 227-241.

34. Jordan (as in note 8), p. 15.

35. C. Kent Osborne et al, "Effects of Tamoxifen on Breast Cancer Cell Kinetics," *Cancer Research*, 43 (Aug. 1983), pp. 3583-3585.

36. "Interactions of Tamoxifen with Cytotoxic Chemotherapy," in Jordan (1994), pp. 181-198.

37. Saul E. Rivkin et al, "Adjuvant CMFVP Versus Tamoxifen Versus Concurrent CMFVP and Tamoxifen," *J Clin Oncol*, 12 (Oct. 1994), pp. 2078-2085.

38. Kathleen I. Pritchard et al, "Increased Thromboembolic Complications with Concurrent Tamoxifen and Chemotherapy," *J Clin Oncol*, 14 (Oct. 1996), pp. 2731-2737.

39. Kathleen I. Pritchard et al, "Randomized Trial of CMF Chemotherapy Added to Tamoxifen," *J Clin Oncol*, 15 (June 1997), pp. 2302-2311.

40. John H. Glick et al, "Meeting Highlights," *J Natl Cancer Inst*, 84 (Oct. 7, 1992), pp. 1479-1485.

41. Bernard Fisher et al, "Chemotherapy and Tamoxifen Compared with Tamoxifen Alone . . . Results from NSABP Project B-16," *J Clin Oncol*, 8 (June 1990), pp. 1005-1018.

42. Rivkin et al (as in note 37), p. 2084. For the ER and PgR levels of B-16 participants, see Fisher et al (as in preceding note), Table 2 on p. 1008.

43. Bernard Fisher et al, "Tamoxifen and Chemotherapy for Node-Negative, Estrogen Receptor-Positive Breast Cancer," *J Natl Cancer Inst*, 89 (Nov. 19, 1997), pp. 1673-1682.

44. Richard D. Gelber et al, "Adjuvant Chemotherapy Plus Tamoxifen for Postmenopausal Breast Cancer: Meta-analysis of Quality-adjusted Survival," *Lancet*, 347 (Apr. 20, 1996), pp. 1066-1071.

45. Aron Goldhirsch et al, "International Consensus Panel on the Treatment of Primary Breast Cancer," *J Natl Cancer Inst*, 90 (Nov. 4, 1998), pp. 1601-1608.

46. Swedish Breast Cancer Cooperative Group, "Randomized Trial of Two Years Versus Five Years of Adjuvant Tamoxifen for Postmenopausal Breast Cancer," *J Natl Cancer Inst*, 88 (Nov. 6, 1996), pp. 1543-1549.

47. "NSABP Halts B-14 Trial: No Benefit Seen Beyond Five Years of Tamoxifen Use," *J Natl Cancer Inst*, 87 (Dec. 20, 1995), p. 1829. See also the published NSABP analysis by Bernard Fisher et al, "Five Versus More than Five Years of Tamoxifen," *J Natl Cancer Inst*, 88 (Nov. 6, 1996), pp. 1529-1542.

48. Douglass C. Tormey et al, "Adjuvant Tamoxifen Beyond Five Years in Node-Positive Breast Cancer," *J Natl Cancer Inst*, 88 (Dec. 18, 1996), pp. 1828-1833.

49. Goldhirsch et al (as in note 45), p. 1606.

50. Jordan (as in note 8), pp. 10-11.

51. Richard R. Love et al, "Effects of Tamoxifen Therapy on Lipid and Lipoprotein Levels in Postmenopausal Patients with Node-Negative Breast Cancer," *J Natl Cancer Inst*, 82 (Aug. 15, 1990), pp. 1327-1332.

52. Susan G. Nayfield et al, "Potential Role of Tamoxifen in Prevention of Breast Cancer," *J Natl Cancer Inst*, 83 (Oct. 16, 1991), pp. 1450-1459.

53. C. C. McDonald and H. J. Stewart, "Fatal Myocardial Infarction in the Scottish Adjuvant Tamoxifen Trial," *Br Med J*, 303 (Aug. 24, 1991), pp. 435-437.

54. Lars E. Rutqvist and Anders Mattsson, "Cardiac and Thromboembolic Morbidity in a Randomized Trial of Adjuvant Tamoxifen," *J Natl Cancer Inst*, 85 (Sept. 1, 1993), pp. 1398-1406.

55. Fisher et al (as in note 47), p. 1534.

56. Frederick S. Kaplan et al, "Estrogen Receptors in Bone," *N Engl J Med*, 319 (Aug. 18, 1988), pp. 421-425.

57. Richard R. Love et al, "Effects of Tamoxifen on Bone Mineral Density in Postmenopausal Women with Breast Cancer," *N Engl J Med*, 326 (Mar. 26, 1992), pp. 852-856.

58. Tommy Fornander et al, "Long-term Adjuvant Tamoxifen: Effect on Bone Mineral Density," *J Clin Oncol*, 8 (June 1990), pp. 1019-1024.

59. Bent Kristensen et al, "Tamoxifen and Bone Metabolism," *J Clin Oncol*, 12 (May 1994),

pp. 992-997.

60. Trevor J. Powles et al, "Effect of Tamoxifen on Bone Mineral Density in Healthy Premenopausal and Postmenopausal Women," *J Clin Oncol*, 14 (Jan. 1996), pp. 78-84. The preclinical experiments with rats are discussed on p. 82.

61. Powles et al (as in preceding note), pp. 82-83.

62. Fisher et al (as in note 47), p. 1540.

63. Bernard Fisher et al, "A Randomized Clinical Trial Evaluating Tamoxifen in the Treatment of Patients with Node-Negative Breast Cancer Who Have Estrogen Receptor-Positive Tumors," *N Engl J Med*, 320 (Feb. 23, 1989), pp. 479-484.

64. Samuel Hellman, "Clinical Alert: A Poor Idea Prematurely Used," *Advances* (1991), pp. 255-257; K. C. Lee and Vincent T. DeVita, Jr., "The 'Clinical Alert' from the National Cancer Institute" (correspondence), *N Engl J Med*, 319 (Oct. 6, 1988), pp. 948-949.

65. "Adjuvant Therapy of Node-Negative Breast Cancer," *N Engl J Med*, 320 (Feb. 23, 1989), pp. 525-527.

66. As explained by former NCI director Vincent T. DeVita, Jr., "The NCI's Clinical Alert," *Advances* (1991), pp. 241-246.

67. "Table 2: Characteristics of Patients" in Fisher et al (as in note 63), p. 480.

68. The NSABP's protocol was critically reviewed by Trudy L. Bush and Kathy J. Helzlsouer, "Tamoxifen for the Primary Prevention of Breast Cancer," *Epidemiol Rev*, 15 (1993), pp. 233-243.

69. Fugh-Berman and Hubbard quoted by Ruth Hubbard and Elijah Wald, *Exploding the Gene Myth* (Beacon Press, 1993), p. 90.

70. For reports of possible ocular effects, see Fritsch and Wolf (as in note 10), p. 246.

71. "Should Healthy Women Take Tamoxifen?" (correspondence), *N Engl J Med*, 327 (Nov. 26, 1992), pp. 1596-1597.

72. "NCI Audit of NSABP" (news article), *J Natl Cancer Inst*, 86 (June 1, 1994), pp. 822-824.

73. This episode is discussed in Chapter Fifteen, pp. 311-312.

74. Susan Jenks, "Congressional Hearing Delves into NSABP Fraud Issues," *J Natl Cancer Inst*, 86 (May 4, 1994), pp. 664-665; "Former NSABP Chief Grilled," *J Natl Cancer Inst*, 86 (July 6, 1994), pp. 963-964.

75. "No Misconduct in Fisher Case," *J Natl Cancer Inst*, 89 (Apr. 2, 1997), p. 472; "Fisher Suit Settled," *J Natl Cancer Inst*, 89 (Sept. 17, 1997), pp. 1336-1337.

76. Paul Recer, "Drug Cuts Chances of Breast Cancer" (Associated Press report), Savannah *Morning News*, Apr. 7, 1998, p. 7A.

77. Dick Thompson, "Beware this Breakthrough!" *Time*, Apr. 20, 1998, pp. 62-63.

78. "When to Take Tamoxifen" (letter), *Time*, Oct. 5, 1998.

79. Bernard Fisher et al, "Tamoxifen for Prevention of Breast Cancer: Report of the NSABP Project P-1 Study," *J Natl Cancer Inst*, 90 (Sept. 16, 1998), pp. 1371-1388.

80. "Table 3: Average Annual Rates" (as in preceding note), p. 1375.

81. "Ischemic Heart Disease, Fractures, Vascular Events" (as in preceding notes), pp. 1376-1379.

82. "Discussion" (as in preceding notes), pp. 1380-1383.

83. "Failure of Tamoxifen Therapy," in Jordan (1986), pp. 512-519.

84. "Tamoxifen in the Treatment of Breast Cancer," *N Engl J Med*, 339 (Nov. 26, 1998), pp. 1609-1618.

85. Hyman B. Muss et al, "High-Dose Megestrol Acetate in Advanced Breast Cancer," *J Clin Oncol*, 8 (Nov. 1990), pp. 1797-1805.

86. Richard J. Santen et al, "A Randomized Trial Comparing Surgical Adrenalectomy with Aminoglutethimide in Advanced Breast Cancer," *N Engl J Med*, 305 (Sept. 3, 1981), pp. 545-551. See also Paul E. Goss and Karin M. E. H. Gwyn, "Aromatase Inhibitors in Breast Cancer," *J Clin Oncol*, 12 (Nov. 1994), pp. 2460-2470.

87. Charles W. Taylor et al, "Goserelin Versus Surgical Ovariectomy in Premenopausal Patients with Receptor-Positive Metastatic Breast Cancer," *J Clin Oncol*, 16 (Mar. 1998), pp. 994-999.

88. William J. Gradishar and V. Craig Jordan, "Potential of New Antiestrogens," *J Clin*

Oncol, 15 (Feb. 1997), pp. 840-852.

89. Daniel F. Hayes et al, "Randomized Comparison of Tamoxifen and Toremifene in Metastatic Breast Cancer," *J Clin Oncol*, 13 (Oct. 1995), pp. 2556-2566; and Tiina Saarto et al, "Antiatherogenic Effects of Antiestrogens: A Trial Comparing Tamoxifen and Toremifene," *J Clin Oncol*, 14 (Feb. 1996), pp. 429-433.

90. Schering advertisement for Fareston in *J Natl Cancer Inst*, 90 (Mar. 4, 1998).

91. "Tamoxifen and Toremifene in Breast Cancer: Comparison of Safety and Efficacy," *J Clin Oncol*, 16 (Jan. 1998), pp. 348-353.

92. Discussion of raloxifene by Gradishar and Jordan (as in note 88), pp. 847-848; advertisements for Evista in *Time*, Apr. 6, 1998, and *N Engl J Med*, 338 (Apr. 30, 1998).

93. Breast cancer prophylaxis with raloxifene cited by Scott M. Lippman et al, "Cancer Chemoprevention," *J Natl Cancer Inst*, 90 (Oct. 21, 1998), pp. 1514-1528 (see pp. 1517-1518); Brian W. Walsh et al, "Effects of Raloxifene on Serum Lipids," *JAMA*, 279 (May 13, 1998), pp. 1445-1451.

94. "NSABP Names Centers for Study of Tamoxifen and Raloxifene" (news report), *J Natl Cancer Inst*, 90 (Oct. 21, 1998), p. 1504.

95. "Antiestrogenic Action of Raloxifene and Tamoxifen," *J Natl Cancer Inst*, 90 (July 1, 1998), pp. 967-971.

96. "Aromatase Inhibitors in the Treatment and Prevention of Breast Cancer," *J Clin Oncol*, 19 (Feb. 11, 2001), pp. 881-894.

97. "Anastrozole Versus Megestrol Acetate in Postmenopausal Women with Advanced Breast Cancer," *J Clin Oncol*, 14 (July 1996), pp. 2000-2011.

98. Per Dombernowsky et al, "Letrozole Compared with Megestrol Acetate," *J Clin Oncol*, 16 (Feb. 1998), pp. 453-461.

99. Manfred Kaufmann et al, "Exemestane Superior to Megestrol Acetate after Tamoxifen Failure," *J Clin Oncol*, 18 (Apr. 2000), pp. 1399-1411.

100. Paul E. Goss et al, "Letrozole in Postmenopausal Women after Five Years of Tamoxifen for Early-Stage Breast Cancer," *N Engl J Med*, 349 (Nov. 6, 2003), pp. 1793-1802.

101. "Letrozole in Breast Cancer" (correspondence), *N Engl J Med*, 350 (Feb. 12, 2004), pp. 727-730.

102. R. Charles Coombes et al, "Randomized Trial of Exemestane after Two to Three Years of Tamoxifen Therapy," *N Engl J Med*, 350 (Mar. 11, 2004), pp. 1081-1092.

103. "Adjuvant Treatment of Breast Cancer with Exemestane" (correspondence), *N Engl J Med*, 351 (July 1, 2004), pp. 100-102.

104. ATAC Trialists' Group, "Anastrozole Alone or in Combination with Tamoxifen Versus Tamoxifen Alone for Adjuvant Treatment of Postmenopausal Women with Early Breast Cancer," *Lancet*, 359 (June 22, 2002), pp. 2131-2139.

105. ATAC Trialists' Group, "Efficacy and Safety Update Analyses," *Cancer*, 98 (Nov. 1, 2003), pp. 1802-1810.

106. ATAC Trialists' Group, "Results of the ATAC Trial after Completion of Five Years' Adjuvant Treatment for Breast Cancer," *Lancet*, 365 (Jan. 1, 2005), pp. 60-62.

Chapter Twenty-three

1. Shorter, pp. 184-188.

2. The efforts of Farber and many later researchers have been ably recounted by Emil J. Freireich and Noreen A. Lemak, *Milestones in Leukemia Research and Therapy* (Johns Hopkins University Press, 1991), and by John Laszlo, *The Cure of Childhood Leukemia: Into the Age of Miracles* (Rutgers University Press, 1995).

3. Freireich quoted in Laszlo (as in preceding note), pp. 140-145.

4. VAMP regimen described in Freireich and Lemak (as in note 2), pp. 77-78.

5. Laszlo (as in note 2), p. 173.

6. "In Memoriam" (obituary of C. Gordon Zubrod), *J Clin Oncol*, 17 (May 1999), pp. 1331-1333.

7. Dr. Li's cure of choriocarcinoma has been recounted by Shorter, pp. 191-192, by John Laszlo (as in note 2), pp. 145-147, 226-227, and by C. Gordon Zubrod, "Origins and Development of Chemotherapy Research at the National

Cancer Institute," *Cancer Treatment Reports*, 68 (Jan. 1984), pp. 9-19.

8. Vincent T. DeVita, Jr., et al, "Hodgkin's Disease," *PPO*, pp. 1819-1858. The B-cell derivation of Reed-Sternberg cells was not established until the mid-1990s. See Theresa Marafioti et al, "Origin of Hodgkin's Disease from Mutated Germinal-Center B-Cells," *N Engl J Med*, 337 (Aug. 14, 1997), pp. 453-458, as well as the accompanying article by Toshiyuki Ohno et al (pp. 459-465) and editorial by Robert S. Schwartz (pp. 495-496).

9. DeVita et al (as in preceding note), pp. 1836-1838. See also John Laszlo (as in note 2), pp. 177, 185-187, and Freireich and Lemak (as in note 2), pp. 80-81.

10. "Thomas Hodgkin and Hodgkin's Disease," *JAMA*, 265 (Feb. 27, 1991), pp. 1007-1010.

11. George J. Bosl and Robert J. Motzer, "Testicular Germ-Cell Cancer," *N Engl J Med*, 337 (July 24, 1997), pp. 242-253.

12. Stephen D. Williams et al, "Treatment of Disseminated Germ-Cell Tumors," *N Engl J Med*, 316 (June 4, 1987), pp. 1435-1440.

13. Survival rates cited by Scott B. Saxman and Craig R. Nichols, "Testicular Cancer," in Skeel, pp. 326-330.

14. Williams, p. 115.

15. Bernard Fisher described the first two NSABP trials in "Systemic Chemotherapy as an Adjuvant to Surgery in the Treatment of Breast Cancer," *Cancer*, 24 (Dec. 1969), pp. 1286-1289.

16. Bernard Fisher et al, "L-phenylalanine Mustard (L-PAM) in the Management of Primary Breast Cancer," *N Engl J Med*, 292 (Jan. 16, 1975), pp. 117-122.

17. Bernard Fisher et al, "L-PAM in Premenopausal Patients with Breast Cancer: Lack of Association of Disease-Free Survival with Depression of Ovarian Function," *Cancer*, 44 (Sept. 1979), pp. 847-857.

18. Gianni Bonadonna et al, "Combination Chemotherapy as an Adjuvant Treatment in Operable Breast Cancer," *N Engl J Med*, 294 (Feb. 19, 1976), pp. 405-410.

19. "Major Advance in Breast Cancer Therapy" (editorial), *N Engl J Med*, 294 (Feb. 19, 1976), pp. 440-441.

20. Gianni Bonadonna and Pinuccia Valagussa, "Dose-Response Effect of Adjuvant Chemotherapy in Breast Cancer," *N Engl J Med*, 304 (Jan. 1, 1981), pp. 10-15.

21. Bonadonna and Valagussa (as in preceding note), p. 15.

22. G. Tancini et al, "Adjuvant CMF in Breast Cancer: Comparative Five-Year Results of 12 Versus 6 Cycles," *J Clin Oncol*, 1 (Jan. 1983), pp. 2-10.

23. International Breast Cancer Study Group, "Duration of Adjuvant Chemotherapy for Node-Positive Premenopausal Patients," *J Clin Oncol*, 14 (June 1996), pp. 1885-1894. See especially "Figure 5: Five-year DFS" on p. 1890.

24. Rose Kushner, "Is Aggressive Adjuvant Chemotherapy the Halsted Radical of the 80s?" *CA*, 34 (Nov/Dec. 1984), pp. 345-349.

25. "Progress Against Cancer?" *N Engl J Med*, 314 (May 8, 1986), pp. 1226-1232.

26. "Correspondence," *N Engl J Med*, 315 (Oct. 9, 1986), pp. 963-968. Dr. Bailar and his colleague Heather L. Gornik continued to voice skepticism about chemotherapy in a 1997 article entitled "Cancer Undefeated." See *N Engl J Med*, 336 (May 29, 1997), pp. 1569-1574.

27. Gianni Bonadonna et al, "Adjuvant CMF in Node-Positive Breast Cancer: The Results of 20 Years of Follow-up," *N Engl J Med*, 332 (Apr. 6, 1995), pp. 901-906.

28. Elaine Blume, "Oncology Professions Transformed in 20 Years," *J Natl Cancer Inst*, 83 (May 1, 1991), pp. 596-598.

29. The Dana-Farber rug fiasco was described by Edward J. Sylvester in *Target: Cancer* (Scribner's, 1986), p. 122.

30. "Doxorubicin" in Skeel, pp. 100-101.

31. Pawan K. Singal and Natasha Iliskovic, "Doxorubicin-Induced Cardiomyopathy," *N Engl J Med*, 13 (Sept. 24, 1998), pp. 900-905.

32. Sandra M. Swain et al, "Cardioprotection with Dexrazoxane for Doxorubicin-Containing Therapy in Advanced Breast Cancer," *J Clin Oncol*, 15 (Apr. 1997), pp. 1318-1332, and "Delayed Administration of Dexrazoxane" (second article), pp. 1333-1340.

33. Aman U. Buzdar et al, "Adjuvant Chemotherapy Trials in Breast Cancer at M. D. Anderson Hospital," *Chemotherapy Consensus*,

pp. 81-85.

34. Aman U. Buzdar et al, "Ten-Year Results of FAC Adjuvant Chemotherapy Trial in Breast Cancer," *American Journal of Clinical Oncology*, 12 (1989), pp. 123-128.

35. "Table 3: Survival of Patients with Stage II Disease," Buzdar et al (as in preceding note), p. 126.

36. CAF regimen described in Skeel, p. 266.

37. "Correspondence," *N Engl J Med*, 315 (Oct. 9, 1986), pp. 963-964; "Achievable Survival in Breast Cancer," *J Natl Cancer Inst*, 84 (May 20, 1992), p. 811.

38. "Adjuvant Systemic Therapy," *Breast Cancer Res Treat*, 14 (Oct. 1989), pp. 3-22.

39. Bernard Fisher et al, "Two Months of AC Compared with Six Months of CMF in Node-Positive Breast Cancer," *J Clin Oncol*, 8 (Sept. 1990), pp. 1483-1496.

40. G. Thomas Budd et al, "Short Course FAC-M Versus One Year of CMFVP in Node-Positive Breast Cancer," *J Clin Oncol*, 13 (Apr. 1995), pp. 831-839.

41. Gianni Bonadonna et al, "Sequential or Alternating Doxorubicin and CMF Regimens in Breast Cancer," *JAMA*, 273 (Feb. 15, 1995), pp. 542-547.

42. "Polychemotherapy for Early Breast Cancer: An Overview of the Randomised Trials," *Lancet*, 352 (Sept. 19, 1998), pp. 930-942. See especially "Figure 7: Absolute Effects of Anthracycline-containing Regimens Compared with CMF" (p. 938).

43. The role of P-glycoprotein has been reviewed by William S. Dalton and Thomas P. Miller, "Multidrug Resistance," *PPO Updates*, 5 (July 1991), pp. 1-13, and by Donna M. Bradshaw and Robert J. Arceci, "Transmembrane Drug Efflux as a Mechanism of Multidrug Resistance," *J Clin Oncol*, 16 (Nov. 1998), pp. 3674-3690.

44. Lori J. Goldstein et al, "Expression of a Multidrug Resistance Gene in Human Cancers," *J Natl Cancer Inst*, 81 (Jan. 18, 1989), pp. 116-124.

45. Sydney E. Salmon et al, "Prediction of Doxorubicin Resistance by P-glycoprotein Staining," *J Natl Cancer Inst*, 81 (May 3, 1989),

pp. 696-701.

46. "Multidrug Resistance in Breast Cancer: A Meta-Analysis of *MDR1* (P-glycoprotein) Expression," *J Natl Cancer Inst*, 89 (July 2, 1997), pp. 917-931.

47. Gregory D. Pennock et al, "Toxic Effects Associated with High-Dose Verapamil Infusion," *J Natl Cancer Inst*, 83 (Jan. 16, 1991), pp. 105-110.

48. Bert L. Lum et al, "Cyclosporine to Modulate Multidrug Resistance," *J Clin Oncol*, 10 (Oct. 1992), pp. 1635-1642.

49. D. J. Boote et al, "PSC833 as a Modulator of Multidrug Resistance," *J Clin Oncol*, 14 (Feb. 1996), pp. 610-618; and Alexander J. Smith et al, "PSC833, Inhibitor of P-glycoproteins," *J Natl Cancer Inst*, 90 (Aug. 5, 1998), pp. 1161-1166.

50. Tom Reynolds, "Research on Drug Resistance Unearths Many Mechanisms" (news article), *J Natl Cancer Inst*, 90 (Aug. 5 and 19, 1998), pp. 1120-1122, 1186-1188.

51. Moscow quoted by Reynolds (as in preceding note), pp. 1121-1122.

52. William C. Wood et al, "Dose and Dose Intensity of Adjuvant Chemotherapy for Stage II, Node-Positive Breast Carcinoma," *N Engl J Med*, 330 (May 5, 1994), pp. 1253-1259.

53. Daniel R. Budman et al, "Dose and Dose Intensity as Determinants of Outcome in the Adjuvant Treatment of Breast Cancer," *J Natl Cancer Inst*, 90 (Aug. 19, 1998), pp. 1205-1211. The statistics quoted are based on Figure 1 ("Disease-free and Overall Survival by Treatment Arm"), p. 1208.

54. Henderson (as in note 38), pp. 4, 8.

55. "Be a Survivor" (book review), *J Natl Cancer Inst*, 91 (Mar. 17, 1999), pp. 558-559.

56. "Chemotherapy in Private Practice" (correspondence), *J Natl Cancer Inst*, 84 (May 20, 1992), p. 810.

57. Van Scoy-Mosher quoted by John Burklow, "Consumerism" (news report), *J Natl Cancer Inst*, 83 (Sept. 4, 1991), pp. 1205-1207.

Chapter Twenty-four

1. Bernard Fisher et al, "Influence of the Interval between Primary Tumor Removal and Chemotherapy on Kinetics and Growth of Metastases," *Cancer Research*, 43 (Apr. 1983), pp. 1488-1492.

2. Bernard Fisher et al, "Effect of Preoperative Chemotherapy on the Outcome of Women with Operable Breast Cancer," *J Clin Oncol*, 16 (Aug. 1998), pp. 2672-2685.

3. Bernard Fisher et al, "Effect of Preoperative Chemotherapy on Local-Regional Disease in Operable Breast Cancer," *J Clin Oncol*, 15 (July 1997), pp. 2483-2493.

4. Gianni Bonadonna et al, "Primary Chemotherapy in Operable Breast Cancer: Eight-Year Experience at the Milan Cancer Institute," *J Clin Oncol*, 16 (Jan. 1998), pp. 93-100.

5. "Nomograms for Determining Body Surface from Height and Mass" (appendix), in Skeel, pp. 695-696. Mark J. Ratain pointed out some of the method's limitations in "Body Surface Area as a Basis for Dosing" (editorial), *J Clin Oncol*, 16 (July 1998), pp. 2297-2298.

6. Drug delivery systems have been ably reviewed by Margaret Barton Burke et al, *Cancer Chemotherapy: A Nursing Process Approach* (Jones and Bartlett Publishers, 1991), pp. 397-423.

7. Janelle M. Tipton and Roland T. Skeel, "Acute Reactions and Short-term Side Effects of Cancer Chemotherapy," in Skeel, pp. 555-573. Extravasation is also discussed by Burke et al (as in preceding note), pp. 383-387, and by Ellen J. Gallina, "Practical Guide to Chemotherapy Administration," *PPO*, pp. 2570-2580.

8. Tipton and Skeel (as in preceding note), pp. 556-559, and Burke et al (as in note 6), pp. 387-388, 393-395.

9. *Winning the Chemo Battle* (W. W. Norton & Company, 1988), pp. 28-29. A similar experience was recalled by Nancy Brinker (as in note 24), p. 51.

10. Burke et al (as in note 6), pp. 114-118.

11. Ajit B. Divgi, "Oncologist-induced Vomiting," *N Engl J Med*, 320 (Jan. 19, 1989), pp. 189-190.

12. The physiological mechanisms behind vomiting have been reviewed by Steven M. Grunberg and Paul J. Hesketh, "Control of Chemotherapy-induced Emesis," *N Engl J Med*, 329 (Dec. 9, 1993), pp. 1790-1796.

13. "Making Chemotherapy Easier" (editorial), *N Engl J Med*, 322 (Mar. 22, 1990), pp. 846-848.

14. Advertisement for Marinol in *J Clin Oncol*, 9 (Feb. 1991); John Bowersox, "PHS Cancels Availability of Medicinal Marijuana," *J Natl Cancer Inst*, 84 (Apr. 1, 1992), pp. 475-476.

15. "Pharmacology and Antiemetic Properties of Ondansetron," *Semin Oncol*, 19 (Aug. 1992), Supplement 10, pp. 1-8.

16. Grunberg and Hesketh (as in note 12), p. 1795.

17. Alison L. Jones et al, "Comparison of Dexamethasone and Ondansetron in Moderately Emetogenic Chemotherapy," *Lancet*, 338 (Aug. 24, 1991), pp. 483-487; and Martin Levitt et al, "Ondansetron Compared with Dexamethasone and Metoclopramide as Antiemetics in Breast Cancer Chemotherapy," *N Engl J Med*, 328 (Apr. 15, 1993), pp. 1081-1084.

18. "Examples of Regimens for Antiemetic Prevention," Tipton and Skeel (as in note 7), p. 564.

19. "Myths of Antiemetic Administration," *Cancer Nursing*, 12 (Apr. 1989), pp. 102-106.

20. "Bitter Pills to Swallow," *N Engl J Med*, 338 (June 18, 1998), pp. 1844-1846.

21. The mechanisms of hair growth and loss have been reviewed by Ralf Paus and George Cotsarelis in "The Biology of Hair Follicles," *N Engl J Med*, 341 (Aug. 12, 1999), pp. 491-497.

22. Robert J. Brooks et al, "Adjuvant Chemotherapy Using Doxorubicin and Cyclophosphamide," *Chemotherapy Consensus*, pp. 136-137. For chemocaps, see Kushner, p. 368.

23. According to Tipton and Skeel (as in note 7), p. 568, "scalp hypothermia is no longer recommended because of concern for scalp

metastases."

24. *The Race Is Run One Step at a Time* (Simon and Schuster, 1990), pp. 139-140.

25. "Bone Marrow Depression" in Burke et al (as in note 6), pp. 50-67. See especially "Expected Time of Drug Nadirs" (table) on p. 52.

26. Frankie Ann Holmes et al, "Phase II Trial of Taxol," *J Natl Cancer Inst*, 83 (Dec. 18, 1991), pp. 1797-1805.

27. Alison Freifeld et al, "Oral and Intravenous Antibiotic Therapy for Febrile Patients with Neutropenia," *N Engl J Med*, 341 (July 29, 1999), pp. 305-311. This issue of the *Journal* also contains a study with comparable findings by Winfried V. Kern et al (pp. 312-318) and a relevant editorial by Robert W. Finberg and James A. Talcott (pp. 362-363).

28. "First-cycle Blood Counts and Subsequent Neutropenia in Breast Cancer Therapy," *J Clin Oncol*, 16 (July 1998), pp. 2392-2400.

29. Nancy Brinker (as in note 24), pp. 51-52; Joyce Slayton Mitchell (as in note 9), p. 142.

30. Denise J. Mahood et al, "Inhibition of Fluorouracil-induced Stomatitis by Oral Cryotherapy," *J Clin Oncol*, 9 (Mar. 1991), pp. 449-452.

31. Sherry Greifzu et al, "Oral Care is Part of Cancer Care," *RN*, June 1990, pp. 43-46.

32. "Diarrhea" in Burke et al (as in note 6), pp. 81-84.

33. For a detailed study of this problem, see Pamela J. Goodwin et al, "Adjuvant Treatment and Weight Gain after Breast Cancer Diagnosis," *J Clin Oncol*, 17 (Jan. 1999), pp. 120-129.

34. "Adjuvant Systemic Therapy for Resectable Breast Cancer," *J Clin Oncol*, 3 (Feb. 1985), pp. 259-275.

35. "Toxicity of Adjuvant Chemotherapy Regimens Containing Doxorubicin," *Chemotherapy Consensus*, pp. 105-109.

36. "Effect of Chemotherapy on Ovarian Function, Fertility, and Birth Defects," *Younger Women*, pp. 125-129.

37. Tom Reynolds, "Preserving Fertility after Chemotherapy" (news report), *J Natl Cancer Inst*, 91 (Apr. 21, 1999), pp. 664-666.

38. "Correspondence," *N Engl J Med*, 321 (Aug. 17, 1989), pp. 472-473.

39. Bernard Fisher et al, "A Randomized Clinical Trial Evaluating Methotrexate and Fluorouracil in Node-Negative Breast Cancer," *N Engl J Med*, 320 (Feb. 23, 1989), pp. 473-478.

40. Bernard Fisher et al, "Eight-Year Results from NSABP B-13 and First Report of Findings from NSABP B-19," *J Clin Oncol*, 14 (July 1996), pp. 1982-1992.

41. Vincent T. DeVita, Jr. (as in note 38).

42. "Sexual Functioning in Women with Breast Cancer after Adjuvant Therapy," *Cancer Nursing*, 19 (Aug. 1996), pp. 308-319.

43. For more information on estrogen replacement therapy after a breast cancer diagnosis, see Chapter Six, pp. 134-135. For androgen therapies, see Chapter Twenty-two, p. 416. Estrogen has not been shown to stimulate the growth of ER-negative tumors, as explained by Melody A. Cobleigh et al, "Hormone Replacement Therapy and High S-Phase in Breast Cancer," *JAMA*, 281 (Apr. 28, 1999), pp. 1528-1530.

Chapter Twenty-five

1. "Bone Marrow and Peripheral Blood Stem Cell Transplantation in the Treatment of Cancer," *CA*, 46 (May/June 1996), pp. 142-164.

2. "Does Bone Marrow Transplantation Confer a Normal Life Span?" *N Engl J Med*, 341 (July 1, 1999), pp. 50-51.

3. Patricia S. Stewart, "Autologous Bone Marrow Transplantation in Metastatic Breast Cancer," *Breast Cancer Res Treat*, 2 (1982), pp. 85-92.

4. William P. Peters et al, "High-Dose Combination Alkylating Agents with Autologous Bone Marrow Support," *J Clin Oncol*, 4 (May 1986), pp. 646-654.

5. Peters et al (as in preceding note). See also Mitchell S. Anscher et al, "Liver and Lung Fibrosis after Autologous Marrow Transplantation for Breast Cancer," *N Engl J Med*, 328 (June 3, 1993), pp. 1592-1598.

6. "High-Dose Chemotherapy and Autologous Bone Marrow Support for Breast Cancer," *Advances* (1991), pp. 135-150.

7. Peters et al (as in note 4).

8. William P. Peters, "High-Dose Chemotherapy for the Treatment of Breast Cancer," *Advances* (1995), pp. 215-230.

9. William P. Peters et al, "High-Dose Chemotherapy and Autologous Bone Marrow Support as Consolidation after Standard-Dose Adjuvant Therapy for High-Risk Primary Breast Cancer," *J Clin Oncol*, 11 (June 1993), pp. 1132-1143.

10. Statistics given by Jean McCann, "ASCO Meeting," *J Natl Cancer Inst*, 86 (June 15, 1994), pp. 892-894.

11. Frank R. Dunphy et al, "Treatment of Breast Cancer with High-Dose Chemotherapy," *J Clin Oncol*, 8 (July 1990), pp. 1207-1216.

12. M. John Kennedy et al, "High-Dose Chemotherapy for Breast Cancer," *J Natl Cancer Inst*, 83 (July 3, 1991), pp. 920-926.

13. Peters (as in note 6), p. 147.

14. Cady quoted in *Ann Surg*, 224 (Oct. 1996), p. 427.

15. "Window of Opportunity" (editorial), *J Natl Cancer Inst*, 83 (July 3, 1991), pp. 894-896.

16. "High-Dose Therapy: Here to Stay or Just Visiting?" (editorial), *J Clin Oncol*, 12 (Jan. 1994), pp. 5-6.

17. Hortobagyi quoted by Kara Smigel, "Women Flock to Autologous Bone Marrow Transplantation for Breast Cancer," *J Natl Cancer Inst*, 87 (July 5, 1995), pp. 952-955.

18. "Efficacy and Cost-effectiveness of Autologous Bone Marrow Transplantation," *JAMA*, 267 (Apr. 15, 1992), pp. 2055-2061.

19. Karen Antman et al, "The Crisis in Clinical Cancer Research," *N Engl J Med*, 319 (July 7, 1988), pp. 46-48.

20. Smigel (as in note 17), p. 954.

21. "Peripheral Blood Stem Cell Transplantation," *Semin Oncol*, 22 (June 1995), pp. 202-209.

22. Diane S. Krause et al, "CD34: Structure, Biology, and Clinical Utility," *Blood*, 87 (Jan. 1, 1996), pp. 1-13.

23. Krause et al (as in preceding note), p. 9.

24. Jerome E. Groopman et al reviewed the decade's work on "Hematopoietic Growth Factors" in *N Engl J Med*, 321 (Nov. 23, 1989), pp. 1449-1459.

25. Monika Engelhardt et al, "Filgrastim (G-CSF) for Mobilization of Peripheral Blood Progenitor Cells," *J Clin Oncol*, 17 (July 1999), pp. 2160-2172.

26. Elizabeth J. Shpall et al cite a cost estimate of $2,266 per apheresis; see their "Randomized Study of Peripheral Blood Progenitor Cell Mobilization in High-Risk Breast Cancer Patients," *Blood*, 93 (Apr. 15, 1999), pp. 2491-2501.

27. Elizabeth J. Shpall et al, "4-HC Purging of Breast Cancer from Bone Marrow," *J Clin Oncol*, 9 (Jan. 1991), pp. 85-93.

28. Stephanie F. Williams et al, "Selection and Expansion of Peripheral Blood CD34-Positive Cells in Autologous Transplantation for Breast Cancer," *Blood*, 87 (Mar. 1, 1996), pp. 1687-1691.

29. Charles H. Weaver et al, "Engraftment Kinetics as a Function of the CD34 Content of Peripheral Blood Progenitor Cell Collections," *Blood*, 86 (Nov. 15, 1995), pp. 3961-3969.

30. William P. Peters et al, "Intensive Clinic Support to Permit Outpatient Autologous Marrow Transplantation for Breast Cancer," *Semin Oncol*, 21 (Aug. 1994), Supplement 7, pp. 25-31.

31. Peters et al (as in preceding note), pp. 28-30.

32. Barry R. Meisenberg et al, "Outpatient High-Dose Chemotherapy with Stem Cell Rescue," *J Clin Oncol*, 15 (Jan. 1997), pp. 11-17.

33. Karen Antman and her colleagues pointed out that between 1989 and 1995 "one-hundred-day mortality decreased from 22% to 5%." See their national survey of "High-Dose Chemotherapy with Stem Cell Support for Breast Cancer," *J Clin Oncol*, 15 (May 1997), pp. 1870-1879.

34. H. Kent Holland et al, "Minimal Toxicity and Mortality in High-Risk Breast Cancer Patients Receiving High-Dose Cyclophosphamide," *J Clin Oncol*, 14 (Apr. 1996), pp. 1156-1164.

35. Carole B. Miller et al, "Impact of Age on Outcome of Autologous Marrow Transplant," *J Clin Oncol*, 14 (Apr. 1996), pp. 1327-1332.

36. Charles L. Shapiro et al, "Repetitive

Cycles of Cyclophosphamide, Thiotepa, and Carboplatin Intensification," *J Clin Oncol*, 15 (Feb. 1997), pp. 674-683.

37. David H. Vesole has reviewed the current applications in Skeel, pp. 144-174.

38. Antman et al (as in note 33) observed that 40% of all "autotransplants" performed in 1995 were for breast cancers.

39. Bernard Fisher et al, "Further Evaluation of Intensified and Increased Total Dose of Cyclophosphamide for Primary Breast Cancer: Findings from NSABP Project B-25," *J Clin Oncol*, 17 (Nov. 1999), pp. 3374-3388. See also the earlier report by Bernard Fisher et al, "Findings from NSABP Project B-22," *J Clin Oncol*, 15 (May 1997), pp. 1858-1869.

40. Vaughn quoted by Smigel (as in note 17), p. 954.

41. W. R. Bezwoda et al, "High-Dose Chemotherapy with Hematopoietic Rescue as Primary Treatment for Metastatic Breast Cancer," *J Clin Oncol*, 13 (Oct. 1995), pp. 2483-2489.

42. Bezwoda's report cited by Antman et al (as in note 48), p. 1703.

43. Abstracts of reports by Edward A. Stadtmauer et al (Philadelphia Intergroup trial) and by William P. Peters et al (CALGB trial), *J Clin Oncol*, 17 (Nov. 1999), Supplement, pp. 21a, 21b.

44. Abstract of Bezwoda's report in *J Clin Oncol*, 17 (Nov. 1999), Supplement, p. 21d.

45. "Misconduct Suspected in South African Study," NCI statement posted Feb. 4, 2000, on the agency's Internet website (http://cancertrials.nci.nih.gov). Bezwoda's admission was quoted in a University of Witwatersrand press release dated Feb. 3, 2000, and posted on the University's website.

46. "Misconduct Suspected" (as in preceding note).

47. Gabriella Stern and Ron Winslow, "Aetna Shifts Policy on Treatment of Breast Cancer," *Wall Street Journal*, Feb. 17, 2000, p. 13B.

48. Karen Antman et al, "High-Dose Chemotherapy for Breast Cancer," *JAMA*, 282 (Nov. 10, 1999), pp. 1701-1703.

49. O'Reilly quoted by Andrew Skolnick, "Some Recommend Hitting Cancers Harder and Earlier," *JAMA*, 265 (May 1, 1991), pp. 2165-2166, 2171.

50. Robert Livingston and John Crowley, "Commentary," *J Clin Oncol*, 17 (Nov. 1999), Supplement, pp. 22-24.

51. "Prognostic Factors for Patients with Metastatic Breast Cancer Undergoing High-Dose Chemotherapy," *J Clin Oncol*, 17 (Oct. 1999), pp. 3064-3074.

52. The NCI's role has been chronicled by Susan G. Arbuck et al, "Clinical Development of Taxol," *Taxol Workshop*, pp. 11-24.

53. "Paclitaxel (Taxol)," *N Engl J Med*, 332 (Apr. 13, 1995), pp. 1004-1014.

54. Arbuck et al (as in note 52), p. 15.

55. "Taxol," *PPO Updates*, 5 (Sept. 1991), pp. 1-10.

56. Carlos Caldas and William P. McGuire III, "Taxol in Epithelial Ovarian Cancer," *Taxol Workshop*, pp. 155-159. For the early results in melanoma and lung cancer, see also pp. 177-179, 185-187.

57. Frankie Ann Holmes et al, "Phase II Trial of Taxol, an Active Drug in the Treatment of Metastatic Breast Cancer," *J Natl Cancer Inst*, 83 (Dec. 18, 1991), pp. 1797-1805.

58. Frankie Ann Holmes et al, "The M. D. Anderson Experience with Taxol in Metastatic Breast Cancer," *Taxol Workshop*, pp. 161-169. The management of side effects has also been reviewed by Leslie B. DeLaPena et al, "Taxol: A Case Study," *Cancer Nursing*, 16 (Dec. 1993), pp. 423-430.

59. Tom Junod, "Tree of Hope," *Life*, 15 (May 1992), pp. 71-76.

60. Saul A. Schepartz, "Supply—Harvest of *Taxus brevifolia*," *Taxol Workshop*, pp. 5-6. See also Joseph I. Song and Mark R. Dumais, "From Yew to Us: The Curious Development of Taxol," *JAMA*, 266 (Sept. 4, 1991), p. 1281.

61. Samuel Broder and Judith E. Karp, "Introduction," *Taxol Workshop*, pp. 1-4.

62. Gordon M. Cragg, "Alternative Sources of Taxol," *Taxol Workshop*, pp. 7-8.

63. Caroline McNeil, "Semisynthetic Taxol Goes on Market," *J Natl Cancer Inst*, 87 (Aug. 2, 1995), pp. 1106-1108.

64. J. S. Abrams et al, "Paclitaxel Activity

in Heavily Pretreated Breast Cancer," *J Clin Oncol*, 13 (Aug. 1995), pp. 2056-2065.

65. Daniel D. Von Hoff, "The Taxoids: Same Roots, Different Drugs," *Semin Oncol*, 24 (Aug. 1997), Supplement 13, pp. 3-10.

66. "Docetaxel" in Skeel, p. 99.

67. Nancy J. Nelson, "Another Taxane Takes Center Stage in San Antonio," *J Natl Cancer Inst*, 90 (Feb. 4, 1998), pp. 189-190.

68. Taxotere advertisement in *J Natl Cancer Inst*, 91 (Jan. 6, 1999), after title page.

69. Vicente Valero, "Docetaxel as Single-Agent Therapy in Metastatic Breast Cancer," *Semin Oncol*, 24 (Aug. 1997), Supplement 13, pp. 11-18.

70. Andrew D. Seidman et al, "Paclitaxel as Second and Subsequent Therapy for Metastatic Breast Cancer," *J Clin Oncol*, 13 (May 1995), pp. 1152-1159.

71. Wyndham H. Wilson et al, "Paclitaxel in Refractory Breast Cancer: Trial of 96-Hour Infusion," *J Clin Oncol*, 12 (Aug. 1994), pp. 1621-1629.

72. Andrew D. Seidman et al, "Weekly One-Hour Paclitaxel Infusions in the Treatment of Metastatic Breast Cancer," *J Clin Oncol*, 16 (Oct. 1998), pp. 3353-3361.

73. Taxol advertisement in *J Clin Oncol*, 12 (June 1994), before p. 1107.

74. Seidman's comments quoted in "Discussion," *Semin Oncol*, 24 (Feb. 1997), Supplement 3, pp. 41-49.

75. Results from NSABP Protocol B-26 discussed by Angelo Di Leo and Martine J. Piccart, "Paclitaxel Activity, Dose, and Schedule," *Semin Oncol*, 26 (June 1999), Supplement 8, pp. 27-32.

76. "Fox Chase Workshop on Paclitaxel," *Semin Oncol*, 24 (Feb. 1997), Supplement 3, and (Oct. 1997), Supplement 17.

77. Frankie Ann Holmes et al, "Sequence-Dependent Alteration of Doxorubicin Pharmacokinetics by Paclitaxel," *J Clin Oncol*, 14 (Oct. 1996), pp. 2713-2721.

78. Luca Gianni et al, "Interaction between Doxorubicin and Paclitaxel in Patients with Breast Cancer," *J Clin Oncol*, 15 (May 1997), pp. 1906-1915. See also Per Dombernowsky et al, "Doxorubicin plus Paclitaxel,"

Semin Oncol, 24 (Oct. 1997), Supplement 17, pp. 15-18.

79. Luca Gianni et al, "Paclitaxel with Doxorubicin in Untreated Metastatic Breast Cancer," *J Clin Oncol*, 13 (Nov. 1995), pp. 2688-2699.

80. Intergroup findings discussed by Di Leo and Piccart (as in note 75), pp. 28-29.

81. Stephen Chan et al, "Prospective Randomized Trial of Docetaxel Versus Doxorubicin in Patients with Metastatic Breast Cancer," *J Clin Oncol*, 17 (Aug. 1999), pp. 2341-2354.

82. Jean-Marc Nabholtz et al, "Docetaxel and Anthracycline Polychemotherapy in the Treatment of Breast Cancer," *Semin Oncol*, 26 (June 1999), Supplement 8, pp. 47-52.

83. Sledge quoted in "Discussion," *Semin Oncol*, 24 (Feb. 1997), Supplement 3, p. 48.

84. Abstracts for NSABP protocols posted on the NCI's website (http://cancertrials.nci.-nih.gov), accessed Feb. 6, 2000.

Chapter Twenty-six

1. "Docetaxel and Paclitaxel in Breast Cancer Therapy," *Semin Oncol*, 24 (Aug. 1997), Supplement 13, pp. 27-44.

2. "Chemotherapy of Breast Cancer: A Historical Perspective," *Semin Oncol*, 24 (Oct. 1997), Supplement 17, pp. 1-4.

3. Paul A. C. Greenberg et al, "Long-term Follow-up of Patients with Complete Remission following Combination Chemotherapy for Metastatic Breast Cancer," *J Clin Oncol*, 14 (Aug. 1996), pp. 2197-2205.

4. *How We Die: Reflections on Life's Final Chapter* (Vintage Books, 1995), p. 260.

5. Newcomer quoted by Susan Jenks, "Does Managed Care Jeopardize Cancer Research?" *J Natl Cancer Inst*, 87 (Aug. 2, 1995), pp. 1102-1106.

6. Folkman quoted by Susan Jenks, "Angiogenesis Research," *J Natl Cancer Inst*, 86 (May 18, 1994), pp. 742-743.

7. Amy R. Nelson et al, "Matrix Metalloproteinases: Biologic Activity and Clinical

Implications," *J Clin Oncol*, 18 (Mar. 2000), pp. 1135-1149.

8. Judah Folkman, "Clinical Applications of Research on Angiogenesis," *N Engl J Med*, 333 (Dec. 28, 1995), pp. 1757-1763.

9. Jenks (as in note 6), p. 742.

10. Giampietro Gasparini et al, "Vascular Endothelial Growth Factor in Node-Negative Breast Carcinoma," *J Natl Cancer Inst*, 89 (Jan. 15, 1997), pp. 139-147. See also the findings on VEGF reported by Barbro Linderholm et al, and by Urs Eppenberger et al, *J Clin Oncol*, 16 (Sept. 1998), pp. 3121-3136.

11. Jan Ziegler, "Angiogenesis Research Enjoys Growth Spurt," *J Natl Cancer Inst*, 88 (June 19, 1996), pp. 786-788.

12. Gina Kolata, "A Cautious Awe Greets Drugs That Eradicate Tumors in Mice," *New York Times*, May 3, 1998, pp. 1, 34.

13. Judith Randal, "Antiangiogenesis Drugs," *J Natl Cancer Inst*, 92 (Apr. 5, 2000), pp. 520-522.

14. Nelson et al (as in note 7), pp. 1143-1144.

15. Fine quoted by Ann Saphir, "Jekyll and Hyde: A New License for Thalidomide?" *J Natl Cancer Inst*, 89 (Oct. 15, 1997), pp. 1480-1481. See also Howard A. Fine et al, "Thalidomide for Recurrent High-Grade Gliomas," *J Clin Oncol*, 18 (Feb. 2000), pp. 708-715.

16. Pluda quoted by Pat Phillips, "Skepticism Toward Hype Over Antiangiogenesis Agents," *JAMA*, 279 (June 24, 1998), pp. 1936-1937.

17. Fidler quoted by Randal (as in note 13), p. 522.

18. Michael S. Gordon et al, "Phase One Trial" (abstract), *ASCO Annual Meeting Highlights* (1998), pp. 10-11.

19. Robert A. Catalano et al, "Breast Carcinoma Metastatic to the Uvea," *JAMA*, 264 (Aug. 22/29, 1990), p. 1032.

20. Kristine A. Nelson et al, "Common Complications of Advanced Cancer," *Semin Oncol*, 27 (Feb. 2000), pp. 34-44.

21. Jay P. Ciezki et al, "Palliative Radiotherapy," *Semin Oncol*, 27 (Feb. 2000), pp. 90-93.

22. Salvatore Veltri, "Critical Care Issues in Oncology and Bone Metastasis," in Skeel, pp. 621-641 (see p. 639).

23. Ralph G. Robinson et al, "Strontium 89 Therapy for Osseous Metastases," *JAMA*, 274 (Aug. 2, 1995), pp. 420-424; Linda Strangio and Carol Brudner, "Strontium 89 for Bone Pain," *RN*, June 1995, pp. 28-29.

24. Mundy quoted by Charles Bankhead, "Bisphosphonates Spearhead New Approach to Treating Bone Metastases," *J Natl Cancer Inst*, 89 (Jan. 15, 1997), pp. 115-116.

25. Gordon J. Strewler, "The Physiology of Parathyroid Hormone-Related Protein," *N Engl J Med*, 342 (Jan. 20, 2000), pp. 177-185.

26. "Bisphosphonates as Anticancer Drugs" (editorial), *N Engl J Med*, 339 (Aug. 6, 1998), pp. 398-400.

27. Merck flyer for Fosamax issued April 1997.

28. Gabriel N. Hortobagyi et al, "Efficacy of Pamidronate in Reducing Skeletal Complications in Patients with Breast Cancer and Lytic Bone Metastases," *N Engl J Med*, 335 (Dec. 12, 1996), pp. 1785-1791.

29. Ingo J. Diel et al, "Reduction in New Metastases in Breast Cancer with Adjuvant Clodronate Treatment," *N Engl J Med*, 339 (Aug. 6, 1998), pp. 357-363.

30. J. J. Body, "Current Use of Bisphosphonates in Oncology," *J Clin Oncol*, 16 (Dec. 1998), pp. 3890-3899.

31. Gary Kao et al, "Pamidronate and Metastatic Breast Cancer" (correspondence), *N Engl J Med*, 336 (May 29, 1997), pp. 1609-1610. See also Bruce E. Hillner et al, "Pamidronate Cost Effectiveness," *J Clin Oncol*, 18 (Jan. 2000), pp. 72-79.

32. Jan Ziegler, "Research on Bone Metastases," *J Natl Cancer Inst*, 89 (June 18, 1997), pp. 841-843.

33. Poe's "For Annie" appeared in 1849.

34. "Cancer Emergencies" in Williams, pp. 135-166. See especially "Spinal Cord and Nerve Root Compression" by J. Sweetenham on pp. 148-152.

35. "MRI of the Central Nervous System," *JAMA*, 283 (Feb. 16, 2000), pp. 853-855.

36. Veltri (as in note 22), p. 623.

37. Martin M. Malawer and Thomas F.

Delaney, "Treatment of Metastatic Cancer to Bone," *PPO*, pp. 2225-2245.

38. "Percutaneous Vertebroplasty," *RadioGraphics*, 18 (Mar/Apr. 1998), pp. 311-320.

39. "Invited Commentary," *RadioGraphics*, 18 (Mar/Apr. 1998), pp. 320-322.

40. Zelig A. Tochner and Zvi Fuks, "Radiation Treatment for Palliation of Metastatic Breast Cancer," in Ariel and Cleary, pp. 393-403.

41. Namita Sood et al, "Acute Respiratory Failure Secondary to Lymphangitic Carcinomatosis," *J Clin Oncol*, 18 (Jan. 2000), pp. 229-232.

42. Edgar D. Staren et al, "Pulmonary Resection for Metastatic Breast Cancer," *Arch Surg*, 127 (Nov. 1992), pp. 1282-1284.

43. Valerie W. Rusch et al, "Cisplatin and Cytarabine in the Management of Pleural Effusions," *J Clin Oncol*, 9 (Feb. 1991), pp. 313-319.

44. Paul T. Vaitkus et al, "Treatment of Malignant Pericardial Effusion," *JAMA*, 272 (July 6, 1994), pp. 59-64. See also Walter D. Y. Quan, Jr., "Malignant Pleural, Peritoneal, and Pericardial Effusions and Meningeal Infiltrates," in Skeel, pp. 642-655.

45. J. Sweetenham, "Superior Vena Caval Obstruction," in Williams, pp. 138-140.

46. Edward Leen et al, "Doppler Perfusion Index," *Lancet*, 355 (Jan. 1, 2000), pp. 34-37; editorial by Yuman Fong on pp. 5-6.

47. Jean McCann, "PET Scans," *J Natl Cancer Inst*, 90 (Jan. 21, 1998), pp. 94-96.

48. For the experimental TAC regimen, see Chapter Twenty-five, p. 513.

49. Sandor Paku et al, "Metastatic Hepatic Tumors: Improved Delivery of Chemotherapeutic Agents," *J Natl Cancer Inst*, 90 (June 17, 1998), pp. 936-937.

50. Robert C. Kurtz et al, "Laparoscopy," *PPO*, pp. 498-499.

51. Steven A. Curley et al, "Radiofrequency Ablation of Unresectable Primary and Metastatic Hepatic Malignancies," *Ann Surg*, 230 (July 1999), pp. 1-8. See also Tom Reynolds, "Researchers Use Radiofrequency Ablation to Destroy Tumors," *J Natl Cancer Inst*, 91 (June 2, 1999), pp. 909-910.

52. David M. Mahvi and Fred T. Lee, Jr., argue the case for cryoablation in "Is Heat Better Than Cold?" (editorial), *Ann Surg*, 230 (July 1999), pp. 9-11.

53. Nelson et al (as in note 20), p. 34.

54. Dr. Kase quoted in "Case Records of the Massachusetts General Hospital," *N Engl J Med*, 322 (June 28, 1990), pp. 1866-1878.

55. Sid Gilman, "Imaging the Brain," *N Engl J Med*, 338 (Mar. 19 and Mar. 26, 1998), pp. 812-820, 889-896. The superior sensitivity of MRI in detecting multiple small lesions has been strikingly illustrated by Andrew Lekos and Michael J. Glantz, "CNS Metastases," *J Clin Oncol*, 15 (Aug. 1997), pp. 3019-3020.

56. Deborah L. Ornstein and Kirt Frederickson, "Meningeal Carcinomatosis in Breast Cancer," *N Engl J Med*, 342 (Apr. 13, 2000), p. 1093.

57. "Breast Cancer Metastases to the Central Nervous System," *PPO*, p. 1323.

58. Tochner and Fuks (as in note 40), pp. 394, 397-399.

59. "Primary and Metastatic Brain Tumors," in Skeel, pp. 372-381.

60. Ciezki et al (as in note 21), pp. 91-92.

61. Jay S. Loeffler et al, "Radiosurgery for Brain Metastases," *PPO Updates*, 5 (Feb. 1991), pp. 1-12. See also Eben Alexander III et al, "Stereotactic Radiosurgery," *J Natl Cancer Inst*, 87 (Jan. 4, 1995), pp. 34-40.

62. Andrea Pirzkall et al, "Radiosurgery Alone or in Combination with Whole-Brain Radiotherapy for Brain Metastases," *J Clin Oncol*, 16 (Nov. 1998), pp. 3563-3569.

63. Paul A. Bunn, Jr. and E. Chester Ridgway, "Paraneoplastic Syndromes," *PPO*, pp. 2026-2071.

64. This syndrome has been ably explained by Deborah Kryspin Meriney, "Hypercalcemia of Breast Cancer," *Cancer Nursing*, 13 (Oct. 1990), pp. 316-323, and by Raymond P. Warrell, Jr., "Hypercalcemia and Osteolysis in Breast Cancer," in Harris et al, pp. 750-761.

65. Warrell (as in preceding note), p. 756.

66. Charles L. Loprinzi et al, "Megestrol Acetate Versus Dexamethasone for the Treatment of Cancer Anorexia/Cachexia," *J Clin Oncol*, 17 (Oct. 1999), pp. 3299-3306.

67. Giovanni Mantovani et al, "Cytokine Activity in Cancer-Related Anorexia/Cachexia," *Semin Oncol*, 25 (Apr. 1998), Supplement 6,

pp. 45-52. See also Michael J. Tisdale, "Biology of Cachexia," *J Natl Cancer Inst*, 23 (Dec. 3, 1997), pp. 1763-1773.

68. John S. Spratt et al, "Autopsy as the End-point to Follow-up," Donegan and Spratt (1988), pp. 586-587.

69. Robert T. Greenlee et al, "Cancer Statistics," *CA*, 50 (Jan/Feb. 2000), pp. 7-33.

70. Crile, p. 155.

71. Kathleen Foley, "A 44-Year-Old Woman with Severe Pain at the End of Life," *JAMA*, 281 (May 26, 1999), pp. 1937-1945.

72. Declan Walsh et al, "Symptom Control in Advanced Cancer: Important Drugs and Routes of Administration," *Semin Oncol*, 27 (Feb. 2000), pp. 69-83.

73. Alejandro R. Jadad et al, "The WHO Analgesic Ladder for Cancer Pain Management," *JAMA*, 274 (Dec. 20, 1995), pp. 1870-1873.

74. Nathan I. Cherny, "The Management of Cancer Pain," *CA*, 50 (Mar/Apr. 2000), pp. 70-116.

75. Ruth Mueller, "Cancer Pain: Which Drugs for Which Patient?" *RN*, May 1992, pp. 38-46.

76. "Morphine Sulfate," *Mosby's GenRx*, 10th ed. (Mosby, 2000), Section III, pp. 1170-1177.

77. Walsh et al (as in note 72), p. 75.

78. Declan Walsh, "Pharmacological Management of Cancer Pain," *Semin Oncol*, 27 (Feb. 2000), pp. 45-63.

79. Walsh (as in preceding note), pp. 49-50.

80. Michael H. Levy, "Pharmacologic Treatment of Cancer Pain," *N Engl J Med*, 335 (Oct. 10, 1996), pp. 1124-1132.

81. "Morphine Sulfate" (as in note 76), p. 1175.

82. Walsh (as in note 78), p. 51.

83. Levy (as in note 80), p. 1126.

84. Walsh et al (as in note 72), p. 78.

85. Levy (as in note 80), p. 1126.

86. Cherny (as in note 74), p. 82.

87. "Now Available" (advertisement for Actiq), *J Clin Oncol*, 18 (Jan. 2000), before p. 1.

88. "Fentanyl," *Mosby's GenRx* (as in note 76), pp. 685-689.

89. Linda Jones and Joseph Brooks, "The ABCs of PCA," *RN*, May 1990, pp. 54-60.

90. Kathleen Foley, "Management of Cancer Pain," *PPO*, pp. 2417-2448 (see p. 2443).

91. Murray F. Brennan et al, "Pain in Pancreas Cancer," *PPO*, pp. 877-878.

92. Cherny (as in note 74), p. 105.

93. Foley (as in note 90), p. 2433.

94. Foley (as in note 71), p. 1938; "Bupivacaine," *Mosby's GenRx* (as in note 76), pp. 187-190.

95. Marian Sue Uram, "A New Delivery System Makes Pain Control Easier," *RN*, May 1992, pp. 46-51.

96. Sally B. Donnelly, "Rounding Up the Usual Suspects," *Time*, Sept. 6, 1999, p. 8.

97. Hugh McIntosh, "Regulatory Barriers Take Some Blame for Pain Undertreatment," *J Natl Cancer Inst*, 83 (Sept. 4 and 18, 1991), pp. 1202-1204, 1282-1284.

98. R. Hillier, "Diamorphine and Morphine," in Williams, pp. 174-176.

99. "Methadone for Treatment of Cancer Pain" (letter), *JAMA*, 275 (Feb. 21, 1996), p. 519.

100. "Easing the Pain of Suffering," Savannah *Morning News*, Mar. 8, 1994, p. 6A.

101. Lewis Thomas, *The Youngest Science: Notes of a Medicine-Watcher* (Viking Press, 1983), pp. 10-11.

102. Timothy E. Quill, "Death and Dignity: A Case of Individualized Decision Making," *N Engl J Med*, 324 (Mar. 7, 1991), pp. 691-694.

103. Timothy E. Quill, "Doctor, I Want to Die. Will You Help Me?" *JAMA*, 270 (Aug. 18, 1993), pp. 870-873.

104. "Final Exit" (review), *N Engl J Med*, 325 (Sept. 19, 1991), pp. 894-895.

105. Nancy Gibbs, "Rx for Death," *Time*, May 31, 1993, pp. 34-39.

106. Adam Cohen, "Showdown for Doctor Death," *Time*, Dec. 7, 1998, pp. 46-47; Julie Grace, "Curtains for Dr. Death," *Time*, Apr. 5, 1999, p. 48.

107. Ann Alpers and Bernard Lo, "Physician-Assisted Suicide in Oregon," *JAMA*, 274 (Aug. 9, 1995), pp. 483-487.

108. David Van Biema, "Death's Door Left Ajar," *Time*, July 7, 1997, p. 30; George J. Annas, "Physician-Assisted Suicide," *N Engl J*

Med, 337 (Oct. 9, 1997), pp. 1098-1103; Robert A. Burt and David Orentlicher, "Sounding Board: The Supreme Court," *N Engl J Med*, 337 (Oct. 23, 1997), pp. 1234-1239.

109. Arthur E. Chin et al, "Legalized Physician-Assisted Suicide in Oregon—The First Year's Experience," *N Engl J Med*, 340 (Feb. 18, 1999), pp. 577-583.

110. Chin et al (as in preceding note), pp. 578-579, 582.

111. J. Sweetenham, "Hypercalcemia," in Williams, pp. 142-143.

112. Burt and Orentlicher (as in note 108), pp. 1236-1239.

113. M. J. Friedrich, "Hospice Care in the United States: A Conversation with Florence S. Wald," *JAMA*, 281 (May 12, 1999), pp. 1683-1685.

114. Ira Byock, "Completing the Continuum of Cancer Care," *CA*, 50 (Mar/Apr. 2000), pp. 123-132.

115. Berry quoted by M. J. Friedrich, "Experts Describe Optimal Symptom Management for Hospice Patients," *JAMA*, 282 (Oct. 6, 1999), pp. 1213-1214.

116. "The Dying Cancer Patient," *Semin Oncol*, 27 (Feb. 2000), pp. 84-89.

Chapter Twenty-seven

1. Lewis Thomas popularized Burnet's hypothesis in *The Youngest Science* (Viking Press, 1983), pp. 203-205. Robert Gallo gave several good reasons for doubting it in *Virus Hunting* (Basic Books, 1991), pp. 255-256, 263.

2. "T Cell-Based Immunotherapy for Cancer," *CA*, 49 (Mar/Apr. 1999), pp. 74-100.

3. Morton quoted by Lisa Seachrist, "Spontaneous Cancer Remissions," *J Natl Cancer Inst*, 85 (Dec. 1, 1993), pp. 1892-1895.

4. Maurice M. Black et al, "Prognosis in Breast Cancer," *Cancer*, 36 (Dec. 1975), pp. 2048-2055.

5. "Pathologic Findings from NSABP Protocol 4," *Cancer*, 46 (Aug. 1980), Supplement, pp. 908-918.

6. The new understanding of genetic immunodeficiencies has been ably discussed by Rebecca H. Buckley, "Immunodeficiency Due to Defects in Lymphocytes," *N Engl J Med*, 343 (Nov. 2, 2000), pp. 1313-1324, and by Julie A. Lekstrom-Hines and John I. Gallin, "Immunodeficiency Caused by Defects in Phagocytes," *N Engl J Med*, 343 (Dec. 7, 2000), pp. 1703-1714.

7. "Mechanisms of Cytolytic T Lymphocyte-mediated Cytolysis," in Abul K. Abbas et al, *Cellular and Molecular Immunology*, 4th ed. (W. B. Saunders Co., 2000), pp. 304-307.

8. The story of Coley's career and of subsequent American attempts at cancer immunotherapy has been told by Stephen S. Hall, *A Commotion in the Blood: Life, Death, and the Immune System* (Henry Holt, 1997).

9. Hall (as in preceding note), p. 57.

10. Coley and the *Journal* editorial quoted by Hall (as in preceding notes), pp. 67-68.

11. Coley's results analyzed by Frances R. Balkwill, *Cytokines in Cancer Therapy* (Oxford University Press, 1989), pp. 81-84.

12. "Tumor Necrosis Factor" in Abbas et al (as in note 7), pp. 240-247.

13. Hall gives an excellent account of the discovery and subsequent development of interferon (as in note 8, pp. 131-208).

14. Florence S. Antoine, "Biological Therapy," *J Natl Cancer Inst*, 83 (Apr. 17, 1991), pp. 530-532.

15. "Interferon Genes and Proteins," Balkwill (as in note 11), pp. 9-10.

16. "Antitumor Action of Interferons," Balkwill (as in note 11), pp. 47-53.

17. Samuel Baron et al, "The Interferons: Mechanisms of Action and Clinical Applications," *JAMA*, 266 (Sept. 11, 1991), pp. 1375-1383.

18. Hoffmann-LaRoche advertisements in *N Engl J Med*, 314 (June 26, 1986) and 315 (July 10, 1986).

19. "Interferon Alfa," *Mosby's GenRx*, 10th ed. (Mosby, 2000), Section III, pp. 904-922; Raymond S. Koff, "Treatment of Chronic Viral Hepatitis," *JAMA*, 282 (Aug. 11, 1999), pp. 511-512.

20. Italian Cooperative Study Group, "Interferon Alfa-2a Compared with Chemo-

therapy for Chronic Myeloid Leukemia," *N Engl J Med*, 330 (Mar. 24, 1994), pp. 820-825.

21.   ECOG trial results given by John K. Kirkwood et al, "Interferon Alfa-2b Adjuvant Therapy of High-Risk Melanoma," *J Clin Oncol*, 14 (Jan. 1996), pp. 7-17; Schering advertisement in *J Natl Cancer Inst*, 89 (Oct. 1, 1997), before p. 1391.

22.   Kirkwood quoted in news release dated Oct. 16, 2000, posted on Internet website of the University of Pittsburgh Cancer Institute.

23.   Study Group (R. A. B. Ezekowitz et al), "Interferon Gamma for Chronic Granuloma-tous Disease," *N Engl J Med*, 324 (Feb. 21, 1991), pp. 509-516; "Interferon Gamma" in *Mosby's GenRx* (as in note 19), pp. 929-930.

24.   Lawrence D. Jacobs et al, "Interferon Beta in Multiple Sclerosis," *N Engl J Med*, 343 (Sept. 28, 2000), pp. 898-904. This issue of the *Journal* also contained a review article on "Multiple Sclerosis" by John H. Noseworthy et al (pp. 938-952).

25.   Jayesh Mehta, "Interferon Alfa-2a," *N Engl J Med*, 331 (Aug. 11, 1994), pp. 401-402.

26.   Stefan Zeuzem et al and E. Jenny Heathcote et al, "Peginterferon Alfa-2a in Chronic Hepatitis C" (two articles), *N Engl J Med*, 343 (Dec. 7, 2000), pp. 1666-1680.

27.   The best source of information on Rosenberg's career has been the book he wrote together with the author John M. Barry, *The Transformed Cell: Unlocking the Mysteries of Cancer* (G. P. Putnam's Sons, 1992).

28.   Rosenberg and Barry (as in preceding note), pp. 66-75; Hall (as in note 8), pp. 232-240.

29.   Steven A. Rosenberg, "Lymphokine-Activated Killer Cells: A New Approach to Immunotherapy of Cancer," *J Natl Cancer Inst*, 75 (Oct. 1985), pp. 595-603.

30.   "Table Ten: Treatment of Pulmonary Metastases with LAK Cells," in Rosenberg (as in preceding note), p. 600.

31.   Steven A. Rosenberg et al, "Administration of Lymphokine-Activated Killer Cells and Interleukin-2 to Patients with Metastatic Cancer," *N Engl J Med*, 313 (Dec. 5, 1985), pp. 1485-1492.

32.   Rosenberg and Barry (as in note 27), pp. 233-236; Hall (as in note 8), pp. 293-297;

"Cancer and Interleukin-2: The Search for a Cure" (cover story), *Newsweek*, Dec. 16, 1985, pp. 60-65.

33.   "Immunotherapy of Advanced Cancer" (correspondence), *N Engl J Med*, 316 (Jan. 29, 1987), pp. 274-276.

34.   "On Lymphokines, Cytokines, and Breakthroughs," *JAMA*, 256 (Dec. 12, 1986), p. 3141.

35.   Steven A. Rosenberg et al, "A Progress Report," *N Engl J Med*, 316 (Apr. 9, 1987), pp. 889-897.

36.   Steven A. Rosenberg et al, "Adoptive Immunotherapy of Cancer with Tumor-Infiltrating Lymphocytes," *Science*, 233 (Sept. 19, 1986), pp. 1318-1321.

37.   Steven A. Rosenberg et al, "Tumor-Infiltrating Lymphocytes and Interleukin-2 in the Immunotherapy of Metastatic Melanoma," *N Engl J Med*, 319 (Dec. 22, 1988), pp. 1676-1680.

38.   LAK cell trial discussed by Hall (as in note 8), p. 307; Robert A. Figlin et al, "Multicenter Randomized Trial of Tumor-Infiltrating Lymphocytes in Metastatic Renal Cell Carcinoma," *J Clin Oncol*, 17 (Aug. 1999), pp. 2521-2529.

39.   "Aldesleukin," *Mosby's GenRx* (as in note 19), pp. 37-40.

40.   Steven A. Rosenberg et al, "Treatment of 283 Consecutive Patients with Metastatic Melanoma or Renal Cell Cancer Using Interleukin-2," *JAMA*, 271 (Mar. 23/30, 1994), pp. 907-913.

41.   Steven A. Rosenberg et al, "Durability of Complete Responses in Patients with Metastatic Cancer Treated with High-Dose Interleukin-2," *Ann Surg*, 228 (Sept. 1998), pp. 307-319.

42.   Rosenberg quoted in "Discussion," *Ann Surg* (as in preceding note), p. 317.

43.   Kimberly R. Lindsey et al, "Response to High-Dose Interleukin-2," *J Clin Oncol*, 18 (May 2000), pp. 1954-1959.

44.   Donald L. Morton and Andreas Barth, "Vaccine Therapy for Malignant Melanoma," *CA*, 46 (July/Aug. 1996), pp. 225-244.

45.   Morton and Barth (as in preceding note), p. 228.

46.   Eddy C. Hsueh et al, "Correlation of Specific Immune Responses with Survival in

Patients Receiving Melanoma Cell Vaccine," *J Clin Oncol*, 16 (Sept. 1998), pp. 2913-2920.

47. Elizabeth M. Jaffee et al, "Allogeneic Tumor Vaccine for Pancreatic Cancer: A Phase One Trial," *J Clin Oncol*, 19 (Jan. 1, 2001), pp. 145-156.

48. "Immunologic Responses," Jaffee et al (as in preceding note), pp. 150-151.

49. Christine E. Weber, "Cytokine-Modified Tumor Vaccines," *Cancer Nursing*, 21 (June 1998), pp. 167-177.

50. Tim F. Greten and Elizabeth M. Jaffee, "Cancer Vaccines," *J Clin Oncol*, 17 (Mar. 1999), pp. 1047-1060.

51. "Role of Costimulators in T Cell Activation," in Abbas et al (as in note 7), pp. 167-169.

52. Protocols for the Phase One trials conducted by Smith et al, Kufe et al, and Disis et al posted on the NCI's website (http://cancernet.nci.nih.gov), accessed Mar. 5, 2001.

53. Elaine Blume, "Time of Truth for Cancer Vaccines," *J Natl Cancer Inst*, 86 (Mar. 2, 1994), pp. 330-331; enrollment prerequisites for "Theratope Vaccine Clinical Trial" as given on Biomira website (http://www.biomira.com), accessed Mar. 5, 2001.

54. "The Major Histocompatibility Complex" (pp. 63-78) and "Antigen Processing and Presentation to T Lymphocytes" (pp. 79-101), in Abbas et al (as in note 7).

55. Greten and Jaffee (as in note 50), p. 1048. See also "Activation of T Lymphocytes" in Abbas et al (as in note 7), pp. 161-181.

56. Jacques Banchereau and Ralph M. Steinman, "Dendritic Cells and the Control of Immunity," *Nature*, 392 (Mar. 19, 1998), pp. 245-252.

57. Banchereau and Steinman (as in preceding note), p. 246.

58. Anita Reddy et al, "Maturation of Human Dendritic Cells," *Blood*, 90 (Nov. 1, 1997), pp. 3640-3646.

59. Michael A. Morse et al, "Generation of Dendritic Cells from Peripheral Blood Mononuclear Cells," *Ann Surg*, 226 (July 1997), pp. 6-16.

60. Jan Baggers et al, "Dendritic Cells as Immunologic Adjuvants for the Treatment of Cancer," *J Clin Oncol*, 18 (Dec. 1, 2000), pp. 3879-3882.

61. Trial protocol posted on NCI website (as in note 52), accessed Mar. 14, 2001.

62. Baggers et al (as in note 60), p. 3880.

63. Michael A. Morse et al, "Preoperative Mobilization of Circulating Dendritic Cells by Flt3 Ligand," *J Clin Oncol*, 18 (Dec. 1, 2000), pp. 3883-3893.

64. "Continuous Cultures of Fused Cells Secreting Antibody of Predefined Specificity," *Nature*, 256 (Aug. 7, 1975), pp. 495-497.

65. Grant Fjermedal described this case in *Magic Bullets* (Macmillan, 1984), pp. 67-69, 224-232.

66. Mark S. Kaminski et al, "Radioimmunotherapy of B Cell Lymphoma with Anti-CD20 Antibody," *N Engl J Med*, 329 (Aug. 12, 1993), pp. 459-465.

67. Bruce J. Gould et al, "Anti-Breast-Cancer Immunotoxin: A Toxic Effect Not Predicted by Animal Studies," *J Natl Cancer Inst*, 81 (May 22, 1989), pp. 775-781.

68. Mulshine quoted by Margie Patlak, "Researchers Get Creative in Solving MAb Problems," *J Natl Cancer Inst*, 84 (May 20, 1992), pp. 748-750.

69. Caroline McNeil, "A New Generation of Monoclonal Antibodies," *J Natl Cancer Inst*, 87 (Nov. 15 and Dec. 6, 1995), pp. 1658-1660, 1738-1739; and Joan Stephenson, "Reengineered Monoclonal Antibodies in Cancer Studies," *JAMA*, 274 (Dec. 20, 1995), pp. 1821-1822.

70. Ken Garber, "Monoclonal Antibody Research," *J Natl Cancer Inst*, 92 (Sept. 20, 2000), pp. 1462-1464.

71. Rituxan advertisement in *J Clin Oncol*, 19 (Feb. 1, 2001).

72. Garber (as in note 70), pp. 1463-1464.

73. Ainat Beniaminovitz et al, "Prevention of Rejection in Cardiac Transplantation with a Monoclonal Antibody," *N Engl J Med*, 342 (Mar. 2, 2000), pp. 613-619; and Peter E. Lipsky et al, "Infliximab in Rheumatoid Arthritis," *N Engl J Med*, 343 (Nov. 30, 2000), pp. 1594-1602.

74. Mark X. Sliwkowski et al, "The Mechanism of Action of Trastuzumab (Herceptin)," *Semin Oncol*, 26 (Aug. 1999), Supplement 12, pp. 60-70.

75. David B. Agus et al, "HER-2/*neu* in Lung, Prostate, and Ovarian Cancer," *Semin Oncol*, 27 (Dec. 2000), Supplement 11, pp. 53-63.

76. Paul Carter et al, "Humanization of an Anti-HER-2 Antibody for Human Cancer Therapy," *Proc Natl Acad Sci USA*, 89 (May 1992), pp. 4285-4289.

77. José Baselga et al, "Phase Two Study of Anti-HER-2 Monoclonal Antibody in Metastatic Breast Cancer," *J Clin Oncol*, 14 (Mar. 1996), pp. 737-744.

78. Melody A. Cobleigh et al, "Multinational Study of Anti-HER-2 Monoclonal Antibody in Metastatic Breast Cancer," *J Clin Oncol*, 17 (Sept. 1999), pp. 2639-2648.

79. Bernhard C. Pestalozzi and Sue Brignoli, "Trastuzumab in Cerebrospinal Fluid," *J Clin Oncol*, 18 (June 2000), pp. 2350-2351.

80. Dennis J. Slamon et al, "Addition of Herceptin to First-line Chemotherapy" (abstract), *ASCO Annual Meeting Highlights* (1998), pp. 6-7.

81. Dennis J. Slamon et al, "Use of Chemotherapy Plus a Monoclonal Antibody Against HER-2 for Metastatic Breast Cancer That Overexpresses HER-2," *N Engl J Med*, 344 (Mar. 15, 2001), pp. 783-792.

82. Slamon et al (as in preceding note), pp. 788, 790. See also Kenneth R. Chien, "Trastuzumab Cardiotoxicity," *Semin Oncol*, 27 (Dec. 2000), Supplement 11, pp. 9-14.

83. Giovanni Pauletti et al, "Methods for Detection of HER-2/*neu* Alteration in Breast Cancer," *J Clin Oncol*, 18 (Nov. 1, 2000), pp. 3651-3664.

84. Sliwkowski quoted in "Panel Discussions," *Semin Oncol*, 27 (Dec. 2000), Supplement 11, pp. 92-100.

85. Hortobagyi quoted in "Panel Discussions" (as in preceding note), pp. 93-94.

86. Mark D. Pegram et al, "Trastuzumab and Chemotherapeutics: Drug Interactions and Synergies," *Semin Oncol*, 27 (Dec. 2000), Supplement 11, pp. 21-25.

87. NSABP Protocol B-31 described on NCI website (as in note 52), accessed Feb. 6, 2000.

88. "Herceptin (Trastuzumab) Prescribing Information" posted on Genentech website (http://www.gene.com), accessed Nov. 25, 2000.

Chapter Twenty-eight

1. Seung Myung Dong et al, "Detecting Colorectal Cancer in Stool with Genetic Targets," *J Natl Cancer Inst*, 93 (June 6, 2001), pp. 858-865.

2. Claus F. Eisenberger et al, "Diagnosis of Renal Cancer by Molecular Urinalysis," *J Natl Cancer Inst*, 91 (Dec. 1, 1999), pp. 2028-2032.

3. Steven A. Ahrendt et al, "Molecular Detection of Tumor Cells in Bronchoalveolar Lavage Fluid," *J Natl Cancer Inst*, 91 (Feb. 17, 1999), pp. 332-339.

4. Thomas L. Petty and Paul S. Frame, "Screening Strategies for Lung Cancer," *JAMA*, 284 (Oct. 18, 2000), pp. 1977-1983.

5. Stephen A. Cannistra and Jonathan M. Niloff, "Cancer of the Uterine Cervix," *N Engl J Med*, 334 (Apr. 18, 1996), pp. 1030-1038.

6. Marianne Berwick et al, "Screening for Melanoma by Skin Self-Examination," *J Natl Cancer Inst*, 88 (Jan. 3, 1996), pp. 17-23.

7. David Plotkin, "Good News and Bad News about Breast Cancer," *Atlantic Monthly*, 277 (June 1996), pp. 53-82.

8. Pamela M. Marcus et al, "Lung Cancer Mortality in the Mayo Lung Project," *J Natl Cancer Inst*, 92 (Aug. 16, 2000), pp. 1308-1316.

9. Arnold L. Potosky et al, "The Role of Increasing Detection in the Rising Incidence of Prostate Cancer," *JAMA*, 273 (Feb. 15, 1995), pp. 548-552.

10. Tim Friend, "New Breast Cancer Odds: 1-in-9 Risk," *USA Today*, Jan. 25, 1991, p. 1A.

11. "Public Health Focus: Mammography," *JAMA*, 268 (July 22/29, 1992), pp. 452-453.

12. Virginia L. Ernster et al, "Incidence of and Treatment for Ductal Carcinoma *in Situ* of the Breast," *JAMA*, 275 (Mar. 27, 1996), pp. 913-918.

13. Unnamed surgeon quoted by Ferris M.

Hall, "Screening Mammography—Potential Problems on the Horizon," *N Engl J Med*, 314 (Jan. 2, 1986), pp. 53-55.

14.   Sam Shapiro et al, *Periodic Screening for Breast Cancer: The Health Insurance Plan Project and Its Sequelae, 1963-1986* (Johns Hopkins University Press, 1988).

15.   "Breast Cancer Cases by Modality of Detection" (table), in Shapiro et al (as in preceding note), p. 76.

16.   Sam Shapiro et al, "Ten-to-Fourteen-Year Effect of Screening on Breast Cancer Mortality," *J Natl Cancer Inst*, 69 (Aug. 1982), pp. 349-355.

17.   Kenneth C. Chu et al, "Analysis of Breast Cancer Mortality and Stage Distribution by Age for the HIP Clinical Trial," *J Natl Cancer Inst*, 80 (Sept. 21, 1988), pp. 1125-1132.

18.   Shapiro et al (as in note 14), p. 63.

19.   Chu et al (as in note 17).

20.   Larry H. Baker, "Breast Cancer Detection Demonstration Project: Five-Year Summary Report," *CA*, 32 (July/Aug. 1982), pp. 194-225.

21.   Baker (as in preceding note), pp. 195-196.

22.   "Cancers Detected during the BCDDP" (table), in Baker (as in preceding notes), p. 216.

23.   "Age-Specific Nonmalignant-to-Malignant Biopsy Ratios" (table), in Baker (as in preceding notes), p. 210.

24.   Baker (as in preceding notes), p. 204.

25.   "Age-Specific Cancer Detection Rates" (table), in Baker (as in preceding notes), p. 208.

26.   "Detected Breast Cancer Categorized by Modality, Lesion Size, and Nodal Status at Surgery" (table), in Baker (as in preceding notes), p. 220.

27.   Alan S. Morrison et al, "Breast Cancer Incidence and Mortality in the BCDDP," *J Natl Cancer Inst*, 80 (Dec. 7, 1988), pp. 1540-1547.

28.   Gerald D. Dodd, "American Cancer Society Guidelines on Screening for Breast Cancer: An Overview," *CA*, 42 (May/June 1992), pp. 177-180.

29.   Dodd (as in preceding note).

30.   "Reduction in Mortality from Breast Cancer after Mass Screening with Mammog-raphy," *Lancet*, Apr. 13, 1985, pp. 829-832.

31.   Dodd (as in note 28), p. 178.

32.   David M. Eddy et al, "The Value of Mammography Screening in Women under Age 50," *JAMA*, 259 (Mar. 11, 1988), pp. 1512-1519.

33.   Dodd (as in note 28), p. 179. See also Amy Suzanne King, "Not Everyone Agrees with New Mammographic Screening Guidelines," *JAMA*, 262 (Sept. 1, 1989), pp. 1154-1155.

34.   ACS advertisement in *RN*, Jan. 1993, before p. 19.

35.   "Screening Mammography" (correspondence), *N Engl J Med*, 314 (May 29, 1986), pp. 1451-1453.

36.   Shapiro et al (as in note 14), p. 87.

37.   Baker (as in note 20), pp. 203-204.

38.   Spratt quoted in "Discussion: Breast Cancer Screening," *Ann Surg*, 186 (Sept. 1977), pp. 359-362.

39.   Peggy L. Porter et al, "Breast Tumor Characteristics as Predictors of Mammographic Detection: Comparison of Interval and Screen-detected Cancers," *J Natl Cancer Inst*, 91 (Dec. 1, 1999), pp. 2020-2028.

40.   Margaret T. Mandelson et al, "Breast Density: Comparison of Interval and Screen-detected Cancers," *J Natl Cancer Inst*, 92 (July 5, 2000), pp. 1081-1087.

41.   Frank D. Gilliland et al, "Biologic Characteristics of Interval and Screen-detected Breast Cancers," *J Natl Cancer Inst*, 92 (May 3, 2000), pp. 743-749.

42.   Anthony B. Miller et al, "Canadian National Breast Screening Study: Breast Cancer Detection and Death Rates," *Canadian Medical Association Journal*, 147 (Nov. 15, 1992), pp. 1459-1488.

43.   Malorye Allison, "Mammography Trial Comes under Fire," *Science*, 256 (May 22, 1992), pp. 1128-1130; Beverly Merz, "Canadian Breast Cancer Study," *J Natl Cancer Inst*, 84 (June 3, 1992), pp. 832-834.

44.   *Time*, May 18, 1992, p. 25.

45.   Letters from Moskowitz, Kopans, and Miller published in "Correspondence: Canadian Breast Cancer Study," *J Natl Cancer Inst*, 84 (Sept. 2, 1992), pp. 1365-1370.

46.   Cornelia J. Baines, "The CNBSS: A Perspective on Criticisms," *Ann Intern Med*, 120

(Feb. 15, 1994), pp. 326-334.

47. Stephen A. Feig, "Methods to Identify Benefit from Mammographic Screening of Women Aged 40 to 49," *Radiology*, 201 (Nov. 1996), pp. 309-316.

48. Anthony B. Miller et al, "The CNBSS: Update on Mortality," in *National Institutes of Health Consensus Conference on Breast Cancer Screening for Women Ages 40-49* (Oxford University Press, 1997), pp. 37-41.

49. The hospital's statistics were published by Adam Stacey-Clear et al, "Breast Cancer Survival among Women under Age 50," *Lancet*, 340 (Oct. 24, 1992), pp. 991-994. Maryann Napoli criticized the General Electric commercial in *Consensus Conference* (as in preceding note), p. 12.

50. Suzanne W. Fletcher et al, "Report of the International Workshop on Screening for Breast Cancer," *J Natl Cancer Inst*, 85 (Oct. 20, 1993), pp. 1644-1656.

51. "Deficiencies in the Analysis of Breast Cancer Screening Data" (editorial), *J Natl Cancer Inst*, 85 (Oct. 20, 1993), pp. 1621-1624.

52. "Screening for Breast Cancer" (letter), *J Natl Cancer Inst*, 86 (Apr. 6, 1994), pp. 558-559.

53. Nancy Volkers, "Board Recommends Changes to Breast Cancer Screening Guidelines," *J Natl Cancer Inst*, 85 (Nov. 17, 1993), pp. 1794-1796.

54. Nancy Volkers, "NCI Replaces Guidelines with Statement of Evidence," *J Natl Cancer Inst*, 86 (Jan. 5, 1994), pp. 14-15; and Charles Marwick, "NCI Changes Its Stance on Mammography," *JAMA*, 271 (Jan. 12, 1994), p. 96.

55. Curtis Mettlin and Charles R. Smart, "Breast Cancer Detection Guidelines for Women Aged 40 to 49," *CA*, 44 (July/Aug. 1994), pp. 248-255.

56. Daniel B. Kopans et al, "Correspondence: Efficacy of Screening Mammography for Women in their Forties," *J Natl Cancer Inst*, 86 (Nov. 16, 1994), pp. 1721-1731.

57. Charles J. Wright and C. Barber Mueller, "Screening Mammography and Public Health Policy," *Lancet*, 346 (July 1, 1995), pp. 29-32.

58. Plotkin (as in note 7), p. 82.

59. Karla Kerlikowske and John Barclay, "Outcomes of Modern Screening Mammography," *Consensus Conference* (as in note 48), pp. 105-111.

60. Maryann Napoli, "What Do Women Want to Know?" *Consensus Conference* (as in note 48), pp. 11-13.

61. "Consensus Statement" and "Minority Report," *Consensus Conference* (as in note 48), pp. vii-xii.

62. "A Surgeon's Challenge," *Newsweek*, Feb. 24, 1997, p. 60.

63. "Mammograms Have Been Oversold," Savannah *Morning News*, Feb. 3, 1997, p. 7A.

64. Nancy J. Nelson, "The Mammography Consensus Jury Speaks Out," *J Natl Cancer Inst*, 89 (Mar. 5, 1997), pp. 344-347.

65. Nancy J. Nelson, "NCAB Considers Mammography Screening," *J Natl Cancer Inst*, 89 (Mar. 19, 1997), pp. 417-418.

66. Peggy Eastman, "NCI Adopts New Mammography Screening Guidelines," *J Natl Cancer Inst*, 89 (Apr. 16, 1997), pp. 538-540. See also Charles Marwick, "Final Mammography Recommendation?" *JAMA*, 277 (Apr. 16, 1997), p. 1181.

67. "Whither Scientific Deliberation in Health Policy Recommendation?" *N Engl J Med*, 336 (Apr. 17, 1997), pp. 1180-1183.

68. Jacquelyn Paykel and William H. Wolberg, "Screening Mammograms," *J Natl Cancer Inst*, 89 (June 18, 1997), p. 889.

69. Kenneth C. Chu et al, "Recent Trends in Breast Cancer Incidence, Survival, and Mortality Rates," *J Natl Cancer Inst*, 88 (Nov. 6, 1996), pp. 1571-1579.

70. Nils Bjurstam et al, "The Gothenburg Breast Screening Trial," *Cancer*, 80 (Dec. 1, 1997), pp. 2091-2099.

71. "Increased Benefit from Shorter Screening Mammography Intervals" (editorial), *Cancer*, 80 (Dec. 1, 1997), pp. 2035-2039.

72. Anthony B. Miller et al, "CNBSS: Thirteen-Year Results of a Randomized Trial in Women Aged 50 to 59," *J Natl Cancer Inst*, 92 (Sept. 20, 2000), pp. 1490-1499.

73. Baines and Smith quoted by Paul Recer, "Study Questions Survival Benefit of Mammography," Savannah *Morning News*,

Sept. 20, 2000, p. 8A.

74.   Peggy Eastman, "Task Force Issues New Screening Guidelines," *J Natl Cancer Inst*, 88 (Jan. 17, 1996), pp. 74-76.

75.   William C. Black et al, "Perceptions of Breast Cancer Risk in Women Younger than 50," *J Natl Cancer Inst*, 87 (May 17, 1995), pp. 720-731.

76.   "Biologic Characteristics of Interval and Screen-detected Breast Cancers" (correspondence), *J Natl Cancer Inst*, 93 (Jan. 17, 2001), pp. 151-152. See also Kelly-Anne Phillips et al, "Breast Carcinomas Arising in Carriers of Mutations in *BRCA1* or *BRCA2*," *J Clin Oncol*, 17 (Nov. 1999), pp. 3653-3663.

77.   Robert A. Smith, "Breast Cancer Screening among Women Younger than Age 50," *CA*, 50 (Sept/Oct. 2000), pp. 312-336.

78.   "Breast Imaging Modalities," *Seminars in Breast Disease*, 2 (Mar. 1999), pp. 1-2. See also "Clinical Prospects for Full-Field Digital Mammography" by Stephen A. Feig and Martin J. Yaffee (pp. 64-73 in this issue).

79.   "Mammography Screening Aid Approved," *JAMA*, 280 (Aug. 5, 1998), p. 410.

80.   Daniel B. Kopans et al, "Mammographic Screening" (correspondence), *JAMA*, 273 (Mar. 1, 1995), pp. 701-702.

81.   Michael Swift et al, "Incidence of Cancer in 161 Families Affected by Ataxia-Telangiectasia," *N Engl J Med*, 325 (Dec. 26, 1991), pp. 1831-1836. See also the correspondence in the *Journal* for May 14, 1992 (Vol. 326, pp. 1357-1361).

82.   Cornelia J. Baines et al, "Impact of Menstrual Phase on False-Negative Mammograms," *Cancer*, 80 (Aug. 15, 1997), pp. 720-724.

83.   "False-Positive Rate of Screening Mammography" (correspondence), *N Engl J Med*, 339 (Aug. 20, 1998), pp. 560-564.

84.   "From the FDA: New Information Regarding Mammography Results," *JAMA*, 281 (Apr. 7, 1999), p. 1164.

85.   Edwin R. Fisher et al, "Pathologic Findings from NSABP Protocol B-17," *Cancer*, 75 (Mar. 15, 1995), pp. 1310-1319.

86.   Paul C. Stomper et al, "Mammographic Detection and Staging of Ductal Carcinoma *in Situ*," *Seminars in Breast Disease*, 3 (Mar. 2000), pp. 26-41.

87.   Monica Morrow and Stuart J. Schnitt, "Treatment Selection in Ductal Carcinoma *in Situ*," *JAMA*, 283 (Jan. 26, 2000), pp. 453-455.

Chapter Twenty-nine

1.   Andrea Walker Gehrke, "Breast Self-Examination: A Mixed Message," *J Natl Cancer Inst*, 92 (July 19, 2000), pp. 1120-1121.

2.   "Clinical Breast Examination for Detecting Breast Cancer" (correspondence), *JAMA*, 283 (Apr. 5, 2000), pp. 1687-1688.

3.   Cornelia J. Baines et al, "Physical Examination: Its Role as a Single Screening Modality in the Canadian National Breast Screening Study," *Cancer*, 63 (May 1, 1989), pp. 1816-1822.

4.   Baines et al (as in preceding note), p. 1818.

5.   Baines et al (as in preceding note), p. 1818.

6.   Mary B. Barton et al, "Does This Patient Have Breast Cancer? The Screening Clinical Breast Examination," *JAMA*, 282 (Oct. 6, 1999), pp. 1270-1280.

7.   Barton et al (as in preceding note), p. 1271.

$\mathcal{I}ndex$

abortion: as disputed risk factor, 85-87

Abrams, Jeffrey, 312, 503-504, 508

abscesses: treatment of, 167

ABVD regimen for Hodgkin's disease, 454

AC regimen for breast cancer: favored by NSABP, 464-465, 468; used before breast surgery, 472-473; NSABP trials test AC regimen in combination with paclitaxel, docetaxel, and Herceptin, 513-514; concurrent Herceptin increases risk of cardiotoxicity, 584-585

acetaminophen, 205, 540-541

acini, 69

ACS: see American Cancer Society

Actiq (brand name), 544

acute lymphoblastic leukemia (ALL), 449-452, 459-461

acute myelogenous leukemia (AML), 452

adaptive (specific) immunity, 559, 579

addiction to opioid drugs, 546-547

adenocarcinoma, 224

adjuvant therapy: definition of, 30, 412

adoptive immunotherapy, 566-571

adrenal glands, 72; surgical removal of glands as hormonal manipulation, 414

adrenalectomy, 414, 440

Adriamycin (brand name for doxorubicin): drug's side effects increased by concurrent radiation therapy, 375; probable favorable interaction with concurrent tamoxifen, 425-426; drug's use in regimens for leukemia and Hodgkin's disease, 452, 454; drug's mode of action and its side effects, 461-462; FAC, AC, and other regimens used in breast cancer, 462-465; meta-analysis reveals slight survival advantage over CMF variations, 465-466; Bonadonna's Milan group tests Adriamycin followed by CMF, 465; P-glycoprotein

linked to drug resistance, 467-468; risk posed by extravasation, 474; drug associated with severe alopecia (hair loss), 479, altered sense of taste, 482, and diarrhea, 483; paclitaxel (Taxol) as second-line therapy, 508; scheduling to avoid negative interactions with paclitaxel, 511; combining Adriamycin with docetaxel (Taxotere), 512-513; NASBP trials test the AC regimen in combination with paclitaxel and docetaxel, 513-514; concurrent Herceptin increases risk of cardiotoxicity, 585

AIDS (Acquired Immune Deficiency Syndrome), 9, 79, 548, 559, 565, 579

Albertini, John J., 329-330

alcohol consumption, 108-111

aldesleukin, 570

alendronate, 524, 536

alkaline phosphatase assay, 379, 390, 530

alkylating agents: risk of carcinogenesis, 319; mustard gas and nitrogen mustard, 449; thiotepa and L-PAM in early NSABP trials, 455-456; cyclophosphamide as cornerstone in CMF regimen, 457-458; effect on ovaries, 485-486; principally dose-limited by marrow suppression, 491

ALL: see acute lymphoblastic leukemia

alleles, 32-33

allocation bias, 603

allogeneic: definition of term, 452, 489-490

alopecia (hair loss), 457, 462, 478-480

ALS: see amyotrophic lateral sclerosis

alternative therapies for cancer, 394-411

alveoli, 56, 69-70

Alzheimer's disease: no protection from conjugated estrogens, 137-138

amenorrhea during chemotherapy, 484-487

American Cancer Society: educational campaign about "Seven Danger Signals," 152, 292;

American Cancer Society—*continued*
George Crile, Jr., objects to cancerphobia, 294-296; Society's dietary recommendations, 403-404; its statistics on cancer mortality, 538; lung cancer screening strategy proves doubtful, 590-591; lifetime risk of breast cancer said to be one-in-nine, 593; Society's guidelines on breast cancer screening, 598-600, 612; listing of patient support services, 619-620
American Pain Foundation, 623
American Society of Clinical Oncology, 461
American Society of Pain Management Nurses, 548
Americans with Disabilities Act, 252
Ames, Frederick C., 385
aminoglutethimide, 440
amitriptyline, 540
amplification of HER-2/*neu* gene, 50-53, 283, 583
amyotrophic lateral sclerosis (ALS), 548, 550
analgesics for cancer pain, 539-548, 554. See also pain control and opioid drugs
anaplastic tumors, 218
anastomosis, 359-360
anastrozole, 443-447, 621
anchorage independence, 26
Anderson, Thomas J., 150
androgen insensitivity, 73-74
androgens, 72-73; their use in breast cancer therapy, 416
anemia during chemotherapy, 480
aneuploidy: definition of, 38; as prognostic factor, 275-276
Angell, Marcia, 348, 351
angiogenesis: essential role in tumor growth, 22, 25; microvessel density proposed as prognostic assay, 221-222; efforts to develop angiogenesis inhibitors, 518-521
angiography: imaging of coronary arteries, 129, of liver, 531, and of brain, 533
angiosarcomas, 232
angiostatin, 519-520
anorexia in terminal cancer, 28, 536-539, 553
anthracycline antibiotics, 461-462, 468, 585
antibody-mediated immunity, 579
anticipatory vomiting, 461-462, 475
antiemetic drugs used during chemotherapy, 475-478

antiestrogens, 413
antigen-presenting cells (APCs), 575-579
antigens, 557-558, 561-562, 579-580. See also tumor-associated antigens
antimetabolites, 450; inclusion of methotrexate and fluorouracil in CMF regimen, 457
antioxidant vitamins, 396-402
Antman, Karen, 490, 495, 504
APCs: see antigen-presenting cells
apheresis, 497-498
aplastic anemia, 490
apocrine glands, 97
apoptosis, 67
Apple, Rima D., 395
Aredia (brand name for pamidronate), 524-525
areola, 56-57
Arimidex (brand name for anastrozole), 443-447
arm exercises after breast surgery, 338
Aromasin (brand name for exemestane), 443-444, 446
aromatase (enzyme), 75, 414, 440, 443
aromatase inhibitors in breast cancer therapy, 440; drugs indicated only for postmenopausal ER-positive patients, 442-443; three available agents, 443-444; ATAC trial compares anastrozole and tamoxifen, 444-446, but mature data lacking, 446-447
aromatization of androgens, 72, 443
around-the-clock (ATC) dosing of opioid analgesics, 541-544
arteriosclerosis, 109
aspirin, 205, 540
ATAC trial, 444-446
ataxia-telangiectasia, 613
ATC dose: see around-the-clock dosing
Ativan (brand name): see lorazepam
atomic bomb survivors, 77-78
atypical hyperplasia, 171-172, 212; tamoxifen seen as effective prophylaxis against malignant progression, 437-439
Auchincloss-type mastectomy, 332-333
autoimmune diseases, 349-353, 557, 559, 582
autologous: definition of term, 488-489
autosomal dominant transmission in hereditary breast cancer, 112
axilla (armpit), 24, 27
axillary dissections in breast cancer surgery: Halsted's view of, 262, 264; NSABP finds no effect on survival rates, 265; sentinel

node sampling wins acceptance, 265-266; axillary dissection never indicated for *in situ* (noninvasive) tumors, 287; rationale behind Halsted's *en bloc* dissection, 290-292; Halstedian tradition still prevailing in 1950s and 1960s, 295-297, but refuted by NSABP experiments and trials, 298-300; combining axillary dissection and lumpectomy, 326; side effects of careless surgery, 327; the three levels of nodes, 327-329; recovery from surgery, 337-340; risk factors for arm lymphedema, 340-341

axillary lymph nodes: their involvement in breast cancer dissemination, 24, 27; function of lymph nodes, 59-62; number and location of axillary nodes, 60; NSABP findings on prognostic significance of positive axillary nodes, 262-265; erroneous Halstedian view of nodes as barriers, 291; management of axillary recurrences, 387; no immune response to breast tumors has been observed in the nodes, 558. See also negative nodes and positive nodes

B cells, 60, 559-560, 571-572, 576, 579-582. See also lymphocytes
Bailar, John C., III, 459
Baines, Cornelia J., 603, 610, 616-617
Baker, Larry H., 597, 601
Baker, R. Robinson, 225, 303
barium enema, 590
Barrett-Connor, Elizabeth, 127
basal cell carcinomas, 407
Baselga, José, 583-585
baseline mammogram, 599-600
basement membrane, 19-25
basic fibroblast growth factor (bFGF), 519
batimastat, 520
Bazell, Robert, 582, 585
BCDDP: see Breast Cancer Detection Demonstration Project
Beatson, George Thomas, 413-414
benign breast disorders: diagnosis and treatment of, 152-170; benign disorders and risk of malignant transformation, 170-172. See also "lump in the breast"
Bernstein, Leslie, 75-76, 85, 107

beta carotene, 396-400, 403
Bexxar (brand name), 582
Bezwoda, Werner R., 502-504
bias in epidemiological studies: types of, 80-81, 603-604
bilirubin, 530
biological response modifiers, 521
biomarkers, 390-391
biopsy of the breast: about 25% of biopsies done for nonpalpable calcifications discover cancer, 192, 194-195; traditional one-step biopsy, 200-201, largely replaced by two-step procedure, 201-203; undergoing outpatient biopsy and recovering from it, 203-205; core-needle biopsy, 206-208; wire localization technique, 208-209; stereotactic needle biopsies, 209-213; difference between excisional biopsy and lumpectomy, 323-324
bisphosphonates, 446, 524-525
Black, Maurice M., 219, 558
Bland, Kirby I., 177, 205, 334, 338, 382
blood-brain barrier, 533, 584
blood cells: differentiation of diverse cell lineages, 488-489
blood clots (venous thrombosis): association with exogenous estrogens, 127-128, 135-139, 141-142, 151; modest risk from tamoxifen therapy, 430, and from Megace, 536-537
bloodstream: close relationship with lymphatic system, 59
body size: association with breast cancer incidence, 97-98
Body Surface Area (BSA), 473
bolus infusions, 474, 513
Bonadonna, Gianni, 263-264, 313, 426, 456-458, 465, 472, 485
bone: anatomy of, 131; preventing fractures in metastatic cancer, 522-527. See also osteoporosis
bone marrow: definition of, 131; detecting breast cancer cells in the marrow, 278-280, 392; differentiation of blood cells in the marrow, 488-489; aspiration and cryopreservation of marrow, 489-491; reasons for growth of disseminated cancer cells in the marrow, 523-524
bone marrow suppression during chemotherapy, 480-482

bone marrow transplantation (BMT): allogeneic BMT potentially curative for adult leukemias and lymphomas, 452, 489-490; autologous "transplants" used for breast cancer, 488-496, are made easier by PBSC technology, 496-500, but clinical trials fail to demonstrate significant benefits, 500-504

bone mineral density: postmenopausal estrogen replacement increases density, 131-133; effect of tamoxifen varies in younger and older women, 430-432; raloxifene preserves density, 442, while aromatase inhibitors decrease it, 444-447

bone scans, 389-390, 392, 522

boost to tumor bed (radiation therapy after lumpectomy): 308, 310, 325, 365-366, 372, 376

Bostwick, John, III, 333

brachytherapy, 529

brain: detection and treatment of metastatic disease in, 390, 532-535

brain tumors (malignant gliomas), 448, 520, 533

BRCA1 gene: implicated in hereditary breast and ovarian cancers, 113-115, 612; screening for inherited mutations, 622-623

BRCA2 gene, 114, 623

breakthrough pain, 542-543

breast (human): anatomy of, 55-62; variations in size and shape, 56, 58; subcutaneous fat, 58; changes during reproduction, 65-71, and after menopause, 71-73; glandular tissues in the male breast, 74-75; division into quadrants, 153, 155. See also mammary gland

breast cancer: conspiracy of silence about, 1-2; Presidential families afflicted, 2; not a single disease, 3, 10; steps in malignant transformation, 18-28; symptoms of, 22, 24-25; systemic therapies for, 29-31; deletion of *Rb* gene, 46; mutations of *p53* gene, 47-48; *nm23* gene seen as metastasis suppressor, 48-49; HER-2/*neu* gene associated with tumor aggressiveness, 49-54; lymphatic dissemination of cancer cells, 58-62; role of hormonal stimulation, 62-64; male breast cancer, 73-75; estrogen imbalances implicated, 75-76; suspected carcinogens, 76-77; risk of radiation

breast cancer—*continued*
carcinogenesis varies by age at time of exposure, 77-78; epidemiological studies of risk factors, 79-82; effect of parity on risk, 83-85, of miscarriage and abortion, 85-87, of breast-feeding, 87-90, of menstrual history, 90-91, and of number of ovulations, 91-93; international variations in disease incidence, 94-95; Japanese and other Asian women at low risk, 95-98; studies of dietary fat prove inconclusive, 98-102; Mediterranean diet seen as protective, 102-103; obesity as postmenopausal risk factor, 104-106; exercise seen as protective, 106-107; smoking inversely associated with disease incidence, 107-108; alcohol consumption as minor risk factor, 108-111; hereditary (familial) breast cancer, 111-116; growing older as unavoidable risk factor, 116-118; early-onset cases often aggressive, 118; heart disease far greater cause of mortality in women, 129; comparatively small risks from postmenopausal estrogen replacement, 133-139, and from oral contraceptives, 143-147, 149-151; most breast symptoms due to benign processes, 152; cancers frequent in upper outer quadrant, 153, 155; malignant tumors produce dominant masses, 154, but so do various benign lesions, 154, 156-162; unilateral breast symptoms always need to be investigated, 162, 167; cancers affecting the nipple-areola complex, 164-166; differential diagnosis of skin symptoms, 167-169, and of breast nodularities, 169-170; benign disorders and subsequent cancer risk, 170-172; symptoms suggestive of malignancy often ignored in younger women, 178-179; mammography indispensable in symptom evaluation, 180-184; radiological characteristics of malignant tumors, 184, 186-197, and why mammograms sometimes fail to detect them, 198-199; the different types of invasive breast cancers, 223-232, and the *in situ* (noninvasive) carcinomas, 233-245; reactions to a cancer diagnosis, 246-247, and the need for second opinions, 247-248; lumpectomy rates vary by

breast cancer—*continued*

geographical region, 248-250; role of support groups, 250; most breast tumors either localized or indolent, 251-252; job security, health insurance, and personal relationships, 252-255; traditional staging of tumors, 256-260; effect on prognosis of tumor size, 260-262, and of nodal status, 262-265; axillary dissection and sentinel node sampling, 265-266; effect of estrogen receptor (ER) levels, 267-271, and of progesterone receptor (PgR) levels, 271-272; assays for measuring tumor growth rates, 272-275, and DNA content, 275-276; detecting breast cancer cells in the bone marrow, 278-280; immunostaining to evaluate *p53* and HER-2/*neu* expression, 281-285; a quiz on prognostic factors, 285-287; earliest recorded mastectomies, 288-289; Halsted's radical mastectomy achieves local control, 289-292; first experiments with lumpectomy and irradiation for breast preservation, 293-294; the debate over radical surgery, 294-297; NSABP trials question effectiveness of radical mastectomy, 298-300, and of postmastectomy irradiation, 300-301; total (simple) mastectomy becomes orthodoxy, 301-303; sporadic (nonhereditary) ductal carcinomas usually suitable for lumpectomy, 304-306; the Joint Center's regimen for irradiation after lumpectomy, 306-309; NSABP finds lumpectomy equivalent to mastectomy in survival rates, 309-312; implications of the NSABP findings, 313-314; the basic indications for mastectomy, 315-316, lumpectomy, 316-319, and irradiation, 319-322; surgical techniques for lumpectomy, 323-326, axillary dissection, 326-327, and sentinel node sampling, 329-331; types of mastectomy, 331-334; surgery and recovery, 334-341; breast reconstruction, 342-362; radiation therapy after lumpectomy, 363-377; surveillance for possible recurrences, 378-380; management of recurrences in the other breast, 381-382, in a preserved breast, 382-384, in the skin flaps after mastectomy, 384-387, and in the regional lymph nodes, 387-389;

breast cancer—*continued*

tests used to search for distant metastases, 389-391, and their limitations, 392-393; possible effect of dietary fat and fiber on outcome, 402-404; history of previous hormonal therapies, 412-416; effectiveness and side effects of tamoxifen, 416-434; NSABP's controversial trial of tamoxifen prophylaxis, 434-439; second-line therapies after tamoxifen failure, 439-442; aromatase inhibitors tested as adjuvant therapy for postmenopausal patients, 442-447; early NSABP trials of cytotoxic chemotherapy, 455-456; the CMF regimen, 456-459, and some skeptical reactions to it, 459-461; Adriamycin-based regimens, 461-466; multidrug resistance seen as main reason for treatment failure, 466-468; full-dose chemotherapy seen as achieving 65% survival in Stage Two disease, 468-471; preoperative chemotherapy aids in breast preservation, 472-473; high-dose chemotherapy with bone marrow support tested for metastatic disease and subsequently for high-risk patients, 488-493, but proves controversial, 493-496; PBSC technology reduces cost and toxicity of high-dose strategies, 496-500, yet clinical trials fail to demonstrate a significant survival benefit, 500-504; paclitaxel (Taxol) and docetaxel (Taxotere) achieve responses in metastatic disease, 506-513; NSABP trials test taxane-based adjuvant regimens, 513-514; long-term prognosis in metastatic disease remains poor, 515-516; systemic therapies for metastatic disease, 516-518; management of metastases in the skeleton, lungs, liver, and brain, 522-535; treatments for hypercalcemia, 535-536; statistics on causes of death, 538; no reliable evidence that breast tumors elicit an immune response, 558; vaccine strategies tested in clinical trials, 574-575, 578-579; Herceptin achieves responses in HER-2-positive disease, 582-587; overdiagnosis associated with screening assays, 592-593, while the death rate remains constant, 593; ductal carcinoma *in situ* leads to treatment dilemmas, 593-594;

breast cancer—*continued*
    estimates of mortality reductions obtainable by screening, 594-598; American Cancer Society urges screening mammography, 598-600, but Dr. Spratt and a big Canadian trial question the strategy's effectiveness, 600-604; experts divided on mammography for women in their forties, 604-608; more convincing data needed to establish mammography's effect on mortality rates, 609-612; practical advice on undergoing mammography, 613-614; rationale and techniques for breast self-examination, 615-618
Breast Cancer Detection Demonstration Project (BCDDP), 596-599, 611
Breast Cancer Prevention Trial (NSABP Protocol P-1), 434-439
breast examination by a physician, 173-174, 182, 594-595
breast-feeding, 55, 71, 87-90
breast-ovarian syndrome, 114-115
breast-prostate syndrome, 115
breast prostheses, 339-340, 620
breast reconstruction: end of radical mastectomy opens new market, 303; specialized mastectomy techniques permitting immediate reconstructions, 333-334; almost all patients eligible, 342; importance of silicone gel implants, 342-345, and the controversy over their safety, 345-346; FDA restriction on silicone gel implants, 347-348, and the ensuing litigation, 349-351; implant risks seem modest, 351-353; immediate reconstruction becomes norm, 353-355; the three steps in reconstruction, 356; tissue-transfer reconstructions, 356-357, using pedicle flaps, 357-359, or free flaps, 359-361; techniques to reconstruct the nipple-areola complex, 361-362
breast self-examination (BSE): recommended by Dr. Spratt, 170, and by CNBSS, 602-604; rationale for BSE, 615-616; techniques for BSE, 616-618. See also palpation of the breast
Brinker, Nancy, 116, 479-480
Brinton, Louise A., 125, 147
broccoli: touted as breast cancer prophylaxis, 2, 82, 404

Broder, Samuel, 400
bronchoscopy, 529, 590
Bruning, Nancy, 349
bupivacaine, 545
Burkitt, Denis, 94
Burkitt's lymphoma, 38, 43
Burnet, Macfarlane, 556, 571
Buzdar, Aman U., 441, 443-444, 462-463

CA 15-3 (assay for recurrence), 391
cachexia in terminal cancer, 28, 537-539
Cady, Blake, 250, 322, 327, 329, 494
CAF regimen for breast cancer, 463
caffeine, 170
calcifications seen on mammograms, 189-195; techniques for biopsy and diagnosis, 208-213; benign calcifications not an obstacle to lumpectomy, 317
calcium: dietary requirement, 132-133; mineral's role in mammary gland, 190
CALGB: see Cancer and Leukemia Group B
Canadian National Breast Screening Study (CNBSS), 602-606, 609-610, 613, 616-618
cancer: definition of, 9-10, 15-18; hereditary (familial) cancer syndromes, 17, 45-48; stepwise development of malignancies, 18-28; curable cancers, 29-31; role of oncogenes, 42-44, and tumor suppressor genes, 45-49; cellular division as prerequisite for malignant transformation, 62-63; international variations in tumor incidence, 94-95; aging as predominant risk factor, 117; "Seven Danger Signals," 152, 292; degree of cellular differentiation as noted on a pathology report, 218; systems of tumor grading, 218-220; *in situ* cancers, 233-234; patient reactions to diagnosis, 246-247; cancerphobia and "ultra radical" operations, 294-297; attempts to develop cancer vaccines, 571-579; value of early-detection screening assays measured by their sensitivity and specificity, 589-592, but their effect on mortality rates is hard to determine, 592-593
Cancer and Leukemia Group B (CALGB): trials of dose-intense FAC, 468-469, 493, and of high-dose chemotherapy, 502-503

Cancer and Steroid Hormone Study (CASH), 86, 144-147, 171
CancerCare organization, 621
cancer personality, 405
cancerphobia, 294-297
Canellos, George P., 456, 494
carboplatin, 500
carcinoembryonic antigen (CEA), 391
carcinogens: examples of, 16-17; in breast cancer, 76-78; in cervical cancer, 81; in lung and oral cancers, 82; examples of DES, 120-121, and of unopposed estrogen replacement, 123-124
carcinomas: definition of, 18
cardiovascular disease, 7, 79, 93, 96, 102-104, 106; moderate alcohol consumption seen as protective, 109-110; controversy over estrogen replacement therapy, 127-131, 134-139; vitamin E seen as protective, 397, but not beta carotene, 400; NSABP finds that tamoxifen does not reduce risk, 429-430, 438
Carlson, Grant W., 331, 333
carmustine, 491-493, 499, 502-503
Carter, Christine L., 171, 260-261
Carter, Jimmy, 17
CASH: see Cancer and Steroid Hormone Study
CAT: see computerized axial tomography
cathepsin D, 276-278
CD20 molecule on B cells, 581-582
CD34 protein expressed by stem cells, 496-497
cell lines: definition of, 26
cell separator, 498
cell-mediated immunity, 571-574
cells: types of, 10-14
centigrays (cGy), 307
central nervous system (CNS): sanctuary site poorly penetrated by many cancer drugs, 452; diagnosis and treatment of metastases in CNS, 532-535
central venous catheters, 474
cereal consumption: association with lower cancer rates, 94-96, 98, 101-103, 403
cerebrospinal fluid, 532-534
cervical cancer, 17, 29, 81, 589, 591
Chabner, Bruce A., 506
Charen, Mona, 547, 608
Chechik, Diane Craig, 179
chemotherapy: a systemic treatment, 29-30;

chemotherapy—*continued*
administration during breast irradiation, 374-375; counterindicated in first trimester of pregnancy, 375-377; drugs are cytotoxic, 412, and typically serve as chemical oophorectomy in premenopausal patients, 424; CMF regimen seen as antagonistic to concurrent tamoxifen, but Adriamycin appears synergetic, 425-427; Saint Gallen guidelines for systemic therapies, 428; limitations of chemotherapy for solid tumors, 448; combination chemotherapy cures childhood leukemia, 449-452; the basic principles of cancer chemotherapy, 451-452; curative regimens developed for choriocarcinoma, Hodgkin's disease, and germ-cell tumors, 452-455; doubling times of cancer cells determine degree of chemosensitivity, 455; early NSABP trials of breast cancer chemotherapy, 455-456, and the Milan trial of CMF, 456-461; the Adriamycin-based regimens, 461-466; three reasons for treatment failure, 466; how multidrug resistance develops, 466-468; dose-intensity seen as beneficial, 468-469; survival rates in node-positive breast cancer, 470-471; the indications for chemotherapy before breast surgery, 472-473; dose calculations and the abbreviations used by oncologists, 473; procedures for outpatient drug administration, 473-475; antiemetic drugs, 475-478; dealing with hair loss, 478-480; bone marrow suppression is greatest threat, 480-482; gastrointestinal side effects, 482-484; coping with adverse effects on fertility and sexuality, 484-487; high-dose "bone marrow" strategies prove controversial, 488-496; PBSC technology reduces cost and toxicity of high-dose therapy, 496-500, but clinical trials fail to document a survival benefit, 500-504; development of paclitaxel (Taxol) and docetaxel (Taxotere), 505-509, and the determination of their side effects, 509-511; clinical trials test paclitaxel and docetaxel in combination with Adriamycin, 511-513, and with the NSABP regimen AC, 513-514; regimens for metastatic disease, 517-518; regional perfusion of the

chemotherapy—*continued*
liver, 531; intrathecal chemotherapy of cerebrospinal fluid, 534; combining the AC regimen with paclitaxel and Herceptin, 584-586. See also side effects of chemotherapy

chest X-rays, 181, 389

childbirth, 69

childhood leukemia: cure of, 449-452

Chin, Arthur E., 551

chlorpromazine, 554

cholera, 80

cholesterol, 79, 85, 102-103; HDL (high-density lipoprotein) cholesterol, 103, 109, 127-131, 135-136; LDL (low-density lipoprotein) cholesterol, 103, 127-131; effect of tamoxifen on lipid profiles, 429-430

choriocarcinoma, 30, 452-453

chromatin, 219-220

chromosomes: definition of, 33-35; karyotyping of, 36-39

chronic granulomatous disease, 565

chronic lymphocytic leukemia, 467

chronic myelogenous leukemia, 29, 37-39, 467, 490, 565-566

Chu, Kenneth C., 595-596, 609

cimetidine, 506

cisplatin, 454, 475, 477, 491-493, 498, 502, 506, 508

Clark, Gary M., 270-272, 276

Clark, Roy M., 321

Cleveland Clinic, 292, 295-296, 320-321, 325

"Clinical Alerts" from the National Cancer Institute, 426, 429, 433-434

clinical trials: importance of, 297-298; finding information on current trials, 620-621. See also Phase One, Two, and Three trials

Clinton, Bill, 2, 608

clodronate, 525

CMF regimen for breast cancer: compatible with concurrent breast irradiation, 375, but not with concurrent tamoxifen, 425-426; Milan trial of classical CMF, 456-458; six cycles prove superior to twelve, 458-459; twenty-year results from the Milan trial, 460-461; CMF compared with AC and other Adriamycin-based regimens, 463-466; Milan statistics on CMF-related amenorrhea, 485

CNBSS: see Canadian National Breast Screening Study

Cobleigh, Melody A., 584-585

codeine, 541

Colace (brand name for docusate sodium), 541

Colditz, Graham A., 127, 146

Coley, William B., 560-562, 566

collagen, 19, 154

colon and rectal cancers, 16; stepwise development of tumors, 44, 47-48; suspected dietary risk factors, 94, 100, 102; possible association with *BRCA1* gene, 115; colostomy bags, 295; reasons for resistance to chemotherapy, 455, 467; screening assays for, 589-590

colonoscopy, 590

colony-stimulating factors (CSFs), 497, 499. See also granulocyte (G-CSF) and granulocyte-macrophage (GM-CSF) colony-stimulating factors

colposcope, 233

combretastatin, 520

comedo subtype of ductal carcinoma *in situ* (DCIS), 235, 238, 240-242, 273-274, 283, 594, 614

Compazine (brand name for prochlorperazine), 476-477

Complete Blood Count (CBC), 10-11, 257, 379

complete responses (chemotherapy for metastatic disease), 490, 492-494

Comprehensive Cancer Centers, 620

compression (mammography), 183, 195

computerized axial tomography (CAT scans), 195-196, 380, 389-390, 392, 531, 533-534, 590-591

condylomata acuminata (genital warts), 9, 565

confounding factors, 81-82, 97-98, 108-109, 128, 137

conjugated equine estrogens: definition of, 122

connective-tissue diseases, 349-353

Consensus Development Conferences on breast cancer: June 1979 Conference endorses total (simple) mastectomy, 302-303; June 1990 Conference finds breast preservation preferable to mastectomy, 312-313; September 1985 Conference endorses systemic therapy for node-positive disease, 422-423, 463; January 1997 Conference fails to recommend mammography screening for women in their forties, 606-608

constipation: during chemotherapy, 484; during opioid analgesia, 541, 553

contact inhibition, 26

contracture around breast implants, 343, 346, 357

contralateral breast biopsy, 304

Cooper, Richard, 456

Cooper's ligaments, 58, 72

Copeland, Edward M., 334

core-needle biopsy, 206-208

corpus luteum, 66-68

cortical bone, 131

corticosteroids: used as antiemetics, 476-478; used to manage spinal cord compression, 527, and intracranial pressure, 534; used to combat anorexia, 536-538; used as adjuvants in pain control, 540-541

costimulatory molecules, 576

Cousins, Norman, 409-410

craniocaudal position (mammography), 183, 595-596

craniotomy, 534

Crile, George, Jr., 202, 295-297, 308, 539

Crile, George W., 292-293, 295-296

cryoablation, 532

Curie Institute, 294

cycles in cancer chemotherapy: rationale for, 451-452; reason that 21-day or 28-day cycles are used, 480

cyclical nodularity, 170

cyclophosphamide: risk of carcinogenesis with concurrent irradiation, 319; most regimens induce ovarian failure in premenopausal patients, 424; possible antagonistic interaction with tamoxifen, 425-426; cornerstone drug in CMF regimen, 456-459; use in FAC regimen, 462, and in AC regimen, 464; patients advised to drink fluids, 475; dosage level determines amount of hair loss, 479; drug's effect on the ovaries, 485; high-dose therapy with marrow support, 490-494, or with PBSCs, 498-500; NSABP reports that dose escalation is ineffective, 501, while CALGB and Intergroup trials of high-dose regimens prove inconclusive, 501-503

cyclosporine, 467, 490

cystic fibrosis, 15, 32, 40

cystosarcoma phyllodes, 231-232

cysts in the breast: common in older premenopausal women, 158-161, 172; identification of cysts, 174-176, 184, 192, 597; treatment considerations, 159, 161

cytokine cascade, 571

cytokines, 41, 537, 563-571, 573-575, 578-579

cytologists, 33

cytology, 166; role in evaluating breast aspirates, 176-178

cytoplasm of the cell, 12-13

cytotoxic T cells, 560, 567, 569, 571-572, 574-575, 579. See also lymphocytes

Cytoxan (brand name): see cyclophosphamide

daclizumab, 582

Daling, Janet R., 87

D'Andrea, Gabriella M., 516

Dashiell, Bessie, 560-561

daunorubicin, 452, 462

DCIS: see ductal carcinoma *in situ*

DCs: see dendritic cells

DDT (pesticide), 76-77

deathbed vigils, 548, 554-555

death rattle, 555

Decadron (brand name): see dexamethasone

delayed-type hypersensitivity (DTH), 573-574

dendritic cells (DCs), 575-579

de novo breast tumors (new primary cancers): as one type of recurrence, 378, 381-383; tamoxifen prophylaxis useful, 421-422, but aromatase inhibitors seen as more effective, 443-445

Depo-Provera (brand name), 148

dermatitis (skin inflammation), 164

DES: see diethylstilbestrol

designer drugs for cancer, 29; Herceptin cited as example, 585

Designer Foods Program, 404

desmoplasia, 217

desquamation, 370

DeVita, Vincent T., Jr., 453-454, 456, 459, 486, 568

dexamethasone, 476-477, 506, 509, 527, 534, 536-538, 540

dexrazoxane, 462

diagnostic bias, 603-604

diagnostic mammography, 180-199; definition of, 180; radiological characteristics of benign and malignant masses, 184-189; calcifications as clues, 189-195; specialized techniques, 195, 197; MRI sometimes superior in imaging densely glandular breasts, 196, 198-199; reasons for false negatives, 198-199. See also mammography and screening mammography

diamorphine, 547

diarrhea during chemotherapy, 483-484

diazepam, 477, 540

Diel, Ingo J., 280, 525

diet as a risk factor for cancer: epidemiological studies subject to bias and confounding, 81-82

dietary fat hypothesis in breast cancer: high-fat diet associated with early menarche, 91, and with elevated incidence of breast, colon, and prostate cancers, 94-95; Japanese low-fat diet seen as protective, 95-97; considerable epidemiological evidence for hypothesis, 98, but results from Nurses' Health Study fail to support it, 99-100; Dr. Willett's objections to it, 101-102; diet of Greek islanders lauded, 102-103; preteen and adolescent fat intake seen as important, but not addressed, 104; dietary fat linked to higher estrogen levels, 402

dietary fiber hypothesis, 100-101, 402-403

dietary strategies as treatment adjuvants, 394; vitamins prove controversial, 398-402, but low-fat, high-fiber diet seen as possibly helpful, 402-404

diethylstilbestrol (DES), 120-121, 139, 415-416

differentiation: process as observed in embryos, 11-12; loss of differentiation in cancer cells, 28; differentiation of mammary gland, 68-69, 84-85; term as used in pathology reports, 218; ongoing process in bone marrow, 488-489

digital mammography, 198, 210, 612-613

digital rectal examination (DRE), 589-590

Dilaudid (brand name): see hydromorphone

dimpling (contour retraction) of breast, 167-168, 174

diphenhydramine, 506

diploid cells, 11, 275

disease-free interval (DFI), 379, 383, 385, 516

disease-free survival (DFS): definition of, 52

distant metastases: see metastatic disease

DNA (deoxyribonucleic acid): deciphering the genetic code of DNA, 35-36; sequencing and synthesizing DNA, 39-41. See also recombinant DNA technology

docetaxel (Taxotere): drug welcome innovation in cancer chemotherapy, 488, 505; developed in France, 508-509; side effects, dose, and scheduling, 509-510; pitted against Adriamycin in metastatic breast cancer, 512-513; NSABP trials combine AC regimen with docetaxel, 514

docusate sodium, 541

dominant masses (breast lumps), 153, 160-161, 169-170; evaluation of, 174-179; mammography of, 184-189; indications for MRI examination of, 196-197; masses sometimes radiologically invisible, 198-199; excisional biopsies usually preferred, 204

Donegan, William L., 152-153, 161, 164-165, 169, 174, 178, 195, 205, 260, 334, 340, 387, 390, 407

dopamine antagonists, 476

dorsal rhizotomy, 545

dose calculation in chemotherapy, 473

dose escalations in chemotherapy, 468, 489-494, 498-504

dose intensity in chemotherapy, 468-469

dose-response curve, 491

double helix of DNA, 35-36

double-lumen implants, 344

doubling times of cancer cells, 455

Down's syndrome, 37

doxorubicin: see Adriamycin

drainage tubes after breast surgery, 337-338

Dressler, Lynn G., 276

Drife, James Owen, 316

drug resistance to chemotherapeutic agents: associated with HER-2/*neu* overexpression, 283-285; as observed in 1942 Yale experiment, 449; multidrug resistance seen as principal reason for treatment failure, 466-468; taxoid drugs seen as non-cross-resistant to other agents, 505; terminal breast cancer characterized by multidrug resistance, 537-538

duct ectasia, 161-163, 192

ductal carcinoma *in situ* (DCIS): development of, 19-23; *nm23* assays possibly prognostic, 49; DCIS usually detected by patterns of calcification seen on mammograms, 192-193; diagnostic limitations of stereotactic needle biopsies, 211-213; DCIS forerunner of invasive ductal carcinomas, but risk of progression varies from case to case, 234-235; DCIS subtypes cited by pathologists, 235-239, 241; treatment options, 238, 240, 242-243; growth rates (S-phase) vary by subtype, 273; palpable DCIS tumors often have spread through the ductal system, 306; extensive DCIS is a risk factor for local recurrence after lumpectomy, 309; tamoxifen prophylaxis found effective, 437-439; mammographically detected DCIS poses treatment dilemmas, 593-594, 607, 610-611; what patients should be told about DCIS, 614. See also comedo subtype of DCIS

ductal papillomas, 165-166, 172, 194

ductography (galactography), 166, 195, 197

ducts of the mammary gland: lined with epithelial cells, 16, 19-25; anatomical arrangement, 56-57; small terminal ducts, 58; cellular reproduction after menopause, 73; obstruction of ductules leads to cyst formation, 159

Dunne-Daly, Carrie F., 369-370

Dupont, William D., 171-172, 234

Duragesic (brand name), 544

dying cancer patient, 554-555

dysphagia, 553

dyspnea, 528-529, 553-554

Early Breast Cancer Trialists' Collaborative Group, 421-422, 465-466

earwax hypothesis, 97

Eastern Cooperative Oncology Group (ECOG), 429

Eberlein, Timothy J., 336, 358

eczema, 164-165

edema, 169, 257-258. See also lymphedema

Eddy, David M., 599-600

Egan, Robert L., 182-184, 186, 188, 190, 192, 194, 317, 594

Ehrlich, Paul, 448

elastomer (flexible silicone in prostheses), 343-345, 349

electric blankets, 76

electromagnetic fields, 76

electron beams, 363

electron microscope, 215

embedding (specimen preparation), 215

embolisms: definition of, 128

emesis: see vomiting

end-of-dose failure, 542-543

endometrial cancer, 29, 107; danger posed by unopposed estrogen replacement therapy, 123-125, is reduced by adding a progestin, 135-136; oral contraceptives found to be protective, 143-145; risk associated with tamoxifen therapy, 418, 421, 432

endometrium, 65-67, 123, 418

endostatin, 520

epidemiologists: their influence on public health policies, 79-80

epidemiology: definition of, 79; common pitfalls in, 80-82; inability to document small risk factors, 82

epidermal growth factor receptor (EGFR), 50, 276-277, 583

epidural analgesia, 336, 545

epidural tumors, 526-527

epirubicin, 462, 468

epithelial cells, 16, 18

ER: see estrogen receptors

erb oncogene, 42, 50

*erb*B-2 gene: see HER-2/*neu* gene

erysipelas, 561

erythema, 370

erythropoietin, 41, 497

Escherichia coli, 40, 563, 582

esophageal cancer, 107

Estraderm (trademark for estradiol patches), 135

estradiol, 75, 85, 97-98, 105-106, 110; as transdermal hormone replacement, 135; as ligand in ER assay, 269; tamoxifen elevates premenopausal estradiol levels, 419

estriol, 75

estrogen: action on mammary cells, 62-63; receptors for, 64-65; role in menstrual cycle, 65-67, and in pregnancy, 68-71; reduced levels after menopause, 71-73; role in male body, 73-74, and in male

estrogen—*continued*
breast cancer, 74-75; types of estrogen, 75-76; serum estrogen lowered by parity, 85; effect of diet and genetics on estrogen levels, 97-98; elevated estrogen levels in obese women, 105-106; alcohol consumption raises estrogen levels, 110-111; exogenous estrogens suspected in carcinogenesis, 119-121; effect of oral estrogens on hepatic (liver) metabolism, 128, 141-142; loss of ovarian estrogen reduces bone mass, 131-132; benefits and risks of conjugated estrogens, 133-139; synthetic estrogens used in oral contraceptives, 141-142, 150. See also estrogen replacement therapy and oral contraceptives

estrogen insensitivity syndrome, 74

estrogen-progestin regimens (hormone replacement), 124-127, 129-130, 135-138

estrogen receptors (ER) in breast cancer medicine, 64-65; measurement of cellular ER levels predicts likely response to hormonal therapy, 267-269; biochemical (ligand-binding) assay, 269-270, regarded as more precisely quantitative than immunostaining assays, 270-271; about one-third of premenopausal breast tumors are ER-positive, 414; positive assay results do not exclude the possibility of ER-negative tumor cells, 424-425

estrogen receptor-negative (ER-negative) breast tumors: more frequent in younger patients, 118, 270; ER-negativity associated with tumor aggressiveness, 268-269, and with failure to respond to hormonal therapies, 269-270; MF regimen tested in node-negative patients, 486-487; estrogen replacement therapy seen as possibly beneficial, 487

estrogen receptor-positive (ER-positive) breast tumors: possibility of some ER-negative cells not excluded, 424-425; ER-positive postmenopausal patients seen as receiving little benefit from chemotherapy, 427-428; tamoxifen prophylaxis found to be effective, 437

estrogen replacement therapy (ERT): concern about possible carcinogenesis, 119, exemplified by DES, 120-121; Premarin comes to dominate market, 121-123; Dr. Wilson's exaggerated claims for ERT, 122-123; risk of endometrial cancer, 123-124, is reduced by adding a progestin, 124-125; early studies of breast cancer risk, 125-127; ERT believed to protect against cardiovascular disease, 127-131; ERT shown to preserve bone mineral density, 131-133; ERT pondered for breast cancer patients, 134-135; new products, 135; results from Women's Health Initiative largely unfavorable, 135-139

"estrogen window" hypothesis, 91-92

estrone, 75, 85, 97, 105-106, 110

estrus, 65

ethinyl estradiol, 141-142

etidronate, 524

etiology (cause) of cancer, 10, 17

etoposide, 502-503

euthanasia, 550, 552

Evista (brand name for raloxifene), 442

exemestane, 443-444, 446

exercise: seen as reducing breast cancer risk, 106-107

exogenous hormones: definition of, 119

expansile growth pattern (pathology report), 217, 224-227

extended radical mastectomy, 295, 311

extensive intraductal component (EIC), 309

extravasation, 474, 532-533

ex vivo generation of LAK cells, 567, of tumor-infiltrating lymphocytes, 569, and of dendritic cells, 576, 578-579

FAC regimen for breast cancer: concurrent administration during breast irradiation seen as problematic, 375; FAC recommended after cutaneous recurrences, 385; ten-year survival rates reported by M. D. Anderson Cancer Center, 462-463; CALGB trial of dose-intense FAC, 468-469; standard FAC regimen written as a prescription, 473; one patient's experience of side effects, 475; risk of amenorrhea by patient age groups, 485; dose-intense FAC used as induction therapy, 493; effect of FAC chemotherapy on Stage Four survival rates, 517

false-negative readings, 589

false-positive readings, 589; appalling number in BCDDP, 597

familial cancer syndromes: see hereditary cancer

Farber, Sidney, 449-450

Fareston (brand name for toremifene), 441-442

fascia, 58

fat consumption: see dietary fat hypothesis

fat necrosis, 154, 156, 186, 293

fecal occult blood (assay for colon cancer), 590

Feig, Stephen A., 603, 609, 612-613

Feldman, Gayle, 116, 209

Femara (brand name for letrozole), 443-444, 446

femtomoles of estradiol binding per milligram (fmol/mg), 269-270

fentanyl, 541, 544

fertility: effect of chemotherapy on, 484-487

fibroadenomas, 156-157, 171-172, 176, 184, 192

"fibrocystic disease," 159, 170, 194, 597

fields (demarcated areas for radiation therapy), 307, 365-368

filgrastim, 497

film-screen mammography, 182-183

Final Exit (book), 549

fine-needle aspiration of breast masses, 176-178; cardinal rule for, 179; often performed before surgery, 205-206

Fisher, Bernard, 202, 263, 265; as influential chairman of NSABP, 298-303, 309-314; 323, 332, 427, 432-433, 435-438, 455-456, 464, 472, 486, 501

Fisher, Edwin R., 219-220, 226, 242, 260, 263-264, 268, 298-299, 305, 381-382, 558

Five-a-Day ("5-a-Day") campaign, 403-404

Five-FU (5-FU): see fluorouracil

fixation (specimen preparation), 215

"flare": phenomenon observed in DES and tamoxifen therapy, 415, 419, 441

Fletcher, Suzanne W., 604-605, 608

flow cytometry: as staging assay, 274-276; as tool to identify hematopoietic stem cells, 496-498

Flt3 ligand, 579

fluid retention syndrome, 509

fluorescence *in situ* hybridization (FISH), 585-586

fluorouracil (5-FU): suspected antagonistic interaction with tamoxifen, 425-426; drug

tested in early NSABP trials, 455; standard element in Milan CMF regimen, 456-458, 479; implicated in stomatitis, 482, and diarrhea, 483

"focal" tumors suitable for lumpectomy, 304-306

Foley, Kathleen, 539, 545

folic acid antagonists, 450

Folkman, Judah, 221, 519-521

follicle-stimulating hormone (FSH), 65-66, 72

follicular phase, 66-67

follow-up after diagnosis and treatment, 379-380, 391-393

Food and Drug Administration (FDA): its restriction on silicone gel implants, 347-348; vitamin products not rigorously regulated, 396; prophylactic tamoxifen approved, 438; written reports on mammographic examinations required, 613-614

Ford, Betty, 1-2

Fosamax (brand name for alendronate), 524

Fox, Maurice S., 267

fractionation in radiation therapy: rationale for, 364-365

fractions (radiation therapy increments), 307-308, 364-365

Framingham Heart Study, 128-129, 133

Fraumeni, Joseph F., 83

free flaps used in breast reconstruction, 359-361

freehand interventional sonography, 206, 208

free radicals, 396

Frei, Emil, 451-452

Freireich, Emil J., 38, 451-452

Frisch, Rose E., 107

frozen section: definition of, 200-201; less accurate with small nonpalpable cancers, 202-203. See also permanent sections

fruit consumption advocated for cancer prevention, 403-405

FSH: see follicle-stimulating hormone

Fugh-Berman, Adriane, 435

galactoceles, 159

galactography: see ductography

Galen, 288, 314

Gambrell, R. Don, Jr., 126

Ganz, Patricia A., 253

G-CSF (abbreviation): see granulocyte colony-stimulating factor

Gelber, Richard D., 427-428

gel bleed, 349

gene probes, 40

genes: as units of heredity, 32; dominant or recessive, 32-33; DNA as genetic material, 35-36; oncogenes, 42-54; gene amplification in breast cancer, 50-53, 283, 583. See also oncogenes, tumor suppressor genes, *p53*, HER-2/*neu*, and *BRCA1*

genetic diseases, 14-16, 40

genetic profile, 3; essential in staging leukemias and lymphomas, 281; genetic mutations seen as determining likelihood of metastasis, 300

genetic tumor markers, 53

genistein, 404

germ-cell tumors, 454-455

germline genetic defects, 15

Giuliano, Armando E., 329-331

Gleevec (brand name for imatinib mesylate), 29

gliomas: see brain tumors

"Glorious Consensus of 1989" (guidelines for screening mammography), 600

GM-CSF (abbreviation): see granulocyte-macrophage colony-stimulating factor

GnRH (abbreviation): see gonadotropin-releasing hormone

Goldwyn, Robert M., 344

gonadotropin-releasing hormone (GnRH), 65-66, 72; GnRH agonists, 93, 424, 441, 516

goserelin, 441

Goss, Paul E., 443-444

Grady, Deborah, 136

graft-versus-host disease (GVHD), 490

granisetron, 477

granulocyte colony-stimulating factor (G-CSF, filgrastim), 497, 499, 507, 510, 512, 514

granulocyte-macrophage colony-stimulating factor (GM-CSF), 497, 573-575, 578-579

granzymes, 560

grays (radiation dose measurement), 307, 365

Greenberg, Paul A. C., 517

Greenspan, Ezra M., 463-465

growth rates of tumor cell populations: assays used to estimate, 272-276

Gump, Frank E., 245, 305-306

Guy's Hospital trial, 307-308

Gy (abbreviation): see grays

gynecomastia, 74-75

Grunberg, Steven M., 476-477

Haagensen, C. D., 161, 243, 245, 257-258, 295, 297, 329, 380-381

hair dye, 76

hair loss during chemotherapy, 457, 462, 478-480

hairy cell leukemia, 564-565

Haldol (brand name), 476

"halo" encircling benign masses (diagnostic mammography), 184-185

haloperidol, 476, 540, 554

Halsted, William Steward, 62, 257, 262, 264; his innovations in surgical practice, 289-290, and his radical mastectomy, 290-292; Halstedian tradition of breast cancer surgery strong in 1950s and 1960s, 295-297, but refuted by NSABP trials, 297-303, 309-314

H and E (H&E) stain (specimen preparation), 216, 265, 329-330

haploid germ cells, 11

Harris, Jay R., 308-309, 313, 321, 366, 534

Hartrampf, Carl R., Jr., 358-359

hCG (abbreviation): see human chorionic gonadotropin

Health Insurance Plan Project (HIP trial), 594-596, 600, 602

Health Professionals' Follow-Up Study, 109-110, 397

healthy user (confounding factor), 137

Healy, Bernadine, 103-104, 130-131

Heart and Estrogen/progestin Replacement Study (HERS), 136

Hellman, Samuel, 302, 308, 320, 433-434, 454

helper T cells, 560, 574-575. See also lymphocytes

hematologic malignancies, 449-452

hematomas, 154, 156

hematopoiesis, 489

hematoxylin and eosin (H&E stain), 216, 265

Hemlock Society, 549

hemoptysis, 528

hemostasis during breast surgery, 204-205

Henderson, Brian E., 88, 92-93, 104

Henderson, I. Craig, 286, 464, 470, 494, 500

hepatic cancer: see liver cancer

hepatic (liver) metabolism of estrogens, 75, 128, 135, 141-142

hepatic (liver) metastases, 530-532

hepatitis, 9, 565-566

HER-2/*neu* gene: associated with aggressive breast tumors, 49-54; overexpression in node-positive ductal carcinomas linked to chemotherapy resistance, 283-285; Herceptin and chemotherapy tested as adjuvant therapy in HER-2-positive breast cancer, 514, 587; protein peptides used in vaccine trial, 575; related HER family receptors, 583; effect of gene amplification on mammary cells, 583; assays for gene overexpression, 585-586

Herbert, Victor, 397-398, 401

HercepTest (brand name), 585-586

Herceptin (brand name for trastuzumab), 29, 521; NSABP's trial of adjuvant Herceptin in node-positive breast cancer, 514, 586; development of drug, 582-583; response rates and side effects, 583-585; necessity of verifying HER-2 status, 585-586; negative interactions likely from concurrent Adriamycin or fluorouracil, 585-586; optimal duration of Herceptin therapy unknown, 586; thirty-minute infusions recommended, 586-587

hereditary (familial) cancer: in President Carter's family, 17; example of retinoblastoma, 45-47; *p53* gene and Li-Fraumeni syndrome, 47-48; male breast cancer, 74; understanding hereditary breast cancer, 111-113; *BRCA1* and *BRCA2* genes implicated, 113-115; testing and surveillance, 115-116; family history as obstacle to lumpectomy, 317-318; listing of resources for counseling and screening assays, 622-623

Hermann, Robert E., 320-321

heroin, 547

heterozygous: definition of term, 32-33

HIP trial of periodic screening, 594-596, 600, 602

Hippocrates, 288, 518

histological grading of breast tumors, 218

Hodgkin, Thomas, 453

Hodgkin's disease, 29, 78, 319, 453-455,

460-461, 489

Holland, James F., 457-458

Holland, Jimmie, 406

Holmes, Frankie Ann, 506-507, 511

homozygous: definition of term, 33

Hoover, Robert, 125

hormonal therapies for breast cancer, 31; ER assays indicate likelihood of response, 267-271; PgR assays also advisable, 271-272; drugs deprive cancer cells of hormonal stimuli, 412-413; oophorectomies and other surgical ablations, 413-415; DES proves effective as additive strategy, 415-416; androgens used for younger patients, 416; tamoxifen found suitable for adjuvant therapy, 416-419; tamoxifen's effectiveness limited to ER-positive disease, 419-424; rationale for combining tamoxifen with cytotoxic chemotherapy, 424-428; side effects of long-term tamoxifen, 428-432; tamoxifen tested in node-negative patients and as prophylaxis, 432-439; progestins and other therapies after tamoxifen failure, 439-441; raloxifene and other SERMs studied, 441-442; aromatase inhibitors outperform tamoxifen in tumor control, but with higher rate of fractures, 442-447; hormonal therapies in metastatic disease, 516-517

hormones, 62-76; dietary patterns linked to steroid sex hormones, 94-98. See also estrogen and progesterone

Hortobagyi, Gabriel N., 423-424, 485, 494, 500, 504, 516, 524, 586

hospice care, 552-555

hospice organizations and referral services, 623

hospitals: ACS database for cancer hospitals, 620

"hot flashes," 72, 120, 122-123, 441; as tamoxifen side effect, 419, 433

Hughes, L. E., 153, 156, 161, 164, 167

human chorionic gonadotropin (hCG), 68-69, 453, 580

human leukocyte antigens (HLA), 490

human papillomavirus (HPV), 17, 81, 589

humoral immunity, 571, 575

Humphry, Derek, 549

Huntington's disease, 40

hybridomas, 580-581

hypercalcemia, 524, 535-536, 539, 552

hyperchromatic nuclei, 218

hyperplasia, 19-22, 123, 194. See also atypical hyperplasia

hypersensitivity reactions during chemotherapy, 474-475, 506, 586

hyperthermia, 386-387

hypophysectomy, 414

hypothalamus, 65

hypoxia, 364

hydromorphone, 541, 543-544

ibandronate, 524

ibuprofen, 540

IL-2: see interleukin-2

immune response to cancer: absence of convincing evidence for, 406-408, 556-558, but spontaneous remissions in melanomas and renal cell carcinomas have been documented, 557-558

immune surveillance hypothesis, 556, 571

immunohistochemistry: see immunostaining

immunostaining, 51; advantages of, 53-54; ability to detect occult cancer cells in axillary lymph nodes, 265-266, and ER protein in small tumor specimens, 270-271; Ki-67 and MIB-1 assays of growth rates, 275; identification of "micrometastases" in bone marrow, 279; *p53* and HER-2/*neu* assays in breast cancer prognosis, 281-285; immunostaining essential for sentinel node analysis, 329-330

immunotherapies for cancer, 556-587; most tumors not antigenic, 557-558; Coley's toxins cure some sarcomas, 560-562; interferon hyped as cancer cure but proves of limited use, 563-566; Rosenberg et al experiment with LAK cells and tumor-infiltrating lymphocytes, 566-569; single-agent IL-2 approved as therapy for metastatic melanomas and renal cell carcinomas, 570-571; strategies for cancer vaccines, 571-575; dendritic cells seen as key to T cell activation, 575-579; development of monoclonal antibodies, 579-582; Herceptin therapy for HER-2-positive breast cancer, 582-587

implants used in breast reconstruction: types of implants, 342-345; controversy over safety of silicone gel implants, 345-350, leads to litigation, 350-351; silicone exposure suspected in connective-tissue diseases, 351-353; role of tissue expanders, 353-355

indoles, 404

infectious diseases: control of, 8-9, 80, 297, 571-572

infiltrating ductal carcinomas: stepwise development of, 22-25; usual diagnosis in male breast cancer, 74; associated with stromal fibrosis, 154, 156, and contour retraction, 167-168; spiculated mass on mammograms is characteristic, 186-187, 194; most common type identified by "NOS" abbreviation, 223-224; HER-2/*neu* overexpression found mainly in NOS tumors and comedo DCIS, 283-285; sporadic (non-hereditary) ductal tumors usually focal and suitable for lumpectomy, 306

infiltrating lobular carcinomas, 229-231; often multicentric and less suitable for lumpectomy, 306; prone to be missed on mammography, 601

infiltrative border (pathology report), 217, 224

inflammatory breast cancers, 24, 169, 227-229, 257-258, 472-473

infliximab, 582

innate immunity, 559

in situ cancers (pathology report), 233-234

interferon: discovery of, 563; the three types of interferons (alpha, beta, gamma) and their therapeutic applications, 564-566

interleukin-2 (IL-2), 558; a potent T cell growth factor, 567; used in controversial experiments with LAK cells and tumor-infiltrating lymphocytes, 567-569; as standard therapy for metastatic melanomas and renal cell carcinomas, 570-571

interleukin-4 (IL-4), 578

internal mammary nodes, 60-62, 295, 301, 387-388

international variations in cancer rates, 94-96

interval-surfacing tumors during screening mammography: not associated with calcifications, 192; reasons why mammograms fail to detect them, 600-602; differences in tumor biology as one explanation, 610, 612

intraductal carcinoma of the breast: see ductal carcinoma *in situ*
intrathecal analgesia, 545-546
Intron-A (brand name), 565
invasive tumors, 18. See infiltrating ductal and lobular carcinomas
in vitro cultivation of cancer cells, 24, 26
irradiation: see radiation therapy
isoflavonoids, 404

Jaffee, Elizabeth M., 573-574, 576
James, Alice, 289
Japanese: their low incidence of breast, colon, and prostate cancers, 94-98
jaundice, 530
Jenner, Edward, 8, 571
Jensen, Elwood V., 64, 267-268
Joint Center for Radiation Therapy (Boston), 306-309, 313-314, 324-326, 365, 368, 372, 374, 383-384, 534-535
Jordan, V. Craig, 417-418, 424, 437-439, 442

Kaposi's sarcoma, 520, 565
karyotyping: definition of, 36-37; role in cancer medicine, 37-39, 45-46, 51
Kessler, David A., 347-348, 350, 352
Kevorkian, Jack, 549-551
Keynes, Geoffrey, 293-294, 296, 307
Ki-67 immunostaining, 275
kidney cancer: see renal cell carcinoma
killer T cells: see cytotoxic T cells
kinetic factors in chemotherapy, 466
King, Mary-Claire, 113-114
Kinne, David W., 174, 245
Klausner, Richard D., 436, 608
Klinefelter's syndrome, 37, 75
Knudson, Alfred G., Jr., 45-46
Koch, Robert, 8, 80
Kopans, Daniel B., 174, 192, 199, 317, 603-606, 612-613
Kurtz, John M., 383
Kushner, Rose, 145, 173, 175, 202, 302, 378, 459
K-Y jelly (brand name), 487
Kytril (brand name), 477

lactation, 55, 69, 71, 74; effect on breast cancer risk, 88-90
Lagios, Michael D., 234, 238, 240, 242-243, 322
LAK cells, 567-570
Langerhans cells, 576
laparoscopic techniques, 531-532
laparotomy, 531-532
laryngeal cancer, 16, 295, 316
Lasser, Terese, 201
Laszlo, John, 203, 218, 406, 408, 452
latissimus dorsi flap, 358
laxatives, 541
LCIS: see lobular carcinoma *in situ*
lead-time bias, 592-593, 595
letrozole, 443-444, 446
leukapheresis, 497-498, 567, 570
leukemias, 18, 29-30, 37-39, 275, 281, 319-320, 449-452, 467, 490, 500, 582
leukocytes (white cells), 556-560, 563-564, 575-576, 579
Levy, Michael H., 543-544
LH: see luteinizing hormone
Li, Min Chiu, 453
Liberman, Laura, 211
Lichter, Allen S., 376
Li-Fraumeni syndrome, 47-48
life expectancy: gains in, 7-9, 63
ligand-binding assay to measure ER levels, 269-270
light microscope, 215-216
linear accelerators, 363
linkage analysis, 113
lipomas, 184
Lippman, Marc E., 64, 228-229, 270, 376
liver cancer, 17, 448, 467. See also hepatic (liver) metastases
liver scans, 390, 531
liver surgery for hepatic metastases, 531-532
living wills, 551-552
loading doses, 527, 534, 587
lobes of mammary gland, 56-57
lobular carcinoma *in situ* (LCIS), 234, 243-245, 305; tamoxifen prophylaxis seen as effective, 437-439
lobular neoplasia (old term for LCIS), 243
lobular tumors (invasive), 229-231, 306, 601

lobules, 56-57, 68-69

"Look Good—Feel Better" program, 480, 619-620

lorazepam, 476-478, 540

Love, Medicine & Miracles, 408-409

Love, Richard R., 419, 429-431

Love, Susan, 159, 608

low-fat diet: see dietary fat hypothesis

L-PAM (abbreviation for L-phenylalanine mustard), 455-456

"lump in the breast": dominant masses usually benign, 152, but also typical presentation of infiltrating cancers, 153-154; characteristics associated with benign masses, 156-157; distinction between lumpiness and lumps (true masses) often hard to make, 169-170; mammographic appearances of benign and malignant masses, 184-189; normal breast "usually lumpy on palpation," 618. See also abscesses, atypical hyperplasia, cysts, duct ectasia, eczema, fat necrosis, fibroadenomas, galactoceles, hematomas, lipomas, mastitis, nipple discharges, papillomas, phyllodes tumors, and sclerosing adenosis

lumpectomy: as treatment for ductal carcinoma *in situ*, 238, 240, 242-243; lumpectomy rates vary by geographical region, 247-250; first experiments with breast preservation and radiation therapy, 293-294; sporadic (non-hereditary) ductal tumors usually suitable for breast preservation, 303-306, but lobular carcinomas often multicentric, 306; Joint Center radiotherapists develop standard regimens for breast preservation, 306-309; NSABP Protocol B-06 finds lumpectomy equivalent to mastectomy in overall survival, 309-312; indications for lumpectomy, 316-320; breast radiotherapy cannot be repeated, 320; NSABP guidelines for lumpectomy, 323-324; importance of cancer-free margins, 324-326; recovery from lumpectomy, 337, and from axillary dissection, 338, 340-341; preoperative chemotherapy increases proportion of eligible patients, 472-473

lumpectomy without radiation therapy: NSABP Protocol B-06 documents increased risk of local recurrence, but no significant differences in overall survival, 309-312; Cleveland Clinic experience favorable, 320-321, but large tumor size and poor nuclear grade associated with local recurrences in breast, 321-322

"lumpy breasts," 169-170, 618

lung cancer, 16, 24, 82, 107, 400, 448, 506, 590-591, 593

luteal phase of menstrual cycle, 66-67, 91-92

luteinizing hormone (LH), 66, 68, 72

lymph: definition of, 59

lymph nodes: function of, 59-60; nodal chains involved in breast drainage, 60-62; not barriers to tumor dissemination, 298-300. See also axillary lymph nodes and axillary dissections

lymphangitic carcinomatosis, 528-529

lymphatic drainage of the breast: role in dissemination of cancer cells, 19-28, 58; explanation of lymphatic system, 59-62; drainage interrupted by breast surgery, 337-338, 340-341

lymphatic invasion as prognostic factor (pathology report), 220

lymphedema of arm after axillary dissection, 295-296, 300, 327; strategies to prevent complications, 329, 340-341

lymphocytes: definition of, 59-60; lymphocyte activity seen as associated with better prognosis, 406-408; three main types of lymphocyte, 559-560; Rosenberg et al attempt to induce lymphocyte reactivity to tumors, 566-569; responses to IL-2 therapy probably mediated by lymphocytes, 570-571. See also B cells and T cells

lymphocytic reaction (pathology report), 217

lymphokines, 564

lymphomas, 18, 29, 38, 43, 232-233, 275, 281, 449, 489-490, 500, 580-582

Lynch, Eileen P., 336

Lynch, Henry T., 111, 114, 622

MAbs: see monoclonal antibodies

MacMahon, Brian, 83

macrophages, 59, 559, 575, 578-579

magnetic resonance imaging (MRI): as supplemental examination to mammography,

196, 198, 317; use of MRI in searching for disseminated disease, 390, 392, and in diagnosing epidural tumors, 527, and brain metastases, 533

magnification mammography, 161, 195, 614

major histocompatibility complex (MHC), 575-576

male breast cancer, 1, 73-75, 114, 153, 228

malignancy: definition of, 10, 15-18

mammary gland: its tiny ducts, 16; stepwise malignant transformation in, 18-25; anatomy of, 55-58; a paired organ, 56; constant activity in premenopausal women, 62-64; why prone to malignancy, 62-64; hormonal responsiveness of, 62-65; changes during the menstrual cycle, 66-67, during pregnancy, 68-71, and after menopause, 72-73; mitotic rates in, 67; differentiation accomplished by full-term pregnancy, 68-69; rudimentary glandular tissues in men, 73-75; suspected carcinogens, 76-77; radiation carcinogenesis, 77-78; effect of parity, 84-85, of abortion, 85-87, of lactation, 88-90, of high-fat diet, 91, and of regular ovulation, 91-93; parenchymal densities seen on mammograms, 98; hormone replacement therapy increases mitotic activity, 125-126, but postmenopausal estrogen not a major cancer risk, 133-134, 139; effect of oral contraceptives on mitotic rates, 150; glandular tissue concentrated in upper outer quadrant and nipple area, 153, 155; calcifications a byproduct of aging, 189, but some patterns suggestive of malignancy, 190-195. See also breast cancer and "lump in the breast"

mammography: its ability to visualize postmenopausal ducts, 73; images affected by high-fat diet, 98, and by hormone replacement therapy, 125-126; how mammography works, 181-182; the three standard exposures, 183; avoiding radiological artifacts, 183-184; interpretation of mammograms, 184-189, and communication of results, 189; calcifications as clues, 189-195; magnification and spot compression, 195; ductography, 195, 197; digital mammography, 198, 612-613; reasons for false negatives, 198-199; changes seen after breast irradiation often suggestive of recurrent cancer, 373; mammographic accuracy highly operator-dependent, 591-592; ways to reduce false negatives and false positives, 613-614. See also diagnostic mammography and screening mammography

Mammography Quality Standards Act, 199

mammoplasty and mastopexy (breast reconstruction), 356

Mansfield, Carl M., 365, 368, 383-384

Margolese, Richard G., 322-324, 326-327

marijuana: as chemotherapy antiemetic, 477

marimastat, 520

Marinol (brand name), 477

mastectomy: still the prevalent surgical therapy in some areas, 248-250; earliest recorded operations, 288-289; Halsted's radical mastectomy, 289-292, eventually replaced by total (simple) mastectomy, 292-303; current indications for mastectomy, 315-316; the different types of mastectomy, 331-334; undergoing surgery, 334-337; postoperative drainage, 337-338, and arm exercises, 338; local tumor recurrences after mastectomy, 384-387. See also radical mastectomy, modified radical mastectomy, and lumpectomy

mastitis (breast inflammation), 161-162, 167, 169

matrix metalloproteinases, 519-520

McClintock, Barbara, 35

McCraw, John B., 356, 358

McGuire, William L., 64, 270, 272, 276, 433-434

MDR: abbreviation for multidrug resistance, 466; *MDR1* gene, 466-467. See also drug resistance

mediolateral position (mammography), 183, 595-596

mediolateral oblique position (mammography), 183, 599, 602

meditation as treatment adjuvant, 406, 410-411

Mediterranean diet, 102-103

medroxyprogesterone acetate (progestin), 124, 130, 135, 148

medullary breast cancers, 188, 217, 225-226

Megace (brand name for megestrol acetate), 440, 443, 516, 536-537

megestrol acetate (progestin), 440. See Megace

melanoma, 16, 48, 329-330, 400, 506; recognized

melanoma—*continued*
as immunogenic cancer, 557-558; 565; documented responses in LAK cell and TIL experiments, 567-569, but single-agent IL-2 becomes standard therapy, 570-571; CancerVax vaccine tested, 572-573; skin self-examination urged for early detection, 591

memory cells, 562, 571-572

menarche, 90-93

Mendel, Gregor, 32-33, 80

Mendenhall, Nancy Price, 366, 368, 373, 375, 385-386

meninges, 532-533; meningeal carcinomatosis in breast cancer, 533-534

meningiomas, 533

menopause, 71-73; advent of estrogen replacement therapy, 121-123

menses, 65

menstrual cycle, 65-67, 85-86, 89-90, 123

menstrual history: as risk factor for breast cancer, 90-93

menstruation, 65, 123

mestranol, 141-142

metastasis: definition of, 18; outmoded belief in mechanical dissemination of cancer cells, 200-201, 291; nonmammary metastases presenting in the breast, 232-233; bone marrow most likely site for breast cancer dissemination, 278-280; lymph nodes not barrier to metastasis, 298-300

metastatic disease (Stage Four breast cancer): development of, 18, 24-28; as the "M" in TNM classification, 258-260; follow-up on high-risk patients, 378-380; Haagensen's statistics on breast cancer metastases, 380; detection of metastases in contralateral (other) breast, 382, and in the lungs, skeleton (bones), liver, and brain, 389-390; CAT and MRI scans ineffective at detecting early systemic disease, 392; multidrug resistance as cause of treatment failure, 466; high-dose chemotherapy with marrow or PBSC support widely used in 1990s, 488-500, but randomized trials fail to demonstrate significant benefits, 500-504; paclitaxel (Taxol) and docetaxel (Taxotere) used for Stage Four patients, 508-513; rules of thumb for assessment of prognosis, 515-516; the indications for hormonal therapy or for chemotherapy, 516-518; prevention of complications from skeletal (osseous) metastases, 522-525, from spinal cord compression, 525-527, and from lung, liver, and brain involvement, 527-535; management of hypercalcemia, anorexia, and cachexia, 535-537; possible causes of death, 538; pain control through analgesics, 539-548; Herceptin tested for HER-2-positive disease, 583-585

Metastron (brand name for strontium 89), 523

methotrexate: early use in leukemia regimens, 450-452, and for choriocarcinoma, 453; incorporated in CMF regimen, 456-457, and in FAC-M, 464-465; patients advised to drink fluids, 475; drug associated with diarrhea, 483

metoclopramide, 476-477

Meyer, John S., 67, 73, 220, 273

MF regimen, 486

MIB-1 immunostaining, 275

microscopy of tissue specimens, 215-216

microtubules, 505

microvessel density as angiogenesis assay, 221-222

microtome, 215

milk secretion, 68-71

Miller, Anthony B., 602-604, 609-610

"minimal" breast cancer, 321-322, 598

Mini-Pills (progestin-only oral contraceptives), 148

miscarriage, 85, 87

Mitchell, Joyce Slayton, 475

mitomycin, 513, 518

mitosis, 19, 33-34, 36, 84

mitotic figures and mitotic indexing, 273

mitotic rates in mammary gland, 67, 69, 84; noticeably higher in tumors with poor nuclear grade, 220

mitotic spindle, 36, 505

mitoxantrone, 502-503, 518

modified radical mastectomy: early use at the Cleveland Clinic, 292-293, 295-296; endorsed by Dr. Urban, 302-303; Patey-type procedure not favored by NSABP, 331-333

Moertel, Charles G., 399, 408, 568

molecular margins, 325-326

monoclonal antibodies (MAbs): development of, 579-580; diagnostic and therapeutic applications, 580-582; chimeric and humanized MAbs, 582; Herceptin first MAb used in breast cancer therapy, 582-587

monounsaturated fat, 100, 102-103

Montague, Eleanor D., 307

MOPP regimen for Hodgkin's disease, 453-454

Morgan, Thomas Hunt, 33-34

morphine, 541-544

Morrison, Alan S., 598

Morrow, Monica, 154-156, 238

Morton, Donald L., 557, 572-573

Moskowitz, Myron, 184, 186, 188, 194-195, 603

MRI: see magnetic resonance imaging

mucin: secretion of, 188, 226

mucinous breast cancers, 188, 226-227, 601

mucins, 575

multicentric breast tumors: definition of, 245; less suitable for lumpectomy, 304-306, 317; higher risk of contralateral tumorigenesis, 382

multidrug resistance (MDR), 466-468, 505, 537-538

multifocal breast tumors, 304-306

multiple births, 85-86

multiple myeloma, 467, 580

multiple sclerosis (MS), 548, 556, 565

Mundy, Gregory, 523-524

muscular dystrophy, 15, 33, 35, 40

mutations: in somatic cells, 15-17, 29, 37-39; in colon cancer, 44, 47-48; in breast cancer, 46-54; during pregnancy, 84; in hereditary breast and ovarian cancers, 111-116

myc oncogene, 42-43, 47

myelogram, 526-527

myeloma, 467, 580

myelosuppression, 489

Mylotarg (brand name), 582

Nabholtz, Jean-Marc, 513

nadir in cytotoxic chemotherapy, 480-481

naloxone, 541

Napoli, Maryann, 607

naproxen, 540

National Breast Cancer Coalition, 621

National Cancer Institute (NCI): its close association with NSABP breast cancer trials, 297-298, 426, 428-429, 433; its role in developing curative regimens for childhood leukemia and Hodgkin's disease, 451-454; listing of NCI patient resources, 620-621. See also Consensus Development Conferences

National Library of Medicine: its Internet-accessible resources, 622

National Surgical Adjuvant Breast and Bowel Project (NSABP): investigates HER-2/*neu* overexpression, 53; emphasizes nuclear grading of breast tumors, 219-220; Protocol B-17 recommends lumpectomy and irradiation for ductal carcinoma *in situ*, 242; Protocol B-04 findings on positive nodes, 262-264, and axillary dissections, 265; NSABP trials intended to resolve issues in breast cancer medicine, 297-298; Bernard Fisher et al overturn Halstedian doctrine on the regional lymph nodes, 298-300; Protocol B-04 ends era of radical breast surgery, 301-303; only 13.4% of "clinically overt" breast tumors found to be multicentric, 305; Protocol B-06 finds lumpectomy to be equivalent to mastectomy in overall survival, 309-312; NSABP position on breast cancer surgery, 313-314, and its guidelines for lumpectomy, 323-324, 326; NSABP finds low risk of contralateral recurrences, 381-382; Protocol B-09 demonstrates value of ER assays, 420, 424; Protocol B-16 recommends AC regimen and tamoxifen for node-positive postmenopausal patients, 426-427; Protocol B-20 finds a small benefit from chemotherapy in node-negative, ER-positive patients, 427-428; Protocol B-14 finds no benefit from extending tamoxifen beyond five years, 428-429, and documents a small risk of thrombosis, 430; NSABP's interpretation of B-14 data sparks a controversy, 432-434; Protocol P-1 finds prophylactic tamoxifen reduces risk of ER-positive breast cancer, 434-439; Protocol P-2 compares tamoxifen and raloxifene in breast cancer prevention, 442; early NSABP chemotherapy trials find benefit only for premenopausal

National Surgical Adjuvant Breast and Bowel Project—*continued*
patients, 455-456; Protocol B-16 finds AC regimen "seems preferable" to CMF, 464-465; Protocol B-18 results on preoperative chemotherapy, 472-473; Protocol B-13 tests MF regimen, 486-487; Protocol B-19 finds CMF superior to MF, 486-487; Protocols B-22 and B-25 find cyclophosphamide dose escalation to be ineffective, 501; Protocol B-26 reports advantages from 24-hour paclitaxel infusions, 510-511; NASBP trials combine AC regimen in several combinations with paclitaxel (Protocols B-28 and B-31) and docetaxel (Protocols B-27 and B-30); rationale behind Protocol B-31 scheduling of Herceptin, 586; Protocol B-35 compares tamoxifen and anastrozole, 620-621

nausea (chemotherapy side effect), 475-478

NCI: see National Cancer Institute

necrosis as marker of tumor aggressiveness, 217, 224, 235, 238, 241

negative nodes in breast cancer: overexpression of HER-2/*neu* and *p53* genes may affect prognosis, 52-53, 281-285; lymphatic invasion seen as identifying patients at risk, 220; nodal status as expressed in TNM classification, 258-259; tumor size affects risk of metastatic spread, 261-262; occult nodal involvement often missed with H&E staining, 265; sentinel node sampling eliminates need for axillary dissection, 265-266; high S-phase as marker of risk, 274; most tumors cured by local therapy, but some risk factors may justify chemotherapy, 286-287; NSABP Protocol B-14 finds modest benefit from tamoxifen therapy, but Dr. McGuire is skeptical, 432-434; VEGF levels seen as prognostic, 519

Nelson, Kristine A., 522, 533, 554-555

neoadjuvant (preoperative) chemotherapy, 472-473, 514

neoplasms, 557

nerve blocks, 545

neu oncogene, 49-50

neuropathies, 507, 581

neuropraxia, 338

neutropenia, 480-481

neutrophils, 480-481, 559, 579

Newcomb, Polly A., 89

Newton-John, Olivia, 2

NIH: abbreviation for National Institutes of Health

nipple: outlet for mammary ducts, 56-57, 164; nipple symptoms often nonspecific, 162, 164-166, but retraction suggestive of pathological process, 164

nipple discharges, 152, 162, 165-166

nipple-areola complex, 164; how affected by Paget's disease, 227-228; reconstruction of, 361-362

nitrogen mustard, 449, 455

nm23 gene, 48-49, 53

nodal skip metastases, 327, 330

nodular densities in the breast, 170, 597. See also "lump in the breast"

Nolvadex (brand name for tamoxifen), 418. See tamoxifen

nonpalpable lesions in the breast: biopsy techniques for, 208-213; nonpalpable invasive cancers usually prove node-negative, 598

nonsteroidal anti-inflammatory drugs (NSAIDs), 540-541

Noone, R. Barrett, 353-355

Norplant (brand name), 148

Northern blot, 51-52

NOS or NST abbreviation (pathology report), 224, 283, 286-287

"Not Self": immune response to, 407

Nowell, Peter C., 37

NSABP: see National Surgical Adjuvant Breast and Bowel Project

NSAIDs: see nonsteroidal anti-inflammatory drugs

NST abbreviation: same as NOS. See NOS or NST abbreviation

nuclear grade (prognostic factor in breast cancer): relationship to HER-2/*neu* overexpression, 53; systems of grading, 218-220; poor nuclear grade correlated with high S-phrase, 273-274

nucleoli, 219-220

nucleus of cell: definition of, 12-13; appearance of nuclei in malignant cells, 19-25; chromosomes visible during mitosis, 33-34; how pathologists evaluate nuclei, 218-220

Nuland, Sherwin B., 518
nulliparity, 83. See also parity
numbness after breast surgery, 340
nuns: their high incidence of postmenopausal breast cancer, 83
Nurses' Health Study, 83-84, 88, 90; controversial findings on the relationship between dietary fat and breast cancer, 99-101; findings on premenopausal obesity, 105-106, on smoking, 107-108, on alcohol consumption, 108, 110, on hereditary breast cancer, 111-113, on estrogen replacement therapy, 127-129, 134, on oral contraceptives, 146, on atypical hyperplasia, 171, on silicone gel breast implants, 351-352, and on vitamin E prophylaxis, 397

obesity: as breast cancer risk factor, 82, 104-106
O'Connor, Sandra Day, 255
oliguria, 536
olive oil, 102-103
oncogenes: carried by retroviruses, 42-43; three-letter names for, 42; emphasis on *ras*, 44; acceleration of cell growth by, 45
oncologists, 17-18, 461; consultations with, 469-471
oncology: definition of, 17
ondansetron, 477
oophorectomy, 93, 125, 129; as hormonal manipulation in breast cancer, 413-415, 423, 440-441
opioid drugs (opioid agonists), 539; their mode of action, 540-541; misconceptions about, 541-542; alternatives to oral morphine, 543-545; misplaced concerns regarding "addiction" hamper pain control, 546-548; drug administration to dying patients, 554
oral cancer, 82
oral contraceptives (OCs): fallacious association with cervical cancer, 81; their mode of action, 140-141; advantages of, 141; different formulations for, 141-142; protective against benign breast lesions as well as against ovarian and endometrial cancers, 143-144; any breast cancer risk limited to young nulliparous users, 144-

151; progestin-only contraceptives, 148-149; elevation of breast mitotic rates seen in nulliparous OC users, 150; identifying women who should not use OCs, 150-151
oral hygiene during chemotherapy, 482-483
orchiectomy, 414-415
Oregon Death with Dignity Act, 550-551
organelles of cell, 12-13
organochlorines, 77
O'Rourke, Mark A., 547
Osborne, C. Kent, 270, 425, 439-440
osseous (skeletal) metastases, 516, 522-527
Osteen, Robert T., 228-229
osteoblasts, 430
osteoclasts, 523-525
osteocytes, 131-133
osteoporosis, 74, 93, 104; estrogen replacement therapy shown to be protective, 131-133, 136, 138-139; tamoxifen probably protective in postmenopausal women, 430-432, 438; raloxifene approved as prophylaxis, 442; alendronate (Fosamax) and other bisphosphonates studied, 524
osteosarcoma, 46, 295, 316, 462
"other breast" (contralateral) tumorigenesis, 381-382; tamoxifen helpful in preventing, 421-422, and aromatase inhibitors even more effective, 444-446
outpatient mastectomy, 336-337
ovarian cancer, 30, 52-53, 114-115, 448; oral contraceptives protective, 142-145; germ-cell tumors curable by chemotherapy, 454; paclitaxel (Taxol) indicated after cisplatin failure, 506, 508
overall survival (OS): definition of, 52
overdiagnosis due to screening assays, 592-593
overexpression of gene product, 50-53
ovulation: associated with increasing breast cancer risk, 89, 91-93; erratic ovulation in obese women linked to reduced risk, 106
oxycodone, 541, 543
oxytocin, 71

p53 gene: see p-fifty-three gene
Pacific yew, 505-508
paclitaxel (Taxol): P-glycoprotein linked to drug resistance, 468; bone marrow suppression

paclitaxel (Taxol)—*continued*
usually transient, 481; drug is innovation, 488; history of its development, 505-508; side effects, 506-507; approved for metastatic breast cancer, 508; experiments with dose and scheduling, 509-511; used with Adriamycin, 511-512, and with NSABP's AC regimen, 513-514, 584-586

Page, David L., 19, 158, 171-172, 218, 230, 234, 242, 245

Paget, James, 164, 227

Paget's disease (presentation of ductal breast cancer), 164-165, 227-228

pain control in advanced cancer: possible causes of pain, 539; types of analgesics and adjuvant agents, 539-540; WHO Analgesic Ladder, 540-541; around-the-clock dosing of morphine and other opioid drugs, 541-543; alternatives to oral morphine, 543-545; neurosurgery, nerve blocks, and spinal opioids, 545-546; governmental restrictions on opioids seen as detrimental, 546-548; aggressive pain management may hasten death, 552; relieving symptoms in debilitated or dying patients, 553-555; American Pain Foundation, 623

palliation: definition of, 516. See also metastatic disease and pain control

palpation of the breast: techniques for, 174; palpation outperforms screening mammography in HIP trial, 594-596, but not in BCDDP, 596-597; CNBSS trial finds palpation equivalent to mammography in mortality reduction, but finding is highly controversial, 602-604, 609-610. See also breast self-examination

pamidronate, 524-525, 536, 540

pancreatic cancer, 17, 448, 545

papillary carcinomas, 166, 227

papillomas, 165-166, 172, 227

Pap smear, 29, 591

paraffin-embedding of permanent sections, 215

paraneoplastic syndromes, 535-537

parathyroid hormone-related protein (PHrP), 523-524, 535

paravertebral block, 336

parity: definition of, 68; protective against postmenopausal breast cancer, 83-85

Parker, Steve H., 210-213

parturition, 69

PAS: see physician-assisted suicide

Pasteur, Louis, 8, 571

Patey-type mastectomy, 332-333

pathologists: their role in cancer medicine, 214-215

pathology report: understanding the terms used, 214-245; recording specimen size, 216-217; central necrosis and infiltrative border seen as ominous, 217; histological and nuclear grading, 218-220; lymphatic invasion, 220-221; assay for angiogenesis, 221-222, and other prognostic assays, 223; types of invasive breast tumors, 223-231; sarcomas and other rare malignancies, 231-233; dilemma posed by *in situ* breast cancers, 233-234; ductal carcinoma *in situ*, 234-243, and lobular carcinoma *in situ*, 243-245

patient-controlled analgesia (PCA), 544-546

Pauling, Linus, 398-399

PBSCs: see peripheral blood stem cells

PCA pumps, 544-546

PCR: see polymerase chain reaction

peau d'orange ("orange skin"), 169, 228

pectoralis major muscle, 58

pectoralis minor muscle, 58

pedicle flaps, 357-359

peginterferon, 566

peptides in cancer vaccine strategies, 574-579

Percocet (brand name), 541

percutaneous vertebroplasty, 527

Perez-Mesa, Carlos M., 226-227, 230, 235, 243

perforin, 560

pericardial effusions, 530

perimenopause, 71-72

peripheral blood mononuclear cells (PBMCs), 578

peripheral blood stem cells (PBSCs), 488; techniques for harvesting PBSCs, 496-498; advantages of PBSCs over bone marrow transplantation, 498-500

permanent sections, 202-203, 215-216

pesticide residues as possible carcinogens, 76-77

PET: see positron emission tomography

Peters, Vera, 293-294, 307

Peters, William P., 490, 492-494, 498-499, 502-503

Petrakis, Nicholas L., 97

Petrek, Jeanne A., 232, 376-377

p-fifty-three—*p53*—gene, 47-48, 53, 281-283, 326, 590, 601, 612

P-glycoprotein (P-gp), 466-468

PgR: see progesterone receptors

phagocytes, 559

pharmaceutical sanctuaries in chemotherapy, 466

Phase One trials, 491-492, 500, 502, 506, 509, 512, 574-575, 578-579; Phase Two trials, 583-584; Phase Three (randomized) trials, 500-503, 575, 582, 584-585

phenothiazines, 476-477

phenotype, 32

Philadelphia chromosome, 37-39

Philadelphia Intergroup trial, 501-502, 504

photodynamic therapy, 387

phyllodes tumors, 158, 231-232

physical activity and breast cancer risk, 91

physician-assisted suicide (PAS), 548-551

physician directories, 622

Pierson, K. Kendall, 219-220, 224-225

Pike, Malcolm C., 86-87, 92, 145

"Pill": see oral contraceptives

pituitary gland, 65, 69, 71, 89; surgical removal as hormonal manipulation, 414

placebo effect, 406

placenta, 68, 71

plasma cells, 579

plasma membrane of cell, 12-13

plastic surgeons, 342-346, 348, 353-355

Platinol (brand name for cisplatin), 454

pleomorphic nuclei, 218

pleural effusions, 529-530

pleurodesis, 529-530

ploidy as prognostic assay, 275-276

Plotkin, David, 591, 606

PMS (premenstrual syndrome), 67

polycystic ovary syndrome, 106

polymerase chain reaction (PCR), 41, 326, 590

polymorphonuclear granulocytes, 480

polyunsaturated fat, 100, 102

polyurethane foam in breast implants, 344-345, 347

point mutations in genes, 47-48

Poisson, Roger, 311-312

portable infusion pumps, 544-546

positive nodes in breast cancer: plausible indicator of metastatic potential, 24, 27; relation to HER-2/*neu* amplification, 52-53; nodal status as expressed in TNM classification, 258-259; NSABP findings on prognostic significance of positive nodes, 262-265; high S-phase as risk factor for recurrence, 274; debate over value of *p53* and HER-2/*neu* assays, 281-285; full-dose chemotherapy seen as essential for optimal survival benefit, 468-470

positive thinking as treatment adjuvant, 394, 408-411

positron emission tomography (PET), 531

Postmenopausal Estrogen/Progestin Interventions Trial (PEPI), 130

Poulson, Jane, 478-479

power of attorney for health care, 552

prednisolone, 490, 540

prednisone, 450-454, 456, 540

pregnancy: effects on uterus and breast, 68-71; protective against breast cancer, 83-86; useless DES prophylaxis, 120-121; scheduling chemotherapy or irradiation during pregnancy, 375-377

Premarin (trademark for conjugated estrogens), 121-123, 125, 130, 134-135, 138-139

Prempro (trademark), 135-136, 138-139

primary lymphomas of the breast, 233

Princess Margaret Hospital (Toronto), 293, 320-321, 325

PRN dose, 542-544

prochlorperazine, 476

progesterone: its effect on mammary cells, 62-63; receptors for, 64-65; its role in menstrual cycle, 66-67, and pregnancy, 68-71; synergistic with estrogen in the mammary gland, 92, but counteracts mitotic stimuli in the endometrium, 123, 126; effect of micronized progesterone on HDL cholesterol, 130

progesterone receptors (PgR) in breast cancer medicine, 64-65, 118, 271-272, 422, 424, 428

progestins, 66; in hormone replacement therapy, 124-127, 129-130, 135-138; in combined oral contraceptives, 141-142, and in progestin-only contraceptives, 148-149; as second-line hormonal therapy for breast cancer, 416, 440

prognosis in breast cancer: see staging and prognosis

prolactin, 69, 71, 85, 89

Proleukin (brand name for aldesleukin), 570

prophylactic mastectomy: hereditary (familial) breast cancer as possible indication, 115-116, 318, 612; Dr. Drife's observations on, 316; total (simple) mastectomy and other procedures, 333-334; free-flap TRAM reconstructions, 360; tamoxifen prophylaxis offers less protection, 437

prostaglandins, 535

prostate cancer, 24, 63, 94-95, 115, 448, 589-590

prostate-specific antigen (PSA), 390-391, 590

proteases, 22, 24

proteins: manufacture directed by DNA, 35-36; abnormal proteins as cause of cancer, 39, 50-51; immunostaining to detect protein abnormalities, 53-54

proton beams, 363

proto-oncogenes, 43-44

Provera (brand name for medroxyprogesterone), 124, 130

pseudo-pregnancy, 85

ptosis, 72

quadrantectomy, 324

quadrants of the breast, 153, 155

Quill, Timothy E., 549

radial scar, 186

radiation absorbed dose ("rads"), 307-310, 365

radiation carcinogenesis, 77-78; risk from mammograms "probably not measurable," 181

radiation therapy, 29-30, 78; possible indications after lumpectomy for ductal carcinoma *in situ*, 240, 242-243; early experiments with breast preservation, 293-294; irradiation after mastectomy seen as having no effect on survival rates, 300-301; the Joint Center's regimen for breast preservation, 306-309; the NSABP finds irradiation after lumpectomy improves local control, but not overall survival, 309-312; side effects of breast irradiation, 319-320; how radiation destroys cancer cells, 363-364; therapy given in fractions to well-delineated fields, 364-368; irradiating large breasts and regional lymph nodes, 368-369; management of skin reactions, 370-371; long-term cosmetic results of breast preservation, 371-372; follow-up after lumpectomy and breast irradiation, 372-373; scheduling breast irradiation during chemotherapy or during pregnancy, 374-377; radiation regimens to control cutaneous (skin) recurrences, 385-387, and regional nodal involvement, 387-388; irradiation used to manage skeletal (bone) metastases, 522-523, and to prevent spinal cord compression, 527; whole-organ tolerance of the lungs limited, but small areas can be irradiated, 528-529; irradiation for palliation of brain metastases, 534-535. See also lumpectomy and lumpectomy without radiation therapy

radical mastectomy: traditional therapy for breast malignancies, 200-201; controversies about, 202-203; observations of treatment failure, 257-258; what was "radical" about Halsted's procedure, 289-292; development of an "extended" operation (Urban procedure), 294-295; George Crile, Jr., attacks radical breast surgery, 295-297; results from NSABP trials end the era of radical mastectomy, 297-303; false rationale behind radical operations, 313-314; locally advanced (Stage Three) tumors seen as possible indication, 331. See also modified radical mastectomy and total (simple) mastectomy

radiofrequency ablation (RFA), 532

radiotherapy: see radiation therapy

radium, 364

rads (abbreviation for radiation absorbed dose), 307-310, 365

raloxifene, 442

Ramazzini, Bernardino, 83

ras oncogene, 42-44, 590

Rb tumor suppressor gene, 45-47

"Reach to Recovery" program, 201, 339, 619

Reagan, Nancy, 2, 316

reassurance: not to be confused with diagnosis, 178-179

"rebounds" in hormonal therapy of breast cancer, 416

recall bias, 81

Recht, Abram, 308-309, 366, 373-374, 383-384

recombinant DNA technology, 40-41, 119, 563

recurrence of breast cancer: the two main categories, 378-379; follow-up surveillance of patients, 379-380; *de novo* tumors in contralateral breast, 381-382; recurrences in preserved breast, 382-384, in skin flaps after mastectomy, 384-387, and in the regional lymph nodes, 387-388; tests used to search for distant metastases, 389-391; intensive surveillance usually not warranted, 391-393; evaluation of metastatic disease, 515-516

red meat, 94-96, 102-103, 403

Redmond, Carol, 314

Reed-Sternberg cells, 453-455

Reglan (brand name), 476-477

renal cell (kidney) carcinoma: reason for resistance to chemotherapy, 467; occasional spontaneous remissions documented, 558; responses in LAK cell experiments, but single-agent IL-2 becomes therapy for metastatic disease, 570-571

rescue dose (PRN dose) of opioid analgesics, 542-544

retinoblastoma, 45-47

retinoids, 400-402

retraction of breast contour, 167-168, 174

ribonucleic acid (RNA), 51-52

"Right-to-Die" controversy, 548-551

risedronate, 524

Rituxan (brand name), 582

rituximab, 582

Rivkin, Saul E., 426-427

Rockefeller, Happy, 1-2, 304

Rockefeller, John D., Jr., 560, 562

Roferon-A (brand name), 564-565

Rosato, Francis E., 164-165

Rose, David P., 101

Rose, Mary Ann, 372

Rosen, Paul Peter, 166, 217, 220, 227, 229-230, 235, 261-262, 282, 305, 381

Rosenberg, Steven A., 566-571

Ross, Ronald K., 75-76, 88, 125

Rotter's nodes, 62, 302-303

Rous sarcoma virus, 42

Russo, Irma H., 69

Sabin and Salk polio vaccines, 9

Saint Gallen conference, 428-429

saline implants, 344, 347-348, 352-355

salvage therapy: definition of, 412

sarcomas: definition of, 18; sarcomas arising in the breast, 231-232; Coley's toxin therapy obtains some cures, 560-562

sargramostim, 497

saturated fat, 96-103

Schatzkin, Arthur, 100, 108

schedule-dependent toxicity (chemotherapy), 511

scheduling of paclitaxel (Taxol) and docetaxel (Taxotere), 509-513

schistosomiasis, 75

Schnipper, Hester Hill, 246

Schnitt, Stuart J., 235, 240, 243

scirrhous ductal carcinomas, 154, 217, 224

sclerosing adenosis, 158, 172, 186, 194, 225

screening asymptomatic individuals for cancer, 589-594

screening mammography, 588-614; definition of, 180, 588; multiple controversies about, 588-589; basics of cancer screening, 589, and the diverse assays used, 589-592; mammography varies in sensitivity and specificity, 591-592; effect on survival rates can be obscured by lead-time bias and overdiagnosis, 592-593; HIP trial finds "23 to 24 percent" mortality reduction obtained by screening, 594-596; BCDDP provides data on mammography's potential, 596-598; American Cancer Society urges mammograms for women in their forties, 598-600; interval-surfacing tumors as worm in apple, 600-602; Canadian National Breast Screening Study finds palpation equivalent to mammography, 602-604; experts divided on screening women in their forties, 604-606; Consensus Development Conference suggests that each women "decide for herself," 606-608; no convincing statistics on mortality reduction obtainable by periodic mammography, 609-610; lack of specificity for nonpalpable lesions seen as troublesome flaw, 611; Public Health Service panel

screening mammography—*continued*
recommends mammography for women "aged 50 to 69," 611-612; mammography seen as questionable protection against early-onset familial breast cancer, 612; emerging digital technologies, 612-613; hints on avoiding pitfalls, 613-614. See also mammography, diagnostic mammography, and palpation of the breast

sedatives, 476-478, 540

Seidman, Andrew D., 510, 516

self tolerance (immunology), 556-557

selection bias, 81, 406

Selective Estrogen Receptor Modulators (SERMs): tamoxifen as prototype, 413; qualities of ideal agent, 441; toremifene approved, 441-442; raloxifene tested in breast cancer prophylaxis, 442

Sendai virus, 563, 580

sensitivity of screening assays, 589

sentinel node identification and analysis (also referred to as sentinel node "dissection" and "sampling"): 27, 257, 265-266, 326; indications for, 329, and techniques used, 329-331

SERMs (abbreviation): see Selective Estrogen Receptor Modulators

seromas, 337-338

serotonin antagonists, 477-478

serum tumor markers, 390-391

Seven Countries Study, 102-103

sex chromosomes, 33, 35-37

sex hormone-binding globulin (SHBG), 105

sexuality: effect of chemotherapy on, 484, 487

Shapiro, Sam, 594-596

Shapiro, Samuel, 82, 145

Shaw, William W., 360-361

sickle-cell anemia, 15, 32, 40, 490

Sickles, Edward A., 195, 605, 613

side effects of chemotherapy: produced by cisplatin, 454; by CMF regimen, 457, 464, 479; by Adriamycin, 461-462, 466, 479; by AC regimen, 464; by dose-intense FAC regimen, 468-469; by cyclophosphamide, 475, 479, 485; by paclitaxel (Taxol), 481, 506-507; by fluorouracil, 482; by high-dose cyclophosphamide with marrow or PBSC support, 490-494, 498-500; by docetaxel (Taxotere), 509; by concurrent

Herceptin and Adriamycin, 584-585. See also chemotherapy

Siegel, Bernie S., 408-409

sigmoidoscopy, 233, 590

signal transduction, 64

silicone: properties of, 343, 347-350

silicone gel implants, 343; their use in cosmetic breast enlargement, 345-346, leads to FDA ban, 347-348; implant ruptures and "gel bleed" suspected in connective-tissue diseases, 348-350; epidemiological studies of risk, 351-353; effect on mammographic imaging, 352-353. See also breast reconstruction

Silvestrini, Rosella, 274, 282

Simontons, O. Carl and Stephanie, 406, 408, 410

simple mastectomy: see total mastectomy

Simpson, Jean F., 19, 158, 172, 218, 230, 245

skeletal (osseous) metastases, 516, 522-527

skin cancer, 232, 407

skin-sparing mastectomy, 333-334

skin symptoms affecting the breast, 167-169

Slamon, Dennis J., 52-54, 283, 583-585

Sledge, George W., Jr., 512-513

Sliwkowski, Mark X., 583, 585-586

solar radiation, 16

smoking: carcinogenic effect of, 16-17, 79, 82; inverse association with breast and endometrial cancers, 107-108

Snow, John, 80, 83, 120

somatic cells, 12-14

Southern blot, 39-40, 51-53

Southwest Oncology Group (SWOG): its trials of concurrent CMF and tamoxifen, 425-426, of a GnRH agonist versus oophorectomy, 441, and of modified CMF versus modified FAC, 464-465

specificity of screening assays, 589

S-phase assays in breast cancer staging, 272-275

spiculated margins (mammography), 186-187, 194, 224, 373

spinal cord compression, 525-527

spinal opioids, 545-546

Spock, Benjamin, 90

spontaneous remissions, 557-558

Spratt, John S., 170, 334, 340, 392, 600-602

staging and prognosis in breast cancer: explanation of staging (Stages One, Two, Three, Four), 256-257; Dr. Haagensen's "grave signs," 257-258; the TNM classification, 259-260; tumor size as prognostic indicator, 260-262, 434; nodal status as weightiest factor, 262-264; ER levels predictive of hormonal responsiveness and probable tumor aggressiveness, 267-272; prognostic value of S-phase (growth rate) and DNA content, 272-276; experimental staging assays, 276-278; detecting cancer cells in the bone marrow, 278-280; immunostaining assays for *p53* and HER-2/*neu* overexpression, 281-285; how prognostic factors determine the advisability of chemotherapy or tamoxifen, 285-287; explanation of Stage Four (metastatic) disease, 515-516

staining (specimen preparation), 215-216

STAR Trial (NSABP Protocol P-2), 442

statistical power, 81, 437

statistics: science of, 80-81; numbers glibly quoted in breast cancer matters, 82

stem cells: in the bone marrow, 488-489, and in the bloodstream, 496-498

stereotactic needle biopsies, 209-213

stereotactic radiosurgery, 534-535

steroids, 64

Stoll, Basil A., 104-105

stomach cancer, 16, 94

stomatitis, 482-483

Stomper, Paul C., 125-126, 614

Strax, Philip, 182, 594

stress reduction as treatment adjuvant, 406-407, 409-411

stroma: definition of, 19-21, 58; stromal reaction in breast cancers, 22-25, 154, 217, 224

strontium 89, 523

subareolar ducts and masses, 161-162, 164-166, 228, 305

subcutaneous mastectomy, 333

syngeneic marrow transplants, 490

support groups for cancer patients, 250, 339, 621

supraclavicular nodes, 62, 388

surgery for cancer, 29; historical mastectomy techniques, 288-292; excessive operations of 1950s, 294-297. See also lumpectomy and mastectomy

surveillance bias, 81

Susan G. Komen Breast Cancer Foundation, 621

Swain, Sandra M., 228-229, 462

SWOG: see Southwest Oncology Group

symptoms of breast cancer: 22, 24-25, 257-258; first described in ancient Egypt, 288; advanced tumors give rise to term *cancer* ("crab"), 288-289. See also "lump in the breast" and diagnostic mammography

T cells, 44, 60, 490, 560, 567, 571-579, 582. See also lymphocytes

TAC regimen, 513

tamoxifen, 31; indications for therapy, 285-286, 413; the drug's development and first use in breast cancer therapy, 416-417; drug works by binding to ER protein in cells, but it is not a pure antiestrogen, 418; standard dosage, 418; side effects of therapy, 418-419; clinical trials document a survival advantage in ER-positive breast cancer, 419-422, but no effect in "ER-poor and PgR-poor" disease, 422; tamoxifen's role in premenopausal patients, 423-424; rationale for adding chemotherapy to tamoxifen, 424-425; negative interaction with concurrent CMF regimen, 425-426; NSABP recommends concurrent AC regimen, 426-427; Saint Gallen guidelines for addition of chemotherapy, 428; tamoxifen therapy beyond five years is debated, 428-429; drug improves lipid profiles, but does not prevent heart attacks, 429-430, 438; drug increases bone mass in postmenopausal women while decreasing it in premenopausal women, 430-432; NSABP Protocol B-14 finds benefit from therapy in premenopausal node-negative patients, 432-434; NSABP's trial of tamoxifen prophylaxis (Protocol P-1) proves controversial, but eventually provides impressive data, 434-439; three possible explanations for treatment failure, 439-440; Megace (megestrol acetate) and other second-line therapies, 440-441; tamoxifen pitted against raloxifene, 442, and against aromatase inhibitors, 442-447; tamoxifen use in metastatic breast cancer, 516-517; NSABP Protocol B-35 compares tamoxifen and anastrozole, 620-621

taxanes, 505

taxoid drugs, 488, 505, 514. See docetaxel and paclitaxel

Taxol (taxoid compound, later brand name): development of drug, 505-508. See paclitaxel

Taxotere (brand name), 508-509. See docetaxel

Taxus brevifolia (Pacific yew), 505-508

telangiectasia, 372

terminal cancer: definition of, 537-539; possible causes of death, 538; "right-to-die" controversy, 548-552; hospice care, 552-554; management of deathbed symptoms, 554-555. See also pain control and opioid drugs

terminal ducts, 58, 224

terminal sedation, 552

testicular cancer, 24, 30, 454-455

testicular feminization, 73-74

testosterone, 63, 73, 487

tetracycline, 529-530

thalidomide, 520

Theratope (brand name), 575

thermography, 22, 175

thiotepa, 455, 500

Thomas, Lewis, 548

Thompson, Merle O'Rourke, 252, 470

thoracentesis, 529

thrombocytopenia, 449, 480

thromboembolism: see embolisms

thrombosis: see blood clots

thymidine labeling index (TLI), 273-274

thyroid cancer, 24

Tigan (brand name), 476

TILs (tumor-infiltrating lymphocytes), 569-570

tissue expanders in breast reconstruction, 354-355

tissue transfers in breast reconstruction, 356-362

tissue-type plasminogen activator (t-PA), 109-110

titration, 543

Torecan (brand name), 476

toremifene, 441-442

total (simple) mastectomy, 234, 295, 301-303; indications for, 332-333

toxins (bacterial) as cancer therapy, 561-562

trabecular bone, 131

transfection of oncogenes, 42, 48

TRAM flaps, 358-360

transillumination, 175

trastuzumab: see Herceptin

trauma to the breast, 154

Trojani, Monique, 158

tubular carcinomas of the breast, 225

tumor-associated antigens (TAAs), 557-558, 572-581

tumor bed (site of primary tumor): radiation boosts to, 308, 310, 325, 365-366, 372-373, 376; recurrences near the tumor bed, 382-384

tumor burden, 470, 536-538, 616

tumor grading, 218-220

tumor-infiltrating lymphocytes (TILs), 569-570

tumor necrosis factor (TNF), 562, 578, 582

tumor size in breast cancer prognosis, 260-262, 434

tumor suppressor genes, 45-48, 113-114

Turner's syndrome, 37

Tylenol (brand name): see acetaminophen

ultrasound: its applications in evaluating breast masses, 174-176, in guiding needle biopsies, 206, 208, and in searching for hepatic metastases, 530-532

undifferentiated cancer cells, 28

unilaterality (breast symptoms), 162, 190

Urban, Jerome A., 295-297, 301-305, 311, 381

Urban procedure, 295

vaccines: notable successes against some viral diseases, 8-9, 571-572, but cancer vaccination far more problematic, 572; whole-cell vaccines tested in melanoma and pancreatic cancer, 572-574; lysate and peptide vaccines, 574; breast cancer vaccines tested, 574-575; postulated role for dendritic cells, 575-579

vaccinia virus, 571, 574-575

vaginal carcinoma, 120-121

vaginal dryness: remedies for, 487

vaginitis during chemotherapy, 487

Valium (brand name for diazepam), 477, 540

valspodar, 467

VAMP regimen for leukemia, 451-452

vascular endothelial growth factor (VEGF),

519, 521

vascular invasion (pathology report), 220-221

vasomotor symptoms, 72, 122-123

VEGF: see vascular endothelial growth factor

vegetable consumption as cancer prophylaxis, 94-98, 101-103, 399-401, 403-405

Veltri, Salvatore, 523, 527

vena cava syndrome, 530

venous access for chemotherapy, 473-474

verapamil, 467

Veronesi, Umberto, 302, 324, 330

vertebral fractures due to metastatic disease, 526-527

vesiculae (blisters), 219

vinblastine, 454, 513, 518

vinca alkaloids, 450, 468, 518

vincristine, 450-454, 456, 502

vinorelbine, 518

viruses and viral diseases, 8-9, 563, 565-566, 571-572

visceral metastases, 516-517, 527-532, 544, 584, 586

vitamin A, 396-401, 403

vitamin C, 394-398; as possible anticancer agent, 398-399, 403; risks of excessive consumption, 401

vitamin D, 104, 132, 395, 401

vitamin E, 396-398, 401

vitamin-deficiency diseases, 394-395

vomiting (chemotherapy side effect), 475-478

Wadler, Joyce, 226

Wald, Florence S., 552

Walsh, Declan, 542-543

Watson, James, and Francis Crick, 35-36, 80

Wanebo, Harold J., 305

Weber, Barbara L., 114

Weidner, Noel, 221-222

weight gain during systemic therapies, 439, 484

Weinberg, Robert A., 42-43, 47, 49

well-differentiated carcinoma of the breast, 225

Weltz, Christina F., 336-337

Western blot, 51-53

White, Emily, 147

whole-brain radiotherapy, 534

wigs during chemotherapy, 479-480

Wilkinson, Edward J., 169, 177, 219-220, 224-225

Willett, Walter C., 83-84, 99-102, 104, 109, 397

Williams, C. J., 455, 526

Wilson, Robert A., 122-123, 135

wire localization of nonpalpable lesions, 208-209

Wisconsin Tamoxifen Study, 429-431

withholding treatment in terminal cancer, 552

Women's Health Initiative: the largest clinical trial, 103-104; projected benefits from estrogen therapy, 134, not confirmed by trial results, 135-139

Women's Health Trial (not conducted), 98-99, 103

Wood, William C., 277, 324, 333, 469

Wynder, Ernst L., 96, 100, 108-109

xeromammography, 182-183

Y-ME National Breast Cancer Organization, 621

Zinecard (brand name), 462

Zofran (brand name), 477

zoledronate, 525

Zubrod, C. Gordon, 451

zygote, 10-12